Sexual Health Promotion

Catherine Ingram Fogel, PhD, RNC

School of Nursing
University of North Carolina at Chapel Hill
Chapel Hill, North Carolina

Diane Lauver, PhD, RNC

School of Nursing
University of Wisconsin at Madison
Madison, Wisconsin

1990
W.B. SAUNDERS COMPANY
Harcourt Brace Jovanovich, Inc.
Philadelphia □ London □ Toronto □ Montreal □ Sydney □ Tokyo

W. B. SAUNDERS COMPANY
Harcourt Brace Jovanovich, Inc.

The Curtis Center
Independence Square West
Philadelphia, PA 19106

Notice

In preparing this text, the authors have made every effort to verify the drug selections and standard dosages presented herein. It is not intended as a source of specific or correct drug use or dosage for any patient. Because of changes in government regulations, research findings, and other information related to drug therapy and drug reactions, it is essential for the reader to check the information and instructions provided by the manufacturer for each drug and therapeutic agent. These may reflect changes in indications or dosage and/or contain relevant warnings and precautions. Attention to these details is particularly important when the recommended agent is a new and/or infrequently employed drug. Any discrepancies or errors should be brought to the attention of the publisher.

Library of Congress Cataloging-in-Publication Data

Sexual health promotion / [edited by] Catherine Ingram Fogel, Diane R. Lauver.

    p.   cm.

1. Hygiene, Sexual.   2. Health promotion.   I. Fogel, Catherine Ingram, 1941–   .   II. Lauver, Diane R. [DNLM: 1. Chronic Disease.   2. Health Promotion.   3. Sex Behavior.   4. Sex Behavior—physiology.   5. Sex Disorders.   HQ 21 S51553]

RA788.S4784   1990   613.9'5—dc20   89–10364

ISBN 0–7216–3799–X

Editor: Thomas Eoyang
Designer: Dorothy Chattin
Production Manager: Peter Faber
Manuscript Editor: Roger Wall
Illustration Coordinator: Lisa Lambert
Indexer: Linda Van Pelt
Cover Designer: Jim Gerhard

Sexual Health Promotion   ISBN 0–7216–3799–x

Last digit is the print number: 9   8   7   6   5   4   3   2   1

Contributors

Linda Bernhard, PhD, RN
Assistant Professor, Department of Life Span Process and Center for Women's Studies, The Ohio State University, Columbus, Ohio.
Gynecological Conditions and Sexuality

Judy Brusich, MN, RN, BSN
Assistant Professor, Parent-Child Nursing, Medical College of Georgia, Athens, Georgia.
Religious Influence and Sexuality

Lora E. Burke, MN, RN
Cardiovascular Clinical Specialist, Collaborative Practice, Cardiology, and Assistant Clinical Professor, University of California, Los Angeles, School of Nursing, Los Angeles, California.
Cardiovascular Disturbances and Sexuality

Michael Carter, DNSc, RN
Professor and Dean, College of Nursing, University of Tennessee, Memphis, Tennessee.
Illness, Chronic Disease, and Sexuality

Joanne Dalton, EdD, MSN, RN
Associate Professor, School of Nursing, University of North Carolina at Chapel Hill, Chapel Hill, North Carolina.
Chronic Musculoskeletal Symptoms and Sexuality

Barbara Derwinski-Robinson, MSN, RN
Associate Professor, College of Nursing, Billings Extended Campus, Montana State University, Billings, Montana.
Infertility and Sexuality

Nancy Sharts Engel, PhD, RN
Assistant Professor, College of Nursing, Villanova University, Villanova, Pennsylvania.
The Maternity Cycle and Sexuality, Sexual Assault

Mary Lyn Field, MSN, FNP
Nurse Consultant/Trainer, Chapel Hill, North Carolina.
Psychosomatic Sexual Dysfunction

Catherine Ingram Fogel, PhD, RNC
Associate Professor, Primary Care Department, School of Nursing, University of North Carolina at Chapel Hill, Chapel Hill, North Carolina.
Sexual Health Promotion, Sexual Health Care, Sex and the Law

Mark E. Fogel, JD, MSEE, BE
Attorney, Raleigh, North Carolina.
Sex and the Law

Judith Erickson Forker, PhD, RN, CS
Nurse-psychotherapist, Raleigh, North Carolina.
Sexual Health Care

P. Allen Gray, Jr., PhD, RN
Associate Professor, School of Nursing, University of North Carolina at Wilmington, Wilmington, North Carolina.
Sexually Transmitted Diseases

Rebecca Ingle, MSN, RN, OCN
Oncology Clinical Nurse Specialist, The Dan Rudy Cancer Center, St. Thomas Hospital, Nashville, Tennessee.
Cancer and Sexuality

Susan H. Kalma, MSN, RNC
Assistant Professor of Nursing, Memorial University of Newfoundland, St. John's, Newfoundland, Canada.
Contraception and Sexuality

Colleen Keenan, MS, RNC
Lecturer, School of Nursing, University of California, Los Angeles, Los Angeles, California.
Multidimensional Aspects of Caring for the Abortion Client

Diane Lauver, PhD, RNC
Assistant Professor, School of Nursing, University of Wisconsin at Madison. Formerly Robert Wood Johnson Clinical Nurse Scholar, University of Pennsylvania School of Nursing, Philadelphia, Pennsylvania.
Sexual Response Cycle, Contraception and Sexuality, Sexually Transmitted Diseases

Ginger Manley, MSN, RN, CSC
Associate Professor and Director, Center for Sexual Health Care, Vanderbilt University Medical Center, Nashville, Tennessee.
Endocrine Disturbances and Sexuality

Elizabeth M. Munsat, MSN, RN, CS
Clinical Nursing Educational Specialist, Psychiatry, North Carolina Memorial Hospital, Chapel Hill, North Carolina.
Mental Illness, Substance Abuse, and Sexuality

Barbara Nettles-Carlson, MPH, SpCIN, FNP-C
Associate Professor, School of Nursing, University of North Carolina at Chapel Hill, Chapel Hill, North Carolina.
Gay and Lesbian Lifestyles

Audrey Rogers, PhD, RN
Chief, Center for AIDS Epidemiology, State of Maryland Department of Health and Mental Hygiene, Baltimore, Maryland.
Drugs and Disturbed Sexual Functioning

Barbara Rynerson, MS, RNC
Associate Professor, School of Nursing, University of North Carolina at Chapel Hill, Chapel Hill, North Carolina.
Sexuality Throughout the Life Cycle

Carol Sackett, MPH, BSN
Clinical Nurse Specialist, Urology, North Carolina Memorial Hospital, Chapel Hill, North Carolina.
Spinal Cord Conditions and Sexuality, Genitourinary Conditions and Sexuality

Victoria Shea, PhD
Clinical Assistant Professor, Department of Psychiatry, University of North Carolina at Chapel Hill School of Medicine, Chapel Hill, North Carolina.
Developmental Disability and Sexuality

Raelene Shippee-Rice, MS, RN
Associate Professor, Department of Nursing, University of New Hampshire, Durham, New Hampshire.
Sexuality and Aging

Linda Schoonover Smith, MSN, ANP
Associate Professor, Primary Care Graduate Program, School of Nursing, University of North Carolina at Chapel Hill, Chapel Hill, North Carolina.
Human Sexuality from a Cultural Perspective, Sexually Transmitted Diseases

Camille Stern, PhD, RN
Associate Professor, Ida V. Moffett School of Nursing, Samford University, Birmingham, Alabama.
Body Image Concerns, Surgical Conditions, and Sexuality

Rebecca Stockdale-Woolley, MSN, RN
Pulmonary Clinical Specialist, Hospital of Saint Raphael, New Haven; Consultant, Pulmonary Rehabilitation, Respi-Care, Section of Pulmonary Medicine, Norwalk Hospital, Norwalk; Clinical Instructor, Yale University School of Nursing, New Haven, Connecticut.
Respiratory Disturbances and Sexuality

Michele Bockrath Welch, WC, MSN
Assistant Professor, College of Nursing, University of Delaware, Newark, Delaware.
Sexual Health Care, Sexual Response Cycle

Preface

Promotion of sexual health is now considered to be a legitimate role for health professionals. Clients have often expressed concerns about sexuality and sexual functioning directly to health professionals and in turn expect sexual information, counseling, or therapy. At the same time, health professionals often wonder how to meet such needs. Even though health professionals have acknowledged the legitimacy of clients' sexual concerns and the appropriateness of addressing such concerns for a number of years, health professionals continue to be ill prepared to incorporate this aspect of care into their practice. They suffer from inadequate knowledge about sexuality and sexual functioning as well as believe many of the myths and misconceptions about sexuality. They may be uncomfortable with talking about sex, may have difficulty assessing a client's sexuality or collecting a sexual history, or may be unsure about specific strategies or interventions.

The purpose of *Sexual Health Promotion* is to provide the essential information needed to build a strong knowledge base from which sexual concerns can be developed. A physiological-psychological-social orientation is used in the presentation of content, reflecting the authors' belief that human sexuality is far more than a biological phenomenon addressed in health care practice and that psychological factors and social conditioning strongly influence the expression of human sexuality. Every effort has been made to treat the topics presented in this text with objectivity and sensitivity. A breadth of research findings, opinions, and interventions are offered so that readers may examine the facts, explore their values, and incorporate this information into their practice.

Part 1 of the book explores sexuality and identifies the components of sexual health care. Concepts basic to an understanding of how diseases and disorders adversely affect sexual functioning and sexuality are examined. Frameworks for practice are suggested, and a framework for organizing interactions with clients experiencing sexual difficulties is offered. The process of sexual assessment, e.g., obtaining a sexual history, and providing care to clients is reviewed. Examples of appropriate interventions with case history material are provided.

Part 2 provides an indepth biopsychosocial approach to sexuality, beginning with a focus on the anatomical and physiological aspects of the normal human response cycle. Physiological, psychological, and social factors of human sexuality are discussed within a developmental context from conception through the older years, with one chapter focusing specifically on the sexuality and sexual behaviors of the elderly. Cultural, legal, and religious influences on sexuality and sexual practices are also examined. The reader needs to be aware that these influences are constantly changing. For example, the most recent Supreme Court decision regarding abortion rights, *Webster v. Reproductive Health Services,* allows states to impose far more restrictive regulations on the abortion process. This underscores the necessity identified in Chapter 8 that health professionals need to stay abreast of legal and political developments in American society. Biopsychosocial issues surrounding homosexuality as well as specific clinical issues pertinent to health care for gay and lesbian clients are discussed.

Part 3 presents information on the sexual well-being of couples throughout the maternity cycle. In addition, contraceptive behaviors and sexuality and contraceptive methods and their effect on sexual behavior are examined. Also covered are the historical background and ethical and legal perspectives of abortion, along with the psychological, developmental, and sociocultural factors that combine to make pregnancy termination a critical life event for women. The multidimensional aspects of caring for abortion clients is included. The causes, diagnostic measures, biomedical treatments, and psychosocial interventions of infertility are examined in relation to their impact on sexuality.

Part 4 provides an overview of diseases, disorders, therapies, and conditions that can adversely affect sexual functioning and sexuality. Included here are chapters on illness and chronic disease, chronic musculoskeletal symptoms, endocrine disturbances, cardiovascular disturbances, drugs, respiratory disturbances, body image concerns and surgical conditions, genitourinary problems, spinal cord injuries, gynecological problems, sexually transmitted diseases, and cancer. Psychogenic explanations of sexual dysfunction and the effects of sexual assault of adults and children are also examined. Unique to this book are chapters on mental illness and addictions and developmental disabilities. Each chapter provides an indepth look at how disorders affect sexuality, as well as specific assessment points, and practical intervention strategies for specific diorders.

C.I.F.
D.L.

Contents

PART ONE

HUMAN SEXUALITY AND HEALTH CARE

1: Sexual Health Promotion

Catherine Ingram Fogel

Sexuality is an important dimension of the human personality. It is an integrated, unique expression of the self that encompasses the physiological and psychosocial processes inherent in sexual development and sexual response. Sexuality is inextricably woven into the fabric of human existence; there are few people for whom sex has not been important at some time. Because sexuality underlies much of who and what a person is, it is a significant aspect throughout life. Expressed positively, sexuality can bring great pleasure, but it also has the potential to cause great pain.

The promotion of sexual health is a legitimate role for health professionals and is an essential nursing function. Clients are beginning to express directly their concerns regarding sexuality to health professionals; they are expecting sexual information, counseling, or therapy. Nurses themselves want to know how to assess a client's sexual functioning and needs, how to collect a sexual history,

and what interventions may be offered to a client experiencing sexual dysfunction.

The purpose of this chapter is to provide nurses with an introduction to pertinent aspects of the nursing role in sexual health promotion. Definitions of sexuality are explored, the components of sexual health are identified, and the influence of sexual value systems is discussed. Concepts basic to the understanding of how diseases and disorders can interfere with sexual functioning and adversely affect sexuality are examined. Finally, the nurse's role in promoting and maintaining the sexual health of clients is analyzed. Frameworks for interventions are suggested.

THE CONCEPT OF SEXUALITY

Although sexuality is a basic fact of human existence, the definitions and descriptions of human sexuality are varied, complex, and, at

1

times, vague. Sexuality has been called the quality of being human, a powerful and purposeful aspect of human nature, and an important dimension of humanness (Fonseca, 1970). Sexuality also encompasses one's most intimate feelings of individuality and the need for emotional closeness with another human being. Sexuality is an ongoing process of recognizing, accepting, and expressing one's self as a sexual being (Shippee, 1979). As individuals change, their sexuality changes; learning about sex is a lifelong process.

Sexuality is not just overt sexual behavior, nor is it only an anatomical assignment of gender. It does not exist only in the young and attractive and is not restricted to partners of the opposite sex. Sexuality exists even when a person is not interacting with another. It is a deep, pervasive aspect of the total human personality, which is present in some degree from birth until life's last moment. Sexuality encompasses an individual's particular way of being male or female. It is communicated in ways that range from bodily movements, to relations with others in everyday encounters, to expressions of the deepest feelings of tenderness and love.

It is necessary to differentiate among sex, sexual activity, sexual functioning, and sexuality. Sex is simply an individual's anatomical assignment. Sexual behaviors are the verbal and nonverbal expressions of sexuality and include both genital and nongenital activities. Sexual functioning refers to natural bodily functions that begin in utero and are in some measure subject to conscious control. Despite the conscious control of some aspects of sexual behavior, some elements of sexual functioning remain involuntary, such as male erection and female vaginal lubrication occurring during sleep.

Because sexuality includes much more than sexual activity or sexual functioning, it underlies the complete range of human experience and contributes to our lives in many ways. A healthy or positively developed sense of sexuality offers the following:

■ Enables a person, through children, to establish a link with the future.
■ Provides a means of physical release and sexual pleasure.
■ Binds people together.
■ Allows us to communicate subtle, gentle, or intense feelings.

■ Provides feelings of self-worth when sexual experiences are positive.
■ Is one of the factors that builds an individual's identity.

To understand human sexuality, nurses must examine biological, psychological, and sociocultural factors. These categories are not mutually exclusive but rather overlap and intertwine—human sexuality is more than a biological phenomenon. Psychological factors and social interactions strongly influence the expression of human sexuality.

Similarly, one nurse theorist, Sister Callista Roy (Roy and Roberts, 1980) views persons as biopsychosocial beings in interaction with their environment. Roy proposes that persons adapt to stimuli, both from their internal and external environment, in four different ways, or modes. These four adaptive modes are labeled physiological, self-concept, role function, and interdependence. The goal of coping in these modes is adaptation or integrity of the person. Integrity encompasses physiological, psychological, and social integrity of the person; it implies meeting goals relevant to survival, growth, reproduction, and self-mastery. The physiological, psychological, and social modes of coping have implications for individual development of sexuality and sexual adaptation following an alteration in health. Following a biopsychosocial perspective and drawing on the adaptive responses identified by Roy, physiological, self-concept, role function, and interdependence are themes that will be highlighted throughout the text.

A biological perspective includes the anatomical and physiological aspects of sexuality: the sex organs, hormones, nerves, and centers of the brain. It examines the ways in which separate parts of the human organism, such as the nervous, muscular, endocrine, and other body systems, contribute to an individual's adaptive response to varied environmental stimuli. Knowledge of how diseases and disorders and their treatments affect sexuality and sexual functioning is important to the biological perspective and will be presented in this book. Other important areas addressed are the human sexual response cycle, the role of hormones on sex differentiation in the prenatal period, the relationship of the brain to sexual feelings, and the effects of hormones on behavior.

A psychological perspective of sexuality encompasses both an individual's intrapsychic dimension and perceptions of interpersonal relationships. A psychological perspective incorporates the important dimension of self-concept to sexuality. Roy maintains that self-concept consists of a person's sense of a physical self and a personal self; the latter includes dimensions of moral self, self-ideal, and self-consistency. This self-concept system is influenced by perceptions of internal stimuli and by social learning. A person's self-concept is reflected in self-descriptions, dress, and actions. Inherent in this description of self-concept is a need to strive for a sense of adequacy (Roy and Roberts, 1980). From a developmental perspective, sexuality is thought to be learned, not a force or instinct imparted at birth, but something acquired through interactions. In tracing the development of an individual's sexuality throughout the life cycle, it is important to understand how the sexual characteristics of adult men and women develop from infancy (and perhaps the prenatal period) and what factors determine the direction of this development. The roots of sexual dysfunction may be found in early childhood experiences. Children who are taught that masturbation or sexual exploration is wrong may, in later life, experience anxiety and guilt with sexual experiences.

The foundations for a healthy sexual life are laid down over a period of many years, from early infancy through puberty. An understanding of what is healthy sexually is essential if effective sex education is to be provided to clients. Considered in this perspective are the concepts of self-concept, body image, and gender identity.

Roy assumes that individuals have a need to be nurtured and to nurture. Individuals strive to balance nurturance and nurturing as well as dependence and aggressiveness by giving and receiving help, attention, and affection. These processes are labeled an adaptive mode of interdependence (Roy and Roberts, 1980) and appear applicable to sexual adaptation to disease.

In addition, the etiology of psychogenic sexual dysfunction is often found in the psychological distress or conflict that individuals experience within themselves or in their relationships. An individual's attitudes and values regarding sexuality, motivations to have or to avoid sexual experiences, and the emotional component of sexuality can affect sexual expression, behavior, and functioning. These components of the psychological di-

mension also affect the client's response to therapies, treatments, or interventions employed to improve sexual functioning.

A sociocultural perspective reflects the beliefs that the culture and society strongly influence how a person develops as a sexual being; society shapes and limits our experiences of sexuality. Roy maintains that role function involves the performance of certain duties in conformance with sociocultural expectations, such as moral standards (Roy and Roberts, 1980). Observed role behaviors are the result of taking in, processing, and incorporating cues and cultural norms. Social interactions, or the process by which societal expectations and normative roles are learned, also govern human sexuality. Because societal expectations regarding sexuality are communicated very subtly, it is often assumed that behaviors are innate or instinctive. Examination of different cultures or other time periods quickly reveals that this is not so; that, in fact, there is a range of sexual behaviors to be found in different societies and cultures. For example, some cultures do not discourage premarital sexual activity among adolescents. In ancient Egypt, marriage between close relatives was mandated for the Pharaohs, something that is abhorrent to most Americans today.

Much of what a society prescribes as correct sexual attitudes and behaviors is directed toward controlling sexual expression and functioning. The reasons for this are the following: (1) the human race depends on sexual drive and reproduction for continuity; (2) sexual interactions affect the establishment, continuity, and preservation of the family; (3) sexual responses can include strong emotions involving the individual and others in intimate relationships; and (4) the force of sexuality induces fear due largely to lack of knowledge. Sexual attraction and sexual behavior are mysterious and powerful and therefore are thought to require restrictive control (Higgins and Hawkins, 1984).

Two aspects of culture that attempt to control sexuality are the religious and legal systems. Moral rules do not develop from the experiences of individual persons; rather, they are imposed by the cultures and subcultures in which we live. Religion, as a major purveyor of moral proscriptions, can have a considerable influence on the development of individuals as sexual beings and on their sexual behavior (Hogan, 1982). Religion often defines what is right and wrong sexual behavior. Various Christian denominations have cited scripture from the Bible to reinforce proscriptions against masturbation and adultery. Generally, societal proscriptions are translated into legal ones. Laws regarding sexual behavior fall into three major categories: sexual offenses; rights to life, property, and privacy; and access to erotic or pornographic materials. An examination of societal religious and legal proscriptions will help nurses to identify the prevailing societal sexual value systems that their clients may espouse.

A sociocultural perspective highlights the ways in which a society influences male and female sexuality as well as gender role behaviors. The inability to assume ascribed gender roles can have adverse effects on sexual functioning. For example, the woman who behaves assertively in a community that defines female roles in a traditional way may find herself labeled as "unattractive and unfeminine" or as someone who the men would not want to date. Similarly, conflicts regarding appropriate role behaviors or periods of rapidly changing sexual role expectations can have a negative impact on sexual relationships and ability to function.

SEXUAL HEALTH

Defining sexual health or healthy sexual functioning is as difficult a task as defining health itself. Health is a value that changes, just as other social and cultural values do. For most people sexual health is not something that is considered until its absence is noticed. The World Health Organization (WHO) (WHO, 1975) developed the following definition of sexual health, which provides a focus for nursing education and nursing interventions.

Sexual health is the integration of the somatic, emotional, intellectual and social aspects of sexual beings in ways that are positively enriching and that enhance personality, communication and love.

This definition may be incompatible with some individuals' view of sexuality because of the use of the word love. Depending on how one views sex, love does or does not have to be present for sexual satisfaction. While some may feel the definition is restrictive, it does have several strengths. The definition encompasses three essential elements:

(1) capacity to enjoy and control sexual and reproductive behavior in accordance with a social and personal ethic; (2) freedom from fear, shame, guilt, false beliefs, and other psychological factors that inhibit sexual response and impair sexual relationships; (3) freedom from organic disorders, diseases, and deficiencies that interfere with sexual and reproductive functions. In short, sexual health may be considered the physical and emotional state of well-being that enables us to enjoy and act on our sexual feelings (Boston Women's Health Book Collective, 1985).

Optimum sexual functioning requires an intact nervous and circulatory system. The experience of sexual arousal depends on myotonia (muscle tension) and vasocongestion; without these the response cycle is impaired. The central nervous system integrates and directs the drive for sexual fulfillment. The subcortical center for sexual pleasure is found in the limbic formations of the forebrain, while the hypothalamus is the center of basic emotions, among them erotic pleasure. The appetite for sex, as well as for food and water, originates in the proximal central neuroanatomical sites, which are linked by numerous neural pathways (Watts, 1979). All physiological changes in the sexual response cycle are mediated by the sympathetic and parasympathetic nervous systems. Perception of changes at the cortical levels requires intact sensory pathways from the periphery of the body to the cortex of the brain. The ability to sexually stimulate oneself or a partner requires intact pathways from the cortex to the appropriate cord level and from there to the effector muscle. Also necessary for sustaining interest in sex is a sufficient level of androgens (Kaplan, 1974).

The psychological aspects of sexual health are crucial to healthy sexual functioning. It is important that biological sex and gender identity be congruent and that personal and social behaviors be congruent with gender identity. When they are not, there is the sense of being a male in a female's body or vice versa; individuals wish to behave as they feel and not as how they appear to the outside world. Further, the individual's personal and social behaviors must be in agreement with their gender identity (Maddock, 1975). This may prove problematic in today's society, in which male and female roles are not as explicitly defined as they once were. There should be a sense of comfort with a range of sex role behaviors. Sexual health also includes the ability to have effective interpersonal relationships with members of both sexes that have the potential for love and long-term commitment. The individual should have the capacity to respond to erotic stimuli in ways that make sexual activity a positive, pleasurable experience (Maddock, 1975). It is important that there be congruence between personal sexual value systems and sexual behavior. Inherent in this is the maturity of judgment to make decisions about sexual behavior that are not in conflict with overall value systems and beliefs about life. If this is not done, the potential for conflict within the individual is great. Sexually healthy individuals must not only be aware of the theoreical aspects of sexual functioning, but more important they must also be cognizant of their own personal feelings. It is only when one is knowledgeable as well as honest with oneself about beliefs and feelings that the potential for sexual fulfillment can exist.

The above description implies that sexually healthy individuals have the following:

- Knowledge about sexual phenomena.
- A positive body image.
- Self-awareness about their attitudes toward sex.
- Self-awareness and appreciation of their feelings about sexuality.
- A well-developed, usable value system that provides input for sexual decision-making.
- The ability to create effective relationships with members of both sexes.
- Some degree of emotional comfort, interdependence, and stability with respect to the sexual activities in which they participate.

Related to the concept of sexual health is the view of sexuality as one of the basic human needs that must be met if health is to be achieved and maintained. Maslow (1954) views sex as one of the basic physiological needs necessary for existence and survival, although in the strict sense, sexual activity is necessary only for species survival. Although sexual activity with another can be deferred for a lifetime, sexuality is an essential ingredient in an individual's need for psychological security, self-esteem, love, and feelings of belonging.

The definition of sexual health provided here recognizes the biological, psychological, and sociological dimensions of sexuality. Implied in this definition is integrity and continuity of the individual, the necessity of incorporating sexual health into the concept of total personal health. The concept of sexual health suggests the importance of a holistic, positive approach to human sexuality. The individual's right to sexual information is viewed as basic. Sexual health care becomes a way in which a person's life and personal relationships may be enhanced (Lion, 1982).

What is Normal?

Definitions of sexual health and normalcy frequently contain value-laden terms susceptible to different interpretations. Cultural norms often dictate what is acceptable behavior. Many individuals assume that what is dictated by their culture or subculture as normal sexual behavior is, in fact, the norm for all people. A review of the recorded history of human sexuality makes it clear that patterns of sexual behavior and morality have taken many different forms over the centuries. Even a cursory cross-cultural examination of sexual practices reveals the variety of forms of sexual expression. Defining normal sexual behavior is a futile exercise. There is no way by which concepts of normal and deviant sexual behavior can be divorced from a society's value system (Marmor, 1971).

The problem of defining normal sexual behavior is made more complicated by the many meanings of the word normal: prevalent, optimal function, distributed in a statistical pattern, fashionable, or socially acceptable (Comfort, 1975). Health professionals need to be aware of how they define normal and abnormal sexual practices, since the term normal may be used in different ways: (1) in a pathological or clinical sense indicating stress and poor adaptation in an individual; (2) using a moralistic model, in which abnormal is the same as evil; (3) employing a cultural frame of reference, in which normal is what the prevailing culture defines as such; (4) using statistical standards (if the majority of a population does it, it is normal); and (5) adopting a personal view, in which others are compared with oneself, with personal satisfaction then becoming the standard for normalcy (Hogan, 1982). There is a problem with the personal view in that many of those who feel content with their points of view may be sexual chauvinists who are convinced that there is only one way to feel, think, and act. For these people, persons who are unlike them are considered abnormal or perverted.

Because it is so difficult to ascertain normalcy, Comfort (1975) suggests the following guide for clinicians to use when considering a particular behavior:

- What does the behavior mean to the individual?
- Does the behavior enrich or impoverish the sexual life of the individual and those with whom he or she shares sexual relations?
- Is the behavior tolerable to society? (Woods, 1984)

Marmor (1971) supports these guidelines, suggesting that there are some extremely deviant patterns of sexual behavior that would be, in all likelihood, considered abnormal in every society. For example, practices that cause serious harm to any of the participants would be considered maladaptive. Additionally, it may be possible, within the context of Western cultural value systems, to identify patterns that are viewed as psychologically optimal and healthy. A note of caution: It is not always possible to distinguish clearly between healthy and neurotic sexual behavior.

Threats To Sexual Health

It is often helpful for the nurse to have a framework with which to categorize factors that constitute threats to sexual health. Three major categories of variables are (1) biological, (2) psychological, and (3) social. Biological factors include events that disrupt anatomical structure, thus altering sexual response, and/or that change physiological function, altering the individual's ability to respond to sexual stimuli, or that modify the physiological mechanisms of sexual response. The amount of derangement and the chronicity of the condition are also important to the extent of interference experienced. Diseases or injuries in which the disease process, trauma, or treatment alter sexual functioning are examples. These include diabetes, angina, spinal cord injury, and myocardial infarction. Also included are handicapping conditions such as blindness, hearing loss, cerebral palsy, and mental retardation. Any visible or hidden change that results in a negative change in body image can be a sexual health risk, as can debilitating chronic disease. Certain events in the life cycle that

have a biological component can influence, threaten, or disrupt sexuality and sexual functioning. These include menarche, pregnancy, menopause, and aging. Often, treatments used to correct organic disease can adversely affect sexuality, either by altering function (e.g., medication for hypertension) or by disrupting anatomical integrity (e.g., prostatic surgery). Prescription, recreational, and street drugs can become risks to sexual health.

There are numerous psychological threats to sexual health. Unconscious conflicts may prevent the individual from responding to sexual stimuli or may result in an inappropriate response. Guilt, anxiety, depression, anger, and fear of failure are often at the root of psychogenic sexual dysfunction. Frequently, lack of knowledge and/or ineffective communication contribute to sexual difficulties.

Environmental influences may interfere with an individual's ability or opportunity to function sexually. Lack of privacy, institutionalization, and distracting stimuli can prevent the full range of sexual activities. Furthermore, lack of social acceptance, such as that experienced by gays, can interfere with sexual expression. Cultural scripting, such as the male as macho and the female as passive, may prevent a full range of sexual expression for both sexes.

CONCEPTS IMPORTANT TO SEXUAL HEALTH

There are certain essential components of psychological sexual health: self-concept, body image, and sexual identity. Often, these elements are adversely affected by disease and disorders, thus having a deleterious impact on sexual functioning and the ability to develop and maintain a healthy sexuality.

Self-Concept

One's sense of self is composed of thoughts and feelings; hopes and strivings; fears and fantasies; a view of what the self is, has been, and may become; and attitudes regarding self-worth (Holmes, 1982). One's identity is closely allied with a sense of self. Self-concept is critical to sexuality and sexual health. It is defined as a "composition of ideas, feelings and attitudes that a person has about his/her own identity, worth, capabilities and limitations" (Urdang, 1983). Central to self-concept is an identification with and acceptance of one's gender role. Individuals will assess themselves against societal standards of masculinity and femininity and make evaluations about their adequacy (Hogan, 1980).

A positive self-concept and feelings of self-esteem are essential for the development of a positive sexuality and sense of oneself as a sexual being. High self-esteem allows an individual to be comfortable seeking pleasure, asking another to help satisfy sexual needs, and determining what is sexually pleasing. Those with a negative sexual self-concept are more likely to experience guilt, shame, and anxiety with sexual activity. These negative emotions are etiological factors in psychogenic sexual dysfunction. The experience of illness and chronic disease, with resulting treatments, altered role behaviors, and possibly surgery and hospitalization, can contribute to lowered self-esteem and adversely affect sexuality.

Sexual self-concept refers to how people value themselves as sexual beings. It is an indicator of the relative compatibility of all the other components of their sexuality (Lion, 1982). As an individual's sexual self-concept develops, it affects the continued development of the other aspects of the person's sexuality. Adolescence is a particularly critical time in the formation of sexual self-concept. At puberty and throughout adolescence, all aspects of sexuality alter and grow rapidly; peer interaction is particularly influential. If one has a negative sexual self-concept, formation of relationships may be impeded or prevented. If sexual self-concept is positive, an individual has a solid foundation upon which to form intimate relationships throughout life.

Body Image

Body image, the mental picture that a person has of his or her body, is a critical element of sexuality. It begins to develop during the first 3 years of life and evolves gradually with growth and development. Body image is central to a sense of self; in part, ego integration depends on having and retaining a realistic perception of one's body. Body image is developed through internal comparisons of self both with others and with cultural ideals and through real and imagined feedback from others.

Body image is influenced through specific social interactions. In this respect, physical appearance is important. Body image is influenced by others' perceptions of and responses to one's body. Body image does not consist of only the physical body but also includes objects in daily use. Clothing, for example, can enhance body image and support body boundaries. Objects that are worn regularly or come in regular contact with the body, such as glasses, a wedding ring, or a uniform, may become incorporated into body image so much so that loss or removal of them becomes a threat to body image.

How a woman feels about her body is related to her sexuality. From a very early age she receives messages about the necessity of attracting a mate and the importance of female physical beauty. The media constantly underline the message that physical attractiveness is essential for a woman, particularly if she is to be successful in attaining the major goal of attracting and keeping a male. Although women have an image of a perfect body, most have some part of their bodies that they do not like and would change if possible. Women with poor body image often have various negative responses to sexual arousal. Conversely, women who feel good about their bodies and are comfortable with them are likely to be comfortable with and enjoy sexual activity.

Men tend to focus less on their bodies than do women. There is little correlation between male physical appearance and role status attainment. As long as a man's body reflects those qualities traditionally associated with masculinity, he is apt to feel comfortable. Loss of physical strength, however, with its association of loss of masculinity, is more apt to damage a male's body image than it would a female's. While body image does not affect male sexuality as readily as it does females', most men do worry about penile size and adequacy in satisfying their partners. The myth of "larger is better," particularly if it is erect and has staying power, is pervasive in our society. When his vigor, staying power, and agility are threatened by disease, a man's body image can suffer. Inability to produce an erection may have devastating effects on self-concept and body image. A corresponding inability to be orgasmic every time may not have the same devastating effect on women.

Body image is everchanging. Disease, therapy, pregnancy, aging, and diagnostic procedures can alter appearance and function and impact on body image. During illness, a person receives different messages about his or her body; these are then interpreted, and perhaps integrated, into body image. Disease and trauma often have a negative impact on body image in general (Reinstein et al, 1978; Fitting, 1978). Body image disorder and sexual dysfunction have also been found to be related even in people without disease (Derogatis, 1980).

Sexual Identity

There are three components of sexual identity: biological sex, gender identity, and gender role orientation. Sexual identity is a major subsystem of the system known as self-identity and is closely tied to a personal sexual value system and sexual self-concept. Sexual identity is not inborn but rather develops through experience. Thus, it has social meaning and is subject to social construction. Sexual identity is formed by personal experience, sexual scripts, and an individual's sexual experiences with others. Also important to the formation of sexual identity is the acknowledgment of the self as a sexual being.

Biological sex refers to chromosomal make-up, external and internal genitalia, hormonal states, and secondary sex characteristics. Conception initiates the process of sexual differentiation, which ends in a firmly established adult gender identity. Much of the activity that establishes biological sex occurs during the prenatal period and puberty. It is during the prenatal period that anomalies of sexual development can occur. These do not affect sexual identity at that time; they are unobserved during fetal development, and, indeed, an individual cannot be said to have a sexual identity prior to birth. Sexual anomalies create problems after birth and later in life, when individuals are seen to be different from what is expected of them for their ages and sex. In order to develop an adequate sexual identity, individuals must meet age-graded and sex-typed norms (Laws and Schwartz, 1977).

Sexual identity is built upon a foundation of gender identity and gender role orientation. Gender identity is the belief individuals have that they are male or female, that is, an individual's awareness of the self as either male or female. Gender or sex role orientation refers to learning and performing the socially accepted characteristics and behaviors for a given sex. While male and female sex role scripts contain many elements that are not sexual, the proscriptions for masculinity and feminity are carried into areas of sexual behavior. Sexual identity is formed through an individual's perceiving himself or herself in roles and reorganizing the continuity of behavior in these roles across situations and time. Thus, the evolution of sexual identity involves an individual's attempt to match his or her experience with available sexual scripts. The language that applies to sex feelings and events is learned, as are societal expectations for individuals of a specific age and sex. Also learned are the reciprocal demeanor, attitudes, and behaviors expected of someone of the opposite sex.

An individual's definition of self as a sexually active person is another important component of sexual identity. In addition, some sources suggest that there is a fourth aspect to sexual identity—sexual orientation, or preference (DeCecco and Shively, 1977; Higgins and Hawkins, 1984; Lion, 1982). One of the sexual characteristics of humans is the tendency to prefer certain kinds of partners for sexual activity.

VALUES

Central to working with clients who are experiencing sexual concerns or dysfunction is the issue of values. All persons have a sexual value system that is integral to their sexuality. Such a system defines sexuality as good or bad, appropriate or inappropriate, and intended for procreation or recreation or both. It is reflected in gender role orientation and how personal relationships are defined and structured. Sexual self-concept is closely interwoven with sexual value system. The degree of congruence between sexual value system and sexual behavior influences, either positively or negatively, a person's sexual self-concept. Sexuality is closely related to a person's basic philosophy, and philosophy is a reflection of values. An individual's sexual value system is an important component of the framework of values, beliefs, and experiences used in making sexual decisions.

The health professional who wants to promote sexual health must have a knowledge of human sexuality. The practitioner must be aware of his or her attitudes and values and how these affect nursing practice. It is necessary to understand one's own experiences, knowledge, convictions, attitudes, and values and test these against those of others.

Values are defined as a "set of personal beliefs and attitudes about the truth, beauty and worth of any thought, object or behavior" (Simons, Howe, and Kirochenbaum, 1972, p 13). They are a person's vision of the good life and determine desires and decisions. Values provide general guides to behavior; they are standards of conduct that a person endorses and attempts to meet or maintain. Values provide a frame of reference through which the individual integrates, explains, and appraises new ideas, events, and relationships (Coletta, 1978).

The development of values is basically a decision-making process that begins with a real or perceived need. Once the need is recognized, responses to the need are sought that will allow the need to be met. These responses are compared, and the response that is felt to best meet the need is chosen. The choice made is one that has the highest value for the individual. Creating values is a process, and seven subprocesses define what becomes a value. In order for something to be considered a value, it must be:

- Chosen freely without coercion
- Chosen from alternatives
- Chosen with a knowledge of the consequences
- Prized and cherished
- Publicly affirmed when appropriate
- Acted upon
- Made a consistent behavior pattern (Simons et al, 1972)

Values may be intrinsic or internalized from an individual's personal situation and experience. Or the value may be extrinsic, derived from society's standards of right and wrong, good and bad.

Hogan (1982) identified six major forces that determine attitudes toward sexuality: (1) sexual interest; (2) development of personality and behavior pattern; (3) societal and cultural influences; (4) immediate environment and the people in it, especially one's home and family; (5) education; and (6) sexual experiences with intense emotional impact, for example, rape, incest, or loss of virginity.

Societal values regarding sexuality are particularly strong, primarily because sexuality is an enormously powerful force. Societal values are constructed to control sexual behavior and are very powerful in themselves. In the United States, freedom of choice is a paramount value; however, this "choice" does not extend to sexuality. Major influences on the restrictive sexual attitudes and behaviors of Americans are many. Remnants of the Judeo-Christian patriarchial view of society, which equated women with property, are still to be seen in traditional male and female duties, state laws on marital rape, and a systemic reluctance to prosecute wife battering. The Puritans, who colonized America, brought with them a stern code of morality that banned lewd thought, ostracized "fallen women," and equated sexual interests and urges with sin. Sexual research has played an important role in shaping sexual attitudes, providing benchmarks for sexual practice, understanding, and fuel for the continuing ideological debates about the right and wrong of sexuality. Table 1–1 is a summary of a number of key reserchers' efforts in the field. The earliest sex researchers "brought sexuality out of its Victorian morass," yet their views of sexuality were based largely on control-repression and drive models (Gagnon, 1975). Freud and his disciples were especially influential in general intellectual matters and probably were most important in the development of twentieth century sexual ideology. Freud's writings, with his observation that sex was an early and powerful influence in peoples' lives, had a tremendous impact in America during the first half of the twentieth century. Although his philosophy supported a movement away from Puritanical and Victorian values and toward sexual freedom, Freud was a product of his times, and his writing reflected the prevailing Victorian ethic of overt prudery and sexual underground. Men were thought to be lustful creatures with sexual desires that required an outlet. Freud's conviction that all women suffered from penis envy and that vaginal orgasms were normal did women a major disservice by labeling clitoral orgasms as neurotic or immature.

Beginning in the 1920s and culminating in the 1940s and 1950s with the work of Alfred Kinsey (1948, 1953), sex research focused on "sexual bookkeeping," which studied the sexual behavior of relatively normal persons. This represented a movement away from case histories and populations that were defined as neurotic or criminal. Many social

TABLE 1–1. A Summary of Key Sex Research Studies

Names of Researchers and the Study	Year	Type of Study	Focus and Scope	Strengths and Weaknesses
Kinsey, *Sexual Behavior in the Human Male* Kinsey, *Sexual Behavior in the Human Female*	1948 1953	Interview survey	Patterns of sexual behavior, the American population	Most comprehensive taxonomic sex survey yet conducted; but the large sample overrepresented certain groups (educated, urban dwellers, young) and underrepresented others (undereducated, older, non-Protestant, rural, and nonwhite).
Masters and Johnson, *Human Sexual Response*	1966	Direct observation	Female and male physiological responses to sexual stimulation	The only major piece of research to observe and record sexual response (over 10,000 completed response cycles); has been criticized because sample was drawn from narrow-based academic community.
Sorenson, *Adolescent Sexuality in Contemporary America*	1973	Questionnaire survey	Male and female adolescent sexual behavior, ages 13–19	Surveys a broad range of sexual behaviors; has been criticized because of nonresponse bias and length of questionnaire.
Hunt, *Sexual Behavior in the 1970s*	1974	Questionnaire survey	Patterns of sexual behavior, the American population	Much information about a broad range of adult sexual behaviors; has been criticized because of high nonresponse, sampling bias from telephone recruitment, and length of questionnaire.
The Redbook Report on Female Sexuality	1975	Questionnaire survey	Female sexuality (behavior and attitudes)	Very large sample size (100,000 women); but sample bias due to fact that respondents were *Redbook* readers, not a true cross section of American women.
The Hite Report on female sexuality	1976	Questionnaire survey	Female sexuality (behavior and attitudes)	Large number of respondents (3019) provided extensive narrative answers to questions; has been criticized because sample volunteers probably overrepresented young liberal women.
The Hite Report on Male Sexuality	1981	Questionnaire survey	Male sexuality (behavior and attitudes)	7239 respondents out of 119,000 questionnaires distributed; strong possibility of volunteer bias, educational levels of volunteers much higher than national average.
Zelnick and Kantner, "Sexual and Contraceptive Experiences of Young Unmarried Women in the United States, 1979, 1976, and 1971"	1971, 1976, and 1979	Questionnaire survey	Pregnancy, use of contraceptives, and premarital sex among unmarried teenage women, ages 15–19 (1979 survey included men, ages 17–21)	Good sampling techniques; but a narrow population of interest.
Bell and Weinberg, *Homosexualities: A Study of Diversities Among Men and Women*	1978	Interview survey	Homosexual lifestyles and sexual practices	Most comprehensive study of homosexuality to date; criticisms have centered on sampling biases from recruitment methods.

TABLE 1–1. A Summary of Key Sex Research Studies *Continued*

Names of Researchers and the Study	Year	Type of Study	Focus and Scope	Strengths and Weaknesses
Bell, Weinberg, and Hammersmith, *Sexual Preference: Its Development in Men and Women*	1981	Interview survey	Causes of sexual orientation	Utilization of sophisticated statistical techniques to produce findings remarkable in what they disprove; sampling biases from recruitment methods.
George and Weiler, "Sexuality in Middle and Late Life"	1981	Questionnaire survey	Changes in sexuality in the older years	Noteworthy for use of longitudinal approach; sample limited by decision to include only married people.
Blumstein and Schwartz, *American Couples*	1983	Questionnaire survey plus some interviews	Current trends in relationships among heterosexual and homosexual couples	Excellent information about a variety of sexual and nonsexual components of relationships obtained from a large national sample; sample underrepresented certain population groups (low socioeconomic, racial minorities, undereducated).

changes were occurring in America at this time; Kinsey documented these and, in doing so, influenced public opinion. Using the data from interviews with individual men and women regarding their sexual behavior, Kinsey corrected misinformation about sexual behavior. Much of what was regarded as abnormal came to be viewed as within the normal range of behavior. For example, Kinsey's (1953) research established that most individuals masturbate and that women were often orgasmic.

Masters and Johnson opened doors to the study of sexual anatomy and physiology by collecting data on sexual response through direct observation, attaching monitors to research subjects during sexual arousal and intercourse and while they watched erotic movies. Masters and Johnson's (1966, 1970) books on normal sexual response and human sexual inadequacy have become classics in the fields of sexuality.

During the 1960s America experienced a sexual revolution and became a more sexually liberated nation. While changes have occurred in a number of areas pertaining to sexuality, these changes are less than revolutionary. Information about and education for sexuality is more available generally; this has relaxed some previously restrictive standards. Greater availability of reliable contraception and the legalization of abortion have

directly influenced societal practices; sexual attitudes and behaviors have become more liberal. Perhaps the most striking change has been the sexual behavior of women, who begin sexual activity earlier, have more sexual partners (Siemens and Brandzel, 1982), and have permission to be sexually responsive. During the late 1960s and 1970s a range of lifestyles became available to men and women.

Currently, the rapid increase in sexually transmitted diseases, in particular the acquired immunodeficiency syndrome (AIDS), is greatly affecting individual sexual attitudes and behaviors. Individuals are electing to restrict their number of sexual partners, to practice celibacy, and to question their sexual partners about lifestyle and sexual practices in a manner not seen before. Women are carrying condoms and refusing to engage in sexual activity with men who will not use them. While these practices are self-protective and thus beneficial to individuals, some of the other results of societal concerns are not so positive. With the onset of the AIDS epidemic has come an increasing homophobia and often violent reaction to those individuals at greatest risk for contracting the disease.

Three value positions on sexuality, sexual behavior, and sexual expression are commonly found today in our society. The traditional value position attempts to deny and repress all sexual expression except among married heterosexuals. Reproduction is thought to be the purpose of sexual behavior, and sexual instincts must be controlled. Sex education may not be condoned. Prostitution and pornography are unconditionally prohibited. Homosexuality is believed to be abnormal and perverse. Masturbation, premarital sex, and extramarital sex are condemned. Proponents of this value position usually have separate codes of sexual ethics for males and females and ascribe to rigid traditional sex roles.

A second value position, one growing in popularity, accommodates a wider range of sexual activities with greater tolerance of deviations from traditional sexual norms. Sexual urges and needs are considered normal, although some sexual activities (such as homosexuality) may be considered evidence of an underlying problem. Masturbation is considered understandable and probably not destructive. Sex education is accepted. Sex is rarely linked with sin or immorality. Contraception is sanctioned, and prostitution, pornography, divorce, and abortion are viewed in a more tolerant manner. Sex is considered to be a form of communication between partners.

The libertarian or hedonistic view represents a third value position, one less commonly encountered. Sexual intercourse is thought to be a positive good within itself, and sex is thought to be essential to a happy life in the same way food, exercise, and rest are. Adherents to this position cultivate their sexuality and believe sexual pleasure is desirable as an end in itself. Sex education is viewed as a tool by which sexual skills and techniques may be developed. Frequently, individuals will incorporate portions of all three value positions into their personal value system.

NURSING AND HUMAN SEXUALITY

Nursing focuses on the human responses to actual and potential health problems (ANA, 1983). The practitioner, educator, and researcher alike emphasize the health of the total person and recognize that human beings constantly interact with their environment. A primary goal of nursing practice is to en-

hance self-care practices that lead to better health (Woods, 1984). Because nursing views clients holistically and because sexuality is a basic human need, sexuality is one of the essential foci of nursing care. There is a growing body of knowledge indicating that problems in human sexuality are "more pervasive and more important to the well-being and health of individuals in many cultures" than had previously been recognized. Further, there are important relationships between sexual ignorance and misconceptions and many diverse problems of health and quality of life (WHO, 1975). Nursing has a responsibility to help clients achieve high-level wellness and a quality of life that includes an integrated, positive sexuality.

Unfortunately, nurses all too often have inadequate knowledge of sexuality and are uncomfortable with both their own sexuality and that of their clients. For many nurses, clients' sexual needs, concerns, or problems are anxiety producing, uncomfortable topics that are best left alone or ignored. Few nurses assume the responsibility for discussing sexuality with their clients except in obvious circumstances in which it is required, such as when a client has a sexually transmitted disease or is seeking birth control.

Societal attitudes are changing, and clients are now asking for help in many areas of sexuality. The sexual rights of those receiving health care were clearly outlined by Mary Calderone (1966), founder of the Sex Information and Education Council of the United States (SIECUS):

We affirm the right of consumers to receive health care by an informed and humane professional whose diagnostic, treatment and human relations skills have been developed by systematic and thoughtful preparation in sexual health care. Such preparation confronts the very nature of a person's sexual beliefs and practices, and should facilitate better understanding of self as well as an appreciation of a more holistic approach to the consumer in need of sexual health care.

Not all nurses need to be prepared as sex therapists; indeed, most clients need nowhere near this level of expertise. All nurses can integrate sexuality into their health care, however, focusing on preventative, therapeutic, and educational interventions that help individuals attain and maintain sexual health.

Preparation

There are three levels of learning that all health care professionals must go through to become capable of caring for clients who have sexual concerns or problems. It is first necessary to overcome any sexual embarrassment that they may feel. This may be done by talking with other nurses about how they feel about discussing sexual concerns with clients, taking human sexuality courses, or participating in values clarification exercises. Next, nurses must develop the ability to recognize, identify, and understand sexual problems. Finally, they must develop the competency needed to deal with sexual problems. In order to accomplish these objectives, it is essential that nurses become aware of their own sexuality, become comfortable with it, and be able to express it.

In order to provide effective sexual health care, the nurse or other health care practitioner must have a sound and comprehensive knowledge of the subject matter. An awareness of one's own beliefs, attitudes, and values is essential, since these are a major determinant in how one deals with clients. Finally, it is neessary to develop assessment, intervention, integration, and communication skills in all aspects of sexual health (Mims, 1977).

Knowledge

Nurses are educated to recognize and care for the physical and emotional aspects of health and illness. Yet, in the past this education included little about human sexuality, graduating health care professionals who were able to deal with no more than a narrow range of sexual behavior and who were ill-prepared to handle many types of sexual dysfunction. In some schools, nursing faculty appeared reluctant or ambivalent about sexuality in the nursing curriculum (Mims, 1977; Walker, 1971). Although there are some nurses who continue to believe that sexuality is not a nursing concern (Zalar, 1982), it is essential to include sex education in nursing curricula (Chaffee, 1984). Without sex education, it is highly questionable whether nurses will have the knowledge and sensitivity to assist clients or the ability to recognize and handle their own feelings. Accordingly, to meet nurses' needs, and hence their clients', several courses and programs have recently been developed (Koch, 1985; Bartscher, 1983; Keller, 1982).

The subject of human sexuality is vast, sensitive, and complex. Basic knowledge includes sexual development; reproduction; sexual expression; sexual dysfunction and disease; human sexual response cycle; sociocultural aspects of sex, marriage, and family development; and the moral, aesthetic, and religious sensitivities of clients. Until recently, information about the effects of illness and disease on sexuality has been lacking, and research in all fields has been scarce. While much research is currently being done in the area of human sexuality with regard to health and disease, very little of this is being done by nurses. There is no special professional group within nursing whose major area of concern is the sexuality of patients. Although there now appear to be many courses on human sexuality in both baccalaureate and master's degree programs (Hott and Ryan-Merritt, 1982), information is not sufficient to fill the gaps. Core content about human sexuality must be identified and built into required curricula in the same way that other concepts basic to nursing practice have been. Existing textbooks, laboratory objectives and guidelines, guides for nursing assessment, nursing diagnosis, and nursing care plans should be reviewed and revised to include sexual health care. Students need opportunities to carry out sexual assessments and to provide care for clients with sexual problems.

Nursing incorporates research as a foundation for practice. The essence of research is contained in the everyday practice of nursing (Diers, 1979), and nursing has not yet looked to everyday practice to generate questions about sexuality that could be evaluated through nursing research. There are many problems that handicap research about human sexuality. Human subjects cannot be placed in the same sorts of experimental situations as animals. Human thought and behavior is extremely complex. Research about human sexuality can be critically evaluated with the following checklist, compiled by Crooks and Bauer (1983):

1. Who conducted the research? Are they reputable professionals?
2. What type of methodology was used? Were scientific principles adhered to?
3. How large was the sample group? Was there bias in the selection procedure?
4. Can the results be generalized to others not in the sample group?
5. Did the methods used bias the findings?
6. Are there other published reports that confirm or contradict the study in question? Sex research should be humanistic and directed toward providing individuals with a

greater measure of freedom, one that is tempered by responsible behavior toward others; should help to dispel myths and taboos that impede fact finding and utilization of knowledge; and should be conducted within a holistic framework (Kirkendall, 1979).

Values

It is imperative that nurses identify their own values in order to understand their feeling about specific sexual practices. The literature illustrates that medical and nursing students lack knowledge of and comfort with sexual feelings, attitudes, values, and beliefs (Zalar, 1982; Lief and Payne, 1975). It is only when one knows oneself that one is able to be nonjudgmental—to be tolerant of another's sexual beliefs, feelings, and behaviors. Health professionals working with clients experiencing sexual difficulties must be able to accept a variety of values, many of which may conflict with their own. Values conflicts can interfere with health care in that inaccurate assessment and subsequent inappropriate interventions can lead to less effective teaching and health care (Lauver, 1980). They should cultivate as high a tolerance level as possible. Characteristics of effective nurse sex counselors include a personal resolution of sexual identity and overall sexual adjustment and the ability to speak openly, honestly, and confidently about any aspect of human sexuality (Krozy, 1978).

Once nurses are aware of their sexual attitudes, it is important to examine how these attitudes affect nursing practice. Do attitudes restrict or enhance practice? A nurse might ask herself: How am I viewed by others? Do patients see me as someone they can talk to? Am I comfortable discussing sexual concerns? What nonverbal messages do I send out? Do I penalize individuals whose beliefs or practices are different from mine?

Values and attitudes can affect a nurse's practice in a number of ways. The nurse with strong religious beliefs about the immorality of certain sexual practices may experience conflict when expected to care for individuals whose practices do not conform to these beliefs. In addition to believing that some behaviors are wrong, nurses may be repulsed, embarrassed, or shocked by sexual behaviors that do not fit their definition of normal. Some nurses have firm convictions that sexuality is a personal matter and that apart from its role in reproduction sexuality is not an area of nursing concern. Because we learn early that sexuality is a taboo subject, many female nurses may find talking about sex difficult, having grown up with the image that "nice girls don't talk about such things." Although traditionally society has been far more apt to sanction men's discussion of sexuality, at least when done in the company of other men, than it has been to sanction women's, there is no indication that male nurses are any more comfortable than female nurses with initiating or carrying out discussions with clients about their sexuality.

Sexual self-confidence is the result of becoming knowledgeable about and comfortable with sexual matters. People who are sexually comfortable have high self-esteem and a positive body image. They have experienced a personal resolution of sexual identity and overall sexual adjustment. They have up-to-date, factual knowledge about human sexuality. They are able to accept the sexual preferences and activities of others without feeling personally threatened or without moralizing or judging the other person. Nurses who are self-assured and comfortable with their own sexuality are able to be sensitive to cues indicating areas of sexual dysfunction from patients. They are able to be sensitive to a client's nonverbal communication and are able to unmask indirect cues. The sexually comfortable nurse can recognize her own strengths and limitations without feeling threatened and can actively search for the knowledge she needs to assist her clients. The self-confident nurse is able to create an environment that facilitates communication.

A major influence on an individual's value system is the culture in which the individual exists. Nurses reflect their cultural background, and this influences all client-practitioner interactions. Nursing is a cultural institution; it is the only helping profession with societal sanction to touch a person's body and to assist with the most private daily needs. This means that nurses are allowed to be concerned about the intimate and bodily functions of others. Because nursing is predominantly a profession of women, it is also subject to the prevailing stereotypes about women as well as those associated with nursing.

NURSING ROLES

Nursing has traditionally been the health profession most concerned with the total person. Nursing has a holistic view of clients that encompasses attention to sexual needs and problems. Clients require a variety of health services, ranging from education at the individual or community level to intensive therapy for complex sexual dysfunction. Who will be able to intervene at each level of complexity will depend on professional preparation. Expertise among nurses will differ. Some will learn only basic information, others will expand their sex education and communication skills, and a small number will receive advanced training, enabling them to provide sex therapy. Figure 1–1 illustrates a model for organizing nursing interventions by levels of increasing complexity. This model is particularly helpful for those who are beginning to explore how sexual interventions can be incorporated into nursing practice.

While a few clients will need intensive therapy for complex sexual dysfunction, many do not need indepth sexual therapy. They want someone to whom they can express their feelings and worries, someone who can offer understanding and support, and someone who can provide accurate information. Basic nursing education will prepare the nurse to intervene at this level if three prerequisites are met: (1) an accurate knowledge base, (2) self-awareness of personal value systems and self-acceptance as a sexual being, and (3) the ability to communicate genuinely and therapeutically with clients. Skills that are utilized in the provision of sex education and counseling range from active listening to sophisticated psychotherapeutic skills. The nurse must be able to employ active listening strategies, use communication techniques to elicit feelings, demonstrate acceptance, and have the ability to set objectives and solve

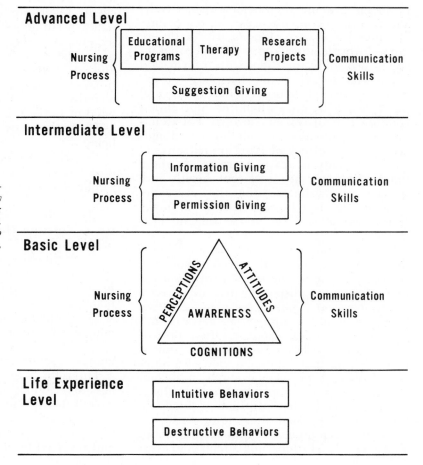

FIGURE 1–1. Mims-Swenson sexual health model. (Reproduced by permission of Mims FH, Swenson M: Sexuality: A Nursing Perspective. New York, McGraw-Hill, 1980, p 5. Copyright by The CV Mosby Co, St. Louis.)

problems. With these skills, knowledge, and awareness, the nurse has a strong foundation for providing sex education and counseling (Woods, 1984). It is not enough to base the provision of sexual health care on life experiences and intuitive responses. While care with such a foundation may be intuitively helpful, it is just as apt to perpetuate incorrect, destructive ideas about sexuality (Mims and Swenson, 1980). Identification of one's own intuitively positive and destructive sexual behaviors heightens sensitivity to the need for discarding and replacing attitudes, beliefs, and behaviors that may limit the therapeutic effect of interventions. This process must be done before providing sexual health care.

In the provision of sexual health care, nurses perform many roles. It is first necessary to create an environment that is supportive of sexual health. A milieu that minimizes the guilt and anxiety that clients feel in connection with expressing their sexual thoughts, attitudes, feelings, and behavior is essential. Only then can clients begin to solve problems, examine their behavior objectively, and realize its consequences within a reality-oriented framework (Woods, 1984). Often, nurses provide anticipatory guidance that involves providing the client with information about what to expect or what phases of experience are likely to occur. There are several points in the life cycle when this intervention is important for sexual concerns. For example, during adolescence, childbirth, and midlife and as the effects of aging are felt, anxiety about sexuality is apt to increase. At these times many persons seek out health care providers for validation that they are experiencing what is to be expected, or "normal." It is essential that the nurse validate normalcy.

Sex education is obviously a major role for the nurse concerned with sexual health care. As a sex educator, the nurse provides accurate information, dispels myths, and corrects misinformation. The degree of information provided should be appropriate to the client's level of concern and interest. Often, providing information limited to a specific topic is more helpful than an exploration of a number of sexual topics. For example, if a client is seeking information about various birth control methods, that information should be provided rather than an indepth discussion of sexual techniques or information about abortion. Sexual counseling attempts to assist the client to alter behavior in order to achieve a preset goal. The counseling process helps clients to reach a more satisfactory level of functioning. While some nurses provide intensive therapy, for most referral is an important component of their nursing practice. Those individuals with complicated sexual dysfunctions may require referral to persons with additional preparation in psychotherapy who have special intervention approaches for dysfunction. Finally, nurses may serve as consultants for the development of sex education programs or community groups. Others may function in a clinical specialty role for individual nurses experiencing specific client-care problems.

SUMMARY

Nursing can have a primary role in promoting and maintaining the sexual health of individuals and groups. Nurses can assess clients regarding sexual concerns and sexuality, accurately identify problems, and intervene effectively. It is not necessary that nurses be sex therapists; however, teaching and education are within the province of all nurses. Nurses have a responsibility to help all individuals achieve sexual freedom as outlined in Jacobsen's (1974) bill of rights:

The right to express yourself as a sexual being.

The right to be self-confident and self-directing in regard to your sexuality.

The right to become the person you would like to be.

The right to select and be with a sex partner of your choice, whether of the same or opposite sex.

The right to be aware of the influence your sexuality can have on someone else and how to use it in a constructive and therapeutic manner.

The right to encourage your peer group members to function as sexual beings.

The right to be accepting and tolerant of another's sexual attitudes and preferences.

The right to assist men and women of all ages to recognize their sexuality as an integral part of their personality, inherited at conception, molded and tempered by environment, sustained by health, threatened by disease, and reversed by choice.

REFERENCES

Adams G: Human sexuality. Recognizing the range of human sexual needs and behaviors. Part 1. Matern Child Nurs J 1:165–169, 1976.

American Nurses Association: Standards of Maternal and Child Health Nursing Practice. Kansas City, American Nurses Association, 1983.

Bartscher PW: Human sexuality and implications for nursing intervention: A format for teaching. J Nurs Educ 22:123–127, 1983.

Beach FA: Human Sexuality in Four Perspectives. Baltimore, The Johns Hopkins University Press, 1977.

Bidgood FE, Burleson DL: A study of sex education in the nursing curriculum. New York, Sex Information and Education Council of the United States, 1973.

Boston Women's Health Book Collective: The *New* Our Bodies, Ourselves. New York, Simon & Schuster, 1985.

Bradshaw CE: Concentrated experiential learning laboratories. J Nurs Educ 22:32–33, 1983.

Calderone MS: Sex education for young people—and for their parents and teachers. In Brecher R, Brecher E (eds): An Analysis of Human Sexual Response. New York, New American Library, 1966.

Chaffee MW: The missing link in nursing education: Sexuality. Imprint 31:43, 1984.

Cias SJ: Some thoughts on being a male in nursing. In Muff J (ed): Socialization, Sexism, and Stereotyping, Women's Issues in Nursing. St. Louis, CV Mosby, 1982.

Cleland VS: Symposium on current legal and professional problems. To end sex discrimination. Nurs Clin North Am 9:563–571, 1974.

Coletta SS: Values clarification in nursing—Why? Am J Nurs 78:2057–2063, 1978.

Comfort A: The normal in sexual behavior: An ethological view. J Sex Educ Ther 1:1–7, 1975.

Crooks R, Bauer K: Our Sexuality. 2nd ed. Menlo Park, Benjamin/Cummings Publishing Company, 1983.

DeCecco JP, Shively MG: Children's development: Social sex-role and the hetero-homosexual orientation. In Oremland EK, Oremland JD (eds): The Sexual and Gender Development of Young Children. Cambridge, Ballinger Press, 1977.

Derogatis LR: Breast and gynecologic cancers. Front Radiat Ther Onc 1:1–11, 1980.

Diers D: Research in Nursing Practice. Philadelphia, JB Lippincott, 1979.

Fitting MD: Self-concept and sexuality of spinal cord injured women. Arch Sex Behav 7:143–156, 1978.

Flemming AA: Sexuality in adolescence. In Lion EM (ed): Human Sexuality in Nursing Process. New York, John Wiley & Sons, 1984.

Fogel CI, Woods NF: The Health Care of Woman: A Nursing Perspective. St. Louis, CV Mosby, 1981.

Fonseca JD: Sexuality—A quality of being human. Nurs Outlook 18:25, 1970.

Gagnon JH: Human Sexualities. Glenview, Scott, Foresman & Company, 1977.

Gagnon JH: Sex research and social change. Arch Sex Behav 4:111–141, 1975.

Hacker S: Student's questions about sexuality. Implications for nurse educators. Nurse Educ 9:28–31, 1984.

Higgins LP, Hawkins JW: Human Sexuality Across the Life Span: Implications for Nursing Practice. Monterey, Wadsworth Health Science Division, 1984.

Hogan RM: Human Sexuality: A Nursing Perspective. Norwalk, Appleton-Century-Crofts, 1980.

Hogan RM: Nursing and human sexuality. Nurs Times 76:1296–1330, 1980.

Hogan RM: Influences of culture on sexuality. Nurs Clin North Am 17:365–376, 1982.

Holmes MA: Lesbian health care. In Sonstegard LJ, Kowalski KM, Jennings B (eds): Women's Health: Ambulatory Care. Orlando, Grune & Stratton, 1982.

Hott RJ, Ryan-Merritt M: A national study of nursing research in human sexuality. Nurs Clin North Am 17:429–447, 1982.

Jacobson L: Illness and human sexuality. Nurs Outlook 22:53, 1974.

Kaplan HS: The New Sex Therapy. New York, Brunner/Mazel, 1974.

Keller MC: Teaching sexuality as a nursing elective. Nurs Health Care 3:311–313, 1982.

Kinsey AC, Pomeroy WB, Martin CE: Sexual Behavior in the Human Male. Philadelphia, WB Saunders, 1948.

Kinsey AC, Pomeroy WB, Martin CE: Sexual Behavior in the Human Female. Philadelphia, WB Saunders, 1953.

Kirkendall LA: Aims and objectives in sexual research and theory. In Bullough VL (ed): The Frontiers of Sex Research. Buffalo, Prometheus Books, 1979.

Koch JJ: Psychotherapeutic techniques and methods applied in teaching human sexuality. J Nurs Educ 24:346–349, 1985.

Krozy R: Becoming comfortable with sexual assessment. Am J Nurs 78:1036–1038, 1978.

Krizinofski MT: Symposium on the patient with long-term illness. Human sexuality and nursing practice. Nurs Clin North Am 8:673–681, 1973.

Lauver D: Recognizing alternatives: A process for health education. Health Values: Achieving High Level Wellness 4:134–138, 1980.

Laws JL, Schwartz P: Sexual Scripts. Hinsdale, The Dryden Press, 1977.

Lief HS, Payne T: Sexuality—knowledge and attitudes. Am J Nurs 75:2026–2029, 1975.

Lion EM: Human Sexuality in Nursing Process. New York, John Wiley & Sons, 1982.

Maddock JW: Sexual health and health care. Postgrad Med 58:52–58, 1975.

Magenity J: A plea for sex education in nursing curriculum. Am J Nurs 75:1171, 1975.

Mandetta AF, Woods NF: Learning about sexuality–A course model. Nurs Outlook 22:525–527, 1974.

Marecek J: Psychological disorders in women: Indices of role strain. In Freize I, Parsons J, Ruble D, et al (eds): Women and Sex Roles: A Social Psychological Perspective. New York, WW Norton, 1978.

Marmor J: "Normal" and "deviant" sexual behavior. JAMA 217:165–170, 1971.

Maslow A: Motivation and Personality New York, Harper & Row, 1954.

Masters WH, Johnson VE: Human Sexual Response. Boston, Little, Brown & Company, 1966.

Masters WH, Johnson VE: Human Sexual Inadequacy. Boston, Little, Brown & Company, 1970.

Mims FH: Sexuality in the nursing curriculum. Nurse Educ 2:20–23, 1977.

Mims FH, Swenson M: Sexuality: A Nursing Perspective. New York, McGraw-Hill, 1980.

Mims FH, Brown L, Lubow R: Human sexuality course evaluation. Nurs Res 28:248–253, 1979.

Money J, Ehrhardt AA: Man and Woman: Boy and Girl. Baltimore, Johns Hopkins University Press, 1972.

Muff J: Socialization, Sexism and Stereotyping, Women's Issues in Nursing. St. Louis, CV Mosby, 1982.

Patterson JM, McCubbin HI: Gender roles and coping. J Marriage Family 46:95–104, 1984.

Payne T: Sexuality of nurses: Correlation of knowledge, attitudes and behavior. Nurs Res 25:286–292, 1976.

Reinstein L, Ashley J, Miller K: Sexual adjustment after lower extremity amputation. Arch Phys Med Rehabil 59:501–503, 1978.

Roy SC and Roberts S: The Roy Adaptation Model: Conceptual Models for Nursing Practice. 2nd ed. Norwalk, Appleton-Century-Crofts, 1980.

Roy SC: Theory Construction In Nursing: An Adaptation Model. Englewood Cliffs, Prentice Hall, 1981.

Schaffer KF: Sex Roles and Human Behavior. Cambridge, Winthrop, 1981.

Schuster EA, Unsain IC, Goodwin MH: Nursing practice in human sexuality. Nurs Clin North Am 7:345–349, 1982.

Shippee RV: Touching and pleasuring behaviors in a well elderly population. Masters thesis. Rochester, University of Rochester, 1979.

Siemens S, Brandzel RC: Sexuality: Nursing Assessment and Intervention. Philadelphia, JB Lippincott, 1982.

Simons S, Howe Z, Kirochenbaum H: Values Clarification: A Handbook for Practical Strategies for Teachers and Students. New York, Hav Publishing Company, 1972.

Urdang L: Mosby's Medical and Nursing Dictionary. St. Louis, CV Mosby, 1983.

Walker EG: Study of sexuality in the nursing curriculum. Nurs Forum 10:19–31, 1971.

Watts RJ: Dimensions of sexual health. Am J Nurs 1979; 1568–1572.

Woods NF: Human Sexuality in Health and Illness. 3rd ed. St. Louis, CV Mosby, 1984.

Woods NF, Mandetta A: Changes in students' knowledge and attitudes following a course in human sexuality: Report of a pilot study. Nurs Res 24:10–15, 1975.

Woods NF, Mandetta A: Sexuality in the baccalaureate curriculum. Nurs Forum 15:294–313, 1976.

World Health Organization: Education and Treatment in human sexuality: The training of health professionals (Report of a WHO Meeting, Technical Report Series, No. 572), 1975.

Zalar MK: Human sexuality—a component of total patient care. Nurs Digest 3:40–43, 1975.

Zalar MK: Role preparation for nurses in human sexual functioning. Nurs Clin North Am 17:351–363, 1982.

2: Sexual Health Care

Catherine Ingram Fogel

Judith Forker

Michele Bockrath Welch

Health professionals draw upon a breadth of knowledge and skills in order to provide sexual health care. These include the following:

1. An awareness of one's own value system and an acceptance of a variety of potentially different value systems. Awareness and acceptance then lead to an understanding of the effect of values and attitudes on the provision of health care.

2. A comprehensive and interdisciplinary knowledge base that incorporates research findings. With a strong knowledge base, professionals are able to use the decision-making process in planning and providing care to clients in a variety of settings.

3. Selected communication skills with which knowledge about the client is obtained and information regarding care communicated.

4. The decision-making process that provides a systematic way of organizing health care and becomes a framework for practice that moves the provider from assessment to evaluation of each client situation.

5. A theoretical framework that guides the decision-making process and organizes the collection of data and selection of interventions.

In this chapter a framework for organizing interactions with clients experiencing difficulties in sexual functioning is offered. The decision-making process is briefly outlined, and its use in sexual health care is discussed.

In addition, the chapter focuses on the assessment phase of the process, specifically obtaining a sexual history. Finally, the intervention phase is examined in detail, with examples of appropriate interventions in sexual health care given.

THE DECISION-MAKING PROCESS

Individuals solve problems in a variety of ways, depending on their knowledge base, clinical experience, and the specific situation. The decision-making process is based on the scientific method of systematically collecting data through the senses and then drawing conclusions through logical analysis of data. The nursing process is used to illustrate how health professionals use the scientific method to provide care for their clients.

The nursing process is a problem-solving, systematic approach to care delivery that requires actions based on judgment (Gordon, 1982). This process standardizes an approach to care while also providing individual service (Bulechek and McCloskey, 1985). A logical method of critical thinking, the nursing process is open, flexible, and dynamic. It is a facilitative process, enabling provision of quality client care, and is cyclical (Fig. 2–1), involving five steps: assessment, diagnosis, planning, implementation, and evaluation.

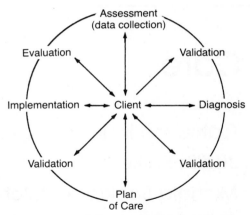

FIGURE 2–1. *A client-centered model of nursing process.*

Although there are several variations, it appears that the original four-step model (assessment, planning, intervention, evaluation) is being replaced by the five-step model. While the steps in the process occur in somewhat linear progression, with more assessment at the beginning of an interaction and more intervention at the end, assessment is ongoing. Participation of both the client and nurse is necessary in all phases, ensuring continuity and individualized care.

Assessment

The nursing assessment begins when the nurse becomes aware of a client's need. The primary source of data is the client, although family and friends may also provide information. Additional data may be obtained from health care records, physical examination, and laboratory tests. Both subjective and objective data are gathered during this phase. Objective data include information from the physical examination, laboratory test results, and the nurse's clinical observations. The interview provides data regarding clients' subjective interpretation of present health status, health history, and reasons for care as well as contextual information about their environment.

Diagnosis

In this step, the assessment data are analyzed, assimilated, and clustered into relevant categories, from which nursing diagnoses may be derived. While there is as yet no universal definition of what a nursing diagnosis is,

Bulechek and McCloskey (1985) have suggested that it is "the identification of a patient's problem that the nurse can treat." More specifically, a nursing diagnosis is a summary statement of analyzed data that defines the nature and extent of a client's health problem, that is within the boundaries of nursing practice, and that meets standards of practice as delineated by the professional association.

Data analysis involves a process of searching for categories in the data that suggest tentative diagnoses. Synthesis of data involves looking for relationships and patterns. The client's ideas about the problem are combined with other data collected to arrive at a diagnosis. It is essential that the diagnoses be validated with the client prior to implementation because without accurate perceptions of the client's problems, there can be no effective interventions.

The North American Nursing Diagnosis Association (NANDA) publishes an annual list of approved nursing diagnoses and nursing diagnoses categories. Examples of nursing diagnoses relevant to sexual health are disturbance in sex role performance related to pregnancy, disturbance in body image related to mastectomy, sexual dysfunction related to spinal cord injury, post-traumatic response related to rape, sexual knowledge deficit related to misinformation and lack of exposure to education, and anxiety related to threat to self-concept due to high-risk pregnancy.

Planning

Each diagnosis is the stimulus for initiating a plan of care. Goals for interventions should be established and clarified with the client whenever possible. Once goals have been established, priorities should be determined on the basis of the immediacy of the problem. Criteria to be used to measure progress toward the goals must also be defined. Finally, actions to assist the client in meeting the goals are identified. These actions may be selected from a repertoire of known interventions or by trial and error with careful evaluation and documentation. It is important to ascertain how the client has coped with similar problems or situations previously. Those techniques that have previously been successful can be incorporated into the care plan.

Implementation

Three types of interventions are used to meet the goals of care—assessment strategies, therapeutic measures, and educational measures. Assessment strategies continue the process of data collection and are used to update the nurse's data base, confirm progress toward the goal, and modify the existing care plan. Therapeutic measures provide treatment for a condition and offer the client comfort. Educational measures are activities that assist in the maintenance or promotion of health. Implementation may also include referral to other health professionals.

Evaluation

Evaluation involves assessing the client's response to intervention and progression toward or attainment of the goals. This is greatly facilitated by the use of outcome criteria or predetermined standards. Evaluation outcomes determine the need for revision of goals, additional data, and/or modification of nursing actions.

A FRAMEWORK FOR PROVISION OF SEXUAL HEALTH CARE

A number of theoretical frameworks are available for organizing care for clients with sexual dysfunctions or concerns. Roy's (Roy and Roberts, 1980) adaptation model of nursing practice is an example of a framework for nursing care. Roy views individuals as constantly adapting to a changing environment through four modes, or methods, of acting: physiological function, self-concept, role function, and interdependence. This framework rests on an assumption of an individual's need for biological, psychic, and social integrity. The physiological mode reflects adaptation regarding exercise and rest, nutrition, elimination, fluid and electrolyte balance, oxygen and circulation, and regulation of temperature, the senses, and the endocrine system. The self-concept mode reflects efforts to achieve and maintain a self-concept, e.g., a person's perceptions of the physical, personal, and interpersonal self. The role function mode reflects efforts to achieve and maintain mastery in social inter-

action and the performance of duties based on one's position in society. The need for social integrity is also emphasized in the adaptive mode of interdependence. The interdependence mode reflects efforts to achieve a comfortable balance between dependence and interdependence in relationships, e.g., seeking and giving help and affection.

Changes in the environment may cause either a greater need or a deficit in adaptive abilities. An individual's process of adaptation is dynamic and is a response to the stimuli to which the person is exposed. Stimuli may be focal (most immediate), contextual (background), and residual (past beliefs, attitudes, or experiences aroused by the present situation).

Human behaviors are, in general, actions within a given context or reactions under specific circumstances or stimuli. Behavior may be external, such as talking with another, or it may be internal, such as heart rate. Further, behaviors are observed, measured, and/or subjectively reported. Behavioral responses in the physiological mode are often identified by clinical observation, physical examination, and laboratory data. They are classified as adaptive or maladaptive according to established norms. Responses in the self-concept, role performance, and interdependence modes are identified by interview as well as clinical observation. Responses that maintain the sexual integrity of the individual, i.e., a positive sense of the self as a sexual being, are adaptive, while those behaviors that disrupt the sexual integrity of the individual are maladaptive or sexually dysfunctional.

ASSESSMENT

The goal of nursing and of all health professions is to promote and support individual adaptation in situations of health and illness. Everyone copes differently with illness and changes in health status. Therefore, health professionals must be able to identify a person's state of adaptation accurately and negotiate with the client about goals, so that interventions designed to alter stimuli and promote adaptation can be initiated. Roy (1980) suggests that nurses begin by assessing individuals' responses in the four adaptational modes: physiological function, self-concept, role function, and interdependence.

Second, nurses should assess the stimuli to which clients are responding. Roy (Roy and Roberts, 1981) defines three classes of stimuli: focal, or the primary, immediate stimuli; contextual, or the additional, background stimuli; and residual, stimuli or beliefs, attitudes and dispositions from prior experiences that may affect the present situation. Finally, nurses intervene by manipulating the actual or perceived stimuli so that a client can adapt and meet the goals of physiological, psychological, and social integrity. The Roy model does not identify or suggest specific interventions. Rather, as a theoretical framework, it guides creative problem solving.

Adaptational Modes

PHYSIOLOGICAL FUNCTION

Three dimensions of sexual adaptation should be assessed in the area of physiological function: sexual response, reproductive capacity, and physical characteristics. The physiological portion of sexual activity is interrelated with other bodily systems. For example, in males, prostatic problems associated with the urinary system may also herald dysfunction in their "sexual prowess." In this instance, a male client might be asked about urinary symptoms such as difficulties in initiating the stream, the quality of the urinary stream, and pain upon urination that might suggest prostatic abnormalities. A female client might be asked about pain during intercourse and its relationship to her menstrual cycle or the presence of any abnormal vaginal discharge or odor. In another example, a high-risk pregnancy may impose restrictions on a woman's sexual activity, as when women who have had preterm labor symptoms are asked not to have sexual intercourse and orgasm. Other examples of assessment of the physiological function are inquiries about the orgasmic experience for both men and women, obtaining a menstrual and obstetrical history from a woman, and determining a couple's fertility history.

Psychological Function

Assessment of sexual adaptation in the area of psychological functioning includes assessment of the self-concept mode or of individuals' sense of wholeness and a sense of physical and personal self (Roy, 1981). Examples

of data to be gathered include a client's view of physical appearance, sense of sexual attractiveness, and the level of confidence in the ability to function sexually.

Role Function

Because role function is concerned with the question "Who am I in relation to others?" assessments of sexual health include evaluation of individual beliefs regarding perceived sex-appropriate roles for men and women and their abilities to fulfill these roles competently. For example, the man who believes that his masculinity and sexual worth are tied to his ability to earn a living may experience sexual difficulties if he is unable to work owing to a chronic illness. The woman whose identity as a female is linked to her reproductive capacities and who is unable to have children may find that she no longer desires intercourse.

INTERDEPENDENCE

Because the underlying need in this mode is for affectional integrity experienced through love, value, and respect, adaptation in this mode may be threatened by illness. Assessment should include client concerns regarding the stability of the marital and/or sexual relationship, whether a partner may leave if a client is unable to perform sexually, partner demands for sexual performance, and partner concerns regarding the effect of sexual activity on the client's health.

Sexual History

Techniques used to gather data in order to assess sexual health and sexual functioning consist of the sexual history and physical examination.

The goal of the sexual history is to ascertain an individual's level of sexual health and sexual functioning. According to Rosalyn Watts (1979), the sexual history should "educate and counsel individuals who raise questions about the sexual aspect of life." Such persons may be those clients who are healthy or others whose feelings about sexuality are distorted because of acute or chronic illness." Obtaining a sexual history, in addition to providing data for assessment, may also be therapeutic. Taking the history gives the message that sexuality and sexual functioning are legitimate and appropriate components of health. The assessment process gives the client an opportunity to discuss concerns while allowing the health professional to provide the client with information and to validate the client's concerns or practices as normal and acceptable.

Woods (1984) suggests that sexual histories be obtained from clients with an initial complaint of sexual dysfunction, from individuals whose illnesses or surgery may affect their sexual functioning, from clients who have sexually transmitted diseases or are infertile or pregnant, and from clients who seek contraceptive counseling. While all individuals have the potential for experiencing sexual problems, some may be more at risk than others. Individuals experiencing maladaptation in one or more of Roy's (1981) modes of adaptation have an increased possibility of developing sexual problems. Further, there are specific problem areas related to sexuality and sexual functioning (Table 2–1) that may place individuals at increased risk.

SUGGESTIONS FOR COLLECTING DATA

Many health professionals and their clients are not completely comfortable discussing sexuality. This discomfort may be exaggerated when two individuals do not know each other, have had little opportunity to establish a trusting relationship, and/or have backgrounds or personal characteristics that are dissimilar. In the extreme, a young female

TABLE 2–1. Problem Areas Related to Sexuality and Sexual Functioning*

1. Frequency or timing of sexual relations
2. Varieties of sexual activity
3. Who initiates; who refuses
4. Concerns about what is normal
5. Myths and ignorance regarding sexual activity, behavior, function
6. Effects of medical conditions on sexuality
7. Sexual expression without a partner
8. Children and sexuality—their own and that of adults
9. Parent and adolescent sexuality
10. Adolescents' own sexuality
11. Effects of aging on sexuality
12. Anxiety and guilt about sexual activities
13. Sexual disorders (e.g., erectile disorders, premature ejaculation, orgasmic disorder)
14. Atypical sexual behavior (e.g., pedophilia, fetishism, sadomasochism)

*Problems are generally listed in order of increasing anxiety-provoking problems.

nurse may be viewed by the older male client as a potential "daughter figure," while a handsome male nurse may generate sexual feelings in the young female client. It is important for health professionals to foster a trusting and professional relationship with their clients as soon as possible (MacElveen-Hoehn, 1985). Attitudes are often communicated nonverbally during an interview. Clients who sense that the health professional is acutely uncomfortable will probably not feel free to discuss sexual problems. It is essential that health professionals communicate their interest and concern for their clients in a kind, straightforward manner, thereby providing an open door for the communication of sexual concerns. When the health professional approaches sexuality comfortably and in a serious manner, the client may be able to share concerns that otherwise would not have been raised (Muscari, 1987).

A sexual history may need to be collected over several meetings. If the client's anxiety level is high at the first interview, the health professional may need to help the client become more comfortable before proceeding with the interview. The history does not have to be completed at the first contact but can be gathered when most appropriate. Often, only the most essential information is collected at the initial interview, allowing trust and rapport to develop prior to soliciting what the client might consider more personal and intimate information. Health professionals should be flexible and should maintain a relaxed tone to the interviews.

The location of the interview as well as the positions of the participants can make the difference between success and failure. Whenever possible, nurses should choose a location where clients will feel comfortable sharing personal information (Chapman and Sughrue, 1987). A hectic, crowded lounge or a busy ward are not the most conducive areas for communication.

The space between practitioner and client can also be inhibitory or facilitative. Eye contact may initially be difficult for clients to establish, and they may prefer that the interviewer not be directly across from them. Others may respond better to continued eye contact (Muscari, 1987), which can facilitate the nurse's empathetic facial expressions and can convey a more accepting attitude. Astute interviewers will be able to pick up the subtle cues that the client gives off and adjust their behavior accordingly.

Certain guidelines must be kept in mind when any health information is gathered but particularly in the area of sexual functioning. Interviewers should be aware of their own feelings; if nurses are embarrassed or feel negatively about the material, their patterns of communication, both verbal and nonverbal, may hinder openness in the client. Usually, more information is obtained if the interviewer starts with open-ended questions, allowing clients to tell their story on their own terms. At the same time, closed questions are appropriate for the collection of a medical history, menstrual history, and drug reactions. Closed questions often follow open questions in order to facilitate the assessment process. The interviewer can guide the assessment process by setting limits if excessive or irrelevant information is offered, directing the client if information becomes tangential, and providing encouragement if progress is slow. Because of the personal nature of the material being collected, clients may sometimes misinterpret the professional's intentions. Clients should be told why the questions are being asked and that the information will assist the nurse in the provision of care. Feelings of prying are most often the concern of the nurse, not the client; however, the nurse must always weigh the value of the information to be disclosed against encouraging the disclosure of unnecessary information. This can be avoided by continuing to treat the client as an individual, by maintaining a professional relationship, and by dealing directly with possible misinterpretation of intentions.

Because a sexual history contains questions of a sensitive nature, it is helpful to start with the less threatening material. This technique facilitates the progression of the interview by increasing the client's comfort with the interviewer and the questions being asked. For example, after the nurse has asked a woman about her obstetrical history and elimination patterns (more acceptable areas of discussion), it may be easier to address more sensitive topics. Or, the interviewer may begin by discussing the client's childhood sexual development and education before exploring current sexual behavior and practices. General guidelines for explicit sexual content might be to begin with questions about the individual's sexual learning history, to proceed to personal attitudes and beliefs about

sex, and finally to assess their actual sexual behaviors.

Use of excessive medical terminology should be avoided during the interview. This may only serve to further distance the client from the health professional. However, use of the most technical language that the client knows and is comfortable with will ensure that both client and interviewer have a similar understanding of the data and that both have an adequate grasp of the client's problem. It may be necessary for either or both of them to define the terms they are using. Euphemisms about sex (e.g., "Have you ever slept with someone?") should be avoided in the interest of clarity.

When conducting an interview, the nurse should pose only one question at a time. Enough time should be allowed for the client to think through what is being asked and to provide the information. Abrupt shifts in topics should be avoided. It is important to set up a logical flow of questions that makes sense to both the interviewer and client. Clients should not be asked statistical questions such as how many times a week they have intercourse or how many orgasms they have. This type of question leaves clients wanting to provide an answer that shows they are normal or average, rather than encouraging accurate answers. Instead, the nurse might say, "Tell me about your sexual activity in a week's time. What sorts of things do you do?" "Universalizing" is a technique that implies that a wide variety of sexual behaviors are acceptable, giving the client permission to answer the question honestly. This technique is helpful in avoiding prompting clients to answer in a way that they think will demonstrate normalcy or that they think the nurse wants to hear. The nurse might say, "Many people have erotic fantasies about someone other than their husband. Is this something that has happened to you?" If health professionals are interested in the masturbation habits of their client, the subject could be approached by saying, "The Kinsey Reports showed that most males (females) start masturbating at an early age. At what age did you begin masturbation?" This signals to the client that the practitioner accepts masturbation and considers it a normal activity. In the individual who has not had an active masturbation pattern, the use of the word "most" in the above example is an indication that their lack of activity is also normal practice. While prefacing a question with the phrase "many people experience" is a useful technique, the health professional should guard against making assumptions about the client's sexual activities or sexual preference. In addition to making clients feel comfortable about their choice of sexual experiences, health professionals must realize and be comfortable with the fact that their own sexual choices may philosophically conflict with those of their clients.

The method by which information is recorded is important to the ease of the interview. If the sexual health history is incorporated into the overall health history, clients may readily accept answers to personal aspects of their life being documented. However, if the interview is more focused, the client may be uncomfortable having responses recorded during the interview. In addition, rapport is difficult to maintain if the interviewer is constantly taking notes. Developing a shorthand system that is thorough and unobtrusive is useful. It is also helpful if the interviewer emphasizes the goal of the interview beforehand and assures clients of the confidentiality of their answers. If the client is still uncomfortable, then a mutually agreed upon strategy for recording the data must be determined.

SEXUAL HISTORY FORMATS

Brief Sexual History

A brief, or screening, sexual history can be incorporated into a total health history. A short format of three questions, as suggested by Woods (1984), enables the nurse to gather information about the client's usual sexual roles, views of the self as a sexual being, and sexual functioning:

1. Has anything (illness, pregnancy, surgery) interfered with your being a (mother/wife/husband/father)?
2. Has anything (illness, medical treatment, surgery) changed the way you feel about yourself as a man or woman?
3. Has anything (surgery, medication, disease) altered your ability to function sexually?

When it is known that sexuality is likely to be affected by a specific illness, treatment regimen, or surgery, it may be useful to gather specific information about sexual functioning. Certain basic questions can be asked in early contacts with clients. It is first necessary to ascertain whether the client is currently sexually active. If sexually active,

clients are then asked to describe their sexual activity to determine the frequency of sexual activity. Next, they are asked whether they are satisfied with their sexual activity. Men are queried about their ability to attain and maintain an erection and about ejaculatory control. Women are asked whether they have difficulty becoming aroused or having orgasm. Both men and women are asked whether they experience any pain with intercourse. The history concludes by asking whether there are any questions or problems the client wishes to discuss with the nurse. Kolodny, Masters, and Johnson (1979) believe that 95 per cent of all sexual problems can be elicited using this format. The information can provide pretreatment baseline data that can later assist in assessing the impact of the disease or treatment on sexual functioning. Further, this information can be used to develop interventions tailored to the individual's and couple's needs. The nurse should also explore the client's knowledge of the diagnosis, disease process, and treatment effects. Questions should explore the meaning ascribed by clients to the illness and diagnosis and the effect of the disease and treatment on self-concept and sexual functioning.

The total health history also provides information relevant to the individual's sexual health. The client's educational level, occupation, religious beliefs, and practices may dictate the level and type of questioning used and will influence the type of interventions that are chosen. Physical and/or psychological disorders and medical interventions should be documented, since many disease processes and pharmacological agents can cause sexual dysfunctions. In addition, specific categories of assessment for females, males, and couples should be designed.

The Female Client

Certain elements of the sexual history are unique to the female client. When assessing a female client's sexual health, it is important to gather information about her menstrual history, including age of menarche, number of days in cycle, characteristics of menstrual flow, and duration of active bleeding. In addition, the nurse inquires about the level of comfort during the menstrual cycle, focusing on ovulatory discomfort and cramping during menses. Questions about intermenstrual bleeding and vaginal discharge, including characteristics and timing, are asked. The method of sanitary protection is often clarified, and the client's level of satisfaction with her chosen protection is ascertained. If the woman is beyond her childbearing years, she is asked when menopause occurred and whether she has experienced any difficulties with sexual functioning. If she has had problems, she is asked how she dealt with them.

Next, the interviewer obtains the obstetrical history. Clients are asked about the number of pregnancies, deliveries, and spontaneous and induced abortions they have had. Difficulties conceiving and any history of infertility are noted. A comprehensive contraceptive history is also gathered, including methods used, how used, and the woman's satisfaction and/or dissatisfaction with each method. Additionally, history of infectious and sexually transmitted diseases are recorded.

Finally, the woman is briefly interviewed regarding her sexual response cycle. It is important to clarify the degree of vaginal lubrication during sexual arousal or of pain with intercourse.

The Male Client

The male client also has unique needs that require assessment. The urinary system is investigated, including frequency of urination, identification of specific times when the frequency may increase or decrease, difficulty in initiating the stream, the quality of the urinary stream, and pain on urination. Any prostatic abnormalities are described as well as interventions utilized to correct the problems. History of testicular trauma is noted. The client is asked about penile discharge, including its characteristics, and any past or present genital infections and their treatment. In addition, the man should be asked about his contraceptive experiences and fertility problems.

As with the female client, the male sexual system is assessed. Desire for sexual activity and the client's erection potential are described, including difficulty in initiating and/or sustaining an erection once sexually aroused, situations of erectile failure, pain on erection, and the volume of ejaculate. If difficulty is assessed, a more indepth discussion includes specific instances during which the dysfunction occurred, possible precipitating factors, and when and if the erection returned. The presence or absence of morn-

ing erections is determined because their presence could be significant in the differentiation between a psychogenic and physiological disturbance.

Both males and females are questioned about their premarital sexual activity (if married). Family experiences with touching and affection are ascertained. The acceptability of masturbation for an individual is determined, and individuals are questioned about their satisfaction with personal sexual response and partner satisfaction.

Information about the individual's present relationship is relevant. Clients can be asked to rate the relationship with respect to communication, affection, sexual needs met, and sexual communication. Additional areas that might be explored are presented in Table 2–2.

Sexual Problem History

A sexual problem history can be used to supplement a brief sexual history. It can be obtained within the context of sexual counseling or therapy. This type of history is intended to collect information to be able to define the character, etiology, onset, severity, duration, and psychosocial effect of a presenting sexual dysfunction. If a problem or disorder is uncovered during the course of a screening sexual history, a detailed sexual history may be indicated. Although the parameters of the sexual problem history may vary with the theoretical framework guiding the health professional's practice, there are commonalities that should be explored regardless of the approach to therapy. The first step is to obtain a description of the problem in the client's own words that is solicited in objective, nonjudgmental terms. The interviewer can ask the client, "How old were you when the problem first started?" and attempt to understand what is being said and what is meant. The second step is to explore the onset and course of the problem. The client is asked to describe the duration, intensity, frequency, and situational circumstances of the problem. Questions include "Does it occur with all partners?" and "Does it happen with activities other than sexual intercourse?" Third, the health professional determines the client's own assessment of the problem, realizing that some may have no idea while others may be quite accurate. The client's concept of the cause and persistence of the problem is very important. Past attempts at treatment

TABLE 2–2. Content Areas for Sexual History: Relationship Aspects

Desire for Sexual Experience
> Increased, decreased, fluctuation, changed patterns.
> Concern about sexual adequacy.
> Feelings about body image and their impact on desire.

Sexual Interaction with Partner

Male and Female
> *Preliminaries of lovemaking*: initiation, extent of communication.
> *Characteristics of love play*: behaviors that detract from the overall erotic encounters, sexual norms within the unit—extracoital options.
> *Extramarital experience*: frequency, duration.

Male
> *Erectile functioning*: quality of erections, situations that precipitate erectile failure, satisfaction with penis size.
> *Orgastic experience*: frequency of climax or orgasm; how achieved—vaginal penetration, by hand, orally; change in quality of experience; concern over partner reaching climax.
> *Coital positions*: degree of experimentation.

Female
> *Facility for vaginal lubrication*: sufficient time for lubrication, rapidity of, increased/decreased, vaginal pain during penile penetration.
> *Orgastic capacity*: achievement of climax; method—masturbation, manual/oral manipulation by partner; description of frequency, situations that inhibit orgasm

and their results represent the fourth area to be assessed. The client's use of books, past professional treatment, personal steps taken, and advice from friends should be noted. Finally, the client's expectations should be ascertained. It is important to know whether the client hopes for a reversal of symptoms, wants to save a relationship, or has a secret desire to fail in the relationship (Elmasia and Wilson, 1983).

An indepth sexual history for sexual dysfunction has been developed by Masters and Johnson (1970). They recommend assessing the following: nature of the presenting distress; statistics of the present relationship; life cycle influences and events in childhood, adolescence, premarital adulthood, and marriage; perception of self; and response to sensory stimuli. This type of format can generate an enormous amount of information, including experiences, feelings, sexual practices, and perceptions of the self and self-concept, although several hours of interview are required. A sexual problem history should only be undertaken by health professionals with extensive training in sexual counseling and/or therapy.

ADDITIONAL AREAS OF SEXUAL ASSESSMENT

Health professionals should assess their clients' understanding of various aspects of sexuality, including reproduction, conception, contraception, sexual anatomy and physiology, and the sexual response cycle. The client's sexual self-awareness should also

be determined and should include the assessment of client understanding and practice of testicular and breast self-examination and client awareness of the symptoms of sexually transmitted diseases.

Sources of the client's sexual education should be assessed as well as the age at which this information was given. Clients should be asked to reflect on how they reacted to the material and whether their initial values and/or beliefs have subsequently been altered. If changes have occurred, the client is asked to identify events that may have precipitated the changes. Examples of questions that can be asked include the following: "When you were a child, how were your questions about sex answered? Where did your sexual information come from (appropriate for teenagers)? When you were a teenager, how were your questions about sex answered (to be used with adults)? How did you first find out about sexual intercourse? How babies were made?" (Mims and Swenson, 1980).

Clients' beliefs regarding gender roles and appropriate sex role behaviors are also assessed. Clients can be asked about their beliefs regarding appropriate ways to interact with members of the opposite sex and to describe their dating patterns and what qualities they value in a partner. Health professionals should keep in mind the influence of religious, educational, social, and economic factors on sex role orientation.

INTERVENTION

Nursing interventions are the means by which nurses assist clients in their efforts to adapt (Randell, Tedrow, and Van Landingham, 1982; Roy, 1981). Nursing interventions to promote sexual health may be simple or complex, preventive or therapeutic. They will vary with each client and are designed within the context of individual needs. Clients may be individuals, families, or groups, and interventions may change according to the site or practice setting. The physiological, psychological, and social aspects of the client's experience of sexuality are the focus of sexual interventions. Through a partnership established between nurse and client, the nurse facilitates the client's sexual adaptation to enhance or maintain health.

Nursing roles in the provision of sexual health care include education, counseling, and therapy. The role of the nurse varies depending on the characteristics of the nurse, the client, and the setting (Woods, 1984). *Nurse variables* essential to effective sexual intervention are a comprehensive sexual knowledge base, awareness of one's own and others' sexual value systems, and a positive self-concept, which, in turn, allows acceptance of others' differing needs and perspectives. Abilities basic to effective intervention in sexual health include open, genuine, therapeutic communication skills; a professional manner that is accepting, supportive, and growth promoting; the use of the decision-making process for ongoing assessment, planning, intervention, and evaluation; and the ability to engage the client in identifying needs, setting goals, and problem solving.

Client variables identified by Woods (1984) include the nature of the client's actual or potential sexual health problem and client characteristics: for instance, whether the client is an individual, couple, group, organization, or community. Client variables are not static. They change in response to interventions; and in the process of change, the client can be more fully understood. As client variables change, indications for intervention may also change.

Setting variables relate to the site where the nurse practices, the characteristics of the particular institution or system, and whether the system allows for and supports the delivery of sexual health care services by nurses. The setting will also to some extent define the client population. The characteristics of the health care facility may determine the age range and socioeconomic status of the clients and the presence of special groups, such as the sexually disenfranchised or stigmatized client or the victims of sexual abuse. Each of these setting variables will then influence the level and nature of nursing interventions.

The PLISSIT Model for Sexual Health Interventions

Annon (1974; 1976) developed a model for ordering levels of interventions for sexual problems that is appropriate for health professionals providing sexual health care (Table 2–3). The Annon model, which incorporates four levels of sexual counseling, has become known as the PLISSIT model (from the first initial of each word in the four levels: permission, limited information, specific suggestions, intensive therapy). In Annon's framework, increasing knowledge and clinical skills are required as the intervention levels of the model increase in complexity. The PLISSIT model is based on principles of learning theory and uses a behavioral approach to the treatment of sexual problems.

Nurses should be able to intervene at the first three levels. Data obtained from a brief or screening sexual history is needed to assess clients' sexual problems, and interventions range from permission giving and providing limited sex education to offering brief sexual counseling or specific suggestions (levels I to III). Nurses providing intensive therapy (level IV) should have postgraduate education as a sex therapist. Sexual problem his-

TABLE 2–3. Annon Model of Approaches to Sexual Concerns

Permission: Providing reassurance that the client is normal and has professional permission to continue what he or she has been doing. It is important that permission not be given for activities that are potentially harmful to the individual.

Limited Information: Providing information directly relevant to the client's concern. This can effect significant changes in the client's attitudes and behavior.

Specific Suggestions: Direct efforts to assist the client to change behavior in order to attain stated goals by providing specific suggestions directly related to the particular problem.

Intensive Therapy: Highly individualized therapy, which is used when brief therapy is not effective.

Adapted from Annon J: Behavioral Treatment of Sexual Problems: Brief Therapy: Vol I. New York, Harper & Row, 1976.

tories are used to assess clients at this level, and interventions may include sex therapy, marital therapy, and psychotherapy.

PERMISSION

At the first level, nurses give clients professional "permission" to continue sexual behaviors that they have been practicing and offer reassurance that their behavior is normal. The client may raise questions about sexual behaviors, such as actions, feelings, fantasies, or dreams. Health professionals are often approached as authorities to clarify behaviors the client is practicing and to determine whether the actions or thoughts, feelings, or fantasies are normal. While anxiety may often be present when the concern is discussed, the person is usually not bothered or limited by the actual behavior. Clients may be concerned, however, about whether there is something wrong or unusual about what they are doing. Giving permission allows the person to continue the behavior and alleviates anxiety about normalcy. According to Annon, this first level of intervention has the potential for prevention because it resolves concerns that otherwise may grow into problems. Permission giving can also be considered a health-promoting intervention, enabling clients to incorporate sexual behaviors into a positive, accepting sexual self-concept. Permission should not be given, however, for behaviors that may be either physically or emotionally harmful to the individual or to the sexual partner.

Permission giving is the least complex of the sexual interventions in the PLISSIT model and requires minimal preparation on the part of the clinician. It can be a less formal mode of intervention, since concerns expressed at this level may be brought up anywhere. Usually, the simple reassurance that the behavior is normal is enough to alleviate the concern.

Inquiries about the effect of developmental changes, illness, or lifestyle alterations on the client's sexuality are ways of giving the client permission to be a sexual being. When a client raises sexual questions or concerns, the nurse's willingness to listen can also communicate the importance of sexual health. No intervention has the potential to enhance sexual health unless it occurs within a respectful, accepting environment, in which permission is communicated and anxiety and guilt are minimized. Specific interventions may

give the client permission to continue current practices, but an accepting therapeutic milieu allows the client to be free to question, grow, or seek help if needed.

Nurses have many opportunities to use permission giving with clients. The following are some clinical examples:

A school health nurse is visited by a 16-year-old girl, Gloria, who seems anxious and distracted while she complains that she has a bad backache.

Nurse: You do seem to be uncomfortable. And you also seem nervous. Is anything else bothering you?

Gloria: All the girls in my group are teasing me because I'm the only one who is still a virgin. They're putting a lot of pressure on to go all the way with Calvin—he's my boyfriend.

Nurse: I can understand how that might make you feel really upset and pressured. No one wants to feel like they aren't like the rest of their friends—like a geek!

Gloria: But I don't want to have sex yet! I like it the way it is.

Nurse: It's okay not to want to have intercourse—to not feel ready for that yet. And, you know, what you're feeling isn't all that unusual. . . . People your age often feel that something is wrong with them if they don't seem to want what everyone else in their group wants.

Gloria: Gosh, I really thought I was the only one. You mean it's okay for me to wait?

Nurse: Yes, it is okay.

After this interaction, Gloria becomes noticeably more relaxed and asks if she can talk with the nurse about how she can get her girlfriends to stop bugging her.

Mr. and Mrs. Lowell have just moved into a nursing home, where they share a room. Although both have accepted that their individual physical limitations necessitated the move to a health care facility, the decision was not an easy one, since they cherish their privacy as individuals and as a couple. About 2 weeks after admission, Mr. Lowell asks the nurse, who is male, to close the door, so that he can talk about a private matter.

Mr. Lowell: There's something that's really been bothering me—well, us, really. Now Shirley says not to talk with anyone about it but . . . I don't know.

Nurse: Mr. Lowell, if there's something

bothering you, it's a good idea to talk about it. Maybe I can help?

Mr. Lowell: Well, you know, when we decided to come in here, we thought it'd be as nice a place as we could find—except a real home, of course. I've got my arthritis, and Shirley can't hear too well—well you know all that. . . .

Nurse: (Nods, encouragingly, aware that Mr. L is anxious about whatever it is he needs to talk about.)

Mr. Lowell: The truth is, what's bothering me is sex. We still do it. I know everybody thinks that once you're over the hill like Shirley and I are, you just don't bother anymore (waits, looking for a response).

Nurse: Actually, Mr. L, interest in sex is lifelong for most people. It's not unusual, and there's nothing strange or wrong about it—it's healthy, even good for you!

Mr. Lowell: (Relieved, shakes head) Well, I'm glad to hear you say that . . . so it's not abnormal, eh? People sure don't talk about it much.

Nurse: It's very normal. Are you concerned about changes in your sex life now that you and Mrs. Lowell have moved here?

Mr. Lowell: Well, like I said, my wife and I still have intercourse; (leaning forward) I'll tell you a little secret, we did last night . . . closed the door, pulled the bedcurtain . . . but Shirley was real worried that they'd catch us. I guess that's what I need to ask you about. Is it okay? I mean we're married and it's our room, isn't it?

Nurse: Yes, it is your room, and you have the right to privacy in it. We can give you a Do Not Disturb sign that you can place on your door when you and Mrs. Lowell want some private time, uninterrupted. How about that?

Mr. Lowell: Oh, I think that'd make both of us feel a lot better . . . like we don't have to sneak around or be ashamed . . . afraid of being caught.

Nurse: No, Mr. Lowell, you don't have to sneak around. Let's see how this works out, if it helps you and Mrs. Lowell feel more comfortable. By the way, I'm glad you felt comfortable enough to talk with me.

Mr. Lowell: Well, it was really bothering me but I feel a lot better now. Thanks a lot!

These situations illustrate the essential characteristics of permission giving in nursing practice settings. In each situation, the client is bothered by concerns about sexual behavior, feelings, or attitudes, although the client's sexual behavior is not actually limited by the concerns. But the client needs permission and reassurance that the behavior is normal. The intervention phase involves recognition that questions of self-concept are valid concerns, acceptance of the appropriateness of sexual expression within role expectation is normal, a direct statement that the behavior is usual or normal, and encouragement to continue the behavior. Positive experiences in the kinds of help-seeking situations described may make the client feel more comfortable about approaching health professionals again in the future.

LIMITED INFORMATION

Giving limited information provides clients with specific facts that are directly related to their area of concern. Directly related information can be helpful in changing potentially negative thoughts and attitudes about particular aspects of sexuality. A list of common concerns and misconceptions about sexuality is found in Table 2–4. Providing information, especially when the content is immediately relevant and limited in scope, can also effect behavioral changes (Annon, 1976). Helping clients to increase their knowledge about sexuality or answering questions about sexual concerns promotes sexual health by preventing or limiting dysfunctional behaviors. This level of sexual intervention requires the health professional to have a comprehensive sexual knowledge base. The greater the health professional's knowledge,

TABLE 2–4. Common Concerns and Misconceptions Regarding Sexuality

Myths regarding the characteristics of male and female sexual experiences.

Notions about what constitutes the body, e.g., "normal" genital size, shape, or form.

Masturbation.

Oral-genital contact.

Myths about menstruation.

Body image changes or sexual functional ability changes related to surgery or chronic illness.

Sexual developmental concerns, particularly during adolescence and in the middle years.

Situational events or processes that alter or affect sexual behavior, such as periods of increased life stress, specific psychological stresses, or crises related to sexuality (unwanted pregnancy, rape, incest, homophobia).

the more comfortable they are likely to feel intervening at this level.

Providing limited information takes more time and requires more knowledge than does permission giving. Frequently, giving limited information directly follows permission giving. In the clinical examples presented, the content of the client's concern focused on the acceptable, the usual, or the normal. Often the concerns arise because the person is not sure what is normal. The client may be struggling to place sexual behavior in the context of normalcy but doesn't know whether the behavior is acceptable, hence, the need for permission. So frequently, there is a need for both permission giving and information giving to clarify misinformation, dispel myths, or provide specific information.

Information giving may take the form of responses to direct questions, in which the nurse presents information to help the client prepare for or adapt to sexual changes brought about through developmental processes, situational events, surgery, and chronic or acute illness. Or an individual, group, or community approach to sex education may be required.

When used appropriately, information giving can enhance positive self-concept, increase role mastery, and facilitate interdependence. Information giving can be anticipatory or at the person's direct request. Assessment of the need and readiness for learning, the nature and extent of the knowledge deficit, and the most appropriate teaching method (demonstration, positive reinforcement, modeling, or verbalization) should be carried out before actual content is shared.

Information giving will only be helpful when the client has a knowledge deficit. Knowing what to expect or that current behavior is appropriate often decreases anxiety and increases the client's adaptation. But information should not be provided simply in the service of "health teaching" or "sex education." At a recent professional meeting, a group of nursing colleagues became involved in laughter and joking about hot flashes and the simultaneous need for air conditioning and heat. The group used humor to recognize common concerns and in doing so, the interaction was at once accepting and supportive. But the anxiety among these group members was not generated by limited knowledge. Had someone intervened and given limited information to this group, they would have been very much put off. In similar clinical situations, accurate assessment is an essential precursor to the provision of limited information.

Assisting couples in their adaptation to illness or surgery that may affect sexual functioning is an important preventive and therapeutic measure. The following example illustrates this point:

> Mrs. Gray is a 40-year-old woman who is about to have a hysterectomy. She would most likely benefit from the following limited information-giving interventions: explaining to her and her partner (if she has one) how the hysterectomy will affect her reproductive capacities and menstrual cycle, clarifying misinformation about the effects of hysterectomies on sexual functioning, dispelling myths that may be contributing to negative attitudes or fears about the surgery, and discussing her or her and her partner's ideas about anticipated changes in physical self-concept or role as a sexual being after the hysterectomy.

Assisting an individual or family to adapt to behavioral changes that occur during normal development is another common area for information giving. While individuals may expect developmental processes to occur, normal milestones and the behavioral changes that accompany them can be a source of anxiety, especially when they relate to sexuality.

Situational stressors may stimulate temporary sexual dysfunction or behavior pattern changes. Efforts to adapt to these situations often include modification of previous behavior patterns as a means of coping with the stressor. Limited information interventions can be used to assist clients in understanding how and why stress affects sexual functioning. The following clinical example illustrates this point:

> Jerry, a 32-year-old engineer, his wife Ann, and their three children were transferred to a new state 1 month ago. Ann, a bookkeeper, is working part-time until the family gets settled in their new environment. Jerry's transfer accompanied a promotion and increased job responsibilities. The company is undergoing a growth spurt, which directly affects Jerry. Although Ann has made a commitment to a temporary career compromise, she is not happy doing part-time work and looks forward to feeling more settled. On his first visit to the employee health service, Jerry confides that he and Ann used to have intercourse three or four times a week; however, since the move,

they fall into bed at night exhausted, too tired for sex, and not really interested. What concerns them both is their lack of interest. They have never experienced this before, and they're afraid that "it's never going to be like it used to be."

Jerry needs to be helped to understand the changes in his sexual interest level. The nurse can first point out the number of stressors he is experiencing. This intervention, a form of permission giving, assures him that his response is normal and not unusual under the circumstances. The nurse can follow up by telling Jerry about the effect stress can have on sexual health. Jerry is likely to be reassured by learning that the changes in the level of sexual interest he is experiencing are probably temporary and that as his stress decreases, more energy will be available, and Jerry and Ann can return to their "premove" level of sexual interest and activity.

In addition to relieving concern and anxiety about sexuality, information giving can help prevent temporary sexual behavior changes, such as the one described above, from becoming permanent modes of adaptation.

SPECIFIC SUGGESTIONS

In certain situations, giving a client direct behavioral suggestions can help to relieve a sexual problem or difficulty. This level of intervention is characterized as being time and problem limited. Typically, one or two sessions of 30 minutes or less are needed to meet the client's needs. The nature of the sexual difficulty treated at this level is also limited in scope. Problems of sudden onset and/or short duration (weeks or months) are most responsive to this form of brief treatment. Sexual dysfunction that is generated by interpersonal conflict or is of long duration cannot be treated by this approach. Behavioral change is brought about by setting clear goals with the client and by identifying specific behaviors that the client can carry out directed at enhancing self-concept, role functioning, and interrelating in terms of sexuality, sexual self-concept, or sexual relations.

Two frequently used approaches to sexual behavior change at this level of intervention are *successive approximation* and *paradoxical intention*. In successive approximation, existing positive behaviors are reinforced as clients, on successive occasions, move closer to the desired behavior they wish to achieve. The following clinical example illustrates this intervention:

Carolyn, a freshman in college, recently had sexual intercourse for the first time and is coming to the clinic for contraceptives. The nurse is taking a brief sexual history.

Carolyn: You know, having sex felt good—I liked it—and it's really nice to feel that close to my boyfriend, but I haven't had an orgasm yet, no matter how hard I try.

Nurse: It is not unusual for young women to not have an orgasm when they first begin having intercourse. Have you had orgasms at other times or in other situations?

Carolyn: Oh yes, I've been masturbating since I was in the ninth grade, and I've also had them when we were messing around. But during intercourse, nothing happens.

Nurse: I understand that this is a real concern of yours. As I said, this is neither unusual or abnormal. Only about 20 to 30 per cent of all women have orgasms with only intercourse because it is more difficult for them to have adequate clitoral stimulation.

Limited information is appropriate, since the client reveals that during intercourse she is "trying hard" to have an orgasm. She might benefit from learning that an orgasm is not a voluntary response achieved by trying hard. The nurse can also point out the discrepancy in Carolyn's report that during intercourse she feels that "nothing happens" yet also describes a very pleasurable feeling of closeness with her boyfriend.

The specific suggestion of successive approximation would be appropriate for Carolyn. Since manual stimulation has been successful for her, a series of steps that incorporates self or partner stimulation with penile entry at the moment of orgasm could be suggested. When orgasm is achieved in this manner, a combination of manual stimulation and penile thrusting could be a next step. If this behavior consistently results in orgasm, an association will be made between thrusting and orgasm. Finally, manual stimulation could be gradually decreased if orgasm is reached more readily through penile thrusting. The nurse could also suggest to Carolyn that she redirect her attention (another form of specific suggestion) during intercourse to focus on the positive sensations in her body rather than the specific goal of orgasm. Since she has already told the nurse that she has positive feelings of closeness with her partner, redirecting her attention from "trying hard" to achieve an orgasm to awareness of other positive physical sensations may help alleviate some of the performance anxiety she is experiencing.

These suggestions can be made within the framework of Annon's specific suggestion format. At the initial session, after assessment, a plan is outlined in detail. This is followed by a limited period (perhaps several weeks) for Carolyn to try out the new behaviors, and then a second appointment for evaluation is scheduled. If Carolyn were to report that she had not reached the mutually agreed upon goal, reassessment and further intervention would then be indicated.

Paradoxical intention is another specific suggestion that can be helpful in reducing anxiety associated with sexual performance. With this approach, suggestions take the form of directing the client to increase the frequency or intensity of the behavior that the client has been avoiding. Consider a couple who seeks help for the man's recently developed difficulty with maintaining an erection during intercourse. They are told, "Between today's appointment and next week, I want you to have at least four 1-hour sessions in which you focus entirely on giving each other sensual pleasure. You can do whatever you find mutually enjoyable, except you are *not* to have intercourse." The object here is to relieve both partners of the pressure to perform: the man, who fears his condition might become a permanent problem, and the woman, who is so involved in worrying about whether her partner will lose his erection again that they are unable to relate to each other or to enjoy sexual activities. By focusing narrowly on their "problem," a limp penis, they are unable to experience any pleasurable sexual feelings. If the situation continues, it can escalate to the point at which sexual intercourse is completely avoided because of the anxiety it generates in both partners. Intervention, in the form of the direct suggestions to engage in sensual and sexual relating without intercourse, shifts the couple's focus to the behaviors they are avoiding—experiencing each other, mutual exploration, stimulation, and increasing arousal. The directive not to have intercourse relieves their performance pressure and allows the couple to begin to take part in previously overlooked or avoided behaviors that have the potential to resolve their difficulty. Frequently, the pleasure and involve-

ment derived from the prescribed sessions provides sufficiently positive reinforcement to relieve the problem, and the couple will proceed to genital intercourse, "disregarding" the nurse's instructions. Movement toward the goal of arousal and erection during intercourse becomes possible because the anxiety associated with the problem has been alleviated by the shift in intention, and the previously avoided arousal-enhancing behaviors are tried out successfully and positively reinforced.

These two examples illustrate several important principles of specific suggestions. In both situations, the client's problem was of recent onset and short duration. Specific goals were stated and agreed upon. Treatment, in the form of specific suggestions, was successful after one or two sessions. Neither client had underlying interpersonal problems, and their anxiety was relieved by following the suggestions.

There are numerous suggestions that can be made to clients, but the behavior prescribed should always be tailored to the individual's needs and particular situation. Specific suggestions may take the form of redirection of attention, relaxation techniques, movement or positional changes, the squeeze technique, or sensate focus exercises. The health professional must be able not only to draw on a variety of approaches to common sexual problems but also be able to formulate individualized suggestions.

The technique of specific suggestions may also be used in settings in which sex therapy is not an aspect of the role of the nurse. The following clinical examples illustrate this point:

> A woman with a recent mastectomy might be counseled to use a side-to-side position during intercourse, since this does not place pressure on the wound. Also, suggesting initiating sexual relations by gentle caressing or pleasing might help both partners in their adaptation to the surgery, since this approach may provide them both with reassurance of each other's continued care and need for sexual intimacy.

After colostomy, the mechanics of intercourse are of great concern. Suggestions such as emptying the ostomy bag just prior to sexual relations, placing a covering over the bag, or using a side-to-side position if the client is concerned about injuring the stoma may be helpful. Any of these actions will help a client or partner adjust to the surgery and encourage re-engagement in sexual relating. This in turn helps to limit feelings of loss and the possibility of depression secondary to the experience of loss. Thus, the nurse will have enhanced the client's level of adequacy through teaching, supporting, and enabling (Randell, Tedrow, and Van Landingham, 1982).

INTENSIVE THERAPY

Intensive therapy is the most complex of the treatment approaches to promote sexual health. It is used when the client's problems have not been resolved by interventions from the first three levels and when the problems are ones in which personal and emotional difficulties are interfering with sexual expression. Usually, a combination of factors are present that necessitate more than the previous three levels of intervention can offer (Poorman, 1988). The therapeutic process at this level of intervention is longer and more involved. While all nurses should be able to screen for sexual dysfunctions and to use interventions drawn from Annon's first three levels, only nurses with advanced training should provide sex therapy to clients. Health professionals who incorporate intensive sex therapy into their practice must be highly qualified. A broad base of sexual knowledge, the ability to use a variety of sex therapy and behavioral therapy techniques, and training in interactional or psychodynamic therapy are essential preparation for this advanced practice role. Sex therapists may come to specialized practice from a variety of professional disciplines, including nursing, psychology, social work, and medicine. In addition to the basic preparation of each of these disciplines, further advanced education is necessary if the health professional is to be well qualified to practice intensive sex therapy.

Sex Therapy

Since the early 1970s, therapeutic approaches to sexual dysfunctions have undergone radical change. Prior to this period, sexual dysfunctions were thought to be the expression of deep psychosexual conflicts that could be traced back to early childhood experiences (Freud, 1962). Based on this psychoanalytic view, the common approach to treatment was long-term psychotherapy directed toward resolution of the client's unconscious conflicts. Traditional psychotherapy required individual insight-oriented psychotherapy several times a week for months or even years. However, movement toward a new understanding of sexual dysfunction began during the 1950s and 1960s, when behavior therapy was used to treat sexual difficulties. Behavior therapy employs directive techniques to focus on changing present cognitive, affective, and relationship patterns. In the late 1960s and early 1970s, the field of sex therapy was profoundly changed with the publication of Masters and Johnson's extensive research on human sexual response (1966) and inadequacy (1970), followed by their development of a program of directive, time-limited strategies for the management of sexual difficulties (Masters and Johnson, 1970).

No one theory or modality is, by itself, sufficient in providing a framework for either the explanation or the treatment of sexual disorders (Hogan, 1978). Currently, most sex therapists practice from an eclectic perspective, utilizing aspects of behavioral therapy and a psychodynamic or interactional focus as well as aspects of Masters and Johnson's framework for the intensive treatment of sexual dysfunction. The strategies or framework used depends to a large degree on the unique needs of the client and the nature of the particular sexual dysfunction. Utilizing an eclectic approach in the treatment of sexual dysfunction allows flexibility in creating individualized treatment plans.

While the current trend in sex therapy is to draw from a variety of theoretical models, consistent characteristics can be identified that are basic to a general treatment approach. These include shortening of treatment period to as little as several weeks (Kolodny, Masters, and Johnson, 1979), prescribing structured sexual experiences (Kolodny, Masters, and Johnson, 1979; Kaplan, 1974), emphasizing education and the use of learning theory (Annon, 1976; Hawton, 1985), and using a couples therapy approach, in which mutual responsibility and interactional patterns are emphasized (LoPiccolo, 1979; Kaplan, 1974; Masters and Johnson, 1970).

PRINCIPLES UNDERLYING THE GENERAL THERAPEUTIC APPROACH

Provision of accurate information is considered a basic component of the sex therapy process. Because lack of knowledge is frequently a contributing factor in the development of sexual dysfunction, treatment necessitates correction of learning deficits, misinformation, myths, and negative attitudes. Teaching focuses on male and female sexual anatomy and response cycles, dispelling myths, and the identification of knowledge deficits that may be contributing to the dysfunctional sexual behavior (Hawton, 1985). Readings are often recommended at this time.

Focus on the Sexual Relationship. Sexual disorders are, by their very nature, shared disorders (Hawton, 1985; LoPiccolo, 1978). Both partners require assistance and share responsibility for change. This emphasis on the couple and mutual responsibility in the treatment of sexual dysfunction first emerged in the work of Masters and Johnson. Their focus emphasized interpersonal relationships as the context for sexual dysfunction (Masters and Johnson, 1970). Active involvement in the treatment process by both partners, focusing on the patterns of sexual relating of both partners, is believed by Masters and Johnson to enhance the effectiveness of treatment. While there is general agreement in the literature on the importance of an approach that emphasizes the partners' mutual responsibility within the sexual relationship (Kaplan, 1974; LoPiccolo, 1978, 1979), LoPiccolo (1978) points out that certain situations or sexual dysfunctions are better addressed by individual or group treatment.

Interpersonal problems are frequently uncovered in the process of exploring a couple's sexual relationship. These issues must be addressed in order to pave the way for changes in the pattern of sexual relating. General training as well as sexual communication skills is an important aspect of treatment.

Structured Sexual Experiences and Specific Techniques. The integration of structured sexual experiences into the therapeutic process is a distinctive characteristic of sex therapy (Kaplan, 1974). The choice of the structured experience and/or the specific technique depends upon the particular sexual disorder. Most often, experiences are graduated, i.e., the couple learns new sexual behaviors by completing a series of homework assignments designed to gradually rebuild the sexual relationship without being overly demanding or anxiety producing. At each step in the process, attention is given to reducing anxiety and building skills. These therapeutic experiences prescribe pleasure as the couple progresses toward their identified treatment goal. This approach, based on principles of learning theory, was adapted to sex therapy by Masters and Johnson and subsequently by Kaplan. Today, it is considered integral to the practice of intensive treatment for sexual dysfunction (Hawton, 1985; LoPiccolo, 1978).

Relief of Anxiety. Kaplan (1974) identified three kinds of anxiety present in sexual disorders: performance anxiety, fear of failure, and the excessive need to please one's partner. Progressive relaxation, self-hypnosis, imagery, and chemical agents are anxiety-reducing measures that can be used in formulating a treatment plan (Hogan, 1978). High levels of anxiety will often interfere with sexual performance. It is not unusual for a cyclical process to occur, in which anxiety precipitates sexual dysfunction, escalates as the dysfunctional behavior pattern is developed and maintained, and re-emerges in the treatment process during the client's attempts to learn new ways of sexual relating. The therapist must intervene directly in situations in which reduction of anxiety is necessary for progress to occur.

TREATMENT MODALITIES

As previously indicated, a number of therapy modalities are presently employed by those working with persons experiencing sexual problems.

Behavioral treatment assumes that human sexual behaviors are learned or conditioned and that specific learned behavior (sexual dysfunction) must be unlearned before the dysfunction will disappear. In the absence of physical pathology, sexual dysfunction is viewed as a learned phenomenon, maintained internally by performance anxiety and externally by reinforcements in the environment. Techniques drawn from learning theory are used and include systematic desensitization or flooding to relieve phobias and the assignment of specific therapeutic sexual tasks such as those described in the section on specific suggestions. Tasks are designed to reinforce more effective sexual responses and to shape sexual behavior gradually toward the goal of sexual competence.

Conjoint sex therapy, or the simultaneous treatment of both partners, is the treatment modality most frequently used today. Developed by Masters and Johnson (1970), it is based on the premise that there is no such thing as an uninvolved partner in a relationship affected by sexual dysfunction. Extended further, this concept sees complete sexual functioning as a reflection of suitable physical and behavioral interaction between two people, and a sexual dysfunction is a shared disorder for which each partner has responsibility for effecting change and achieving resolution (LoPiccolo, 1978). Conjoint therapy may also use a dual-therapist approach.

Dual sex-therapy, developed by Masters and Johnson, provides a same-sex therapist for each partner in conjoint therapy and encourages each partner to identify with this therapist. This approach is based on two assumptions: that women and men cannot fully understand each other's sexuality or dysfunctions and that each person is more likely to feel "represented" and understood by a therapist of the same sex. The therapists act as educators and interpreters as well as providing clients with support. Masters and Johnson believe that this dual-sex therapy approach enhances communication and mirrors the client relationship in a way that can be used to illustrate communication or interactional patterns. Increased education, permission giving, and modeling behaviors are benefits of the dual sex-therapy approach.

Kaplan's approach to sex therapy combines a dynamic interaction of specific sexual techniques and psychotherapy (Kaplan, 1974). The basic conceptual framework is eclectic and multicausal; sex therapy is viewed as a task-centered form of crisis intervention with an opportunity for rapid conflict resolution (Poorman, 1988). In order to achieve resolution, sexual tasks, insight therapy, marital therapy, supportive therapy, and other psychiatric techniques may be used. The initial purpose of therapy is to modify the immediate causes of dysfunction and defenses against sexuality; more remote issues are dealt with only to the extent necessary to relieve the sexual symptom and prevent the disorder from recurring. Kaplan's method does not require a dual sex-therapy approach; individual therapists of either gender may be used.

Group therapy has been successful in treating individuals, and some therapists use this method to treat couples as well. Benefits of a group approach include economy, social reinforcement and support, a variety of role models in addition to the therapists, and the opportunity to share problems and to learn that one's experiences are not isolated or unusual. An example of a group program that has been frequently utilized in the treatment of a specific dysfunction is that of Barbach (1974), who has outlined a group approach for women with orgasmic disorder. The group setting has also been used successfully in the treatment of erectile dysfunction (Lobitz and Baker, 1979; Zilbergeld, 1975) and premature ejaculation (Kaplan, 1974; Zeiss, 1978).

Referral as an Intervention

The referral process is an essential component of sexual health care. When the nurse's level of preparation is insufficient to meet the client's need for care, if the nurse has intervened but the client has not responded successfully or if more intensive interventions are needed, referral is indicated. Health professionals may also refer clients when their practice setting prevents adequate time or resources for intervention. The health professional's level of sexual health practice may dictate the need for a referral. In some instances, a client's current or prior psychiatric history or the existence of significant intrapersonal conflicts will necessitate a referral. Finally, referrals may be appropriate if the relationship is highly conflictual or if the problem is long-standing or complex.

Dysfunctional nurse-client relationship patterns may interfere with the nurse's ability to provide sexual health care. If the client behaves seductively toward the nurse, the nurse dislikes the client, or the nurse has strong sexual feelings toward the client, the nurse may be unable to intervene effectively, and referral may be indicated.

When clients are educated about the need for further treatment and nurses accept and explore clients' fears or negative attitudes about seeking help, the potential for successful referral is greatly enhanced. The health professional's approach to the referral process can help the client to seek treatment that is needed to alleviate sexual distress or dysfunction. The direct suggestion that the nurse thinks a client will work well with a particular sex therapist or that the client would benefit from further treatment or counseling will often help solidify the client's resolve to seek needed help.

Before making a referral, the health professional should be familiar with the sexual health or sex therapy resources available in the community. If possible, clients should be referred to colleagues with whom the health professional has an ongoing professional relationship. This provides a basis for knowing the therapist's preparation and qualifications and for referring clients to a professional who is able to meet their particular sexual health care needs.

SUMMARY

Nurses and other health professionals intervene with clients about sexual issues daily. The extent of their role in promoting sexual health will depend on their level of preparation, the needs of the client, and the characteristics of the practice setting. This chapter has provided information to enable nurses and other health professionals to better meet their clients' needs for sexual health care. The decision-making process guides the provision of health care in a systematic way, which moves the provider from assessment to evaluation of each client. Specific tools with which to gather data about clients' sexual problems allow the health professional to assess client needs appropriately, and the framework for intervention suggested allows health professionals to intervene at a level appropriate to their preparation. Familiarity with the techniques and processes basic to assessment and intervention furnishes the health professional with a variety of possibilities for maximizing clients' potential for sexual health.

REFERENCES

Annon JS: The PLISSIT Model: A proposed conceptual scheme for the behavioral treatment of sexual problems. J Sex Educ Ther 2:1–15, 1976.

Annon JS: Behavioral Treatment of Sexual Problems: Brief Therapy. New York, Harper & Row, 1974.

Barbach LG: Group treatment of pre-orgasmic women. J Sex Marit Ther 1:139–145, 1974.

Barnard MU, et al: Human Sexuality for Health Professionals. Philadelphia, WB Saunders, 1978.

Bulechek GM, McCloskey JC: Nursing Interventions: Treatments for Nursing Diagnosis. WB Saunders, 1985.

Campbell SJ: Sexuality Assessment. Nursing Assessment: A Multidimensional Approach. In Bellack J, Bainford PA (eds): Monterey, Wadsworth Health Sciences Division, 1984.

Chapman J, Sughrue J: A model for sexual assessment and intervention. Heal Care Women Inter 8:87–99, 1987.

Elmassia BJ, Wilson RW: Assessment and diagnosis of sexual problems. Nurse Pract June:13–15, 19, 22, 1983.

Freud S: Three Essays on the Theory of Sexuality. New York, Avon, 1962.

Green R: Human Sexuality: A Health Practitioner's Text. Baltimore, Williams & Wilkins, 1975.

Green R: Taking a sex history. In Green R (ed): Human Sexuality: A Health Practitioner's Text. Baltimore, Williams & Wilkins, 1975, pp 9–19.

Gordon M: Nursing Diagnosis: Process and Application. New York, McGraw-Hill, 1982.

Group for Advancement of Psychiatry: Assessment of sexual function: A guide to interviewing. GAP Report No. 88, Committee on Medical Education. New York, GAP, 1973.

Hawton K: Sex Therapy: A Practical Guide. Oxford, Oxford University Press, 1985.

Hogan DR: The effectiveness of sex therapy: A review of the literature. In LoPiccolo J, LoPiccolo L (eds): Handbook of Sex Therapy. New York, Plenum Press, 1978.

Kaplan HS: The New Sex Therapy. New York, Brunner/Mazel, 1974.

Kolodny RC, Masters WH, Johnson VE: Textbook of Sexual Medicine. Boston, Little, Brown & Co, 1979.

Krozy R: Becoming Comfortable with Sexual Assessment. Am J Nurs 78:1036–1038, 1978.

Lion EM: Human Sexuality in Nursing Process. 3rd ed. New York, John Wiley & Sons, 1982.

Lobitz WC, Baker EL: Group treatment of single males with erectile dysfunction. Arch Sex Behav 8:127–138, 1979.

LoPiccolo J: Treatment of sexual concerns by the primary care male clinician. In Green R (ed): Human Sexuality: A Health Practitioner's Text. 2nd ed. Baltimore, Williams & Wilkins, 1979.

LoPiccolo J: Direct treatment of sexual dysfunction. In LoPiccolo J, LoPiccolo L (eds): Handbook of Sex Therapy. New York, Plenum Press, 1978.

MacElveen-Hoehn P: Sexual assessment and counseling. Semin Oncol Nurs 1:68–75, 1985.

Masters WH, Johnson VE: Human Sexual Response. Boston, Little, Brown & Co, 1966.

Masters WH, Johnson, VE: Human Sexual Inadequacy. Boston, Little, Brown & Co, 1970.

Mills KH, Kilmann PR: Group treatment of sexual dysfunctions: A methodological review of the outcome literature. J Sex Marit Ther 8:259–296, 1982.

Mims FH, Swenson M: Sexuality: A Nursing Perspective. New York, McGraw-Hill, 1980.

Munjack DJ, Oziel LJ: Sexual Medicine and Counseling in Office Practice. Boston, Little, Brown & Co, 1980.

Muscari ME: Obtaining the adolescent sexual history. Pediatr Nurs 13:307–310, 1987.

Poorman SG: Human Sexuality and the Nursing Process. Norwalk, Appleton & Lange, 1988.

Randell B, Tedrow MP, Van Landingham J: Adaptation nursing: The Roy conceptual model applied. St. Louis, CV Mosby, 1982.

Reznoy M: Taking a sexual history. Am J Nurs 76:1279–1282, 1976.

Reznoy M: The young adult—taking a sexual history. Am J Nurs 76:1279–1282, 1976.

Rosenbaum M: Treatment of sexual concerns by the primary care female clinician. In Green R (ed): Human Sexuality: A Health Practitioner's Text. 2nd ed. Baltimore, Williams & Wilkins, 1979.

Roy SC: Theory Construction in Nursing: An Adaptation Model. Englewood Cliffs, Prentice-Hall, 1981.

Roy SC, Roberts S: The Roy Adaptation Model: Conceptual Models for Nursing Practice. 2nd ed. Norwalk, Appleton-Century-Crofts, 1980.

Sexuality in the Medical School Curriculum: A Series of Audio-visual Teaching Aids. A series of films dealing with interviewing patients and couples with sexual problems. Produced and distributed by Ortho Pharmaceuticals, Raritan, NJ.

Siemens S, Brandzel RC: Sexuality: Nursing Assessment and Intervention. Philadelphia, JB Lippincott, 1982.

Watts R: Dimensions of sexual health. Am J Nurs 179:1568–1572, 1979.

Woods N: Human Sexuality in Health and Illness. 3rd ed. St. Louis, CV Mosby, 1984.

World Health Organization: Education & Treatment in Human Sexuality: The Training of Health Professionals. Report of a WHO Meeting, Technical Report Series No. 572, Geneva, WHO, 1975.

Zeiss RA: Self-directed treatment for premature ejaculation. J Consult Clin Psychol 46:1234–1241, 1978.

Zilbergeld B: Group treatment of sexual dysfunction in men without partners. J Sex Marital Ther 1:204–214, 1975.

PART TWO:

A BIOPSYCHOSOCIAL APPROACH TO SEXUALITY

3: Sexual Response Cycle

Diane Lauver

Michele Bockrath Welch

The human sexual response is a rich example of the interplay of physiological, psychological, and social influences in determining behavior. The importance of psychological factors, such as self-concept and body image, and of sociocultural influences, such as gender and sex roles, to sexual expression cannot be overemphasized. However, the focus of this chapter is on the anatomical and physiological aspects of the normal human sexual response. Other chapters will highlight psychosocial aspects of sexual expression in relation to specific alterations in health status.

A basic understanding of the anatomy and physiology involved in sexual response is important to the promotion of sexual health. Myths and misconceptions about sexual response can contribute unnecessary anxiety and tension to sexual expression. The well-informed health professional is in an ideal position to offer clarifying accurate information on the sexual response when questions arise. This information can correct misconceptions, reduce tensions, and promote sexual health of individuals and couples.

THE SEXUAL ORGANS

Male

In both males and females, some reproductive organs are located internally, while others are located externally. A rough differentiation between the two suggests that the internal structures function more for reproduction while the external structures function more for physical pleasure.

In the male, the external reproductive organs are the penis, scrotum, and testes (Fig. 3–1). The penis has two parts: the shaft, or the proximal part of the penis, and the glans, the rounded distal portion. The glans is important because it is a highly sensitive and

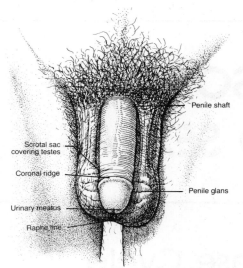

Penile shaft

Scrotal sac
covering testes

Coronal ridge

Penile glans

Urinary meatus

Raphe line

FIGURE 3–1. Typical adult male external genitalia. The penis has been circumcised, exposing the glans and coronal ridge. Penis shape, length, and position while flaccid are different for each man. Scrotal size in relation to penis varies among men. Notice indentation caused by the raphé line, asymmetry of the scrotal sac, and the indication of the vas deferens flanking the penile shaft. The pubic hair extends up the abdomen in the typical male pattern. (Reproduced by permission of Pierson EC, D'Antonio WV: Female and Male Dimensions of Human Sexuality. Philadelphia, JB Lippincott, 1974.)

erotic area. The glans is richly supplied by nerves, explaining its tactile sensitivity. In uncircumcised males, the foreskin (or prepuce) covers a portion of the glans. Normally, the prepuce is retractable and causes no interference with sexual pleasure. A substance called smegma is produced under the foreskin. Smegma does not serve any known function.

The penis is composed of three cylindrical bodies of erectile tissue. The two cavernous bodies, the corpora cavernosa, are located dorsally. The spongy body, the corpus spongiosum, is located ventrally and contains the urethra (Pettit, 1984) (Fig. 3–2). Erectile tissue consists of an irregular network of potential vascular spaces; these spaces are connected to arteries and veins. In the flaccid state, these vascular spaces are empty. With excitement, blood usually flows into these spaces as a result of arteriolar dilation and increased hydraulic pressure. After orgasm, the tissues return to a more flaccid state as a result of venous outflow exceeding arterial input. (Kolodny, Masters, and Johnson, 1979.)

The external male genitalia also includes the scrotum, a thin sac of skin forming a

pouch. The outermost layer of scrotal skin is darker than the body and contains sweat glands. An inner layer is composed of involuntary muscle that contracts with exercise, cold, or sexual excitation; it relaxes in particularly hot weather. This contracting and relaxing serves an adaptive, protective function because sperm, which are made within the scrotum, are sensitive to extreme changes in temperature (Kolodny, Masters, and Johnson, 1979; Pettit, 1984).

The scrotal sac is partitioned into two compartments, each composed of a testis, epididymis, and spermatic cord. The spermatic cord supports the testis; it includes the vas deferens and an abundant supply of blood vessels, nerves, and muscle fibers. The vas deferens is the duct or passage through which the sperm travel from the scrotum to an ejaculatory duct.

The testes* are responsible for the production of sperm and the secretion of the male hormone, testosterone. More specifically, spermatozoa are produced in the seminiferous tubules. This system of tubules is several hundred yards long. Sperm leave the testes to mature in the epididymis, located just superior and posterior to the testes. Sperm exit the epididymis via the vas deferens. The vas enter the abdominal cavity, pass posterior to the bladder, and empty into the ejaculatory duct. Roughly 20 per cent of the ejaculate is from the vas deferens (Pettit, 1984).

Testosterone is made in Leydig cells that are located in between the seminiferous tubules in the scrotum. It is important to note that the production of testosterone is independent of a dysfunction in the seminiferous tubules. However, spermatogenesis is dependent upon normal testosterone production (Kolodny, Masters, and Johnson, 1979).

In addition, there are three internal organs related to male sexual functioning: the prostate, seminal vesicles, and bulbourethral glands (See Fig. 3–2). The prostate gland is located inferior to the bladder. It produces a prostatic fluid that is alkaline in nature. This fluid constitutes about 20 per cent of the semen, or ejaculate. The alkaline nature of this fluid is important in protecting sperm from the acidity of the vagina.

Seminal vesicles are a pair of vesicles that

---

*Testes comes from a Latin word associated with an ancient custom of placing one's hand over the genitalia when taking an oath. The word testify shares a common root (Pettit, 1984).

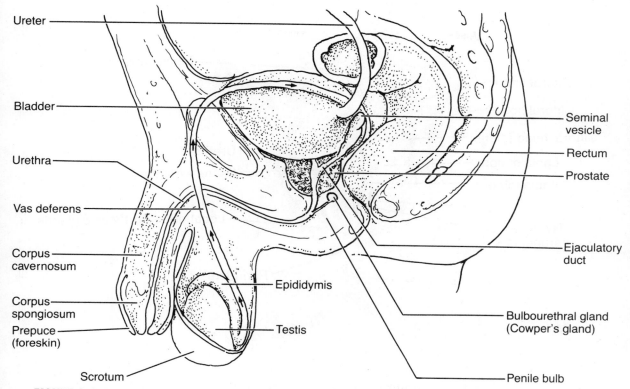

Ureter

Bladder

Urethra

Vas deferens

Corpus cavernosum

Corpus spongiosum

Prepuce (foreskin)

Scrotum

Epididymis

Testis

Seminal vesicle

Rectum

Prostate

Ejaculatory duct

Bulbourethral gland (Cowper's gland)

Penile bulb

FIGURE 3–2. Internal male anatomy. Midsagittal section of the male pelvis and external genitalia. The locations of the erectile tissue (corpus spongeosum and corpus cavernosum) are indicated. (From Jacob SW, Francone CA, Lossow WJ: Structure and Function in Man. 5th ed. Philadelphia, WB Saunders Co, 1982, pp 536, 597.)

are located posterior to the prostate; the vesicles join at the vas deferens to form the ejaculatory duct. These produce a seminal fluid that constitutes 60 per cent of semen. The seminal fluid consists of an activating principle, fructose, and prostaglandins. Activating principle serves to transform sperm from an immobile to a mobile state, while fructose provides energy for sperm. Prostaglandins may stimulate uterine contractions to facilitate sperm migration to the fallopian tubes (Pettit, 1984).

The bulbourethral, or Cowper's glands, are located inferiorly to the prostate. These glands secrete a small amount of an alkaline preejaculatory fluid. This fluid is important in protecting sperm from the acidity in the urethra. Because of this protective, neutralizing action, it is possible that isolated sperm (e.g., from previous ejaculate) may be present in the preejaculatory fluid and could cause pregnancy (Pettit, 1984).

Female

It is surprising to some persons that many of the anatomical structures of the female are comparable in origin and development to those of the male. The external female genitalia are collectively labeled the vulva, meaning covering; it has been previously referred to as the pudendum, meaning a thing of shame. The vulva refers to the mons pubis, the labia majora and minora, the vaginal orifice, and the clitoris (Figs. 3–3 and 3–4). The mons pubis is a fatty tissue covering the pubic bone. This fatty padding accentuates this area of the female anatomy and becomes more pronounced with puberty when a fine layer of dark genital hair appears. However, the amount and distribution of pubic hair can vary widely among women.

The labia majora, or outer lips, are folds of skin that cover the entrance to the vagina.

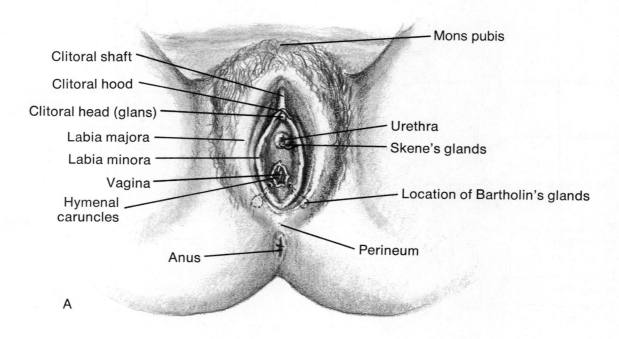

Mons pubis

Clitoral shaft

Clitoral hood

Clitoral head (glans)

Labia majora

Labia minora

Vagina

Hymenal caruncles

Anus

Urethra

Skene's glands

Location of Bartholin's glands

Perineum

A

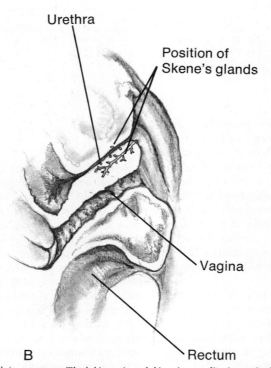

Urethra

Position of Skene's glands

Vagina

B

Rectum

FIGURE 3–3. A, *Visible pelvic structures. The labia majora, labia minora, clitoris, vaginal opening, hymen fragments, Bartholin's glands openings, and perineum can be visualized. B, Skene's glands. (Copyright 1981 Catherine Ingram Fogel and Nancy Fugate Woods. Used with permission.)*

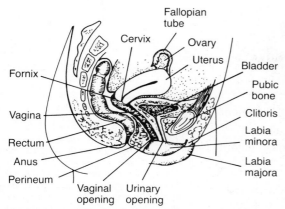

FIGURE 3–4. The vaginal canal is a potential rather than a real space and inclines posteriorly at about a 45-degree angle. The cervix pierces the anterior superior wall of the vagina. The recessed portion of the vagina adjacent to the cervix is the fornix. (Copyright 1981 Catherine Ingram Fogel and Nancy Fugate Woods. Used with permission.)

The labia majora are more prominent anteriorly, in the area of the mons pubis. They continue posteriorly to the anal region, where they become less distinctive and appear to become part of the surrounding tissue. Following puberty, the labia majora are covered laterally by hair. On the lateral and medial aspects of these labia, sweat and sebaceous glands are found. Internally, these labia are composed of fat tissue and a thin layer of smooth muscle. The labia majora provide protection for the urethra and vagina (Kolodny, Masters, and Johnson, 1979).

Between the labia majora are structures referred to as the labia minora, or inner lips of the vagina. Anteriorly, the labia minora converge to form the hood, or prepuce, over the clitoris. Just posterior, and slightly deeper, is a portion of the labia minora called the frenulum, or lower fold of the clitoris. The labia minora also cover the urethral orifice, vaginal opening, and the openings of the Bartholin's glands; they do not cover the anus. These labia are not covered by hair but do contain sebaceous glands that provide some lubrication. These labia are composed of vascular, spongy connective tissue and have many tactile nerve endings, making this area very sensitive. (Field, 1986; Kolodny, Masters, and Johnson, 1979.)

The clitoris, from the Greek word meaning key, is a particularly sensitive and erotic area for women. It has two parts, the body and glans; it is about one-half to one inch long (Figs. 3–5 and 3–6). The clitoris is histologically similar to the penis, being composed of erectile tissue, or corpora cavernosa. The clitoris also contains many nerves and blood vessels. When a female is sexually stimulated, the rich supply of nerves and blood vessels cause the clitoris to become engorged. Being highly sensitive to stimulation, the clitoris serves to provide sexual pleasure. The female is uniquely endowed with the clitoris, which has, as its single purpose, sexual excitement; the male has no such counterpart (Masters, 1987). Like the penis, the clitoris also produces smegma.

The female genitalia has three orifices. The first opening, located anteriorly, is the urethra, which serves for the passage of urine. The second opening is the vaginal orifice, or introitus. It is usually visible only when the labia majora and minora are separated. Sometimes this is not so, such as after childbirth. The third and posterior orifice in the female is the anal opening.

At the vaginal entrance is a membrane called the hymen. This membrane is normally perforated to allow for menses. The hymen is visualized as an irregular narrow fold around the introitus, forming a hymenal ring (Field, 1986). The hymen serves no physiological purpose but over the years has taken on considerable emotional and cultural significance. According to myth, women who possess an intact hymen are sexually inexperienced or virginal, while those whose hymens are torn are nonvirginal. This idea is not true; the hymen can be broken by vigorous exercise or remain intact even with sexual intercourse.

There are two sets of glands in the female genitalia: Bartholin's and Skene's. Bartholin's glands are located at the posterior surface of the vaginal introitus (See Fig. 3–3). These glands are analogous to Cowper's glands in the male. There is debate whether these glands secrete a mucus to moisten the vagina or a fluid to offer lubrication during intercourse (Field, 1986; Pettit, 1984). These glands are important because their opening ducts can be the site of a painful cyst secondary to retention of fluid; such a cyst can develop into an abscess. Skene's glands or ducts are also called paraurethral glands. Located on either side of the urethra, these glands do not appear to have a specific purpose (See Fig. 3–3B). However, they are a site for possible infection, for example, gonorrhea (Field, 1986).

The internal female reproductive organs consist of the ovaries, fallopian tubes, uterus,

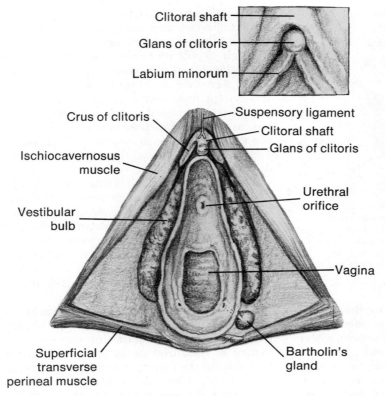

FIGURE 3–5. The clitoris. The sole purpose of the clitoris is the reception and transformation of sexual stimuli. The glans and two corpora are held in place by a suspensory ligament and two ischiocavernosus muscles. The glans is exquisitely sensitive and increases in size with sexual stimulation, as does the shaft of the clitoris. (Copyright 1981 Catherine Ingram Fogel and Nancy Fugate Woods. Used with permission.)

and vagina (See Fig. 3–4). The vagina is the genital opening connecting the internal and external structures. When not stimulated, the walls of the vagina collapse; with sexual excitement, they become more distended. The vagina is multilayered; the innermost layer is a mucosal surface that has a rich blood supply and is affected by hormonal levels. Premenopausally, the texture is fleshy and soft; postmenopausally, the lining becomes more thin and fragile. The middle layer is composed of muscle fibers, especially during the childbearing years, allowing for contraction and expansion. The outer covering is a thin mucosa. Of note, the vagina does not contain secretory glands. It has been widely believed that the vagina does not have a rich nerve supply; this could explain why vaginal sensations during intercourse may be minimal and why second stage labor pains are bearable (Field, 1986).

It is noteworthy that although much is known about many body parts and functions, there remains a question about whether the vagina is erotically sensitive. Predominant beliefs have held that the vagina, particularly

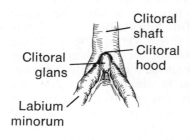

UNSTIMULATED
BASELINE

EXCITEMENT
PHASE

PLATEAU
PHASE

FIGURE 3–6. The clitoris. The arrangement of the labia minora around the clitoris makes it possible for traction on the labia to indirectly stimulate the clitoris. (Adapted from Masters W, Johnson V: Human Sexual Response. Boston, Little, Brown & Co, 1966.)

the upper two thirds, is not sensitive and that women only experience orgasm through clitoral stimulation. However, more contemporary data from case reports and direct laboratory observations support the idea of erotically sensitive areas in the vagina (Alzate and Hoch, 1986). If further research validates the existence of such sensitive areas in the vagina, the idea that some women have orgasms through vaginal stimulation, or vaginal orgasms, would be supported.

One area of the vagina that may be particularly sensitive in some women is called the G-spot, after Dr. Gräfenberg who identified it. The G-spot has been described as located in the anterior vaginal wall near the urethra. It has been reported (Bullough et al, 1984; Heath, 1984) that some women experience vaginal orgasms secondary to stimulation of the G-spot, casting doubt on the idea that women only have clitoral orgasms. However, some researchers find evidence for such an anatomical spot inconclusive (Alzate and Hoch, 1986).

Although there is much controversy about the existence and function of the G-spot, it has been suggested that it is an analogue to the male prostate, as based on historical and case reports (Belzer, 1981), direct observations (Alzate and Hoch, 1986), and interviews about an expulsion of fluid, like an ejaculate, during some women's orgasms (Bullough et al, 1984). Reports have suggested that stimulation of the G-spot results in both orgasm and fluid emission. However, because some women report emission of a fluid with clitoral rather than vaginal stimulation, the link between stimulation of the G-spot and a female ejaculate is questioned (Bullough et al, 1984).

Although most women do not emit a fluid with orgasm, for some women this is a usual occurrence (Alzate and Hoch, 1986; Belzer, 1981; Bullough et al, 1984; Heath, 1984). There are some reports of this fluid being chemically similar to prostatic fluid (Heath, 1984; Zaviacic, 1987). However, there are other reports of this fluid being more similar to urine; two researchers conclude that the nature and source of this fluid is still unknown (Alzate and Hoch, 1986).

The internal female reproductive system includes the two ovaries. The ovaries have a dual function: They produce the ova, or female germ cells, as well as secrete the female hormones estrogen and progesterone. What is unique about the development and passage of the ova is that they do not follow

a direct tubular course. Rather, their release occurs by a rupturing of the ovarian wall with subsequent movement out of the ovary. Like the male testes, the ovaries have numerous follicles in various stages of maturation. Approximately once each month after puberty, a follicle matures, ruptures, and discharges from the ovum cell. The remaining empty follicle is labeled the corpus luteum. After producing progesterone for 12 to 14 days, it eventually decomposes in the body.

The paired fallopian tubes lay between the ovaries and the uterus. The ovarian end of the fallopian tube does not actually connect with the ovary but rather possesses fingerlike projections in close proximity to the ovaries. After release from the ovary, an ovum migrates toward the uterus. Facilitating ovum passage through the fallopian tubes are cilia with hairlike projections and wavelike motions that line the entire segment of the tube. However, the fallopian tubes serve more than to provide the route for ova transport; it is in the uterine end of the tube that actual fertilization takes place.

The uterus, or womb, is a hollow muscular structure that houses the embryo if impregnation occurs. The uterus consists of several portions, with the major portion called the body. When the uterus is in the midline without flexion, the fundus is the uppermost portion of the uterus, at the level of the opening of the fallopian tubes. The more narrow portions are the isthmus and cervix, leading into the vaginal canal. The cervix is the lower portion, or neck, of the uterus.

The uterus is multilayered in structure. The innermost layer, the endometrium, is composed of a rich network of glands and blood vessels; it is this layer that is cyclically developed and then shed with menses. The next layer, composed of muscular tissue, is referred to as the myometrium. During menses or orgasm, these muscular fibers contract. It is these contractions that propel the fetus outward during the birthing process. The outermost layer of the uterus is called the perimetrium.

Except for uterine contractions that may be observed with orgasm, the role of the uterus in sexual expression is negligible from a physiological perspective. However, the uterus is important from a psychological and sociocultural perspective. The uterus may be symbolic of being a woman, because of its association with menses, and of being a mother, because of its association with pregnancy.

Another potentially erotic structure in the female and the male is the breast. The breast is composed of glandular, fibrous, and fatty tissue. The nipple is highly endowed with innervation. The erectile tissue of the nipple responds to sexual excitation, cold, or friction, making it more rigid and prominent (Field, 1986).

PHYSIOLOGY OF REPRODUCTION

Hormones play an important role not only in maturation of the reproductive systems but also in facilitating conception. This discussion will introduce the sex hormones that pertain directly to sexual expression. A more indepth discussion of these and other hormones is found in Chapter 17, Endocrine Disturbances and Sexuality. The two main hormones that stimulate the reproductive organs are follicle-stimulating hormone (FSH) and luteinizing hormone (LH). These hormones are secreted by the anterior pituitary gland.

In the male, FSH serves to stimulate the seminiferous tubules to initiate and maintain spermatogenesis. It does not stimulate production of testosterone. In the female, FSH serves to stimulate a primary ovarian follicle to mature into a graafian follicle (Vick and Schindler, 1984).

In the male, LH serves to stimulate the Leydig, or interstitial, cells of the testes and to synthesize and secrete testosterone. In the female, LH stimulates (1) an ovarian follicle to mature, (2) the theca internal cells to synthesize and secrete estrogen, and (3) ovulation of the follicle. Following ovulation, LH serves to develop the corpus luteum from the ruptured follicle. The luteal cells of the corpus luteum, in turn, synthesize and secrete progesterone and estrogen (Vick and Schindler, 1984).

The pituitary hormones FSH and LH herald adolescence in both the male and the female. As a result of the action of LH and FSH in males at puberty, testosterone production is increased; this stimulates the development of male secondary sex characteristics. This includes development of a longer and wider penis, scrotal rugae, and the darker color of the genitals. It also stimulates the growth and pattern of scalp, pubic, and axillary hair, the deepening of the voice, sebaceous gland activity, and greater muscle mass. In men, hair distribution increases on the body and decreases on the scalp.

Similarly, the secondary sex characteristics of females are the result of increasing estrogen and some androgens at puberty. Estrogen serves to stimulate maturation of the breast and female genitalia as well as the distribution of fat on the hips and thighs. The distribution of scalp, pubic, and axillary hair development is stimulated by androgens. In contrast to the male, scalp hair is promoted and body hair minimized.

FSH and LH play critical roles in the menstrual cycle. In response to FSH, a developing follicle secretes estrogen; this stimulates a positive feedback loop, producing more estrogen. Estrogen stimulates the proliferation of uterine endometrium, maturation of the ovum, and increased clear, stretchy cervical secretions (Vick and Schindler, 1984). At midcycle, the cervical mucus is particulary supportive of sperm penetration (See Chapter 11, Contraception and Sexuality). This preovulatory phase of the menstrual cycle is called the follicular phase, because of ovarian activity, or the proliferative phase, because of the endometrial activity.

Ovulation, the release of a secondary oocyte or ovum, occurs as a result of the positive feedback of estrogen and an LH surge. The second phase of the menstrual cycle is marked by the production of progesterone and estrogen from the remains of the follicle, the corpus luteum. Progesterone serves to mature and develop secretory glands in the endometrium and the lobules and alveoli in the breast (Vick and Schindler, 1984). This phase of the cycle is called the secretory phase because of endometrial activity, or the luteal phase, because of ovarian activity. If conception does not occur, the end of this phase is marked by a drop in the production of progesterone from the corpus luteum; the corpus luteum only functions for 14 days plus or minus 2. Without hormonal support, the endometrium sloughs, menses occurs, and this cycle begins again.

Although certainly not true for all women, for some women the latter part of the luteal phase and the beginning of menstruation is characterized by a time of perimenstrual distress (Woods, Most, and Dery, 1982). Premenstrually, women may experience water retention, tender breasts, irritability, depression, fatigue, and, to a lesser degree, headache or back or uterine discomfort (Brown and Zimmer, 1986; Heitkemper, Shaver, and Mitchell, 1988; Woods, Most, and Dery, 1982). With menses, some women experience cramping, backache, irritability, fatigue, and, to a lesser degree, water retention (Woods, Most, and Dery, 1982; Heitkemper, Shaver, and Mitchell, 1988). During the premenstruum and menstruation, with such concomitant symptoms women often decrease usual activities (Brown and Zimmer, 1986) and may decrease sexual activity (Harvey, 1987). However, for some women, menstruation is perceived as a safe time for intercourse, and orgasm may relieve cramping.

There is debate about how the menstrual cycle affects women's sexual desire and behavior. Harvey (1987) has studied the effect of phase of menstrual cycle on sexual behavior. She conducted her study over 2 to 3 months' time, measuring ovulation with basal body temperatures and sexual behavior with diaries. Sexual behaviors included arousal, pleasure, and female initiation of heterosexual activity and autosexual activity (i.e., fantasy and masturbation). From 66 normally menstruating young women, the data revealed that sexual arousal and sexual pleasure were highest in the ovulatory and premenstruum phases but lowest in the menstrual phase. Although autoinitiated activities were higher at ovulation, heterosexual, female-initiated activities were not. The author suggests that masturbation may be initiated at ovulation because of some fear of pregnancy. Interestingly, the data revealed that male partners of these female subjects initiated intercourse more during ovulation than during other phases of the menstrual cycle. The author suggests that the male-initiated activity could have been in response to greater behavioral messages of arousal from his partner. Or possibly, these males responded to secretion of pheromones by the female, which may be perceived as arousing by the male.

Hoon, Bruce, and Kinchloe (1982) also studied the effect of phase of the menstrual cycle on sexual arousal. These authors also used basal body temperatures to measure five menstrual phases; they used a self-report measure of arousal and three physiological indices of arousal (labial temperature, vaginal blood volume, and vaginal pulse amplitude). No differences either in self-reported *or* in physiological arousal were observed in rela-

tion to phase of the menstrual cycle in 13 women exposed to erotic stimuli in a laboratory setting. How well these findings can be generalized to women not in a laboratory setting may be questioned. The differences in findings about menstrual cycle phase and sexual arousal in the two studies cited reflect some of the inconsistency of results in this area.

SEXUAL RESPONSE CYCLE

Commonly occurring phases of the human sexual response cycle have been identified. These phases, on a continuum of sexual response, follow a similar sequence in both males and females regardless of sexual orientation. However, within specific phases there are some characteristic differences between the sexes. Despite commonalities in sexual response, there is great individual variation as well.

At the present time, there are different approaches to labeling the phases of the sexual response cycle (SRC). Four phases of the cycle are identified in the revised Diag-

TABLE 3–1. Sexual Response Cycle

Desire	Influenced by a wide variety of environmental stimuli, including psychosocial and cultural factors and physiology; that which causes one to initiate or be receptive to sexual activity.
Excitement	Develops from any bodily or psychic stimuli; with adequate stimulation, intensity increases rapidly; may be interrupted, prolonged, or ended by distracting stimuli.
Plateau	A consolidation period, with maintenance of stimulation; sexual tension becomes intensified to orgasm; may be affected by distracting stimuli.
Orgasm	Involuntary climax of increased sexual tension; usually only a few seconds; vasocongestion and myotonia are decreased; greater variation of intensity and duration of orgasm among females; total body is involved, with focus in the pelvic area.
Resolution	Involutional changes return body to preexcitement state; female, when adequately stimulated, may begin another sexual response cycle before sexual excitement totally resolves; male, during refractory period, cannot be restimulated.

nostic and Statistical Manual of Mental Disorders III (1987): appetitive, excitement, orgasm, and resolution. These four phases appear to be an integration of phases identified by leading sex researchers. Masters and Johnson, who were pioneers in this area, identified four physiological phases in the SRC as excitement, plateau, orgasm, and resolution (Kolodny, Masters, and Johnson, 1979). Taking a different physiological perspective, Kaplan (1974) described a biphasic SRC, one characterized by two fundamental and relatively discrete events: genital vasocongestion, marked by penile erection and vaginal swelling with lubrication, and reflex contractions, characteristic of orgasm. Using a biopsychological perspective, Kaplan (1979) later categorized the SRC by three phases: desire, excitement, and orgasm.

Each of these perspectives of the SRC highlights aspects of human adaptation from a resting state to one of sexual arousal and satisfaction and then a return to the resting state. The inclusion of a desire, or appetitive, phase of the SRC is important; it recognizes a psychological dimension to the sexual response. It also identifies an area in which there may be disorders of response. The subsequent section will begin with discussion of the desire phase of SRC and will subsequently review four phases of the SRC: excitement, plateau, orgasm, and resolution (Table 3–1).

Desire

Sexual desire may be influenced by a physiological drive from activation of specific parts of the brain (Poorman, 1988), by mood states, by psychological perceptions of oneself (e.g., self-concept and body image), and by sociocultural factors (e.g., role expectations and images of attractiveness). Sexually explicit visual images, sounds, or fantasy may elicit arousal. Sexual desire may be thought of, regardless of its source, as the stimulus that causes one to initiate or to be receptive to sexual activity (Poorman, 1988).

Because sexual fantasy can affect desire, it is important to reflect on factors that may affect sexual fantasy. It is commonly recognized that certain sociocultural or religious attitudes may cause one to feel guilty about sexual thoughts and to be somewhat sexually inhibited. In a study of factors influencing sexual fantasy (Follingstad and Kimbrell, 1986), persons with more guilt about sex wrote sexual fantasies that were shorter and less varied in content than those with less guilt. Those with more sex-related guilt reported greater embarrassment and less sexual arousal when asked to write about their sexual fantasies. It was also found that women reported more sex-related guilt than men. Thus, guilt may play a role in sexual fantasy and arousal, particularly among persons like those studied, who were college students.

It is commonly believed that males may feel more free to engage in sexual fantasy because of sex role socialization. In the study mentioned previously (Follingstad and Kimbrell, 1986), the effect of gender on reports of sexual fantasy was also studied. As expected, men wrote about sexual fantasies that were longer, more specific, and more varied in content than did women. These findings support the idea that the socialization of males and females continues to affect aspects of sexual behavior.

In one study (Beggs, Calhoun, and Wolchik, 1987), commonly reported descriptions that were sexually arousing for 19 female volunteers included sexual acts such as hugging, kissing, breast stimulation as well as oral genital stimulation, and intercourse. Common descriptions of stimuli that were both pleasant *and* arousing for these women included slow timing of activity, positive experiences with alcohol, positive aspects of the environment, and partner attractiveness. Common descriptions of stimuli that were both anxiety provoking *and* arousing included hurried timing, lack of control, negative moods, physical pain, partner unattractiveness, and lack of privacy. The authors make the point that some stimuli are sexually arousing in general, independent of pleasantness or anxiety. Although it is questionable how well these findings can be generalized to nonvolunteers and males, they do reflect aspects of pleasant and anxious sexual encounters that are commonly reported by women in health care settings.

Excitement

Tactile stimuli such as touch, warmth, and pressure as well as psychogenic stimuli may cause excitement. These stimuli alone may not result in excitement but depend on psychological readiness (Diamond and Karlen,

TABLE 3–2. Physiological Changes in Four Phases of Human Sexual Response

Male	Female
Excitement Phase	
1. Penile erection (within 3 to 8 seconds) as phase is prolonged.	1. Vaginal lubrication (within 10 to 30 seconds) as phase is prolonged.
2. Thickening, flattening, and elevation of scrotal sac.	2. Thickening of vaginal walls and labia.
3. Partial testicular elevation and size increase.	3. Expansion of inner two thirds of vagina and elevation of cervix and corpus.
4. Nipple erection (in about 30 per cent of men).	4. Tumescence of clitoris.
	5. Nipple erection (in all women).
	6. Sex flush (in about 25 per cent of women).
Plateau Phase	
1. Increase in penile coronal circumference.	1. Orgasmic platform in outer one third of vagina.
2. Testicular tumescence (50 to 100 per cent enlarged).	2. Full expansion of vagina.
3. Full testicular elevation and rotation (orgasm inevitable).	3. Uterine and cervical elevation.
4. Purple hue to corona of penis (inconsistent).	4. Discoloration of labia minora.
5. Mucoid secretion (perhaps from Cowper's glands).	5. Mucoid secretion (perhaps from Bartholin's glands).
6. Sex tension flush (in 25 per cent of men).	6. Withdrawal of clitoris.
7. Carpopedal spasm.	7. Sex flush (in 75 per cent of women).
8. Generalized muscular tension.	8. Carpopedal spasm.
9. Hyperventilation.	9. Muscular tension.
10. Tachycardia (100 to 160 bpm).	10. Hyperventilation.
11. Increased blood pressure (20 to 80 mm Hg systolic; 10 to 40 mm Hg diastolic).	11. Tachycardia.
	12. Increased blood pressure (20 to 60 mm Hg systolic; 10 to 20 mm Hg diastolic).
Orgasmic Phase	
1. Ejaculation.	1. Pelvic response.
2. Contraction of accessory organs of reproduction (vas deferens, seminal vesicles, ejaculatory duct).	2. Contraction of uterus from fundus toward lower uterine segment.
3. Relaxation of external bladder sphincter and contraction of internal bladder sphincter.	3. Minimal relaxation of external cervical os.
4. Contractions of penile urethra (0.8-second interval for three to four contractions).	4. Contractions of orgasmic platform (0.8-second interval for 5 to 12 contractions).
5. Anal sphincter contractions.	5. External rectal sphincter contraction.
6. Specific skeletal muscle contractions.	6. External urethral sphincter contractions.
7. Hyperventilation (up to 40 breaths/minute).	7. Hyperventilation (up to 40 breaths/minute).
8. Tachycardia (up to 180 bpm).	8. Tachycardia (up to 180 bpm).
9. Increased blood pressure (40 to 100 mm Hg systolic; 20 to 50 mm Hg diastolic).	9. Increased blood pressure (30 to 80 mm Hg systolic; 20 to 40 mm Hg diastolic).
Resolution Phase	
1. Refractory period with rapid loss of pelvic vasocongestion.	1. Ready return to orgasm with retarded loss of pelvic vasocongestion.
2. Loss of penile erection is a two-stage response: 50 per cent loss rapidly; gradual loss of rest of erection.	2. Loss of flush in labia minora and orgasmic platform (rapid).
3. Sweating reaction (30 to 40 per cent of men).	3. Remainder of pelvic vasocongestion slow.
4. Hyperventilation.	4. Loss of clitoral tumescence.
5. Tachycardia decreases.	5. Sweating reaction (30 to 40 per cent of women).
	6. Hyperventilation.
	7. Tachycardia decreases.

Sources: Masters and Johnson, 1966; Fogel and Woods, 1981; Woods, 1984.

1981). The excitement phase is characterized by reflexive vasocongestion in both sexes. In the male this results in penile erection or tumescence. In the female, vasocongestion results in vaginal lubrication, or sweating; this is technically transudation rather than secretions from any particular glands (Kolodny, Masters, and Johnson, 1979).

Additional changes are observed in the excitement phase (Table 3–2). In the male, the skin of the scrotum becomes smoother (secondary to vasocongestion), and the scrotum flattens. The testes become somewhat elevated as the spermatic cords shorten. In the female, the labia majora flatten, the cervix becomes somewhat elevated, and the inner two thirds of the vagina expand or balloon. In addition, vasocongestion causes clitoral enlargement or tumescence (See Fig. 3–6).

In both sexes, erection of the nipples may occur. However, nipple erection occurs in nearly all women, while in only about 30 per cent of men. A sex flush, or measlelike rash, may appear on the skin over the breasts and epigastric area; this, too, is more common in women than in men, in blonds and redheads, and in warmer climates (Diamond and Karlen, 1981; Kolodny, Masters, and Johnson, 1979). Many of these changes can be viewed as functional adaptations to facilitate penile-vaginal intercourse.

Plateau

The plateau phase identified by Masters and Johnson (1966) represents an increase and leveling off of sexual tension (Fig. 3–7). Some experts would incorporate this phase within the excitement phase because it is a continuation of processes stimulated by sexual excitement. For example, vasocongestion continues, as marked by penile and testicular enlargement and by engorgement of the outer third of the vagina (called the orgasmic platform).

The changes in the vagina with sexual arousal have important implications. Because the outer third of the vagina swells to grip the penis and because this area has many sensory nerves, the actual size of the penis is not critical to vaginal stimulation. The ballooning of the inner two thirds of the vagina and the relative absence of nerve endings in this area further support the idea that penile size is not essential to vaginal stimulation (Kolodny, Masters, and Johnson, 1979). Important to clitoral stimulation and female satisfaction is the fact that the clitoris may be difficult to identify during the plateau stage. This is because the clitoris retracts against the symphysis pubis and because the surrounding labia become engorged. In spite of its location, the clitoris remains highly sensitive to stimulation (See Fig. 3–6).

Other changes also develop in the plateau phase. Minimal secretions, perhaps from the male Cowper's and the female Bartholin's glands, occur. Sex flush may progress. In women, breasts increase in size, and the areola engorge. Generalized skeletal muscle tension occurs along with hyperventilation and tachycardia (Kolodny, Masters, and Johnson, 1979).

Orgasm

Orgasm is characterized by feelings of heightened excitement, a peaking of subjective pleasure, and subsequent release of sexual tension. In the orgasmic phase, awareness of other sensual experiences is diminished, and individuals become very self-focused (Masters, 1987). Both males and females experience involuntary contractions and myotonia, or increased muscle tension, during this phase. Tension may be felt and seen in the mouth, neck, fascial grimaces, buttocks, thighs, and toes. Carpopedal spasm and contraction of arms and limbs occur with orgasm (Diamond and Karlen, 1981). Both males and females have increases in breathing, heart rates, and blood pressure.

In the male, the prostate, seminal vesicles, and vas deferens rhythmically contract, often at intervals of 0.8 second. Then, emission, or the emptying of semen into the prostatic urethra, usually occurs. This is often experienced, perhaps more easily in younger men, as ejaculatory inevitability. Ejaculation occurs as semen is discharged from the urethra by rhythmic contractions of the prostate, perineal muscles, and shaft of the penis. The internal sphincter of the bladder is closed at this time; urine is not passed with semen (see Table 3–2) (Diamond and Karlen, 1981; Kolodny, Masters, and Johnson, 1979)

In the female, contractions of the outer third of the vagina (the orgasmic platform), the uterus, and rectal sphincter occur, often at 0.8-second intervals. Women's orgasmic contractions may continue longer than those of men. Also, women can experience multiple orgasms in close succession, whereas men cannot. However, women's experiences of orgasm are quite varied.

Resolution

The resolution phase is characterized by the body's return to its resting, or preexcitation, state as vasocongestion is relieved. In the male, this is signaled by a loss of erection, which occurs quickly secondary to penile contractions with orgasm; total resolution occurs more slowly with the return of normal blood

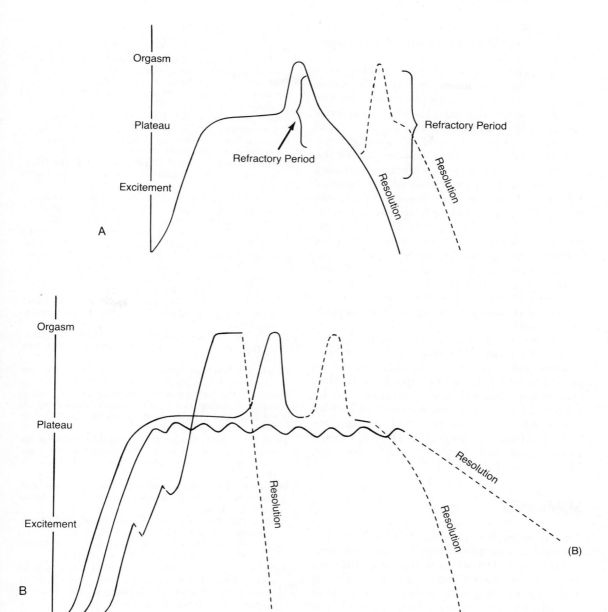

FIGURE 3–7. Sexual response cycle by sex. A, Male sexual response cycle. B, Female sexual response cycle. (Reproduced by permission of Masters W, Johnson V: Human Sexual Response. Boston, Little, Brown & Co, 1966.)

flow. In addition, the scrotum descends, and testes decrease in size.

In the female, the clitoris decreases in size, and the orgasmic platform disappears. The uterus descends into the pelvis to its usual position; the vagina decreases in width and length (Kolodny, Masters, and Johnson, 1979). In both men and women, heart rate and blood pressure return to resting rates. Also, in both men and women, a sexual experience without orgasm may result in pelvic or genital discomfort when vasocongestion is not relieved.

Although the phases of the sexual response are the same for males and females, there are differences within the phases that are sex specific. Males characteristically experience one pattern of orgasm, consisting of a rapid excitement phase, followed by a short plateau period, orgasm, and then resolution. For the female, there are several patterns of orgasm, but three patterns are commonly recognized. In the first pattern, the woman experiences multiple orgasms with a fairly rapid resolution period (see Fig. 3–7A) In the second pattern (see Fig. 3–7B), the female does not achieve total orgasm but rather achieves several peaks in the plateau phase with a longer resolution period. For the third pattern (see Fig. 3–7C), the female's sexual excitement is interrupted, followed by an intense orgasm and a rapid resolution.

The second difference in sexual response is refractory period. Immediately after ejaculation, the male experiences a refractory period in which he is not capable of further ejaculation, although partial erection may be present. The female has no such refractory period; she may have repeated orgasms before experiencing resolution. However, most women are not multiorgasmic (Kolodny, Masters, and Johnson, 1979).

SUMMARY

This chapter has focused primarily on the anatomical and physiological aspects of sexual response. However, sexual response also involves one's psychological and sociocultural make-up, which may, in many instances, play a significant role in sexual satisfaction. It is within the role of the health professional to support and facilitate healthy sexual expression, and accurate knowledge of the normal sexual response cycle is important to this role. Explaining aspects of the sexual response to clients, when appropriate, can sometimes dispel their myths and concerns about abnormalities in sexual response. Future chapters will address specific alterations in health and how such alterations can affect sexual response.

REFERENCES

Alzate H, Hoch Z: The "G spot" and "Female ejaculation": A current appraisal. J Sex Marital Ther 12:211–220, 1986.

Beggs VE, Calhoun KS, Wolchik, SA: Sexual anxiety and female sexual arousal: A comparison of arousal during sexual anxiety stimuli and sexual pleasure stimuli. Arch Sex Behav 16:311–319, 1987.

Belzer E: Orgasmic expulsions of women: A review and heuristic inquiry. J Sex Res 17:1–12, 1981.

Brown MA, Zimmer PA: Personal and family impact of premenstrual symptoms. JOGNN 15:31–38, 1986.

Bullough B et al: Subjective reports of female orgasmic expulsion of fluid. Nurs Pract 9:55–59, 1984.

Diagnostic and Statistical Manual of Mental Disorders. 3rd ed, rev. Washington DC, American Psychiatric Association 1987.

Diamond M, Karlen A: The sexual response cycle. In Lief HI (ed): Sexual Problems in Medical Practice. Monroe, American Medical Assoc, 1981, pp 37–52.

Field ML: The female reproductive system in health and illness. In Kneisel CR, Ames SW (eds): Adult Health Nursing. Menlo Park, Addison Wesley, 1986.

Fogel CI, Woods NF: Health Care of Women: A Nursing Perspective. St. Louis, CV Mosby, 1981.

Follingstad DR, Kimbrell CD: Sex fantasies revisited: An expansion and further clarification of variables affecting sex fantasy production. Arch Sex Behav 15:475–486, 1986.

Harvey SM: Female sexual behavior: Fluctuations during the menstrual cycle. J Psychosom Res 31:101–110, 1987.

Hatch JP: Psychophysiological aspects of sexual dysfunction. Arch Sex Behav 10:49–64, 1981.

Heath D: An investigation into the origins of a copious vaginal discharge during intercourse: "Enough to wet the bed" that "Is not urine." J Sex Res 20:194–210, 1984.

Heitkemper MM, Shaver JF, Mitchell ES: Gastrointestinal symptoms and bowel patterns across the menstrual cycle in dysmenorrhea. Nurs Res 37:108–113, 1988.

Hoon PW, Bruce K, Kinchloe B: Does the menstrual cycle play a role in sexual arousal? Psychophysiol 19:21–27, 1982.

Kaplan HS: Disorders of Sexual Desire. New York, Simon & Schuster, 1979.

Kaplan HS: The New Sex Therapy. New York, Quadrangle/The New York Times Book Co, 1974.

Kolodny RC, Masters WH, Johnson VE: Textbook of Sexual Medicine. Boston, Little, Brown and Co, 1979.

Masters WH, Johnson VE: Human sexual response. Boston, Little, Brown & Co, 1966.

Masters WH: Sexuality in perspective. Trans Stud Coll Phys Phila 9:45–57, 1987.

Pettit GW: Human sexual function. In Vick RL (ed): Contemporary Medical Physiology. St Louis, CV Mosby, 1984.

Poorman SG: Human Sexuality and the Nursing Process. Norwalk, Appleton & Lange, 1988.

Vick RL, Schindler WJ: The gonads and gonadotropins. In Vick RL (ed): Contemporary Medical Physiology. St Louis, CV Mosby, 1984.

Woods NF: Human Sexuality in Health and Illness. St Louis, CV Mosby, 1984.

Woods NF, Most A, Dery GK: Prevalence of perimenstrual symptoms. Am J Public Health 72:1257–1264, 1982.

Zaviacic M: The female prostate: Nonvestigial organ of the female. A reappraisal. J Sex Marital Ther 13:148–152, 1987.

4: Sexuality Throughout the Life Cycle

Barbara Rynerson

To discuss sexuality throughout various stages of lifelong growth and development, it is necessary to clarify the term life cycle. Life cycle implies a cyclic nature of development from conception to death and connotes not only repetition but also progression in all areas of human development. The research regarding the development of sexuality is inconclusive and often conflicting, particularly in the area of sex-linked behavior (behavior that is specifically attributed to either males or females). One reason for this is that most biological research involves lower animals and primates, owing to the nature of sexual research. Human studies are frequently confined to those subjects who have genetic and gender defects. Once a normal child is born, it is difficult to separate the biological variables from the psychological and social ones that influence typical male or female sexual behavior.

In this chapter, physiological, psychological, and social factors of human sexuality are discussed in the context of current knowledge about progression from conception through old age. The intent is to facilitate the nurse's understanding of what constitutes the range of normal sexual behavior and the characteristics of healthy sexuality during each stage of life. Sexuality, as a major component of a person's identity, is explored in terms of issues unique to both individuals and to relationships. Guidelines are presented for the nurse to determine where deviations and problem areas in sexual growth and development might arise. Nursing interventions are suggested to provide the client with education and anticipatory guidance in achieving sexual maturity, responsibility, and satisfaction.

PHYSIOLOGY AND SEXUALITY

The biological basis of human sexuality is the genetic determination of gender at the moment of conception when either the X or the Y chromosome in the sperm unites with the X chromosome of the egg. The XX chromosomal combination produces a female and the XY combination a male. The most recent knowledge of chromosomal study indicates that the testes-determining genes are localized in the Y chromosome, and the only established effect of the Y chromosome is to determine maleness. There is further evidence of the Y chromosome's direct influence on body growth, skeletal muscle maturation, and dental development; the genes of the Y chromosome directly affect the slower growth rate in boys (Kahn and Cataio, 1984). All fetuses, at conception, are considered dimorphic; that is, they have both female and male rudimentary elements and the potential to develop as either sex. The chromosomal linkage, the establishment of genetic sex, is the first of three stages in the process of sexual differentiation.

It was once thought that the determination of sex through the XX and XY chromosomes was absolute in the later formation of female and male sex organs. However, it is now known that hormone action has an effect on genetic programming even at this level of differentiation and may lead to abnormalities. Hines (1982) reports this hormonal action as primarily affecting the male (XY) sometime between the fourth and eighth week after conception when testosterone is secreted by the embryo's rudimentary testes. If it is not secreted, the embryo will develop as a physical female. If secreted by accident (for example, should the mother take certain drugs at this stage), the result may be an ambiguous genitalia in the infant, with some characteristics of both male and female.

The second phase of sexual differentiation, the establishment of gonadal (genital) sex, occurs by about the tenth to twelveth week of gestation. The male-determining factor in the Y chromosome leads to the development of the internal testes from the gonad medulla; without the male factor, there is development of the internal ovary from the gonad cortex (Bancroft, 1983).

The third phase of differentiation is the establishment of phenotypic sex, when the additional internal and external genital organs develop (Kahn and Cataio, 1984) and result in the actual characteristics of biological sex. The wolffian duct system is the structure that in the presence of testosterone gives rise to the epididymis, the vas deferens, and the seminal vesicles in males. The müllerian duct gives rise to the fallopian tubes, the uterus, and the upper part of the vagina in the female. This is also a critical time in sexual differentiation, since each fetus has both the wolffian and the müllerian duct systems, one of which must develop while the other must regress to produce actual male or female external genitalia. Further, prenatal sexual and body structure development proceeds through a complicated series of events and is dependent upon continuous feedback between the production of sex hormones by the ovaries and testes and the adrenal cortex and the control in the brain by the hypothalamus and the pituitary gland (Kahn and Cataio, 1984). Figures 4–1 and 4–2 illustrate the differentiation of the internal and external genitalia.

We have progressed considerably from the time when the myth that genital (and genetic) "anatomy is destiny" was believed to determine sexual differences in development and manifestations of later gender behavior.

However, on the basis of animal brain research and identifiable differences in human intelligence, cognition, moral development, and behavior, we have to respect findings that do indicate differences in the male and female brain. There are more questions than answers regarding the biological, or more specifically the biochemical, influence on the brain and how it affects male-female differentiation and differences in gender-typical behavior. What we do know is that the human brain is dimorphic, just as there is genital dimorphism in the developing fetus (Kahn and Cataio, 1984; Gagnon, 1977). The details of the processes by which these differences occur are beyond the scope of this chapter, but basically, sex hormones influence sexual differences in the brain in much the same way as they influence sexual organ differentiation. As reported in Kahn and Cataio (1984), it is speculated that the brain of the fetus is female unless influenced by the male hormones. Testosterone acts on the brain during the early months of pregnancy to sensitize the brain as male. In the fully developed male brain, testosterone activates the brain to produce male-typical behavior. Sensitization *must* occur, or later activation will not result in male-typical behavior.

The mechanism by which this sensitization occurs has been researched more definitively in animal studies (Kahn and Cataio, 1984); however, studies of children with adrenogenital syndrome (AGS) and Turner's syndrome substantiate animal findings to some degree. In AGS, an excess amount of androgens causes masculinization of the female fetus and precocious pubertal development in males. Ehrhardt, in collaboration with Money (1967) and Baker (1974), reported distinct behavioral differences in higher levels of physical energy expenditure, aggression, rough and tumble outdoor play, and less interest in dolls in AGS females as compared with normal girls and unaffected siblings. In Turner's syndrome there is an unmatched X chromosome, and thus no endogenous gonadal hormones are present; yet, female sex differentiation occurs (Unger, 1979). Money and Ehrhardt (1972) determined that these Turner's syndrome females tended to identify themselves as female on the basis of their external genitalia despite the absence of central nervous system influence by gonadal hormones.

Another difference in the male and female brain is in the functional asymmetry of the

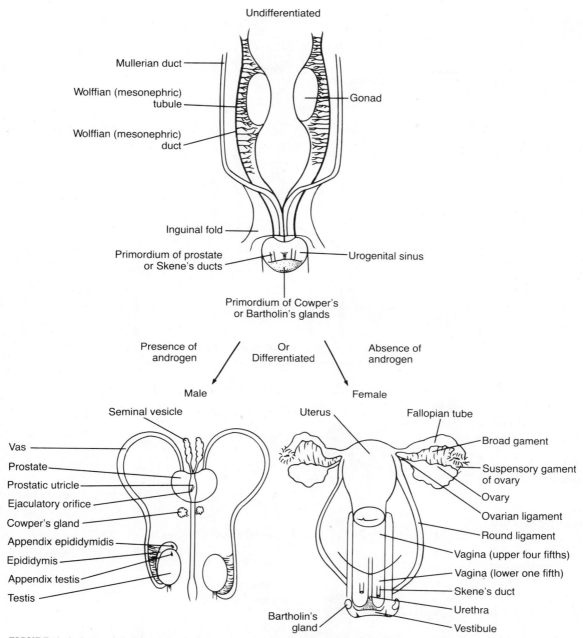

FIGURE 4–1. Internal male and female genitalia: development from undifferentiated into differentiated stage. (From Human Sexuality, *3rd Brief Ed, by SP McCary and James L. McCary © 1984 by SP McCary and LP McCary. Reprinted by permission of the publisher, Wadsworth Publishing Co.)*

cerebral hemispheres, which accounts for dominant sidedness in individuals. In right-handed people, the left cerebral hemisphere is dominant for language and motor functions, and the right hemisphere is more dominant for nonverbal functions such as perception of spatial relationship. In their review of the research literature, Kahn and Cataio (1984) reported that there were significant differences between the sexes in the lateralization of cognitive functions. In the adult female brain, language and nonverbal functions are represented in both hemispheres, but in adult males both functions occur in only the left hemisphere of the brain; thus, language and spatial functions are more lateralized and localized in males.

Numerous studies have been conducted to

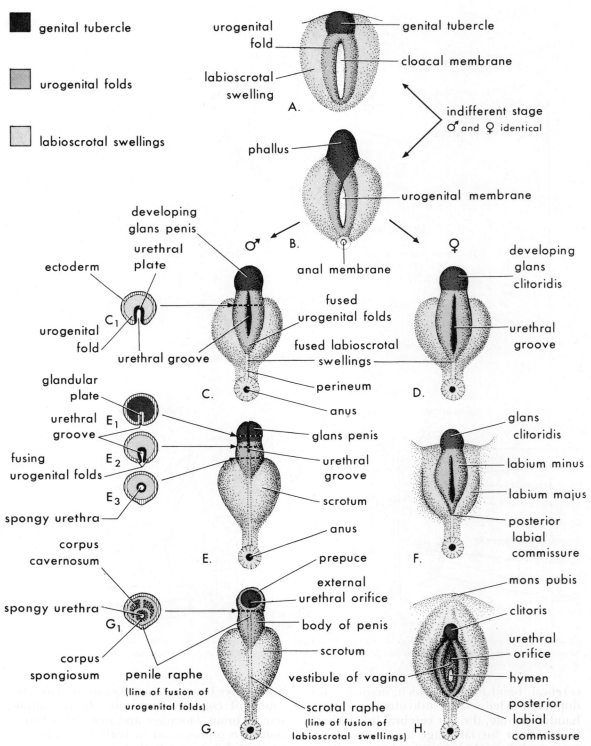

FIGURE 4–2. A and B, *Diagrams illustrating development of the external genitalia during the indifferent stage (fourth to seventh weeks). C, E, and G, Stages in the development of male external genitalia at 9, 11, and 12 weeks, respectively. To the left are schematic transverse sections (C_1, E_1 to E_3, and G_1) through the developing penis, illustrating formation of the spongy urethra. D, F, and H, Stages in the development of female external genitalia at 9, 11, and 12 weeks, respectively. (Reproduced by permission of Moore KL:* The Developing Human. *4th ed. Philadelphia, WB Saunders, 1988).*

determine sex-typical cognitive, emotional, and spatial abilities and physical capacity behaviors as a result of both cerebral hemispheric difference and the influence of testosterone in males. While differences between the sexes in each of the areas have been demonstrated, many of the differences are eliminated, or at least become closer in similarity, through learning and socialization that ignores sex stereotyping. A characteristic that tends to be associated with the right-left brain function is the difference between male and female typical response styles. The most enduring difference is in the greater male aggressiveness (potential and actual), which even exists cross-culturally (Bancroft, 1983; Kahn and Cataio, 1984). The nature-nurture controversy regarding male and female behavioral differences is not yet resolved.

Nursing Care

In the prenatal stage of sexual differentiation there are many implications for nursing care. Nurses expend a good deal of effort in working with pregnant women and their families in activities such as prenatal diet, exercise, and maternal health care to ensure a maximally healthy in utero environment for the developing fetus. Indeed, these are very important aspects of nursing for the total physical health of the unborn infant as well as for physical sexual differentiation to occur, especially since appropriate biochemical actions are vital in preventing sexual anomalies. However, an important dimension of prenatal nursing care relevant to sexual development and yet often overlooked is an assessment of parental attitudes and expectations regarding the sex of the unborn child. Many parents-to-be will say that they wish for a healthy baby, no matter which sex. While this statement expresses a very natural desire, it is typically only part of parental hopes. Is the father hoping for a boy who will follow in his footsteps (for example, take over family business or carry on family traditions) or accomplish athletic, professional, or intellectual goals that the father had hoped for himself but has not achieved? Does the mother have her heart set on a girl to be the Miss America she was not? Or, perhaps more relevant, do the parents each hope for the same-sex child to raise in each of their own images?

A holistic nursing approach to sexuality should include a discussion with the parents regarding their dreams, hopes, and expectations regarding the sex of their children. This information will assist the nurse in understanding the existent parental attitudes toward sexuality generally and may provide clues to parental needs for knowledge and anticipatory guidance. For example, a nurse made a home visit to parents in their late 20s after the birth of their first child. The mother asked the nurse how "fragile" her girl infant was as compared with a boy. When the nurse responded that healthy infants are pretty sturdy, no matter what the sex, the mother further volunteered that her husband was hesitant to pick up the child or to spend much time in assisting her in child caring activities. The nurse inquired about what expectations the father had prior to birth, and the mother said he had really anticipated having a son. The nurse encouraged the mother to discuss with the father his initial disappointment about having a girl and to allow him to share any other feelings he may be experiencing, so that she could better understand his behavior.

Since it is now possible to determine the sex of an unborn child using reproductive technology, parents may desire to know the fetus' sex, particularly if one or both parents has a strong desire for a particular sex child. When their hopes are not to be realized, this information will provide the nurse an opportunity to assist parents in working through their feelings toward acceptance and establishment of a relationship that is not distorted by preconceptions.

PSYCHOSOCIAL FACTORS AND SEXUALITY

Gender Identity

Upon the birth of a child, there is typically the pronouncement of "It's a girl!" or "It's a boy!" Since these statements are based on observation of the external genitalia, the initial assignment of gender to a normal infant is indeed based on its anatomical structure. Due to this initial assignment, along with society's existing images of masculinity and femininity, the assumption frequently exists that sex determines gender. However, gender identity is a phenomenological concept, being a result of introspection and the subjective awareness of being female or male (Hoenig, 1985). Gender refers to "socially learned responses, meanings, and cues that are taken as reflections of society's conceptions of masculinity and femininity" (Petras, 1978, p 96). Petras (1978) further describes gender, as distinguished from biological sex, which is body linked, as a series of meanings regarding definitions of the self and behavior toward others. Gender is a framework within which one is able to interpret the responses of the body.

According to Bee (1985), gender identity is the first of three stages of the development of the gender concept and is accomplished between 15 and 18 months of age. The second stage is gender stability, the understanding that one stays the same gender throughout life, which occurs by 4 years of age. The third stage is gender constancy, or a fully developed concept of gender, and occurs by age 5 or 6. Gender constancy is the recognition that one stays the same gender even though he or she may appear to change; for example, a girl may wear typically boy's clothes without experiencing a change in her feminine gender (Bee, 1985).

Gender Role

Gender role (or sex role) is the behavior and appearance that one presents in terms of what the culture considers to be masculine or feminine (Hinsie and Campbell, 1975). Although cultures vary in the specific tasks and characteristics expected of men and women, the majority ascribe different characteristics and behaviors to each sex (Schaffer, 1981). Gender role is typically congruent with gender identity and may or may not be congruent with biological sex.

Sexual Orientation

Sexual orientation refers to the preference an individual develops for a partner, in essence physical and emotional attraction to another person. While certain groups may share certain characteristics, each individual is probably unique in his or her preference pattern. Sexual preferences exist along a continuum, ranging from complete orientation to the same sex, through bisexuality, to complete orientation to the other sex (Kinsey, Pomeroy, and Martin, 1948, 1953). Such qualities as body shape, face, age, certain types of body movement, personality traits, and behaviors influence sexual attraction.

The exact mechanism by which sexual orientation occurs is not yet clear; however, data from the Institute for Sex Research appear to suggest that sexual preference is established early in life and is so deeply ingrained that it is not subject to dramatic modification in later life. Societal beliefs and attitudes dictate the relative acceptability of the various partner preferences.

Theoretical Frameworks

Psychosocial aspects of sexuality are even more complex than biological ones. Research in the various psychosocial theories and sociocultural ideologies of sex has led to our understanding of human growth and development. Given that there are theoretical biases, most studies acknowledge that sexuality is influenced by interacting psychological, social, cultural, and religious forces. The psychoanalytical theories of Freud and Erikson are basic to understanding sexuality, even though in contemporary scientific literature there is considerable questioning of their value because of the male superiority orientation. Nevertheless, the psychoanalytic approach integrates inborn physiological and psychological qualities and social factors as they relate to psychosexual development.

Early Freudian theory has its basis in instinctual drive. It postulates that all behavioral development—cognitive, interpersonal, and social—is motivated, directly or indirectly, by the service and expression of two basic drives: self-preservation (an aggressive drive) and species preservation (a love, or binding together, drive) (Eagle, 1984). Psychic energy connected with sensual and somatic satisfactions is said to be sexual energy, or libido (Hinsie and Campbell, 1975). This energy, in pursuit of satisfaction of the drives, participates in ultimate personality development by being attached to bodily areas of primary significance through the five stages of psychosexual development. According to this early view, the child's identity emerges as internally motivated needs are gratified through objects external to the self; the major focus is on the aim of the instinctual drive, rather than on its object (Bellak, Hurvich, and Gediman, 1973).

Particularly crucial for an intrapsychic

sense of sexual identity is the resolution of the oedipal conflict. As libidinal energy shifts to the genital zone, the male child develops an incestuous craving for his mother and a resentment toward his father as the rival for his mother's attention. For the girl, the symbiotic existence with the mother is broken as she finds a love object in her father, who tends at this stage of development to be warm and affectionate toward her. Anxiety occurs as erotic feelings toward the opposite-sex parent are aroused and as children fantasize about replacing the same-sex parent. The resolution of the conflict occurs as parents maintain their parental role and as the child accepts the reality of the basic bond between the parents. Feelings of jealousy are shifted to an identity with the same-sex parent, thus beginning masculine or feminine identities (Lidz, 1968).

The contemporary view of psychoanalysis is an object relations theory, which began with the work of Melanie Klein (1948, 1957). Since her work, many more theorists have added their own variations. No attempt is made in this chapter to cite or critique each contribution; rather, it summarizes the salient points of object relations theory because of its relevance to current thinking about the development of sexuality and gender-typical behaviors.

In object relations theory, the instinctual drives of the infant are satisfied throughout stages of development as the infant comes in contact with his or her environment. As Rubin (1984) points out, "objects" is a crude word to describe people and relationships; however, the intent is that objects are the internal representations or mental images that occur as a result of the infant's inner experiencing of his transactions with people and the environment. Considering the infant's total reliance on the mothering person, this view indicates that (1) the nature of this symbiotic relationship must be complementary and is crucial for later healthy psychic development and (2) the early experiences of the infant in the preoedipal phase have more importance in developmental life than the resolution of the oedipal conflict (Bellak, Hurvich, and Gedman, 1973; Rubin, 1984). Thus, in object relations theory the focus is on self-other differentiation that occurs during the process of separation-individuation in this preoedipal phase (Eagle, 1984). Object constancy implies that the individual not only establishes a healthy sense of self-identity

through this separation process but also comes to see others as whole, separate individuals with both positive and negative characteristics that affect the child's continuing development of the self. Rubin (1984) discusses the mental images (of objects) as being formed differently at different stages of life, creating in the developing individual a layering effect about the variations in relationships with an individual as well as about the relationships with different individuals. The result in a psychically healthy individual is the ability to then sustain love for another person and to have a realistic perception and representation of another with a minimum of distortion. As Bellak and colleagues state, the "two major aspects of object relations are the ability to form friendly and loving bonds with others with a minimum of inappropriate hostility and the ability to sustain relationships over time with little mutual exchange of hostility" (Bellak et al, 1973, p 142).

Additional insights regarding the meaning of object representations, or mental images, for both men and women have come from feminist literature and recent studies on gender issues. As reported in Rubin (1984), for the first time questions that are extremely relevant to the development of healthy sexuality and gender-typical behaviors are being asked, such as "What is the effect on human development of the fact that only women mother?" and "Is the fact that women are primary caretakers of developmental significance?" (Rubin, 1984).

From a psychoanalytical basis, Erikson (1950) postulated his eight ages of man, which, along with contemporary psychosocial perspectives, will be discussed in relation to similarities and differences between the sexes in each of the life cycle phases.

SOCIOCULTURAL FACTORS

In the social sense, sexuality or sexual behavior should not be separated from all other forms of social behavior. For example, the sexual revolution did not occur apart from other revolutionary changes in society. Prevailing attitudes about sexuality are thus consistent with the existing moral, political, economic, and social values.

Throughout history a particular attitude regarding sexuality typically focuses on sexual response behavior rather than on the broader view of sexuality as a wide range of gender-typical behaviors. Masculine or feminine behaviors, as manifestations of sexuality ascribed by social and cultural standards, reflect the former view.

Our sociocultural heritage of sexuality is Victorian-Puritanical, in which a relationship between sexuality and morality was taken for granted. Petras (1978) refers to this as the sacred ideology, or the conceptualizing of one's sexuality in terms of religious standards. This ideology has played a major role in generating feelings of guilt about our bodies (Petras, 1978).

A second ideology, according to Petras (1978), was the scientific, which began with psychoanalysis. Studies were concerned with relationships among behavior, sexual repression, and childhood expression. Kinsey and Masters and Johnson are credited for their contributions to the scientific ideology. Eventually, sociocultural variables became a part of the gestalt of human sexual behavior, leading to the entire area of sexuality being closer to the everyday life behavior of individuals in society. This is the current ideology, referred to as secular. "The strength of the secular ideology in its role of defining our thinking about sexuality is found in its ability to reinterpret and thus reincorporate the religious and scientific ways of thinking about sexuality into its own context" (Petras, 1978, pp 81–82).

Speaking of sexual conduct, Gagnon (1977) refers to changes in purposes over time from limited (for procreation) to multiple purposes (for procreation, pleasure, expressions of joy and love) and from collective (what was done for social groups) to individual purposes. The individuality of sexuality is consistent with current secular ideology of society in general. A part of this perspective is the idea of sexual liberation, which began in the 1970s, and embodies not only to sexual practices but also how each individual views and expresses sexuality. Perhaps the time has come to understand that everyday life determines sexuality and not that anatomy determines sexuality.

The status, roles, and functions of the sexes are continuing rapid transitions. The interrelated societal changes in (1) technology; for example, work, household composition, contraception, and longevity; (2) economy; for example, an increase of women in the labor force and in traditional men's jobs, men entering the job market later owing to the need for increased technical training, and altera-

tions in work weeks; (3) family; for example, nuclear, single parent, blended (parents with children who remarry and combine their families into one), and convergence of functions and roles of men and women in the family; and (4) marriage customs; for example, later-life marriages, greater female independence, childless marriages, and single households, have significant implications for contemporary understanding of sexuality (Lee and Sussman, 1976).

Pierson (1974) reports two cultural norms in transition that will profoundly affect sexuality and gender development. The first is attitudes about masturbation, from the traditional view of its being evil to the acknowledgment that not only is it *not* harmful but also that it may even be helpful or simply pleasurable. The second norm involves the double standard regarding different expectations of males and females in sexual behavior outside of marriage; in essence, traditionally it was acceptable for men but not women to have pre- or extramarital sexual experiences. This particular change recognizes the natural proclivity for sexual activity in both males and females.

The emerging concept of androgyny has important implications for both male and female sexuality, especially in adolescents and adults. Androgyny (from the Greek, meaning male and female) is an anthropological term describing the exhibition of male and female characteristics in the same individual. As Wallum (1977) and Bee (1985) point out, this allows both sexes to express compassion and independence and gentleness and aggressiveness or to be passive or active or instrumental or expressive in accordance with the requirements of the situation. The popular beliefs that masculine and feminine are on opposite ends of a continuum and that sex typing is good for individuals and society have been challenged. The potentially wide range of behavior and experiences for both men and women that androgyny connotes will be discussed in adolescent and adult stages of sexuality. Bee (1985) indicates that research on androgyny in children is lacking and suggests that it is uncommon in early ages. She further postulates that a rigid schema for sex roles in young children is normal and may even be essential; however, a blurring of these sex-type rules may be an important process in adolescents.

Cultures vary in their perspectives of sexuality, especially in regard to rites of passage to becoming an adult (mature) sexual being, to what is considered acceptable gender-typical behavior (including sexual expression), and to masculine and feminine role patterns. In most Western cultures, adolescence and its characteristic physiological changes signals that individuals are now sexual persons (Gagnon, 1977). This pronouncement may be a very formal one, such as the Jewish Bar Mitzvah for the male child or the debutante ball for the female child of the aristocratic culture, or the transition may be no different or more noticeable than any other event in the life of an individual. Some cultures have very rigid gender behavior and roles ascribed as masculine or feminine, and others accept a blend of both genders in all individuals. Any effort to educate and promote healthy sexuality must take into consideration the practices of the culture in which the individual has been socialized.

LIFE CYCLE AND EMERGING SEXUALITY

Infancy and Childhood

Infancy, from birth to 1 year, is the oral phase of development (Freud) and the stage of trust versus mistrust (Erikson). The stage of infancy is primarily a time for acquiring a sense of self, which forms the basis for later manifestations of healthy sexuality. Object experiencing and need satisfaction are met by sucking and taking in nourishment, touching a soft blanket or the skin of another person, and exploring with the eyes. A sense of trust is established through these experiences when needs are satisfied as they occur and within an environment that is nurturing as well as nourishing. Mistrust in the environment occurs when there are prolonged delays, inconsistency, or lack of nurturing in attending to the infant's needs. Attachment to a nurturing person and his or her complementary warm, loving, and caring responses must occur. Contact comfort was demonstrated in Harlow's monkey experiments to be the vital force in the child's thriving and in the fundamental development of a secure sense of self (Bellak et al, 1973; Eagle, 1984).

Sex differences in temperament (personality characteristics) and physical activity in infancy are few, and most of the differences reported are the result of the parent's stereotypical perceptions of gender. In some aspects of physical maturity, girls develop somewhat ahead of boys, and the bodies of males are greater in muscle tissue than those of females (Bee, 1985).

Most authors agree that since the infant is in a symbiotic or undifferentiated self-inner state, there is also little *awareness* of gender differences. Efforts on the part of the infant to explore his or her body, including the genitals, are random, and we have no way of knowing if there is any sense of self-experiencing as masculine or feminine. However, it is important to acknowledge that the infant's environment is not gender neutral, that parents and others interacting with the infant certainly influence gender-typical responses. For example, Gagnon (1977) reports that mothers tend to talk to and look at girls and respond to their crying more immediately than they do boys. By 6 months of age, boys are touched less frequently, played with more roughly, and are generally encouraged to be more independent according to the stereotypical view that males are supposed to explore and master their world. While these are not deliberate attempts to influence gender behavior, roles, and attitudes, they nevertheless reflect general societal attitudes that social behaviors of males and females differ. Because of the totally dependent nature of the infant, he or she is the passive recipient of whatever interactions occur.

The next stage of early childhood, occurring about ages 1 to 3, is known as the anal stage (Freud) and the stage of autonomy versus shame and doubt (Erikson). During this stage the lower trunk becomes more developed and more under voluntary control, and the anal region becomes the center of pleasure. Allowing the child sufficient anal exploration and pleasure fosters the successful completion of this stage (Bee, 1985). The events of toilet training and the greater involvement of the father (viewed as the disciplinarian) influence self-control, discipline, will power, and orderliness in the developing child (Gagnon, 1977). Physical skills such as grasping and walking, which are more purposeful movements, and the beginning of speech are the basis for autonomy or active seeking of what the child desires and, thus, the child's sense of a separate identity. The child also experiences a continuing sense of security and sensual pleasure from hugging and kissing, and healthy relationships are established when this occurs among family members of both sexes.

During this stage the child's sense of sexuality is manifested in what is observed as self-stimulating behaviors such as touching and exploring the genitals, pelvic thrust movements, and even sexual arousal and orgasm that parallel adult sexual behavior. However, to the child, these activities are pleasurable and sensuous and not eroticism as evidenced in adults (Lion, 1982; Hogan, 1980). Shame and doubt occur if the parents respond in such a way that displays disgust or discomfort toward the infant's movements, giving him or her the sense that this part of the body is somehow dirty, untouchable, or undesirable.

As previously mentioned, there is a great deal of interest among contemporary researchers regarding the formation and pervasiveness of gender-typical behaviors and attitudes during these two stages of development. Chodorow (1974) and Rubin (1984) discuss the mothering role, which is universally assumed by women, as having the greatest consequences for gender-typical behaviors of men and women. Using the separation-individuation concept of psychoanalysis, Chodorow states that females experience this process within an ongoing relationship and "experience themselves as like their mothers, thus fusing the experience of attachment with the process of identity formation" (Chodorow, 1978, p 150). Females emerge from this stage with a capacity for empathy (a strong basis for experiencing another's needs and feelings) built into their primary self-definition. In contrast, boys must separate their mothers from themselves to define themselves as masculine, which breaks the primary love and sense of empathic tie, and consequently, a clearer individuation and ego boundaries that are defensive (against the primary attachment to the mother). She further postulates that because girls are parented by a person of the same gender there is no need to define themselves by denying the preoedipal relational modes to the same extent that boys must. Girls are therefore "less differentiated than boys, more continuous with and related to the external object world, and differently oriented to their inner object world as well" (Chodorow, 1978, p 167).

Gilligan (1982) adds that this difference in separation-individuation is what profoundly affects the determination of gender-typical behaviors, particularly regarding relationship and dependency issues. Masculine gender identity, being dependent upon separation from the mother, is threatened by intimacy, and males experience difficulty in relationships. For females, gender identity is not dependent on separation from the mother nor on the progress of individuation; therefore, for females gender identity is threatened by separation, and they experience difficulty with individuation. Since most developmental achievements in traditional psychological literature depend on increasing separation and independence, the consequences for females are great in that problems of separation become perceived as failures in development; therefore, the notion of female inferiority is perpetuated throughout life.

The third stage of development, which occurs at ages 4 to 5 is the phallic or genital stage (Freud) and the stage of initiative versus guilt (Erikson). The fact that the child's genitals increase in sensitivity (Bee, 1985) means that the focus of pleasure and object experience is in the genital zone. This physiological phenomenon and the concomitant intrapsychic experiences of resolving oedipal issues (discussed previously) result in the child's emergence as a clearly separated individual. The child's recognition of an identity, including a clear concept of gender, now focuses attention on the kind of person he or she is to become.

Erikson (1950) states that three strong developments lead to initiative: (1) the greater mobility of the child, (2) increasing perfection of language and cognitive skills enabling the child to understand and inquire about many things, and (3) expanding imagination as a result of the first two developments. As children take advantage of these skills, they vigorously test environmental boundaries, and behavior may even be viewed as aggressive. A sense of guilt develops if parents are either too rigid in their restriction or punishment of the child's exploration or overly permissive, so that the child takes more risks than he or she is capable of handling. Guilt may also be experienced because of oedipal conflicts (Bee, 1985).

Not only do children at this stage know their own bodies, but they are very aware that the bodies of the opposite sex are different. The child develops a sense of pride in his or her genitals through fondling, which becomes more purposeful and may even result in genital arousal. Masturbation is a natural developmental occurrence at this time. Children experience curiosity regarding genital activity, reproduction, and bathroom activities of the opposite sex. Childhood sex play, such as playing doctor, is a means of exploring the genitals of others.

The next stage of development, occurring from about age 6 through 12, is the latency stage (Freud) and the stage of industry versus inferiority (Erikson). Freud postulated that because this is a time of very rapid physical growth and the environment of object experiences becomes greatly expanded, the whole body becomes the focus of pleasure, and psychosexual development is held in abeyance. Industriousness occurs as the child participates in a broader range of socializing activities, including school, peer group play, and athletic and other social events. Winning acceptance and approval through developing abilities for being productive and social becomes paramount. If for any reason the child does not develop the skills necessary to actively participate and establish himself or herself with peers or is not accepted, a sense of inferiority develops (Bee, 1985).

Gender differences are very apparent during these latter two stages, and both physiological and psychosocial experiences have a great impact on sexuality and the continuing development of gender identity and role. Following separation-individuation, identification with the same-sex parent (or appropriate surrogates) is the major influence on masculine and feminine behavioral development; in essence, the role playing the child does with age mates resembles the models the child has witnessed. Through games in middle childhood, children increasingly practice cognitive and interactional skills, learn rules of games (and of society), and the roles of the opposite sex. In later childhood they learn to negotiate, compete, and compromise through their interactions with others. Macoby and Jacklin (1974) present a fairly comprehensive research review of the variability between males and females during this time, although they indicate the evidence remains weak and unconvincing. They report the following sex-typical behavioral differences: females exhibit greater (1) sensitivity to touch, (2) timidity or anxiousness, and (3) compliant and nurturant behavior. Males tend to be more (1) active, (2) competitive, and (3) concerned with dominance in their relationships.

From studies of gender differences in intellectual functioning of school age children, Woods (1984) reports the following: Girls initially test higher on intelligence, learn to read sooner, pay more attention to detail, make better grades, and are better at grammar, spelling, and word fluency. Boys perform better in math reasoning and spatial and analytical abilities and by age 10 equal the intelligence testing and reading ability of girls.

During the school age years, the influence of early gender personality formation becomes apparent. The major source of socialization is peer play. Gilligan (1982) discusses the differences between boys and girls in moral issues that are manifested in play behaviors. She cites a study of 181 fifth grade, white, middle-class children and the structure and organization of their playtime activities. Boys, more often than girls, played out of doors in large and age-heterogeneous groups and in competitive games, and their games lasted longer. The most significant phenomenon observed was that throughout their play, boys' games required a higher level of skill, were less boring, and when disputes arose, boys resolved them and went on with their play with minor interruptions. In contrast, girls' games ended when quarrels arose.

Citing the works of Piaget and Kolberg, Gilligan (1982) further discussed the implications that boys thus learned elaboration of rules and fair procedures for resolving conflicts, which are appropriate skills for leading large groups of people and achieving corporate success. Since girls' games, like hopscotch and jump rope, are turn taking and less competitive, the opportunities for learning to resolve arguments are less. In competitive games, quarrels ended the game, and any processes for resolving problems were not elaborated. "Girls subordinated the continuation of the game to the continuation of relationships" (Gilligan, 1982, p 10).

Among the numerous biological changes that occur during infancy and childhood are the development of body structures and certain physical capacities relevant to gender identity. Every body system, except the reproductive system, which remains quiescent until the onset of puberty, grows rapidly (Woods, 1979). Since body image is the basis for how one views oneself as a sexual being, all the characteristics that foster general health and development are important to healthy sexuality. These include nutrition, cleanliness, mobility, and protection from disfiguring injury and disease, to the extent possible.

NURSING CARE

In making use of developmental theory, there are some general considerations for nurses. First, the age range for each given developmental period is somewhat flexible, and variations in each child and family will account for some overlap in tasks, emotional responses, and activities of the child. In healthy children and environments, development will proceed according to the theoretical premises. The child's successful achievements during each stage have major implications for both physical and psychosocial development, positive self-concept, and ultimately healthy sexuality. First time parents especially may ask the nurse many questions regarding physical and psychosocial aspects of sexual development. The nurse who is aware of developmental tasks and progressions during these early stages of development, has a framework for assessing, educating, and guiding parents and children in their roles and responsibilities. The nurse should be prepared to discuss the developmental tasks of each stage and their implications for development of healthy sexuality.

A second factor that the nurse must consider is that extremes in parental behavior and environmental influences may interfere with healthy progression and have negative consequences that will be manifested later in life. For example, on a home visit to a new mother a nurse observed that the infant's crib was in the middle of the living room, the room temperature was uncomfortably hot, and the mother was hovering over the crib, which she acknowledged was the way she spent much of her time. The nurse immediately recognized a problem of overprotection and excessive concern in relation to the infant's dependency needs. Such extremes are not difficult to detect; however, what is more difficult is assessment of and guidance regarding which behaviors and interactions are appropriate. Most people rely on a combination of knowledge, experimentation, and intuition to guide them.

The nurse must also realize that developmental theories presume the presence of two parents. In contemporary society, this is no longer a given, since there are currently many family constellations. No matter what

the situation, the environment and interactions should in no way give the child or parent(s) the impression that development or sexuality is necessarily adversely affected. In single-parent families, for instance, it may take a surrogate, an extended family member, or some creativity on the part of the single parent to provide for the interactions of the missing parent.

In working with parents of infants, nurses should first observe and assess maternal attachment, including tone of voice in responding to the infant, gentleness, and promptness (within reason) in attending to infant needs, and provision of a secure, safe, and comfortable environment. Any physical abnormalities should be noted and, depending on the nature and severity, referred for treatment.

Even at this early stage of development the nurse might initiate conversation with parents regarding their concept of gender identity and inform the parents that their child's gender concept is being influenced by the way in which they interact with the infant. For example, in bathing and touching the infant, the genitals should be treated no differently than other parts of the body so that the infant "senses" and integrates them as a total body concept. It is also important that genitals be kept clean and infection free. Infants of both sexes need a caring and caressing kind of attention to develop a sense of basic trust in people and the environment; in essence boys need the same kissing and hugging as girls and from both parents.

Early childhood is the time when gender differences become more apparent to the developing child. The child's exploration of his or her body, including the anal region and genitals, should definitely be allowed, and the nurse should assess parents' reactions to this exploration, as well as to what might appear as orgasms in the child. Assisting parents to understand that such reactions are normal, pleasurable, and important to gender identity is a nursing responsibility. When the child is physiologically ready, toilet training should be fostered as a natural occurrence and not forced, punished, or treated with embarrassment or disgust by the parents. As verbal language develops, children should be taught proper language for body parts, such as penis and vagina, and for bathroom activities. Again, parental voice tone and nonverbal expressions that indicate normalcy of these labels will discourage the child's associating shame and guilt with them.

The child's autonomy and separation-individuation can be observed in increased physical activity and in the expanded space the child occupies. To prevent the child's risking doubt or danger, the safety and security of the environment is important. For example, the young child may alternately play alone with toys and seek the security of the parent's lap. Loving words or gestures will reassure the child that he or she is still being nurtured. Discipline, as well as nurturing behaviors, should be shared by both parents and should be the same for both male and female children. Such equality of interactions helps to develop a healthy self-concept and may discourage feelings of gender superiority or inferiority.

An important achievement of this early childhood stage of autonomy is a feeling of being adequate and self-reliant as well as being able to use the guidance of others whom the child has come to trust. In this process, negativism and frustration may be displayed. Rejections of guidance and restrictions ("No, I won't!" or "I don't want your help") are very frequent. Girls usually display more negativism than boys. Physical limitations of the child in making certain choices, such as an inability to reach objects, account for the frustrations experienced. Parents should be encouraged to allow whatever choices the child is capable of, provide assistance as needed without calling undo attention to it, and help the child to accept necessary restrictions. Consistency in what is allowed and what is forbidden is the key to successful guidance in assisting the child to learn the proper ratio of cooperativeness, willfulness, and initiative without loss of self-esteem. Parents may seek support from nurses to be tolerant of the stormy and seemingly inconsistent behavior in their children at this age. Parents often become anxious owing to conflicts between providing safety and giving children opportunities to explore and master the external world. The nurse may also encourage talking with other parents or others who have already guided children through this stage for reassurance that both children and parents survive.

Parents may need assistance in understanding the intrapsychic turmoil surrounding oedipal conflicts as well. Both genders have fantasies of possessing the opposite sex parent and simultaneously experience guilt and fear of punishment. It is important to teach parents that children's possessions are important to them and may become objects for displacing frustrations; that is, hostile actions toward toys, dolls, and other inanimate objects are healthy outlets.

In working with parents or children the nurse must answer questions about sex (and sexuality) truthfully and without anxiety. It is important to understand the latent or interpersonal issues, meaning oedipal wishes, seductive competition, and guilt, in sexual discussions. Children may ask questions about intercourse and the birth process in a provocative manner to elicit punishment, which parents must avoid. Frank, simple answers to questions keep the discussion from deteriorating into negative responses (Strean, 1983). In assessing a 6-year-old boy, referred to the school nurse because he was "hanging out" in female restrooms in school and looking underneath girls' skirts on the playground, the nurse discovered that the father could only discuss the child's problem with much embarrassment and great difficulty. If a parent is inhibited to this extent, referral to a physician or a counselor for greater ease in communicating about sex is warranted. Strean (1983) indicates that children will not misuse sexual information if it has not been transmitted to them in a distorted manner. There are numerous educational books for children of varying ages with which the nurse could become familiarized and suggest to parents for use with children.

While children learn from parental verbal communication, they also learn from nonverbal behaviors and do need to witness loving behaviors between parents. It is most healthy to impart to the child that males and females both receive and give love and that intercourse is pleasurable for both sexes. Under the guise of sexual freedom, parents may feel nudity in the presence of their children is acceptable. However, it may be experienced by the child as seductive and should be discouraged.

School age children will be exposed to values different than parental values and to same-sex peer bodies of differing sizes and shapes. These will arouse greater curiosity in the child as well as the use of sexual slang terms. Nurses and parents need to maintain and reaffirm the values they initiated with the child and to clarify perceptions that are grossly distorted. For example, a child who does not know about an erection may misconstrue what he has heard from a school friend about how large his father's penis is.

The child should also be taught the rationale for culture-specific beliefs about sexuality and sex-role behaviors to enhance his or her understanding and to maintain a commitment to their beliefs. This teaching, as well as acknowledgment of feelings, is imperative, especially if the child discovers significant differences in others with whom he or she socializes. The viewing of other's bodies, such as in gym classes, enhances the child's notion of a range of gender (and genital) normalcy and helps to solidify gender identity.

Nurses are called upon to participate in sex education in schools, which can be both enlightening and anxiety provoking. The nurse is obligated to obtain explicit expectations regarding what is to be taught and to what level of students, recognizing that it is impossible to be prepared for all the questions that might get asked. Questions such as, "What do my mom and her boyfriend do when they are in the bedroom together and shut the door?" from early school age children and "Will I bleed to death when I have my period?" from older school age children are typical. The nurse should refer the former question to the child's mother and certainly answer the latter question. The rationale behind this decision is to respond to private (family, relationship) questions for which the nurse has no factual information by referring them to the person from which the question arises and to respond to public information questions with accurate data both to inform and clarify misconceptions. Age-appropriate audio-visual aids greatly enhance learning about sex, and familiarity with their content will add to the nurse's comfort in presentation.

The nurse should realize that there is little consistency regarding sex education, whether it is school curricula, home teaching by family members, peer transmittal of information, or mass media. Given the abundance of information available to a child, and its sometimes exploitative or stereotypical presentation of gender (especially female gender), it is best for the nurse to elicit from the child some ideas about the information he or she has and, if possible, some clarity regarding the expected answer. In teaching, there is an excellent opportunity to assess children's responses to sexual content and to identify the ones who need additional information and/or guidance in comprehension. In such instances, follow-up with the child, teacher, and/or parents is a nursing responsibility.

Many parents try to learn about what is being taught in schools and will assist their child in integrating this teaching with their own. For those who do not, nurses should be active in publicizing school subjects as well as other educational programs that have potential benefit. A broader nursing role would be to screen programs for accuracy and advocate policies that ensure availability of sex education.

In relation to gender role socialization, currently there is a wide range of athletic opportunities such as little league baseball and soccer for both boys and girls. Girls particularly should be encouraged to engage in competitive sports according to their interest. Boys should be supported in creative endeavors (for example, art, writing poetry, and dancing) and should not be ignored or labeled sissies because of their interest in these areas. In contemporary society there is greater acceptance of behaviors and activities in childhood for both sexes that were once thought to be typically masculine or feminine. Parents, particularly those who have been raised in more rigid environments, could benefit from listening to their children talk about their peer activities to aid their understanding of current norms in play. When parents question the nurse regarding child's play activity, an appropriate response would be to have them talk about what their children are saying to them. This will not only help to answer questions but will also facilitate assessment of the kind of communication between parents and their children.

In later childhood, same-sex friendships serve many purposes, including expanding sex role behaviors, coping with physical sexual inadequacy, and initiating activities that indicate sexual preference for a partner. Private conversations and secret activities are typical in "chum" relationships, which frequently lead to parental anxiety about the nature of the intimacy shared. The nurse can teach parents that this same-sex attachment is a means of seeking security in a peer world and is protection from engaging in premature sexual activities. Experimentation in homosexual behaviors is normal at this developmental level and will be intermittent, short lived, and undisclosed. If a child does have a homosexual orientation, which will indeed begin to be manifested in later childhood, parents will need much guidance in accepting and adapting to the situation. Given that such an orientation is not likely to change, this will be a traumatic time, as society has not yet accepted homosexuality carte blanche.

Small group peer activities at the later childhood stage help children of both sexes to experience frustration, tolerance, mutuality, negotiation, compromise, and problem solving, which are necessary characteristics of confidence and competence in increasing maturity. Slumber parties, camping trips, athletic and social events, and numerous other group outings are healthy outlets to meet the needs of later childhood.

Adolescence

Adolescence is currently recognized not merely as a phase between childhood and adulthood but as a distinct stage of development with concomitant pubertal-induced behavioral and identity changes, a second parent-child separation process, peer group processes, and other phenomena specific to, or peaking in, adolescence. (Chilman, 1983; Pierson, 1974). This developmental phase spans a 10-year period, beginning with puberty. As a physiological phenomenon, adolescence currently begins at an earlier age because of improved nutrition and health practices in developed societies, and because of current economic, work, and family systems, it lasts longer. Youth are not needed in the work force as they once were, and with current technology, a longer period of occupational preparation is supported. According to Pierson (1974), adolescence is a sociocultural construct and is defined and limited by roles, particularly occupational roles, rather than age and sex performance ability; in essence, an individual is not considered an adult until he or she performs an economic role as an established member of society's work force.

Puberty refers to the hormonal and physical changes leading to maturation of reproductive capacity (Chilman, 1983). These events underlie characteristic psychological changes in mood, gender role, peer activity, and modified relationships with parents and other significant adults (Strean, 1983). In Freudian theory, the hormonal changes and concomitant maturation of the sexual organs have led to the identification of adolescence as the genital stage of development. In terms of psychosocial development, there is a re-emergence of oedipal issues, which are worked out at a different level; sensuous and affectional attachments are directed away from the same-sex parent (and parents in general) toward peers of the opposite sex (Lidz, 1968). Adolescence is the stage, according to Erikson, in which individuals need to emerge with a clear identity—gender identity as well as a sense of purpose toward being a contributing member of society. To not accomplish the developmental tasks necessary for achieving adulthood is to suffer identity or role diffusion: an uncertainty of self-concept, indecisiveness, and a clinging to the more secure dependencies of childhood.

In seeking gender identity, the most significant feature in the lives of adolescents is the development of the sociocultural meaning of sexuality. Today's society nurtures this emerging sexuality increasingly more in isolation from adult gender roles. Educational environments are more adapted to the adolescent ways of life and encourage young people to question traditional views of sexuality and gradually develop their own (Pierson, 1974). Evidence of the ways in which the images of both genders are changing can be seen in variations in hair length in males and in unisex jeans as universal adolescent wearing apparel.

Adolescence is frequently labeled as a time of trouble and turmoil and is viewed by society with ambivalence, anxiety, and often lack of positive sanctions. Psychosocial achievement expectations along with tremendous physiological activity give some credence to this labeling and view. However, most youth experience the events of this stage without overt trauma and concern. The negative connotation is more perpetuated by adult perceptions of adolescent behavior inconsistencies and mood swings, which can cause negative self-fulfilling prophecies. Rapid physiological changes accompanied by great alterations in sex differences do create havoc with emerging self-identity as well as with every relationship system. The conflicts that adolescents face are due largely to the anxiety they experience during the wide range of years in which physical maturation begins.

PHYSIOLOGICAL FACTORS

Figure 4–3 illustrates the physiological sexual differentiation that occurs during adolescence. On average, females reach puberty at about 10 to 12 years of age, 2 years earlier than males. With the onset of puberty, fe-

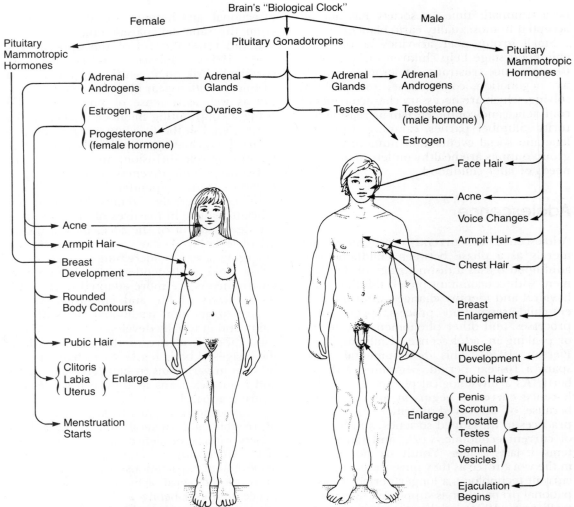

FIGURE 4–3. Effects of sex hormones on pubertal development. (From Human Sexuality *by John H. Gagnon. Copyright ©*
1977 by Scott, Foresman and Co. Reprinted by permission.)

males' breasts begin to develop, and pubic
hair appears. At the same time, growth of
the uterus and vaginal canal occurs, and
there is enlargement of the labia and clitoris.
Menarche (onset of menstruation) is a definitive and mature stage of uterine development and occurs after the peak of the female
growth spurt.

Since female sexual organs are basically
internal, the clitoris is not as easily stimulated
as is the penis, and there is potential for less
awareness of sexual arousal. Thus, females
are inclined to view sexuality in dualistic,
ambivalent, self-protective, and more emotionally dependent terms than males (Chilman, 1983).

Sexual maturation in males begins at about
age 12 or later, with an increase in the rate

of growth of the testes and scrotum and the
development of pubic hair. These events are
followed by increased growth of the penis,
increase in body height, breast and nipple
sensitivity, and marked increase in hormones
released by the endocrine glands. For males,
androgens are most important at this stage,
as testosterone is necessary for activating the
prenatal masculinization of the brain. Breast
and nipple sensitivity may be a source of
anxiety for males if they fear it to be a sign
of femininity. Boys experience a growth
spurt at about age 13 that lasts 2 to 3 years.
During this spurt, height, weight, facial features, body hair, and muscular strength alter,
resulting in body contour changes. The un-
even growth rate, causing lack of coordination, is a source of embarrassment (Chilman,

1983). The onset of nocturnal emissions (wet dreams) follows the maturation of the prostate gland and seminal vesicles. The male sexual organs, because they are external, are more easily stimulated (by clothing or other contact), leading to an increased awareness of sexual arousal. Thus, the male view of sex is pleasure oriented, exciting, assertive, achieving, unitary, and less personal (Chilman, 1983). Kinsey's studies indicate that it is during this time that sex drive and orgasmic capacity increase rapidly in the male (Kinsey, Pomeroy, and Martin, 1948). However, Chilman (1983) reports that the heightened need for sexual gratification in males during this stage of development is a result of a combination of physiological, cultural, and social learning influences, and given current cultural norms male and female differences are less likely.

PSYCHOSOCIAL FACTORS

The psychosocial development in adolescence is focused on self-concept issues, specifically, gender and occupational identity. Identity is referred to as an existential position and is defined by Marcia as a self-structure consisting of "internal, self-constructed, dynamic organization of drives, abilities, beliefs, and individual history" (Marcia, 1980, p 159). The importance of identity in the adolescent, different from the process of self-object differentiation in the infant, is that physical, cognitive, and social skills exist simultaneously. The late adolescent has the ability to synthesize and integrate all previous identity experiences toward a well-developed (including flexibility and openness to changes) identity structure in adulthood (Marcia, 1980).

In terms of gender, there is inconclusive evidence that the pattern of identity development for females is more blurred than that for males and that girls find it more difficult than boys to obtain a separate identity. The separation issue for females is congruent with contemporary studies indicating the lack of need in females to separate completely from their mothers in order to identify with them. The greatest influence on gender role identity for both sexes continues to be the same-sex parent, although peers, heroines, and stars from mass media do influence gender behaviors. Also true for both sexes, feelings of sexual adequacy throughout life, and in particular the self-concern and preoccupa-

tion with body image manifested in adolescence, play a significant role in gender identity (Chilman, 1983).

Even though the research on androgyny is just beginning to emerge, preliminary reports provide important insights on adolescent identity in contemporary society. Bee (1985) reported that about 25 to 35 per cent of high school students consider themselves androgynous; however, there were more females in the masculine category than males in the feminine category. In addition, an androgynous or masculine concept of self in both sexes correlate with high self-esteem. This means that girls who display traditional sex role behaviors may be at risk for lower self-esteem and poorer relationships with peers, but for boys, traditional male role behaviors still correlate with high self-esteem and success in peer relationships. Wallum (1977) provides similar information from several studies regarding androgyny and mental health: Girls and women high in femininity showed high levels of anxiety, low social acceptance, and poor social adjustment; adolescent males high in masculinity had better psychological and social adjustment than those low in masculinity.

In summary, the achievement of a clear gender identity is different for males and females. Girls tend to have more difficulty obtaining a separate identity, seeking it progressively through families, boyfriends, and then a significant mate. Their energy is directed toward the expressive role of achieving interpersonal skills, including acceptance, security, and support. Thus, identity becomes linked to intimacy, the task of the next stage of development. The male focus of energy is on the more instrumental areas of independence and achievement, including autonomy from parents and conformity to peer group values, which lead toward an occupational identity (Chilman, 1983).

ROLES

The changing view toward androgynous gender role behaviors has many positive benefits in terms of gender identity but poses dilemmas for both sexes. Society has not yet fully accepted the concept of androgyny. Nevertheless, there appears to be no basis, biologically or psychosocially, for the stigma of female inferiority; and marriage and motherhood are no longer the set pattern for a female life style (Chilman, 1983; Pierson,

1974). The consequences for males seem to be greater, especially since late adolescent and adult males have been socialized in traditional ways. Dilemmas for men involve threats to power, aggressiveness, and sexual prowess—assets they can no longer count on for survival in a technological and interpersonal society. Contemporary researchers agree that a major focus of both research and socialization ought to be on legitimizing androgyny, predicting that people and society will be much richer for the diversity (Chilman, 1983; Wallum, 1977).

In addition to individual identity issues, the many socio-cultural influences on the adolescent are often viewed as pressures to grow and progress toward adult competency. Conflicts occur with regard to socioeconomic status (variations in backgrounds of the peer group) and in relation to establishing intimate relationships, specifically sexual intimacy. Chilman (1983) indicates that middle-class families retain a more traditional role socialization for their offspring, and the upper-class tends toward more equality in sex role socialization. Certainly, the conflict over sexual intimacy centers around the fact that while attitudes toward greater sexual expression for both sexes may be changing, such behavior is still a moral issue as well as a health and potentially life-threatening issue (because of the existence of the acquired immuno-deficiency syndrome).

The role socialization process in adolescents centers around dating in preparation for mate selection. The progression is from cliques of intimate friends, to intimate same-sex friendships, to formation of couple relationships (Chilman, 1983). During the formation of same-sex relationships, homosexual activities are common. Anytime during the surge of sexual physiology, masturbation may be engaged in; boys are more comfortable with this practice than girls (Chilman, 1983). Dating serves the purpose of freedom of choice, with the adolescent testing out ideas about the self and opposite-sex partners, ultimately experiencing the pleasures of heterosexual acts (Pierson, 1974). Chilman (1983) reports that by age 15, adolescents are vulnerable to inadequacies in interpersonal relationships. In particular, girls are highly sensitive to these inadequacies, as sensitivity, empathy, and acceptance are extremely important; their frustrations, jealousies, and conflicts are over friends. Boys disagree and argue about activities, property, and girlfriends.

Recent studies focus attention on the effects of single-parent families on dating. Chilman (1983) reported that girls without fathers living at home had more difficulty interacting appropriately with males and spent much time seeking male company and engaging in sex-related behaviors. Boys whose fathers were absent had difficulty in sex role development and adjustment to their peer group.

There is voluminous literature on adolescents who engage in premature or premarital sexual intercourse. Two trends are that adolescents of both sexes are engaging in non-marital intercourse at an earlier age and that more females are sexually active than in previous years. Several studies report that female motivation is the need for affection and closeness (Doctors, 1985). Perceptions and attitudes toward this practice vary widely, from those who believe that sexual experimentation is optimal for a person's development (Strean, 1983) to those who retain self-denial and anticipation as a means of satisfaction (Pierson, 1974). For both males and females there are powerful emotions surrounding the sexual act, and adolescents in particular struggle in handling them. Most authors agree that for both sexes intercourse in the context of a meaningful relationship is still the norm. A most interesting issue is that mothers and fathers (as well as health professionals) are very good at teaching and modeling sex role behaviors in relation to being men and women (identity and roles) but do very poorly when it comes to teaching about being lovers and mates (relationships). Sexual intimacy should include a mutual sharing of feelings, hopes, attitudes, memories, and all else that makes a relationship have value and worth (Strean, 1983).

NURSING CARE

Physiological Factors

Nurses have numerous opportunities to influence the positive development of sexuality in adolescents. Since the age of onset of puberty is so variable, there will be teenagers who will consider themselves early or late maturers. For those groups specifically, and all adolescents generally, a thorough physical assessment and health history are very important to detect any pathophysiological process needing treatment. For most healthy adolescents, a combination of genetic, physical, nutritional, and psychosocial factors determines pubertal processes. The nurse can offer reassurance by sharing with the adolescent client adequate information regarding physical health, progress of development, and the highly individual nature of the pubertal process. The adolescent's focus on the self and body renders him or her extremely open to straightforward information pertaining to physiological sexuality. For both adolescents and their parents, knowing the sequence of physiological events and predicting changes ease anxieties; for example, suggesting a jock strap to the adolescent boy to increase comfort in sports activities can make him more comfortable with genital development. Nurses may suggest that a single parent with an adolescent child of the opposite sex find a respected confidant of the same sex with whom the adolescent can share concerns. Pierson (1974) points out that no matter how knowledgeable the parent is, he or she is never fully prepared to handle matters in the same way as the parent of the same sex.

Dispelling myths, such as the myth that the larger one's breasts or penis the greater capacity for sexual enjoyment, is definitely a nursing responsibility. Initial questioning of adolescents can reveal their beliefs and any erroneous information they have received. Accepting whatever the adolescent discloses and discussing sexual development in a rational, nonthreatening manner will facilitate the nurse-adolescent client relationship. Adolescents often prefer talking over concerns with an objective adult prior to or in place of parents, who are often more emotional and tend to misinterpret. Assisting parents to understand the totality of adolescent sexual issues rather than the narrow focus of the erotic will certainly facilitate parent-child communication.

Psychosocial Issues

Countering the often negative and stereotypical images of gender identity pervasive in television is a vital role for the nurse. For example, informing males that macho behavior is less popular and supporting male gentleness and sensitivity may provide the adolescent comfort and security to deal with identity struggles. By the same token, teaching assertiveness training, will ease the pain

of conflict in a female who is striving for a career when peers and family question why she has not yet selected a steady mate.

In the adolescent's effort to practice adult behaviors or cope with all that is occurring in his or her life, the use of drugs and alcohol is a major concern. The most important information in ensuring sexual health is that misuse of these chemicals interferes dramatically with both physical and emotional processes; the risk is that the adolescent will enter adulthood with inadequate social and emotional skills to participate in adult tasks and relationships. Alcohol, taken in excess, negates the experience of sex.

Adults view dating experiences of adolescents in their own terms of what their experiences were as adolescents. There is no real clarity about what is right and wrong regarding current adolescent sexual activities except what particular cultural practices dictate. Nurses can help parents understand that crises, such as an unwanted pregnancy, can be avoided if the adolescent has some parental guidance, interest, and instruction about dating, rather than leaving their learning totally up to chance or the peer group. Adolescents still need behavioral parameters with rewards and punishments in the process of learning what is best for them. Most adolescents who have been raised in an atmosphere of trust, love, and openness in communication continue to respect their families' values and will need support to persist in maintaining these values when contradictory situations arise. At no other time in human development is the openness of parent-child communication so vitally important. Nurses often serve as sounding boards for both parents and adolescents as they express frustrations and attempt to resolve their many struggles in accepting conventional societal standards. Listening attentively, acknowledging feelings, and providing accurate information are useful nursing skills in working with families in which there are adolescent members.

Working in high schools consistently or through consultation is a role the nurse assumes. Teachers as well as students need assistance in sorting out the nature of adolescent issues, specifically accurately determining whether a problem is truly physical or a physical manifestation of a psychosocial concern. The latter is a frequent occurrence, since the adolescent is not always aware of the physical manifestations of emotional turmoil. For example, on three consecutive days during an afternoon class, one female student developed a headache and asked to be excused. The student was seen by the school nurse who discovered she had not been eating lunch on those days because a classmate had told her she looked heavier than usual. The student's missing lunch, resulting in an afternoon headache, was related to a behavioral and emotional response to a "heavy" self-image. When a student is referred to the nurse for consultation, as in the above example, guided discussion of the immediate parameters of the problem and questioning about antecedent situations or interactions will be helpful to the nurse in determining intervention. Sometimes empathic listening and suggesting possible alternatives for problem solving may be all that is needed. Problems beyond the scope of the nurse's ability should be referred to the appropriate professional. It is essential to obtain the adolescent's permission before informing parents of needed attention, or at least the nurse must tell the student that parents will be informed. School guidance counselors can be the nurse's allies in this endeavor. For example, one student member of a drug prevention skills group was talking about suicide and had visible scratches on her wrists. During the nurse's discussion with the student, she learned that the girl had a continuing conflict with her stepfather and did not feel as though her mother was listening to her. The nurse, with the assistance of the guidance counselor, held a family conference at the school, and the entire family was referred to juvenile services for family counseling. The student was much relieved by this action.

High school curricula currently include courses such as those in family relations, which facilitate social and interpersonal learning. When nurses are asked to teach these type classes, they have an excellent opportunity to expand the concept of sexuality, demystify sex, and engage students in discussions about dating behaviors. Other kinds of classroom activity may involve conducting life skills groups that address such topics as communication, assertiveness, problem solving, and values clarification.

Adolescents are fun to work with because they are very sensitive and eager to learn. When given the proper respect, care, serious attention, and essential facts, they often reward the nurse by their generous display of appreciation.

Adulthood

Having survived the vicissitudes of adolescence, healthy individuals arrive at adulthood with at least an identity oriented toward a purpose in life, gender constancy, and a notion about gender roles, however clear or confused those might be in today's society. No distinguishing biological developments define an age range for this stage of growth in sexuality. Adulthood begins at the end of adolescence, or when men and women begin to establish themselves as autonomous members of society, particularly in the work force.

Erikson describes the stage of adulthood as characterized by developing intimacy, meaning the capacity for love and mutual devotion, and a commitment to a social ideology. During early adult years there is the capacity for full sexual expression, both in physical union with a partner and in gender role behaviors. This is a period of maximum sexual self-consciousness (Woods, 1984). The primary tasks are developing a satisfactory life style, including work, social relationships, educational pursuits, and geographic location. Sheehy (1974) describes early adulthood as a time to build a structure for the future, with dilemmas centering around establishing a *set* or a *tentative* structure in which to experiment and explore numerous opportunities in both work and relationships. If one has not been adequately prepared to make commitments, permanent or tentative, the consequence is isolation.

Typically during this early stage of adulthood, individuals are making numerous decisions about roles and living arrangements: being single (and for how long), selecting a mate or a sexual partner, being a parent or not, combining and accomplishing a number of roles simultaneously, selecting a particular role to the exclusion of others. Each decision has its rewards and consequences. A clear trend in U.S. society is that individuals are allowing more time for making decisions, as evidenced by later marriages, deferring families several years into marriage, and increased numbers of single households for both sexes. Another advantage of this extended time for decision making is that role choices are being made more rationally and in the context of a wide variety of background experiences.

Ribal (1973) identifies four significant developments at this time: (1) formation of stable and meaningful relationships; (2) avoidance of incompatible persons; (3) changes in ways sexual behavior fit into people's lives, i.e., greater responsibility and self-control; and (4) sex as a medium for expressing love. He further indicates that this can be a time of social and sexual unlearning; that is, expanding the social process established by elders and desiring something different from life. He describes male behavior as more genuine, learning and acting more rationally, displaying an increased concern for the needs and rights of others, and seriousness in planning the future. Female behavior is less marked by major changes in expression of sex roles, except for those roles that emphasize the equal status of women (Ribal, 1974).

Middle adulthood, according to Erikson, is a time of generativity and, assuming the adult has made a commitment to a life goal, a time in which energy is devoted to productivity, including work, family, relaxation activities, creative endeavors, and assumption of a broader social role. Stagnation, or being in a rut, is the consequence of not assuming the developmental tasks of this life stage. Sheehy (1974) says it is a time when persons truly disinherit the imagery and strong pull to be like parents and integrate aspects of their selves previously hidden, often through trying out new roles. She implies that these different yearnings may be part of the reason marriages break up, especially for couples who married young. While life may become more complicated, there is also a new richness.

Much of the developmental literature on adolescence centers around individual identity. As is evident in forming social peer groups and in dating experiences, people are increasingly aware of the interpersonal dimension of identity, that is, defining themselves partly in terms of the extent to which they understand and are emotionally sensitive to others. Inherent in the tasks of adulthood, and indeed in the concept of intimacy itself, are the processes of interacting and establishing relationships. As Marcia (1980) indicates, during all of adulthood the opportunities are great for growing in self-identity and increasing individual and social integration.

Whatever the experience of sexual differences for males and females during adolescence, sensitivity to these differences increases drastically in adult interactions.

Negotiating and reconciling these differences toward mutual satisfaction and goal achievement along with continuing self-actualization lead to genuine and mutual psychological intimacy. The women's liberation movement generated a number of studies about women's struggles toward a more egalitarian and androgynous life style and the effects of this on relationships, but information about men's experiences is still scarce. Both men and women, socialized in traditional gender roles, have become increasingly discontent in intimate relationships during adulthood. Many relationships do not survive, as evidenced by the escalation in the divorce rate.

Self-concept of adult men and women is influenced by societal expectations as well as individual needs. The attractiveness or beauty of youth that seems to be a characteristic of women's sexuality diminishes with aging. On the other hand, competence and competitiveness, the valued characteristics of men, improve with age (Petras, 1978). However, women still do not receive adequate social support for striving toward autonomy and achievement (Rubin, 1984; Gilligan, 1982) and therefore experience self-doubt. Wallum (1977) reports studies indicating that adults who were highly sex role typed exhibited behavior congruent with sex role characteristics; when tasks required behaviors more appropriate and sensitive to the situation, they succeeded poorly. Mental health relative to gender in later adulthood is manifested very differently in men and women. More women than men in every age group and in every population suffer from depression. Women generally tend to have higher rates of mental illness, attributed to traditional subordinate roles as well as secondary economic status. Men use and abuse alcohol, commit more crimes, and have a higher suicide rate, the latter occurring beyond the age of 35 and into the 80s with increasing frequency. Married men tend to be more mentally healthy than single men and married women.

Females, having experienced difficulty with identity and autonomy during adolescence, enter adulthood with a clearer idea than males of what constitutes intimacy, including a greater ability for introspection and sensitivity to others. For men intimacy is associated with danger, based on separation-individuation from the mother early in life (Gilligan, 1982). This is the basis of conflict in most relationships, in which men elaborate facts and rights, while women attend to the emotional and relational aspects of problem situations. In Rubin's (1983) interviews of both partners in intimate relationships, men constantly misunderstood or were antagonistic toward women's emotionality, and as a result had minimal ability to communicate. Women discussed the incessant rationality, intellectualization, and insensitivity of men as barriers to communication and therefore barriers to true intimacy. Rubin (1983) states that for men who have been socialized into highly stereotyped sex roles that emphasize repression and denial of their feelings, fears, and fantasies, the emotional side is truly not consciously available to them. An interesting conclusion in a study by Komarovsky (1976) of male seniors in an Ivy League college was that these men believed that they experienced psychological intimacy with females because they could disclose themselves more freely with women than with men. However, the women involved with these men still criticized their reserve and lack of full self-disclosure.

Schwartz (1979) takes the position that mature loving in adulthood must transcend sex role values through cognitive restructuring toward androgyny. Love must involve sharing and meeting of psychosexual needs based on egos with positive self-esteem, which for both sexes have the characteristics of openness to tenderness, nurturance, assertion, passion, and empathy.

Both sexes are often confused and bewildered by role changes. Rubin (1983) cites personal difficulty when in middle adulthood her husband wanted to quit his job and pursue a writing career. She was in a position to support the family and agreed to allow this transition. She describes in detail her lack of preparation for the feelings that ensued, especially threats to security and dependency needs, which had not been a source of anxiety prior to this time. In a study reported by Bem (1976), highly sex role–typed males and females were given cross-sex tasks to perform (nailing and ironing) and displayed anxiety and nervousness in performing the activity. Further studies found that androgynous persons of both sexes were more flexible and more successful in both independent and nurturing activities. Females displayed "masculine" independence under pressure to conform, and males displayed "feminine" nurturance when interacting with a kitten.

In discussing the life patterns of adult males and females, Sheehy (1974) indicates that whatever their traditional life patterns have been, all people end up with some dissatisfaction and discontent regarding the roles they have played and desire something more or different in middle adulthood. As changes in gender roles and relationship structures continue, there is increasing awareness that both males and females have the same needs for love and belonging. Currently, men's struggles constitute an effort to be more effective in getting these needs met in relationships, and women's struggles are about obtaining an accepted equal position in whatever their choice of roles happens to be, homemaker, caregiver, or member of the labor force.

Almost all of developmental literature discusses stage-related crises that both men and women encounter, and these become particularly obvious in middle adulthood. Midlife crises revolve around what Davis (1980) refers to as losses in "critical life exchange values." Physiological changes in the process of aging and challenges to the American value systems of youth and beauty, considered women's issues, and money and power, considered men's issues, must be reconciled. Biological changes include a decrease in height, muscle mass, strength, and cardiac power (Woods, 1984), and in part because of these changes, health risks increase. Menopause in women, because of a lower amount of estrogen secretion, is accompanied by atrophy in both breasts and genitalia. In men there is a more insidious decline in androgen-dependent tissues, resulting in changes in the penis and scrotum (Woods, 1979). These physiological changes also mean concomitant alterations in sexual response capacity; however, there is such a variety of individual differences in both men and women that the psychosocial dimensions of sexual responsiveness certainly must be considered along with loss or decline in physical sexual functioning.

Regarding both relationships and decline in physical status, a word about affairs is necessary because some authorities see them occurring as a means of coping with midlife crises. An appropriate definition of an affair in the context of contemporary society is any encounter, either sexual or intensely emotional, that occurs outside of marriage, cohabitation, or other commitment to another person. A perusal of the personals columns in magazines and newspapers, which include advertisements stating "married person (man or woman) desires discreet companionship," bears witness to the extent to which these interactions are occurring. Reasons stated in the literature as to why affairs occur include the need in both sexes to reconfirm sexual identities, a wish to relieve boredom in primary relationships, companionship, improved sexual experiences, revenge, and changing needs (Denoltz, 1981). Another reason could be either mental or physical illness in a partner that stifles their full participation in a relationship. Affairs are experienced very differently by males and females, depending on the configuration and intent of the dyad. For example, in the married man–single woman affair, the woman invariably waits for the man's marriage to end and fantasizes about her ultimate union with him; the man typically is quite satisfied with the way things are and has no intention of altering the situation. In this and other dyad arrangements, the temporariness and continual conflict are more sources of frustration than relief unless there is some resolution that is mutually satisfying. It is important to understand that affairs are, at best, ways to avoid dealing with crises, and when discovered, are painful for all involved.

In terms of the psychosocial crises of midlife, most authorities agree that the worst enemy for both genders is denial that they exist. When each individual faces crises without false assurance or overconcern, the dilemmas become manageable. Davis (1980) suggests a prescription for making middle age transitions less traumatic through recognizing realities, confronting issues in manageable parts, taking respite as needed, discerning the facts, avoiding blame of others, and accepting help from others.

NURSING CARE

Adult sexuality issues are complex and multifaceted. It is unreasonable to expect the nurse to be competent in assessing and intervening in every situation that arises. Therefore, some general areas of nursing responsibility in interacting with the adult population are presented here followed by a model that provides guidelines for assessing the development and characteristics of adult heterosexual relationships. Certainly, physical health and body image are important factors in adult sexual health. Making assessments in these areas and assisting people to identify the origins of concerns regarding sexuality should be a primary consideration.

In addressing adult sexuality concerns, the nurse, more so than in any other developmental stage, must be aware of his or her own concept of gender, including thoughts and feelings about gender role. Whether or not the nurse believes in androgyny, the literature demonstrates this to be a desired and mentally healthy style of behaving for both genders; therefore, the nurse has an obligation to increase her or his own knowledge about the effects of androgyny on adults. The nurse should take advantage of any opportunity to raise public consciousness of androgyny and clarify what is known. Education would include dispelling myths, such as that androgyny will lead to a unisex society in which gender differences are so blurred they will be nonexistent. With many adult individuals, the nurse can assist in coping with gender role stereotypes through anticipatory guidance and enhancement of problem-solving skills. Nurses may also actively initiate, act as consultant to, or participate in a wide variety of adult groups whose goal is support of persons as they attempt to make individual changes.

Many individuals seek therapy, or feel they should, for assistance in dealing with adult crises or for assurance that they are not crazy in making choices not yet generally favored by society. The nurse's empathic listening and counseling skills will be helpful in assisting both males and females to sort out specific problems needing more expert counseling from those that simply require acceptance, understanding, and a sounding board to resolve. For example, a nurse counseled one young woman who had just graduated from college and had been steadily dating a non-college graduate who is loving, kind, considerate, nonassertive and apparently content with his life and works in a blue collar job. The woman, in contrast, is very career oriented, highly motivated, and energetic and not currently interested in a permanent commitment. The messages—that she will "never find anyone that will be as good to her"—she receives from family, friends, and even some peers convey very traditional female role expectations. Continued support from the nurse for the woman's own values and striving as a woman is most helpful at this time, as the nurse has demonstrated the ability to face and work through similar gender issues.

If the nurse decides referral for mental health counseling is warranted, assisting in the selection of an appropriate professional counselor is a very important nursing role. Studies indicate that professionals steeped in traditional sex roles are more of a hindrance than a help in resolving gender difficulties, especially those who view women's role strains as indicative of emotional problems (Boverman et al, 1970). The nurse is obligated to know the strengths and specialties of referral sources.

ASSESSMENT OF ADULT HETEROSEXUAL RELATIONSHIPS

Stiles' (1979) developmental sequence in intense relationships can be used as the basis for a framework for assessing the development and characteristics of heterosexual relationships. The premises of Stiles' developmental model are the following:

1. Certain emotional or interpersonal issues are confronted by persons in the relationship at each stage of development. The issues are focused around the central task Erikson determined as belonging to each developmental level.

2. As participants in the relationship invest in the central issue of each stage (e.g., trust), there is experiencing of the negative characteristic (e.g., mistrust), around which individual and relationship conflicts or crises arise.

3. As these conflicts become resolved, the central issue becomes synthesized as an integral part of the relationship (the participants have developed a basic sense of trust), and there is positive growth.

4. Once the central task is synthesized, it leads to experiencing the negative characteristic of the central task in the next developmental stage (shame and doubt), and the cycle is repetitive throughout all of the stages.

Stage One

In the initial stage, a couple's energy is invested in forming the relationship and establishing a sense of *trust* in each other. Basic virtues of drive and hope lead to openness to experience in general. Curiosity and interest are easily aroused. People need consistency of experience and congruence in verbal communication and behavioral follow through. Consideration and gentleness are important in physical contact, which typically includes hand holding, hugging, and kissing as expressions of affection. In this process, sexual arousal may occur as a part of the excitement and stimulation of investing emotional energy in another individual. If self-pleasure has been taboo in early individual development, sexual union may occur prematurely, that is, before the couple is ready for either the depth of commitment or the handling of emotions that accompany sexual involvement.

Behaviors indicative of mistrust are suspiciousness, wariness, and withdrawal from contact. If there is sound rationale for not trusting and both partners are basically secure, they will validate or clarify their suspicions. If inconsistencies are deemed greater than trusting behaviors, the persons involved may decide not to proceed with the relationship.

Assessment. From the interview ask the following questions: How was the relationship initiated and by whom? Describe the early stages, sequence of relationship events, and individual interests. In what ways were each of the partners considerate of each other's needs and feelings? Was the identity of each of the individuals blurred or compromised, that is, did either one deny parts of him- or herself to cater to the wishes of the other? If there are concerns about trust, attempt to determine the legitimacy of incongruence. (For example, unexpected work obligations may prevent one partner from not keeping a planned meeting.) Another factor is an individual one, stemming from personal lack of trust in relationships in general.

Intervention. Ask the individuals to share what previous experiences each brought to the new relationship. There may be unresolved trust issues or feelings from other relationships that are being displayed inappropriately in the current relationship. If so, the person will need to reach closure or resolution of the old issues and feelings to prevent interference in the current relationship.

If one partner is insecure, the individual may suggest to the other what behaviors will overcome the mistrust in the new relationship; for example, a phone call with an explanation or alternate plans when a planned meeting cannot be kept. Discuss what behaviors can be substituted for the sexual act to prevent engaging in it prematurely. Referral for individual or couple counseling is certainly an alternative to discontinuing a relationship based on lack of trust.

Stage Two

The second stage is *autonomy*. The characteristics of autonomy are establishing clear and separate identities, exercising self-control and will power, actively seeking what one desires from another, and believing that each individual is responsible for his or her own behavior. Within the context of a healthy relationship, a person's individual identity is not blurred or compromised in an identity as a couple; some individual control may be relinquished in terms of negotiating the relationship; in mutual decisions, both partners have the right to seek need fulfillment, both inside and outside of the relationship; and both individuals assume responsibility for actions or decisions as a couple.

Talking becomes important, especially self-disclosure, seeking what each individual wants from the relationship, and negotiation for rights and respect. There is also a degree of mutual dependency in that neither partner will exploit disclosures nor use what is shared against each other. Some frustration and inhibition is a normal part of this process because of the newness of the relationship and dependency. Decision-making begins to be integrated into the relationship about activities as well as relationship issues. Spending time alone as a couple may lead to experiencing some social constraints and demands on their time and energy from friends and family.

Elements of shame and doubt may appear in one or the other person in the form of being embarrassed about what has been disclosed, a feeling that a person is not "good enough," and continuing to act in terms of what an individual is "supposed to do" rather than spontaneously acting according to desire and trust in the self.

Assessment. Assess ways and examples of how the dyad communicates, both verbally and nonverbally. Do they (1) give and receive feedback about interpersonal and sexual interactions and satisfactions, (2) have adequate words to describe themselves and their feelings, (3) understand the differences in connotations of words, (4) understand that the context of what is being discussed may be different for males and females, and (5) talk for each other, or does each person state his or her own opinions? Determine each partner's negotiation and decision-making abilities; look for assertiveness as opposed to aggressiveness or threats. When level of disclosure is low, elicit what is inhibiting the couple from being real or genuine.

Intervention. Teaching some communication skills, such as effective listening, may be warranted. Also, modeling feeling statements, especially with men, will facilitate discussion.

Role playing in which the nurse is an observer is a very effective means of facilitating communication and disclosure. This allows each person to try out new behaviors and obtain feedback, and each can discuss how it feels in a safe environment.

With regard to pressures outside of the couple, elicit what it is they would like or like to do along with the risks and benefits. For example, decisions about where holidays are to be spent are frequently problematic, whether the decision focuses on spending them with one or the other partner's family, with special friends or even alone. Reassurance that decisions agreed to mutually generally withstand outside pressure and eventually may receive respect and understanding is helpful.

If either individual exhibits compulsive self-restraint, compliance, or defiance, individual counseling may be necessary.

Stage Three

The third relationship stage is *initiative*, in which there is a realistic sense of purpose and an ability to evaluate an individual or a couple's own behavior and its consequences. In taking some initiative and independent action there is the implication of personal responsibility; in essence, a risk of getting into something that may not be acceptable or worthy. Individual efforts may be in the form of trying to "be good," whatever that is perceived to be, and are usually based on social, religious, and moral values.

Themes of inclusion and intrusion become apparent; that is, each wants to be with the other without being invasive. Feedback from both peers and partner is important for individuals to frame their own ways of behaving and experiencing. Feedback may need to be solicited.

Normal guilt may be experienced based on real or fantasized disapproval (of autonomous actions) from others. To gain genuine initiative involves confidence that each person's intentions are good, that initiatives are acceptable, and that the other is a desirable person. Acceptance is expressed in a need for closeness through another's self-disclosure. Both partners can discuss differences, roles, pleasures, and displeasures without intimidation.

Once this process is underway in the relationship, it may be experienced as elation, in which there is a feeling of confidence, enthusiasm, and a sense that activities are worthwhile. There is a positive outlook in the relationship; each person believes in his or her own goodness and that of the other, and each can be an individual and still be close and intimate without a sense of clinginess.

Assessment. Continue to assess methods of communication between the dyad and observe for signs of extreme anxiety when each individual is increasing self-disclosure and attempting new ways of behaving. Observe for signs of guilt that may be manifested in shyness or "I wonder if I should have said that" kinds of statements. Determine whether values within the dyad are discrepant and, if so, whether satisfactory compromises are reached in decision making. This also may be a time when couples will seek personal information from the nurse, and what they typically want to know are qualifications for making assessments and intervening.

Intervention. Encourage and support effective behaviors in the couple's interactions. Support may be in offering reassurance that anxiety will decrease as they continue to engage in self-disclosure without exploitation. Help individuals to look at each of their own reactions when behaviors are inappropriate and do not achieve the desired response rather than focus on what others do or say. This will facilitate the individual's own ability to discriminate which behaviors work for them and which ones do not. Ask individuals to discuss with each other which behaviors feel invasive and have them offer suggestions regarding which behaviors would decrease the threat to privacy. Teaching assertiveness skills to both men and women may be needed in this stage. Provide positive feedback, when deserved, to enhance self-confidence.

Stage Four

The fourth stage is *industry*. Achieving self-confidence raises the question of competence, especially since when one takes initiative in relationships, or anything else, there must be follow through to some kind of resolution. When one does not have prior experience and/or skills, the follow through can become

threatening. The following may be experienced: (1) feeling inferior—failure becomes a risk; (2) feeling unequal to expectations—questioning whether the goals of the relationship are attainable and thus backing off to some extent from working at the relationship; and (3) becoming uncertain about what to do next. Individuals may need to ask for assistance in obtaining the skills or knowledge that are missing in order to keep working at their relationship.

Evidence of the couple's working in the relationship will be an attitude of perseverance, increasing individual openness and willingness to learn, and increasing verbal communication and feedback, especially about what is and is not working toward the fulfillment of goals. Other evidence will include more freedom in trying out new behaviors, risk taking, and persistence in a selected area of the relationship to really give it a chance. For example, relationship issues get raised and not dropped, there is a sense of harmony and resonation within the couple, a heightened sensitivity and responsiveness to each other's needs will occur, and independent interests and activities get pursued and accepted and serve to enhance the relationship.

Signs of degeneration within the couple will be manifested as a retreat to superficiality, game playing, and an attitude of "things will take care of themselves." Individuals or the couple may fantasize about or look for solutions in magical or supernatural powers, rather than build on the skills they do have.

Assessment. A primary assessment will be of genuine competitive issues in the dyad relationship versus competitive one-upmanship. Detect avoidance behaviors such as complacency or magical thinking that things will take care of themselves if ignored. Ask each individual what he or she thinks the real issues are when tensions rise. It may be easier for each one to relate negative feelings to an objective nurse for some clarity before sharing with a partner. Assess the expectations each has of his or her partner. Assist each one to determine if they are realistic or if there are too many. This assessment may be especially relevant if both partners are actively pursuing careers that are demanding of their time and energy.

Intervention. Teaching clients about relationship development might be done in any stage but is especially pertinent at this time. In time of retreat following openness and initiative particularly, feelings of rejection tend to occur when there is lack of understanding as to the reason.

Help individuals to discuss feelings of inadequacy. Provide information that one cannot be dominant in all areas of functioning and that current social norms are more toward equal partnerships in a number of areas. (Middle age men and persons of lower socioeconomic levels have more trouble accepting the concept of an equal partner—equal partner dyad.) For those individuals who are highly sex role typed, they could try teaching each other some aspects of the opposite role behaviors.

The Cinderella, or romantic affect, is not omnipresent as it was in the initial stages of the relationship, and the couple's risk is in expressing negative feelings or giving constructive feedback. Offer support and give suggestions about how to fight or negotiate fairly.

Stage Five

The fifth stage is *identity*. Sensitivity and responsiveness of the partners from the previous phase increase awareness of the implicit demands each makes of the other. In order to please each other, a need to comply with often conflicting demands may be felt, especially in today's complex society in which both partners play a number of roles. Physical strength and health are essential for having energy available for the various roles. Time alone and privacy become issues.

Most demands are perceived as external to the relationship and are usually crisis points in most relationships. This is a time when, if the couple is married or committed to each other, a spouse or partner will seek extramarital satisfaction, or one partner will seek another person as a confidant to escape the demands of the relationship. Anger will get expressed and be misinterpreted.

Struggles to negotiate and compromise are sometimes manifested in moodiness, negativism, and other forms of acting out that seem out of character, such as overindulgence in alcohol, drugs, or any other escape mechanisms. Independence and responsibility may be asserted inappropriately to the point that an individual will seem like two different people at different times. Even more drastic will be denying a partner sexual experience and pleasure. A provisional sense of identity may be achieved in making adult commitments in order to decrease anxiety about making irrevocable ones.

The resolution of identity issues is similar to that of autonomy, especially when a partner must overcome a kind of dependency. Autonomy concerns the ability to act as a separate person (change in locus of control), and identity concerns the ability to decide which of several actions is best (change in locus of evaluation from external to internal). The couple may engage in an active search for role models who seem to have successfully resolved identity issues.

Synthesis of identity will occur as the couple looks inward (within oneself and within the partnership) rather than outward for a system of values. They begin to attend to their own needs and feelings in deciding a course of action. There is less need to please others as the couple's actions fit with what they have internalized as values and interests and what is self-satisfying and yet not at the expense of the partner. There is some risk of offending friends: "We cannot go to the movies with you because we have other priorities"; offending extended families: "We will not be spending the holidays with you this year"; and even children: "We need time together as a family so you can't go with your friends this time."

The identity stage is a crucial time in relationships. Many people stay stuck here, as they cannot tolerate the pain in the battle, do not see an end to it, and give up. Other options are to regress or to move on to the intimacy stage. They may need external objective support to cope, as friends and family do not understand what is occurring and see the couple's behavior as rejection rather than a working out of all sorts of relationships, primarily the couple's own relationship and particularly in the area of making choices.

Assessment. Determine what needs each partner is attempting to obtain from the other and the ways in which requests are made. Many couples lack understanding of what compromise really is; genuine give and take requires some practice plus a lot of internal emotional struggle. Too often individuals feel the need to give up part of themselves and give in. This is the basis for real difficulties later in the relationship. Explore with the couple which of the above is really happening.

Intervention. Men and women both need some knowledge about ways they experience relationships, that both experience them differently. Assist them to understand that active listening and clarifying will prevent discussions from deteriorating into accusations and irrelevant digressions. Teach the couple negotiating skills and the effect of quid pro quo (something for something) in getting needs met. Assist the couple in sorting out the pros and cons of various choices and actions in establishing an identity as a couple. Assist the couple in determining who they can relate to that has weathered this adolescent turbulence. A wise mentor who is not family is helpful to spend time with. Men have some difficulty with genuine male relationships; encourage men to seek a peer group such as the Rotary Club or church men's groups or suggest they have breakfast with male friends as a support group. The nurse may be the objective support person for listening and reassuring the couple that their struggles are normal. Referral for short-term counseling may be appropriate when identity struggles become overwhelming.

Stage Six

The sixth stage is *intimacy*. As the couple makes choices about which relationships to continue and affirms their own values, others often feel alienated. The couple must recognize the choices they have made may lead to isolation and feelings of loneliness. However, reassurance can be found in realizing that decisions were made on the couple's own integrity rather than on an inability to relate and that previous close friendships were based on incomplete understanding of the differences in value systems.

As a temporary or permanent avoidance of intimacy, people may change jobs or frequently latch onto new partners. Both men and women are vulnerable to attention received outside of the primary relationship and may perceive it to be more manageable. Based on the avoidance of intimacy, these relationships are impersonal and superficial rather than committed. This situation is referred to as an isolation dependence, in which one person may look to another for planning a life or life style that appears impossible in the current situation.

In terms of commitment, this stage may be a time when marriages, engagements, and intimate relationships terminate realistically and with agreement that values, desires, and needs are not compatible, especially if one or the other simply cannot compromise. For example, the concept of an open marriage, including sexual interaction, outside of the committed dyad may be objectionable to one partner and not the other. If termination does occur, the individuals are freed to seek other relationships in which these values are more shared. What each partner needs to realize also is that there is no completeness in intimacy but that certain limits and priorities as to what will be tolerated can be established without revenge or degradation.

The achievement of intimacy is thus not through a perfect match but by valuing and accepting another's uniqueness equally as one's own. There is mutual respect and love of another while maintaining one's own individuality. Roles and goals become clear and distinct, not fixed and rigid. Problems get solved in the here and now and within a context of caring. Individuals and couples do not bring past events or hurts into current situations.

Assessment. When there is a decision to give up a personal or social connection, a grieving process occurs just as in any loss. This may account for some acting out behaviors in the dyad relationship. The nurse should assess if this process is occurring and which stage of grieving is being manifested, such as denial, anger, or sadness. In this stage also, issues may need to be clarified, so continued assessment of communication skills is warranted. Assess the developmental task level of each of the individuals; in essence, are both partners equally mature in their ability to observe and describe a particular situation and feelings about it? Observe for increased use of alcohol or other avoidance behaviors.

Intervention. Assist the couple to understand grieving the loss of friendships as just that and not necessarily an attack on the relationship. If extended families feel alienated, they cannot be forced to accept the couple's resolution of their relationship. Accepting the feelings family expresses without retaliation and allowing them time to adjust are helpful. Assist the couple in clarifying their own ideology, life style, and career goals. In discussion with the couple, assist them to stay focused on sharing relevant information pertinent to present circumstances.

If the relationship is in the process of termination, assist each person to work through his or her feelings, including any guilt or blame that may be experienced. People often feel that justification for breaking a commitment is in finding fault with the other person rather than acknowledging differences as irreconcilable.

A wide gap in maturity levels between the partners is an indication that one individual needs to seek counseling to work through personal issues that interfere with the relationship. The intent of personal counseling should not necessarily be perceived as preserving the relationship, because as personal issues are disclosed and worked through, there may be more clear evidence of genuine incompatibility and the need to separate from it.

Stage Seven

The seventh stage is *generativity*. Having achieved at least a sense of the characteristics of intimacy, the question for the couple becomes "Now what?" Generativity literally means to "generate" something new through productivity and creativity. There is an urge to expand an individual's and couple's own horizons and to follow interests and to enjoy privileges of life without making envious comparisons.

To accomplish the tasks of this stage, the couple may alternately experience crises and restabilization phases, in which they adjust to what they have accomplished and what they want to accomplish and determine what they can still accomplish. They may become invested in greater social responsibilities, pursue vocations and avocations in a more relaxed manner, and work toward realizing goals that were stifled in earlier stages of the relationship. In generativity, the primary relationship takes on a new meaning. There is a renewed sense of intimacy and sharing and a real sense of what the rest of life together is all about.

However, if prior knowledge, skills, and strengths are not used for continued growth both inside and outside of the relationship, there is a risk of stagnation. Stagnation is manifested in a focus on mundane everyday matters, and there may be minimal, novel stimulation for maintaining interest in each other. The experiencing of waning mutual interest may present a dilemma once again about continuing the relationship. This is often seen among couples who decide to separate after having been together for 20 or 30 years. Many others decide to stay together out of convenience, but primary individual socializing occurs outside of the relationship as a means of coping.

Assessment. Observation of the couple's interactions will provide cues to growth-enhancing behaviors versus boredom and stagnation. Manifestations of the latter might include minor complaints about not feeling loved, preoccupation with work or household tasks, a decrease in quantity and quality of communication, and even physical complaints (tiredness and minor aches and pains).

Assess what the couple perceives as life goals as well as ways in which they have arrived at their decisions. Is there mutual respect for the uniqueness of each individual in exploring new opportunities and tolerance for novel plans introduced into the relationship? Determine whether there is a decreased feeling of stress in the relationship; for instance, is there an ability in both partners to find humor in some of the dilemmas they encounter. In discussing the possibility of terminating the relationship, explore with the individuals and couple the strength of the desire to do so versus willingness to consider other options.

Intervention. Encourage a couple to engage in the process of introspection as a basis for gaining a realistic perspective about future plans in relation to the progress they have accomplished. The nurse might explore with the partners ways to take some initiative in reviving the romance of earlier stages of the relationship. For example, for one couple who was experiencing boredom in their relationship, it was suggested that they renew "courtship" behaviors, such as sending flowers to each other for no apparent reason.

Reaffirming or altering life goals may induce some anxiety in the relationship. The nurse should assist the couple to use past strengths in problem solving and suggest resources that the couple might not have thought of. For example, altering goals may cause financial strain, and consulting a financial planner may be the means toward reworking plans.

Suggest methods for relieving stress. These may include relaxation activities or taking a different view of the current situation that makes it more tolerable. Support and accept realistic decisions about termination or facilitate the couple's exploration of options.

Stage Eight

In the final stage—*integrity*—adjustments to changes lead to an acceptance of the worth and uniqueness of life; a sense of continuity of past, present, and future; and a sense of satisfaction and completeness. Each partner acknowledges the impact of relationship issues on each participant's life and the satisfactions derived from the investment in each other. The ultimate expression of gentleness, caring, and silent acknowledgment of one another is experienced in nonverbal communication. Verbal communication may focus on sharing information about external events of mutual interest or in alluding to private jokes or intimacies that are special to the relationship.

Prior to achieving integrity, there may be a sense of despair in anticipation of death. This certainly is more relevant in the older age couple as they cope with numerous losses. In working together there is a sense of real fulfillment that people do not want to give up. There is also attention to what has not been accomplished and a feeling of unfulfilled potential that may never be. Part of the process of integrity is reconciling these disparaging factors with the idea that there will always be "more" and it is unrealistic to expect all that is hoped for.

Assessment and Intervention. Once the stage of integrity has been reached, the relationship should be considered genuinely healthy. The nurse's role is to support and encourage continuing progress toward whatever life has to offer the couple. Another role is in assisting them to understand and accept that intermittent feelings of despair are appropriate to this stage. Pervasive despair is usually a result of incomplete or inadequate completion of the tasks of previous stages. Counseling may be necessary to assist the couple to attend to previous tasks or to accept the situation as it is with greater ease.

Older Adulthood

A concept of what constitutes the older adult varies according to both social and cultural contexts. Again, technology and improvement of health status serve to redefine the aging process; there are more persons making up the elderly population, and more elderly persons are living longer. Given that there is a great variation in time of onset and rate of progress of physical changes of aging (Strean, 1983), a time span from postclimacteric to death is referred to as older age.

Erikson identifies the central task of this group as being integrity, defined as acceptance of self-worth; adjustment to changes; a sense of continuity of past, present, and future; and body transcendence. Failure to accomplish older age tasks is to experience a sense of "nothingness" and loss known as despair.

Aging has been viewed as having many negative qualities, in part because of the realization that numerous losses are the fate of aging persons. Indeed, life itself is terminal, and we are a death-denying society. Research has enlightened the public toward a better understanding of the interplay of physical and psychosocial factors inherent in the aging process and has contributed a great deal toward fostering a more favorable perspective.

PHYSIOLOGICAL FACTORS

In general, the physiological processes in aging persons continue to decline. Weg (1983) reports studies indicating that men in their 50s and 60s experience a climacteric consisting of an abrupt loss of general well-being, involving emotional (anxiety and depressive symptoms), physical (fatigability, poor appetite, and weakness), and sexual complaints (reduced libido or impotence). These are all insults to masculinity as traditionally defined. Actual physical changes are a continuation of those mentioned in middle years but seem to become more apparent and interfere with sexuality in older age, especially atrophy of sexual organs and decline in sexual response, decrease in muscle tone and strength, and, due to enlargement of the prostate gland, susceptibility to all sorts of genitourinary dysfunctions. In aging women, changes along with menopause include alteration in body contours related to decreased muscle tone, skin elasticity, and misplaced fatty bulges; atrophic changes in genital, muscular, and skeletal systems; and estrogen deficiency, which according to recent studies is the basis for much of the affective and psychological problems experienced by women. Double-blind studies have shown that anxiety, depression, and headaches are responsive to estrogen replacement (Weg, 1983).

In terms of the capacity for sexual response, there is a wide variation of experiences and variables in aging persons of both sexes. In general, both sexes experience a gradual diminishing in intensity and duration of response to sexual stimuli. Men experience an increase in the time involved in each phase of the sexual response cycle: An erection takes longer to achieve but can be sustained longer than in earlier years before ejaculation, and there is less force of ejaculate expulsion. These factors may be advantageous in male sexual satisfaction (Weg, 1983; Woods, 1979). Aging women generally respond in a similar fashion as younger women. Cessation of sexual activity is *not* associated with menopause, and many women, freed from the risk of conception, seek intercourse and report heightened sexual satisfaction. However, the vaginal wall is thinner and dryer, causing discomfort, and, especially for those women who do not engage in regular intercourse, it is very painful without additional lubrication.

As Weg summarizes, "Although a number of anatomical and physiological changes do take place in the genital and related organ systems, there is nothing in the changing biology that warrants the prevalent image of sexless, neutered, loveless aging" (Weg, 1983, p 61). For a number of aging persons, sexual desire, physical love, and sex continue to be integral parts of their lives, and intimacy is expressed in addition to intercourse through closeness, touching, and body warmth; in essence, caring and gentleness in loving activities may be more important (Weg, 1983; Strean, 1983).

General physical health is an important factor in aging and sexuality. It is a myth that most older people are infirm. The reality is that bodily defenses in all other systems are affected in the aging process, leaving older people more vulnerable to illness; when illness does occur, they recover more slowly. Attractiveness in women and strength and virility in men are physical qualities of sexuality more difficult to sustain in older age and even more difficult if one is generally in poor health or has a chronic illness. Therefore, health-enhancing practices in older people are vitally important to maintaining a sexual self-concept.

PSYCHOSOCIAL FACTORS

The greatest inhibitor of positive sexuality in aging persons is their own integration of the negative views toward aging projected by the rest of society (Robinson, 1983; Strean, 1983; Woods, 1979). There are numerous stigmas and misunderstandings associated with old age that are increasingly being debunked through research. Knowing some current facts may sensitize everyone toward greater acceptance of elderly people as the sensual, sexual human beings they are.

Livson (1983) provides a fairly comprehensive survey of studies about gender identity and role behaviors in the elderly. With regard to gender identity, men may be viewed as "early maturers" in autonomy and independence, which results in more stress and rigidity later in life. Women more fully actualize later in life (when their own parents' authority is no longer an issue), and the reward is greater flexibility. Women whose self-concept has been focused around physical appearance experience narcissistic injury in response to skin wrinkling, and men whose esteem is related to physical strength feel vulnerable and depressed (Strean, 1983).

Some mental health trends in aging are that highly feminine women are more vulnerable in widowhood and divorce and more dependent on family members for successful adaptation; androgynous women over 55 are less critical of themselves, more psychologically healthy, and tend to value themselves for what they do rather than whom they attract. Men report a sense of control over self and environment at age 50, a decline in psychic distress, more mellowness, less ambitiousness, less restlessness, and more self-acceptance after age 60 (Livson, 1983).

ROLES

Several authorities concur that roles in aging transcend gender role stereotypes in which a psychological androgyny is integrated into a repertoire of behaviors in both sexes. As children leave home, occupational goals change, and retirement is imminent, the demands of women's nurturant role and men's achieving role decrease, allowing greater freedom and flexibility in sex role development (Livson, 1983). Livson (1983) reports the following behaviors supportive of this transcendence: men become less power oriented, more focused on communal concerns, more receptive to women, more passive in mastery, more tolerant of their nurturant and affiliative impulses, and more expressive and giving while they maintain ambitious and assertive behavior. Women become more power oriented in domestic settings (more likely to become the boss in the family), move from passive to active mastery, are more tolerant of their aggressive and egocentric impulses, and less sensitive to human relations. They depict themselves as robust and energetic.

These role behaviors are labeled as the most complex level of gender development attributed to factors of increased capacity for resolving conflict, changes in life tasks, and less conflict between masculine and feminine role norms (Livson, 1983). Healthy older men and women engage in a wide variety of activities, such as volunteering, traveling, and pursuing hobbies and recreational activities with much vigor. The more androgynous and self-actualized individuals seem to display more comfort in both being together and engaging in separate activities, thus contributing to the enrichment of their lives.

Relationships and intimacy take on a different quality in older age than in younger years. Weiss (1983) discusses Loewinger's ego development theory, which posits that with increased age or maturity, there is an increase in competence and interpersonal style; that is, people move away from dependent, manipulative, and superficial kinds of interactions toward more conscientious, responsible, and considerate modes of relating. It is probable that older persons will more closely approximate the qualities of knowledge, respect, concern, and responsibility that Fromm (1956) describes as necessary for success in all relationships. Weiss (1983) reports that there is a definite shift toward lower levels of intimacy in older adults; men successively decrease intimacy level from high school to retirement; women displayed an increase in intimacy upon marriage, a drastic reduction in intimacy when children left home, and an increase in intimacy again during retirement. While older persons may have lower intimate intensity in their relationships, they perceive their relationships to be closer, more important, more meaningful, and more mutually satisfying than do younger persons (Weiss, 1983).

With regard to life stress, adaptation, and levels of intimacy, for older persons the presence of a confidant or intimate companion seemed to be a buffer against the gradual losses experienced in aging, especially the social losses in interactions and roles and the more traumatic losses of widowhood. Men valued respect, comfort, and ease in friendships with other men, while women emphasized emotional support, acceptance, de-

pendability, and reciprocal affection in friendships. Both men and women valued emotional attraction and the elements of tenderness, caring, and passionate feelings in intimate spouse relationships. Weiss (1983) reported that intimacy with a spouse in older age had a mediating effect with regard to morale and degree of satisfaction among men and to both morale and psychosomatic symptoms among older women.

Relationships in older age are vulnerable to some of the same factors that affect relationships in middle age. For example, there are many more older women than men due to the shorter life span of men. It is fortunate in this regard that women are experienced in sustaining friendships throughout their lives (Weiss, 1983), as it is through these companionships that single or widowed women find some respite from loneliness. For some men, either from boredom in their primary relationship or inability to face their own mortality, marrying or seeking extramarital companionship of younger women is a respite. Older women generally do not engage in extramarital sexual activities (Robinson, 1983).

In summary, it is apparent that there is much potential in our aging population for manifesting healthy sexuality in a variety of ways. Having been socialized in very traditional gender roles and attitudes about sexuality in general they are limited in selecting the many options open to them (for example women initiating relationships with younger men). Within the next 2 decades, it will be very interesting to learn in which ways they will be affected by the women's liberation movement.

NURSING CARE

From the literature on aging and sexuality, two nursing role priorities emerge. One is education and consciousness raising with both the elderly and the rest of society regarding attitudes and values in older age sexuality. Apart from the negative views of themselves that older people adopt, the second most discussed inhibitor in expressing sexuality are the children of the elders, who seem to think any type of sexual experience in their parents is nonexistent or even repulsive. Older people themselves expect their sexual drive to diminish and cease, and education about normal aging, physical health, physiological processes, and possible options for relationships would have a freeing effect in all intimate interactions. Assessment of the values and attitudes of elders would be prerequisite to individual teaching, as some may be threatened by new knowledge. For example, in the absence of an intimate partner, masturbation may be an important way to enhance potency and genital lubrication (Weg, 1983). However, if this elicits guilt, it will not be helpful. The nurse's own attitude must be positive in any communication about sexuality in aging, as older persons will be very sensitive to negative messages, both verbal and nonverbal.

Promotion of group activities, in the community or in institutions, will divert older persons' attention from loss and loneliness. During a Christmas carol songfest conducted by a nurse at a geriatric nutrition site, behavior and facial expressions of the participants changed drastically from inertia and apathy toward animation and smiles. There are many activities that both men and women enjoy; the nurse should take every opportunity to encourage heterosexual mixing. It is difficult to motivate some elders who are in a depressed or apathetic state, and encouraging activities regardless of apparent lack of interest may be more stimulating than lengthy focusing on feelings. Also, cognitive restructuring or helping elders find a different meaning in their experiences is helpful.

In any interaction with elderly persons the nurse should attempt to promote their self-concept. Offering support for the positive qualities displayed in both genders and ignoring the negative ones are helpful. Acceptance and respect for individual uniqueness, just as in any other age group, will discourage negative self-views.

The second priority for the nurse relates to physical health promotion. Aging people seem to go to two extremes regarding their health: either they avoid health care professionals, attributing every complaint to "just old age" or a serious illness about which nothing can be done, or they overuse a variety of health services in an effort to get needs met and receive minimal continuity of care. First, through interview and physical assessment the nurse can discern more precisely what their needs are and, second, can assist them in seeking a caregiver best suited to their needs. For women, at least an annual visit to a trusted physician for detection of signs of breast and genital cancers is recommended. For men, annual checkups are important, owing to increased risks of both cardiovascular and genitourinary problems. Nurses can alleviate many fears about aging and sexual potency by discussing what can be expected in the natural process of aging and what preventive measures will facilitate greater comfort and ease. Older people are very vulnerable to the blatant advertising of remedies for disguising aging or for alleviating symptoms they sometimes do not even know they have. Some remedies are harmless and do nothing, while others are potentially dangerous. One elderly diabetic woman in a public health case load was desperately trying to lose weight and succumbed to the pressure of the Dexatrim ads as a magical solution. She was totally unaware of the deleterious effects on the regulation of her diabetes. Helping persons such as her make wise and economic choices of products is very much a prerogative of the nurse.

Since there is a decreasing sensitivity in all five senses in aging, helping persons to adapt or obtain appropriate aids (glasses, hearing aids) may make a tremendous difference in the quality of their interactions. People are often too proud to display these signs of aging overtly and need a great deal of understanding by the nurse before they are amenable to taking advantage of the aid that is available. Helping them to appreciate that many persons who are not old have glasses or hearing aids for their impairments will separate their need from the context of aging.

REFERENCES

Bancroft J: Human sexuality and its problems. New York, Churchill Livingstone, 1983.

Bee H: The developing child. New York, Harper & Row Publishers, 1985.

Bellak L, Hurvich M, Gediman HK: Ego functions in schizophrenics, neurotics and normals: A systematic study of conceptual, diagnostic and therapeutic aspects. New York John Wiley & Sons, 1973.

Bem SL: Probing the promise of androgyny. In Kaplan AG, Bean JP (eds): Beyond Sex-Role Stereotypes: Readings Toward a Psychology of Androgyny. Boston, Little, Brown and Company, 1976.

Boverman K, Boverman M, Clarkson E, et al: Sex-role stereotypes and clinical judgments of mental health. J Consult Clin Psychol 34:1–7, 1970.

Chilman CS: Adolescent Sexuality in a Changing American Society. New York, John Wiley & Sons, 1983.

Chodorow N: Family structure and feminine personality. In Rosaldo MZ, Lamphere L (eds): Woman, Culture and Society. Stanford, Stanford University Press, 1974.

Chodorow N: The Reproduction of Mother. Berkeley, University of California Press, 1978.

Davis AE: Whoever said life begins at 40 was a fink or, those golden years—phooey. Inter J Women Stud 3:583–589, 1980.

Denholtz E: Having It Both Ways: Married Women with Lovers. Briarcliff Manor, Stein & Day, 1981.

DeFries Z, Friedman RC, Corn R: Sexuality: New Perspectives. Westport, Greenwood Press, 1985.

Doctors SR: Premarital pregnancy and childbirth in adolescence: A psychological overview. In DeFries Z, Friedman RC, Corn R (eds): Sexuality: New Perspectives. Westport, Greenwood Press, 1985.

Eagle MN: Recent Developments in Psychoanalysis. New York, McGraw-Hill Book Company, 1984.

Ehrhardt A, Baker S: Fetal androgen, human CNS differentiation and behavior sex differences. In Friedman RC, Richard RM, and Vander Wiele RL (eds): Sex Differences in Behavior. New York, John Wiley & Sons, 1974.

Ehrhardt A, Money J: Progestion-induced hermaphroditism: IQ and psychosexual identity in a study of ten girls. J Psychosex Res 3:83–100, 1967.

Erikson EH: Childhood and Society. New York, WW Norton, 1950.

Freud S: Outline of Psychoanalysis. New York, WW Norton, 1949.

Fromm E: The Art of Loving. New York, Harper & Row, 1956.

Gagnon JH: Human Sexualities. Chicago, Scott, Foresman and Company, 1977.

Gilligan C: In a Different Voice. Cambridge, Harvard University Press, 1982.

Hines M: Prenatal gonadal hormones and sex differences in human behavior. Psycholog Bull 92:56–80, 1982.

Hinsie LE, Campbell RJ: Psychiatric Dictionary. Oxford, Oxford University Press, 1975.

Hogan R: Human Sexuality: A Nursing Perspective. Norwalk, Appleton-Century-Crofts, 1980.

Hoenig J: The origin of gender identity. In Steiner BW (ed): Gender Dysphoria, Development, Research, Management. New York, Plenum Press, 1985.

Kahn AU, Cataio J: Men and Women in Biological Perspective. New York, Praeger Publishers, 1984.

Kinsey A, Pomeroy W, Martin C: Sexual Behavior in the Human Male. Philadelphia, WB Saunders, 1948.

Kinsey A, Pomeroy W, Martin C, Gebbard A: Sexual Behavior in the Human Female. Philadelphia, WB Saunders, 1953.

Klein M: Contributions to Psychoanalysis, 1921–1945. London, Hogarth Press, 1948.

Klein M: The Psycho-Analysis of Children. London, Hogarth Press, 1957.

Komarovsky M: Dilemmas of Masculinity: A Study of College Youth. New York, WW Norton, 1976.

Lee PC, Sussman RS: Sex Differences: Cultural and Developmental Dimensions. New York, Urizen Books, 1976.

Lidz T: The Person. New York, Basic Books, 1968.

Lion E: Human Sexuality in Nursing Process. New York, John Wiley & Sons, 1982.

Livson FB: Gender identity: A life span view of sex role development. In Weg RB (ed): Sexuality in Later Years, Roles and Behavior. New York, Academic Press, 1983.

Luria Z, Rose D: Psychology of Human Sexuality. New York, John Wiley & Sons, 1979.

Macoby EE, Jacklin CN: The Psychology of Sex Differences. Stanford, Stanford University Press, 1974.

Maherly ER: Psychogenesis and the Early Development of Gender Identity. Boston, Routledge & Kegan Paul, 1983.

Marcia JE: Identity in adolescence. In Adelson J (ed): Handbook of Adolescent Psychology. New York, John Wiley and Sons, 1980.

Money J, Eharhardt A: Man and Woman, Boy and Girl. Baltimore, John Hopkins University Press, 1972.

Oaks WW, Melchiode GA, Ficher I: Sex and the Life Cycle. Orlando, Grune & Stratton, 1976.

Petras JW: The Social Meaning of Human Sexuality. Newton, Allyn & Bacon, 1978.

Pierson EC, D'Antonio V: Female and Male: Dimensions of Human Sexuality. Philadelphia, JB Lippincott, 1974.

Ribal JE: Learning Sex Roles. New York, Canfield Press, 1973.

Robinson PK: The sociological perspective. In Weg RB (ed): Sexuality in Later Years, Roles and Behavior. New York, Academic Press, 1983.

Rubin LB: Intimate Strangers. New York, Harper & Row, 1984.

Schaffer KF: Sex Roles and Human Behavior. Cambridge, Winthrop Publishers, 1981.

Schwartz AE: Androgyny and the art of loving. Psychother Theory Res Prac 16:405–408, 1979.

Sheehy G: Passages. New York, EO Dutton, 1974.

Stiles WB: Psychotherapy recapitulates ontogeny: The epigenesis of intensive interpersonal relationships. Psychother Theory Res Behav 16:391–404, 1979.

Strean HS: The Sexual Dimension. New York, The Free Press, 1983.

Unger RK: Female and Male: Psychological Perspectives. New York, Harper & Row, 1979.

Wallum LR: The Dynamics of Sex and Gender. Skokie, Rand McNally 1977.

Weiss LJ: Intimacy and adaptation. In Wen RB (ed): Sexuality in Later Years, Roles and Behaviors. New York, Academic Press, 1983.

Weg RB: Sexuality in Later Years, Roles and Behavior. New York, Academic Press, 1983.

Woods NF: Human Sexuality in Health and Illness. St. Louis, CV Mosby, 1984.

5: Human Sexuality from a Cultural Perspective

Linda Schoonover Smith

Every culture guides the rate and direction of sexual development of its members. The meaning of a given act, be it sexual or otherwise, can only be fully understood when it is examined within the cultural context in which it occurs. The culture of a society also determines the expression of sexuality by defining what is sexual and what is not. This is achieved by transferring the sexual code of rules, definitions, expectations, sanctions, and taboos from older to younger members of the society. The sexual code ("blueprint" for sexual conduct and practice) is transmitted at different ages by different methods in different societies; the society's culture dictates how information is passed from one generation to another. Younger members receive messages of appropriate sexual behavior, internalize them, and generally apply those values to personal practice. Thus, sexuality is structured, regulated, and controlled through society (Davenport, 1977). Society defines the sexual nature of dress, speech, action, posture, physical attributes, food, and dance. A cross-cultural analysis of different peoples reveals tremendous cultural diversity in sexual beliefs and practices. No two cultures are similar. Each society's sexuality is created by different values, ideas, beliefs, and environments. The practice of sexuality in a particular culture is interdependent on the beliefs and rules about marriage, family, kinship, social responsibilities, and religion.

This chapter will describe cultural influences on sexuality, cite methodological prob-

lems of cultural sexual research, contrast intercultural variations in sexual behavior, discuss culture-specific sex practices, and present an overview of the knowledge on sexual behavior across cultures.

PROBLEMS OF RESEARCH AND PUBLICATION OF CULTURAL INFLUENCES ON SEXUALITY

Many serious and severe problems of data collection, analysis, and publication of research on sexual practices of different societies currently exist. Most descriptive ethnologies from anthropology contain voluminous detail about social organization, kinship, and religion but have little on matters of sex and sexuality. Sexual matters in most societies are private, which makes accessibility to information by the anthropologist difficult. Ethnographies also suffer from masculine bias, as most ethnographers are men. The traditional participant observation field technique used by anthropologists may be limited by information bias, since informants may manipulate their stories toward successful or dramatic outcomes in this area. Suggs and Marshall (1971) explain that the lack of anthropological literature on sexual practices is due to a reluctance by publishing houses to publish investigations and a scarcity of research funds. They note the difficulty of using the quantitative approach in the study of sexual behavior of societies and also lament the different field techniques of study among anthropologists, which precludes rigorous comparisons of sexual behavior between societies. Other research problems such as lack of operational definitions, lack of rigorous methodology, diverse reporting styles, and different levels of detail make comparisons between cultures impossible. They claim that there is not general consensus among anthropologists on the direction that research on cross-cultural sexuality should take. Brink (1987) describes the difficulty in obtaining reliable data on sexual beliefs and customs in sexually repressed societies or in societies in which sexual freedom is not sanctioned. A paucity of data about sexuality and sexual behaviors across cultures still exists today.

Intercultural Variations in Sexual Behavior

Two societies are described in this section to illustrate the wide variations in sexual behavior that may be found in the society of man. John C. Messenger (1977) conducted a study from 1958 to 1966 of a small agrarian Irish Island Community, Ines Beag (renamed for anonymity), and sampled all 350 inhabitants on the island. The method of study included open-ended interviews, guided interviews, participant observation, life histories, cross-checking histories, photography, and ethnography. The majority of the data was collected from observation and unguided interviews.

Messenger classified Ines Beag as a sexually repressed society. Through the ages, multiple historical, religious, and psychological factors created a sexually repressed culture. Sexes were segregated in this island community from early life to adulthood and were separated within family, church, and school. Bathing and swimming places, playgrounds, school classrooms, and church pews all separated persons according to sex. All adolescent and adult activity was segregated. Male solidarity existed before and after marriage. For example, men interacted mostly with men during a typical day. Men were more socially active than women, since the latter were more restricted in their social interactions by island norms. Men attended parties,

went to dances, frequented the pubs, played cards at others' homes, visited homes of male friends, and wandered the entire island and surrounding sea in pursuit of their economic goals. During these occasions, men felt a common bond of affection and understanding with each other. They felt comfortable with each other and enjoyed their outings, whether they were for social, religious, or economic purposes. Women did not share the same feeling of solidarity, since they were more socially isolated and restricted to attending church, visiting relatives, and attending winter parties. A typical day for a woman consisted of household chores and light farm jobs, such as milking the cows. Thus, women did not receive the same social benefits of frequent social interactions among other female islanders.

Unlike many other societies in which marriage is for love, the men and women in Ines Beag married for economic and reproductive reasons. The average age of marriage for females was 25; for males it was 36.

During courtship, premarital coitus was rare. After marriage, sexual activity was generally initiated by the husband. Marital coitus was limited to foreplay (kissing and fondling of buttocks) and consummation. The male superior position was predominant. Intercourse generally occurred with clothes on, and orgasm was generally achieved quickly.

Members of both sexes in Ines Beag were sexually secretive. Sex was never discussed openly in homes with youth or between adults. Both adults and young persons generally lacked knowledge about sexuality. Sexual misconceptions were common. For example, most people believed that men were more libidinous than women. Males believed sex was debilitating, a common belief in primitive societies. No sexual advances were made to women soon after childbirth or during menstruation, since females were considered dangerous to men at that time. Women were taught to endure sexual advances. The female orgasm was not described by either male or female islanders to anthropologists. Sexuality was not generally integrated into the folklore of songs, poems, and stories. The common tradition of dirty jokes found in most societies was absent. Other behaviors, not perceived as sexual in many societies, were deemed so here; for example, nudity and evacuation were thought to be highly suggestive of sexuality. Islanders were embarrassed to be caught barefoot and all clothing was changed in private to prevent embarrassment at being seen nude. Men were unwilling to go to the island nurse when ill, because it might have necessitated disrobing in front of her. Men also never learned to swim, although they spent much of their life at sea in a canoe. One of the reasons for a high prevalence of nonswimmers in this society was an unwillingness to expose their bodies and put on bathing clothes, which is a prerequisite to learning to swim.

Ines Beag was a community of sexually naive islanders due to lack of education about sexuality, multiple false beliefs, and primitive myths. In contrast are the Mangaians, a society exhibiting sexual openness. Anthropologist Donald S. Marshall described the open sexual society of the Mangaians in his Polynesian ethnology "Sexual Behavior on Mangaia" in *Human Sexual Behavior: Variations in the Ethnographic Spectrum* (1971). Mangaia, a southern Cook Island in Central Polynesia, South Pacific, was characterized by sexual liberation and freedom.

To study the Mangaians, Marshall used the traditional anthropological participant observation methods and obtained kinship status in a principal family on the island. He interviewed full-time informants of various levels and segments of society and also did extensive linguistic analysis of the language. Since most of his informants were male, his study contained masculine information bias.

His study documented that the Mangaians were a sexually open society: Mangaians were comfortable with their sexuality from birth to death, and sexuality was a prevalent theme in social life, folklore, and religion. Mangaians grew up in homes that contained kin clustered in one room. Public privacy was practiced in these homes. The male Mangaian copulated in a room in his hut that contained all of the family. All sexual acts occurred without notice by family or kin. Everyone else was busy doing something else and looking in another direction, which granted personal privacy.

Regularity of sexual practice occurred throughout an individual's lifetime. Exploratory sex play of same- and different-sexed children was widely tolerated by parents. Masturbation by both sexes at 7 to 10 years of age was advocated and practiced. Premarital sex was also accepted and widely practiced. Married sexual relationships were mutually fulfilling, since orgasm was universally achieved among both sexes. Extramarital relationships were common.

The practice of Motoro ("sleep crawling") was used by male youths to win future brides. The young suitor generally crawled into the living room of his girlfriend's hut at night when all the family was asleep. The entrances and exits were predetermined by the boy. The girlfriend generally was persuaded by romantic compliments to engage in coitus during the night. Parents permitted this to occur under the roof because they believed it an opportunity for their daughter to secure a husband. So parents feigned sleep, and the male suitors believed the parents were sound sleepers.

For the Mangaians, the major emphasis on sexuality was action. The prolongation of sexual activity was the goal of coitus, unlike in Western cultures, which place higher value on orgasmic experience. However, generally all women experienced orgasm because they learned from older males who were concerned for their partner's pleasure in order to preserve one's reputation. The norm among women was active participation. Passivity was thought to be deviant. Sexual intercourse preceded personal intimacy between partners, unlike in Western cultures such as the United States, in which personal intimacy generally precedes intercourse in adult sexual relationships.

Thus, this society demonstrated freedom of sexual expression by norms that reinforced active, frequent, and assertive sexual behavior. The serious nature and importance of sexuality in the Mangaians' lives was found in the vivid description of detailed sexual acts in folklore, romantic practices of the lavish use of flowers and scents, graphic explicit sexually provocative local dances, and severe superincisionism (see the following) practices that symbolized the rite of passage to adult sexual life.

Culture-Specific Sex Practices

Sexual practices that are unique and specific only to a particular society evolve over time. Puberty rites, defloration ceremonies, body beautification, sexual partnerships, and circumcision are examples of culture-specific sex practices. Examples of each will be described to give the nurse an appreciation of the diversity of culture-specific sex practices.

The puberty rite of an adolescent Mangaian was a severe, dramatic rite that symbolized passage to adult sexuality. Superincision was practiced in the society (incision of the entire length of the penis) as the ritualistic passage. As the father noted the onset of adolescence (13 years of age), he asked an older relative to provide sexual education for the youth. Youths were instructed by the older relative on how to be a successful sexual partner and bring the female to orgasm. Later, a priest and a surgeon performed the painful incision. Afterwards, the older relative arranged for an experienced older woman to provide lectures, stories, and practice in coitus. She gave feedback on his technique, especially style, timing, and position. Upon completion of the sexual instruction, the father gave a feast. The son was now a man, and was sanctioned by the community to engage in active sexual adult practices (Marshall, 1971).

Girls may also be subjected to mandatory rituals during rite of passage ceremonies. Janda and Klenke-Hamel (1980) described Samoan defloration marriage ceremonies in the South Pacific. Defloration of young girls by the chief priest occurred in public. Family and friends cheered at the drops of blood, which proclaimed the purity of the bride. The girl then walked around the visitors to exhibit the evidence of virginity. In societies in which girls must be virgins on their wedding night, girls who were not virgins often selected the last day of their menstrual cycle, or injected some drops of blood from doves into the vagina to mimic the breakage of the hymen on the wedding night (Janda and Klenke-Hamel, 1980).

Female body beautification is another form of sexual expression among specific cultures. During 1959–60, the Bala (Basongye) people of the Belgian Congo traditionally covered females with keloids (scars) from above the chest to the groin. The keloids were made at 4 to 5 years of age by the girl's mother or older sister with a razor blade during 1 day. Charcoal was then rubbed in the wounds to provide greater inflammation, causing more prominent scarring. It was deemed shameful to cry despite the extreme pain. The purpose of body designs was to make the female become more decorative and feminine and did not connote rank, social position, or other status. Symmetry of geometric markings was considered beautiful. No one but the husband was allowed to see the markings. The men were fond of fondling the markings prior to coitus (Janda and Klenke-Hamel, 1980).

Another culture-specific sexual practice is polygamous sexual partnerships. Although Western society generally practices monogamy, or the legal marriage of one man to one woman, other societies practice polygamy. For example, the Yolngu tribe of Aborigines of Elcho Island in Arnhem Land on the shore of the Arafura Sea of the Northern Territory of Australia have a polygamous culture in which men are permitted to have more than one wife at a time. In that society, a girl between the ages of 12 and 16 is married to her promised husband, who is often in his 40s. She would be the fifth or sixth wife. Frequently, her own sisters were among the other wives. Wives lived with their cowives and their children under the same hut or around the camp fire. Wives received the husband's sexual affections as he chose (Money and Musaph, 1977).

Three misconceptions about polygamy are common in our society. Westerners often believe that (1) the purpose of polygamous marriages is to satisfy the sexual drives of the male, (2) that the wives are often believed to be treated as slaves by the husband, and (3) that jealousy among the wives is common in polygamous marriages. In most societies that practice polygamy, the men desire male heirs to continue the family line. Men may also desire male children to orchestrate economic advantages for the family in traditional community life. The possibility of family arguments are decreased by placing the wives in order of rank. The first wife has the most authority. All household work is evenly distributed among the wives. Separate houses or sleeping quarters are provided for each wife. The husband maintains a rotational system for conjugal visits, giving each wife equal access to sexual encounters. In primitive societies in which polygamy is practiced, the legal marriage of a man to one or more wives is perceived by all members of the society to be desirable, functional, and natural.

Female circumcision is practiced by many cultural and religious groups, with more than 74 million women and female children mutilated by female genital operations in Africa alone (Hosken, 1981) (Table 5–1). Two types of operations are practiced in Africa today. Excision or clitoridectomy may include excision of the clitoris, the labia minora, and the

TABLE 5–1. Geographical Distribution of Female Genital Mutilation

Asia
  Indonesia
  Malaysia

Arab Peninsula
  United Arab Emirates
  Oman
  Bahrein
  Southern Yemen
  Saudi Arabia

Africa

Ethiopia	Nigeria	Mauritania
Sudan	Ghana	Liberia
Somalia	Burkina Faso	Togo
Kenya	Ivory Coast	Benin
Egypt	Mali	Cameroon
Uganda	Guinea	Zaire
Tanzania	Sierra Leone	Chad
Djibouti	Senegal	Niger
Central African Republic	The Gambia	

Adapted from Hosken FP: Female genital mutilation in the world today. Inter Heal Serv 11:420, 1981.

labia majora. Infibulation is intentional closure of the vagina immediately after excision. The vaginal walls are held together with sutures, thorns, or paste so that a wall is formed to close the upper part of the vaginal vault. A small opening is left by inserting a stick into the wound to allow for elimination of urine and menstrual blood.

The immediate complications of female circumcision are urinary retention, hemorrhage, infection, and shock. About 25 per cent of women who have female circumcision experience one or more complications. Long-term complications include chronic pelvic inflammatory disease, chronic urinary tract infection, inclusion dermoid cysts, sexual difficulties, genitourinary tract fistulas, and problems with labor and delivery (Cutner, 1985). Major complications in obstetrics from infibulation occur during the second stage of labor. Loss of perineal elasticity causes problems with normal fetal descent and contributes to the incidence of stillbirth and vesicovaginal fistulas. In women who have had infibulation, physical examinations to assess labor progress are difficult. Preventive gynecological care is made difficult, as performing a Papanicolaou's test, cervical cultures, and examinations to screen for malignancies is impossible.

The operations are performed on young children, often only a few days old, by lay midwives or traditional birth attendants, usually in primitive conditions without asepsis. The social and traditional rites that used to

accompany the operations are rapidly disappearing, but the physical mutilations continue. The surgery decision is usually made by the head of the household, who pays for the operation. However, in some families, the operations are planned by well-meaning and loving mothers or aunts who believe that they are ensuring their daughters' economic and social security (Cutner, 1985). Case reports from Egyptian women who experienced female circumcision have common themes of ignorance about the procedure, lack of emotional preparation for surgery, misinformation about the rationale for the procedure, deception as a manipulation to consent to surgery, physical restraint during the surgery without their consent, painful surgery without any anesthesia, fear of subsequent intercourse, and lack of physical enjoyment of intercourse (Assad, 1980).

The reasons for sexual mutilation vary from culture to culture, with the most common being economic factors, sexual control, perception of positive effects on childbirth, and religious beliefs. Female circumcision via infibulation guarantees the bride's virginity and thus, inheritance of property cannot be questioned. Proof of virginity is an important prerequisite to marriage in patrilineal cultures. Female circumcision is believed to have other advantages—to reduce the female's sexual desire and vulnerability to temptation. It reinforces the woman's passive-receptive sexual role. Since polygamy is often practiced in the same areas, reduced sexual desire in wives is considered necessary. Shaw (1985) reports that some cultures believe that the female genitalia produce adverse effects during childbirth. For example, some cultures believe that if the clitoris touches the baby's head during childbirth the infant will die. Other cultures believe that if a nursing mother has intercourse, sperm will contaminate her milk and cause fetal death.

The more severe forms of female circumcision are mainly performed in Muslim cultures today. The operations are not required, but optional, and considered "a commendable deed by Allah" (Hosken, 1981, p 419). Genital mutilation in Islamic countries symbolizes the status of women in those countries. The status of women is inferior to men in the political, educational, physical, social, and legal arenas of life. For example, in Islamic countries, men practice polygamy with up to four wives. Divorce is a prerogative of men alone. Property and inheritance rights are exclusively in favor of men over women. The wife's share of property is usually less than 10 per cent. Penalties for murdering a man are twice that for murdering a woman. Custody of children goes to the father, not the mother, in case of divorce. Women in Islamic countries are expected to do the menial tasks and to do the domestic laborers and child care providers, while everything else is delegated to men to do (Cutner, 1985).

Efforts to eliminate mutilation of female genitalia have historically met with resistance in spite of the health care burden it imposes on societies. In 1980, the World Health Organization (WHO) and the United Nations Children's Fund (UNICEF) unanimously decided that all forms of female circumcision should be abolished (Assad, 1982). Yet developing countries do not have the capabilities to enforce community-based preventative education programs, and thus the practice continues, probably at the same rates.

Shaw (1985) surveyed a group of 11 circumcised women to determine their perception of their needs for health care in America. The women were concerned about the health provider's lack of knowledge about female circumcision and cultural beliefs. They wanted women health care providers because Muslim women are forbidden to have any physical contact with a man other than their husbands, except in an emergency. They were very concerned about modesty and wanted their modest views respected. The husband or father must grant permission for the woman to be examined or receive treatment in their culture. Women were fearful that American obstetricians were not competent to give them prenatal, labor, delivery, and postpartum care because of their different anatomy and structural changes after surgery. A few were unaware of signs of infection after delivery and delayed seeking treatment.

Shaw (1985) recommends that the circumcision scar be incised during the second stage of labor. An episiotomy may also be performed then if needed. After delivery, the two edges of the wound are approximated and sutured together in one layer. The wound is given the same care as that for an episiotomy. If voiding is problematic, the patient should be catheterized. After delivery, the woman may wish to be reinfibulated and should discuss the advantages and disadvantages with the obstetrical team.

Nurses need to be sensitive to the patient's perception of the value, use, and need for genital surgery as defined by her religion and/or culture. Nurses may have difficulty in accepting the practice or its continuation in our culture and should strive to understand the reasons for the client's continuation of the practice. The patient needs a sensitive nurse who respects her choices and values.

Nurses should serve as agents of change for the next generation of women by introducing these women patients to health education, which includes the physical, emotional, and social complications of human-made damage to female children. Female sexuality should be discussed in detail with an emphasis on the function of the parts of the genitalia that are removed. Sexuality in marital relationships may be explained. The anatomy and physiology of female and male reproductive systems should be understood by clients. Women patients should understand that genital mutilation does infringe upon human rights and may cause disfigurement, disharmony in marital relationships, and physical, obstetrical, and psychological complications.

COMPARATIVE ANALYSIS OF SEXUAL BEHAVIOR ACROSS CULTURES
Childhood Sexuality

Wide variation exists from society to society in the beliefs about childhood sexual behavior. In certain societies with liberal and permissive attitudes toward sexuality, sexual behavior in children is tolerated, accepted, and even encouraged. Members of some preliterate societies still believe that childhood sexual behavior will encourage adult fertility and/or successful adult sexual behavior. In other more restrictive societies, childhood sexual practices are not promoted or encouraged. Western countries generally tend to be more restrictive in their beliefs about childhood sexual behavior, and children are not encouraged to explore their sexual nature or engage openly in childhood sex play.

The Mangaians believed that sexuality is natural and beautiful, even during childhood. Mangaian children had many opportunities to observe parental sexual behavior, since they slept in the same room at night.

Marshall (1971) reported a pervasive permissive attitude among Mangaians about youthful sexual behavior. Young children were permitted to engage in masturbation in private areas. The children also received extensive education about sexual matters, even at young ages. Young Mangaian children had a descriptive, detailed vocabulary for sexual behavior, such as a complete knowledge of the anatomy and function of the male and female genital organs. Many of the other island societies of the South Pacific were also permissive about childhood sexual activity. Children were often permitted to practice masturbation and engage in sex play with other children. Childhood sex play often included manual manipulation of sex organs, oral-genital contacts, and possibly coitus (Crooks and Bauer, 1983).

William Davenport described a society that was not tolerant of childhood sexual play in his ethnography of East Bay (pseudonym) on the Melanesian Island in the South Pacific (1977). In East Bay, boys and girls were separated after birth and not allowed to play with or even talk to each other. While heterosexual childhood sexual play was thus restricted, male masturbation was permitted during adolescence and was the primary sexual outlet of boys aged 13 to adulthood. Prior to adolescence, Davenport described limited childhood sexual experience in that society.

Adolescent sexuality is dependent upon the cultural norm of parental sexual education and behavior to their children. For example, DeSantis and Thomas (1987) found a difference in parental attitudes toward adolescent sexuality in Haitian and Cuban immigrants. Cuban mothers believe that they are able to influence the child's sexual behavior and adopt a discussion-based teaching method of explaining sexuality to their children. Parents participate in sexual education of their children, and there is discussion between the generations about sexuality. Haitian mothers use more physical punishment and less dialogue to teach social values and attitudes. Haitian children do not usually discuss sexuality with their parents, as this would be seen as disrespectful. As a result, there is less discussion of sexuality in Haitian families.

Premarital Coitus

A wide variety of societal attitudes exists about premarital coitus. In Ford and Beach's *Patterns of Sexual Behavior* (1951), 190 preliterate societies were surveyed by the authors about patterns of premarital coitus. Most societies fell between the two extremes of complete restriction of premarital coitus to enthusiastic endorsement of premarital coitus. The majority of societies tended to combine formal cultural prohibitions with informal tacit acceptance of premarital coitus, as long as the behavior was conducted away from public eyes.

Premarital coitus was often encouraged in preliterate societies, whose members believe that premarital coitus will offer the woman an opportunity to obtain a husband. It was also encouraged by societies who believed that coitus was a set of learned skills that were acquired through appropriate instruction and practice. The Mangaians and the Marquesans both openly encouraged coitus before marriage.

In other more restrictive societies, sexual intercourse before adulthood and/or marriage was not encouraged. It was believed that only adults (as symbolized by the newly wed adult) were sexually and emotionally mature and able to be allowed sexual freedom. In societies that prohibited premarital coitus, prohibitions against sexual intercourse occurred during puberty and continued until betrothal or marriage. Methods used by societies to prevent premarital sexual activity during adolescence included segregation of the sexes, strict chaperonage of adolescent girls, and threats of physical punishment or disgrace to offenders. There were few societies in which these methods of control appear to have been completely effective in preventing intercourse among young unmarried couples.

Marital Coitus

Marital coitus is the most common form of adult sexual activity in all societies. There is a wide variation in both the frequency of sexual intercourse and in the types of coital positions used in societies. Most of the ethnographic descriptions focus on the frequency of marital intercourse. However, frequency of marital intercourse is an unreliable outcome measure owing to the provisional nature of the reported data, which is subject to a great number of potential information and measurement biases. According to Gebhard (1971), behavioral trends in marital coitus across cultures include the following:

1. The husband initiates most of the coital events.

2. Marital coitus occurs predominantly at night at home just prior to sleep.

3. Marital coitus is not practiced during the menses or the last portion of pregnancy.

4. Frequency of marital coitus generally declines with age.

5. Great intercultural variation in frequency of marital coitus exists across societies.

Extramarital Coitus

Most societies have more restrictive taboos about premarital coitus than extramarital coitus and also allow men greater freedom than women in extramarital affairs. In the 1951 Ford and Beach survey, approximately 40 per cent of all preliterate societies surveyed tolerated some form of extramarital coitus for wives. Some societies even informally legislate the conditions and nature of the extramarital coitus. Community rules may condone extramarital coitus during special tribal or religious ceremonies or as a form of sexual hospitality. For example, aborigines of Australia's Arnhem Land endorse extramarital sexual relationships. Both marital partners participate in extramarital sex, and their extramarital partners are assigned the status of tribal wives or husbands (Crooks and Bauer, 1983). Such relationships are welcomed and sanctioned by the members of this society, who believe that such a practice decreases the monotony of same partner sex and increases sexual interest and variety, which in turn increases the strength of the primary marital union. The trend in most societies is for the occurrence of extramarital coitus to raise complex social issues and questions for the involved couple. Issues that are usually raised by the event and faced by the individuals involved may include some of the following:

■ Does extramarital coitus constitute a defiance of the spouse?

■ Does it involve a disruption of the primary bond between husband and wife?

■ Will it decrease one's self-esteem and/or social status?

■ Will it result in pregnancy?

■ Will it weaken spouse love and intimacy?

■ Will it be a sin against the religious belief of the community?

Female Orgasm

Anthropologists note that males from all societies experience orgasm as part of coitus. However, many anthropologists believe that the capacity to achieve orgasm for the female is culturally determined. In some societies, such as in Mangaia, adolescent females rapidly learn to achieve orgasm and experience orgasm in most of their sexual encounters thereafter. In this society, women were valued, and much esteem was given to men who could please women sexually. Most male sexual partners wanted their female partners to achieve more orgasms than they did. There were other sexually repressed societies, however, that did not value women or put much emphasis on their sexual pleasure. In Ines Beag, the female orgasm was never mentioned or described and appeared to be virtually nonexistent. The United States, along with other Western countries, has had a long tradition of considering the female orgasm as insignificant. Recent influences from the women's liberation movement have caused a shift in prevalent attitudes about the equality, value, and importance of females to society. This shift in attitude has also been changing attitudes about sexual practices among partners. A proportion of the female population in this culture is changing by becoming more vocal and assertive about their sexual preferences, and a proportion of the male population is also changing by being open, receptive, and valuing female pleasure.

Homosexuality

Some form of sexual behavior between same-sex adults is permitted in nearly two thirds of preliterate societies (Ford and Beach, 1951). The incidence of homosexuality varies with the society. Ford and Beach described that same-sex behavior was never the predominant form of sexual behavior for adults in any of the societies that they studied, that more males than females tended to be involved in same-sex behavior in these preliterate societies, and that regardless of the society's endorsement or nonsanction of homosexuality, same-sex behavior occurred in at least some individuals in the society. Later,

Davenport (1977) reviewed cross-cultural data on homosexuality and concluded that the data were scarce, of dubious quality, and difficult to interpret. There was a diversity of belief and opinions about homosexuality among societies. For example, male homosexuality was an accepted behavior in East Bay culture. Same-sex male relations were legitimized and considered normal and acceptable. Same-sex contacts between adolescent and adult men were legitimate forms of sexual expression. For older men without partners, same-sex contacts were viewed as an acceptable alternative mode of sexual expression. Other cultures do not legitimize same-sex contacts. In these societies, individuals who participate in same-sex behavior often have less status in the community.

SUMMARY

In most societies there is an explicit and well-defined view about the nature of human sexuality. A highly individualized erotic code exists in every society and consists of an inventory of signs and acts that suggest or enhance sexuality. Various odors, fragrances, foods, speech, colors, posture, and behavior, such as sexual speech, songs, poetry, and sexual jokes, symbolize eroticism in the society. Societies also regulate the sexual behavior of their members. Each society explicitly defines the rights, responsibilities, and obligations of the members of a sexual relationship. The conditions of a sexual union and the legal nature of different kinds of sexual unions are all prescribed in each society. Societies also engage in culture-specific sexual practices, or sexual practices that are unique and specialized to a specific culture. As one meditates on the differences in sexual behavior across cultures, the first impression is of the tremendous variety of sexual behaviors. Each society shapes, structures, and guides the sexual development and expression of all its members and develops a unique sexual expression that is based on the internal values, needs, and logic of the culture. Thus, there is tremendous diversity of sexual behavior, rules and regulations, symbols, sanctions, and taboos across societies. Nurses need to appreciate and develop an awareness of cultural diversity in human sexual expression. Variations in the ethnographic spectrum of sexual behavior demand a tolerance for differences. Nurses also need to convey a complete acceptance of different beliefs, attitudes, behaviors, and values of patients from different cultural backgrounds. Each sexual attitude, action, or belief of a person can only be fully and completely understood by an examination of the cultural context in which it occurs.

It is helpful for the nurse to understand the American culture's affect on sexuality and sexual behavior. Brink (1987) notes that heterosexuality is the dominant acceptable sexual pattern in the United States. In our country, coitus between consenting and married adults is socially endorsed. Sexual liaisons between nonmarried partners are not valued. Sex between nonconsenting adults, sex between children and adults, and sex between adults and animals is not condoned. American culture emphasizes the individual's rights and consent in a sexual relationship. However, other cultures do not operate according to our rules, and many of the former behaviors or rules are tolerated or sanctioned in other cultures.

Effective nursing practice requires being free of cultural prejudice and bias. The professional nurse often finds it difficult to view health as laypersons do, but if the nurse wishes to work effectively with different groups of people, he or she must overcome cultural bias and learn to see health and beliefs from the patient's perspective. Cultural health practices affect all domains of life. Nurses should strive to understand the influence of the client's culture on sexuality. The sexual health of the client should be promoted by individual and community education on male and female sexuality and sexual relationships as well as a sensitive concern for the individual cultural variations in sexual behavior.

REFERENCES

Assad MB: Female circumcision in Egypt: Social implications, current research, and prospects for change. Stud Fam Plann 1980, 11:3–16, 1980.

Assaad F: The sexual mutilation of women. World Health Forum 3:391–394, 1982.

Brink PJ: Cultural aspects of sexuality. Holistic Nurs Pract 1:12–20, 1987.

Crooks Baur K: Our Sexuality. Redwood, Benjamin-Cummings, 1983, pp 64–66.

Cutner LP: Female genital mutilation. Obstet Gynecol Surv 40:437–443, 1985.

Davenport WH: Sex in a cross cultural perspective. In Beach FA (ed): Human Sexuality in Four Perspectives. Baltimore, The John Hopkins University Press, 1977, pp 115–163.

DeSantis L, Thomas JT: Parental attitudes toward adolescent sexuality: Transcultural perspectives. Nurse Pract 12:43–48, 1987.

Gebhard PH: Human Sexual Behavior: A Summary Statement. In Marshall DS, Suggs RC (eds): Human Sexual Behavior: Variations in the Ethnographic Spectrum. New York, Basic Books, 1971.

Ford CS, Beach FA: Patterns of Sexual Behavior. New York, Harper & Row, 1951, pp 174–195.

Hosken FP: Female genital mutilation in the world today: A global review. Inter J Heal Serv 11:415–430, 1981.

Janda LH, Klenke-Hamel KE: Human Sexuality. D. Van Nostrand Company, 1980, pp 209–210.

Marshall DS: Sexual behavior on Mangaia. In Marshall DS, Suggs RC (eds): Human Sexual Behavior: Variations in the Ethnographic Spectrum. New York, Basic Books, 1971, pp 103–162.

Marshall DS, Suggs RC: Human Sexual Behavior: Variations in the Ethnographic Spectrum. New York, Basic Books, 1971, pp 220–229.

Messenger JC: Sex and repression in an Irish folk community. In Beach FA (ed): Human Sexuality in Four Perspectives. Baltimore, The John Hopkins University Press, 1977.

Money J, Musaph H (eds): Handbook of Sexology. Excerpta Medica, 1977, pp 519–540.

Shaw E: Female circumcision. Am J Nurs 6:685–687, 1985.

6: Sexuality and Aging

Raelene Shippee-Rice

I can remember the first time Eddie kissed me. I felt a thrill down my back and it was like I was sixteen again. (Shippee, 1979)

The above quote was obtained from a 73-year-old woman in an interview that was part of a research project. She said that she wanted to marry Eddie but that he was jealous. He would get angry whenever she talked to her male friends at the senior center they both attended. "I can't marry him if he is going to be like that even if I do love him. And no one else will ask me out because they all think of me as 'Eddie's girl.'"

During the same research project, a woman in her sixties shared: "I have been having an affair with the man next door, but I felt so guilty about it I just recently broke it off. Sex was such an important part of my marriage, and since my husband died I have really missed it. How long will these feelings last?" And finally, from an 82-year-old woman: "It is so good to talk about what it was like when we were married. I haven't talked about it to anyone in years." She described how she used to sit in her husband's lap every night in the rocking chair and he would rock her back and forth. "It brings back such pleasant memories."

Rarely do we think of elders experiencing intimacy and sexuality concerns similar to those just described. These anecdotes reflect some of the needs the elderly have in relation

The author wishes to acknowledge the assistance of Ann Kelley, Associate Professor of Nursing, University of New Hampshire, for her thoughtful suggestions and valuable comments; Dale W. Rice for his assistance in editing and preparation of this manuscript.

to their sexuality and sexual activities; concerns about relationships, feelings, memories, morality, and lack of knowledge. Although all the above-mentioned anecdotes are about women, men have concerns, too. A man in his seventies wanted to talk to his wife about experimenting with oral/genital sex. He wanted to know if he was "sick" or being unreasonable. "Am I normal?" he asked. Another man said, "Oh, we gave that (sexual intercourse) up years ago. What can you expect at our age? But I still think about it sometimes."

Sexuality is a part of our selves, our beings: It is a deep and pervasive aspect of the total human personality. It is intertwined with our identity as a man or a woman, with our feelings of self-esteem, and with our relationships to others. It begins at birth and continues throughout life. The ability to express and to enjoy one's sexuality leads to feelings of pleasure and well-being—feelings that are essential at any age if our human needs for intimacy and belonging are to be satisfied (Maslow, 1970; Shippee, 1979). Many of the physiological, psychological, and social changes elders experience influence their sexuality and thus their ability to meet the basic human needs for intimacy and self-actualization (Maslow, 1970). Education about these changes and their influence on sexuality is a critical element in promoting the health and well-being of aging clients (Harp, 1984). To be effective health educators, especially in the area of human sexuality, nurses need a knowledge base from which to implement the nursing process. In addition, nurses must develop a sensitivity and awareness of the effect their personal values have on their own perceptions and interpretations of sexual issues and concerns. Similarly, nurses need to be sensitive to the effect that clients' values have on sexual beliefs, practices, and concerns. This is especially true when addressing issues of sexuality in aging.

This chapter will examine the factors that are important to the discussion of sexuality and sexual behaviors in the elderly. A conceptual model of sexuality is used to provide a framework for the discussion of age changes that influence elders' sexuality. The final section of this chapter contains recommendations for nursing assessments and interventions that may be useful in helping elders identify or adjust to changes in their sexuality.

Before further discussion, the following terms warrant clarification: aged or elder, sexuality, and sexual behaviors. Elders or the aged refers to persons over age 65. It is important to note that this group of persons is a very heterogeneous population. Although we generalize about "the aged" or "elders," we must keep in mind that elders have a lifelong history of unique individual and cohort experiences. They are less homogeneous in their beliefs, attitudes, and life styles than younger age groups. This is especially true in regard to experiences as personal and intimate as expressions of sexuality.

Although the terms sexuality and sexual behaviors are often used interchangeably, they are not synonymous. In this chapter, sexuality is defined as an ongoing process of recognizing, accepting, and expressing oneself as a sexual being (Shippee, 1979). Sexual behaviors are the verbal and nonverbal expressions of sexuality and include both nongenital and genital activities. The term sex is a generic word and will be used to refer to any activity, behavior, or attitude that carries a sexual connotation.

The next section will review some of the critical research on sexual behaviors in the elderly and will also address some of the probable causes for the limited amount of research available on sexuality in the aged.

LITERATURE ON SEXUALITY
Introduction

The literature on sexuality and the aged is less prolific than the research on sexuality in younger groups. Several reasons have been cited for this. A major one is the view of elders as "old, wrinkled, and ugly" (Starr and Weiner, 1982). In our modern society, sexuality, feeling sexy, and participation in intimate or sexual activities is assumed to be only for those who are young and beautiful. This common myth is reflected in the following statement by a young man:

> But how can I tell an elderly male patient to be excited about his wife when I think about how unexciting it must be to think of and see flabby breasts, an unshapely body, and an old face? (Starr and Weiner, 1981, p 3)

A second reason for the lack of research on sex and aging is the incest taboo (Comfort, 1963; Pfeiffer, 1977). Children, even those in middle age, have difficulty accepting their parents as sexual beings involved in sexual intercourse or any other overt sexual activity. For the average adult, elders represent the parental generation. Many researchers, therefore, have difficulty asking elders about their sexual life styles and behaviors. Another factor that has limited sexuality research is the commonly held myth that elders are uncomfortable talking about sex as a result of their Victorian background. To protect elders from feeling embarrassed or insulted, it is assumed that such questions should be avoided.

The same factors that prevent researchers from studying sexuality and aging may contribute to the reluctance of professionals to ask elderly clients questions that pertain to sexuality or sexual behaviors. Statements such as "I don't want to embarrass Mr. Jones," "Mrs. Smith is a widow so it won't make any difference to her," or "It [sex] isn't important for them anymore at that age" may indicate discomfort with the topic itself or with the topic in relation to the older age group. Family members and institutions or organizations that provide services to elders reflect societal attitudes through their reluctance to approve research projects that involve talking to elders about sexuality, claiming that such research "will upset them [the elders] too much" (Pfeiffer, 1977).

Researchers who have asked elders about sex report that elders are usually willing and even eager to talk about their sexual feelings, values, beliefs, and behaviors. Elders report there is little information available to them about sex and that health care providers are hesitant to talk to them about it. When someone does express an interest, elders respond positively, not only because they have questions themselves, but also because they want to share their knowledge and experiences to help others learn (Shippee, 1979; Starr and Weiner, 1982).

Most of the literature about sexuality and aging is based on the work of the classic triad: Alfred Kinsey (1948, 1952), Eric Pfeiffer and associates in the Duke Longitudinal Studies (1968, 1972), and Masters and Johnson (1966). These major contributions built the foundation for most of the current literature on sexual behaviors and variables that influence those behaviors in the aged. They are the standard by which new research findings are measured for evidence of change.

Although the work of Kinsey on sexual activities and the studies of Masters and Johnson on sexual physiology are considered the classics on sex and aging, these studies have limitations, and their findings must be carefully evaluated. First, neither of these studies had a large subject population of elders: Of the 8000 men and 6000 women surveyed by Kinsey and associates, only 126 men and 56 women were over age 60. Masters and Johnson observed only 31 men and women over age 60, of which only nine were over 70 years old. The sample in the study by Masters and Johnson consisted primarily of well-educated, upper middle-class elders. Caution must be used when applying the findings from such a small sample to the general population of elders.

Second, the work on sexual behavior was done 20 to 50 years ago. Kinsey's research was done in the 1930s and 1940s. The Duke Longitudinal Studies reported by Pfeiffer and associates began in 1953 and covered a period of 10 years, ending in 1964. Those who were over 65 during these studies were a very different cohort than the current generation of elders over 65. Cultural and social attitudes about sexuality and sexual behaviors have changed from those of the 1930s, 1940s, and 1950s. (The sexual revolution of the 1960s had not yet occurred.) The current generation of elders who are now in their sixties and seventies were in their twenties and thirties when Kinsey did his research.

A critical question must be asked: Are the findings of early research on sexual activities in the elderly applicable to elders today? It is important to determine whether Kinsey's findings of differences in sexual behaviors between age groups were only a reflection of developmental changes or were they also a reflection of the mores and expectations of the generation. Despite the different time periods in which the two studies were done, the work of Kinsey and Pfeiffer and associates at Duke produced similar results. The next section will examine some of the findings of these classic studies.

The Classic Triad

Kinsey's research shattered many commonly held myths about the sexual activities practiced by men and women in the United States. One of these myths was that elderly men and women who were sexually active were "perverted." Shattering this myth was a significant first step in making sexual activity by elders acceptable. He reported that although elderly males continued to be sexually active, their level of sexual activity decreased with increasing age. The incidence of male impotence (currently referred to as erectile dysfunction) increased rapidly after age 55. Kinsey (1948) reported that 25 per cent of 70-year-old males complained of impotence; this figure increased to 75 per cent by age 80.

Kinsey himself did not publish much information on the sexual activities of the aged female, but the data were later analyzed and published by Newman and Nichols (1960). Women's frequency of sexual intercourse was influenced by the male partner. Women with older aged husbands or who were widowed experienced less frequent sexual intercourse than did women whose husbands were younger. For women, the lack of a sanctioned male partner, i.e., a marital partner, was a major barrier to sexual relationships. Only a few women practiced masturbation. Those who engaged in masturbation were better educated and had a higher socioeconomic status than women who did not.

Kinsey found that the type and number of sexual outlets in which men and women engaged were closely related to their decade of birth. Persons born in earlier decades engaged in only a few types of sexual outlets, whereas those who were born later engaged in a wider variety. For example, those born in later decades (1930s) were more apt to indicate that they had engaged in masturbation, orgasm, nudity, and premarital sex at some time in their lives than did those who were born in 1900. This is probably a reflection of changes in society's attitudes toward sexual activities and the decreasing influence of the so-called Victorian attitudes. Kinsey noted that continued sexual interest and activity in later years was closely related to the level and satisfaction of sexual activity in younger years; that is, those couples who had a high interest and satisfaction with their activity level during their youth continued to be more sexually active as they grew older.

The Duke Longitudinal Studies represented a significant piece of research on aging in general. The work is of special interest because of its longitudinal design: The same subject population is studied over a period of years to identify changes that occur in each individual as a result of time. The original subject population consisted of 254 men and women aged 60 to 90 years. The Duke studies examined many different aspect of aging, of which sexual activity was only one small section. Of the entire psychosocial questionnaire administered to the study subjects, only seven items related to sexual activities.

The results of the Duke study supported a finding from earlier studies: Sexual activity declined with advancing age, usually as a result of the male's decision. Reasons most commonly given for the cessation or decrease in sexual activity were poor physical health and decreased social interactions secondary to mental health changes. The sharpest decline was noted in men during their midseventies.

An unexpected finding was that the level of interest in sexual activity remained high even though the actual activity level decreased. This was true in *both* sexes. The researchers did not anticipate that elders would retain an interest in sexual expression if they were not still actively engaged in it. At first glance this assumption appears reasonable. However, with further thought it loses credibility, and the finding of continued interest makes sense: If people marry in their midtwenties, as the majority of this cohort did, and are studied when they are 60, 70, or 80 years of age, it can be assumed that individuals had been sexually active for 40 to 50 years on average. Sexual activities may include more than just sexual intercourse. Hugging, sleeping in the same bed, holding, kissing, and so on may all be viewed as sexual activities (Shippee, 1979). If a person has engaged in an activity for a major part of his or her life and if it can be assumed that some level of pleasure was associated with the activity, it should not come as a surprise that

the person retains an interest in the activity, even if no longer engaged in.

In 1972, Pfeiffer and associates conducted a second longitudinal study to examine the relationship of sexual behavior in the middle years with sexual behavior in later years. For men, the most significant determinants for the maintenance of a continued active sex life were age, health status, and life satisfaction. Men who were older, whose health was deteriorating, or who experienced a low level of life satisfaction tended to be less active sexually. For women, the significant determinants of sexual activity were marital status and age. Past satisfaction and frequency of sexual activity in youth and middle years were important determinants for both men and women in continuing sexual activity in later years. The results of Kinsey's work and the Duke studies lend support to the idea that the frequency of sexual activity decreases with increasing age. This decrease is probably a result of the biological aging process rather than of a cohort or social phenomenon. However, the samples are small, and both studies took place before the sexual revolution occurring in the 1960s. Further research is needed on different generations to compare the relationship of biological effects and cohort effects on sexuality in aging.

The work of Masters and Johnson (1966) on the human sexual response advanced our understanding of human sexuality considerably and added a much needed dimension to human sexuality research. Previous sexuality research only asked questions about sexual behaviors; Masters and Johnson actually observed them and documented the physiological responses that occurred during sexual arousal and activity. They documented that men and women were similar in their sexual responses and that these responses remained essentially unchanged even into the later years.

Masters and Johnson, in the first part of their study, conducted extensive sex histories on 140 women and 225 men over age 50. The second part of the study involved the documentation of physiological changes during sexual activity. Of the total aging subject population, only 11 women and 20 men over 60 years of age participated in the second phase of the study. The authors clearly state, "The material to be presented must be accepted in the light of an admittedly inadequate study-subject population" (Human Sexual Response, 1966, p 248). The information they gathered from the sex histories and physiological observations is crucial to our knowledge of sexual responses in the elderly male and female.

Masters and Johnson documented physiological changes in the sexual organs of both men and women that are associated with aging. These changes did not interfere with the actual ability to experience the sexual response cycle, but they did influence the time frame of the cycle and the intensity of the response. Men experienced a longer excitement phase, decreased intensity of orgasms, decreased quantity of ejaculate, and a shorter resolution phase with a longer refractory period. Women experienced less change in the time scale of the cycle but had fewer orgasms of less intensity and less vaginal lubrication during excitement and plateau. Based on these findings, Masters and Johnson concluded that men and women who maintained a regular schedule of sexual activity in their later years experienced fewer physiological changes than those who were sexually inactive for long periods of time.

More Recent Findings

Two large-scale studies of sexual activity in the aged were completed in the 1980s (Starr and Weiner, 1982; Brecher, 1984). Starr and Weiner interviewed over 800 volunteers about their attitudes toward sexuality and the frequency and quality of their sexual activities. These interviewees were 60 to 91 years of age and living at home. Consumer Union asked its readers of *Consumer Reports* to respond to a questionnaire on love, sex, and aging. The majority of subjects in both studies indicated a high level of satisfaction with their sexual activity. Starr and Weiner reported that subjects in this sample reported more frequent orgasms than those studied in the Kinsey Report. Respondents in both studies generally held positive or at least accepting attitudes toward nudity, oral/genital intercourse, and masturbation. Elders continued to maintain an interest in sex that was not related to the frequency or type of sexual activity. Subjects generally felt positive about themselves and their own sexuality. Many of them indicated they believed sexual expression to be important for a continuing sense of mental and physical well-being. An unexpected number of men and women in their seventies, eighties, and nineties responding

to the Consumer Union survey reported nonmarital sexual activity. Many of those interviewed by Starr and Weiner stated that the quality of the sexual expression became more important than the frequency as the years progressed. Hand holding, hugging, and kissing continued to be an important aspect of physical activity even though the frequency of sexual intercourse decreased. Elders stated that these affectional touching activities were an important contribution to their continued sense of well-being and satisfaction (Starr and Weiner, 1981).

Related Research

The issue of touch has special significance for looking at sexuality and aging. Montagu (1971) has described touch as a psychobiological hunger that must be satisfied to provide growth, development, and stability in the human person. The awareness and identity of the self is maintained through the sense of touch with one's own body or through the touch of another (Montagu, 1971, Burnside, 1975). Affective touch, that is, touch that conveys caring and warmth, provides a medium for intimacy and sharing. One study found that healthy (self-defined) elderly persons living in the community experience less affective touch as they age (Shippee, 1979). This loss of affective touch is even more common for elders who live in nursing homes, especially those who are cognitively impaired or perceived as unattractive or unsociable. Men in nursing homes receive less affective touch from staff members than do women. This is probably because of the association of affective touch with sexual overtones.

The importance of touch in our lives is evident in our everyday language. We speak of "being touched" by someone's experience. We are "touched" by sadness, joy, and anger. We use the word touch, or touched, to indicate that an emotional and physiological response has been elicited by the experience.

Touch is such a strong influence on a person's well-being that it has come under investigation as a therapeutic technique (Krieger, 1975). Although the technique of therapeutic touch includes both physical and nonphysical contact, the actual laying on of hands is most closely associated with the nursing profession.

Touch has always been the special mark of the

nursing profession—its way of making its unique and special presence felt by those in need of comfort and care. (Fanslow, 1983)

Therapeutic touch has been shown to increase nutritional intake in elders with organic brain syndrome (Eaton et al, 1986), decrease anxiety level in hospitalized patients (Heidt, 1981), and reduce the heart rate (Drescher et al, 1980).

All the literature on touch points to its importance as an affirmation of caring and communication when used judiciously. It is through touch that we come to know ourselves, to know others, and to know the world around us. The lack of touch or its abuse may not only impair a person's emotional and physical well-being but may also lead to an increased number of physiological problems (Franks, 1957) and even death (Talbot, 1941).

In summary, research has shown that many elders continue to be interested in expressing their sexuality through sexual and nonsexual physical behaviors as well as nonphysical behaviors. Variables that influence the frequency of sexual activity include age, health status, and the availability of a socially sanctioned partner. The qualitative dimension of sexual behavior in aging is closely related to the level of satisfaction with the sexual activity experienced in young and middle adulthood. The next section will present a model of sexuality as a framework for identifying additional variables that may affect sexuality and sexual behavior in the aged.

A CONCEPTUAL MODEL OF SEXUALITY

Figure 6–1 depicts a conceptual model of sexuality designed by the author during a research project on sexuality and aging (Shippee, 1979). The model reflects the belief that sexuality is a multidimensional, interactional concept that does not develop or exist in a vacuum. The model is also based on the assumption that the individual strives for a wholeness of the self and attempts to balance the biological, psychological, and social dimensions of the self within a complex everchanging environment. Therefore, anything that significantly affects the individual's internal or external environment impacts on sexuality, on other dimensions of the self, and on other persons. The structure in Figure 6–1 represents four broad areas that are essential to the development and continuation of the self as a sexual being: the *self*, the *components of sexuality*, the impact of *significant others*, and *environmental variables*.

At the center of the model is an individual's *self*, composed of body, mind, and spirit. This triangle represents the synthesis, or integrity, of the individual as a whole, combining the physical, mental, and spiritual aspects of being. Surrounding and interacting with the *self* is the circle labeled *components of sexuality*, which are the processes and behaviors that affect the development and maintenance of the self as a sexual being. The components identified are trust, intimacy, touch, interactions with others, self-concept, consensual validation, and sexual identity.

The circle labeled *significant others* represents those people, past and present, who positively or negatively contribute to a sense of the sexual self. The influence that significant others exert on the *self* varies, depending on the growth and development stage of the individuals involved and on the strength and importance of the relationship, that is, the intimacy level. Intimacy, in this model, is defined on a continuum consisting of emotional, intellectual, and physical dimensions. Each dimension has its own independent continuum, and the level of intensity of the particular dimension shifts along that continuum over time. For example, a student and a mentor may share intellectual intimacy but experience very low levels of emotional or physical intimacy. Another example would be of an older married couple who may have developed a high level of emotional intimacy while only experiencing moderate levels of intellectual and physical intimacy.

The variables on the outermost circle represent *environmental variables* that affect the development and maintenance of a sexual self. The social, cultural, religious, and physical environments in which an individual matures and lives bias the attitudes and beliefs a person develops about sexuality and the types of behaviors that are considered acceptable.

The interactions among the variables are represented by a series of circles and lines. The double circles around the *self* and the *components of sexuality* represent a circular feedback process among the body, mind, and spirit and among the processes that are the components of sexuality. In other words, these processes are not unidirectional but

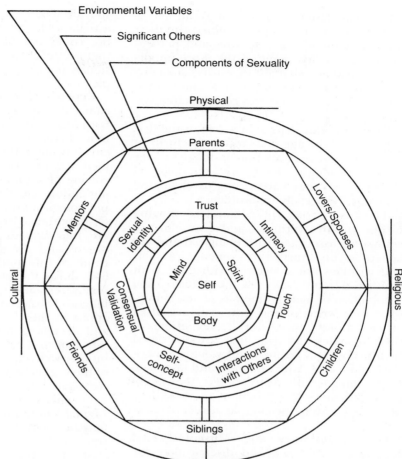

Environmental Variables
Significant Others
Components of Sexuality

FIGURE 6–1. A conceptual model of sexuality. (Shippee-Rice, 1986).

bidirectional, flowing in both directions. The double lines connecting the circles around the *self* with the *components of sexuality* and connecting the circles around the *components of sexuality* with *significant others* designate a two-way interaction. The single lines from the *environmental variables* indicate a stronger unidirectional influence. Although there is interaction in both directions, the influence of the *environmental variables* on the elements in the inner circles is stronger than the influence of the inner circle elements on the *environmental variables.*

A change in any single dimension in the conceptual model at any point in time can lead to temporary or permanent alterations in sexuality. Barriers and facilitators to a client's sexual self can be identified by looking at these multiple dimensions. By examining each of these dimensions of sexuality, we can identify the way each variable may inhibit or

facilitate a client's feeling of positive sexuality.

SEXUALITY AND AGING

Aging is a universal, intrinsic, progressive, and decremental process. It happens to each of us biologically, psychologically, and socially but at different rates and in different ways. This section will discuss how aging affects the variables identified in the conceptual model of sexuality. The discussion of the conceptual model will start from the inner circle, *self,* and move outwards to *environment variables.*

Self: The Inner Circle

BODY

Many changes occur in the body as part of normal growth and development. Changes that occur from normal aging can be as important as those due to illness in their influences on sexual responses and perceptions of sexuality. Some of the more important normal age changes that affect sexuality are those that occur in the skin, the musculoskeletal system, and the reproductive system.

Skin and Hair. The skin is one of the first organs to show age changes in the form of wrinkles and the development of age or liver spots. Although these are physiological changes, they may have strong psychological overtones, especially for women.

There is a strong double standard of aging in our culture. Wrinkles and gray hair are commonly associated with being old and are labeled as unattractive in women. Gray hair and wrinkles are associated with the loss of youth and beauty, sex appeal, and decreasing recognition of aged women as sexual beings. Men with wrinkles and gray hair are often viewed as attractive, worldly, experienced; their wrinkles and gray hair are associated with distinction. As men and women experience skin and hair changes and associate these changes with attractiveness, they begin to alter their views of themselves as sexually appealing or unappealing, as sexual or asexual.

Cardiorespiratory and Musculoskeletal Systems. Both aging and disease alter the cardiorespiratory and musculoskeletal systems. Changes associated with cardiac output and lung function can increase fatigue levels, decrease activity endurance, and interfere with a sense of well-being. Movement may be impaired secondary to arthritis and to decreased flexibility of muscles with associated physical discomfort. As a result, both physical and psychological energy levels may be reduced. The loss of energy may interfere with the individual's sexuality, with an associated lack of interest or participation in sexual behaviors. Significantly, the reverse can occur. The inability to engage in sexual behaviors due to discomfort or energy reduction may cause the individual to experience an altered sexuality. For example, a 72-year-old woman attended a feminist sexuality workshop in a wheelchair. She told the group that she and her husband both had severe arthritis and that sexual relations were no longer possible. No one had talked to either of them about different positions or alternative sexual activities other than the traditional "missionary position" of sexual intercourse. As a re-

sult, they had given up all intimate physical activities. She missed their intimate relations but could not think of a way to continue them. Intervention from health care professionals might have been helpful to this couple.

Reproductive System. The onset of the climacteric is a major transition period for both men and women. Although there is more knowledge about the changes that occur in women, there is reason to believe that men also experience a transition period involving physical and emotional changes during middle age. The menopause is the major physiological event in the female climacteric. Of importance to the older man and woman are the changes that occur in the sexual organs and the sexual response cycle as a result of this midlife biological event. Table 6–1 shows the physiological changes in the sexual response cycle in the aged male and female. These changes are the result of alterations in the circulation to the genital area and decreased hormone levels. The loss of estrogen in the female creates specific involutionary changes in the vagina. The mucosa of the vagina becomes very thin, loses its well-corrugated appearance, and changes to a light pinkish color. There is a shortening of vaginal length and width. As a result, coitus may be painful, especially during the penetration phase or with prolonged thrusting. Postcoitus, some women complain of vaginal burning and/or dysuria as a result of the mucosal thinning in the vagina. Urinary urgency after intercourse secondary to mechanical irritation of the urethra is a common complaint. In women who have regular sexual activity, that is, one to two times a week, vaginal irritation is less of a problem.

In males, major age changes in sexual function include erectile ability and the change in the character of ejaculation. Penile erection is less firm and requires more stimulation and a longer time period to achieve. Once penile erection occurs and is lost without ejaculation, many older men are unable to attain a second erection immediately. The amount of ejaculate and intensity of ejaculatory pressure is diminished with age. For many men, the ejaculatory process is closely linked with orgasm. The diminished ejaculatory response may decrease the qualitative satisfaction associated with orgasm.

MIND

The concept of the mind is difficult to define. In this model, the mind refers to "the seat of

TABLE 6–1. Physiological Changes Associated with Aging

Male	Female
Excitement	
Requires more direct stimulation and longer time period to attain full penile erection	Decreased vaginal lubrication
Penile erection less firm	Time required for vaginal lubrication lengthened
Sex flush less frequent	Vasocongestion of labia minora decreased
	Vaginal ballooning delayed
	Vasocongestion of breasts diminished
Plateau	
Testicular elevation diminished	Elevation of labia majora decreased
Scrotal wall vasocongestion reduced	No sex flush present
	Levels of muscle tension decreased
	Vaginal barrel does not elongate or widen
Orgasm	
Ejaculatory strength decreased	Vasocongestion of orgasmic platform decreased
Number of penile contractions decreased	Number of vaginal contractions decreased
Sensation of ejaculatory inevitability diminished	Uterine contractions may be intense or even painful
Psychosexual pleasure of orgasm with ejaculation diminished	
Resolution	
Rapid penile detumescence	Delayed areolae detumescence
Prolonged refractory period	Rapid shrinking of vaginal balloon
	Possible urinary urgency immediately postcoitus
	Increased complaints of dysuria

Adapted from Masters WH, Johnson VE: Human Sexual Response. Boston, Little, Brown & Co, 1966.

consciousness, thought, volition, and feeling," as defined in the Concise Oxford Dictionary, and to the rational intelligence and emotional responses of an individual (Shippee, 1979). The mind includes both the anatomical and physiological functions of the brain and the dimensions of personality.

The effects of aging on the mind are not clearly understood. Anatomical changes that occur include loss of neurons, loss of brain weight, and alterations in neurotransmitters. Exactly how these changes affect the mind, personality, and abilities of elders is still under investigation. In the past there were two separate views on personality and aging. One view is that personality remains relatively stable throughout adulthood and may even become rigid with age. The other view is that personality tends to change over time as a result of life experiences. Current research suggests that there is individual variation, and therefore both views are valid. It is unclear from the research how intellectual abilities change with age and how they may influence personality. In the past, some theorists posited that intellectual abilities decreased with age. More recent research, however, suggests that some intellectual abilities remain relatively stable while others may actually show growth. The changes associated with the mind and aging influence sexuality as an expression of the self. An individual's perception of holistic health and well-being are closely related to the integrity of the mind. One factor that may affect the mind and the sense of well-being of the aged person is the experience of loss. Losses may include friends and family members, feelings of productivity and purpose, status, income, and previous roles. These losses may have cumulative effects over time and lead to feelings of uselessness, loneliness, and diminished self-image. Depression or anxiety may also result from the losses and stresses associated with aging. Changes in mental status or cognitive functioning due to disease are a major cause of loss of marital intimacy and sexual activity. They may also cause the aged person to lose sexual inhibitions and lead to overt or public displays of sexual behaviors.

The mind can also support positive changes and coping strategies. Elders who are motivated and interested can adapt their sexual activities to meet new situations. They can change previously held attitudes and beliefs and develop new patterns of sexual behaviors. They often have a greater understanding and tolerance of others and a willingness to compromise. Many elders, especially those who have lost a sexual partner, choose to channel their sexual energies into other creative areas of their lives, including, but not limited to, helping others, learning new skills, and participating in different social activities.

SPIRIT

Spiritual needs are an integral part of a person's self. The spiritual needs reflect the desire for meaning in life. Erikson (1963) describes aging as a time when there is a sense that life has had meaning and has been a source of satisfaction or as a time of despair and a sense that there has been little to appreciate. If the spirit or sense of purpose in life is missing, the energy to experience the self is also missing. The loss of the spirit can profoundly interfere with the ability to feel one's sexuality. For the aged person who views this part of life as a time of freedom to express the spirit or essence of his or her self, the sexual self and the spiritual self can work together to be a creative life force.

Components of Sexuality: The Second Circle

TOUCH

The experiences and beliefs associated with the components of sexuality are altered with age. The skin can be considered the largest sex organ because it is through the skin's receptors that we receive our sense of touch. Persons maintain a need for tactile communication for affirmation throughout our life span. "Tactile communication may be even more important to the older individual as other sensory processes are altered with age" (Burnside, 1975).

Many elders experience a decrease in the quantity and quality of touching behaviors as they age (Shippee, 1979). There are a number of reasons for this. As we age, we are touched less frequently by others. The aged, i.e., those over age 65, are not seen as physically attractive. Research on nurses' touching of elders has shown that elders who are confused or unattractive receive little affective touch and are touched only to carry out physical nursing care. One reason given for not using touch with the aged is the unfounded assumption that the social milieu in which elders were raised did not encourage affective touching. As a result, health professionals are afraid that elders might be offended if they were touched by a nonfamily member. Elders themselves are very sensitive to the labels of "dirty old man" or "dirty old woman"; thus, they are often hesitant to initiate touch with persons who are younger or of the opposite sex. Elders often wait to be touched even by members of their own families.

Touching is usually associated with some degree of intimacy. Intimacy may be defined as the sharing of one's self with another (Shippee, 1979) and is an important variable in the development and maintenance of sexuality.

INTIMACY AND TRUST

Intimacy is based on trust. It develops between individuals over a period of time as a result of shared experiences, beliefs, and values. Physical intimacy may include a continuum of behaviors from hand holding to sexual intercourse or oral/genital intercourse. However, some intimate relationships are only emotional or intellectual interactions with little or no physical sharing involved. As one ages the number of individuals with whom one is intimate decreases. Intimate friends or loved ones die or move. Elders may be hesitant to develop new intimate relationships. The threat of another loss or the required investment of time and energy to develop intimacy may be too great. A major question surviving elders may ask is, "Who's left to hold and to share the tender moments of life?" This question is poignantly addressed in the lines from the following poem:

> MINNIE REMEMBERS
> How long has it been since
> someone touched me
> Twenty years?
> Twenty years I've been a widow.
> Respected. Smiled at.
> But never touched.
> Never held so close that
> loneliness was blotted out.
> (Swanson, 1976)

SEXUAL IDENTITY, SELF-CONCEPT, CONSENSUAL VALIDATION

The components of sexual identity, self-concept, and consensual validation are closely interrelated. The ways in which a person perceives him- or herself as an aging individual is a reflection of the validation that is received from friends, family, and society in general. The validation is based on the verbal and nonverbal communication and results in an agreement or consensus of perspectives. If the validation of the aging person as an individual is positive, self-esteem is maintained or even enhanced. As a man or woman ages, questions about sexual identity or the masculinity or femininity of the individual may arise. Questions about one's attractiveness, behaviors, and role identification may be important: "Am I too old?" "Will people tell me to 'act my age'?" or "No fool like an old fool?" Answers to such questions may support or negate the individual's expressions of sexuality. Validation that one is still a man or woman and a sexual being contribute to a positive sexual identity.

Significant Others: The Third Circle

As people age, their significant others may change. Those who had major significance at one point may become less important later on, or they may take on new significance. The dynamics of the relationships that existed between an individual and his or her significant others throughout the life cycle will strongly influence the quality of those relationships in later life.

A group that may achieve new significance for aging individuals is their adult children. Aged parents may seek the opinions of their adult children and follow their advice. Adult children may in turn attempt to control their parents' life style. This may be a major issue in areas of sexuality. The adult children may express strong opinions on ways elder parents express their sexuality in dress, behaviors, and relationships. They may or may not support their parents' need for sexual activity or the establishment of new intimate relationships. Aged parents may give up their intimacy with others if the children are not supportive or express disapproval. This influence of children on parents is often seen when the parent has experienced the loss of a spouse or partner through death or divorce.

The loss of a spouse or significant other is a common experience among aged persons. This loss usually creates a major impact on the life style and well-being of the survivor. For many elders, the loss of a partner or spouse heralds the end of one's sexual activity. Among the current generation of older women, sexual activity is strongly linked to the presence of a marital partner. For these women, and for the men who have similar value beliefs, social activities, volunteer work, or other energy-expendable activities may be used to fill the void. The redirection of sexual energies into other aspects of life is a successful coping mechanism for many elders,

but for others there may be a lingering sense of dissatisfaction or discontent.

Environment: The Outer Circle

SOCIAL, CULTURAL, AND RELIGIOUS ENVIRONMENTS

The social, cultural, and religious environments in which one lived during childhood and any changes in those environments throughout adulthood may strongly influence expressions of sexuality. The social and cultural milieu defines expectations of sexual role and determines the boundaries of acceptable expressions of sexuality. Men of the present older generation associated their sexuality with a dominant role in relationships. The male was expected to be the aggressor in sexual relationships, set the tone of sexual interactions, and be the primary wage earner for the family. Women were expected to take a passive role in relationships, to be the receiver of sexual attentions, and to be the homemaker. For some elders in this age group, their environment did not encourage couples to discuss with each other or with others their sexual activities or concerns. These previously defined expectations and the lack of an ability to communicate create barriers to the development of new patterns of sexual relationships. For example, women who were socialized to be passive participants in sexual relations may find it difficult to take an active role and provide direct penile stimulation as part of foreplay.

Masturbation is an example of how social, cultural, and religious environments may influence an individual's attitudes at one point in life but not at another. In the early 1900s (when many of today's elders were children), masturbation was referred to as the "secret vice" or "self-abuse" and was strongly discouraged, particularly in children. One medical text of the period stated, "[This] secret sin [masturbation] ruins more constitutions every year than hard work, severe study, hunger, cold, privation, and disease combined" (Jefferis and Nichols, 1922, pp 294, 346). Remedies to cure this "affliction" included covering the organs with a cage, circumcision for young boys, and the application of pure carbolic acid to the clitoris in girls (Jefferis and Nichols, 1922). Since the mid 1960s, masturbation has become a more acceptable form of sexual behavior. Texts on sex therapy even recommend masturbation as a treatment for sexual dysfunctions, including preorgasmic states in women and erectile dysfunctions in men, also commonly referred to as impotence. The literature on aging women and sexuality suggests masturbation as an alternative sexual outlet when a partner is not able or willing to engage in sexual activity or is unavailable. Elders, however, who were raised under the belief system that masturbation was a sin or a vice may find it difficult to overcome old messages. Attitudes can change and new behaviors can be utilized, but it requires time and the support of others to facilitate the adaptation.

PHYSICAL

The physical environment and living arrangements of the elder may create barriers to expressions of sexuality. Elders who live with family members other than the spouse or in institutions may not have the level of privacy necessary to allow sexual activity to occur or intimate relationships to develop (Kaas, 1978). In some living situations, husbands and wives or significant others may not have the option to sleep in the same bed or even in the same room. Accessibility to a private space when significant others visit may be limited if an elder is not living independently.

We express our sexuality by the way we dress, the hair styles and make-up we wear, and the toiletries we use. Elders may be restricted either by their living situations or by the unavailability of sufficient funds to purchase toiletries, have their hair done, or buy the type of clothing they want. Persons residing in institutions may not have opportunities to go shopping, or their funds may be spent on their care, with little left over for personal use. Limited transportation services in rural areas for elders who do not or cannot drive may also restrict access to shopping, significant others, and social events.

Sexuality is a process of personal expression of the self as a sexual being. It is a multidimensional process that includes the physical, psychological, social, and spiritual self in relation to other persons. Throughout the life span, changes in each of these dimensions occur that influence the individual's perception of his or her sexuality. Many of these changes occur as a result of the aging process and life experiences that affect the ability of the aged person to express him- or herself as a sexual being. Frequently, health care professionals can be instrumental in helping elders to adapt to these changes and to maintain a positive sense of the sexual self. In the next section, implications for nursing practice in the sexual health of the aged are addressed.

NURSING IMPLICATIONS

Taking a sexual history should be part of routine client care (Steinke and Bergen, 1986; Renshaw, 1985). This statement has been a consistent theme in the nursing and health care literature for the past 10 to 15 years. However, attitudes about sexuality and beliefs about the acceptability of sexual behaviors in the elderly strongly influence whether or not the nurse includes a sexual history as part of a client's data base. If the nurse does not consider sexual expression an important aspect of the elder client's mental or physical health, a sexual history may not be instituted.

The belief that a client is responsible for initiating sexual concerns may inhibit nurse-client interactions about sexuality. Elders who do have concerns may not raise them for one or more reasons, including: previous rebuffs by health care professionals, questions about the appropriateness of discussing the topic, fears of being labeled a dirty old man or woman, fear of embarrassing such a "sweet young person," or feeling that they do not have the correct terminology and their use of slang or vernacular may not be accepted. It is the nurse's responsibility to anticipate such concerns and to ensure open discussions of sensitive and personal issues through careful listening when taking a client's history. For nurses who are uncomfortable with discussions about sexual issues, one way to overcome the discomfort is to actually initiate the conversation. Avoidance does not increase comfort for either nurse or client. Workshops, seminars, and conferences are a good way to begin to talk openly about sexual attitudes and information. It is often helpful to talk with close friends and practice doing sexual assessments until one begins to feel at ease with the words and the questions. It is helpful to remember that clients appreciate the message that sexuality is an issue that may be discussed in an open supportive atmosphere. Simply identifying a sexual issue or question as a legitimate concern can relieve anxieties about normalcy and self-esteem. The nurse's attitude and openness may be of greatest value in helping client's identify and discuss sexual issues. The following story may illustrate the importance of listening and asking questions about sexual issues even when there may not be an obvious connection.

Sharon Moss was caring for Ms. Sayles, a 68-year-old woman. During her care for Ms. Sayles, Sharon inadvertently exposed her for a brief moment. Sharon Moss apologized, saying "I'm sorry." Ms. Sayles responded, "Oh, one gets used to that in the hospital. Privacy doesn't seem to mean very much here." Sharon commented, "I know it certainly seems that way at times. However, it does seem important to try and protect someone's privacy as much as possible." Ms. Sayles was silent for a few minutes. She then said, "I've always been a very private person. I've always changed my clothes in the closet where no one can see me." The nurse heard something in Ms. Sayles voice, a slight inflection for which she did not know the cause. Sharon wanted to clarify the reason for the inflection. She said, "How did you feel about changing your clothes that way?" Ms. Sayles responded with a little laugh and said, "Oh, I don't know, but my husband never really liked it very much." Sharon felt there was a real concern underlying the casual conversation. She asked Ms. Sayles if she would like to talk more about it. Ms. Sayles went on to discuss a number of issues: She was raised not to let others see her body, her husband had never seen her naked but often said how much he would like to, she now wanted to feel free to expose herself to him but was self-conscious and did not know how to begin. Perhaps she was too old. What would he think if all of a sudden after all these years, she were to suggest such a thing? The nurse listened very carefully, validated that those were reasonable concerns, and supported Ms. Sayles in her wish to be more open with her husband. The nurse and the client worked out several ways in which Ms. Sayles could carry out her desire to begin being more open with her husband and eventually even undressing in front of him and being nude around him. Ms. Sayles expressed relief at being able to talk with someone about wanting to change her behavior and how silly she felt. She realized that maybe she wasn't being "an old fool" and that it was not too late to change.

Later, Sharon Moss related the story to the author. She said, "I was so afraid she would think I was meddling or, even worse, that she really wasn't talking about sexuality when I thought she was. I thought what if I'm wrong and I've embarrassed her? But then I thought, well I'll leave it open and see what she wants to talk about. If she doesn't want to talk about it any more right now, she'll at least know I'm concerned and willing to talk with her if she wants to discuss it later. And it felt good to be someone with whom she could share her concerns and discuss ideas about how to begin changing."

Clients often want to discuss sexual issues and concerns but do not know how to begin. Only by taking the risk to ask questions and to be open will nurses become aware of their clients' concerns.

Assessment

The conceptual model of sexuality gave us a framework from which to institute the nursing process. The nursing assessment must include a careful history of the elder client's physical and mental health, previous experiences and attitudes regarding sexuality, self-concept and self-esteem issues, and environmental conditions. Although an extensive sexual history may not be part of the admission or initial interview, the subject of sexuality or sexual concerns can be raised. This initial discussion gives the message that sexual issues are important and sets the stage for a more extensive assessment. The assessment data enable the nurse to identify a problem if one is present. Table 6–2 provides a guide for the identification of some of the issues that may affect sexual health. This is only a guide and is not meant to be all-inclusive. The nurse needs to be sensitive to the implicit and explicit cues given by the client that indicate areas of concern and suggest the need for further investigation. Frequently, with the client's permission, it is useful to take a history from the sexual partner if one exists. In addition to the assessment information listed in Table 6–2, a health history and physical assessment must be included.

Diagnosis and Planning

It is important to recognize that an alteration in sexuality patterns due to aging may not necessarily indicate a problem. Many elders may have adapted to changes in their sexual activity or accepted the alterations and not wish to make any new changes. Reassurance

TABLE 6–2. Assessment of Sexual Health

Sexual Satisfaction
Have you experienced any changes in your sexual relationships recently?

To what do you attribute this change?

What types of sexual activities have you usually enjoyed the most, including things such as hugging, kissing, sleeping together, intercourse, masturbation, and so on?

Do you or your partner take any prescription medications? What are they? How often do you take them? Have you experienced any changes in your level of energy since you started them? What about overall feelings of well-being? Any changes in sexual desire or activity?

Have you had any problems using the same positions for sexual activity that you have used in the past?

For Men:
Have you noticed any changes in the intensity of your ejaculations, orgasms, or ability to attain/maintain an erection?

Have you ever had orgasms without ejaculations?

Has your level of enjoyment with sexual relations altered as a result of these changes?

Have you had any problems with urethral discharge or urination?

For Women:
Have you experienced any vaginal soreness or irritation after sexual intercourse? How long does it last? Any problems with urgency or burning on urination after intercourse? Have you experienced abdominal contractions or back pain after intercourse?

Have you had any problems with vaginal discharge or itching?

Have any of these problems interfered with your sexual pleasure?

Have you or your partner experienced any changes in your health status recently? How have these changes affected your sexual relationship?

How did the menopause affect your sexual activities?

Alterations in Self-Perception
How has growing older changed your life style or things you enjoy doing?

How has the change in your health or your partner's health altered your life style or your goals?

How do you rate your general health?

On a scale of 1 to 10 how would you describe your satisfaction with your life?

On a scale of 1 to 10 how would you describe your satisfaction with your sexual relationships?

Relationship with Others
Have you ever discussed sexual topics with your spouse, friends, family, or health care professional?

Do you have close friends of your same sex? Of the opposite sex?

Who do you talk to when you have problems of any kind or just want someone to talk to?

Who do you go to social activities with?

Who makes you feel good?

Environment
With whom do you live?

Do you have a chance for privacy? To be alone? To talk with others privately if you want to?

Are you able to get to shopping areas when you want to?

Have you ever experienced any conflict between your sexual desires and the teachings of your religion?

Note: The sexual health assessment should be complemented by a general health history and general physical examination.

that their patterns of sexuality and responses to associated changes are reasonable and acceptable may be helpful in supporting the elder client's self-esteem and may be an important intervention. Otherwise, for these individuals, the issues of sexuality or sexual activity are not of concern and therefore do not require any interventions.

After the nursing history and physical assessment have been completed, the nurse summarizes the findings and affirms areas in which there may be a need for help. In making a nursing diagnosis, it is absolutely critical that there be no sense of failure, deficit, or blame associated with it. Clients experiencing concern about sexual functioning, behavior, or attitudes are highly sensitive to the idea that somehow it is "my fault or your fault" whether such blame is implicitly or explicitly stated. The nurse must protect the potentially fragile self-esteem of the client experiencing alterations in sexuality. Therefore, it is important to validate that the client also sees a need for help and agrees that a problem requiring intervention is present. After validating findings with the client, the nursing diagnosis is developed. Suggestions for nursing diagnoses associated with alterations in sexuality of the aged include the following:

Knowledge Deficit Related To:
1. Effects of normal aging on sexual functioning.
2. Concerns about what are normal sexual practices.
3. Effects of altered health states on sexual activity.
4. Secondary effects of therapy on sexual functioning (e.g., medications, surgery).

Alterations in Sexual Pleasure Related To:
1. Loss of partner or significant other.
2. Changes in living arrangements (indicate what they are).
3. Alterations in physical health (indicate the alterations).
4. Alterations in mental health (indicate alterations).
5. Decrease in self-esteem.
6. Attitudes of significant others (state who and what).

Many elderly clients are not familiar with the process of working with a health care professional to develop a plan of care. They may have been socialized through previous experiences with the health care system to be passive recipients of care. Elders may follow the directions of the professional without questioning the reason or the result. A comment frequently heard is, "Whatever you (or the doctor) says." This response may reflect a condition of learned helplessness, in which the client feels no control over the directions of care. The nurse needs to be sensitive to this possibility and to explain carefully the value of the client's active participation when-

ever possible in identifying and selecting intervention strategies. The client needs to recognize, especially in issues of sexual functioning, that the situation is not hopeless and that change can occur. The level of change may be smaller and occur more slowly than that with younger clients. Elders need to be aware of this limitation and not associate slow change with failure. It is often more helpful to focus on short-term, concrete goals or objectives. Problems of sexuality are rarely limited to the individual and usually occur in the context of relationships with significant others or within the social, emotional, spiritual, or physical environment. Significant others who are involved should be included in the planning process but only with the client's permission. The following is an example of a frequently encountered nursing diagnosis with related long- and short-term goals (objectives):

Nursing Diagnosis
Alteration in sexual pleasure related to effects of normal aging: decreased vaginal lubrication.

Long-term Goal
Client will state she experiences less physical discomfort during sexual intercourse within the next month as a result of increased vaginal lubrication through a natural response to changes in sexual stimulation or through application of a lubricate.

Short-Term Goals
1. The client and partner will describe the effects of decreased vaginal lubrication as a result of normal age changes on sexual function prior to initiation of other short-term goals.
2. The client and partner will engage in activities associated with pleasurable foreplay as identified by the client to assess whether such activity increases vaginal lubrication.
3. The client and partner will apply a water soluble lubricating jelly to the outer two thirds of the vaginal barrel and the penis prior to every intromission.
4. Client will indicate whether these interventions are personally agreeable or cause mental and/or physical discomfort.

Interventions

Nursing interventions need to be tailored to the values and preferences of the client (and partner if one is available) and to the nursing diagnosis and objectives agreed upon. Alterations in sexuality may require a number of different interventions, including education, support, attentiveness, sensitivity, medical and pharmacological treatment, and insight-oriented psychotherapy to name a few. Usually, a combination of approaches is required (Eckert, 1984). This following section presents suggestions for interventions to assist clients with alterations in sexual health.

KNOWLEDGE DEFICIT

If the nursing diagnosis is a knowledge deficit, information and teaching directed at dispelling myths and misinformation may be all that is necessary. Discussion of changes in physiological function due to normal age changes often alleviates concern about changes in sexual functioning and enjoyment. Reassurance and supportive words of encouragement can do wonders in alleviating elders' fear about normalcy and the appropriateness for older persons to be interested in sex. This can be accomplished through direct teaching by the nurse or by providing clients with popular books and magazine articles or other written information. If written information is utilized, the nurse can provide follow-up information as necessary if further clarification is still needed. Table 6–3 lists suggestions for interventions to alleviate common problems associated with age changes in sexual response.

Attitudes of family members, particularly

TABLE 6–3. Interventions for Age-Associated Changes in Sexual Functioning

Female: Problems associated with vaginal changes
1. Regular sexual activity that includes intromission one to two times a week.
2. Vaginal lubrication with water soluble jelly.
3. Adequate time provided for foreplay or pregenital activities.
4. Control of when intromission occurs during sexual intercourse in collaboration with partner.

Male: Problems associated with penile erection
1. Direct penile stimulation by manual, oral, or mechanical (e.g., vibrator) contact.
2. Regular sexual activity.
3. Avoidance of alcohol prior to intercourse.
4. Sexual activity when energy levels are highest.

adult children, may interfere with an elder's ability to develop new intimate or sexual relationships after the loss of a spouse. The nurse may act as an advocate for the older adult and help the family to recognize and accept the basic human need for intimacy and caring.

ALTERATIONS IN SEXUAL PLEASURE

Any primary physical or mental health problem needs to be corrected or addressed prior to focusing on the sexual issue itself. Frequently, alterations in sexual functioning occur as a result of interventions to correct an underlying health problem. Although all clients need to be given anticipatory guidance about the potential effects of therapy on sexual functioning, this is of special importance in the aged client. Elderly clients often attribute changes in sexual functioning to old age. They may not even question whether changes in sexual feelings or response are caused by therapy. If the nurse does not ask specifically about changes in sexual response, the secondary problem of sexual alteration may go undiagnosed. When giving anticipatory guidance, the nurse needs to be sensitive to the self-fulfilling prophecy concept; that is, if one expects something to happen, it will. Reassurance that the secondary effects are only a possibility and that specific identification of what those effects are may help to prevent the self-fulfilling prophecy. Examples of common situations in which anticipatory guidance is needed are the development of retrograde ejaculation after a transurethral resection and erectile dysfunction or inhibited sexual desire secondary to antihypertensive medications. There is little that can be done to eradicate the problem of retrograde ejaculation, but it is important that the client know that orgasm can still occur even though penile ejaculation may not. A change in medication or adjustment of the dosage may decrease the problem associated with antihypertensive treatment. However, before suggesting that the client seek a change in medications, the nurse must carefully assess the situation. Sexual alterations secondary to medications may be either a direct result of the action of the medication or a psychological response to the disease, decreased energy levels, or self-fulfilling prophecy. The self-fulfilling prophecy is the result of the client's anxiety that an alteration in sexuality will occur, and therefore it does.

Before initiating an intervention, the cause of the change must be carefully identified.

If correction of the underlying health problem does not resolve the sexual concerns, alternative interventions can be developed. These may include the use of assistive devices such as penile implants for permanent physiological erectile dysfunction. For elders with physical disabilities, modifications in clothing that allow them to continue to dress attractively and in style may promote a positive sexuality. Other adaptations include changes in position for sexual intercourse and alternative sexual practices. Persons with cardiorespiratory disorders or musculoskeletal changes often find that changes in positions of sexual intercourse minimize energy expenditures and physical discomfort. The side-lying position with the couple facing each other is one position that decreases energy expenditure and promotes comfort. Another way to enhance sexual pleasure and decrease fatigue or energy expenditure is to engage in sexual activity when energy levels are high, for example, in the early morning after the couple is rested.

If sexual intercourse is not an available option, other sexual outlets such as mutual or self-masturbation, use of a vibrator, or oral/genital intercourse can be suggested for consideration. Elders who have lost a spouse or significant other as a sexual partner may need help in identifying alternative sexual outlets or meeting needs for intimacy and touch. Previously held attitudes and beliefs about alternative sexual outlets and sanctioned relationships must be explored before suggesting interventions. Sexual activity is not limited to sexual intercourse. Many elders find that being together, sleeping in the same bed, kissing, holding hands, or hugging promotes intimacy, sexual satisfaction, and a sense of well-being. Some sex therapists recommend body massage as a satisfactory alternative for providing touch, warmth, and intimacy. One widow stated, "Yeah, I'd like someone to go out with once in a while. Maybe even to hold my hand. But that's it. I don't want someone all over me."

Clients who have long-standing relationship problems or who have histories of dissatisfaction with sexual experiences may be helped to achieve more satisfactory life styles. It is important for the nurse to realize that elders who have not had a satisfactory sexual relationship in the past are able to change and achieve pleasurable sexual activity. The nurse may not have adequate preparation to deal with complex sexual problems but can be a resource person and refer clients to a certified sex therapist. Information on certified sex therapists can be obtained from the American Association of Sex Educators, Counselors, and Therapists, Washington, DC.

Evaluation

The criteria for evaluation are established during the planning and goal development stage of the nursing process. An evaluation criterion for the nursing diagnosis alterations in sexual pleasure is an increase in the level of sexual pleasure experienced by the client. Criteria for the short-term goals include the ability of the client to describe age-associated changes, the increase in the time spent in foreplay and the pleasure and comfort associated with that activity, the amount of vaginal lubrication resulting from foreplay, the use and correct application of lubricating jelly if vaginal lubrication does not occur from increased foreplay, and the level of physical comfort associated with intromission. Follow-up assessments need not only focus on the effectiveness of the interventions in meeting these criteria but also on the feelings and attitudes experienced by the client in relation to the interventions themselves and their outcomes. Short-term goals attained are evaluated in terms of progress toward the long-term goal. If any of the short-term goals are not met, the assessment will provide data on barriers that may have been present to interfere with goal attainment. During the evaluation process, it is necessary to avoid the implicit message that there has been a failure. It is during this stage that elders must be supported and the message reinforced that the time frame for change may be longer in elders than in younger age groups. Elders may find it difficult to state that goals have not been met and attempt to avoid discussion of the situation. Another area that elders may have difficulty discussing is dissatisfaction with the interventions. This may be due to a desire to protect the nurse from feeling badly because they did not like her suggested interventions. The nurse's attitudes may provide the encouragement for the elderly client to continue with current plans for care, adapt the interventions as needed, or lead the elder to give up on the goal. In working with issues of sexuality, it is important for the nurse to stress that the process is as important as the result.

Change in Living Arrangements

Elders living in long-term care institutions such as nursing homes and chronic disease hospitals have limited opportunities for sexual expression. Sexual activities require privacy, which clients in institutions have limited access to. Elders who are not interested in sexual relationships do not want to be confronted by the sexual behaviors of others. Staff members often feel that they should not have to provide opportunities for sexual activity or to be confronted by it when they enter a room. Although only about 5 per cent of elders live in nursing homes at any one point in time, approximately 20 per cent of all aged persons will spend some portion of their lives in a long-term care institution. Problems and concerns associated with sexuality of the institutionalized elderly are complicated by the perceived frailty of the population, the environment, and the organizational structure of the institution.

In 1974, a federal regulation was passed that stated, "the patient may associate and communicate privately with persons of his choice" (Federal Register, 1974). Some patient rights advocates interpreted this statement to mean that rooms should be set aside in institutions for residents to engage in sexual activity in private, but few institutions initiated any policies to carry out this regulation. Part of this reason for their failure to comply was the concern about ethicolegal problems as well as a lack of appreciation of the needs of elder residents by those associated with the institution. Although many elders are institutionalized because of alterations in cognitive functioning, they may still retain a need for intimacy and even sexual activity. It is unclear whether elders with cognitive dysfunction are capable of giving consent for sexual relations by legal definitions. There is a concern that these elders are at risk for sexual abuse by other residents or even a family member, notably a spouse.

One example may serve to highlight the dilemma. An elderly woman with mental retardation resided in a chronic disease hospital. She frequently tried to get in bed with another resident (male), who encouraged her actions. The staff of the hospital was torn between the recognition that this woman went to the other person's room apparently willingly and appeared to enjoy the experience and their concern that she was not competent to make decisions based on her level of cognitive impairment. They were also concerned about the legal liability associated with this woman's activities as well as the moral issues involved. Their concern for her centered on whether she was being taken advantage of by a person who was not as impaired as she. The situation is not unique and is faced by staff members in many institutions. What are the legal implications overlying the moral dimensions?

The courts are beginning to recognize that cognitive impairment due to either developmental or acquired disabilities is not sufficient grounds for mental incompetence in making treatment decisions. This is true even though the impaired person may be declared mentally incompetent for making other types of decisions. It would seem that if mental impairment does not preclude a client from making decisions about treatments that involve their physical health, it should not preclude their ability to make decisions about their sexual health. These questions have not been adequately addressed by either the gerontological literature or the legal system. There is little information in the research literature on sexuality in long-term care institutions except statements that it is an important topic and should be addressed.

Nurses can play a key role in long-term care settings through their acceptance of expressions of sexuality as a basic human need. Clients need a place where they can be alone or have privacy to meet with visitors. One way to meet this need, if there are no privacy rooms, is to place a "Do Not Disturb" sign on the closed door of a room when a resident has visitors. If the room is shared, the roommate can be asked to sit in another area for a while. If the roommate cannot or will not leave the area, curtains or screens should be placed around the bed area to provide privacy to those who request it.

A common question by those who work in long-term care institutions is what to do about the resident who masturbates or exposes his or her genitalia in public. These behaviors may be disconcerting, upsetting, or, as indicated by staff in one study, seriously disturbing (McCartney et al, 1987). Nursing staff and residents may respond to these behaviors with embarrassment and anger. The resident is often chastised publicly. Other residents and nurses begin to avoid the resident and prevent him or her from engaging in social activities because of their fear that the resident will publicly masturbate or expose him- or herself. Residents need to be included in the social world of the long-term care institution. Social deprivation only increases their isolation, leading to increased withdrawal, regression, and mental and physical impairments.

A positive approach to the resident who publicly masturbates or exposes him- or herself is to move the resident from the public area to a private area in a calm quiet manner without bringing attention to the incident. When the masturbatory activity ceases, the resident can be returned to the social or public activity and be included. The nurse's acceptance of the need for masturbation without accepting its public display can serve as a model for members of the staff and for the other residents. Discussions with other residents about their feelings and how they can help enables the residents to be more accepting of the person and more willing to continue including him or her in social activities.

Nurses can encourage men and women in long-term care institutions to congregate socially. Many nurses help elders to dress in attractive clothing and apply make-up and after-shave lotions as expressions of their sexuality. Expressions of intimacy, warmth, and caring can be promoted through the use of affective touch between residents and staff and among residents to whom it is acceptable. Family members who are concerned about an elder member's relationship with another resident can be helped to accept the elder's need for companionship. Living in an institutional setting does not take away the basic human needs for love and affection. Nurses can assume the role of resident advocate in issues of sexual relationships and behaviors.

SUMMARY

Sexuality is a holistic process that includes more than physical sexual behaviors. It becomes and remains an important part of self-identity throughout the life span. Changes associated with the aging process influence the way a person expresses his or her sex-

uality but not its existence. The nurse who is knowledgeable and accepting about sexuality in the aged serves as an advocate to enhance clients' ability to meet their needs for intimacy and sexual expression.

REFERENCES

Brecher E: Love, Sex, and Aging: A Consumer Union Report. Boston, Little, Brown, & Co, 1984.

Burnside IM: Sexuality and the older adult: Implications for nursing. In Burnside IM (ed): Sexuality and Aging. Los Angeles, University of Southern California Press, 1975.

Comfort A: Sex in Society. New York, Citadel, 1963.

Drescher VM, Gantt WH, Whitehead WE: Heart rate response to touch. Psychosom Med 42:559, 1980.

Eaton M, Mitchell-Bonair IL, Friedmann E: The effect of touch on nutritional intake of chronic organic brain syndrome patients. J Gerontol 41:611, 1986.

Eckert JW: Clinical perspectives on sexuality in older adults: Discussion. J Geriatr Psychiatry 17:183, 1984.

Erikson EH: Childhood and society. New York, WW Norton, 1963.

Fanslow CA: Therapeutic touch: A healing modality throughout life. Top Clin Nurs 5:72, 1983–84.

Federal Register. Skilled Nursing Facilities. 1974. 39:139, 1974.

Franks LK: Tactile stimulation. Genet Psychol Monogr 56:235, 1957.

Harp A: Intimacy and sexuality in the elderly: Discussion. J Geriatr Psychiatry 17:161, 1984.

Heidt P: Effect of therapeutic touch on anxiety level of hospitalized patients. Nurs Res 30:32, 1981.

Jefferis BG, Nichols, JI: Safe Counsel. Tulsa, Joseph Nichols, 1922.

Kaas M: Sexual expression of the elderly in nursing homes. Gerontologist 18:372, 1978.

Kinsey A, Pomeroy WB, Martin CE: Sexual Behavior in the Human Male. Philadelphia, WB Saunders, 1948.

Kinsey A, Pomeroy WB, Martin CE: Sexual Behavior in the Human Female. Philadelphia, WB Saunders, 1952.

Krieger D: Therapeutic touch: The imprimatur of nursing. AJN 75:784–787, 1975.

Lynch JI, Thomas SA, Mills M: The effects of human contact on cardiac arrythmia in coronary care patients. Heart Lung 88:160, 1974.

Maslow A (ed): Motivation and Personality. 2nd ed. New York, Harper & Row, 1970.

Masters WH, Johnson VE: Human Sexual Response. Boston, Little, Brown & Co, 1966.

McCartney JR, Izemon H, Rogers D, Cohen N: Sexuality and the institutionalized elderly. J Am Geriatr Soc 35:331, 1987.

Montagu A: Touching: The Human Significance of the Skin. New York, Columbia University Press, 1971.

Newman G, Nichols CR: Sexual activities and attitudes in older persons. JAMA 73:33, 1969.

Pfeiffer E: Behavior and Adaptation in Later Life. Boston, Little, Brown & Co, 1977.

Pfeiffer E, Davis GC: Determinants of sexual behavior in middle and old age. J Am Geriatr Soc 20:151, 1972.

Pfeiffer E, Verwoerdt A, Wang HS: Sexual behavior in aged men and women. Arch Gen Psychiatry 19:753, 1968.

Renshaw DC: Sex, age, and values. J Am Geriatr Soc 33:635, 1985.

Shippee RV: Touching and Pleasuring Behaviors in a Well Elderly Population. Master's thesis. Rochester, University of Rochester School of Nursing, 1979.

Shippee RV, Rice DW: A Conceptual Model of Sexuality. Presented at the American Association of Sex Educators, Counselors, and Therapists, March 1980.

Starr BD, Weiner MB: Sex and Sexuality in the Mature Years. Briarcliff Manor, Stein and Day, 1982.

Steinke EE, Bergen MB: Sexuality and aging. J Gerontol Nurs 12:6, 1986.

Swanson D: Minnie Remembers. Baltimore, Mass Media Ministries, 1976.

Sykes JB (ed): The Concise Oxford Dictory of Current English. Oxford, Oxford University Press, 1982.

Talbot F: Discussion. Transcript American Pediatric Society 62:469, 1941.

7: Gay and Lesbian Lifestyles

Barbara Nettles-Carlson

Until the mid 1970s, research and clinical information addressing the health needs of lesbians and gay men was almost nonexistent in medical and nursing texts and journals. Lesbians were especially ignored. Remarkably, a survey of 100 gynecologists indicated that over half had never knowingly treated a lesbian, and 90 per cent of those surveyed had knowingly treated three or less (Good, 1976). Until recent years most clinical and research data about homosexuality appeared in the psychiatric and social science literature. Not only were nonpsychiatric clinicians unlikely to read this literature, if they did, they were likely to receive a negative picture of gay people as tortured individuals who seek health care mostly for treatment of venereal diseases. Thankfully, this picture is changing, and articles in nursing journals and texts are now addressing the needs of gay people in a positive, holistic way (Laurence, 1975; Pogoncheff, 1979; Gillow & Davis, 1987; Olesker & Walsh, 1984; Brossart, 1979, 1982; Irish, 1983; Noyes, 1982; Nursing Grand Rounds, 1983; Hogan, 1985; Siemans and Brandzel, 1982; Woods, 1984). Nevertheless, the traditional health system as a whole retains a strong heterosexual bias.

According to Brossart (1982), there are several reasons for the failure of the traditional health care system to meet the special needs of lesbians and gay men, beginning with many providers' lack of awareness of gay men and lesbians in their patient population. Health professionals who are heterosexual may believe the traditional stereotypes of gay people and therefore may reflect in their practice the societal norm of nonacceptance of gays. In its extreme form, nonacceptance may be described as homophobia, i.e., an irrational intolerance and fear of same-sex sexual behavior (Woods, 1984). In addition, the lack of gay role models in the health care delivery system tends to foster homophobia, which in turn stimulates homosexual professionals and clients to remain invisible. Moreover, the emergence of the acquired immunodeficiency syndrome as a major public health problem may also foster homophobia among health professionals (Douglas, Kalman, and Kalman, 1985; Young, 1988). Understandably, gay men and lesbian women approach the traditional health care system with negative expectations. Many choose alternative services. Some delay care or rely heavily on self-help methods. What can be done to remedy this situation?

Improving the quality of health care for lesbians and gay men must begin with the health professional becoming more knowledgeable about homosexuality in the context of our society and with our being willing to examine critically the extent to which personal feelings, values, and stereotypes about gay people influence professional practice. Therefore, this chapter deals with the biopsychosocial issues surrounding homosexuality as much as with the clinical issues.

HOMOSEXUALITY AND SOCIETY

They gave me a medal for killing 10 men and 10 years for loving one. —*A gay male*

Few phenomena have been associated with as much social ambivalence, varieties of social control, and degree of public stereotyping as homosexuality. Being gay has been called a sin, a crime, an illness, a behavior disturbance, a way of life, and a normal variant of human sexual behavior (Bullough, 1979).

Incidence

Despite varying degrees of social control, homosexuality, as far as history shows, has always existed—in ancient Egypt, in the Tigris-Euphrates Valley, in ancient China, and in India. Modern anthropologists have observed homosexual behavior in many societies (Bullough, 1979). A classic cross-cultural and cross-species comparison of patterns of sexual behavior based on reports from 190 primitive societies and extensive zoological observations suggested that homosexuality, while never the predominant type of sexual activity for adults in any society or in any species, may be an inherent biological tendency in mammals and humans (Ford and Beach, 1951).

Whitam (1983) offers some tentative general conclusions about homosexuality and society based on an extensive review of the cross-cultural literature as well as his field work in male homosexual communities in the United States, Guatemala, Brazil, and the Philippines.

1. Homosexuals appear in all societies.

2. The percentage of homosexuals in all societies seems to be the same and remains stable over time.

3. Social norms do not impede or facilitate the emergence of homosexual orientation.

4. Homosexual subcultures appear in all societies, given sufficient aggregates of people.

5. Homosexuals in different societies tend to resemble each other with respect to certain behavioral interests and occupational choices.

6. All societies produce similar continua from overtly masculine to overtly feminine homosexuals (Whitam, 1983, p 209).

Since not all societies were in Whitams study, he may have overgeneralized by claiming universality in his conclusions. Nevertheless, the study is provocative and offers evidence that same-sex orientation is not a creation of social structure but is rather a fundamental form of human sexuality, acted out in different cultural settings.

The landmark studies of Alfred Kinsey and his associates (1948, 1953) provide the first scientific estimates of the incidence of homosexual behavior in the United States. A nonrandom sample of 5537 males and 5608 females, most of whom were white and college educated, were interviewed about many aspects of their sexual behavior. About 38 per cent of males and 13 per cent of females reported at least one homosexual experience. About 11 per cent of males and 4 per cent of females reported extensive homosexual experience—21 or more partners and/or 51 or more experiences (Gebhard and Johnson, 1979). These responses indicate that homosexual experiences are more common than anyone, including the researchers, had previously thought.

Throughout history ambivalence has marked societal and religious attitudes toward same-sex sexual behavior. For example, the Greeks idealized love between an older male mentor and a younger male student, while the ancient Jews had strong scriptural sanctions against sex between males. The earliest specific mention of same-sex sexual behavior in the Bible is in Leviticus 18:22: "You shalt not lie with a man as with a woman: That is an abomination" (King James Version).

Sociologists differ with regard to the influence of religion on public attitudes toward same-sex orientation. Bullough (1976, 1979) asserts that religion has been the most important historical force shaping negative Western attitudes. Other historical analyses (Boswell, 1980; Greenberg and Bystryn, 1982) argue, however, that sanctions against homosexuality as a life style was not a major tenet of Judeo-Christian theology. Rather, early scriptural prohibitions had to do with avoiding sexual excesses and conserving male sperm. Same-sex affection was not proscribed, and biblical accounts praise the deep devotion of David and Jonathan and Ruth and Naomi. Boswell (1980) concludes that strong religious attitudes against same-sex sexual behavior began with the emergence of corporate states in the Middle Ages and reflected increased societal intolerance of all minority groups by both secular and religious institutions.

Intolerance of homosexuality may be viewed as one example of society's response to deviance from normative sexual behavior. In this century, social control mechanisms have extended to persecution, as in Germany between 1933 and 1945, when a kiss or embrace between males became a felony (Lesbianism was ignored as being of no consequence!), and death was the penalty for members of the same sex caught in homosexual activity. A record or conviction of homosexuality led to the concentration camp, where gays were identified by a pink trianglar insignia. Pink-triangle prisoners more frequently had difficult work assignments, a higher death rate, and lower survival rate upon release than did other political prisoners (Lautmann, 1981).

Throughout history, with few exceptions, lesbians have been either ignored or tolerated, while male homosexuals have received most of the condemnation. According to Bullough, "This double standard may have existed so long because the males who have dominated the writing of history and the making of laws have assumed that women were nothing without men, and that no sex could take place without a penis involved" (Bullough, 1979, p 3).

How do we respond to homosexuality today? Current attitudinal research as well as changes in the official stance of various groups and institutions indicates that as a society we are in a period of relative tolerance, though not full acceptance, of gay people.

Public Opinion

A 1982 national Gallup poll indicated that a majority of Americans (59 per cent) believed homosexuals should have the same job opportunities as heterosexuals. However, an almost equal number (51 per cent) were opposed to hiring homosexuals as elementary school teachers or clergy. These findings suggest that the issue of equal job rights for gays is conditional and influenced by stereotypical fears. According to the same poll, about one quarter of the American public accepted gays on legal, moral, and social grounds. This group was largely college educated, young (age 18 to 29), Catholic, living in the east or far western United States, and, to a slightly lesser degree, female. Another one quarter of the adults sampled were intolerant of gays. Heavily represented in this group were those age 50 and older, persons with an elementary education, Protestants, and Southerners. The remaining one half of Americans were ambivalent. The largest portion of this group,

representing about one fourth of the public, reportedly found homosexuality morally and legally acceptable but felt it was not a socially acceptable alternative life style (Gallup Report, 1982).

Religion

In answer to the question, "In your opinion, can a homosexual be a good Christian or a good Jew, or not?" 53 per cent of the adult population said yes, 32 per cent said no, and 15 per cent had no opinion. These figures were virtually unchanged since the 1977 national Gallup poll, indicating no recent change in the public's mixed feelings about religion and homosexuality. Individual ministers and laypersons have advocated for gay rights, and Quakers were one of the first groups to support gay rights publicly. The emergence of organizations such as Dignity, for gay Catholics, and Integrity, for gay Episcopalians, indicates a degree of denominational recognition, as do positive statements on homosexuality from the Episcopalians, Unitarians, Universalists, Presbyterians, and Lutherans. Fundamentalist groups, however, remain strongly antihomosexual (Moses and Hawkins, 1982).

Law

A full discussion of homosexuality and the law is beyond the scope of this chapter. However, because of the importance of laws as indicators of public attitudes, a few examples of legal inequities will be given. Today, in the United States, private consensual sexual activities between adults of the same sex are criminal offenses in 29 states. The laws range from prohibition of sodomy to forbidding "gross indecencies between two men" and "gross indecencies between two women." These "crimes" are often felonies punishable by up to 20 years in prison (Rivera, 1982). It is important to note that a criminal record can justify the refusal to hire or the denial of apartment rental, professional licensure, or admittance to the military. Since 1949 the armed forces have had a clear policy of discharging men or women discovered to be gays or lesbians. Although this issue is presently being litigated, known homosexuals may still be denied entrance to the military and may be discharged upon discovery (National Gay Task Force, 1988; Rivera, 1982). The areas of life in which homosexuals face discrimination are multiple and include employment (especially teachers), child custody rights, and immigration. Inequitable laws and regulations, though often not enforced, tend to legitimate public stereotypes and reinforce other kinds of discrimination against homosexuals.

Health Professionals

What are the attitudes of health professionals toward homosexuality? Medicine has long been dominated by the psychoanalytic model of homosexuality as either a disease or a deficiency (Weinberg, 1973; Moses and Hawkins, 1982; Nass, Libby and Fisher, 1984). Until 1974, the diagnostic manual of the American Psychiatric Association (APA) classified homosexuality as a mental disorder, and negative attitudes of mental health professionals, including psychiatric nurses, have been well documented in the literature (White, 1979).

The present picture is encouraging, however. Recent policy statements, official publications, and the professional literature reflect a marked trend toward viewing homosexual behavior as a sexual variant not necessarily requiring any intervention (Committee on Adolescence, American Academy of Pediatrics, 1983; Gonsiorek; 1988, Council on Scientific Affairs, American Medical Association, 1982; Brossart, 1982; National Institutes of Mental Health, 1976). Acceptance among clinicians, however, is by no means universal (Douglas, Kalman, and Kalman, 1985). The APA vote to remove homosexuality from the diagnostic nomenclature was won by a narrow margin only after heated debate within the organization and strong political pressure from gay activists (Bayer, 1981).

The topic of health professionals' attitudes will be discussed further, from the client's point of view, in the section Homosexuals and the Health Care System.

DEFINITIONS AND LABELS

Both gays and straights must stop thinking of homosexuals as primarily sexual beings. Everyone, gay or straight, is several things before he or she is gay or straight. I'm a human first, then a man, then a teacher, then a Christian, then an American, a political liberal, and a lover before I'm gay. Heterosexuals are guilty of pointless bigotry, of course, but we homosexuals should take our minds off our genitals long enough to achieve the wholeness and harmony characteristics of well-integrated personalities (Spada, 1979, p 301).

Homosexuality has been defined in multiple ways—on the basis of fantasy content, erotic preference, overt behavior, and self-reported homosexual identity. Kinsey (1948) suggested a compromise that took into account both the degree of *preference* for partners of one's own gender and the degree of sexual *activity* with those of one's own gender. He devised a useful scale of sexual orientation ranging from exclusive heterosexual response/experience (0) to exclusive homosexual response/experience (6). Bisexuals, who describe themselves as relating sexually to both sexes, fall into the middle range between 2 and 4 on the Kinsey scale (Fig. 7–1). Other writers use the term "obligatory" to describe exclusive erotic same-sex orientation and the term "situational" to describe homosexual relationships that develop in same-sex environments such as prisons, boarding schools, and the military (Ovesey, 1969; Socarides, 1970).

For the purposes of this chapter, a definition of Judd Marmor and Richard Green, psychiatrists who have researched and published extensively in the field of human sexuality, will be generally used. Acknowledging the multiplicity of definitions, they proposed as a working definition that homosexuality be described as "a strong preferential attraction to members of the same sex" (Marmor and Green, 1977, p 1052). However, in this text, the term 'orientation' will be used rather than 'preference' to avoid the implication of choice associated with the latter term.

Even those persons who openly acknowledge their same-sex orientation and activities differ in the labels they prefer for themselves. Some prefer the word "homophile," which comes from two Greek words, meaning "same-loving." They feel this word avoids the narrowly explicit sexual meaning of "homosexual" (Spada, 1979). Among women who predate the gay liberation movement, the terms "homosexual" and "female homosexual" are often used. Many younger women prefer "lesbian" because of its exclusively female associations, indicating solidarity with the women's movement and separation from gay males (Nass, Libby, Fisher, 1984). "Gay"

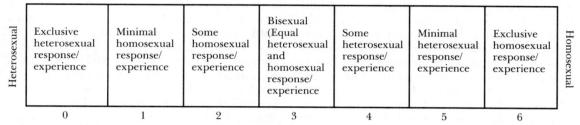

FIGURE 7–1. Kinsey continuum of heterosexuality-homosexuality. (From Sexual Choices: An Introduction to Human Sexuality. 2nd ed, by GD Nass, RW Libby, and MP Fisher. Copyright 1984, 1981 by Wadsworth, Inc. Reprinted by permission of Wadsworth Health Sciences Division, Monterey, California 93940.)

is still commonly used as a generic term referring to both male and female homosexuals. For many females, however, this term is a reflection of historic male dominance, analagous to using "mankind" to refer to all humans. Probably the most widely used and accepted terms today are lesbian and gay male. Bisexuals often refer to themselves as being "bi."

Labeling includes at least two elements: how we label ourselves and how others label us. "Coming out" is an example of self-labeling; it is important to consider the degree to which an individual has defined his or her own sexual orientation. For example, a study of men who were both fathers and gay distinguishes among *trade* (furtively engaging in homosexual acts but considering themselves heterosexual), *homosexual* (seeing themselves as gay but trying to maintain a heterosexual public image), *gay men* (revealing their preferences only to a small audience such as the gay community), and *publicly gay men* (acknowledging their homosexuality to everyone) (Nass, Libby, Fisher, 1984).

How others label us may be illustrated by our responses when individuals fail to conform to gender role expectations. Effeminate men and aggressive women are often assumed to be gay. In a study on perceptions regarding male and female homosexuals, 103 adults in a randomly drawn sample were asked to rate the prevalence of a number of personality attributes in "men," "women," "male homosexuals," and "lesbians." Respondents described male homosexuals as "needful of others approval, not runners of the show, helpful to others, expressive of tender feelings." Lesbians were described in the opposite terms. In this study persons labeled as homosexual were those who exhibited characteristics *opposite* to their expected gender role, suggesting that labeling and stereotyping of homosexuals as behaving like the opposite sex still exists (Taylor, 1983).

A growing body of research clearly contradicts these stereotypes (Bell and Weinberg, 1978; Masters and Johnson, 1979; Ross, 1983). Bell (1975), in a wide-ranging discussion of the homosexual as client, argues that there is no such thing as "the homosexual," and little can be predicted about an individual based on this label.

Although definitions may be necessary, and sometimes useful, it is well to recognize their arbitrariness. The task of the helping professional is to put aside labels and to relate to each person as an individual.

ORIGINS OF HOMOSEXUALITY

The origins of homosexuality remain as cloudy as the various definitions and labels that are applied to homosexual behavior. Attempts to find a single reason for the emergence of homosexual orientation in some people and heterosexual orientation in others remain inconclusive. There is a recent trend toward an interaction model, acknowledging the mutual influence of biological, psychological, and sociological factors responsible for the emergence of sexual preference. Most theories of development and research efforts, however, fall somewhere along the nature/nurture continuum, with some writers favoring biological and others psychosocial variables.

Research Bias

Our understanding of homosexuality is limited not only by its complexity but also by several research problems (Nass, Libby, Fisher, 1984). Obvious sources of bias occur when researchers apply normative societal values such as heterosexual behavior and male dominance. Heterosexual bias has been documented in much psychological research (Morin, 1977), which uses the mental illness model to study homosexuality. The dominance of male norms is evident in the paucity of research on female homosexuality. Further, gays in some studies do not constitute representative samples. For example, subjects in a number of studies have been either psychiatric clients or members of homophile societies, neither of which represents a cross-section of the homosexual population.

The wide occurrence of homosexuality throughout the human species and in animals suggests a biological basis. Freud himself believed all persons were inherently capable of a bisexual response, which seemed to him to be a natural part of the developmental process leading toward adult heterosexuality. He found evidence for this in childhood same-sex explorations and "crushes" as well as in homosexual fantasies in the dreams of heterosexual adults (1953).

The observation that many homosexual adults recall childhood awareness of their emotional same-sex orientations also invites a biological explanation. A study involving pairs of monozygotic male twins (Kallmann, 1952) suggested strongly that if one twin is homosexual the other will be, too. Although Kallmann's methodology has been criticized, the conclusions remain provocative. Pillard, Paunadere, and Carretta (1982) found that in both twin and family history studies homosexual subjects have more homosexual siblings than do heterosexual subjects. They also found that in a pilot study of 36 male homosexuals 25 per cent of the brothers of subjects were homosexual or strongly bisexual but that this was true of only 6 per cent of the sisters of subjects.

Other researchers have investigated biochemical causes of homosexuality. Levels of testosterone, androgen, and estrogen have been compared in male homosexuals and heterosexuals with conflicting and inconclusive results (Kolodny, 1971; Pillard, Rose, and Sherwood, 1974; Doerr, 1973; Dorner, 1975). Endocrine studies of female homosexuals have been practically nonexistent (Marmor and Green, 1977).

A promising area of biological research involves prenatal hormone influences. There is some evidence to suggest that prenatal sex steroid levels might effect postnatal behavior.

For example, a young female rhesus monkey exposed in utero to testosterone was born with a penis and subsequently behaved more like a male than a female, i.e., became a "tomboy" monkey (Young, 1964). Similarly, in humans, females born with adrenogenital syndrome have been found to be more "tomboyish" than normal controls (Ehrhard and Baker, 1974). A study of 10 boys with idiopathic adolescent gynecomastia found an increased association with homosexual behavior as compared with a control group. The researchers argue that common biological prenatal factors may be precursors of both (Money and Lewis, 1982).

Many childhood psychosocial factors have been linked with the later development of homosexuality. These include abnormal parental relationships, early negative or traumatic sex experiences, disturbed gender identity, cross-gender dress and play activities, and disturbed peer group relationships. It is important to remember that until recent years theories about the origins of homosexuality have been based largely on data derived from samples of adult homosexuals seeking psychiatric treatment. The work of Freud is a case in point. Freud viewed homosexuality as arrested psychosexual development in the clients he treated, resulting from the individual's failure, in early childhood, to achieve identification with the same-sex parent. Freud's theories of psychosexual development set the direction for the medical model of the treatment of homosexuality as a mental illness. In all fairness to Freud, it should be said that his attitudes toward the homosexual individual were much more accepting and tolerant than he is usually given credit for today. In a letter written in 1935 in response to a worried mother of a son who was homosexual, Freud reassured her, "Homosexuality is assuredly no advantage, but nothing to be ashamed of, no vice, no degradation; it cannot be classified as an illness: we consider it to be a variation of the sexual functions produced by a certain *arrest of sexual development*" (Freud, 1951).

Psychosocial theories about the causes of homosexuality based on research with psychiatric clients were further developed by the work of Irving Bieber. For example, in one study Bieber (1962) found that a majority of neurotic homosexual clients had seductive, overprotective mothers and weak, detached or hostile fathers. Neurotic heterosexual clients might have had similar family histories. However, Bieber's and similar studies had no comparison groups. The research of Evelyn Hooker (1957) was a landmark in a move away from the mental illness model because she was the first to compare normal (i.e., not in therapy) homosexual and heterosexual males on various psychological scales. Her conclusions and those of subsequent researchers indicate that homosexuals are no more likely to be psychologically maladjusted than heterosexuals (Hooker, 1957; Wilson, 1982; Harry, 1983; Siegelman, 1972).

Some social scientists have tried to explain homosexuality as a reaction to early negative personal experiences such as learned fear of the other sex based on abuse or rape. Even though such events may contribute to some person's homosexual orientation, research in this area has not supplied evidence to support a causal relationship. (Nass, Libby, and Fisher, 1984).

A considerable body of research has established a correlation between homosexuality, gender identity disorders, and cross-gender behaviors in childhood. These include childhood play activities, "tomboy" and "sissy" designations by parents and peers, and cross-dressing. Many adult gay males report having exhibited during childhood a variety of interests and orientations characteristic of girls (Bullough, Bullough, and Smith, 1985). Lesbians also report childhood cross-gender behavior, though not as marked. The difference may be due to the fact that being a "tomboy" is more socially acceptable than being a "sissy" and thus may not be remembered or brought to the attention of a clinician (Green, 1974, 1975, 1979; Grellert, 1982; Harry, 1983; Whitam, 1977).

The controversy between nature and nurture rages on. In a 1981 retrospective study sponsored by the Kinsey Institute and based on interviews with 979 homosexual and 477 heterosexuals of both sexes, adult sexual orientation showed no consistent linkage to early childhood experiences or parental or peer relationships. The researchers concluded that the only possible explanation for homosexual behavior rests with as yet unknown biological factors (Bell and Weinberg, 1981). Herman (1983) calls for an interaction theory such as that proposed by Green (1979) in which biological and psychological and social factors could be viewed as affecting each other and the child as development proceeds.

THE GAY EXPERIENCE: A LIFE CYCLE APPROACH

I'm not a "lesbian" mother! I pay the nursery bills, and I take the baby to the doctor, and he's had the chicken pox, and he's been in the hospital. And when it all happens, you don't hold him in your arms and think "I'm a lesbian mother." You think, "That's my child, and I love him." (Nass, Libby, and Fisher, 1984, p 167)

As human beings, we are united by a great many common experiences and events. By and large, a major difference between the homoerotic and the heteroerotic experience of life events seems to be the impact of deviation from social roles and norms and the corresponding lack of any social script to express homosexual orientation. Instead of trying to explain the causes of homosexuality (often with the assumption that homosexuals are heterosexuals gone awry), many social scientists are now interested in how gay men and lesbians experience life events and processes. These include role models, intimate roles and relationships, coming out, parenthood, health and illness, aging, and the impact of the gay liberation movement.

Role Models

There are few role models for gay people, and those available are typically either famous or notorious. "Average" gay people who could serve as role models rarely disclose their sexual orientation publicly. This means that anyone who grows up or becomes gay is unlikely to know how to go about being gay in the same way a nongay person knows how to go about being a heterosexual. There are nongay models for the roles of wife, mother, husband, lover, and father and for nongay male and female behavior toward people of the same and opposite gender. No comparable models exist for gays. Therefore, many gays follow the nongay model in public and develop a second identity when they are around other gays (Moses and Hawkins, 1982).

Early Awareness

For females, there is often a gap of a year or more between recognizing that one may be a lesbian and acting on that belief by having sex with a woman; the average age for the latter is 20 or 21 years. Affectionate relationships with women may become sexual but are not defined as such. For females, more so than for males, heterosexual sex may precede or be concurrent with lesbian relationships; however, these women report their principal emotional attraction is toward other women. They recognize, nonetheless, that a lesbian identity may mean denial of major cultural goals for females: marriage and parenthood (Wolf, 1979).

For males, homosexual activity usually begins earlier, at about age 14, and more frequently excludes previous heterosexual contact. Nevertheless, many males who participate in these activities do not label themselves homosexual. Instead, they classify their behavior as "masculine." Some common patterns are maintaining a dominant but emotionally uninvolved role, pretending that one is only responding to another's desires, seeing sex with males as a phase one will outgrow, and believing that one is experiencing the sexual expression of a unique love or special friendship (Saghir and Robins, 1973; Tripp, 1976). Compared with females, males report greater difficulty accepting homosexual behaviors in themselves or in others. The reason may be that feeling masculine is a major element in male self-esteem. Because homosexuality is popularly defined as *impaired* masculinity, it threatens the self-esteem of those acknowledging their homosexual orientation (Nash, Libby, and Fisher, 1984).

Coming Out

Given the risks of acknowledging one's homosexual identity (even to oneself), it is not surprising that the average lesbian and gay male, except in a few urban areas or tolerant communities, remains rather invisible. Several researchers have identified sequential landmarks in the "coming out" process. These are initial awareness of same-sex attraction, same-sex acts, self-designation as homosexual, initial involvement in a long-term relationship, self-disclosures to significant others, and acquiring a positive gay identity (Dank, 1971; DeMonteflores and Schultz, 1978; Kus, 1985).

A study of 199 self-defined male homosexuals (McDonald, 1982) will be reported in some detail because it also illustrates the diversity of individual experiences within the overall linear pattern of coming out. Participants reported an awareness of same-sex feelings at an average age of 13, with first sexual experiences and understanding of the word homosexual occurring simultaneously on average 2 years later. Self-labeling occurred 4 years later at an average age of 19. Disclosure of sexual orientation to a significant nongay person took place at age 23, 4 years after self-labeling. It is noteworthy that 10 per cent of the sample (mean age 31) had never disclosed their sexual orientation to anyone other than another known gay person. Respondents also reported acquiring a positive gay identity (i.e., were glad to be gay) at age 24, an average 5 years after self-labeling. Also of note is that 15 per cent of the sample had not acquired a positive gay identity. Other significant findings included 18 per cent who labeled themselves homosexual in the absence of any overt same-sex experience and 23 per cent who adopted homosexual self-definitions only after a long-term relationship with another man (McDonald, 1982).

Persons who are homosexual may experience coming out in a variety of ways, from profound relief to intense anxiety. The concept of coming out can be broadly understood as giving up a neurosis, dropping a façade, or, in Jungian terms, removing the mask, or "persona," which is our public face (Fordham, 1982).

In one sense we are all in the process of either coming out or going back into our closets. To live as social human beings we constantly resort to wearing various facades. Only in relatively few situations can we truly be open, spontaneous and honest with ourselves. (Gershman, 1983, p 129)

Unfortunately, the dilemma of whether and when to drop the "persona" is magnified many times for the homosexual person in our society.

Intimate Relationships

For a long time, psychiatrists and the general public thought that homosexual relationships were either pathetic caricatures of conventional masculine and feminine roles or furtive, brief, and purely sexual encounters. In the past decade a growing body of research has largely debunked these myths.

Bell and Weinberg (1978) in a study of homosexual individuals (574 males and 227 females) found that about one third of males and one half of the females were coupled in quasimarital relationships. "Close-coupled" pairs had few sexual problems, high psychological adjustment, and little regret about being homosexual. Overall, gay males were more likely than females to have brief and frequent sexual encounters. In the Bell and Weinberg study, 84 per cent of the males but only 7 per cent of the females had more than 50 partners. In a study of 1000 gay males of all ages and background, 90 per cent of the respondents preferred sex with affection; the majority considered the ideal human relationship as having a best friend with whom one can also have sex (Spada, 1979).

Friendship and sexual fidelity seem to be more typical of lesbian than gay male relationships. Frequently, the first significant same-sex love relationship grows out of friendship, and there is an overlap between self-definitions of "friend" and "lover" (Peplau 1982; Vetere, 1982). Satisfaction in lesbian relationships has been associated with equality in both power and involvement (Peplau, Padesky, and Hamilton, 1982). Finally, although some lesbians and gay men report patterns of behavior that resemble conventional gender roles (i.e., in division of housework, sexual expression, decision-making), homosexual couples generally exhibit and value androgyny in their relationships (Jones and DeCecco, 1982; Maracek, Finn, and Cardell, 1982; Peplau, 1982; Harry, 1983).

Sexual Behavior

For many heterosexuals, there is an aura of mystery and taboo surrounding homosexual acts. The assumption is that by not having genital parts that naturally "fit" together, homosexuals must be limited in their choices or else do some unusual things. Actually, homosexuals do many of the same things heterosexuals do. Males and females engage in mutual masturbation. Cunnilingus is a favorite technique of lesbians, fellatio and anal intercourse for gay males. Partners typically share insertor and insertee roles, although one role may be preferred by a particular partner (Nass, Libby, and Fisher, 1984).

Masters and Johnson (1979) in their laboratory observations of sexual response found no physiological differences in the sexual response of homosexuals and heterosexuals.

A major behavioral difference they did find was that the homosexual couples they observed spent more time in the arousal phase of the sexual act. Both males and females seemed to enjoy prolonging pleasure rather than racing toward orgasm. Homosexuals may have sex problems just like heterosexuals; Masters and Johnson (1979) concluded that sexual problems among homosexuals can and should be treated with the same psychotherapeutic techniques, professional personnel, and objectivity with which heterosexual dysfunctions are treated.

Parenthood

Lesbians and gay men who are or want to be parents face many legal and social difficulties. Coming out may mean loss of parental rights. The courts have repeatedly ruled that a mother will lose custody and visiting privileges if she lives with a female partner, is affiliated with a lesbian community, or discloses her lesbianism to her children (Rand, Graham, and Rawlings, 1982). The evidence on whether children raised by a gay parent are more likely to be gay is inconclusive. Case reports and uncontrolled studies suggest that children raised by lesbian and transsexual parents have an appropriate psychosexual development and a heterosexual orientation (Green, 1978). There is some evidence suggesting that being a single parent, rather than being gay, may be more of a psychiatric risk factor for the child (Golombok, Spencer, and Rutter, 1983). Both lesbian and gay male parents have reported feelings of acceptance upon disclosing their sexual preference to their children, and there is no evidence that homosexuals are less effective as parents than heterosexuals. Overall, there is a lack of data to support the present social and legal limitations on gay parenthood (Hanscombe, 1983; Hotvedt and Mandel, 1982).

Developmental Issues

Aging presents some special problems for gay people. If a couple is in a long-term relationship, and one partner is institutionalized, the other may not be recognized as family or even receive full visiting privileges. When one partner dies, there may be little social support for the bereaved partner. The birth family may claim inheritance and property rights despite will provisions to the contrary (Kelly, 1980).

Youth is highly valued in the gay male subculture; the stereotype of the pathetically effeminate old queen still persists. One study of elderly gay women and men reported that the males were more concerned than females over loss of physical attractiveness. Both sexes reported that their closest friend was of the same gender. They also reported active involvement with family members, including children, and community groups. Loneliness is a problem for many but perhaps no more so than for the elderly in general.

Gay Liberation

The emergence of the gay liberation movement within the broad stream of the civil rights and women's movements has profoundly influenced the experience of many gay people. It has promoted public acceptance, helped gays have a more positive self-image, and perhaps most important called public attention to many forms of discrimination that were formerly hidden. The role of gay activists in institutional change should not be underestimated. One major example is the removal of homosexual orientation per se from the psychiatric taxonomy (Bayer, 1981).

Another recent aspect of gay liberation is increased public disclosure by gays in all walks of life, beginning with the formation of homophile societies: the Mattachine Society in 1950 and the Daughters of Bilitis in 1955. In more recent years some gay persons in the health professions have chosen to identify themselves openly. There are now gay groups within the ranks of medicine, nursing, public health, psychology, and social work. It should be emphasized, however, that the majority of homosexuals, in and out of professions, prefer to remain unidentified.

HOMOSEXUALS AND THE HEALTH CARE SYSTEM

Homosexuals as Health Care Professionals

As in other institutions in our society, gay men and lesbians in the health professions tend to be largely invisible. Considering the longstanding illness model of homosexuality, it is not surprising that most remain undisclosed to their colleagues and patients. A substantial minority of Americans (38 per cent) still believe that homosexuals should not be hired as doctors (Gallup Report, 1982). The public perception of nursing as an appropriate occupation for gay people was not investigated in this study. Since nursing is so strongly identified with females, public opinion is probably more favorable toward lesbians, and perhaps gay men, in nursing than in medicine.

The homosexual health professional's invisibility is based on the need for self-protection, avoidance of harassment, or possible loss of employment. For some, public disclosure is worth the risk (Messer, 1975). It is sad that potential gay role models among nurses and physicians are still so few (Brossart, 1982). In "Glad to be Gay?" a nurse gives a moving account of his development as a gay person and his decision not to reveal his sexual orientation (1983).

Homosexuals As Clients

In recent years, several studies have been reported exploring health care utilization patterns and attitudes, experiences, and perceptions of homosexual persons toward their primary health professionals (Dardick, 1980; Reagan, 1981; Johnson et al, 1981). The results of these studies, while preliminary, have direct implications for nursing care and will be discussed in some detail.

Dardick (1980) surveyed 622 individuals via a questionnaire sent to subscribers to a gay newspaper. The respondents were predominantly male (73 per cent), white (91 per cent), young (78 per cent were between 22 and 41 years old), urban (68 per cent), and well educated (73 per cent had college degrees). Most had received some medical care during the past year, and 91 per cent identified that they had an identified care provider. Of these, 69 per cent designated a physician and 19 per cent a nurse practitioner as their health professional.

Only half of Dardick's sample group had explicitly identified themselves as homosexual to their health professional, and another 11 per cent assumed their professional knew. The feeling of having dealt with a prejudiced health professional was common, especially among women. The commonest answer to an open-ended question on improving overall health care was related to overcoming such prejudice. Specifically, respondents suggested that health professionals avoid not only explicit but also implicit expressions of prejudice, such as assuming the need for birth control during a routine examination. Not surprisingly, the feeling that a prior professional was prejudiced was associated with a current preference for a same-sex or declared homosexual provider. The primary reason given by 70 per cent of the 356 who preferred a homosexual professional was comfort and ease of communication (Dardick, 1980).

Factors associated with coming out to one's health professional included being male, being exclusively homosexual, having come out to family and peers, and perceiving that the health professional's attitude toward homosexuality was supportive. Those who disclosed their gay identity were much more satisfied with their health professionals and rated them as more medically competent. For men, there was an association between quality of medical care received and having come out to the professional. Specifically, three quarters of those who had been explicitly open received venereal disease screening compared with less than half (44 per cent) of those who had not.

Reagan (1981) conducted an exploratory study of the relationships and attitudes of 38 lesbians to the health professionals they had seen during the previous 2 years. The author recruited subjects from a local gay discotheque, from a lesbian organization, and from among her students. Twenty-nine of the women reported delay in obtaining care for symptoms because of apprehension concerning their sexual orientation. Only 13 women had come out to their professional; of those who had, the most common reason was that counseling about relationships had required some disclosure. For those who had come out, the health professionals' responses to being informed were more positive than the subjects had expected. This finding implies that an active effort on the part of the professional to acknowledge the lesbian client might overcome fears and promote increased trust and communication. Whether the examination was physical or psychological, lesbians were more comfortable with a woman professional. Regardless of the sex of the professional, the pelvic examination and counseling were most stressful because of the presumption by the professional that the client was heterosexual.

Johnson and associates (1981) conducted a larger exploratory study of lesbian women's health care utilization, their gynecological and obstetrical problems, and their attitudes toward physicians. They surveyed 117 women, again recruited from a local lesbian organization. One hundred were exclusively homosexual and 15 bisexual. The majority were white, educated, and between 19 and 59 years old. Most were highly satisfied with their sexual orientation. With regard to frequency and regularity of gynecological care, about half had yearly physical examinations while 53 per cent sought care only when problems arose. Physicians were the most frequent source of care, although a substantial minority (20 per cent) used alternative services exclusively. Forty per cent of the group thought their present care would be adversely affected if their physicians knew of their sexual orientation. Of importance, a majority said they would be more likely to disclose their sexual orientation if they were assured that it would not be made part of the medical record. Ninety-four per cent would prefer a female homosexual physician if one were available.

In addition to these studies more recent reports also indicate that health professionals' attitudes toward homosexuals are still a major concern to the respondents (Smith, Johnson, and Guenther, 1985; Raymond, 1988). The extent to which the lack of openness between professional and client affects quality of medical treatment is unclear, although intuitively one would suspect there to be an association. Furthermore, these studies may overestimate the openness of homosexual men and women with their health professionals, given that most subjects had come out to some extent in gay organizations. It seems reasonable that given nonjudgmental professionals and assurance of confidentiality, many homosexual clients would prefer to disclose themselves, thereby receiving more individualized, quality care.

Health Problems

By and large, gay men and lesbians seek health care for the same types of problems heterosexual people do. Homosexual people have colds, get the flu, break bones, and develop high blood pressure. There are, however, some specific medical problems that are related to male homosexual behavior or that have a greater prevalance in a male homosexual population.

Gay men tend, as a group, to have more sexual contacts than heterosexual persons and as a result have a higher incidence of sexually transmitted diseases, including anal and oral gonorrhea, herpes, and syphilis. Shigellosis, amebiasis, and giardiasis also are more prevalent among gay man than in the general population (Mintz and Drew, 1983; Webster, 1983). Other problems related to anal intercourse can include proctitis, rectal trauma, foreign bodies in the rectum; and hepatitis A and B (Council on Scientific Affairs, 1982; Barone, 1983; Goodell, 1983). Knowledge of a client's sexual history and current behavior can help the clinician in considering client needs and medical diagnoses that might otherwise be overlooked (Owen, 1986).

Acquired immunodeficiency syndrome (AIDS) is an obvious and tragic medical problem that has been primarily associated with male homosexuals. As of May 1988, physicians and health departments in the United States had notified the Centers for Disease Control (CDC) of 60,852 clients meeting the case definition for national reporting (CDC, 1988). The human immunodeficiency virus (HIV) is transmitted through exchange of saliva or semen during sexual contacts, by parenteral exposure to blood or blood products, and from mother to child during the perinatal period.

For a complete discussion of AIDS, the reader is referred to Chapter 23. It is important to point out here that homosexual clients now face an added stigma because of the AIDS epidemic and the often irrational fears of both the public and health professionals (Bayer, 1983; Nursing Grand Rounds, 1983). The CDC has investigated occupational transmission of HIV infection and confirmed that the risk of transmission to health care workers from clients is extremely low (CDC, 1985; 1987a). CDC has also published recommendations for prevention of HIV transmission in health care settings (CDC, 1987b).

In contrast to gay men, lesbians do not experience increased health risks associated with sex practices. In fact, the classical sexually transmitted diseases, gonorrhea, syphilis, and herpes, are rare among lesbians. *Candida vaginitis* may be transmitted between female partners, and therefore both partners should be treated. Johnson (1981) documented three cases of trichomoniasis among lesbians who reported exclusive homosexual contact at the time. The incidence of cervical dysplasia in this study was low (1 per cent) and was limited to bisexual women. Compared with heterosexual women, lesbians as a group have a theoretically lower risk of cervical cancer due to less sexual contact with men and others carrying sexually transmitted diseases. Theoretically, they have a possibly higher risk of breast and ovarian cancer due to lower parity (Brossart, 1982).

Other health differences between lesbians and heterosexual women include fewer contraceptive and pregnancy-related needs and a greater demand for artifical insemination (Brossart, 1982). Although some lesbians who want children may purposefully choose a father and have intercourse, others prefer not to have any sexual contact with men. As the technology of artificial insemination has been refined, there is a growing demand for it among lesbians.

IMPLICATIONS FOR NURSING

When gay men and lesbians enter the health system, they not only face disclosure and the societal stigma attached to their sexual orientation, but they also must cope with the inherent decreased personal autonomy and increased vulnerability of the "patient role." Clients who are invested in hiding an important part of their life may be doubly vulnerable. The perception of vulnerability and negative expectations can result in delay in seeking health care. There are several things nurses can do to decrease perceived vulnerability and to improve the quality of care delivered to gay people. A number of nursing implications have already been discussed; here are some guidelines and general suggestions to increase one's awareness of a gay life style, foster gay clients' sense of acceptance by nurses, and support communication between gay clients and nurses.

1. *Demonstrate a positive attitude toward homosexuality as an alternative lifestyle*—to your clients, colleagues, friends, students, and family. Start consciousness raising first with yourself. Whether you are homosexual or heterosexual you have been exposed to myths and stereotypes about gay people. Increase your knowledge of homosexuality in history, law, literature, and all aspects of society. Talk

to gay people, read some gay literature, and visit a gay bar. Stereotypes can be changed with exposure to information. Consider coming out if you are a lesbian or gay man in the health professions; you may be a role model for someone. If a member of your family is gay, acknowledge this fact in a positive manner.

An important way that a professional can demonstrate a positive attitude to a homosexual client is to assume, unless indicated otherwise, that the client is satisfied with being homosexual and does not desire to change. Too often the professional may assume that functional disorders or psychosocial problems that the gay person may have are caused by homosexuality. An inappropriate and unwanted referral may result. Another negative, insulting assumption is that a gay person seeking health care must be there for treatment of venereal disease (Brown, 1976; Gonsiorek, 1988; Borhek, 1988).

2. *Avoid heterosexual bias* in your care of clients. Bias can occur from lack of knowledge or lack of sensitivity or both. For example, lack of knowledge of certain problems seen frequently in homosexual males may result in omission of laboratory tests needed for diagnosis of these conditions. For females, the question "What do you use for birth control?" assumes that the person is both sexually active and heterosexual. If, for example, a woman has pelvic pain and pregnancy needs to be ruled out, the question, "When was the last time you had sexual relations?" assumes heterosexuality. When a client is offended by the professional's assumption of heterosexuality and cannot or will not risk self-disclosure, inadequate care may result. Lack of sensitivity of the professional raises barriers not faced by heterosexual clients, such as when hospitalized homosexual clients are denied the emotional support of visits from lovers and friends (Owen, 1986).

3. *Make explicit assurances of confidentiality and honor them.* Indicate specifically that sexual information, including sexual orientation, will not appear on the medical record unless this is specifically validated with the client. The client has no obligation to reveal sexual orientation. Coming out is a difficult process, sometimes associated with alienation of family and friends, embarrassment, or loss of employment. You can be supportive during this process by providing an atmosphere of acceptance without pressures. Do not be a

crusader if your own views on homosexuality are liberal. Remember, the client has a lot more to risk from self-disclosure than you do.

4. *Examine policies and practices in your institution.* Is heterosexual bias reflected in visiting policies? Is the staff treating for homosexuality instead of the admitting diagnosis? If so, follow your conscience in calling attention to these deficiencies and in actively working toward change (See Pogoncheff, 1979).

5. *Use appropriate terms when referring to sexual orientation.* Language is very important in revealing stereotypes, norms, and dominance issues. Obviously, words like fag and queer and deviant and pervert are objectionable. Most homosexual women prefer to be called lesbians not homosexuals or gays. Most homosexual men prefer to be called gays rather than homosexuals.

6. *Be a knowledgeable professional.* Explore the resources available for lesbians and gay men. If you feel uncomfortable interacting with homosexual clients, develop access to appropriate referral channels. In many communities there are clinical screening facilities that specialize in medical problems of homosexuals. Be aware of current guidelines on HIV testing (CDC, 1988) and know the resources for HIV testing in your community. The National Gay Health Education Foundation (PO Box 834, Linden Hill, NY 11354) sponsors a National Gay Health Care Conference and publishes the *National Gay Health Care Directory* listing physicians and clinical facilities that serve the gay community. The Gay Caucus of the American Psychiatric Association (1700 18th St., NW, Washington, DC 20009) maintains a listing of psychiatrists who specialize in problems of sexual orientation. The Gay Nurses Alliance (PO Box 17593, San Diego, CA) provides support and information and is actively involved in promoting a positive image of gay people. Many campuses have active gay student organizations.

There are also a variety of gay mental health professionals in private practice. Their important commonality, according to Brossart (1982), is that they can be relied on to help the client work on the actual problems and not to assume that all problems stem from the client's homosexuality.

CONCLUSION

A nursing perspective is one that supports development of the whole person toward healthy ways of being. The premise in this chapter has been that a healthy sexuality is determined by factors other than sexual orientation.

In general, the health needs and concerns of lesbians and gay men both as individuals and as a minority group have largely been ignored by the traditional health system. In general, health professionals have, as does society, a heterosexual bias. For the majority, heterosexuality is normative and thus "healthy."

Knowledgeable, effective, and nonjudgmental care for this population must be based on (1) an understanding of homosexuality in a historical and societal context; (2) an appreciation of the phenomenon of labeling and the label preferences of gay and lesbian people; (3) knowledge of various theories on the origins of homosexuality and the limitations of such research; (4) an appreciation of the gay and lesbian experience as it emerges in the life cycle, from the early development of sexual preferences to adult roles and relationships; (5) knowledge of the expressed concerns and health problems of gay and lesbian people—as professionals and as clients—in the health care system; and (6) positive interventions that demonstrate an affirmation of homosexuality as an alternative form of sexual expression.

REFERENCES

American Psychiatric Association. Press release. Washington, DC, The American Psychiatric Association, Dec 15, 1973.

Barone JE, Yee J, Nealon TF: Management of foreign bodies and trauma of the rectum. Surg Gynecol and Obstet 156:453–457, 1983.

Bayer R: Homosexuality and American Psychiatry: The Politics of Diagnosis. New York, Basic Books, 1981.

Bayer R: Gays and the stigma of bad blood. Hastings Cent Rep 13:5–7, 1983.

Bell AP: The homosexual as patient. In Green R (ed): Human Sexuality: A Health Practitioner's Text. Baltimore, Williams & Wilkins, 1975.

Bell AP, Weinberg MS: Homosexualities: A Study of Diversity Among Men and Women. New York, Simon and Shuster, 1978.

Bell AP, Weinberg MS, Hammersmith SK: Sexual Preference—It's Development in Men and Women. Vols I, II. Bloomington, Indiana University Press, 1981.

Bieber I: Homosexuality: A Psychoanalytic Study. New York, Basic Books, 1962.

Borhek MV: Helping gay and lesbian adolescents and their families: A mother's perspective. J Adoles Health Care 9:123–128, 1988.

Boswell J: Christianity, Social Tolerance, and Homosexuality: Gay People in Western Europe from the Beginning of the Christian Era to the Fourteenth Century. Chicago, University of Chicago Press, 1980.

Brossart J: The gay patient: What you should be doing. RN 42:50–52, 1979.

Brossart J, Lapierre E: From self-help to health: Alternative services for gay men and lesbians. ANA Publications (G-157):65–76, 1982.

Brossart J (ed): National Gay Health Directory: A Compendium of Health Services for Lesbians and Gay Men. 3rd ed. Linden Hill, National Gay Health Education Foundation, 1982.

Brown DF: The health service and gay students. J Am Coll Health Assn 24:272–273, 1976.

Bullough B, Bullough V, Smith RW: Masculinity and femininity in transvestite, transexual and gay males. West J Nurs Res 7:317–332, 1985.

Bullough V: Sexual Variance in Society and History. New York, John Wiley & Sons, 1976.

Bullough V: Homosexuality: A History. New York, Meridian Books/New American Library, 1979.

Centers for Disease Control: Evaluation of HTLV-III/LAV infection in healthcare personnel. MMWR 34:38, 1985.

Centers for Disease Control: Update: HIV infections in health care workers exposed to blood of infected patients. MMWR 36:19, 1987a.

Centers for Disease Control: Recommendations for prevention of HIV transmission in health care settings. MMWR 36:2S, 1987b.

Centers for Disease Control: Public health service guidelines for counseling and antibody testing to prevent HIV infection and AIDS. MMWR 36:31, 1988.

Centers for Disease Control: Personal conversation with Brenda Garzo Staff, Weekly Surveillance, May 6, 1988.

Committee on Adolescence, American Academy of Pediatrics: Homosexuality and adolescence. Pediatrics 72:249–250, 1983.

Council on Scientific Affairs, American Medical Association: Health care needs of a homosexual population. JAMA 248:736–739, 1982.

Dank B: Coming out in the gay world. Psychiatry 34:180–187, 1971.

Dardick L, Grady KE: Openness between gay persons and health professionals. Ann Intern Med 93:115–119, 1980.

DeMonteflores C, Schultz S: Coming out: Similarities and differences for lesbians and gay men. J Soc Issues 34:58–72, 1978.

Doerr P: Plasma testosterone, estradiol and semen analysis in male homosexuals. Arch Gen Psychiatry 29:829–833, 1973.

Dorner G: A neuroendocrine predisposition for homosexuality in men. Arch Sex Behav 4:1–8, 1975.

Douglas CJ, Kalman CM, Kalman TP: Homophobia among physicians and nurses: An empirical study. Hosp Community Psychiatry 36:1309–1311, 1985.

Ehrhard A, Baker S: Fetal androgens, human central nervous system and behavior sex differences. In Friedman R, Richard R, Vande Wiele R (eds): Sex Differences in Behavior. New York, John Wiley & Sons, 1974.

Ford CS, Beach FA: Patterns of Sexual Behavior. New York, Harper & Row, 1951.

Fordham F: An Introduction to Jung's Psychology. New York, Penguin Books, 1982.

Freud S: Three Essays on the Theory of Sexuality. In Strachey J (ed, trans): The Standard Edition of the Complete Psychological Works. Vol VII. London, The Hogarth Press, 1953, pp 125–243.

Freud S: Letter to an American mother. Am J Psychiatry 107:786–787, 1951.

Gallup Report. Homosexuality. 205:3–19, 1982.

Gebhard PH, Johnson AB: The Kinsey Data: Marginal Tabulations of the 1938–1963 Interviews Conducted by the Institute For Sex Research. Philadelphia, WB Saunders, 1979.

Gershman H: The stress of coming out. Am J Psychoanal 43:129–139, 1983.

Gillow KE, Davis LL: Lesbian stress and coping methods. J Pyschosoc Nurs Ment Health Serv 25:28–32, 1987.

Glad To Be Gay? (anonymous) Nurs Mirror 156:33–34, 1983.

Golombok S, Spencer A, Rutter M: Children in lesbian and single-parent households: Psychosexual and psychiatric appraisal. J Child Psychol Psychiatry 24:551–572, 1983.

Good RS: Gynecologist and the lesbian. Clin Obstet Gynecol 19:473–482, 1976.

Goodell SE et al: Herpes simplex virus proctitis in homosexual men. N Engl J Med 308:868–871, 1983.

Gonsiorek JC: Mental health issues of gay and lesbian adolescents. J Adoles Health Care 9:114–122, 1988.

Grellert EA, Newcomb MD, Bentler PM: Childhood play activities of male and female homosexuals and heterosexuals. Arch Sex Behav 11:451–477, 1982.

Green R: Adults who want to change sex; adolescents who cross-dress; and children called "Sissy" and "Tomboy." In Green R (ed): Human Sexuality: A Health Practitioners Text. Baltimore, Williams & Wilkins, 1975.

Green R: Sexual Identity Conflict in Children and Adults. New York, Basic Books, 1974.

Green R: Sexual identity of 37 children raised by homosexual or transsexual parents. Am J Psychiatry 135:692–697, 1978.

Green R: Childhood cross-gender behavior and subsequent sexual preference. Am J Psychiatry 136:106–108, 1979.

Greenberg DF, Bystryn MH: Christian intolerance of homosexuality. Am J Soc 88:515–548, 1982.

Hanscombe G: The right of lesbian parenthood. J Med Ethics 9:133–135, 1983.

Harry J: Defeminization and adult psychological well-being among male homosexuals. Arch Sex Behav 12:1–19, 1983.

Herman SP: Gender identity disorder in a five-year old boy. Yale J Biol Med 56:15–22, 1983.

Hogan R: Human Sexuality: A Nursing Perspective. 2nd ed. Norwalk, Appleton-Century-Crofts, 1985.

Hooker E: The adjustment of the male overt homosexual. J Project Tech 22:33–54, 1957.

Hotvedt ME, Mandel JB: Children of lesbian mothers. In Paul W et al (eds): Homosexuality: Social, Psychological and Biological Issues. Final report of the SPSSI Task Force on Sexual Orientation. Beverly Hills, Sage Publications, 1982.

Irish AC: Straight talk about gay patients. Am J Nurs 8:1168–1170, 1983.

Johnson RJ et al: Factors influencing lesbian gynecologic care: A preliminary study. Am J Obstet Gynecol 140:20–28, 1981.

Jones RW, DeCecco JP: Femininity and masculinity of partners in heterosexual and homosexual relationships. J Homosex 8:37, 1982.

Kallmann F: Comparative twin study on the genetic aspects of male homosexuality. J Nerv Ment Dis 115:283–298, 1952.

Kelly J: Homosexuality and aging. In Marmor J (ed): Homosexual Behaviors: A Modern Reappraisal. New York, Basic Books, 1980.

Kinsey AC, Pomeroy WB, Martin CE: Sexual Behavior in the Human Male. Philadelphia, WB Saunders, 1948.

Kolodny R: Plasma testosterone and semen analysis in male homosexuals. N Engl J Med 285:1170–1174, 1971.

Kus RJ: Stages of coming out: An ethnographic approach. West J Nurs Res 7:177–198, 1985.

Laurence J: Homosexuals, hospitalization and the nurse. Nurse Forum 14:305–317, 1975.

Lautmann R: The pink triangle: The persecution of homosexual males in concentration camps in Nazi, Germany. In Licata SJ, Petersen RP (eds): Historical Perspectives on Homosexuality. New York, Haworth Press, 1981.

Marecek J, Finn SE, Cardell M: Gender roles in the relationships of lesbians and gay men. J Homosex 8:45–59, 1982.

Marmor J, Green R: Homosexual behavior. In Money J, Musaph H (eds): Handbook of Sexology. New York, Excerpta Medica, 1977.

Masters W, Johnson V: Homosexuality in Perspective. Boston, Little, Brown & Co, 1979.

McDonald GJ: Individual differences in the coming out process for gay men. J Homosex 8:47–59, 1982.

Messer HD: The homosexual as physician. In Green R (ed): Human Sexuality: A Health Practitioners Text. Baltimore, Williams & Wilkins, 1975.

Miller B: Unpromised paternity: Lifestyles of gay fathers. In Levine N (ed): Gay men: The sociology of male homosexuality. New York, Harper & Row, 1979.

Mintz L, Drew WL: Sexually transmitted viral infections in homosexual men. Med Clin North Am 67:1093–1094, 1983.

Money J, Lewis V: Homosexual/heterosexual status in boys at puberty: Idiopathic adolescent gynecomastia and congenital virilizing adrenocorticism compared. Psychoneuroendocrinology 7:39–346, 1982.

Morin SF: Heterosexual bias in psychological research on lesbianism and male homosexuality. Am Psychol 32:629–637, 1977.

Moses AE, Hawkins RO: Counseling Lesbian Women and Gay Men: A Life-Issues Approach. St. Louis, CV Mosby, 1982.

Nass GD, Libby RW, Fisher MP: Homosexual and bisexual orientations. In Nass GD, Libby RW, Fisher MP (eds): Sexual Choices: An Introduction to Human Sexuality. 2nd ed. Monterey, Wadsworth, 1984.

National Gay Task Force: Personal communication with headquarters. May 1988.

National Institutes of Mental Health: Task Force on Homosexuality: Final Report and Background Papers. Livingood JM (ed). HEW Publication No. 1 (ADM) 76–357, 1976.

Noyes LE: Gray and Gay. J Gerontol Nurs 8:636–639, 1982.

Nursing Grand Rounds: Caring for the AIDS patient fearlessly. Nursing 83 Sept:50–55, 1983.

Olesker E, Walsh LV: Childbearing among lesbians: Are we meeting their needs? J Nurse Midwife 29:322–329, 1984.

Ovesey L: Homosexuality and Pseudohomosexuality. New York, Science House, 1969.

Owen WF Jr: The clinical approach to the male homosexual patient. Med Clin North Am 70:499–535, 1986.

Peplau LA: Research on homosexual couples: An overview. J Homosex 8:3, 1982.

Peplau LA, Padesky C, Hamilton M: Satisfaction in lesbian relationships. J Homosex 8:23, 1982.

Pillard RC, Paumadere JP, Carretta RA: A family study of sexual orientation. Arch Sex Behav 11:511–520, 1982.

Pillard R, Rose R, Sherwood M: Plasma testosterone levels in homosexual men. Arch Sex Behav 3:453–458, 1974.

Pogoncheff E: The gay patient: What not to do. RN 42:46–49, 1979.

Rand MA, Graham DLR, Rawlings EI: Psychological health and factors the court seeks to control in lesbian mother custody trials. J Homosex 8:27–39, 1982.

Raymond CA: Lesbians call for greater physician awareness, sensitivity to improve patient care. JAMA 259:18, 1988.

Reagan P: Interaction of health professionals and their lesbian clients. Patient Counsel Health Educ 1:21–25, 1981.

Rivera R: Homosexuality and the Law. In Paul WP et al (eds): Homosexuality: Social, Psychological and Biological Issues. Beverly Hills, Sage Publications, 1982, pp 323–336.

Robinson BE, Skeen P: Sex-role orientation of gay fathers verses gay nonfathers. J Percept Motor Skills 55:1055–1059, 1982.

Ross MW: Femininity, masculinity and sexual orientation: Some cross-cultural comparisons. J Homosex 9:27–36, 1983.

Saghir MT, Robins E: Male and Female Homosexuality—A Comprehensive Investigation. Baltimore, Williams & Wilkins, 1973.

Siegelman M: Adjustment of male homosexuals and heterosexuals. Arch Sex Behav 2:9–25, 1972.

Siemens S, Brandzel RC: Sexuality: Nursing Assessment and Intervention. Philadelphia, JB Lippincott, 1982.

Socarides C: Homosexuality and medicine. JAMA 212:1199–1202, 1970.

Smith EM, Johnson SR, Guenther SM: Health care attitudes and experiences during gynecologic care among lesbians and bisexuals. Am J Pub Health 75:1085–1087, 1985.

Spada J: The Spada Report: The Newest Survey of Gay Male Sexuality. New York, Signet Books, 1979.

Taylor A: Conceptions of masculinity and femininity as a basis for stereotypes of male and female homosexuals. J Homosex 9:37–53, 1983.

Tripp CA: The Homosexual Matrix. New York, McGraw Hill, 1976.

Vetere VA: The role of friendship in the development and maintenance of lesbian love relationships. J Homosex 8:51–65, 1982.

Webster SB: Dermatologic diseases of the sexual revolution: Newer aspects and disease associated with male homosexuality. Primary Care 10:429–441, 1983.

Weinberg G: Society and the Healthy Homosexual. Garden City, Anchor Press/Doubleday, 1973.

Whitam FL: Childhood indicators of male homosexuality. Arch Sex Behav 6:89–96, 1977.

Whitam FL: Culturally invariable properties of male homosexuality: Tentative conclusions from cross-cultural research. Arch Sex Behav 12:207–226, 1983.

White TA: Attitudes of psychiatric nurses toward same sex orientations. Nurs Res 28:276–281, 1979.

Wilson ML: Neuroticism and extraversion of female homosexuals. Psychol Reports 51:559–562, 1982.

Wolf DG: The Lesbian Community. Berkeley, University of California Press, 1979.

Woods NF: Human Sexuality in Health and Illness. 3rd ed. St. Louis, CV Mosby, 1984.

Young EW: Nurses' attitudes toward homosexuality: Analysis of change in AIDS workshops. J Cont Educ Nurs 19:9–12, 1988.

Young W, Goy R, Phoenix C: Hormones and sexual behavior. Science 143:212–218, 1964.

8: Sex and the Law

Mark E. Fogel
Catherine Ingram Fogel

In every society there are norms regulating sexual behavior, some of which will become law. Laws attempt to regulate human behavior so as to protect individuals and property and to ensure the continuation of society. Sex laws attempt to meet these purposes and are established to lend teeth to generally accepted morality. Examination of the laws regulating sexual behavior may provide insights about a society's attitudes on sexuality. Such insights will help health care providers identify the societal norms that have shaped their views regarding acceptable sexual behavior. In this chapter, the battery of U.S. criminal statutes enacted to regulate sexual behavior is discussed to improve health professionals' understanding of the sexual laws in the society in which they live.

Individuals responsible for the delivery of health care need information regarding laws that regulate their professional practice. Situations may arise in which the health care provider may play an important role in the enforcement of criminal laws dealing with sexuality. This chapter provides information on legal issues affecting health care practice and the delivery of health care.

A major intent of this chapter is to provide the reader with sufficient information to review present day legal statutes critically in order to determine whether changes in the law are necessary, wise, or prudent. Health professionals should be aware of current public debates surrounding sexually related behavior. A framework for viewing current laws regulating sexuality that distinguishes between levels of acceptance is presented. There are those acts believed to be so harmful to the victim that they are beyond the level of tolerance of our society, those acts that may be classified as psychological disturbances, and those acts that are victimless and probably accepted as normative by large segments of society. Additionally, information on abortion, although not a sexual activity per se, is presented, since this is an area in which knowledge of the law is critical for the health professional.

THE SOCIAL CONTEXT OF LAWS REGULATING SEXUALITY

The laws regulating sexuality are concerned primarily with transgression. With certain exceptions they are not laws commanding one to do something but rather laws prohibiting one from doing something. Examples range from laws against rape to laws against adultery and fornication. For at least the past decade scholars have argued over the legal regulations of sexual conduct on the basis of protection of citizens against injury (with special regard to the safeguarding of children) versus regulation of sexual conduct based on moral principles.

Those espousing the former position have based their views on principles stated by John Stuart Mill in 1859. In his seminal work, *On Liberty,* Mill urged

that the only purpose for which power can be rightfully exercised over any member of a civilized community, against his will, is to prevent harm to others. . . .

Mill also asserted that

liberty of taste and pursuits . . . of doing as we like, subject to such consequences as may follow: Without impediment for our fellow creatures so long as what we do does not harm them even though they should think our conduct foolish, perverse, or wrong.

The issue for those questioning the current basis (i.e., religious and moral precepts) for regulation of sexual conduct, often called "Mill supporters," is not whether sex should be free of all regulations or rigidly restricted but rather which restrictions are necessary and which may be discarded. The role of criminal law should not be to regulate individuals' private sexual lives, except to repress conduct injurious to society or highly injurious to the persons engaging in it. A distinction is made between persons whose conduct may be offensive (e.g., exhibitionists and minor lewd offenders) and those whose conduct is dangerous and aggressive (e.g., rapists, sex slayers, and those damaging to young children). It is believed important to separate sex activities that are nontraumatizing or a nuisance from activities that are traumatizing or a menace (Slovenko, 1965).

The Mill supporters further argue that placing emphasis on nontraumatizing sexual acts detracts from the law's capacity to regulate traumatizing sexual behavior. While it is agreed that the law should protect society from the dangerous and aggressive individual and protect children and adolescents from sexual assault or persuasion, proponents of this position oppose labeling as a crime such activities as prostitution, fornication, adultery, or homosexuality between private consenting adults. Where laws restrain violent as well as consensual activity, it is argued that all laws may then be held in mockery.

A modern version of Mill's principles is found in the recommendations of the Wolfenden Committee. In 1957 in England, the Wolfenden Committee was established to review the laws governing prostitution and homosexuality. Recommending repeal of a statute punishing acts of homosexuality between consenting adults, the Committee held that criminal regulation's function should be limited to preservation of the public order, protection of citizens against offense or injury, and the safeguarding of children and other vulnerable groups against harm. In particular, the Committee stressed "the importance society and the laws ought to give to the individual freedom of choice and action in

matters of private morality" and concluded that "there must remain a realm of private morality and immorality which, in brief, is not the laws' business" (Grey, 1983, p 4).

A morality-based view of the law's role in regulating sexual conduct can be found in the words of Lord Devlin. In 1958 Lord Devlin criticized the theoretical premises of the Wolfenden Report, arguing against the delineation of a sphere of private morality that would remain outside the concern of criminal law. In his view, the health of a society rests on its firm adherence to a binding moral code; the entire system of prevailing moral beliefs must be subject to legal enforcement, although prudence may suggest limits on morals legislation.

British legal philosopher H. L. A. Hart entered the dispute with his 1963 book entitled *Law, Liberty, and Morality.* Hart placed the controversial Wolfenden Report in the wider context of the century-old debate surrounding Mill's writings. At the same time, Hart offered a modern revision of Mill's principles. Lord Devlin responded, expanding his original position and criticizing Hart's views in the enforcement of morals. The Hart-Devlin debate has since attracted the attention of a wide variety of scholars and writers on both sides of the Atlantic.

A key aspect of the Devlin position is the belief that the question of whether or not to have a particular piece of morals legislation is an open-ended matter of policy, to be decided by weighing all factors that might seem relevant in the circumstances. Those ascribing to Mill's principles argue that there is a definite limitation upon such legislation.

The recent Attorney General's Commission on Pornography, Final Report (1986), or Meese Commission Report, stated that "where there is an identified harm, then governmental action ought seriously to be considered." The Meese Commission Report stated that the question of harm as it relates to the moral environment is a significant issue. Careful reading of the Meese Commission Report conveys the impression that the Report upholds the belief that protection of society's moral environment is a legitimate purpose of societal enforcement mechanisms. Although charged with determining the extent and impact of pornography on society, the Meese Commission extended this mandate by viewing the entire issue of sexual morality as an essential part of the social fabric. Whether the Meese Commission Report reflects a momentary aberration or a prediction of the future outcome of the debate remains to be seen.

Within the United States, the Hart-Devlin debate has translated into controversy over the legitimacy and content of the constitutional "right to privacy" developed by our courts since the mid 1960s (Grey, 1983, p 39). The right to privacy issue raises the question of whether matters of sexual conduct are better left to regulation by individual states responding to local considerations, including morality, or whether sexual conduct should be regulated at a federal level based on constitutional principles of rights to privacy where no harm to others is involved. Abortion represents the most current example of this debate: Should the right to an abortion be afforded by the constitutional right of privacy or be left to be decided by individual state legislators?

Opinions regarding the content of the right of sexual privacy range from advocating the protection of matters considered within the context of traditional family life to adopting a position of protecting all matters of a sexual nature.

The right to privacy doctrine originated in 1965 in *Griswald* v. *Connecticut* (1965). In this case, the Supreme Court recognized the existence of a constitutional right of privacy within the context of the marital relationship. The court held that a state cannot prohibit married couples from using contraceptive devices and that such a prohibition invades the "intimacy of the marriage bed; a preserve that the state may not constitutionally enter" (Barnett, 1973).

The major problem with defining the scope of the constitutional right of privacy is determining at which point it stops. There is no question that its parameters have been defined over a period of time and on a case by case basis. The next step in the development of the privacy doctrine after the Griswold ruling occurred in *Stanley* v. *Georgia* (1969). In this case, police officers had discovered pornographic films in the bedroom of the defendant's home. The Supreme Court held that the mere possession by an individual of obscene material cannot constitutionally be labeled a crime. Justice Thurgood Marshall's opinion in the case clearly indicated the existence of a right to privacy, with no implication of the right being in any way restricted to married couples or only to homes occupied by such couples. *Stanley* v. *Georgia* provided a basis for development of a broader right of privacy than the marital right spelled out in the Griswold decision.

Two more recent decisions extended the right of privacy to single persons as well as to married couples. In *Isenstadt* v. *Baird* (1974), the Supreme Court affirmed a general right of free choice in matters of procreation, reversing a conviction for public distribution of contraceptive foam to an unmarried person, an act violating Massachusetts state law. In *Cary* v. *Population Services International* (1977), the court invalidated prohibitions on the sale of nonprescription contraceptives by persons other than licensed pharmacists to persons under age 16, stating that "the decision whether or not to beget or bear a child is at the very heart of the right to privacy." Finally, in the case of *Roe* v. *Wade* (1973), decided January 22, 1973, the Supreme Court struck down the Texas anti-abortion law on the grounds that it violated the right to privacy of an unmarried pregnant woman.

To this date, however, the Supreme Court has not held that the constitutional right of privacy is absolute. In the recent case of *Bowers* v. *Hardwick* (1986), decided June 30, 1986, the Supreme Court ruled that the right of privacy does not extend to homosexuals engaging in acts of consensual sodomy. Thus, notwithstanding the rights conferred previously in the areas of family relationships, marriage, and procreation, the court has not upheld constitutional rights of privacy for all individuals.

While the rights to privacy have been expanded in some areas, sexual behavior that violates prevailing societal norms remains a matter of social control through criminal law. Even if one accepts regulation of social conduct based on society's moral precepts, however, continually changing views of acceptable morality pose a number of difficult questions.

The remainder of this chapter, which describes current regulation of sexuality, can be viewed in the context of society's struggle with the different points of view just discussed. The reader is advised to bear in mind that societal regulation of sexuality is dynamic and everchanging and that changes reflect a new equilibrium between these two opposing camps.

CURRENT LAWS REGULATING SEXUAL BEHAVIOR

An examination of current American criminal statutes regulating sexual behavior provides important information regarding past and present sexual norms in our society. Crime, as currently defined in the United States, consists of acts that violate the penal code of a government jurisdiction that is punishable by the criminal courts of the government. Thus, any sexual act defined by the penal code as criminal becomes a crime. This has resulted in a battery of laws regulating criminal acts such as rape and child molestation and defining adultery, seduction, and many forms of sexual intercourse as criminal. While many of the current laws are obsolete and unenforced, they reflect traditional American values, in which monogamous heterosexual marriage is considered the norm and all other expressions of sexuality are morally deviant.

MacNamara and Sagarin (1977) have suggested that the criminal regulation of sexuality can be best understood by assigning sexual acts to groups according to the degree to which conduct can be tolerated in a permissive society without resort to criminal statutes and punitive sanctions. MacNamara and Sagarin generally classified sexual criminal acts as follows:

Category I. Sexual acts that clearly require criminalization and enforcement in order to protect society. Sexual molestation of children and rape would be included in this category.

Category II. Sexual acts that have a psychopathological component. Here, criminalization and enforcement would be accepted on the grounds of the potential for victimization. The possibility of the offender committing more serious acts exists alongside the possibility of facilitating treatment of the offender. This category would include exhibitionism and voyeurism.

Category III. Sexual activities that are on the borderline between acts considered morally reprehensible and those that result in clear victimization. Acts in this category include prostitution and adultery.

Category IV. Sexual acts that are purely private consensual decisions by adults. Sexual activities in this category include consensual homosexuality and, specifically, the criminalization of acts such as sodomy.

Category V. Behaviors that are nonsexual in nature but are either criminalized or considered to be sex crimes. Activities in this category include abortion, the use of contraception, and the sale and distribution of pornography to adults.

Category I sexual acts are those that arouse the greatest indignation and public concern and for which the greatest consensus exists regarding the appropriateness of criminal statutes for regulation. However, many persons may feel that society's response to the sexual acts defined in category II should be therapeutic rather than punitive. Individuals believe that the sexual behaviors encompassed by category III should be discouraged by nonpunitive means, if at all. Sexual behaviors described in categories IV and V are, for many, not inherently wrong or antisocial and therefore not subject to regulation by criminal statutes.

RAPE AND OTHER SEXUAL ASSAULT

Rape is the fastest rising violent crime among the FBI's major crime categories (Geer, Heiman, and Leitenburg, 1984). In the United States, it is estimated that a rape is committed every 7 minutes (FBI, 1979). While more women are reporting rape than in past decades, many rapes still go unreported. In the majority of cases, women are the victims and men the offenders (Geer, Heiman, and Leitenburg, 1984).

Definitions

Rape is usually considered to be a sexually aggressive crime and is generally defined as "the act of sexual intercourse with a female person without her lawful consent." And as defined in most penal codes, rape refers to "a completed sexual assault by a male upon an adult female." This definition is typically restricted to forceful sexual intercourse and implies female resistance. However, the definition is also assumed to include females who did not resist but were so young or so mentally or intellectually impaired that they were incapable of giving consent.

Historically, the only intercourse with a female above the age of consent that could be termed rape was that which employed force. Over time, however, judicial decisions have held that intercourse with a female (except a wife) who is insane, drugged, intoxicated, asleep, or unconscious is also a type of forceable rape. In these cases, whatever effort however slight that was needed for penetration is presumed by the court to satisfy the requirement that there was carnal knowledge by force. In each of these cases, the law presumes that the female would not consent to coitus. For an act to be considered rape, penetration of the female genitalia by the penis is necessary; however, neither full penetration, rupture of the hymen, or ejaculation of seminal fluid is needed to support the charge of rape. If the male succeeds in penetrating elsewhere, regardless of the other crime committed (e.g., sodomy, sexual assault, carnal abuse), legally and technically the act is not prosecutable as rape. If the man uses his tongue, fingers, a dildo, or some other instrument rather than his penis, the crime is considered assault and/or attempted rape.

In addition to this definition, there are a number of other legal terms used to delineate specific types of rape: Statutory rape is sexual intercourse with a female below the age of consent. While different states specify different ages of consent, the age range is 13 to 18. The term statutory rape is used even if both parties agree to the act and no force is involved.

Attempted rape is the effort to commit violent or forceful rape, in which the male does not succeed in penetration because of resistance by the woman, interruption during the struggle, loss of erection, or fear of apprehension. In order for an individual to be convicted under the rape statute, the act must go past the attempted stage. Prison sentences for attempted rape are often half the length of sentences for a completed act of rape.

Sexual assault is the term used to describe uninvited touching of the erogenous zones, such as the breast, buttocks, or genitalia, of another person's body. The term is not interchangeable with attempted rape, in which force and violence are used, but penetration does not occur.

Consent

Men who have been accused of rape and who have denied their guilt have generally offered two types of defense: mistaken identity and participation in consensual sexual intercourse. Consent is an absolute defense to rape (Bessmer, 1984).

Rape prosecution is complex when the accused has admitted that he had sexual intercourse with the woman but insists that the act was mutual and voluntary. The issue of consent raises two major questions: "How much resistance must a woman put up for the act to be defined as rape?" and "How much of a woman's prior sexual history is admissible evidence?" The latter question has frequently been linked to the credibility of the rape victim and to the truthfulness of her testimony in relation to lack of consent.

The question of how much resistance a woman must offer and at which point her lack of or decreased levels of resistance can be interpreted as acquiescence becomes critical when there is no overt evidence of physical violence. For some, the man's very presence, particularly if he is a stranger, may be sufficient to frighten a woman into submission. Others have been skeptical of the ability of a man to insert his penis into the vagina of an unwilling woman (MacNamara and Sagarin, 1977). It is important for health professionals to know what standards of resistance are enforced in their jurisdiction, so that relevant evidence necessary for prosecution may be collected during the rape victim's initial contact with the health care system. For example, recording the victim's exact words of how frightened she was may help establish her reason for submitting to the act of rape.

Until about 1940, laws required women to resist to the "utmost." This requirement, called the "utmost or uttermost" standard, is no longer used because resistance could seriously endanger the victim's life. There are now two other standards used for determining resistance. The "reasonable" resistance standard demands that the female do only what is reasonable given the circumstances of the case. The "fear" standard is employed when the female does not resist, if she can show that her submission was due to fear for her life or of grave bodily injury. In this instance the rapist must have threatened to harm physically the woman or a third party.

Under the fear standard, a rapist can be convicted even when the victim's resistance does not meet the reasonable resistance standard, if it can be shown that her failure to resist was due to fear. Although the fear standard may be employed today, it is not unusual for a woman to find herself in the position of not having physically resisted, having no physical evidence of bodily harm, not having screamed because she was frightened, and then being confronted in court with her inability to produce evidence that she was an unwilling partner. For this reason repudiation of the resistance standard is needed.

Chastity/Rape Shield Laws

Traditionally, evidence of a woman's prior nonmarital sexual experiences was allowed at trial because it was thought to be relevant to the issue of her consent to the sexual act and to her credibility as a witness. It was assumed that nonmarried women who were sexually active were more likely to consent to a man's sexual advances. A further assumption underlying the use of such testimony was that the primary societal injury from the act of rape was the loss of chastity (Bessmer, 1984). Evidence of prior nonmarital sexual experiences thus negated the loss of chastity. It was also assumed that an unchaste woman would probably consent and that such a woman was also more dishonest than her chaste sister. The Kinsey Reports of the 1950s, which documented that almost 50 per cent of the married women interviewed had engaged in premarital sex, provided some of the first evidence of changing societal mores. As society's attitude toward nonmarital sexual intercourse has evolved, so has the law.

States have responded to the changing relevance of a rape victim's sexual history with a variety of "rape shield" statutes. In all states with rape shield statutes a woman's sexual behavior may not be used to show consent or lack of credibility in a rape case. Additionally, it is now recognized that sexual conduct may prejudice the case in the eyes of the jury. A classic legal study has shown that there is a direct relationship between the rape victim's perceived respectability and the degree of punishment imposed on the defendant by the jury (Kalven and Zeisel, 1966).

At one end of the spectrum, some states give the trial judge discretion in admitting evidence of sexual history after an in-camera (in his private chambers) hearing. At the other end of the spectrum, some courts prohibit evidence of a sexual history except in a few specific situations and only after an in-camera hearing has determined its admissi-

bility. A very small number of states do not have rape shield statutes of any type.

Currently, the rape shield statutes enacted permit the introduction of evidence that shows that the woman had had previous sexual intercourse with the defendant. Regardless of society's prevailing sexual norms, the woman is presumed to be more likely to have consented to the alleged rape if she previously has engaged in intercourse with the man. Some rape shield statutes also permit evidence of the victim's sexual history to be introduced if there is a highly unusual pattern of sexual behavior that seems to indicate consent to the act of intercourse. For example, prior patterns of sexual behavior resembling the defendant's version of the alleged encounter tend to prove that the victim consented to the act. Finally, because the rape charges have sometimes been shown to have been fabricated, many statutes permit expert testimony showing that the woman may have fantasized the alleged rape.

In all these instances, there is a potential for conflict between the defendant's right to a fair trial and the woman's right to have her claim to protection of the law vindicated without invasion of her sexual privacy. In many cases, this conflict may be without solution. However, careful monitoring by trial judges of both cross-examination and jury arguments can do much to preserve the rape complainant's sexual privacy without detracting from the fairness of the trial. Closed hearings can be used to determine the relevance of any evidence, testimony, or cross-examination that may involve the victim's sexual history. The determination of relevance should be stated by judges on the record with their reason for the decision.

Spousal Rape

In the past it was legally presumed that a man could not rape his wife. This presumption is now being disputed by feminists, libertarians, and legal scholars. Traditional law exempting a husband from legally raping his wife is based upon the presumption that a wife consents to be her husband's sexual partner when she marries him. A more egalitarian concept of marriage, however, would state that the timing and circumstances of sexual activity should be a choice made by both partners.

Currently, in less than one half of the

states, if a woman resists the sexual advances of her husband and he beats her into submission, he is technically not committing rape, although he can be prosecuted on an assault charge. The courts have ruled, however, that a woman who is divorced or legally separated can be raped in the legal sense by her estranged husband. If a forceful sexual attack occurs that meets all other criteria for rape, it would not fall outside the definition by reason of their former marital relationship (MacNamara and Sagarin, 1977).

Spousal rape is one of the frontier issues that the law is still pondering. At the present time, more than half the states and the District of Columbia have discarded the legal exemption for marital rape, although in practice if the couple is not separated it is hard to bring such a case to trial. According to the National Clearinghouse on Marital Rape, Berkeley, California, prosecution of this type remains a relatively rare event, with only 100 prosecuted cases nationally. Most have ended in convictions, often after acrimonious testimony (*Newsweek*, May 25, 1985).

The American Law Institute has suggested that a model statute on rape and related offenses continues to exclude the possibility of marital rape. The Institute would not only exclude a husband from prosecution on the charge of rape or other offenses of a sexual nature (which would be considered criminal if committed against someone other than a wife) but would also extend this exclusion "to persons living as man and wife regardless of the legal status of their relationship" (American Law Institute, 1985). The American Law Institute would make the exclusion inoperative if the man and woman were living apart "under a decree of judicial separation." In the authors' opinion, this position of the Institute represents an example of the law's attitude toward the sanctity of the marital unit. On the other hand, traditional attitudes toward women's roles in marriage may have shaped the policy. In either case, the position reflects current perceptions and attitudes, which can be expected to modify over time.

Statutory Rape and Related Nonviolent Rapes

Like rape, sexual contact between adults and children receives little or no institutional support in most societies. Since rape is defined as nonconsensual sexual intercourse, it is reasoned that a minor, no matter how willing or eager, cannot give consent because she is below the age at which she has either the legal right or the social maturity to offer it. Moreover, this right is not vested, as are certain others, in parents or guardians. No one has the right to consent to a sexual act as the agent or on behalf of a minor. Statutory rape is a part of the general problem of child sexual abuse and is discussed more thoroughly in the next section.

Legally, statutory rape includes only sexual relations with a minor in which intercourse has taken place or penetration occurs. The crucial determining factor, which varies from state to state, is the age of consent. A second factor that has become relevant in a small number of jurisdictions, and is being considered by others, is the age difference between the female and the male. The issue of "near/peer" offenders is another area in which laws are currently undergoing changes.

In general, the concealment of age by the younger of the partners in a willing relationship has been an unacceptable legal defense in cases involving minors. Especially unacceptable are cases in which one partner is a child (usually defined as under 12 years of age).

Because the age of consent is the crucial factor in statutory rape, chastity is not a legally relevant consideration; however, many judges take it into account as a mitigating factor in determining the punishment to be imposed on the male. The age the victim presents to the perpetrator and the male's motives and intentions have also been significant in determining the punishment.

Cases involving child prostitution present complex problems for which equitable solutions are difficult to find. Use of mistaken age, as a defense in statutory rape by arguing that the man reasonably believed the female to be over the age of consent, has been allowed in some courts. The American Law Institute has suggested that the mistaken age defense should be unacceptable if the female is under age 10; if she is above age 10, but below the legally established age of consent, it would be up to the defendant to prove that he reasonably believed the female to be above the critical age. Health professionals should find out what the statutes are in the state in which they practice. Incest, which can be statutory rape if the victim is a minor, is discussed later in this chapter.

Intervention

It is clear that society's value systems allow a female who is sexually active the right to say "no." This may seem an absurd statement in the 1980s; however, less than a generation ago, that proposition was arguable. Issues of resistance, consent, and prior sexual behavior still have relevance in every court system. Health professionals must understand the relevance of these issues in order to ensure that care provided immediately after episodes of sexual violence results in the obtaining and documenting of all possible physical, medical, and emotional evidence.

Holmstrom and Burgess (1980) in their study of 146 rape victims who they followed through the health care and criminal justice systems uncovered several problems with documentation in patients' records, including the exclusion of helpful information such as the presence of bruises or the patient's emotional state and the inclusion of evidence such as the victim's past sexual history, the presence of previous vaginal infection, contraceptive use, or such comments as "patient uncooperative." The authors pointed out the double bind in which health professionals are placed: The information is essential to provide appropriate health care, yet the public often discredits rape victims who might be described as promiscuous. Many health professionals were ignorant of the value of certain evidence, such as the victim's clothing, pubic hair combings, or fingernail clippings.

Generally, the first encounter between the nurse and the victim will occur in an emergency room setting. Initially, support and reassurance should be provided, with the goal of making the victim feel as safe as possible and in control. Additionally, it is important to prepare the victim for examination. The nurse should obtain the required authorizations for emergency room rape examination (Fig. 8–1) and release of rape information and specimens to appropriate law enforcement officials.

The physical examination can provide important sources of evidence of consent/resistance. Any physical indication of force should be carefully noted by the health professional, including bruises, welts, puncture wounds, lacerations, abrasions, fractures, signs of abdominal injury, or human bite marks. Health professionals should carefully chart any physical signs of the rape itself, such as evidence of semen on the victim's clothing, genitalia, or anal area and signs of bruising or bleeding in the external genitalia, vaginal, and anal area. During the physical examination and collection of evidence, vaginal secretions and fluids are obtained, all affected organs are carefully examined, and samples of pubic hair and material from under the fingernails are gathered. Vaginal secretions and fluids, pubic hair combings, and fingernail samples are potential evidence that may be helpful in identifying the assailant. Hair, sperm, and other secretions are typed in a similar fashion to blood. The nurse should also ensure that clothing is collected as evidence. Finally, it may be helpful to take photographs of the physical damage.

Under the legal rules of evidence, any records kept in the usual course of business may be admitted as evidence, making meticulous record keeping all the more valuable. Nurses should record all information from the client's physical examination and any treatment instituted. The woman's emotional state should be carefully noted on the admitting documents as well as any and all statements made by the victim. The information obtained from the victim's statement as well as the physical examinations should be carefully documented in a sexual assault report form. Such forms are frequently prepared in conjunction with law enforcement officials. A model sexual assault report form is provided in this section (Fig. 8–2).

In many jurisdictions, collaborative efforts between medical and law enforcement personnel have created what are commonly known as rape evidence collection kits. Such kits provide a set of receptacles and containers for needed evidence in rape prosecution cases. These include sacks for the preservation of relevant clothing samples, containers for the victim's pubic hairs, head hairs, pubic hair combings, and blood and saliva samples as well as vaginal and anal swabs. In all cases, the nurse should initial and seal each article to be placed within the rape kit as well as the outside of the box. After signing the chain of evidence form, the nurse should give the kit and chain of evidence form to the law enforcement officials. This is done only when the victim has signed the necessary release forms.

As part of the treatment phase, the nurse administers medication for the prevention of sexually transmitted disease. Nurses should also assist these clients in personal hygiene

Department of Obstetrics & Gynecology
School of Medicine
University of North Carolina
Chapel Hill, N. C.
27514

I hereby give permission to Dr. _____ to perform
a complete physical examination including pelvic examination and for that
physician to collect appropriate specimens of vaginal secretions, blood,
hairs and other related specimens for laboratory examinations. I also
consent to treatment related to my present condition, including penicillin
and/or other antibiotics.

_____ Date

_____ Date _____ Age: _____
Patient's Signature (in all cases)

_____ Date _____
Guardian's Signature (if appropriate)

_____ Date Witness

FIGURE 8–1. Authorization for emergency rape examination. (From North Carolina Memorial Hospital Rape Crisis Program, Chapel Hill, North Carolina.)

after the examination, such as showering and brushing their teeth. Clients should be given wound care instructions and information about return appointments and referrals. Most important, they must be offered continued support and reassurance. The nurse should remain with the victim until she is discharged and has support systems available. The reader is referred to Chapter 26, Sexual Assault, for an indepth discussion of intervention.

SEXUAL ABUSE OF CHILDREN

In the past 10 years the reported incidence of sexual exploitation of children has increased markedly (Geer, Heiman, and Leitenburg, 1984). Although historically considered taboo, various writings have suggested

that the manipulation of children for a variety of sexual purposes has long existed. However, the recent and substantial increase in reported sexual abuse of children has alarmed both the public and public officials (Shouvlin, 1981).

The actual incidence of child sexual abuse is difficult to measure, since it is one of the most underreported forms of crime. It is estimated that only 10 to 20 per cent of sexual abuse incidents are actually reported. Until recently, it was not even specifically covered by many state mandatory abuse-reporting laws. Now, however, most jurisdictions include sexual abuse in their reporting statutes. Fear, embarrassment, and concern about the possible response of social, medical, and legal agencies most likely contributes to underreporting.

Although the number of reported cases of

General Information

Name _____ Unit No. _____

Date of Birth _____ Date _____ Time _____

Personnel

Physician _____ Nurse _____

Psychiatrist _____ Rape Counselor _____

Law Enforcement _____ Other _____

Assault History

Incident (Give an account of assault and description of attacker using patient's own words; use back if necessary.)

_____

_____

_____

_____

_____

_____

_____

_____

_____

Date _____ Time _____ Location _____

Physical Surroundings (describe where rape occurred) _____

_____

_____

_____

Number of Assailants _____ Race _____ Sex _____

Assailant _____ Known _____ Unknown _____ Relative

Violence: Physical

              Restraints ☐ Yes ☐ No   Type _____

              Weapons ☐ Yes ☐ No   Type _____

              Blindfold ☐ Yes ☐ No   Type _____

        Other _____

	Oral	Anal	Vaginal	Digital	Foreign Body (describe)
Type of Sex	____	____	____	____	_____
Penetration	____	____	____	____	_____
Ejaculation	____	____	____	____	_____

Loss of consciousness ☐ Yes ☐ No   Comments _____

Forced use of alcohol and/or drugs ☐ Yes ☐ No

    Describe _____

FIGURE 8–2. Sexual assault report form. (From North Carolina Memorial Hospital Rape Crisis Program, Chapel Hill, North Carolina.)

Ejaculation, urination, or defecation on body ☐ Yes ☐ No

    Describe _____

_____

Condom used ☐ Yes ☐ No ☐ Unknown

Since the assault have you (circle the appropriate response)?

    Bathed   Gargled   Drunk   Washed Hair   Douched   Urinated

    Defecated   Eaten   Changed Clothes   Brushed Teeth

    Other _____

Were medication, drugs, or alcohol taken before or after the

assault? ☐ Yes ☐ No

    Explain _____

_____

Past Medical History

    Parity G _____ P _____ A _____ LMP _____ NML _____ Abnormal _____

    Serious medical illness/hospitalizations _____

_____

_____

    Allergies _____

    Present medications _____

    Use of contraception (method) _____

    Last Pap smear _____

_____

    History of STD or other gynecological illness _____

_____

Physical Examination

  A. Vital Signs Temperature _____ Pulse _____ Respirations _____ B/P _____

  B. Emotional Assessment (describe behavior) _____

_____

_____

  C. Systems Examination (describe if abnormal, check [√] if normal)

    Head ( )   Back ( )   Eyes ( )   Nose, Throat, and Mouth ( )

    Neck ( )   Chest ( )   Breasts ( )   Abdomen ( )

    Extremities   Upper ( )   Lower ( )   Neurological Examination ( )

    Skin examination to search for semen (with Wood's light) (describe)

_____

_____

_____

_____

FIGURE 8–2 Continued

Illustration continued on following page

Treatment (check [√] as appropriate)

  A. **STD Prophylaxis**   ☐ Yes ☐ No

      ( ) Amoxicillin 3.0 g orally and probenecid 1 g orally

               -or-

      ( ) Vibramycin 300 mg orally immediately and repeat in 1 hour

               -or-

      ( ) 4.8 million units IM procaine penicillin and probenecid 1 g orally

  B. **Pregnancy Prophylaxis**   ☐ Yes ☐ No

      ( ) Ovral 2 tablets immediately and repeat in 12 hours

               -or-

      ( ) Ethinyl estradiol 5 mg every day for 5 days

               -or-

      ( ) Premarin 7.5 mg four times a day for 5 days

      ( ) Phenergan suppositories 25 mg every 6 hours PRN nausea

      ( ) Other

          ( ) None (patient using contraception)

          ( ) Wait, if miss next expected menses, pregnancy test followed by therapeutic abortion

          ( ) Schedule menstrual extraction now

  C. **Tetanus Toxoid (if indicated)**   ☐ Yes ☐ No

Follow-up and Referrals

  A. **Medical Follow-up**

      Name of physician _____

      Date of appointment _____

  B. **Referrals**   (check appropriate ones)

      ( ) Rape Crisis   ( ) Department of Social Services

      ( ) Mental Health   ( ) Other

      ( ) Law Enforcement

Disposition of Evidence   (check appropriate ones)

  A. ( ) Law Enforcement

          Agency _____

          Officer _____

  B. ( ) Hospital Security

          Officer _____

  C. ( ) Evidence Kit Sealed by _____

Physician _____   Nurse _____

Date _____   Date _____

FIGURE 8–2 Continued

sexual abuse of children has increased dramatically in the past few years, this may not represent actual increases in abuse incidents. More likely, this phenomenon probably represents the result of increased mandatory reporting statutes, better community awareness programs, and simply better record keeping.

All forms of sexual abuse of children are a crime in every jurisdiction. The term "sexual abuse of children" encompasses a wide range of acts committed against minors. It may be defined in a state criminal code by incest or sex crime statutes, or a separate definition may appear in a state child abuse reporting law or juvenile courts act. It may encompass sexual acts perpetrated by family members or persons in a position of authority over the child as well as acts by acquaintances and strangers. There is no uniformity in state statutes and prohibitions.

Sexual misuse or exploitation of children includes three distinct activities: sexual abuse, child prostitution, and child pornography (Shouvlin, 1981). Sexual abuse of children is usually defined as sexual activity between children and individuals occupying a position of authority. Child prostitution and child pornography most often involve runaway children and their use by strangers (Rush, 1980). In the past, terms such as "sexual misuse of children" or "sexual contact or interaction between adults and children" have also been used. The term "sexual abuse or sexual victimization of children" is more appropriate, however, since children in this society are taught to obey adults and are protected by them. Sex between an adult and a child is abusive, regardless of who initiated it or if it were consensual.

Available data indicate that in 1978, 15.4 per cent of all children for whom reports of abuse were substantiated were found to be sexually abused. When the victims of sexual abuse are both girls and boys, sexual abuse of girls is reported at a much higher rate than that for boys. Recently, however, the number of boy victims seen in treatment programs has increased. The average age of abused children is between 11 and 14, although there are reports of children as young as age 2 or 3 being abused. Some of these cases are detected because the children have contracted gonorrhea. In a large percentage of incest cases, the offense is repeated over periods of time ranging from weeks to several years, and force or threats of bodily harm

are rarely present. More often, the psychological pressures for affection and of dependence upon the adult are played upon and abused (Sloan, 1983).

Prior to 1976, few states had legislation specifically prohibiting sexual abuse and sexual exploitation of children. Until then, rape and incest indictments were relied upon to punish those who sexually abused children. This has proved virtually useless in dealing with a more broadly defined concept of sexual abuse. These laws were not broad enough to provide protection of children from all forms of sexual abuse.

What is needed is a broadly written sexual abuse statute that would apply to a wide range of sexual relationships. Such a statute would bar any person who poses as an authority figure or a responsible adult from engaging in sexual relations with a child, including fondling a child's genitals, intercourse, or forcing the child to perform oral sex. Unlike almost all current state legislation, this type of legislative act would define child sexual abuse more broadly and would make it clear that all forms of sexual activity with children are illegal. A comprehensive statute would also apply to anyone in a custodial or supervisory relationship to the child and especially to all persons trusted by the child, including the child's parents, adult friends of the parents, coaches, teachers, and babysitters (Shouvlin, 1981).

Readers are encouraged to find out what their jurisdiction presently defines as criminally punishable child sexual abuse. In most jurisdictions, proscriptions would be found in separate areas of the criminal statutes covering the subjects of rape, lewd and lascivious conduct, or sometimes indecent assault of a minor. This fragmented type of approach is generally not effective in dealing with sexual abuse by a parent or by someone in a position of authority.

Child Pornography and Prostitution

Child pornography and child prostitution are becoming increasingly recognized as a part of the general problem of child sexual abuse. Any individual engaging in sex for money or loitering and soliciting for that purpose is considered a prostitute and is subject to arrest. Although arrests of male homosexual prostitutes are on the rise, they are still low, and in some states only women can be found guilty of prostitution. Prostitution and the debate surrounding its criminalization are addressed later in this chapter; this section is limited to a discussion of child prostitution.

The incidence of child prostitution greatly increased in the 1960s and 1970s in the United States. Contributing to its growth is the continuing trend of enormous numbers of children who run away from home. There may be as many as 2 million young children who run away from home or who are left homeless each year (*US News and World Report*, June 9, 1980).

Few avenues of profitable, legitimate labor are open to the runaway child. As a consequence, many homeless youths turn to theft or prostitution (Shouvlin, 1981). However, most profits are not retained by the child, for few child prostitutes operate without a pimp. Pimps find customers; collect, manage, and control the profits; and protect their prostitutes from the harassment of other pimps and prostitutes. In child prostitution, the pimp may also initially provide emotional security to the child, who is often lonely and frightened. Pimps do not always directly entice a child into prostitution; however, they certainly play a role in ensuring that a child does not leave the life.

The customer represents the critical cog in child prostitution machinery. It is clear that without customer demand, child prostitution would not exist. The customer, unlike the child molester, must contact the child in public and thus runs a greater risk of discovery. However, few customers are punished for engaging prostitutes, either young or old (Campagna and Paffenberger, 1988). Ordinarily, criminal statutes have focused on punishing the prostitute rather than the customer.

Legislation is not an ideal approach for dealing with child prostitution but if specifically directed toward child prostitution may have some effect on curbing this form of child sexual abuse. However, the most effective means of reversing the trend of child prostitution lies in preventing the problem of runaways by altering the stability of children's home life and environment.

Criminalization of child prostitution is not the answer. Legislation that makes the crime of promotion of child prostitution (pimping) a more serious offense is a necessary step. This can be done by increasing the minimum

punishment levels. The object of any legislation designed to accomplish this is to punish pimps harshly for their contribution to the sexual exploitation of children. Statutes should not allow pimps to claim ignorance of the child's age and should therefore be similar to provisions dealing with statutory rape.

Statutes should also be designed to punish the customer of child prostitutes. At present, only a few states punish the customers of prostitutes. Creating statutes specifically designed to punish users of child prostitutes could serve as a deterrent. One approach might be to punish the patron with greater severity if the prostitute is below a legally designated minimum age.

Currently, most jurisdictions impose only a fine on child prostitutes. This has the effect of encouraging the child to return to the streets to "earn" the fine. Rather than fining the child, legislation should be designed to place these children in treatment facilities in anticipation of the child rejoining a secure family unit, such as foster care or the family of origin.

Child pornography is a further example of adult victimization of children. Child pornography is a flourishing industry, probably grossing profits in the billions. Child pornography depicts children being molested, raped, and otherwise exploited. It has been reported that there is a direct relationship between child prostitution and child pornography. Once recruited and committed to a prostitution ring, child members may help recruit other children, be involved with the filming and production of pornography, perform sexual services, and help set up a network of clientele (O'Brien, 1983).

It is currently unknown how frequently child pornography activity occurs. There are neither national reporting systems nor statewide data collection procedures to establish accurate statistics on this subject. It has been estimated that a significant percentage of the 700,000 to 1 million runaway children are involved each year in pornography and/or prostitution (Hearings before U.S. Congress, House Committee on Education and Labor, Sexual Exploitation of Children, Hearings before Subcommittee on Select Education, 95th Congress, First Session, 1977, pp 39–71, US Code Cong & Ad News, 1978).

Ideally, state legislation should broadly prohibit any activity that contributes toward child pornography. Most statutes presently reserve the stiffest penalties for producers;

however, enticers, producers, and distributors should all be punished with equal severity. Although enticers and producers have direct contact with the child, all three are equally responsible for the child's exploitation. The Supreme Court recently made the control of child pornography easier by holding that states may prohibit distribution of child pornography whether or not the material is legally obscene (see the section on pornography). This will strengthen the power of legislators and law enforcement to control this problem.

Law enforcement officials in many cities have developed strategies to help eradicate child pornography. These strategies include community education and media cooperation as well as enforcement of child pornography laws.

Reporting Child Sexual Abuse

According to Sloan (1983), sexual abuse is not often identified through physical indicators alone. Frequently, a child confides in a trusted teacher, counselor, or nurse that he or she has been sexually assaulted or molested by a caretaker; this may be the first sign that sexual abuse is occurring. There are, however, physical signs that health professionals should look for. These include sexually transmitted diseases, bruising of or pain in the vaginal or anal area, and pregnancy. In addition, there are certain behavioral signs that may be indicative of sexual assault. These include changes in personality, withdrawal, sexually provocative behavior, and play activities utilizing age-inappropriate sexual knowledge.

Today, almost all states include sexual abuse in their child abuse reporting law definitions. However, states differ in their definitions of the sexually abusive acts to be reported. Some states refer to their criminal sexual offense statutes; other states specifically list which act or acts constitute sexual abuse for the purpose of the reporting statute, while other states refer to definitions found in the state's family court acts. Health professionals should be familiar with their state's definition of sexual abuse and reporting statutes. Some states do not limit reportable abuse to that caused by a parent or person responsible for the child's care. Some

states, in addition, require reporting of parental or caretaker neglect as well as sexual abuse. Health professionals should determine the identity of the abusing party and know whether parental neglect triggers the reporting statute in their jurisdiction.

All jurisdictions require a nurse to report suspected child sexual abuse even if not specifically named by the statute. Nurses must take immediate action in reporting such findings once they have identified a child suspected of being sexually abused. A state may require either an oral or written report. Health professionals must report to the agency or agencies responsible for the receipt and subsequent investigation of reports of child sexual abuse and be acquainted with the agencies in their jurisdiction.

Some state statutes allow discretion in the decision of whether to file a report. Health professionals should determine whether such discretion is given in their jurisdiction and understand the criteria for its exercise. It is important for health professionals to know, however, that the great majority of jurisdictions impose a criminal penalty (generally a misdemeanor) for failure to report known sexual abuse. Further incentive to report sexual abuse is the potential for medical malpractice liability for damages caused by the health professional's failure to report.

All states with reporting statutes provide health professionals with immunity from civil or criminal liability when a report has been made in good faith under the statute. Many jurisdictions presume that all reports are made in good faith, and statutes provide absolute immunity for any health professional making such a report.

Gathering Evidence to Support Child Sexual Abuse Cases

Health professionals will often be called upon to provide evidence in child abuse or neglect hearings. The nurse may be the first professional to assess the physical signs of sexual abuse. These must be carefully assessed and documented. Documentation should include careful clinical notes, appropriate photographs, x-rays, and laboratory tests. The importance of careful record keeping cannot be overemphasized. A health professional may not be called upon to testify for weeks, possibly even months, after the client was seen. Records should therefore include sufficient detail to refresh the health professional's memory at the time of judicial proceeding.

In addition, any physical evidence, such as stained underpants or samples of fluids taken from the victim's genital or anal areas should be meticulously preserved for analysis. The health professional should carefully record any statements made by the victim or the suspected abuser. Such statements can be used as evidence in a judicial proceeding.

The health professional is often the first professional with the ability to make accurate observations who has contact with a sexually abused child. The observations and actions taken can well determine whether the child will ultimately receive treatment and protection or whether the cycle of abuse will continue.

ABORTION

Although not technically considered an aspect of sexuality, abortion has, since January 1973, been at the center of a legal debate of monumental proportions. Because health professionals often find themselves both personally and professionally in the midst of this debate, it is important to discuss thoroughly the legal aspects of abortion.

Historical Perspective

Although one purpose of the law is to protect the rights of the people under its jurisdiction, legal sanctions often reflect prevailing social values or beliefs of influential individuals. The laws and sanctions governing abortion are no different.

Prior to 1800, there was no legal prohibition against abortion in the United States or England. Abortion prior to "quickening" (by definition 20 weeks) was accepted by common law (Cohen and Parry, 1981). In 1803, abortion became illegal in England (Pritchard and McDonald, 1976). In the mid 1800s, prevailing Victorian mores and the influence of the Catholic church led to more restrictive legislation. In 1821, Connecticut passed the first antiabortion legislation in the United States, and by 1860 most states had similar statutes (Marrieskind, 1980). In 1873, the Comstock Law was enacted; this law "banned from the mails any drugs, medicines, or articles for

abortion or contraceptive purposes, forbade their advertisement through the mails, and outlawed their manufacture or sale in the District of Columbia or federal territories" (Cohen and Parry, 1981).

In 1869, the Roman Catholic church declared that the soul entered (the body of) the fetus at conception. In this view, to abort a fetus would be murder, and Catholic participants would be excommunicated. Thus, protection of the unborn became a reason for banning abortion. The American Medical Association followed suit by declaring abortion unlawful and unprofessional in 1871 (Cohen and Parry, 1981).

Historically, abortion had been restricted to prevent maternal deaths, since anesthesia, blood transfusions, and antibiotics were not available (Lyon, 1980). However, as these social, religious, medical, and, ultimately, legal sanctions against abortion came into existence, their result was to restrict severely women's choices, particularly in the absence of reliable contraception. In addition, such sanctions helped create negative associations and guilt about issues related to sexuality.

In 1962, the American Law Institute formally published a more relaxed penal code toward abortion as part of a model penal code. This code proposed that abortion be legally permitted in cases when (1) the woman's physical or mental health was endangered by the pregnancy, (2) the pregnancy resulted from rape or incest, or (3) the fetus was likely to be born with a serious physical or mental defect (Romney et al, 1975). Decriminalization of abortion was advocated to protect not only the woman seeking an abortion but also the physician performing the procedure.

By 1970, the civil rights and women's liberation movements had created an environment supportive of individual rights, including women's right to decide freely what to do with an unwanted pregnancy. Medical advances, including antibiotics and anesthesia, had made relatively safe abortion medically possible. In 1970, New York State passed legislation permitting abortion at the woman's request until 24 weeks' gestation. Since 1970, a number of significant court decisions have positively influenced the accessibility and availability of abortion services. Health professionals should be acquainted with their legal rights and obligations in order to play a role in providing accurate information to the public and in dispelling myths.

Today, the state's right to regulate abortion is circumscribed by the famous case of *Roe* v. *Wade*, announced on January 22, 1973. In that case, the Supreme Court struck down the Texas abortion law, which prohibited all abortions except as necessary to save the life of the mother. The court recognized women's fundamental constitutional right to choose abortion, which may be restricted only when the state has a compelling interest, for example, during the third trimester, at which time the Supreme Court held a state had a compelling interest in protecting the fetus.

As a result of *Roe* v. *Wade*, a woman is now legally free to seek an abortion in the first 12 weeks of pregnancy in all states. The 1973 Supreme Court ruling stated the following:

1. During the first trimester of pregnancy, the abortion decision must be left to the pregnant woman and her physician. Thus, the state may not interfere with either a woman's choice to keep or abort the pregnancy or with the physician's right to perform or refuse to perform an abortion.

2. During the second trimester of pregnancy, the woman is still free to decide whether to terminate her pregnancy, but states are permitted to regulate abortion procedures to the extent that these are reasonably related to maternal health. Thus, how and where an abortion is performed may be influenced by the state.

3. In the third trimester, or after fetal viability, the state has a compelling interest in protecting the fetus and, therefore, has the right to limit abortion to situations in which preservation of the life or the health of the pregnant woman is an issue.

Third Party Consent

A husband cannot legally prevent a woman from obtaining an abortion. In 1976, in *Planned Parenthood* v. *Danforth* (1976), the Supreme Court ruled that states may not require a married woman to obtain third party consent for an abortion, deciding that it could not grant a husband power it did not itself possess.

States may, however, require that a woman notify her spouse before obtaining an abortion. In Florida, state law requires pregnant women to notify and to consult with their husbands prior to an abortion. This law was determined to be constitutional by the United States Court of Appeals for the Fifth Circuit in its decision in *Schienberg* v. *Smith* (1981). The court of appeals' opinion hinged upon the fact that the statute required notice and not consent. The court found that the statute encouraged rather than discouraged marital consultation and held that intrusion into a woman's ability to exercise freedom of choice was less than in the *Danforth* case. The court's ruling suggested that the consultation requirement would not substantially impair a woman's freedom to decide whether to have an abortion.

The issue of parental consent for minors was addressed in *Planned Parenthood* v. *Danforth* (1976), in which the Supreme Court ruled that requiring parental consent for all minors seeking abortions was unconstitutional (Bernstein, 1981). In most states, minors may seek and obtain an abortion without their parents' knowledge, although several recent cases have caused some confusion. In *Bellotti* v. *Baird* (1979), the Supreme Court decided on a standard for state statutes involving court approval of a minor's abortion that would allow a minor to go directly to court without consulting her parents. If satisfied that the minor is well enough informed to make the decision to have an abortion, the court may authorize her to proceed without parental involvement or notification. If the court is not convinced of the minor's understanding, it must nevertheless allow the minor to demonstrate that the abortion would be in her best interest. A judge does not have veto power over the abortion. Only the minor who lacks understanding *and* whose best interest, in the judge's view, would not be served by having the abortion would be turned over to her parents for the ultimate decision (Bernstein, 1981).

In the 1983 Supreme Court opinion *City of Akron* v. *Akron Center for Reproductive Health* (1983), the court again declared it unconstitutional to consider all minors under 15 years of age too immature to make a decision regarding abortion. This was decided on the grounds that each minor's case deserves to be considered individually. In another opinion issued the same day, *Planned Parenthood Association of Kansas City* v. *Ashcroft* (1983), the Supreme Court ruled that a juvenile court cannot deny a minor's request for an abortion unless it does not find her mature enough to make a decision. Similarly, in *Bellotti* v. *Baird* (1979) it was deemed constitutional to require third party consent from a parent or judge for an immature minor in the interest of the minor's protection. However, a judge's veto of a mature minor's decision would be an unconstitutional intrusion of the rights of the minor.

Third party consent requirements create barriers between a minor and a desired service. Parents may disagree about abortion while minors often lack an understanding of the legal system. These barriers may unnecessarily delay early, safer abortion. In addition, such requirements have moral implications. Whether someone should decide what is in another person's "best interests" raises questions about the justification of paternalistic interventions.

The Supreme Court appears to have decided, however, that a statute requiring parental notification by a nonemancipated "immature" minor seeking an abortion is constitutional. The court's reasoning in *H.L. v. Matheson* (1981) was that a statute requiring notification does not impose the same degree of burden upon rights to abortion privacy as parental consent requirements. With the ruling directed toward dependent, immature minors, the statute requiring parental notification was not found to be unconstitutional. It is not known how the courts will react to situations in which a similar statute is applied to a "mature" minor.

Governmental Financing of Abortions

While medically indigent pregnant women may in principle receive financial aid for an abortion, in reality this is not always the case. Although adult women have the right to an abortion, women do not have an unqualified right to receive federal funds for abortion. In *Beal* v. *Bolton* (1973) and in *Maher* v. *Roe* (1977) it was decided that states are not constitutionally required to participate in Medicaid programs that pay the expenses of nontherapeutic abortions for indigent women on the basis of previous policy calling for payment of childbirth expenses for indigent women (Marrieskind, 1980). The Hyde Amendment, part of a Department of Health, Education, and Welfare appropriations bill in 1976, stipulated that federal funds may not be used to pay for abortion except when the life of the mother would be

endangered if the fetus were carried to term or in the case of rape or incest. An Illinois statute refused state funding of abortions except when the life of the mother is endangered. Both of these laws are constitutional (*Harris* v. *McRae*, 1980; *Williams* v. *Zbaraz*, 1980).

Medical Regulation of Abortion Practices

Legislative restraints on abortion practice are allowed in some circumstances. During a woman's second trimester of pregnancy, states may regulate abortion procedures if regulation is reasonably related to maternal health. There are also constitutionally permissible state regulations setting minimum standards for abortion clinics. However, a requirement that all abortions carried out after the first trimester be performed in a hospital was determined to (unreasonably) infringe upon a woman's right to abortion in *City of Akron* v. *Akron Center for Reproductive Health* (1983). As a result of improved safety and medical technology, clinics can provide abortions as safely as hospitals through 16 weeks' gestation.

In *Doe* v. *Bolton* (1973), the Supreme Court ruled it unconstitutional to require that two physicians concur prior to an abortion. States do not place such constraints on other surgical procedures.

Informed Consent

As for any surgical procedure, informed consent is required for abortion. In *City of Akron* v. *Akron Center for Reproductive Health* (1983), however, the Supreme Court ruled that there need not be a 24-hour waiting period between the signing of an abortion consent form and the performance of an abortion. Further, provisions requiring vivid descriptions of fetal development, fetal perceptions, adoption, and childbirth were ruled unconstitutional. Such descriptions have been deemed an unreasonable intrusion of physician discretion and a form of harassment. With regards to client education, the court ruled it unreasonable and unnecessary to insist upon a lengthy and inflexible list of physical and emotional implications of abortion in the process of informed consent. More important for nurses, it was decided that it is unreasonable to assume that only physicians are competent to provide the information and counseling relevant to informed consent.

Right to Refuse Participation

The question of whether health professionals who find abortion abhorrent must participate in abortion procedures has been addressed by some states in so-called conscience clause statutes, which attempt to provide protection for employees refusing to carry out abortions. Most of these statutes give medical personnel and others the right to refuse to participate or assist in abortions. Some states specifically forbid discriminatory hiring on the basis of attitudes toward abortion, while others allow employees to refuse on moral, ethical, or religious grounds. And other states allow individuals to refuse to participate regardless of the grounds for refusal. In some instances, statutes may not extend this right of refusal to certain situations, such as emergency treatment.

Just what constitutes participation in abortion procedures is not currently well defined. Whether it includes activities above and beyond participation in the actual procedure is a function of the particular statute's language. Further, whether a statute has the right to exclude a nurse's refusal to care for an abortion patient, based on the protections of the state's conscious clause statute, is not known at the present time.

Nurses should determine for themselves what rights exist for refusal to participate in abortion procedures. Medical facilities' need for flexibility in staffing and health professionals' right to refuse to participate represent a conflict that is likely to continue for some time.

LAWS AFFECTING SEXUAL EXPRESSION BETWEEN TWO CONSENTING ADULTS

In every jurisdiction in the United States there are laws that proscribe certain consensual sexual behaviors between adults performed in private. For some, these behaviors are matters of private morality, while others believe that sexual behavior is a matter of public morality and should be encoded in the law. This section reviews these laws, identifying some problems associated with their enactment and enforcement and recommending changes.

Laws relating to consensual sexual behavior vary, sometimes dramatically, from state to state. Acts included under this rubric are fornication, adultery, lewd and open cohabitation, extracoital heterosexual acts, and so-called crimes against nature.

Fornication

The term "fornication" legally refers to sexual union between unmarried partners. It does not include conduct involving violence, children, or public sexual displays. It is therefore consensual heterosexual intercourse between two unmarried adults.

In some states the crime of fornication requires habitual intercourse in the manner of a husband and wife before the offense may be charged. Other states allow a single act of illicit sexual intercourse to be considered sufficient for charges of fornication. Fornication is generally labeled a misdemeanor, punishable by small fines and/or up to 6 months in prison.

In the states in which a single act of illicit sexual intercourse does not constitute fornication, the length of the individual's association is immaterial if habitual intercourse is established. While fornication is seldom prosecuted, the potential for harassment is always present. Several states, as well as the Model Penal Code of the American Law Institute, have decriminalized adult nonmarital sexual behavior.

Adultery

Laws penalizing adultery were designed to protect the marital unit and to ensure that children would only be born in wedlock. Adultery differs from fornication in that one or both of the parties are married but not to each other. In some states only the married party can be charged with adultery, while the other party may often be charged with fornication. In other states both parties can be charged with adultery.

As with fornication, a single act of illicit sexual intercourse can in some states constitute adultery, while in others the offense must be habitual in the manner of husband

and wife. Again, duration of the association is immaterial if habitual intercourse is established.

Conviction for fornication or adultery does not require that even a single act of illicit sexual intercourse be proved by direct testimony. Acts of intercourse may be inferred from the circumstances presented in evidence. For example, a jury could infer the act from two healthy adults spending several hours in a hotel. Although adultery is not approved by society, there is no longer any serious movement to maintain its criminal character (MacNamara and Sagarin, 1977). However, the adultery laws that remain on the books provide tools for harassment, a license for blackmail, and the threat of discriminatory enforcement by law enforcement officials.

Lewd and Open Cohabitation

A number of states have laws prohibiting adults of the opposite sex from engaging in lewd and open cohabitation. Situations such as trial marriages and older persons living together for convenience and tax advantages can potentially be subject to the lewd and open cohabitation statutes. In reality these laws are enforced very infrequently (Barnett, 1973). Even if no evidence of sexual connection is present, a male and female living together without benefit of marriage may be prosecuted for illicit cohabitation.

Extracoital Heterosexual Acts

There are laws in a majority of states that prohibit "unnatural" sexual acts between consenting men and women. These laws are commonly found under sections dealing with "offense against public morality and decency," such as:

If any person shall commit the crime against nature, with mankind or beast, he shall be punished as a felon. (General Statute of North Carolina)

Not all penal codes define the terms "crimes against nature" and the definitions that exist are often from judges' written opinions in specific cases. Activities commonly criminalized under crimes against nature laws are fellatio, cunnilingus, anal intercourse or sodomy, and any other type of insertion or contact usually included under the heading of extracoital. These laws generally consider such activities criminal even when performed in private.

The often-stated purpose of such laws is to punish persons who "undertake by unnatural and indecent methods to gratify a perverted and depraved sexual instinct which is an offense against public decency and morality" (State v. Adams, 1980). Such crimes have also been pronounced "contrary to the order of nature."

All 50 states have witnessed some degree of legislative or judicial modification decriminalizing extracoital sexual relations, depending on the consensual nature of the relationship, the relationship of the participants, and the level of privacy in which the activities take place. A small number of states exclude prosecution of married couples for such conduct. This parallels the right of privacy decisions of the United States Supreme Court in matters relating to abortion and contraception. Even in states that have not decriminalized extracoital sexual activity between married couples, judicial decisions have consistently held that they cannot be the subject of criminal prosecution, although such behavior by unmarried individuals is still considered a crime.

Private extracoital sexual acts between adults of the opposite sex are rarely, if ever, the subject of criminal prosecution. The very small number of arrests and prosecutions of heterosexual extracoital activity is almost always accompanied by allegations that the activity took place in a public or semipublic environment.

Penalties traditionally associated with such laws are severe: In most cases the acts are considered felonies, and some carry lengthy prison sentences. Historically, attempts to remove these laws from the books have proved unsuccessful. Although in private, many legislators would agree that the laws do not reflect present mores and, in fact, lessen respect for the law, they do not want to publicly vote to remove laws that have traditionally been associated with public morality.

Constitutional scholars have raised questions as to why consensual extracoital activity should be constitutionally permitted between husband and wife and yet barred to other adults (Barnett, 1973). They argue that Gris-

wald v. *Connecticut* and *Roe* v. *Wade* have opened a massive breach in the wall of traditional constitutional wisdom surrounding the sodomy laws. However, constitutional protection for such persons and activities should not be considered absolute. Indeed, recent Supreme Court decisions seem to indicate that there are limits to the Constitution's power to regulate state legislation dealing with private consensual activity of adults. Accordingly, then the means to decriminalize such acts will have to take place on a state by state basis. Decriminalization of all consensual sexual behavior between adults in private promises to be a lengthy and difficult process.

Consensual Homosexual Relation

There are no laws expressly prohibiting homosexuality, but there are statutes regarding "crimes against nature" that directly affect sexual practices between consenting homosexuals (Slovenko, 1965).

There is little doubt that the gay liberation and sexual freedom movements of recent decades have focused attention on the issue of criminalizing sexual contact between homosexual adults. Same-sex behavior between consenting adults is a classic example of a crime without a victim. Subjecting adult homosexuals to a risk of criminal sanctions for their sexual activity is perhaps one of the most significant issues in American criminal jurisprudence today.

These laws are claimed to express the moral sentiment of the community. However, individuals have argued that independent of morality the constitutional right of privacy implies that there should be no crime where there is no victim. Those adopting this position also maintain that criminal law has no place in the privacy of a citizen's bedroom.

It is apparent that the laws dealing with crimes against nature have been interpreted and enforced as antihomosexual acts and do not have as a primary or even secondary purpose the regulation of consensual heterosexual behavior. Infrequently, unmarried heterosexual couples are prosecuted under one of these laws when crackdowns on prostitution or motel raids are carried out.

The United States Supreme Court has upheld the constitutionality of antihomosexual laws. In the case of *Bowers* v. *Hardwick* (1986),

the Supreme Court found that a Georgia statute that made sodomy a criminal offense when applied to an admitted homosexual was constitutional. The Supreme Court in this case made it clear that the Constitution does not confer any fundamental right on homosexuals to engage in acts of sodomy, even in the privacy of their home. Thus, the Supreme Court upheld states' rights to regulate private consensual activity between adults under some circumstances. It appears that regulation of sexual activity between married partners and in the area of contraception is not considered within the province of the state, but it is equally clear that states may regulate sexual activities between homosexuals. The question of regulation of sexual activity between nonmarried heterosexuals has not yet been resolved.

Although the laws described in this section generally do not mention public or semipublic display of the proscribed activity as being essential to criminal charges, in fact, enforcement seems to occur predominantly when such acts have been carried out in public or semipublic surroundings. Study of a number of appellate decisions in crimes against nature cases reveals that enforcement took place when the participants could be and were viewed by others. Constitutional limitations on visual surveillance by police would seem to mandate that only confession by one or more of the participants is legally admissible as evidence when the activities have been carried out in private. However, constitutional theories and enforcement realities often diverge, as can be seen by the number of legal opinions that addresses the definition of privacy.

The Need for Reform

Society's mores are changing. The majority of the American public would probably agree that laws criminalizing any aspect of private sexual activity between consenting adults should not be the subject of the criminal justice system. Such laws can be used by law enforcement officials selectively to harass homosexuals or unmarried adults engaging in otherwise accepted behaviors. Individuals discovered violating criminal laws may also be subject to blacklisting or blackmail.

Continued criminalization of these sexual acts between consenting heterosexual adults will lead to disregard of and lessened respect for the law. When great segments of the population consistently violate the law and are neither frightened nor concerned about the consequences, negative attitudes toward the entire criminal justice system may develop.

Rights of privacy and human rights include the rights of adults to engage in all forms of sexual activity in which force is not used and which is carried out in privacy.

SEXUAL CONDUCT— UNRESOLVED VICTIM STATUS

A number of acts grouped under the umbrella term "sexual crimes" have engendered discussion as to whether victims are involved. Among the activities in this category presently dealt with by criminal law are prostitution, obscenity, and the minor nuisance crimes such as exhibitionism and voyeurism.

Prostitution

The penal codes of all 50 states, except some counties of Nevada, define and proscribe prostitution. While there are probably 50 variations in the definition and legal construction of the term, in general, prostitution includes the offering or receiving of the body for sexual intercourse for hire. In addition, in many jurisdictions the person patronizing a prostitute is also committing an illegal act. Finally, the third party often associated with the act of prostitution (the pimp) commits criminal acts in all jurisdictions when he or she procures, solicits, or in any other way aids in committing the act of prostitution.

Depending on the jurisdiction, the criminal definition of prostitution may or may not be applicable to a male offering his body for hire. In some states, statutes specifically include the fact that the recipient of the fee can be either a male or a female for the purpose of the act of prostitution. In some instances both male prostitution and homosexual prostitution are criminalized.

In general, statutes outlawing prostitution do not have serious penalties associated with them. Often, penalties are light, with the amount of fines considered trivial by the prostitute or pimp. Although patronizing prostitutes is illegal, few customers are arrested. The laws against prostitution are primarily directed against public displays of this activity, and most "busts" actually result from antiloitering campaigns.

Over time, the question has arisen as to whether prostitution should be made legal but not public. Most persons strongly condemn prostitution; however, it has been argued that prostitution serves some redeeming social values while, in fact, being a victimless crime. Others argue that prostitution leads to certain social problems, e.g., sexually transmitted diseases, and often includes one or more victims in its wake.

Proponents of the legalization of prostitution and those favoring its removal from the streets believe that regulating its practice will lead to reduced spread of sexually transmitted diseases. Proponents also argue that prostitution exists because there is a sufficiently strong market for its product and that the customer who purchases such services might be tempted to obtain them from an unwilling victim if they were unavailable (Davis, 1937).

Those opposing decriminalization of prostitution argue that even with registration and regulation, decriminalization would give society's stamp of approval on the commercialization of sex and that prostitutes often victimize their customers by robbery, assault, and blackmail. Studies have not demonstrated, however, that decriminalization of prostitution has any effect on the incidence of forceable sexual crimes (MacNamara and Sagarin, 1977).

Pornography

Pornography has come to be considered the equivalent of obscenity. Historically, however, pornography was associated with the term "erotica" and implied pleasurable life instincts derived from the libido. Over time, pornography became more connected with the term "obscenity," meaning "dirt or filth." This association of pornography with obscenity has taken on legal significance as it becomes a matter for criminal regulation.

The First Amendment to the United States Constitution provides that "Congress shall make no law . . . abridging the freedom of speech or the press." Over time, however, the Supreme Court has determined that certain categories of speech are not protected by the First Amendment and may therefore be regulated, or even proscribed by the states.

One of these unprotected categories includes "obscene" material. The problem of defining obscenity to distinguish it from the rights of speech and press protected by the First Amendment has occupied the Supreme Court for many years. The most recent definition of obscenity is to be found in the case of *Miller* v. *California* (1973). Under the test of the Miller case, an obscenity statute "must be limited to works which, taken as a whole, appeal to the prurient interest in sex, which portray sexual conduct in a patently offensive way, and which taken as a whole, do not have serious literary, artistic, political, or scientific value."

Further, in the Miller case, the court attempted to clarify for the first time what is meant by "patently offensive." It was held that the state must be precise in setting out the type of materials falling into the definition of obscenity. Patently offensive representations or descriptions of ultimate sexual acts, normal or perverted, actual or simulated; masturbation; excretory function; and lewd exhibition of the genitals were given by the court as examples that state statutes may define for regulation. The essence of this part of the test is that only hard-core pornography may be subject to obscenity laws. Whether the work under scrutiny for obscenity is patently offensive must be determined by contemporary standards in the community in which the decision is being made. It is interesting and important to note that the Miller case rejected the use of a national standard community value, previously adopted by the Supreme Court. Thus, what is obscene may differ in Los Angeles, California, and Raleigh, North Carolina.

The issue over time has been whether to regulate pornography by denying access to pornographic materials to individuals who find them satisfying or for any reason desirable. Related to this issue of access are questions of social harm or potential for harm.

From a societal point of view, the major concern about pornographic materials is the possibility that they may encourage the behaviors portrayed, e.g., rape, group sex, child sexual abuse, and sadomasochism (Geer, Heiman, and Leitenburg, 1984). Research has supported both sides of the debate as to whether pornography is a causal factor in antisocial behavior (Presidential Commission on Obscenity and Pornography, 1970). The recent Attorney General's Commission on Pornography, Final Report (1986) characterized pornographic materials as falling to three classes:

1. Sexually violent materials. In this instance, the Commission found "a causal relationship" between this type of material and protrayed behaviors, although not necessarily in every individual exposed to such materials.

2. Nonviolent materials depicting degradation, domination, subordination, or humiliation. The Commission here stated that evidence supports the conclusion that substantial exposure to this type of material increases the likelihood that an individual will experience attitudinal changes.

3. Nonviolent and nondegrading material. Here the Commission manifested substantial disagreement over the effects of such material and stated that the fairest conclusion to be drawn is that the available evidence does not support an association between these materials and acts of sexual violence. It is interesting to note, however, that the Commission found that even the materials in the final category were considered to "harm the moral environment."

Some suggest that there seem to be cogent arguments for the uncensoring of pornographic materials. It is argued that many citizens obtain sexual, literary, or artistic pleasure from pornography. In addition, obscenity statutes provide justification for selective prosecution. The local nature of the community standards test provides local law enforcement officers with almost arbitrary power to deal with written and pictorial materials. Such power can conceivably result in selective harassment of individuals and censorship of ideas not related to sex under the guise of censoring obscenity. While obscene materials can and should be kept away from children, it is felt by some that adults ought not and need not be restricted in order to protect youth from pornography.

A different viewpoint is held by many feminists. While having few illusions about the possibility of truly effective legal control, they view legal proscriptions as serving very important symbolic functions (Schur, 1984). The moral statements made by legally banning pornography outweigh the possible risks incurred by censorship. As Lederer said, "It is better to have it underground than to see it flourish as an accepted part of our culture" (Lederer, 1980, p 29).

MISCELLANEOUS NUISANCE SEXUAL BEHAVIORS

A subset of sexual behaviors remains that appears to be harmless, or at most, has slight potential for harm except to the perpetrator. Individuals exhibiting behavior considered atypical when compared with normal sexual behavior fall into this category. Examples of such behavior are exhibitionism and voyeurism. Both acts contain an element of psychopathology in the individual. The question thus arises as to whether these types of behavior are best addressed by a therapist or by the criminal justice system. As with obscenity and prostitution, discussion has centered on whether these acts are truly victimless crimes, whether victimization actually results, and whether, as offenses against the public order and morality, they should be regulated by the criminal justice system. An example of exhibitionism and voyeurism will highlight the issues raised.

Exhibitionism is defined as the deliberate exposure of the male genitals to unsuspecting females without intention of sexual contact (Geer, Heiman, and Leitenburg, 1984). This act is committed for the purpose of obtaining sexual gratification through the exhibition itself. The line between normal exposure of the genitals and what would be described as pathological exhibitionism is not clear in this era of revealing clothing.

Whether or not persons classified as exhibitionists pose a danger to society has been questioned. Gebhard, Gagnon, and Pomerroy (1965), who conducted classic research on sexual offenders, believed that exhibitionists on the whole "ought to be pitied rather than feared." Currently, this seems to be the generally accepted conclusion among experts. Some authorities suggest, however, that the exhibitionist may be demonstrating hostility or even sadistic tendencies toward the viewer and that therefore risk of rape or assault exists (Ellis and Brancale, 1956).

Criminalization of the exhibitionist should not be decided on the basis of whether the act offends public morality. Should harmlessness be proved, other ways should be found to handle such deviant behaviors. Inappropriateness should not be synonymous with criminality. Treatment would appear to be more appropriate than imprisonment in dealing with such persons.

Voyeurism is defined as a compulsive desire to observe women partially or completely nude without the consent of the female. Voyeurism is almost exclusively associated with males. As with exhibitionism, there is a gray area in which law enforcement has had to distinguish between the "ordinary" person ogling a female and the one who is violating a criminal statute. The law refers to uninvited looking, but both behaviors are, in fact, uninvited.

The criminal justice system generally labels the voyeur a nuisance, perhaps psychopathological, rather than a criminal. As in exhibitionism, there is some disagreement as to whether voyeurs ultimately pose a threat to society. As long as they remain undetected, voyeurs bother no one, although they are violating the privacy of others. There is some question, however, whether voyeurs "graduate" to violent, aggressive crimes. Most research to date suggests that the voyeur is a harmless, if disturbed, individual (Geer, Heiman, and Leitenburg, 1984).

If voyeurism's only effect is an invasion of another's privacy and it does not lead to other antisocial acts, there is doubt as to whether it can be the subject of criminal proscription. While such behavior is certainly unacceptable, it may not be sufficient to label such individuals criminal.

HUMAN IMMUNODEFICIENCY VIRUS

The human immunodeficiency virus (HIV) and the acquired immunodeficiency syndrome (AIDS) have become critical issues in legal and health fields. Between 1981, when AIDS was first reported by the Centers for Disease Control (CDC), and the present, bodies of law and legal scholarship have developed in the following areas related to law, sexuality, and health care: (1) personal liability for the transmission of the virus, (2) criminal law, and (3) liability of hospitals for the spread of AIDS.

AIDS and Liability

The AIDS epidemic has raised a number of new questions regarding the consequences of sexual contact. Is an HIV-positive individual liable for exposing a sexual partner to the virus? Are there legal defenses that the person transmitting the HIV virus will be able to raise? Does a sexual partner have the right to assume that the other partner does not have the HIV virus? Does a legal duty exist to disclose such a disease to a sexual partner? Does a legal duty exist to disclose at-risk life style to a sexual partner?

While there are, at present, no definitive answers to these questions, Baruch (1987) has presented a theoretical framework that suggests answers to the questions. In Baruch's view, liability exists when the following conditions are met: (1) an individual is HIV positive or has AIDS-related complex (ARC) or AIDS and knows it, (2) sexual contact of the type that can transmit the virus takes place, (3) an infected person takes part in sex without telling his or her partners, and the virus is transmitted. Knowing also legally applies to individuals considered at high risk who do not choose to take the HIV antibody test. The law ascribes liability based on what the transmitter should reasonably know. If transmitters knowingly misrepresent the truth to their partners, liability for the results of the transmission will certainly exist.

If the sexual partner is aware of the defendant's condition or should have been aware of it, the law in many states would say that liability does not exist based on the theory of contributory negligence; that is, if the plaintiff knowingly engaged in sexual activity with an individual who was HIV positive or had ARC or AIDS, liability is not present. If the plaintiff knows or should have known of the defendant's condition and insisted upon the use of "safe sex" practices, the question of contributory negligence becomes more muddled. In many states, the doctrine of comparative negligence exists, mitigating the harsh effects of contributory negligence. In these states, liability would be found, but the total amount of damages would be reduced by some ratio of the comparative negligence of the two parties.

There is little question that the dramatic rise in the number of reported AIDS cases presages a corresponding rise in litigation related to AIDS transmission. The law relating to liability in the transmission of AIDS must still be written.

A final topic related to liability for AIDS transmission is the potential liability of physicians for not disclosing a patient's condition to others likely to have sexual contact with him or her. The medical community is divided over whether such a duty exists; therefore, liability for failure to comply with such a duty is yet another chapter to be written in the saga of AIDS and the law.

AIDS and the Criminal Law

AIDS hysteria has reignited homophobic attitudes and has given opponents of gay rights new grounds on which to stand. In several recent cases, AIDS has been offered as a justification for sodomy statutes. For example, in *Bowers* v. *Hardwick* (1986), one of the briefs suggested that the AIDS epidemic provides compelling justification for sodomy statutes (Brief for Petitioner at 37).

Previously discussed consensual sexual activity, including sodomy, should not be a matter of government regulation. However, the state's interest in preventing transmission of AIDS would seem to be a compelling one. States have an overarching interest to protect the public health. The question arises as to whether regulation of certain activities in the interest of public health is conducted in a "legal manner." The courts have developed certain criteria to test the legitimacy of statutes designed to protect the public health. These are the following:

Does the health statute under consideration bear a rational relation to the objective? Is the statute arbitrary to capricious? If legislative classifications result, are such classifications rationally related to a legitimate state interest? Does the scope of the statute go beyond what is required to achieve the objective? Is either a suspect classification (e.g., race or sex) or a fundamental right involved? (If so, there must be a compelling state interest in the matter.)

The criminal law could treat the transmission of AIDS as a crime. This may be preferable to a renewed criminalization of sodomy in that it would focus on a cuprable act rather than on a consensual act between two adults. The transmission of AIDS to another individual causing death could be treated as a crime of murder, manslaughter, or negligent homicide. If the victim does not die, the crime could be assault. For a more complete treatment of these crimes the reader is referred to the recent article "AIDS and the Criminal Law" by Field and Sullivan (1987).

There is a long history of states criminalizing the transmission of sexually transmitted diseases. There have been so-called exposure statutes making it a crime to expose willfully another person to certain diseases (e.g., veneral diseases). Issues of what represents exposure of another person will have to be carefully studied so that activities that are not at risk are not included.

How will laws with criminal sanctions related to involuntary physical examinations, reporting requirements, quarantine, and isolation and/or voluntary hospitalization of carriers of HIV fare under the previously cited criteria to test the legitimacy of public health statutes? We have seen, for example, the criminalization of gay bath houses in New York City upheld as legal (*City of New York* v. *The New Saint Mark's Baths,* 1986).

These are not easy questions. Issues of personal privacy and individual rights and laws created or enforced that are designed to control a legitimate public health problem, rather than regulate morality, are at the forefront of the discussion. Where these lines are drawn will be a historical test of the United States criminal justice system.

Liability of Hospitals in the Spread of AIDS to Staff, Visitors, and Other Parties and CDC Guidelines

Many hospitals out of concern for liability due to the potential spread of AIDS from patients to staff and other patients and visitors have refused to admit patients known to be infected with HIV (NYC Commission on Human Rights, Report on Discrimination Against People with AIDS—November 1983 to April 1986). No legal determination has been made of hospitals' medical obligation to persons with AIDS or to individuals coming in contact with them, including staff, visitors, and other patients. This uncertainty, along with the enormous drain on medical resources that treatment of AIDS implies, will continue to cause hospitals to be cautious in their formulation of AIDS policy and may more often than not result in a policy of excluding people with AIDS from the institution.

A recent study entitled "Hospital Liability in AIDS Treatment, the Need for a National Standard of Care" (Hermann and Gorman, 1987) argues for a national standard of care for the treatment of AIDS patients based on the Centers for Disease Control (CDC) guidelines (see the CDC's recommendations and guidelines concerning AIDS, published in *Morbidity and Mortality Weekly Report,* 1982 to 1986).

If the CDC guidelines were adopted as a national standard of care, liability for exposure of other patients, health care workers, and others to the virus associated with AIDS would be based on a known standard of care.

In addition, hospitals meeting their duty under the guidelines could feel comfortable with respect to liability. The CDC's *Morbidity and Mortality Weekly Report* (MMWR) and other CDC publications provide the most current guidelines for the treatment and care of persons with AIDS. Guidelines are also continually updated by the CDC as new medical advances become known. Thus, they provide a continually updated standard of care over time.

It almost goes without saying that all health professionals involved in the treatment of AIDS should be aware of the latest CDC guidelines in order to provide optimal care for patients and to protect themselves and third parties. All health professionals have a clear duty to use the most comprehensive and up-to-date infection control measures presently available with respect to AIDS as outlined in the CDC guidelines.

AIDS is likely to represent a major test of our society's ability to deal, from a legal point of view, with issues of human sexuality. How the law will choose to respond to some of the issues described in this section remains to be seen.

CONCLUSION

The United States possesses criminal statutes designed to regulate every form of sexual expression other than traditional coitus between married individuals. It proscribes activities regardless of whether victimization has occurred, whether the activity took place in the privacy of the home, or whether the activity meets with the normative approval of a majority of citizens. Conceptually, this has been done on the grounds that the purpose of the law is to proscribe activities that offend the general public morality. The debate over whether the law should prevent victimization or enforce prevailing moral beliefs is continuing and as yet unresolved.

This chapter has shown that in the area of sex and the law, certain behaviors clearly have victims requiring protection; other areas are clearly victimless; finally, in certain areas the issue of victimization has not been resolved. Health professionals should use this chapter as a springboard for further study.

Health professionals may find themselves playing an important role in the enforcement of criminal laws dealing with sexuality. These range from the treatment of victims of sexual crimes to the professional's role in the highly controversial and emotional area of abortion. Health professionals may provide care to the victim as well as be responsible for gathering evidence to be used in the prosecution of the accused.

Finally, the reader is urged to consider where the outer bounds of an individual's right of privacy should lie, where the use of criminal law is appropriate, and therefore, what level of decriminalization should take place in the area of human sexual behavior.

REFERENCES

American Law Institute: Model Penal Code, Proposed Official Draft of Comments, 1985.

Attorney General's Commission on Pornography, Final Report (Meese Commission Report). Washington, DC, US Government Printing Office, July 1986.

Barnett, W: Sexual Freedom and the Constitution. Albuquerque, University of New Mexico Press, 1973.

Baruch D: AIDS In-court, Tort Liability for Sexual Transmission of AIDS. Tort and Insurance Law J 22:2, 1987.

Bernstein A: The legal right to abortion: What's left. Hospitals 59:41–42, 92, 1981.

Bessmer S: The Laws of Rape. New York, Praeger Publishers, 1984.

Birchfield J: AIDS—the legal aspects of the disease. Med Law 6:407–425, 1987.

Campagna DS, Paffenberger DL: The Sexual Trafficking in Children: An Investigation of the Child Sex Trade. Dover, Auburn House, 1988.

Cohen M, Parry J: Abortion on demand: Policy and implementation. Health Soc 6:65–72, 1981.

Davis K: The sociology of prostitution. Am Sociol Rev, 1937.

Devlin P: The Enforcement of Morals. Oxford, Oxford University Press, 1965.

Ellis A, Brancale R: The Psychology of Sex Offenders. Springfield, Charles C Thomas, 1956.

Ferguson RW: Constitutional law—A new standard for states battle against child pornography. Wake Forest Law Review 10:95–117, 1983.

Field M, Sullivan K: AIDS and the criminal law. Law Med Health Care 15:46–60, 1987.

Gebhard P, Gagnon J, Pomeroy W: Sex Offenders: An Analysis of Types. New York, Harper & Row, 1965.

Geer J, Heiman J, Leitenburg H: Human Sexuality. Englewood Cliffs, Prentice Hall, 1984.

Grey C: The Legal Enforcement of Morality. New York, Random House, 1983.

Hart HLA: Law, Liberty, and Morality. Stanford, Stanford University Press, 1963.

Hermann D, Gorman R: Hospital liability for AIDS treatment, The Needs for National Standards of Care, U.C. Davis Law Review 15:36–45, 1987.

Holmstrom LL, Burgess AW: Sexual behavior of assailants during reported rapes. Arch Sex Behav 9:427–439, 1980.

Kalven H, Zeisel H: The American Jury. Chicago, University of Chicago Press, 1966.

Kroselchell LJ: Criminal Law—The Constitutionality of North Carolina's Rape Shield Law. Wake Forest Law Review 17, 781–800, 1981.

Lederer L: Take Back the Night. New York, William Morrow, 1980.

Lyon T: An abortion prospective: Legal considerations. Minn Med 63:659–661, 1980.

MacNamara D, Sagarin E: Sex, Crime and the Law. New York, Free Press, 1977.

Marrieskind H: Women in the Health System, Patients, Providers, and Programs. St. Louis, CV Mosby, 1980.

McGuigan S: The AIDS dilemma, public health and the community law. Law Tranquility 4:545, 1987.

Mill JS: On Liberty. New York, Penguin, 1859.

National Commission.for Preventing Child Abuse: Basic Facts About Sexual Child Abuse, 1978.

O'Brien S: Child Pornography. Dubuque, Kendall Hunt, 1983.

Presidential Commission on Obscenity and Pornography. New York, Bantam Books, 1970.

Pritchard J, McDonald P: Williams Obstetrics. Norwalk, Appleton-Century-Crofts, 1976.

Romney S, Gray MJ, Little A, et al: Gynecology and Obstetrics: The Health Care of Women. New York, McGraw-Hill, 1975.

Rosenblatt C, Pariente B: The Prostitution of the Criminal Law. American Criminal Law Review, 1973.

Rush F: The Best Kept Secret: Sexual Abuse of Children. New York, McGraw-Hill, 1980.

Schur EM: Labeling Women Deviant. New York, Random House, 1984.

Shouvlin D: Preventing the Sexual Exploitation of Children. Wake Forest Law Review 17, 1981.

Sloan E: Child Abuse: Governing Law and Legislation. Dobbs Ferry, Oceana, 1983.

Slovenko R: Sexual Behavior and the Law. Springfield, Charles C Thomas, 1965.

Wolfenden Report, Home Office, Scottish Home Department: Report of the Committee on Homosexual Affairs and Prostitution, 1963.

Case Citations

Beal v. *Bolton,* 432 U.S. 179, (1973)

Bellotti v. *Baird,* 443 U.S. 622, (1979)

Bowers v. *Hardwick,* 92L Ed. 2d, (1986)

Cary v. *Population Services International,* 431 U.S. 679, (1977)

City of Akron v. *Akron Center for Reproductive Health,* 462 U.S. 416, (1983)

City of New York v. *The New Staint Mark's Baths,* 497 NYS 2d 979 NY Sup Ct, (1986)

Doe v. *Bolton,* 410 U.S. 179, (1973)

Griswald v. *Connecticut,* 381 U.S. 479, (1965)

Harris v. *McRae,* 448 U.S. 297, (1980)

H.L. v. *Matheson,* 450 U.S. 398, (1981)

Isenstadt v. *Baird,* 405 U.S. 438, (1974)

Maher v. *Roe,* 932 U.S. 464, (1977)

Miller v. *California,* 413 U.S. 15, (1973)

Planned Parenthood Association of Kansas City v. *Ashcroft,* 462 U.S. 476, (1983)

Planned Parenthood v. *Danforth,* 428 U.S. 52, (1976)

Roe v. *Wade,* 410 U.S. 113, (1973)

Schienberg v. *Smith,* 659 F.2d 476, (1981)

Stanley v. *Georgia,* 394 U.S. 557, (1969)

State v. *Adams,* 264 S.E. 2d, 46, (1980)

Williams v. *Zbaraz,* 448 U.S. 358, (1980)

9: Religious Influence and Sexuality

Judy Brusich

Sexuality, although basically the same component of our human nature in any culture, is experienced and expressed in a multitude of ways, depending on the cultural context in which it is found. Religion, as a component of a particular culture, is usually involved in specific and nonspecific ways with the experience and expression of sexuality. Geoffrey Parrinder says:

Sex and religion are two of the commonest concerns of mankind. Often opposed as physical and spiritual, temporal and eternal, they seem to occupy different and clearly defined territories yet they are always crossing the frontiers. . . . (R)eligion takes all the world as its province and turns its eyes upon the slightest manifestations of sex. . . . (Parrinder, 1980, p 1)

Specific religious doctrines influence sexuality by prescribing or prohibiting certain behaviors, such as premarital intercourse or abortion, but in general religion has an effect on sexuality by how it shapes a person's concept of him- or herself as a sexual being, i.e., as essentially good or bad. Sexuality is affected by religion to the extent that religion influences most people's decisions about what they *do* and perceptions about who they *are*.

Religious symbols can have strong influences on social and sexual roles. For example, Eve may serve as a symbol either of women's subordination to men or of women's equality with men, depending on the biblical interpretation. It is important that health professionals are conscious of how religious symbols may affect sexual attitudes and behaviors in both negative and positive ways (LaChat, 1988).

In terms of religion, Judeo-Christian beliefs and teachings dominate American culture. Consequently, any of the commonly accepted sexual values and practices of Americans are influenced by the sexual beliefs taught by the Jewish, Catholic, and Protestant faiths. This chapter will primarily discuss the teachings of these three religions. Because not all Americans subscribe to these religions, a brief overview of the beliefs guiding sexual practices of Islam, Hinduism, and Buddhism will also be provided. While this chapter is not an exhaustive review of all religious teachings about sexuality, the author hopes to sensitize the reader to the religious influences that may operate in clients' sexual self-perceptions and sexual decision-making. Some knowledge of the teachings of each religion about sexuality should assist health professionals and nurses to accept and to demonstrate understanding attitudes toward clients with different religious backgrounds.

JEWISH BELIEFS AND TEACHINGS

In modern practice, there are three main branches of Judaism: Orthodox, Conservative, and Reform. Orthodox Judaism holds the most traditional beliefs, Reform Judaism the most liberal beliefs, and Conservative Judaism beliefs that are in between those of the Orthodox and the Reform branches. Consequently, individual Jewish clients' beliefs may be somewhat different, depending on which branch they belong to.

Judaism views sexuality as part of our God-given nature and therefore something inherently good. While the pleasure and joy people experience from being sexual creatures and behaving in a sexual manner is considered legitimate, and indeed holy in some instances, Judaism does hold a basic tenet "that marriage and marriage alone is the proper framework for sexual experience" (Gordis, 1978, p 98).

Contrary to what has been a pervading philosophy in Christianity for many centuries, Judaism does not see marriage as a "concession to the lower instincts, but, on the contrary, the ideal human status because it alone offers the opportunity for giving expression to all aspects of human nature" (Gordis, 1978, p 98). Sharing the pleasure of sex in marriage is so encouraged in Judaism that there is a biblical reference (Deuteronomy 24:5), indicating that a man was deferred from the military draft during the first year of marriage so that he may "rejoice with his wife." Ancient Jewish law also asked men to plan business and military trips so that they would be at home during the time when sexual activity with their wives was acceptable, 12 to 13 days after menstruation (Dyck, 1978). Some Judaic teachings go beyond merely encouraging the enjoyment of marital sex and mandate certain sexual behavior. "The talmudic injunction that scholars and their wives have conjugal relations on Sabbath eve is explained by Rashi on the ground that the Sabbath is 'for pleasure, rest, and physical enjoyment'" (Gordis, 1978, p 101).

Interestingly, the responsibility for providing sexual pleasure in a Jewish marriage falls primarily on the man. "Marital relations are seen as the duty of the husband and the privilege of his wife" (Dyck, 1977, p 287). This particular teaching is commonly superseded in American culture by the idea that sexual relations are a woman's duty to her husband.

Also in support of the Judaic acceptance of sexuality as an innately good component of our humanity is the fact that "sexual asceticism was never accorded the dignity of a religious value in Jewish law" (Dyck, 1977, p 287). Gordis (1978) emphasizes this by stating that there is no Jewish counterpart to the Christian monastic orders.

Thus, Judaism engenders a positive concept of the self as a sexual being. While Orthodox Jews today still subscribe to a number of stringent regulations of sexual practices, most Conservative and Reform Jews feel relatively free from excessive proscriptions over the conduct of their sexual lives.

Jewish tradition, including rabbinic rulings themselves, has a great respect for individual conscience, and when it comes to deciding what is right and wrong, it is fair to say that each Jew is ultimately his own rabbi. (Dyck, 1977, p 286)

Basic teachings of the Torah include injunctions against judging others and advice about treating our fellow beings with compassion (Matt, 1978). Consequently, even when one does not follow the sexual teachings of the faith exactly, the attitude of rabbis and other members of the congregation is not necessarily condemnatory. There are no prescribed punishments for failure to live up to religious commandments. Sin of a sexual nature is not treated with any special emphasis or harshness in Judaism, as it has sometimes been in Christianity.

In general, when caring for Jewish clients the nurse should anticipate that the clients will hold positive, accepting attitudes about themselves as sexual beings and that they may base their sexual practices, in part, on certain ancient laws and teachings. The Jewish faith does not teach feelings of guilt or shame about sexuality, which are sometimes encountered in clinical practices. The following section examines the Jewish perspective on a number of issues regarding sexuality.

Contraception

Judaism holds that the purpose of marriage is twofold, procreational and relational, with these two aspects having equal value. Therefore, sexual relations may legitimately be motivated by either the desire to have a child or the expression of love between husband and wife. Both motivations need not be present for sexual activity to be considered acceptable, but Jewish tradition encourages the couple not to neglect the relational aspects of sexual interaction. Based on this philosophy, teachings about contraception are not extremely explicit, but there are certain guidelines about this issue.

Interpreted in its literal sense, Jewish law mandates procreation (Dyck, 1977). Some schools of thought state that this obligation is technically and minimally met with the birth of two children, while more conservative schools of thought state that the birth of two sons is required to fulfill this duty. However, concession to this law is made for serious reasons, such as the health of the mother. While childless marriage is not the ideal of Jewish teachings, many modern rabbis, especially of the Conservative and Reform branches, will participate in the marriage ceremonies of couples who have no procreational intent. This is one example of the way in which Judaism as an organized religion provides certain guidelines about behavior but also supports individual freedom. Prevention of procreation may be accomplished by any means acceptable to the couple. Abstinence is not called for as a method of preventing pregnancy, as this would subvert the relational aspects of sexuality.

Responsible parenthood is seen as a more important issue for Jewish families than which method of contraception they choose or when they choose to use contraception. This is especially true after they have two children. Responsible parenthood implies considering a multitude of factors, such as the ability to care for and educate children properly, the harmony in the home, the health of the mother, the effect of another child on children already in the family, and the effect of another child on the environment in which the child must live. All these are considerations Jewish couples may use in making contraceptive decisions rather than relying on specific prewritten laws. Thus, the quality of the lives of the mother and present children are respected and are of concern.

While specific laws about contraception are not abundant, there are a few principles that Judaism holds about the use of contraception. First, there are times when use of contraception is expected, e.g., by a minor to protect his or her own health or by a nursing mother to protect her offspring (Dyck, 1977). Second, the motivation for preventing procreation should not be of trivial, vain, or purely selfish reasons. For instance, a woman who has endured, in her opinion, unusual pain giving birth to one child is not obligated to bear another. But a woman (or a man) should not use contraception simply to avoid the possibility of "marring her beauty" (Dyck, 1977). Third, conservative interpretations of Judaic law indicate that withdrawal may not be a legitimate form of contraception in that it constitutes "improper emission of generative seed." Other interpretations concerning withdrawal hold that it is sinful only in the context of autoerotic or nonheterosexual activity (Dyck, 1977).

Dyck (1977) states that a number of studies have shown that in actual practice a large percentage of Jewish couples utilize contraception and do so very effectively. When counseling Jewish couples regarding contraception, the nurse should be aware that the couple may face no religious taboos on the practice of contraception. The major influence the religion has on the decision about contraception relates to responsible parenthood. Consequently, a major role for the nurse may be to help the couple resolve what responsible parenthood means in their lives. This may include providing information on growth and development or sibling rivalry, so that the couple may make an informed decision about the effect of a newborn on children they already have. It may also include acting as a sounding board for a woman working through decisions about career versus motherhood, or about how to adjust to the stresses and demands of both.

Abortion

Among Jewish scholars the generally accepted definition for the beginning of life is at the time of birth. Gordis states that "the Halakah explicitly recognizes that the foetus is not a viable being while it is in its mother's womb since its life can not be sustained outside its natural shelter there" (Gordis, 1978, p 140). Dyck (1977) discusses the range of conservate to liberal ideas within the Jewish faith on the issue of abortion:

One school assumes no real prohibition against abortion except, perhaps, in the most advanced stages of pregnancy, and then proceeds to build up safeguards against indiscriminate abortion. The second school sees abortion as akin to homicide, permissible for saving the life of a pregnant woman and then, in its consideration of various cases, embraces grave threats to health as a justification for abortion. (Dyck, 1977, p 305)

The liberal view stems from compassion, especially for the woman. Consequently, a primary rationale for abortion may not necessarily include the knowledge that a child may be born with major defects. Rather, a primary rationale may be concern for the mother's anguish over the abnormal condition of her potential child.

When caring for a woman having or contemplating an abortion, the nurse's first responsibility is to assess the woman's feelings about the abortion. Depending on the degree of conservatism or liberalism in her religious beliefs, as well as other influences in her decision, the woman may feel varying degrees of psychological or emotional discomfort.

Homosexuality

"The relatively few passages in the Torah-text that clearly refer to homosexuality do so in negative terms" (Matt, 1978, p 13). Matt discusses the Jewish view of same-sex sexual behavior by citing numerous biblical references to its sinfulness. Also, the natural order of creation emphasizes heterosexual relationships, which God initiated by creating woman as a complement to man. Gordis (1978) says that homosexuality is contrary to God's will, since it is not consistent with the "natural" relationship between man and woman described in Genesis.

While both these authors (Matt, 1978; Gordis, 1978) represent a Jewish perspective of homosexuality's being sinful, Matt (1978) examines various motivations for homosexuality and their implications for how the Jewish congregation should respond to homosexual individuals. He states that within Jewish thought, those who do forbidden acts without completely free choice are judged more leniently than those who act with complete freedom. Assuming that psychologists and sociologists indicate that the majority of homosexuals are homosexual by some inherent drive rather than by completely free choice, Matt (1978) encourages the church and its members to take a compassionate stance toward homosexuals. While he recognizes that it is not likely that Jews will ever view homosexuals as behaving according to the ideal law of God, Matt (1978) recommends that homosexuals be welcomed into synagogues and temples as an expression of human companionship and the compassion God desires of us.

Sex Outside of Marriage

Marriage is a valued, sacred institution in Judaism. Gordis states that if it is to survive, "it must be endowed with one unique attribute characteristic of it and of it alone—it must be the only theater for experiencing the most intimate interplay of love and sex" (Gordis, 1978, p 170). Sexual intimacies with no intention by the partners to marry are formally opposed by Judaism.

Similar to the accepting attitude Matt (1978) proposes toward homosexuality, Gordis (1978) acknowledges that Judaism generally does not take a punitive attitude toward those who engage in premarital sexual intimacies. This leniency is most pronounced in cases in which the couple is already engaged. In fact, during the Middle Ages, the Jewish rituals of marriage were altered by rabbinic authorities in acknowledgment of the great possibility of engaged couples' having intercourse. Originally, Jewish ritual provided for a ceremony at the time of betrothal. This proclaimed the couple as engaged but gave them no authorization for any kind of intimacies. The actual marriage ceremony took place several months later. However, certain parts of the world, such as Judea, did allow the engaged couple some "private companionship." This laxity in attitude eventually became so pervasive that authorities chose to hold both ceremonies simultaneously, thus removing couples from those "tempting few months" between the engagement ceremony and the marriage ceremony. In practice, a child born to an unmarried woman is not considered illegitimate (Gordis, 1978).

Extramarital sex or adultery, on the other hand, is viewed with much severity. "In the past adultery was always regarded as the most heinous offense in the realm of sexual conduct" (Gordis, 1978, p 177). There are, of course, several biblical references that offer quasilegitimate status to concubinage or "secondary wives." Jewish scholars are still unclear about the acceptability of extramarital sex in biblical times; it has not been condoned in postbiblical times. Jewish law does consider a child conceived by a married woman of a man other than her husband to be illegitimate. By law, such children are under the penalty of not being accepted into the congregation. However, Gordis (1978) points out that the kind of proof of guilt required is virtually impossible to produce, for not even confession of guilt is admissible. It is therefore extremely improbable that a child would ever have to suffer such a penalty.

Should the nurse care for a Jewish couple who have experienced marital infidelity, the nurse must be cognizant of the seriousness of this in their religion. Of course, the way clients respond will be influenced by a variety of factors, including how devoutly they hold to Jewish teachings.

Divorce and Remarriage

Gordis makes a clear distinction between Jewish *attitude* toward divorce and Jewish *law* regarding divorce:

The attitude in life toward divorce is strict, thus underscoring the need for the couple to strive earnestly for the permanence of the marriage bond, but the law on divorce is liberal, offering release where life together proves truly intolerable. (Gordis, 1978, p 121)

Gordis maintains that traditional Jewish life has many powerful sanctions in favor of marriage as a permanent union. Jewish couples, in order to function as a normal part of the social community in which they live, may undergo extraordinary efforts to make even the most difficult marriages last. Once it becomes obvious that irreconcilable differences exist, "judaism recognizes that the union has lost its sanction and its sanctity, for love and mutual respect are the only marks of God's presence in a home" (Gordis, 1978, p 120).

The permissibility of divorce is supported in several biblical references and in the Talmud. One conservative school of Jewish authorities limits the reason for divorce to adultery. Other more liberal schools recognize a plethora of reasons as acceptable. While most scholars' interpretations of the original laws indicate that it was easier for a man to divorce his wife than vice versa, the laws did provide women with a variety of legal reasons to divorce husbands. The reasons listed as justifiable included such trivial ones as the husband having bad breath or an unpleasant disease or the wife's not liking his occupation. Men could divorce their wives if they found someone else they preferred. These complaints in themselves may hardly seem worthy of the granting of a divorce, but the law interpreted them as signs of more serious incompatibilities between the husband and wife (Gordis, 1978).

While today's divorce rates soar, Jewish philosophy remains basically the same as it was in biblical times. It is seen "not as a punishment for a crime, but simply as the frank admission of a failure" (Gordis, 1978, p 120). Thus, rabbinic authorities urge their faithful to regard marriage as a serious commitment and make every effort to preserve any union entered into. If irreconcilable differences develop, divorce is viewed as the appropriate action to take.

The Jewish tradition holds no absolute taboos to divorce. Depending on a variety of factors, a Jewish couple may not feel pressure against divorce, or they may live closer to the Hebrew tradition and feel strongly about maintaining a marriage. Whichever is true, it is helpful for a nurse to recognize the Hebrew tradition when assisting a Jewish couple facing divorce.

The Status of Women

The Bible makes reference to women in a variety of ways: Women are portrayed as vigorous, resourceful human beings, such as Sarah, Rebecca, Leah, and Rachael. They are also portrayed as evil creatures, leading to the destruction and ruination of men. Jezebel, the harlot, is perhaps the most infamous of all biblical women. Biblical stories also portray women as chattel belonging to their fathers or husbands. Because of the numerous ways in which women are portrayed, the status of women in the Jewish tradition is not clearly revealed by biblical study.

Gordis (1978) reviews the traditional status of women in Judaism by examining both the official laws and the customary laws, or the normative behaviors of traditional Jewish communities. Official Jewish law placed women in clearly different status from that of men. Women could be sold into marriage against their wills, they could not inherit property, their vows could be broken by their husbands or fathers, they could not testify in court, and if sexually violated, it was their fathers who received monetary compensation for the injustice done.

Gordis (1978) believes that while it is difficult to substantiate, customary law was significantly kinder to women. The evidence he cites includes the following examples: Job left his daughters an inheritance. The book of Ruth relates Naomi selling property that belonged to her dead husband and sons. The very nature of matrimony itself called for respect of the wife.

Jewish custom has afforded women a special place in many important rituals, such as the Passover seder. These roles, while highly valued in Judaism, were restricted to the home. Women's participation in religious functions in public was severely restricted. Until 1975 they could not be counted for the "minyan," or the Jewish quorum for prayer. The Rabinnical Assembly voted in 1975 to allow women to be counted in this quorum, but congregations are not compelled to do so, and many still do not. The rationale for the minyan tradition is that women were exempt from "commandments that must traditionally be performed at specific times" (Gordis, 1978, p 206). Gordis feels this may have been logical in historical times owing to the domestic, childbearing, and childrearing responsibilities women carried. But in today's world of more equitable division of labor and of labor-saving devices in the home, he contends that it is no longer valid. An important trend in recent years is the increasing numbers of women who have been ordained as rabbis by the Reform and Conservative branches, demonstrating a tremendous improvement in the status of women.

With the evolution of the feminist movement and other rapid social change, how a woman feels about her gender, whether she accepts herself as an inferior person or strives for equality, is powerfully influenced by factors other than religion. The general tone of Jewish teaching about the status of women is most likely to lead a woman to accept her gender positively. Older or conservative Jewish women may define their particular roles in a more traditional fashion than younger or liberal Jewish women. The nurse must bear in mind that traditional roles have their own value and worth. It is imperative that the nurse be sensitive to the client's own role definition.

In summary, when dealing with Jewish clients, the nurse may anticipate attitudes that convey acceptance of one's sexuality. It is in keeping with the Jewish tradition of compassion to accept sexual matters with a nonjudgmental demeanor.

CATHOLIC BELIEFS AND TEACHINGS

The official doctrine of the Catholic church has represented different perspectives regarding sexuality at different points in its 2000 year history, leading to some ambiguity about sexual morality for today's Catholic theologians. Christ discussed sexuality only briefly but did show compassion for those who had broken the sexual laws of the time, such as in the biblical story of the woman accused of adultery (John 8:3–7).

While some scholars believe that St. Paul's writings have been misconstrued and read out of context, Pauline writings have been utilized by both Protestants and Catholics to devalue sexuality. The vision of sexuality as something sinful stems from the writings about the difference between spiritual interests and worldly interests. Sexuality is a worldly interest, and Paul advised that it is far better to devote one's energies to the spiritual interests than to the carnal. He wrote in Galatians 5:17 that "the flesh lusts against the spirit, and the spirit against the flesh; and these are contrary the one to the other" and in Romans 8:6 that "to be carnally-minded is death; but to be spiritually-minded is life and peace." This philosophy was expanded and integrated into Christian doctrine by St. Augustine, who grappled with his own sexual desires for many years. He preached that "temptations of the flesh follow from a falling away from God" (Noss, 1949, p 634).

Bruce (1971) addresses a possible misinterpretation of the terms "the flesh" and "the spirit." It is Bruce's contention that Paul used "flesh" to refer in global terms to ideas, beliefs, laws, and practices that predated one's acceptance of Christ. The "spirit," on the other hand, meant life as it is lived by one who has accepted Christ. Interestingly, the importance of living within prescriptive and proscriptive laws was greater under "the flesh" than under "the spirit." While Paul has been often quoted to condemn and limit sexual activity, perhaps his intention was to place sexuality in the context of a spiritual life.

For example, St. Paul's text has been used to support existing social mores. He wrote that women should be completely subservient to their husbands, which was consistent with the beliefs and customs of the time and place in which he wrote. However, he was also the first Christian writer to indicate that women shared equally in eternal life offered by Christ. This idea, which was radical for his time, is seldom discussed.

While interpretations of Paul and other

early Christian writers have influenced Catholic thought about sexuality, Catholicism does have some positive attitudes toward the sexual aspect of humanity. For instance, marriage is considered a holy sacrament equal to Communion or Ordination:

sexual intercourse, for the Christian, is a sacred act from beginning to end. It is an act that involves the passionate self-offering and commitment, not only of two human persons, but of Jesus Christ as well. (Knight, 1979, p 196)

Perhaps the very emphasis Catholicism places on sexual matters is an indication of the extreme value attributed to human sexuality. It is unfortunate that proscriptions about sexuality have been emphasized more than an underlying philosophy.

Johnson and Weigert (1980) identified that the most frequently confessed sins among Catholics attending the confessional were sins related to sexuality. In a study in which Italian journalists posed as confessors, Johnson and Weigert analyzed various responses of different priests. They found that the priests could be divided into basically three categories: Those who represented the most orthodox views would not grant absolution for things such as sexual relations between engaged couples: "The merely natural is morally suspect and ambiguous . . ." (Johnson and Weigert, 1980, p 373). However, a second category of priests "view as legitimate all non-destructive physical acts which 'naturally' flow from close interpersonal relationships which the individuals define as good" (Johnson and Weigert, 1980, p 374). A third set of priests attempted to legitimize partially sexual sins when "social conditions allow few other alternatives" (Johnson and Weigert, 1980, p 377).

The attempts by some priests to interpret sexual teachings more leniently than in the past coincide with an entire movement in the Catholic church for the past 10 to 20 years. There have been efforts to redefine the Catholic church's teachings in the context of modern reality. In a review of *Human Sexuality: New Directions in American Catholic Thought*, Ruether states that this work, commissioned and approved by the Catholic Theological Society of America, "represents a major effort to shift the basis of sexual ethics from act-oriented to person-oriented principles" (Ruether, 1977, p 682). This book takes a more liberal view of sexual matters than Catholicism traditionally has held. It repre-

sents the views of a growing body of Catholic theologians and lay believers. However, it has caused controversy in the Catholic church; most conservative priests have argued with it.

Because the Catholic church is in a state of change about sexuality, the nurse is likely to encounter Catholic clients whose feelings about sexuality are ambiguous. It is difficult to state the kinds of attitudes the nurse might anticipate among Catholic clients. Two health issues that have been widely debated within the Catholic church during the past 20 years are contraception and abortion.

Contraception

The Catholic religion very strictly defines marriage as the only appropriate relationship in which sexual intimacies may take place. It has traditionally seen the only valid purpose of sexual intercourse within marriage as procreation. In the past 20 years papal encyclicals (official statements from the Pope) have recognized the relational aspects of marital sexual intimacies as equally important, but this in no way deemphasizes the significance of procreation. While the Catholic church accepts the reality that for some very serious reasons, such as the health of the woman, some marriages should not be procreative, these marriages are expected to be virginal (Selling, 1981). However, such an arrangement must be reached after the marriage takes place. A marriage entered into with the intent to be nonprocreative is, by Canon law, considered invalid.

The familiar phrase, "what God has joined together let no man put asunder," is a traditional part of many marriage ceremonies. It is usually interpreted to mean that the man and woman joined in marriage may not be separated by man. Catholic theology has an additional explanation of that phrase: God has joined procreational potential and sexual intercourse; anything that divides the two is contrary to God's will (Kelly, 1979). This interpretation not only makes contraception unacceptable but also other acts that divide the natural union of procreative potential and sexual intercourse, such as artificial insemination, even by the husband, or in vitro fertilization.

Sexuality in Our Time: What the Church Teaches (Kelly, 1979) is a compilation of essays about sexuality written by Catholic authorities. There is agreement among those writers that children are a blessing from God and should be welcomed into any marriage. They state that the evil of birth control is that it prevents the fulfillment of the "primary natural purpose" of marriage (Kelly, 1979, p 31). These theologians also feel that accepting whatever children God sends is an expression of Christian generosity and selflessness.

The publication of *Humanae Vitae* by Pope Paul VI in 1968 created conflict within the Church. *Humanae Vitae*, a papal encyclical on birth control, acknowledges the relational aspects of marriage as equally important to the procreative aspects of marriage. Despite concern among Catholic leaders about responsible parenthood, the Pope's encyclical candidly reaffirmed the traditional doctrine that contraception by means other than abstinence is unacceptable. Some authorities believe this encyclical has been ignored, as no other papal encyclical has ever been (Kelly, 1979).

Indeed, the numbers of Catholics who practice contraception is high. In 1965, 3 years before the encyclical was issued, approximately 55 per cent of Catholic women under age 45 were using non–church-approved methods of contraception. Two years after the encyclical, there was an overall 4 per cent increase in contraception use, including an increase of 14 per cent in contraceptive pill use. These figures include women who appeared to be religious; for example, those using the pill were more likely to receive Holy Communion at least once a month than were those who practiced rhythm or no contraception at all (Greeley, 1976).

Dyck reports that not only do some Catholic laity oppose the birth control encyclical but also some Catholic officials:

Within two weeks following the publication of *Humanae Vitae*, the *National Catholic Reporter* published the text of a statement by American Catholic theologians disagreeing with Pope Paul's ban on artificial birth control. In less than two months, more than 600 Catholic theologians and philosophers had signed it (Dyck, 1977, p 281)

While the official stance of the Catholic church on the question of contraception remains that artificial methods are unacceptable, the reality of what some Catholics practice is different. Many of those practicing technological contraception do so without condemnation from their parish priests.

From the preceding discussion, the nurse may anticipate Catholic clients who practice contraception with little or no guilt, those who practice contraception but suffer guilt over it, and those who, in keeping with church doctrine, refuse contraception at any cost. The nurse is likely to be called upon to serve as a sounding board for those grappling with guilt or for those who endure personal hardship as a consequence of their refusal to use contraception. The role of the nurse is to be accepting and supportive of the decision the individual or couple reaches, regardless of the nurse's personal beliefs.

Abortion

Officially, the Catholic church takes the position that abortion is sinful because it is destruction of human life. The church has been politically active in recent years, contributing time, money, and efforts to influence legislation to make abortion illegal. Some Catholic laity disagree with this political involvement and have organized to make the statement that immorality and illegality are not the same and that each woman should have a legal choice about whether to abort an unwanted fetus. Indeed, some Catholic laity are not willing to classify abortion as immoral. For instance, Kohlbenschlug (1985, p 182) writes, "A responsible new ethic must certainly take into account the primacy of personal conscience and of women's experience, as well as the effects and consequences of reproductive choices on the common good."

Interestingly, the Catholic church's present stand against abortion has only existed since 1869, when it was declared by Pope Pius IX. Before that time there had been several different papal positions on the issue. During the fourth century, abortion was condemned at any stage of pregnancy, as it is now. During the sixth century, concessions were made for abortions to take place during the first 40 days of pregnancy, based on the medical opinion of the day that life did not exist until the fortieth day. This position was maintained for approximately 10 centuries, until it was reversed in a decree by Pope Sixtus V in 1588. Only 3 years later this decree was rescinded by Pope Gregory XIV. This position was upheld until 1869 when the current doctrine was introduced, which is founded on the belief that human life, or personhood, begins at the moment of conception. The nurse should keep in mind that the official stance of a religion is not necessarily consistent with the behavior of members of that religion. For example, for a variety of reasons, Catholic women do choose to have abortions. The nurse should be sensitive to the fact that a Catholic woman having an abortion may suffer some degree of guilt. She may not receive adequate support from friends or family. If so, she may need support and acceptance of her decision, which a nurse can offer.

Celibacy

Catholicism is the only major American religion that expects celibacy of its priests. Some authorities describe celibacy as a sacrifice that is given out of love for God. Celibacy is questioned by some in the Catholic church today, but recent papal encyclicals uphold the traditional position on this issue (Liebard, 1978).

As lifelong celibacy is a less common occurrence in American culture, a nurse may have feelings of curiosity or uneasiness if caring for celebate individuals. Celibacy should only become an issue, however, if the client poses it as a problem.

Homosexuality

The Catholic religion denounces homosexuality as sinful. Among other passages, Leviticus 20:13 is frequently cited against same-sex sexual behavior: "[Y]ou shall not lie with a [human] male as with a woman; it is abomination" (King James Version) or "If a man has intercourse with a man as with a woman, they both commit an abomination" (New English Bible).

An alternative perspective taken in *Human Sexuality: New Directions in American Catholic Thought* is that sex was created by God for social and relational purposes. However, traditional church authorities argue against this position; if the primary purpose of sex were to foster relationships, God might just as well have created only men, they argue. Because sex is not necessary to human relationships or to combat loneliness and because God did create woman to be man's companion, some

authorities reason that sex other than that between a man and a woman is naturally wrong (Kelly, 1979).

Masturbation

Based on similar principles that lead Catholic doctrine to denounce sexual expression outside of marriage, homosexuality, and contraception, Catholicism defines masturbation also as sinful. It is seen as carnal activity that is outside the natural order of potentially procreative, marital sexual intercourse. Masturbation was explicitly condemned in Church writings as early as the eleventh century (Kelly, 1979). Another rationale for naming masturbation as sinful is the philosophy of "improper emission of seed." In Genesis 38, Onan follows the tradition and commandment of taking his deceased brother's widow as his wife. But in order to avoid providing her with a child, which would by law be considered his brother's heir, he "spilled it [his seed] on the ground. . . . And the thing which he did displeased the Lord." While this passage refers to withdrawal as a contraceptive practice, it is often cited against the practice of masturbation as well. The rationale is that any "waste" of human generative potential is unacceptable. Other theologians feel that God was displeased about Onan not obeying his request and not displeased about withdrawal.

Perhaps an area in which this belief would influence nursing care is pediatrics. As part of the discussion of normal growth and development, a nurse is likely to advise parents not to be unduly concerned over masturbation in young children. However, some clients may be unable to accept this advice if they subscribe to the belief that masturbation is sinful.

Incest and Bestiality

Two other topics on which Catholicism takes a clear stand are incest and bestiality. The opinion that both of these practices are sinful is founded repeatedly in scripture taken primarily from the Old Testament. Incest is described by a number of different relationships, all of which are sexually taboo, in Leviticus 18. The wording of these proscriptions is "thou shalt not uncover the nakedness of thy father or the nakedness of thy mother . . .," and continues with proscriptions against uncovering the nakedness of other family members. Leviticus 18:23, Exodus 22:28, and Deuteronomy 27:21 are classic scriptural references against bestiality: "Neither shalt thou lie with any beast . . ." (Leviticus 18:23) and "Cursed be he that lieth with any manner of beast" (Deuteronomy 27:21). The nurse is not often likely to encounter situations involving bestiality, but incest is more common than most persons realize. This practice is so shrouded in other social taboos that the religious beliefs behind these social injunctions are sometimes not apparent. It may be that religious and social connotations against incest contribute to clients' difficulty in facing such a problem. While not condoning the practice, a nurse can still be accepting of an individual or family for whom incest is a problem.

Sex Outside of Marriage

Catholicism condemns premarital and extramarital sexual intimacy. The Sixth and Ninth Commandments constitute the first official statements regarding sexual behavior (Kelly, 1979). The Sixth Commandment states, "Thou shalt not commit adultery," and the Ninth Commandment states, "Thou shalt not covet thy neighbor's wife." The implication is that not only is the actual commission of adultery sinful but so too is the desire. The proscriptions against premarital sex are based on Old and New Testament condemnations of fornication as well as the philosophy that procreative possibility and sexual intercourse are never to be separated.

The nurse will find Catholic clients who vary in their beliefs and practices, from those who fall well within the conservative interpretations of doctrines, to those who reject the official doctrines of the church. It is crucial that the nurse assess how the individual client feels about the particular question of premarital or extramarital sexual activity. The nurse cannot assume that a Catholic client believes and practices the official moral teachings of Catholicism.

Divorce

Catholic theology teaches that marriage is indissoluble; divorce is considered a sin. Until recently, attempts to remarry were grounds for excommunication from the church. Most Christian theologians quote Matthew 5:31–32 to support condemnation of divorce. In this passage Jesus says that even though the law allows a man to put away his wife, doing so causes her to commit adultery. Catholic theologians state that marriage is not governed by earthly law for it is a gift coming directly from God and is therefore under no law except his (Kelly, 1979).

In recent years the Catholic church has taken a more forgiving attitude toward those whose marriages dissolve. Some parishes have special services in which the divorced receive individual consideration. In order for a divorced Catholic to remarry, an annulment must be granted. Annulments may still be difficult to obtain, as they are granted only after provision of proof that a valid marriage never existed.

Status of Women

Just as in the Jewish religion, history indicates that the Catholic religion has viewed women in a multitude of roles, both positive and negative. Catholicism holds the Virgin Mary as being the mother of God and therefore ultimately holy. Thus, the Virgin Mary commands the utmost reverence and worship. There are also a number of female Catholic saints. However, actual participation as equals in the Church hierarchy is still not a reality for Catholic women. Women may be admitted into religious orders but not the priesthood. Individual parishes have the freedom to decide in which areas they allow females to serve. Many now have women on parish boards and councils, have women eucharistic ministers passing communion, and have girls participating as altar servers along with boys, but none of this is mandated by the official Catholic church.

Because of the role granted women in the Catholic church, some Catholic women may express themselves in ways that others might label as "unliberated." As long as this is not problematic for the client, it is not the nurse's domain to question the client's self-expression.

The nurse is challenged to assess the effect of individual religious beliefs regarding sexuality when caring for Catholic clients. Given the dissension within the organized church regarding sexual issues, it is not sufficient to know that the client is Catholic, for this information may provide little insight about the client's particular attitudes. However, because many of the proscriptions of Catholicism conflict with contemporary social views regarding sexuality, the nurse may be likely to encounter feelings of ambivalence toward some sexual issues among some Catholic clients.

PROTESTANT BELIEFS AND TEACHINGS

Just as Catholicism cannot be examined without some reference to Judaism, because of their common roots, so too Protestantism cannot be examined without acknowledging its kinship to Catholicism. Protestantism began in the sixteenth century. As its name implies, it was a protest against many of the teachings and practices of the Catholic church at the time. Consequently, many of the basic precepts of Catholicism and Protestantism are similar, but interpretations vary widely. It is difficult to describe definitively the Protestant view of human sexuality because "there are 239 religious groups within the United States, most of which are Protestant" (Dyck, 1977, p 291). This section will focus on mainstream writings of Protestants, which are generally viewed as liberal, espousing attitudes of acceptance toward alternative expressions of sexuality. The American fundamentalist movement of the 1980s has developed more conservative positions on sexual issues. The contrasting opinions of liberal and fundamentalist Protestants have caused tensions within churches and within individuals.

In general, most Protestant denominations take a positive view of human sexuality in their official statements. The Presbyterian Church in the United States believes that "because our sexuality is part of God's good creation, it is to be not only accepted but positively affirmed and even celebrated" (Sheek, 1982, p 57). The Presbyterian church attests to the full humanity of Jesus Christ; it suggests that he was fully aware of his own sexuality:

there is no evidence to suggest that he denied this aspect of his humanity in the manner of some of his later followers. The morality of his relationship

with others was enviably positive, rooted as it was in concern for their well-being rather than in anxiety about his own purity. (Study Document, 1970, p 896)

The African Methodist Episcopal Church takes the stand that "our identity and nature as sexual beings—is the will of God from the beginning and not an accident" (Sheek, 1982, p 33).

While a positive perspective about sexuality is formally stated in Protestant documents, the attitudes of many Protestant sects and individuals do not always reflect the same openness. A division of the carnal self from the spiritual self has colored earlier Protestant attitudes about human sexuality and continues to influence attitudes today. "Our tradition has been marred by dualisms between mind or soul and body" (The Nature and Purpose of Human Sexuality, 1980, p 6). Again, the nurse is cautioned against making assumptions about an individual client's beliefs or practices based on knowledge only of the official doctrine of a client's espoused religion.

Marriage

Protestant religions universally see marriage as a sacred union. Most hold that it is the only legitimate relationship in which sexual intimacy should occur; all agree that it is the preferred arena for full sexual expression, as indicated in the statement, "Human sexuality is made holy in the married state" (Sheek, 1982, p 16). Protestants differ from Catholics in their perspective of the purposes of marriage, placing much more emphasis on the relational aspects than the procreative aspects of marriage. The Anglican Church of Canada states that

the purposes of marriage are mutual fellowship, support, and comfort, the procreation (if it may be) and the nurturance of children, and the creation of a relationship in which sexuality may serve personal fulfillment. (Sheek, 1982, p 16)

The Reformed Church in America believes that marriage is for fellowship, human fulfillment, and family and community faith (Sheek, 1982).

Marriage is not seen as a carte blanche to satisfy carnal appetites, however. For example, the Presbyterian Church in the United States believes that "people sin sexually within marriage, not so much because of the performance of forbidden acts as because of the violation of sacred relationships" (Sheek, 1982, p 32). The American Lutheran Church states that "sexual behavior that violates human dignity and integrity is sinful" (Sheek, 1982, p 30). The Church of the Brethren says that "when sexual intercourse is detached from love and covenant, intimacy quickly dissipates" (Sheek, 1982, p 31).

Adultery

As marriage is seen as something holy, fidelity in marriage is important to many Protestant groups. Adultery is condemned as a behavior, as is the feeling of lust. "Lust is not a passing fantasy but an untamed craving. Unless *eros* is infused and counterbalanced with *agape*, attitudes become adulterous" (Sheek, 1982, p 31).* This statement expresses the notion that adultery is not limited only to having sexual intercourse with others outside marriage but also includes any breach of the marriage covenant.

Many churches espouse clear opinions that while laws against adultery in Old Testament times were to protect the "property rights" of men, such interpretations are unjust and inapplicable in today's world. "Jesus applied the prohibition of adultery to husbands and wives on an equal basis" (Sheek, 1982, p 31). The United Methodist Church "reject(s) social norms that assume different standards for women than for men in marriage" (Sheek, 1982, p 36).

As in Judaism, Protestantism infuses much forgiveness into its teachings about what is sinful. This is true for adultery. The Church of the Brethren state that "although adultery is a sin, neither Jesus nor Paul suggests that it is unforgivable" (Sheek, 1982, p 31).

Divorce and Remarriage

Protestants intertwine an acceptance of what is intended by God with an acceptance of the human state of affairs when they make judgments about divorce. Most agree that

*Eros is a Greek word meaning love but in a sensual and sexual manner. Agape is also a Greek word meaning love but in a respecting and caring manner, without sexual expression.

marriage is intended to be a lifelong commitment. However, they recognize that numerous circumstances in life often make maintenance of a marriage a source of great suffering. Protestant religions call for compassion in these situations and are not totally condemnatory toward those who choose to dissolve their marriage.

The doctrine of the Church of the Brethren states that "divorce as a tragedy is not to be judged, but is to be seen with sorrow and compassion" (Sheek, 1982, p 41). The Brethren believe that rather than to allow a destructive relationship to continue to do personal damage to human beings, legal termination of the marriage is required. The breakdown of the relationship is seen as the problem, not the divorce itself, which is only a consequence (Sheek, 1982). The Reformed Church in America feels that sins in this area are neither more grievous nor less forgivable than any other sins and calls upon lay members and ministers to be nonjudgmental and supportive to divorced members (Sheek, 1982). The United Church of Canada adopts the philosophy that "rules are helpful because they are specific. They are not helpful when they are literally and simplistically applied" (Sheek, 1982, p 60).

Only a few churches speak clearly to the issue of remarriage, but most of those who do speak positively. The Church of the Brethren in 1964 decided that divorced individuals do have the freedom to enter subsequent marriages with the blessings of the church (Sheek, 1982). The Anglican Church of Canada grants permission for divorced persons to remarry provided certain criteria are met. These criteria basically involve provision for caring of children by the previous marriage(s) and establishment of reasonable faith that the new marriage can be sustained as a lifetime commitment (Sheek, 1982).

The doctrine of the American Lutheran Church states that

the pastor deals with the problem of remarriage not in isolation but in the context of the church's total stewardship of the Gospel. He takes into account relevant factors involved in the lives of the two individuals. (Sheek, 1982, p 48)

The Lutheran Church in America advises individuals and pastors to focus on the potential of the new marriage rather than on the collapse of the first marriage when considering the rightness or wrongness of remarriage (Sheek, 1982).

Premarital Sex

Most Protestant religions see premarital sexual activity as sinful but consider circumstances before passing judgment on the seriousness of the sin. Forgiveness of this transgression is encouraged just as it is with adultery and divorce. The statement of the Presbyterian church is exemplary of this approach.

The church advocates the reserving of total intimacy for the relationship of total commitment which marriage is supposed to be, but not all premarital sex acts are rendered equally irresponsible because they fail to meet that standard. It does matter what motives, intentions, and concerns for consequences are present in the persons involved. (Sheek, 1982, p 73)

The Church of the Brethren recognizes the sexually difficult situation modern society poses for young people. They acknowledge that sexual maturity is reached by about the age of 13, yet marriage does not usually occur until approximately 23 years of age, creating a 10-year period in which sexual drives are strong but in which legitimate relationships for the expression of these drives are not available. However, they advise young people that the religiously responsible thing to do is to resist the temptation to engage in premarital sexual intercourse. They cite the problems of teenage pregnancy, venereal disease, and impairment of emotional development rather than biblical teachings as rationale for this advice:

Sexual relations between unmarried, consenting adults are not explicitly prohibited in the Bible. . . . The New Testament makes numerous references to sexual immorality but no direct reference to premarital sexual relationships. (Sheek, 1982, pp 74–75)

The main objection that most Protestant religions have against premarital sexual intercourse is based on the dehumanization that may occur in indiscriminant sexual relations. The Presbyterian church, recognizing that more than one third of American adults are single, looks very carefully at the individual's motivations when becoming involved in a sexual relationship outside of marriage.

The relationships may not be seen as permanent, but the parties in them may be acting out of love, respect, and a concern for mutual growth. . . . The difference between merely casual and exploitative relationships and these is marked and significant. (Sheek, 1982, p 57)

As with other sins, Protestants caution against judging one another on the issue of premarital sexual activity. "Only God can ultimately judge the degrees of moral responsibility of particular acts and decisions" (Sheek, 1982, p 57).

Contraception

Protestants value responsible parenthood more than procreation in and of itself. This valued responsibility encompasses not only concern for the individual family but for humanity at large. "Restraint in regard to procreation is a responsibility to the needs and conditions of the world around us" (Study Document, 1970, p 908).

Dyck (1977, p 293) states that "the Southern Baptists and the United Methodist Church urge upon their members a small-family norm." Some Protestant churches have taken political stances recommending increased governmental involvement to deal with overpopulation. One of the major recommendations in this area is that all restrictions regarding the dissemination of contraceptive information be stricken from legal records (Dyck, 1977). Several Protestant denominations specifically include single persons among those who have a right and a responsibility to obtain contraceptive knowledge.

The Anglican Church of Canada believes that decisions about procreation are matters of individual conscience, and furthermore "not all married couples have, nor should have, children" (Sheek, 1982, p 77). This statement is fairly representative of the Protestant denominations that address contraception in official documents.

Not surprisingly, Protestants, in general, tend to have the most liberal views on sterilization as a means of contraception. They have also utilized this method of contraception more frequently than those of other religious beliefs (Dyck, 1977). The United Methodist Church recommends that "the individual, after counseling, be given the right to decide concerning his or her own sterilization" (Dyck, 1977, p 309).

Abortion

Protestantism approaches abortion with the same consideration for circumstances and motivations that it does with other sexual issues. Protestantism is careful to point out in documents that while individual denominations may uncategorically define abortion as sinful, judgment is not the jurisdiction of persons or churches. A sense of forgiveness among fellow members is encouraged for this transgression just as it is for adultery, premarital sex, and other sexual sins. For instance, the American Lutheran Church takes the following position:

We view abortion as a fundamentally inappropriate means of birth control. Indeed, willful abortion—the sacrifice of a fetal life—is always an offense against God and the human spirit. There are, however, some circumstances under which abortion may represent a course of action that is more responsible than are other options. (Sheek, 1982, p 78)

Among Protestant denominations, there are those who believe that only threats to life or to the health of the mother are sufficient justification for abortion while there are others who favor abortion upon request (Dyck, 1977). Representing one of the most conservative of Protestant views is the African Methodist Episcopal Church, which states that human life begins at conception and destruction of that human life is a violation of the sanctity of human life. However, in cases in which the life of the mother is threatened, abortion is a life-saving measure, and the church's counsel is for prayer that the Lord's will be done in each individual case (Sheek, 1982). Conversely, the United Methodist Church does not consider the fetus to be a person; they believe that personhood requires more than physical existence (Dyck, 1977). Consequently, they support the legal availability of abortion under proper medical supervision (Sheek, 1982).

In recent years, the father's right to participate in abortion decisions has received some legal and ethical attention. Harris (1986) discusses a woman's moral obligation to respect the father's rights to "legitimate" pursuit of procreation. As this issue receives more attention in the media, theologians will no doubt continue to grapple with the ethical questions surrounding the moral right and obligations of mothers, fathers, and fetuses. Many laity will seek guidance and influence in making their own personal decisions in this area.

Homosexuality

The United Methodist Church makes a statement that "nowhere in the Church's considerations of human sexuality is there more confusion, embarrassment, and even self-hatred evident than in the current discussions about homosexuality" (Sheek, 1982, p 85). Verification of this statement is readily available when one reads the positions of different denominations regarding homosexuality. The United Methodist Church refuses to specify the normalcy of heterosexual or homosexual behavior. It supports the belief that homosexuals have a right to Christian fellowship but states that same-sex sexual practices are against the law of God (Sheek, 1982). The Presbyterian church states that homosexuality "seems to be contrary to the teaching of scripture. It seems to repudiate the heterosexual process which gave us life" (*The Nature and Purpose of Human Sexuality*, 1980, p 14).

The United Church of Canada defends homosexuals as persons who need the nurturance and support that others need and receive from Christian congregations. They support homosexual couples with a commitment to each other in adopting children. They discuss the possibility of ordaining gay ministers and acknowledge that there are already gay ministers ordained without the church's knowledge of their sexual preference (Sheek, 1982). In contrast, some Protestants espouse more conservative, fundamentalist views on homosexuality. Some fundamentalists have spoken publicly and vehemently against homosexuality, viewing homosexuality as one factor contributing to the deterioration of the moral fiber of America.

Hochstein (1986) studied the degree of homophobia among a group of pastoral counselors, most of whom were Protestant. Approximately 50 per cent of the sample described themselves in ways that indicated significant homophobia. Most of the theoretical cases who were refused as counseling clients were homosexual men or lesbians. Of the theoretical cases accepted by this sample for counseling, the most serious diagnoses were assigned to subjects who were homosexual. This kind of research is extremely important in nursing, as well as among pastors. Recognizing one's own feelings about homosexuals is essential. This becomes more necessary as there is an increase in cases of acquired immunodeficiency syndrome (AIDS), a disease prevalent among homosexual men.

Masturbation

As might be expected, Protestantism expresses more concern over motivations and feelings associated with masturbation than with the act itself. The sects discuss masturbation from the perspective of psychological well-being, stating that the guilt religious statements have caused in the past about masturbation is unhealthy in itself. Protestantism objects, in general, to masturbation if it becomes obsessive or if it is chosen over heterosexual activity as a means of avoiding interacting with others.

Celibacy

Protestants value family life in such a way that they encourage their ministers to partake of family life as do other members of the congregation. It is uncommon to find a Protestant minister who is unmarried or who does not have children. The Presbyterian church expresses the commonly accepted Protestant philosophy on abstinence by saying that it is appropriate if it is chosen as a "positive affirmation rather than a negative judgment on sex" (Sheek, 1982, p 99).

Status of Women

Protestant sects are, within their organizations, taking affirmative steps to rectify discrimination against women. This is reflected by the fact that most denominations have women in ordained positions as ministers as well as in prominent positions among lay leadership. Presbyterians and Methodists have ordained women as ministers since the 1950s. These sects have also issued official statements against legal and social sexual discrimination. The Presbyterian Church in Canada urges members and the organization as a whole to "press for just economic policy and equality before the law" (Sheek, 1982, p 15). The United Methodist Church believes that narrow interpretation of biblical teaching has been responsible for encouraging the socially accepted view of women as sex objects and chattel. They now state that such narrow interpretations seriously distort the true Christian message of respect for all humans (Sheek, 1982). The Reformed Church in America says, "Our sex does not determine our status before God. It should not determine our status with one another!" (Sheek, 1982, p 117).

There are, however, exceptions to this general movement of women gaining equal status with men within the Protestant church. Southern Baptists have recently discussed whether or not to ordain women as ministers, with a conservative element influencing the organization to continue to ordain only men. Again, the fundamentalist movement of the 1980s contends that the role of women should be in the home.

In summary, when caring for Protestant clients, the nurse may anticipate that these clients might base their sexual decisions on principles respecting personhood rather than absolute rules or laws. The overall Protestant attitude toward sexuality is positive and accepting. There are still, in practice, some attitudes against certain forms of sexual expression, which might stimulate feelings of guilt about certain behaviors.

Protestant organizations in recent years have formally asked their followers to be open minded about sexual matters and to extend understanding and forgiveness to those who do not always live their sexual lives by ideal prescriptions. Consequently, a nurse may deal with Protestant clients who have such attitudes toward themselves and others. Or, a nurse may find Protestant clients who still hold sexual sins to be more serious than sins of other natures, expressing a great deal of guilt about their own sexual "failings" or judgment toward the "failings" of others. As always, the nurse is called upon to accept the client unconditionally and the client's attitudes nonjudgmentally.

OTHER RELIGIOUS TEACHINGS
Hinduism

Hinduism contains both extremes of asceticism and eroticism that seem contradictory to Western thinking. Yet this combination is not dichotomous to Hindus; both are seen as forms of energy. Extremes of asceticism or eroticism were to be avoided, and a regulated sensual life was to be developed. Priests as well as lay persons marry in Hinduism. Those ascetics who choose celibacy may do so for limited periods of time rather than as a lifelong commitment (Parrinder, 1980).

Sexual intercourse is viewed in Hinduism as something spiritual as well as physical. This belief is partially responsible for the writing of sex manuals, the most famous being the Kama Sutra. This describes erotic rituals, all unhurried approaches to sexual interaction between men and women (Parrinder, 1980).

There were, in contrast to the Kama Sutra and other documents describing sexually pleasurable practices, books of laws restricting certain sexual behaviors. Intercourse was to be practiced in private, never in the open air. Oral sex was forbidden, as was rape and homosexuality. Lesbianism was punished much more severely than was male homosexuality. Interestingly, sexual relations with a teacher's wife were strictly forbidden. Yet temptations must have been great in this domain, for among a student's responsibilities included helping his teacher's wife bathe and dress! Incest was also taboo and was defined not only as sex with family members but also as sex with wives of a friend or son (Parrinder, 1980).

While some women in Hindu mythology were portrayed as being as amorous as men, women are generally treated poorly in Hinduism. The masculine dominance of the religion is reflected in the innumerable artistic representations of the phallus and of worship of the "linga" or phallus. Women were given in marriage against their will and were to be totally faithful and obedient to their husbands, even after death. A woman was honored and protected in some ways within the home by her father, husband, or sons but was never seen fit for independence; she was always under the rule of a man. Widows were not allowed to remarry because it was their eternal obligation to worship their husbands. In fact, from about the tenth century until it was abolished by the British in the nineteenth century, widow burning was not an uncommon practice in India. The widows of the deceased were expected to jump, or were thrown, into their husbands' funeral pyre (Parrider, 1980). Although such Hindu teachings about marriage and the status of women are not necessarily followed among the more educated, or even by all, Hindus, cultural attitudes about the subservient or traditional role of women may persist.

Prostitution as practiced by courtesans, who were highly educated women, was acceptable, but ordinary prostitution as practiced in brothels was condemned. The "devadasis" or "god-servants" were extremely high class prostitutes who practiced their trade in temples. They were technically married to one of the gods, but were "trained in erotic arts and made available to temple visitors, for a price" (Parrinder, 1980, p 27). They were sometimes so numerous and so persistent in their offers that the righteous complained that they interfered with their attempts to worship.

It must be remembered that Hinduism is the oldest of the world's major religions. The teachings, writings, and practices of Hindus vary from time and place in the secular context. Sometimes the erotic aspects have been given greater emphasis, while at other times the ascetic aspects have dominated. Today's Hinduism reflects centuries of interpretation and reinterpretation of ancient writings and is not necessarily followed in exactly the same format in which it was thousands of years ago.

Buddhism

Early Buddhism was primarily a religion for highly dedicated monks. Asceticism was strictly required "Early Buddhism had no priests, said little about marriage and nothing positive on sexual life" (Parrinder, 1980, p 45). Indeed, sexuality had such a negative connotation that Buddha's mother is reported to have committed suicide 7 days after giving birth so as to avoid having to submit to future sexual intercourse. Women were considered so dangerous a threat to a man's spiritual life that a monk was not to look at one if possible and was never to touch one. Even if his own mother fell into a ditch, to help her out he could not offer his hand but only his stick. Monks were not even allowed to handle female animals or sleep under the same roof with them. These efforts to protect themselves from women were based on the idea that sexual relations might distract the monk from the search for liberation. If children resulted, a man might be further encumbered with worldly responsibilities (Parrinder, 1980).

The formation of female orders of ascetics was not automatic, and it is legend that the Buddha's widowed aunt asked for admission and was refused three times. Upon her fourth request one of Buddha's chief disciples spoke in her behalf. At the time of her admission it was prophesied that the order would have lasted 1000 years without women but would last only 500 with them. Ironically, Buddhism is now over 2500 years old.

Eventually, Buddhism grew to include lay followers, and marriage and family laws were developed. As in Hinduism, marriages were arranged by the woman's father, but Buddhist women had a slightly greater degree of influence in choosing their mates. Female infanticide, which was practiced in many parts of the world at the time Buddhism was establishing itself, was never an acceptable practice to Buddhists (Parrinder, 1980). Both parties in a marriage could own property. Husbands as well as wives had responsibilities. The husband's responsibilities to his wife included "respect, courtesy, fidelity, giving her adornments, and allowing her authority in the household." A wife's obligations were "doing her duties well, . . . being hospitable to relatives of them both, . . . fidelity, watching over his good, and industry in all her business" (Parrinder, 1980, p 55). While it seems that women faired much better under Buddhism than Hinduism, there was still a Buddhist axiom that a woman has "five kinds of incapabilities and three kinds of subordination" (Yuichi, 1982, p 55).

As with all ancient religions, what was written originally and what is actually practiced by its adherents at the present time vary, depending on the cultural interpretation and the devoutness of the individual. Consequently, one might find numerous variations of these laws being followed by different Buddhist sects.

Islam

Islam is a religion based on the writings of the prophet Mohammed and has received attention in the Western world recently for its view and treatment of women. On one hand, Mohammed said that women were to be treated with consideration. This was because they were created from Adam's rib,

and attempts to straighten a crooked rib will break it. On the other hand, principles of Islam state many rules that indicate a subservient status for women:

A wife should not be whipped like a slave and then subjected to intercourse, but when a man called his wife to satisfy his desire she should go to him even if she was occupied at the oven. On the other hand, a wife should not tell others of her marital affairs. Being asked what rights a woman could demand of her husband, the Prophet was reported as saying, "That you should give her food when you eat, clothe her when you clothe yourself, not strike her on the face, and not revile her or separate from her." (Parrinder, 1980, p 164)

Early Islamic teachings gave women considerably more freedom than they have had in later years. This curtailing of independence has been as much social as religious in origin (Parrinder, 1980). For instance, veiling of women is not specifically called for in the Koran. This custom probably developed as a consequence of the wives and daughters of Mohammed being considered so revered that men were not supposed to see them or talk to them except through a veil (Parrinder, 1980). Harems, or the sequestering of women away in separate quarters, is an exaggeration of the concept of women not being seen by men other than their husbands. Harems were also thought to control jealousy between those wealthy enough to have several wives and those unable to support more than one wife or no wife at all.

Polygamy was acceptable in ancient Islamic teachings and has been practiced by many Muslims until very recent times. The original rationale behind the institution of polygamy may have been a protection for women. The region of the Middle East, where Islam had its roots, had endured numerous bloody wars at the time the Koran was written, leaving many widows and women taken by the victors as slaves. Some scholars believe that Mohammed encouraged men to marry as many women as they could support and treat fairly so as to avoid leaving the widows and captive women at the mercy of the world. It was stressed that a man should not take more wives than he could treat equitably, and if he could not justly divide his resources, energies, and emotions among several women, he should take only one. It is this teaching that has led modern Muslims to abandon polygamy. Most agree that it is impossible to meet the criteria for treating several wives justly (Parrinder, 1980).

There are a number of strict taboos in formal Islamic teaching. Nakedness is to be avoided whenever possible, homosexuality and heterosexual anal intercourse are prohibited, and sex outside of marriage is forbidden. Sex between two unmarried people is thought to be less serious than adultery. Whether or not the original laws forbid contraception is a matter of interpretation, but Mohammed is reported as saying that it does not matter what we do because any souls who are intended to be born will be.

Divorce has always been possible under Islamic law but is strictly regulated. Only men could seek divorce, and a separation of 3 to 4 months was required before official dissolution of the marriage. This was to ensure that the woman was not pregnant at the time. If she were, the couple was obligated to stay together. Divorced women were given their dowries at the time of the divorce. It is interesting to note that Muslim women were only allowed to marry the same man three times unless she married someone else in the intervening time (Parrinder, 1980). This practice suggests that perhaps serial monogamy was as common as simultaneous polygamy.

While many of the punishments prescribed for sexual offenses are extreme, such as 100 lashes and a year's banishment for fornication or being stoned to death for adultery, Islam also teaches that it is better to "make a mistake in forgiving than to make a mistake in punishing" (Parrinder, 1980, p 165). Consequently, not all offenses are dealt with the same severity. However, there has been a movement in many Islamic states to return to strict adherence to the laws as they are written.

CONCLUSION

While nurses cannot know all the beliefs about sexuality espoused by various religions, they must be aware that religion can be a powerful influence in the arena of human sexuality. Assessment of potentially relevant religious beliefs and feelings should be a part of a thorough nursing data base. It is also necessary for nurses to be aware of their own religious beliefs about sexuality. Religious teachings may not always predominate attitudes about sexuality, but a nurse must be

sensitive to religious influences as a part of the sociocultural make-up that affects clients' attitudes. Having some didactic knowledge of the various religious philosophies regarding sexuality can assist the nurse in assessing data and reaching valid conclusions upon which to plan the client's care.

As one example, a nurse may be called upon to counsel an adolescent about contraception. The client's developmental stage, cultural influences of the peer group, and religious beliefs are all factors that need to be considered in planning the counseling.

An example of how a nurse's personal religious attitudes might influence care is if he or she holds strongly to the belief that homosexuality is a sin. In such a case it would be best to arrange for another nurse to care for the homosexual client.

The importance of nurses demonstrating an accepting, nonjudgmental attitude toward all clients cannot be overemphasized. This does not necessarily imply acceptance of a belief or practice but the acceptance of the individual's right to ascribe to a particular belief. Acceptance of individual diversity is essential in order to provide professional nursing care.

REFERENCES

The Holy Bible. Philadelphia, The National Bible Press, 1958.
Bruce FF: Romans: An Introduction and Commentary. London, The Tyndale Press, 1979.
Dyck AJ: Population policy and ethics. (ed. by Veatch, R. M.) New York, Irvington, 1977.
Gordis R: Love and Sex: A Modern Jewish Perspective. League for Conservative Judaism, 1978.
Greeley AM: Council or encyclical? Rev Religious Res 18:3–24, 1976.
Harris G: Fathers and fetuses. Ethics 96:594–603, 1986.
Hockstein L: Pastoral counselors: Their attitudes toward gay and lesbian clients. J Pastoral Care 40:158–165, 1986.
Human Sexuality: New Directions in American Catholic Thought. A Study Commissioned by the Catholic Theological Society of America. New York, Paulist Press, 1977.
Johnson CL, Weigert AJ: Frames in confessions: A social construction of sexual sin. J Sci Study Relig 19:368–381, 1980.
Kelly GA: Sexuality in Our Time: What the Church Teaches. Boston, Daughters of St. Paul, 1979.
Knight D: The Good News About Sex. Cincinnati, St. Anthony Messenger Press, 1979.
Kolbenschlag M: Abortion and moral consensus: Beyond Solomon's choice. Christian Century 102:179–182, 1985.
LaChat M: Religion's support for the domination of women—Breaking the cycle. Nurse Pract 13:31–34, 1988.

Liebard OM: Love and Sexuality. Wilmington, McGrath, 1978.

Matt HJ: Sin, crime, sickness, or alternative lifestyle: A Jewish approach to homosexuality. Judaism 27:13–24, 1978.

McFadden TM: Theology Confronts a Changing World. West Mystic, Twenty-third Publications, 1977.

The Nature and Purpose of Human Sexuality. Atlanta, The Presbyterian Church in the United States, 1980.

Noss JB: Man's Religions. New York, Macmillan 1949.

Parrinder G: Sex in the World's Religions. New York, Oxford University Press, 1980.

Ruether RR: Time makes ancient good uncouth: the Catholic report on sexuality. Christian Century 94:682–685, 1977.

Selling JA: The childless marriage: A moral observation. BIJRAGEN 42:158–173, 1981.

Sheek GW: A Compilation of Protestant Denominational Statements on Families and Sexuality. 3rd ed. New York, National Council of Churches, 1982.

Study Document (Church and Society). Atlanta, The Presbyterian Church in the United States, 1970.

Yuichi K: Women in Buddhism. Eastern Buddhist 15:53–70, 1982.

PART THREE

SEXUALITY DURING THE REPRODUCTIVE YEARS

10: The Maternity Cycle and Sexuality

Nancy Sharts Engel

The process of pregnancy and birth is an obvious reflection of the sexuality of the new parents. Recognition of this fact influences how the new mother and father regard themselves and each other as well as how they interact with friends and relatives. Consideration of sexuality during the maternity cycle has often been overlooked by health care professionals except, perhaps, for some perfunctory instruction on when to stop and when to resume intercourse before and after birth.

For this reason, it is important for nurses to examine issues related to sexuality throughout the maternity cycle, so that they can better understand the vast range of feelings expressed by new parents and their significant others, assist new parents to process the experience of pregnancy and birth in

a way that enhances their self-concept, and promote or enhance resumption of a positive sexual relationship between the new parents.

There is perhaps no opportunity more golden for assessing sexual well-being than during the antepartal or postpartal periods. Discussion of reproduction in general, changes in the woman's body in particular, and the relationship between the partners throughout the peripartal year can be a quite natural outcome of the process of birth. It is likely, given the opportunity, that both partners have questions or feelings that they would like to discuss with an authoritative health professional.

This chapter is directed toward helping the nurse understand various concepts and issues that relate to the sexual well-being of couples throughout the maternity cycle.

These include, in order, factors relating to the decision to parent; physical and psychological changes experienced by the pregnant woman, including changes in sexual responsiveness; common factors that may alter couples' patterns of sexual activity; sexual implications of birth and the postpartum phase; and finally, application of the nursing process to this area of well-being. While reading this material will not qualify the nurse as a sex therapist, it should facilitate assessment and basic intervention skills, including detection of problems that need referral.

PARENTHOOD AS AN OPTION

Evolution of the Freedom to Parent

Giminez (1980) described ours as a *pronatalist* society; that is, women are expected to marry and reproduce as their primary responsibility, even now. In fact, she criticized the current feminist literature for not emphasizing women's basic choice of whether or not to parent; rather, Giminez believes, feminists still tend to assume that most women will choose to parent, and they focus instead on options related to timing, marital status, alternative families, and continuation of careers after childbearing.

Marriage and childbearing are still cultural norms throughout American society. Even as the divorce rate climbs, so too does the marriage rate, although the age of first marriage has gradually risen over the past 2 decades from 20.3 years for women and 22.8 years for men in 1960 to 22.0 years and 23.9 years, respectively, in 1981 (Gough, 1979; U.S. Department of Commerce, 1984). Once married, couples experience overt or covert pressure from peers and families to have children (Rosen and Benson, 1982).

Yet, particularly for upwardly mobile professional women, the options related to childbearing have multiplied over the past 20 years. In her book *The Feminine Mystique* Betty Friedan (1963) described the inevitability for college-educated women of the postwar years of marrying, and when the babies started coming, of giving up their careers and moving to the suburbs. If boredom set in, many of these women and their spouses thought that another baby was the cure. Surveying the changes in society in the years since her book was published. Friedan (1983) notes that now, although 90 per cent of young adults still marry, they have options for a solitary life or forms of group living, for conceiving or not, for carrying a pregnancy to term or not, and for child care and simultaneous career development, which were unimaginable in the early 1960s. Friedan takes it as a measure of the success of the women's liberation movement that many young women today, particularly those who are not economically disadvantaged, take these choices for granted. As rigidly polarized sex roles have been broken down, a diversity of patterns of task sharing has emerged. She, among others, noted that professional women are tending to delay childbearing until their careers are established, well into their 30s or even 40s, and many women choose to bear fewer children.

Public and private organizations that have emerged to ensure that such options exist for the greatest possible number of American women include city or county public health departments, Planned Parenthood, women's health cooperatives, Legal Aid, and child care agencies as well as the increasing number of universities and technical schools interested in recruitment of adult students. In addition to the more typical emphasis on contraception and maternity care, services for the assistance of couples who are unable to conceive are now proliferating.

This is not to ignore the fact that such options are limited in certain segments of society, including poor urban and isolated rural settings, as well as among selected ethnic or religious groups. But for most Americans the current degree of sexual self-determination, and its impact on the structure of the family and alteration of men's and women's roles, is great. With such freedom may come stresses unknown to prior generations of couples as they deal with such choices as whether to cohabit before marriage; whether to marry; whether the wife should maintain her own name and financial accounts; whether both partners should continue their careers; where they should reside in the best interest of both partners; whether to bear children and if so, when and how many; how to divide domestic responsibilities; what child care arrangements should be made; and what religious, cultural, and social values they wish to impart to their children.

With families choosing to bear fewer children, their investment in each is greater. The payoffs for such arduous deliberations include increased flexibility, an increased potential for self-actualization by both partners, and the satisfaction of self-determination. Individuals can choose to continue in traditional family patterns, but are not forced to if it is disadvantageous.

Gender roles evolved in the preindustrial family in accordance with survival needs (Gough, 1979). The family evolved as an economic unit characterized by males hunting and by females gathering and tending the slow-to-mature human offspring. The birth of many children was desirable to ensure adequate labor and prosperity in old age. But the technology and social institutions of today render old sexual divisions of labor generally unnecessary.

THE PARENTAL ROLE

Developmental and Role-Related Issues

Major developmental theorists have described the normal attainment of adulthood in terms of marriage and parenthood (Deutsch, 1944; Erikson, 1963; Levinson, 1978; Lidz, 1976). Duvall (1977) noted that the arrival of the first child forces young parents to take the last major step into the adult world, as they become totally responsible for another person. Pregnancy also signifies to the prospective grandparents the end of their children's primary relationships with them and the need to accept their children as sexual adults (Howells, 1972).

Briggs (1979) has noted that prospective parents may believe that instinctive care-giving skills will emerge with the birth of their child, and they tend to romanticize the baby as a "bundle of joy." In fact, the transition to parenthood involves a growing complexity of the nuclear family, from a single-dyad unit to a unit comprising three dyads. The individuals will be forced to acknowledge their novice status and to turn to experienced others for support and assistance. As a transitional period, this represents a developmental crisis accompanied by "emotional upheaval and additional pressure for readjustment as well as increased potential for learning and growth" (Briggs, 1979, p 70).

Rossi (1968) characterized the transition associated with parenthood as occurring in phases. In her taxonomy, the *anticipatory phase* begins with a couple's commitment to each other, formally through marriage or informally by mutual agreement. It ends with the birth of the first child. Even before pregnancy the couple is engaged in redefining their roles vis-à-vis each other and in defining the rules of their relationship. The ease with which this occurs supplies clues as to their readiness to parent (Briggs, 1979). The length of time the couple allows for the anticipatory phase, through the use of birth control, is another potential index of parenting readiness. Couples can, although they might not, use their child-free time together to learn to know each other in a variety of circumstances, to develop their own identities, to develop their ability to be intimate, to develop trust, and to become an interdependent unit. The development of functional behavioral patterns during this time, such as conflict resolution, will better equip the couple to cope with a child.

To turn to Erikson's (1963) framework, healthy progression through his eight stages of development includes the capacity for establishment of an intimate relationship in early adulthood. When this is accomplished, the individual then feels compelled to focus on the next generation, through parenthood, mentorship, or other modes of giving of one's self. While Erikson saw parenthood as occurring in the stage of establishment of intimacy, the characteristic of feeling that one has something to give to the next generation is probably important to individuals deliberating over whether or not to become parents. Other criteria of sufficient maturity might include the ability to delay gratification, patience, flexibility, and an identity that is well-enough established so it is not obliterated when the new role of "parent" is added (McBride, 1976).

Money, as elaborated on by Frank and Scanzoni (1982), viewed pair-bonding in a sexual relationship as occurring in three stages, beginning with the *proceptive* or *exploratory* stage, characterized by the erotic process of attraction, and culminating in the *conceptive* or *commitment* phase, during which the couple is committed and the potential for parenthood exists. The intermediate phase, the stage of *acceptance* or *expansion,* is marked by increasing sexual enjoyment after the initial coitus takes place. Within each phase the decision whether to proceed depends on the *context* of the relationship, i.e., available resources, self-esteem levels for each partner, gender role preferences, the physical milieu, and mutuality of the relationship; on the *processes* of the relationship, both explicit and implicit, particularly regarding coitus and contraception; and on the *outcomes* of each phase.

These stages are negotiated in an individualistic manner. For example, one maternity client shared that she and her husband had determined when they wished to have their two desired children and had selected names before their marriage took place. This demonstrated a high degree of commitment to parenthood early on. Another maternity client stated that she felt ready to become a mother only after a courtship of 4 years and 8 years of marriage. Culture influences these patterns. For example, in Japan the decision to marry is usually equivalent to the decision to become a parent within the year.

Campbell, Townes, and Beach (1982) offer an empirically based classification of values considered by couples in deciding whether to parent. Values centered on *self and spouse* include those making up *personal identity,* such as physical well-being, growth and maturity, self-concept, and educational-vocational values; those constituting *parenthood values,* such as caring for children, the role of parents in education, and the nature of the parent-child relationship; and those affecting the *well-being of the family,* including material and nonmaterial considerations. Values centered on the *children* include those about family size and gender of offspring, age of parents, health and well-being of children, sibling relationships, the prospective children themselves, and the effects of society on children. Values centered on *significant others* include those about family and relationships with relatives, family traditions, friends, and society at large.

To this framework, Fox, Fox, and Frohardt-Lane (1982) would add variables of a *sociohistorical nature,* such as the occurrence of war or state of the economy; variables of an *institutional nature,* such as work, church, or the media; variables regarding the *families of origin;* and *individual attributes,* such as one's sex role concept, sexual experiences, personality traits, birth order, and aspirations.

Thus, the decision to parent is a complex one, and many variables can influence it. Most couples probably do not give overt consideration to all of them.

Choosing to Parent: Factors and Consequences

A couple may become pregnant before the decision to parent is made, they may decide and then become pregnant, or they may decide but then be unable to conceive.

When the decision to parent occurs after conception, the couple may or may not have been actually attempting to avoid pregnancy, and they may or may not be receptive to an unplanned pregnancy. Decision-making after pregnancy occurs is necessarily time limited: If abortion is an option for the couple, it must be performed within the first two trimesters in some states and within the first trimester in others. If abortion is not an option, then the couple will continue through birth. At this point they still have a choice—to place the child for adoption or to keep it. Even among unmarried couples the choice of placing a child for adoption has declined in popularity in the past 2 decades as social prohibitions against single parenthood have diminished. Still, institutions such as schools, workplaces, or hospitals may encourage single parents to place their babies for adoption or at least to place them in foster care. Married women who chose this route were, in the experience of this author, severely censured by health care personnel and others.

When parenthood is a more deliberate choice, factors such as those previously delineated are taken into consideration but perhaps not conjointly. One review of the literature reported that prior to 1970 at least one third of couples surveyed did not discuss desired family size or contraception (Rosen and Benson, 1982). Wives tended to believe that their husbands wanted larger families than they actually did. Family planning research overall tends even now to report only wives' attitudes. More recently, Rosen and Benson observed that couples seemed to demonstrate greater joint consideration. Still, women tended to report having children to enhance relationships with their relatives more than men did, and men tended to demonstrate greater consistency among desired family size, size of family of origin, and actual fertility than women. Although women seem to make the immediate decision to become pregnant, these authors noted that husbands tend to get their way in terms of desired family size or else leave the relationship.

An additional issue for some couples having made the decision to parent is the distaste for coitus on schedule to coincide with ovulation. One client described feeling as though he were being bred. Pressure can build particularly if conception does not occur within the first few cycles.

Another alternative outcome is that a couple may decide to become parents but then fail to conceive. While the topic of infertility is too broad to discuss in this context, it should be noted that this outcome can severely undermine the self-concepts of both partners and their relationship. That their reproductive systems are not performing as planned may result in diminished self-esteem in each partner and concern about their masculinity or femininity.

Choosing Not to Parent: Factors and Consequences

Little research, if any, has focused on the attitudes of husbands in child-free marriages, but some interesting information has been compiled on the characteristics of the wives.

Married women in child-free marriages tend to be less traditional in their attitudes toward gender roles than women who are delaying parenthood or their age-mates who are mothers (Bram, 1984). Such women are more likely than their peers to hold professional or doctoral degrees. Not only are they more likely to be working, but they are also more likely to be employed in male-dominated fields than other women. They are more likely to plan to work until retirement and are more likely to view working as equally important as marriage and a family.

Child-free couples demonstrate more mutual, or egalitarian, relationships than child-delaying or parenting couples (Rosen and Benson, 1982). Companionship is more often identified as the most positive aspect of the marriage, whereas congruent values and shared activities are less likely to be identified.

The women in such marriages are less likely to rate themselves as conventional, dependent, or good with children and are more likely to regard themselves as dominant and competitive.

To interpret these results, one may speculate that these women are gratified by careers in which they have heavy investments and thus do not feel the creative or generative urge to parent. Or, perhaps they may choose not to parent, even though they would like to, so as not to interrupt their careers. Both these studies included wives who were still fertile, and no data were found in the literature that addressed changes in family-planning decisions of these women as their reproductive lives drew nearer to an end. Most nurses in maternity settings have encountered "elderly primiparae" either who never planned to parent or who reconsidered their decision as they felt the time for parenting was running out. This would make a fascinating study population from which to determine responses to unanticipated pregnancy, decisions to continue the pregnancy, or, in the case of women who planned their pregnancies, couple-related factors that made them do so.

Finally, some women have stated that they enjoy their marriages but do not believe the relationship could tolerate children. Others have expressed reluctance to experience the loss of intimacy or change in life style that parenthood brings.

Parenthood and Alternative Families

Many different forms of family or group living have emerged in the United States. Two that occur with increasing frequency will be discussed here: the case of the unmarried mother and the case of the gay or lesbian parent.

In the United States almost 2 million couples are living together outside of marriage. In general, such couples have reached the age of majority. Some decide to bear children. In addition, teenagers are becoming evermore sexually active (Zelnic, Kantner, and Ford, 1981). With this increase in sexual activity has come growing numbers of single mothers giving birth. In one small community hospital known to the author, over half the women giving birth in the last year were unmarried. In addition to the issues raised previously relative to married couples' decision to parent, single parents may deal with such issues as bearing the total responsibility for child care, having fewer financial resources than their married counterparts, and having a reduced support system. If they pursue jobs or further schooling or if they attempt to maintain a social life, they must first assure child care. Some unmarried couples are committed to long-term monogamous relationships. It is the author's view that in such cases particular care should be taken to document legally joint parentage of the child in order to protect him or her should the relationship terminate.

Adolescents who become parents face the additional strain of their own incomplete physical maturation. They are competing with their infants for nutrients for growth; this, coupled with the tendency for young people to eat a less than optimal diet, contributes to their higher than usual incidence of obstetrical complications. Young mothers are also often denied the benefit of psychosocial maturity. Depending on the attitudes of their family, the pregnancy may precipitate a crisis at home. In large maternity care settings the problem of a young client having no place to live after her parents turn her out is not uncommon. Pregnant teens may experience social isolation from their peers. Still, the establishment of support services such as high school programs for young mothers that supplement graduation requirements with content on child care, nutrition, and related topics has yielded cases of fairly mature young women taking good care of healthy babies. Rather than condemnation, these clients need extra information and support from health care providers.

Another example of an alternative parenting situation is the gay or lesbian parent. In one maternity setting in a large urban teaching hospital, three lesbian couples gave birth over the course of 4 months. In all three cases pregnancy was actively sought, in one instance by artificial insemination, in one case by the new mother's engaging in coitus with her lover's brother, and in the third situation by the new mother's engaging in coitus with casual dates until pregnancy was achieved. It is to the credit of the nursing staff that although they exhibited anxiety about these clients, they provided courteous, professional care that included both partners as it would have in other cases. It may be that there are particular needs of gay and lesbian parents that have not yet come to light. It seems much more difficult for gay men to undertake parenting, since they cannot bear their own children. Occasionally, cases in which gay or lesbian parents seek to adopt children or gain custody of their own children during divorce proceedings make newspaper headlines. The courts generally demonstrate reluctance to permit these arrangements.

Nurses who come into contact with infants and children and their families may well eventually find gays or lesbians among their clients, both as single parents and as couples. They will need support with the usual crises of parenting as well as with the issues related to their sexual life style, including social stigma, the persistent threat of loss of custody, and gender role socialization of their children (Steinhorn and Weiss, 1984). Nurses who have contact with gay and lesbian clients may also be in a position to help those who are unable to parent come to terms with this fact.

THE EXPERIENCE OF PREGNANCY

Physiological Function

A complete presentation of the anatomy and physiology of pregnancy is not within the scope of this book, but a brief review will help the reader better understand the psychological and sexual changes experienced by women and their partners.

FIRST TRIMESTER

Pregnancy affects every system of the body. Some women experience few or none of the related symptoms, whereas others experience many and may find such changes uncomfortable.

An early change that is considered a presumptive sign of pregnancy is the suppression of menstruation after fertilization takes place. The vascular uterine lining that is prepared in each cycle for the nourishment of a conceptus is now needed. As the blastocyst implants in the uterine wall, uterine, cervical, and vaginal vasculature increases markedly under the influence of elevated levels of sex hormones. This will be observable as Chadwick's sign. This increase continues throughout pregnancy to ensure nutrition and oxygenation of the embryo and is also reflected in other organ systems by such signs as increased perspiration and urine production.

The cervix begins to hypertrophy, becomes

edematous, and softens early in pregnancy. This may result in minor bleeding after coitus as pregnancy progresses. Mucus production is increased.

The uterus itself begins to grow by the eighth week, and connective tissue softens. The fundus may be palpable above the symphysis pubis as early as the twelfth week of gestation. Uterine contractions may be noticed early after conception. This is a mechanism that promotes uterine circulation. It also reflects hypertrophy and expansion of uterine muscle fibers. Growth of the uterus causes it to stretch the bladder, resulting in the frequent urge to urinate. Hormonal effects on the adrenals result in an altered water balance in the body, with increased fluid retention.

Within the first few weeks after conception, the woman may experience changes in her breasts similar to those of the premenstruum. After the second missed period, heaviness, increased sensitivity, and tingling or throbbing progress as milk glands start to develop. Veins become more prominent, and the nipples and areola darken. By the tenth week a watery secretion can be expressed. Upon palpation the breasts will feel nodular. Striae begin to appear.

The woman is expected to gain 3 or 4 pounds during the first trimester. But alterations in hormone levels, especially an increase in human chorionic gonadotropin, lead to changes in metabolism, particularly of carbohydrates. This can cause the woman to experience nausea and vomiting. Additionally, progesterone-mediated relaxation of smooth muscle can result in constipation. The marked increase in anabolic processes may contribute to feelings of lethargy.

SECOND TRIMESTER

During this trimester, from week 12 to about week 26, the abdomen expands noticeably in most women to accommodate the continued growth of the uterus. By about week 20 the fundus reaches the level of the umbilicus. By about the fourth or fifth month of pregnancy the presence of the fetus can be detected by ballottement. Quickening occurs toward the end of the fifth month. By the end of the second trimester the uterine wall has thinned, and the fetus has developed to the point at which the fetal outline can be palpated. Its activities and position can be felt by the mother and even visualized through changing configurations of the abdominal wall. The vagina becomes more engorged, and the vaginal folds become flattened.

The breasts are ready for lactation by about 19 weeks, when colostrum starts to exude from the nipples. They are less tender but feel quite heavy.

As the uterus rises out of the pelvis, the frequent feeling of the need to urinate is relieved. The entire digestive system is relaxed, so that constipation persists. Additionally, eructation, flatulence, and heartburn or esophageal reflux may become noticeable. Venous pressure from pelvic organs leads to the development of hemorrhoids. Some women salivate more.

Some changes in the integumentary system are hyperpigmentation, including chloasma, the development of vascular spiders, and the darkening of the linea nigra; the increased appearance on breasts, the abdomen, and hips of striae gravidarum; a heightened cutaneous allergic response; the continuation of increased perspiration; and increased sebaceous activity. The woman may notice a difference in the growth, increased or diminished, and texture of her hair. Fat is deposited subdermally particularly in the upper arms, hips, thighs, and buttocks. Some women experience nosebleeds. Edema is noticeable, and toxemia can develop toward the end of this trimester.

Cardiovascular changes include a 47 per cent blood volume increase, marked by increased cardiac output, and increased venous blood pressure in the legs, which can result in painful and unsightly varicosities. Blood pressure drops as the vascular bed expands then rises, usually not more than 15 mm Hg both systolically and diastolically after the first half of pregnancy. A pseudoanemia occurs as blood volume increases faster than red blood cell production.

Sensory changes may occur in the legs as a result of nerve compression or venous stasis. Posture changes as the center of gravity shifts, and the resulting dorsolumbar lordosis can cause muscle aches or painful nerve traction or compression.

Hypocalcemia can lead to muscle cramps. Joints, particularly those of the pelvis, relax under the influence of maternal hormones. Pelvic or hip pain may result. Weight gain in the second trimester is about 12 to 14 pounds.

THIRD TRIMESTER

Weight gain during the third trimester is about 8 to 10 pounds. The changes of the second trimester become more pronounced. The uterus continues to grow until the fundus is within 1 to 2 cm of the xiphoid process, at which time the mother's umbilicus is everted. The growth in the uterus has caused dyspnea and a shift to thoracic breathing. The thorax has widened. Lightening occurs in the last 2 weeks in nulliparous women. Lightening offers relief, but it exacerbates ankle edema and varicosities, and urinary frequency recurs. Braxton Hicks contractions become palpable toward the thirtieth week. The placenta has started to show signs of aging already by the seventh month. The cervix is maximally soft and totally or partially effaces within the last few weeks (Boston Women's Health Collective, 1985; Pritchard and MacDonald, 1980).

Psychological Function

THE MOTHER

Caplan (1957) observed that pregnancy is like puberty and menopause in that it is a period of increased susceptibility to other stresses, a time of disequilibrium. Even couples who have well-adjusted patterns of communication may now experience inexplicable changes in these patterns, including crying, anger, or withdrawal (Stichler, Bowden, and Reimer, 1978). The pregnant woman may experience erratic mood swings over which she has no control. These are believed to be hormonally mediated. In addition, these new behaviors may reflect psychological processes undergone by the woman as she comes to terms with impending motherhood. The psychological tasks of early pregnancy are to incorporate the pregnancy as a real fact of life and to begin planning for the future. The fatigue and morning sickness of early pregnancy may be accompanied by depression. During this time many fears, fantasies, and wishes may preoccupy the pregnant woman. Caplan (1957) interpreted this as a reworking of old conflicts. Indeed, he asserted that all psychological development to date is reworked during pregnancy. Fears that tend to surface most often have to do with the health of the woman's baby and her own survival. One of the meanings of pregnancy for many women is that it is a rite of passage into adulthood.

Reva Rubin (1967) has described how the maternal role is assumed by the new mother-to-be. Mimicking and role play reflect the *taking-on* process; fantasy work reflects the *taking-in* process; and grief work is a form of the *letting-go* process, as former roles are abandoned. All three processes have to do with the woman's relationship with her own mother. While she may find herself identifying more strongly with her mother *as a mother*, she must, at the same time, reprocess old conflicts she had with her while growing up and come to a reconciliation. Finally, she must let go of the role of girl. It is hoped that the woman emerges from this process with a sense of herself as a competent adult and as a mother, separate from her own mother (Ballou, 1978).

Some women, even those who desire and plan for it, feel trapped by their pregnancy. It evokes for them negative aspects of woman's lot in life, and they are unable to find much about it to enjoy (Colman, 1983). These women may experience the childbearing years as discontinuous with their sense of self, and their anxiety abates only when they return to work. This reflects a fear of the loss of self-hood and independence.

Pregnancy also forces the woman to deal with the public statement that she and her partner are sexual beings. Pregnancy, according to Falicov (1973), represents for many women proof of their womanhood and mature acceptance of their femininity. Additionally, pregnancy serves to help shed old inhibitions in relation to bodily functions and to promote marital intimacy. Colman observed that the idea that sexual activity can create a baby adds pleasure and meaning to the sex act for some people. She also describes the conflict that our culture perpetuates, that motherhood is pristinely sacred and asexual. This makes it difficult for a woman to acknowledge feeling "sexy and maternal at the same time" (Colman, 1983, p 11).

As pregnancy progresses, the woman usually accepts the reality of it, particularly after quickening, and she directs energy toward preparations for the baby's arrival and care. At the same time, as physical changes are more pronounced, the woman may feel sloppy, unattractive, and out of control of her body. In a study of 50 women, Hollender and McGehee (1974) found an increase in the desire to be held during pregnancy, largely as reassurance that in spite of their appearance their husbands still love them (Fig. 10–1). Over half thought that their husbands thought their bodies were more attractive than they themselves did. This reaction is understandable in a culture in which thinness and adolescent beauty are prized in women. The distortion in body image that the woman must acknowledge when she can no longer wear her clothes is experienced as a distortion in her self (Weinberg, 1978). The way that she experiences a distorted body image will be influenced by the degree to which she is invested in her appearance, by her acceptance of pregnancy, by the values of her ethnic group, by the response of significant others, and particularly by the response of her mate. The importance of self-concept of the mother for perinatal outcome is suggested in a study that showed a direct relationship between mothers' negative scores on self-concept and neonatal perception and negative scores on a parenting instrument (Lee, 1982). The author undertook this study to provide support for observations documented in the literature of a relationship between maternal self-esteem and child abuse potential.

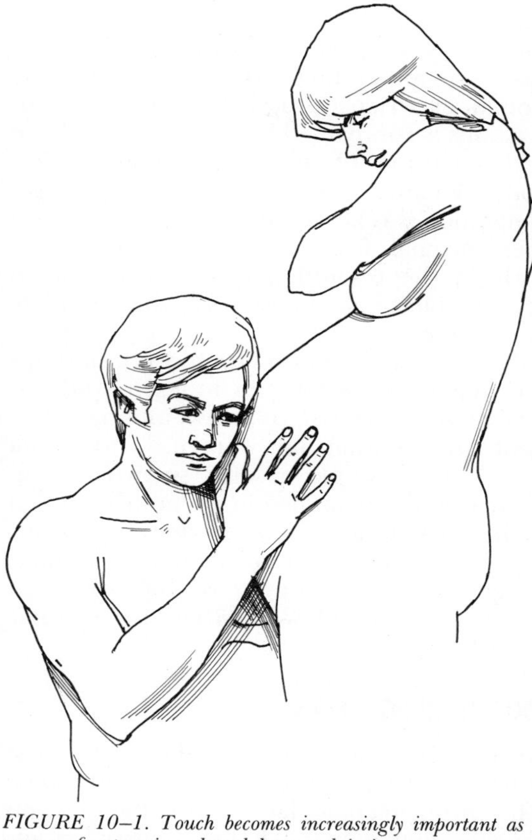

It is quite common for the pregnant woman to become introverted, or withdrawn, and narcissistic. This is congruent with Rubin's (1967) description of the *taking-in* process as preparation for taking on the role of mother. Time and energy spent focusing on her own and her infant's needs now prepare her to direct herself to caring for the infant at her own expense later (Rubin, 1961).

It should be apparent by now that pregnancy is, under optimal conditions, a stressful transition. Other life changes may be triggered by pregnancy and birth, including moving, altered sleep patterns, and altered career patterns. In a study of over 300 pregnant women, Semmens (1971) observed a relationship between stress in the life situation as a whole and the occurrence of nausea, vomiting, and excess weight gain. Thus, the nurse needs to consider pregnancy in the context of a couple's total life.

THE FATHER

Until recently, little attention was paid to the response of the man to impending fatherhood. But along with the women's liberation movement has come more flexible roles and greater efforts to integrate fathers into the process of birth.

Some fathers are appalled by the changes in their wives' bodies (Bing and Colman, 1977). Others find their wives' changing shapes to be quite enjoyable. The man is at a disadvantage in that he cannot know firsthand what it is like to be pregnant. Some men feel overwhelmed by their wives' super-femininity.

In our society the expectant father lacks a clearly defined role (Antle, 1975). While women are the recipients of advice on child care, new maternity clothes, frequent health care contacts, showers, and other forms of attention, there is little to mark the pregnancy for men. This may make the transition to parenthood even harder for them than for women.

Some concerns that expectant fathers may have include the withdrawal of their mates, an alteration in the couple's former pattern of sexual behavior, his own anxiety about labor and delivery and his ability to "take" being present for the birth, and his height-

FIGURE 10–1. Touch becomes increasingly important as a means of expressing shared love and intimacy as pregnancy progresses.

ened dependency needs and nurturant emotions.

What women want of their husbands includes enthusiasm; active interest in the pregnancy, birth, and infant; empathy; assurance that they are still attractive; accompaniment to prenatal clinics and classes; and presence during delivery (Bennett, 1981). But the father-to-be must cope with his *own* anxieties in order to provide support for his mate. He too may experience ambivalence when he learns of the pregnancy. It is proof of his potency and a source of pride; yet it also represents increasing economic and social demands (Stichler, Bowden, and Reimer, 1978). Clients often report that their husbands take on additional jobs for extra income during the pregnancy or undertake home renovations. Many men seem to feel that their ability to adjust well to pregnancy and birth depends on the quality of their marriage (Hangsleben, 1983; Porter and Demeuth, 1979).

Like his mate, the prospective father may begin to relive his experience with his own parents, reprocessing old conflicts and coming to some kind of reconciliation (Briggs, 1979). In addition to having to deal with these issues, it is commonplace for men to be baffled or upset by their wives' behaviors and mood shifts during pregnancy. They may respond by withdrawing from their wives. Many men react to feelings of exclusion from pregnancy and these other issues by becoming more dependent and less dependable (Bing and Colman, 1977; Stichler, Bowden, and Reimer, 1978).

There are societies in which rituals have been established to mark the man's transition to fatherhood. These are termed *couvade* experiences. In our society there is little formal recognition for this rite of passage other than, perhaps, the sharing of cigars or drinks with friends and colleagues after the birth. Some new fathers have admitted that they experienced physical symptoms during their wives' pregnancies, probably either as a manifestation of envy or of identification (Antle, 1975).

Fawcett (1978), building on reports of men's experiences of such symptoms as nausea and vomiting, syncope, lassitude, leg cramps, weight gain, and backache, studied perceived body space in 50 couples during and after pregnancy. Husbands, like their wives, demonstrated a perceived increase in body space as pregnancy progressed and a decrease in the first few months after birth. Colman and Colman (1971) reported that one in ten fathers shared symptoms, while Liebenberg (1969) found that 65 per cent of a group of first-time fathers reported such experiences. Antle (1975) asserts that men who demonstrate such symptoms may be more nurturant after the baby is born. The phenomenon is common enough that it should be included in anticipatory guidance of couples.

PREGNANCY AND SEXUAL FUNCTION

Physiological Function

The physiological cycle of response to sexual stimulation comprises four phases. In the first, the *excitement phase,* the woman experiences genital vasocongestion, vaginal lubrication, and distention of the vaginal barrel in response to sexual stimulation. If stimulation continues, she progresses to the *plateau phase.* The vagina and the labia minora become engorged to form the orgasmic platform. The subjective perception is that orgasm is impending. During *orgasm,* the woman experiences vaginal and uterine contractions accompanied by a feeling of release and suffusion of warmth throughout her body. Finally, during *resolution,* the vasocongestion is relieved, and genitalia return to their normal size and configuration. Very early in the resolution phase most women are capable of reexperiencing the complete response cycle.

Masters and Johnson (1966) were perhaps the first to undertake an indepth study of deviations in sexual response among pregnant and postpartum women. Their data represent a sample of only six women, so caution must be applied in generalizing from their work (Fig. 10–2). It does, however, represent a good start in this area of inquiry. In addition, they conducted interviews on this topic with 111 women and 79 of their husbands.

EXCITEMENT PHASE

During sexual stimulation women in the first trimester report severe breast tenderness. This problem abates later in pregnancy when sexual stimulation no longer causes an appreciable increase in breast size.

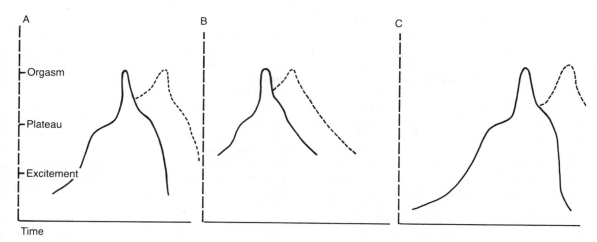

FIGURE 10–2. Comparison of the sexual responses of women at various stages of the maternity cycle. A, Prepregnancy response, B, Antepartal response, C, Postpartal response. (Based on Masters WH, Johnson VE: Human Sexual Response. Boston, Little, Brown & Co, 1966.)

The main genital effect of pregnancy is the progressive increase in pelvic vasocongestion. This may be experienced as a marked increase in sexual interest. In multiparous women the labia majora are quite engorged and occasionally edematous. Vaginal lubrication is more copious than in the nonpregnant state and is more rapid. The labia minora, in response to sexual stimulation, continue to enlarge by a factor of one or two during the first two trimesters, but by the third trimester they are engorged, so that no additional increase is detected.

PLATEAU PHASE

In nulliparous women, localized vaginal engorgement is so marked that about 75 per cent of the vaginal lumen is obtunded. In multiparous women, upon prolonged sexual stimulation, the vaginal barrel often appears completely obtunded. During prolonged sexual excitement, the lateral walls actually come together, and as pregnancy advances, the rate at which the orgasmic platform develops is increased. After the first trimester when the uterus rises out of the pelvis, the uterine-elevation response is not noted. It is not known whether additional vasocongestion occurs in the uterus during pregnancy.

ORGASM

During the first two trimesters orgasmic platform contractions are observable. In the third trimester, the outer vagina is so chronically congested that the orgasmic contractions ap-

pear minimal, although they are experienced by the women. During the last month or so, women may experience uterine spasm lasting as long as a half hour at orgasm rather than a series of contractions. Masters and Johnson did note a transitory slowing in fetal heart rate. Women in the third trimester may secrete colostrum at orgasm.

RESOLUTION

In contrast to women's experience in the nonpregnant state, resolution is transitory. The pelvis is chronically vasocongested, and orgasm does not clear the tissues. As pregnancy progresses, this becomes more pronounced. In a second trimester primigravida it may take 10 to 15 minutes for labial and vaginal vasocongestion to return to the non–sexually excited state, and in multiparous women this may take 30 to 45 minutes. In the third trimester, vasocongestion may not be relieved regardless of the intensity of the orgasm.

All of this may be experienced by the woman as heightened sexual tension, which is not relieved for a significant period of time by orgasm.

EFFECTS OF PREGNANCY ON ADAPTATION
Patterns of Sexual Activity During Pregnancy

Findings of various investigators regarding alterations in patterns of sexual activity during pregnancy are summarized in Table 10–1. These findings can be considered only tentative, owing to serious shortcomings in the studies, which often reflect the sensitive nature of the topic and the resultant difficulties in recruiting participants in the research.

It appears that most women experience a gradual decrease in sexual interest and activity over the course of pregnancy. They may have some resurgence in the second trimester. Yet there were, in three studies, groups who experienced increased interest and responsiveness over nonpregnant levels, particularly in the second trimester. In the third trimester inactivity appears to reflect medical prohibitions of sexual intercourse. Husbands may also experience diminished sexual interest and decreased sexual activity over the course of pregnancy. Husbands may experience increased need for coitus along with the decrease in activity, but their interest may shift toward different partners.

To conclude, a wide range of sexual feelings is within normal limits for men and women during pregnancy. Sexual interest and activity may increase, decrease, or remain stable in either partner. Whatever a couple's feelings, if they are supported in sharing them, they can generally be assured that they are not unusual.

Factors That Affect Patterns of Sexual Activity

Pregnant couples often experience anxiety, arising from a variety of sources, about sexual activity during pregnancy (McGinnis, 1982). Such concerns may be invalid, yet may inhibit couples from engaging in coitus, an important means for them to feel close and to satisfy dependency needs.

One of the most difficult factors to deal with is the personal values of the couple. In many cultures, sexuality has negative associations: It may be considered base and shameful. Various religious groups have advocated sex solely as a means for procreation and not recreation. Or, young people may be taught before marriage that sex is "dirty" and then have difficulty accepting its wholesomeness after marriage. Young girls may be taught that sex is something they have to tolerate, and pregnancy and birth may be cast as women's punishment for Eve's having seduced Adam, as one interpretation of the Old Testament story states.

Sex under any circumstance may be conflict laden for individuals who have grown up with such messages, and pregnancy can intensify conflicts, as it emphasizes the Madonna-seductress dichotomy of woman that arises from such a values system. Even among couples who do not subscribe to such values, conflicts may have to be resolved regarding the wife's assumption of the role of mother and her partner's feelings about his own mother. Resolution of the oedipal conflict in early childhood demands that the child learn that his or her opposite-sex parent is sexually off limits.

Over the years, such feelings have been supported by such "scientific" writing as that of Dr. William Alcott (1972), the brother of the author Louisa May Alcott. He warned that coitus during pregnancy is reckless to the fetus, weakens the mother, and violates the precepts of Christianity. According to Alcott, if nervous women demonstrate a sexual appetite during pregnancy, their mates must respond with aid and sympathy, nutritious food, and mental discipline.

Fear of harming the fetus or the mother is a common concern among pregnant couples and has been the focus of several studies. Solberg, Butler, and Wagner (1978) reported that 27 per cent of their research participants who reported a change in sexual activity during pregnancy were motivated to do so by fear of harm to the baby. Of this group of 260 women, 19 gave birth prematurely. None of these births occurred immediately after coitus or orgasm, and no relationships were demonstrated within the entire group of infants among birth weight, gestational age at delivery, Apgar scores, and maternal sexual activity during the third trimester.

Grudzinskas, Watson, and Chard (1979) observed a *lower* than expected rate of early delivery in relation to orgasm at all stages of pregnancy among 155 pregnant women. However, they did note a positive trend between maternal coitus in the last month of pregnancy and such indicators of distress as Apgar score of 6 or less and meconium staining.

In contrast with the above findings, Goodlin, Keller, and Raffin (1971) noted a significantly higher incidence of orgasm after 32 weeks' gestation in patients who subsequently delivered prematurely than in those who delivered at term. Only 24 per cent of women who delivered at term experienced orgasm after 32 weeks' gestation versus 50 per cent

TABLE 10–1. Patterns of Sexual Activity During Pregnancy

Author	Subjects	First Trimester	Second Trimester	Third Trimester	Pregnancy as a Whole
Masters and Johnson (1966)	101 women 79 men	Decreased sexual tension and activity among primiparas, no change among multiparas.	Most women experienced marked increase above prepregnant levels in desire and activity.	All women demonstrated marked decrease in activity; half of husbands reported decreased interest.	
Falicov (1973)	19 primiparae	14 of 19 experienced decreased desire and activity compared with prepregnant levels.	Twelve of 19 experienced decreased desire and activity over prepregnancy levels but an increase over first trimester levels.	Eleven of 17 reported decreased interest; 15 abstained last 2 months.	
Tolor and DiGrazia (1976)	54 first trimester, 51 second trimester, and 56 third trimester women	Decreased desire in 39%; decreased activity in 15%; and increased activity in 20%.	Decreased desire in 47%; preferred activity level less than usual in 10%; and increased preferred activity level in 21%.	Decreased desire in 54%; preferred activity level less than usual in 21%; and increased preferred activity level in 32%.	
Solberg, Butler, and Wagner (1978)	260 postpartum women				Trend toward decreased orgasmic response and interest; increased responsiveness in small proportion. Linear decrease in activity throughout pregnancy.
Kumar, Brant, and Robson (1981)	119 British primiparae				Linear decrease in activity throughout pregnancy.
Ellis (1980)	15 couples				Decreased enjoyment of sex throughout pregnancy for both men and women. Increased need for sex and interest in other women among men. Decreased desire among one third of women. Desire for more touch and masturbation among men and women.

of the women who delivered prematurely. Twenty-six per cent of the women who delivered prematurely experienced orgasm within 50 hours of the onset of labor. Four women agreed to achieve orgasm at a specified time. Of these, three were admitted in labor within 9 hours of orgasm, and the fourth had a bout of false labor. These authors believe that if women are not willing to forego coitus, they should be cautioned to avoid orgasm if their cervix is ripe at 31 weeks or if they have a poor reproductive history.

Naeye (1979) observed a significant relationship between coitus and amniotic fluid infection. However, this finding must be questioned on the basis of reliability because he used interview data gathered while women were in active labor. Pugh and Fernandez (1953) found no relationship between third trimester coitus and sepsis in their study of 500 women.

A third type of risk is fetal bradycardia. Masters and Johnson noted the occurrence of transient fetal bradycardia during maternal orgasm. Goodlin, Schmidt, and Greevy (1972) saw no deleterious effects as a result of fetal deceleration in a case study in which a couple achieved multiple maternal orgasms while fetal monitoring was performed. Still, one cannot generalize from a single case, and readers are cautioned that this issue remains unresolved.

Physicians and others have tended to be conservative in giving advice about coitus during pregnancy. In Solberg, Butler, and Wagner's 1978 study, 9 per cent of the women altered their sexual practices based on the advice of physicians or others. In Falicov's (1973) group of 17 third-trimester women, 15 had stopped sexual intercourse: Five were following medical advice, and the other 10 had read or heard that they should stop at this time. In a survey of 23 obstetricians (Clark and Hale, 1974) it was found that 11 regarded intercourse as permissible throughout pregnancy, six recommended abstinence during the last 3 weeks of pregnancy, five recommended abstinence during the last 6 weeks, and one recommended abstinence throughout the entire pregnancy. In general, the traditional advice has been to abstain from coitus during the last 4 to 6 weeks of pregnancy even though under normal circumstances there is probably no need to do so before the membranes rupture (Pritchard and MacDonald, 1980).

Women who *should* refrain from genital sexual and/or orgasmic activity include those who are habitual aborters, those experiencing vaginal bleeding, those who are experiencing abdominal pain, those whose amniotic membrane has ruptured, and those whose cervix has begun to efface and/or dilate after 24 weeks. Other complications of pregnancy such as preeclampsia may necessitate restraint.

Other factors demonstrating an impact on women's sexual activity during pregnancy include symptoms described previously, such as fatigue, nausea, heartburn, backache, self-consciousness about appearance, the tendency to withdraw, and the awkwardness of their increasing abdominal girth and weight. As discussed earlier, it is common for women to experience diminished interest in sex. Husbands, too, may report a decreased interest in sexual activity or, while still interested in sex per se, a gradual sexual withdrawal from their spouse (Masters and Johnson, 1966; Solberg, Butler, and Wagner, 1978).

On the other hand, many couples report that their sex lives get a real lift during pregnancy because of elimination of the pressures to conceive or to use contraception, increased awareness of the woman's body, celebration of their accomplishment, and of increased desire and responsiveness due to the physiology of pregnancy (Bing and Colman, 1977; Masters and Johnson, 1966).

Among couples whose sexual interest has not diminished, actual frequency may be less because of uterine cramping at orgasm, unsatisfactory resolution in the female, discomfort or cervical bleeding caused by penetration, and vena cava compression when the woman is in the supine position. Some of these problems can be resolved by the use of alternate sexual positions. This will be elaborated in the following section.

Alternative Modes of Sexual Expression

When coitus is uncomfortable or when couples' levels of sexual desire are incongruent, mutual or solitary masturbation is an alternative. Bing and Colman (1977) reported on a number of women with increased sexual desires during pregnancy, for whom frequent masturbation was an important outlet, as well as in couples who used this technique together. One example cited concerned a woman who had such profound vaginal swelling that her partner was unable to penetrate. For this couple, masturbation may be a desirable choice as the woman reaches her maximum size. Women who must avoid orgasm for the reasons cited previously should be advised that masturbation is contraindicated.

Massage is an important mode of expression, particularly when sexual activity leading to orgasm is restricted. Couples report that touch and cuddling grow in importance throughout pregnancy, whether or not coitus is contraindicated (Bing and Colman, 1977; Hollender and McGehee, 1974). Not only does this convey reassurance to the woman that she is still lovable, but it signifies to the man that his mate is still interested in him and not solely in the baby.

Oral sex is an activity enjoyed by many couples. Fellatio may be an acceptable form of expression when the woman's coital activities are restricted. Many husbands who normally enjoy cunnilingus, however, report that they are "turned off" by it during pregnancy, possibly because of the changing taste and odor of the woman's vaginal secretions (Bing and Colman, 1977). In fact, there is some risk: At least two cases have been documented in which pregnant women died as a result of air emboli from air blown into the vagina (Aronson and Nelson, 1967; Benjamin, 1946). Comfort (1972) advises that partners should *never* blow air (aeroculpus) into body orifices. Therefore, it may be prudent to advise couples to avoid cunnilingus during pregnancy or to apprise them of the risk, as this practice could lead to the partner inadvertently blowing into the woman's vagina.

BIRTH AND SEXUALITY

Birth, Orgasm, and Lactation: Parallel Events

Niles Newton (1971, 1973) has done the most to elucidate the sexual nature of the birth process (Fig. 10–3). She observed that during both female orgasm and undrugged childbirth, the following parallels can be observed:

1. *Breathing* becomes deeper during labor contractions and during sexual arousal. During the second stage of labor and during orgasm, breathing is interrupted.

2. *Vocalizations* such as grunts or gasps occur in the second stage of labor and at orgasm.

3. A *facial expression* of intense strain characterizes both phenomena.

4. *Uterine contractions* characterize both phenomena.

5. The *cervix* opens for the release of the baby before or during labor and for the intake of sperm at orgasm.

6. *Abdominal muscles* contract during labor as well as during sexual excitement.

7. The *position* assumed by the woman for birth and coitus is the same in our culture, generally supine with legs abducted and knees flexed.

8. *Behaviors and expressions* become less inhibited under both circumstances, and there is a tendency to become oblivious to surroundings.

9. The *emotional response* is one of joy and well-being after both birth and orgasm.

10. Additionally, *clitoral engorgement* may accompany both events.

Newton has observed additional parallels between the processes of orgasm and lactation, pleasurable sensations that she believes evolved to ensure the frequent occurrence of both:

1. *Uterine contractions* occur during both nursing and orgasm.

2. *Nipple erection* occurs with both; additionally, breast stroking and nipple stimulation are included both in lovemaking and in preparing to nurse. Newton notes that the infant may respond to nursing with rhythmic movements and penile erection.

3. *Skin changes* during sexual excitement include a sexual flush. During lactation, breast skin temperature rises.

4. The *milk-ejection* reflex is triggered during both events.

5. Finally, women subjectively report *sexual arousal* not only during lovemaking but also during lactation, even to the point of orgasm. Women who breastfeed have been characterized as having more open attitudes in other areas of sexuality.

Newton suggests that all three processes, birth, orgasm, and lactation, are mediated by closely related neurohormonal processes. The *oxytocic hormones* appear to play prominent roles in each. All three processes are inhibited by environmental disturbance, at least in their initial phases. This may reflect the organism's need for security in order for the fight or flight response to be overridden. Further, all three processes reinforce or trigger care-taking behaviors that are essential for survival of the species.

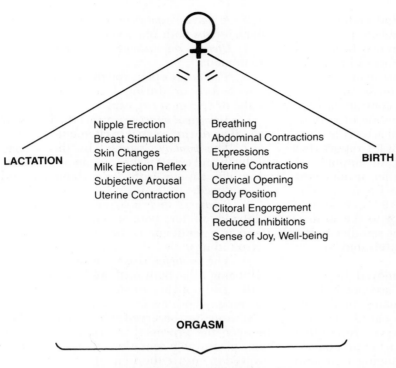

LACTATION

- Nipple Erection
- Breast Stimulation
- Skin Changes
- Milk Ejection Reflex
- Subjective Arousal
- Uterine Contraction

- Breathing
- Abdominal Contractions
- Expressions
- Uterine Contractions
- Cervical Opening
- Body Position
- Clitoral Engorgement
- Reduced Inhibitions
- Sense of Joy, Well-being

BIRTH

FIGURE 10–3. Newton (1971, 1973) has identified parallels among the processes of orgasm, lactation, and birth. Evolving as a means of promoting reproduction of the species and care-giving, these experiences have been suppressed by social institutions.

ORGASM

OXYTOCIC HORMONAL MEDIATION

Newton believes that social norms that control sexual behavior in general have caused inhibition of these natural, enjoyable processes. Women seldom experience birth orgasm in our society, and many women either find breast-feeding distasteful or are concerned if they experience sexual arousal when they nurse. She observes that institutions have interfered with these processes through such practices as medication in intrapartum, physical restraint of laboring women, separation of mothers and their newly delivered infants, and enforcement of rules about the frequency and duration of nursing.

Birth As a Couple-Strengthening Event

While pregnancy and birth are *not* advocated as a means of salvaging a tenuous relationship, sharing a birth can profoundly enhance a loving and supportive one. Newton has stated, "What occurs on the delivery table is very pertinent to what will transpire later in the marital bed" (Newton, 1973, p 78). Bing and Colman (1977) related moving testimonials of couples who had shared undrugged birth experiences.

Richardson (1979) noted that women feel a rising sense of vulnerability as the time for labor draws near and that the woman may demonstrate erratic swings from needing someone to be near to intolerance of contact. Upon analysis of various behaviors of 24 women in labor, she concluded that visual and postural approach behaviors decreased and intrusive procedures were decreasingly tolerated as labor progressed. Yet the women increasingly sought contacts through verbal and tactual behaviors such as calling out to others in loud, demanding voices and grasping persons with increasing forcefulness.

Bing and Colman's (1977) work helps to put Richardson's observations into a couple-focused perspective. They describe the care rendered by the husband, such as massage, offering ice chips, praise, and coaching, as acts of love at a time when nature forces the woman into a state of dependency.

It is postulated that in order for a woman to give birth she must relax and open up and that the marital relationship may be the best indicator of whether or not this will happen optimally (Bing and Colman, 1977). In a good relationship the husband can create a secure environment for birth. For the woman to show herself to her partner in this light, sweating, facially contorted, and anatomically distorted, requires great trust. The positive relationship between relaxation and letting go and ease of labor has some empirical support (Morris, 1979; Scott-Palmer and Skevington, 1981; Spielberger and Jacobs, 1979; Vellay, 1979).

Observations made of 31 men during their first-time experiences with childbirth have showed that they felt it was important to nurture their wives during labor (MacLaughlin and Taubenheim, 1983). Many of the men subsequently reported that being able to comfort and help their wives through labor heightened the experience for them. Their own physical needs were deemed unimportant in comparison to those of their wives, and they were committed to staying by their wives throughout the whole process. The men reported feeling a sense of achievement from helping their wives and were concerned about doing a good job as a labor coach. Most of the men acknowledged that a sense of control in this situation was important to them, although they expressed a desire to be able to depend on the nurse if they could not meet specific needs of their wives. A positive relationship exists between taking on the role of labor coach and enhanced self-esteem (Gabel, 1982). Wives often subsequently described their husbands in the labor coach role in glowing terms. Women, too, experience a sense of accomplishment after giving birth.

Health professionals who have worked in birth settings are familiar with the "high" experienced by many new parents in the immediate postpartum period. Birth, the culmination of a shared sexual moment and a shared pregnancy, will be a peak experience for the couple who can share it while letting go of their fears and anxieties. It can serve to promote more active involvement by the father in the life of his child after birth (MacLaughlin and Taubenheim, 1983; Phillips and Anzalone, 1978).

POSTPARTUM
Physiological Changes Related to Sexual Functioning

Two of the most marked physiological changes in the early postpartum period are the immediate uterine discharge, *lochia,* and the transition of colostrum to *breast milk* by the second or third day. Lochia starts as *rubra,* mostly blood, for 3 or 4 days, then changes to pink *serosa,* followed by *alba* from about the tenth day through the third or fourth week.

Masters and Johnson (1966) continued their study of six women through the third postpartal month. Three of these mothers nursed their infants through the fourth postpartum month.

By the fourth or fifth week pelvic examination showed well-healed episiotomies, cessation of lochia, closure of the cervix, and continued elevation of the uterus into the abdomen, although involution was more advanced among the lactating women.

The vaginal tissue demonstrated steroid starvation: The walls were quite thin, normal patterns of rugae were diminished or absent, and the vaginal walls were light pink. This also was more marked among nursing mothers.

This pattern prevailed at the 6- to 8-week examination, but by the end of the third postpartum month all six women showed return of ovarian hormone production, although this was more marked among nonnursing mothers. Vaginal rugae were once again evident, and the uterus had returned to its usual position.

There are numerous other changes that occur (Pritchard and MacDonald, 1980). The uterus contracts rhythmically as involution progresses. This is more noticeable, even painful, immediately after delivery in multiparous and lactating women. The cervix should be nearly closed by the end of the second week. The external os will appear as a slit in the parous woman, and the surface may show depressions where lacerations occurred. The vagina approaches its usual size and shape by the sixth to eighth week, although a complete return to the original dimensions may never occur. The pelvic floor may be weakened owing to scar tissue formation. Hematomas may be present but resorb within 10 days to 2 weeks. The introitus should return to the nulliparous state.

Menses resumes in nonlactating women by 6 to 8 weeks. The first couple cycles may produce heavier than usual flow, and the first cycle may be anovulatory. However, this is somewhat unpredictable, and contraception should be practiced from the time intercourse is resumed by women seeking to avoid another pregnancy. Resumption of ovulation and menstruation are more variable among lactating women, but in general they are delayed.

The postpartum mother who has lost 500 ml or more of blood during delivery is considered to have hemorrhaged and is most prone to orthostatic hypotension. Normally, blood volume returns to usual levels by 1 week. Within the first few days the mother will diurese 2 to 3 liters of extracellular water. In addition, hormonal fluctuations will be experienced as hot flashes. Tension on the urinary tract during birth, edema, and increased bladder capacity may make voiding difficult within the first 24 hours. Lactose is found in the urine in early postpartum and during lactation. Acetone may be found in early postpartum as well.

The abdomen remains flabby until skin elasticity is regained over time and through exercise. This physical state coupled with the presence of hemorrhoids, episiotomy tenderness, and decreased food intake can make bowel evacuation difficult during the first few days. Over time the linea nigra disappears and striae fade.

Obstetrical traumas other than those identified previously may include vaginal varicosities, tears to the vaginal bulbar system, which can reduce orgasmic response, and perineal tears or stretching that widens the vaginal orifice (Woods, 1979). A positive effect of pregnancy is increased pelvic vascularization, which persists and, for many women, facilitates orgasmic response (Masters and Johnson, 1966).

Mothers who have undergone cesarean birth generally experience most of these changes in addition to an abdominal wound and the effects of general anesthesia. They are at risk for other postoperative complications such as pneumonia, wound infection, and thromboembolic disease.

Sexual Responsiveness After Birth

Masters and Johnson (1966) noted among their subjects a reduction in speed and intensity of sexual responsiveness during the early postpartum period. Vasocongestive reactions of the labia majora and minora were often delayed until well into the plateau phase. Lubrication developed slowly and in reduced quantity. Vaginal distention in the inner two thirds of the vaginal barrel was less pronounced.

At the plateau phase the orgasmic platform developed to a lesser extent than before pregnancy. Immediately before orgasm there was about a 33 per cent occlusion of the vaginal lumen. The color change of the labia minora was less vivid than before pregnancy. Orgasmic contractions were less intense and lasted for a shorter duration. These patterns were observed again during the 6- to 8-week checkup. Subjectively, the women described their sexual tensions as being at prepregnant levels. Masters and Johnson attributed the altered performance to steroid deprivation.

Their subjects demonstrated a fairly complete return to nonpregnant patterns of responsiveness by the end of the third postpartum month. Subjectively, the subjects were unable to define significant differences between their orgasmic experiences of earlier postpartum versus those occurring around the third month checkup.

Postpartum Patterns of Sexual Activity

Studies of postpartal patterns of sexual activity are summarized in Table 10–2. Reversing the general trend for women to experience diminished sexual desire and activity during the course of pregnancy, most women studied returned to prepregnant levels between the second and twelfth month after delivery. In a study of 194 postpartum couples Fischman and associates (1986) found that the couples resumed intercourse approximately 6 weeks after delivery. However, even though sexual activity was resumed, couples reported declines in the frequency of and desire for sexual activity when compared with sexual activity before the infant's birth. Decreases in activity and desire were related to the woman's physical discomfort with sexual intercourse, decline in physical strength, fatigue that interfered with sex, and dissatisfaction with her bodily appearance. Marked variations from this pattern were also reported, such as early increase in desire and activity surpassing the prepregnant levels or delay in the return to prepregnant levels for as long as a couple years after birth. Couples need to be supported in sharing their feelings in this area and need to be reassured that their concerns have been experienced by others.

TABLE 10–2. Postpartum Patterns of Sexual Activity

Author	Subjects	Findings
Masters and Johnson (1966)	101 women 79 men	Full return to sexual activity by 6 to 8 weeks, earlier among lactating women. About half reported lower sexual tension, while the rest of the women reported prepregnant or higher levels.
Falicov (1973)	19 women	Two resumed coitus within a month; 10 resumed coitus by 6 to 7 weeks. Most had more difficulty achieving orgasm than before pregnancy. By 7 months, 10 had less frequent intercourse than before pregnancy. Fifteen reported no change or increased desire; nine reported increased capacity for arousal and orgasm.
Kumar, Brant, and Robson (1981)	119 British primiparae	Decreased frequency throughout first year. Those who rated sex as enjoyable rose from 67% at 12 weeks to 80% at 1 year. Orgasmic function returned to prepregnant levels by 1 year. At 12 weeks, 57% had less than prepregnant libido and 10% reported more.
Bing and Colman (1977)	Not reported	Variable patterns of sexual interest and activity ranging from immediate marked increase in desire to diminished levels of desire and activity for up to 2 years following birth.
Grudzinskas and Atkinson (1984)	144 women	No consistent birth-related factors associated with time of resumption of coitus except excess lochia and third or fourth degree perineal laceration; 100 women had no distress with coitus by 5 to 7 weeks; and 90% used contraception, especially condoms and oral contraceptives.
Fischman, Rankin, Soeken, and Lenz (1986)	68 couples at 4 months postpartum 126 couples at 12 months postpartum	Decline in frequency of and desire for sexual activity, especially for women. Physical discomfort, decline in physical strength, dissatisfaction with bodily appearance, and fatigue contributed to decline in desire.

Factors Associated with Postpartum Patterns of Sexual Activity

Research on postpartum patterns of sexual activity was consistent in identifying factors that had an impact on couples' sexual lives. One of the major factors was the traditional medical advice that coitus should be restricted for the first 6 weeks or until after the postpartum checkup, even though there is no demonstrable need to do so (Pritchard and MacDonald, 1980). The rationale is to allow for healing to occur without the risk of infection and to allow the physician to prescribe contraception. One study of the merit of this practice showed no increased risk in resuming intercourse after 2 weeks, except for dyspareunia (Richardson et al, 1976). Bing and Colman (1977) cited anecdotes of couples who complied with their physicians' advice despite intense feelings of sexual desire as well as those who ignored this advice without ill effect. This author vividly recalls her experience in a postpartum setting during the Vietnam war. An understanding postpartum staff occasionally had to provide conjugal privacy for couples, the husbands of which had only been granted a 48-hour leave of duty to visit their wives and babies. It was important to some of these couples that they experience sexual intercourse during their limited time together.

Physical discomfort may inhibit sexual interest (Fischman et al, 1986), and weakness, fatigue, perineal pain, and vaginal discharge are common complaints in early postpartum. Even when other symptoms abate, many women are surprised by vaginal or perineal discomfort (Hetherington, 1988) when they attempt intercourse due to the physical changes already described. Nurses can provide numerous suggestions for relief of this problem. Use of sitzbaths to promote healing and comfort, the use of surgical lubricating jelly during coitus, gentle manual massage of the vaginal outlet to relax the muscles prior to penetration, the use of sexual positions in which penetration is shallower or in which the woman controls penetration, such as side lying or woman superior, and sensitivity and gentleness on the part of the husband all can alleviate postpartum dyspareunia. The decision to resume intercourse should be mutual, and communication lines between the partners need to be open.

Some women, or their partners, are concerned by the increased size of the vaginal orifice. This can diminish pleasure for both. *Kegel exercises* practiced regularly can help resolve the problem. This technique for strengthening the pubococcygeus muscle can be taught by instructing the woman to contract her pelvic muscles while she is urinating, so that she stops the stream. She then holds back her urine for 10 seconds. This should be repeated, building up to 10 times in a row. The sequence can be performed five to ten times per day, whenever the woman thinks of it, throughout the rest of her life. It helps to prevent relaxation of pelvic support as women age.

As noted earlier, sexual interest may be diminished in postpartum women, and they may experience delayed sexual responsiveness. Bing and Colman (1977) interviewed some new fathers who also felt a decrease in sexual interest after birth. This decline in interest may reflect physiological processes, psychological processes involving the transition to parenthood, and fatigue.

Caring for, and particularly nursing, a newborn 24 hours a day, in addition to her own physical recuperation, can be surprisingly exhausting for the new mother. The husband, too, may experience interrupted sleep if he awakens when the baby cries or more actively shares night-time infant care duties.

Some couples are sexually inhibited by the presence of another person in or near their bedroom. They are afraid of waking the baby. Other relatives may be present in the home to help out, thus limiting spontaneity. Many women report that they are so wrapped up in meeting the needs of their infants that they have little of themselves to share with their partners; what they really want is time alone to "regroup." Some husbands withdraw as a response to feelings of jealousy toward the intruder on their marital relationship. Women also have reported that their needs for touch and intimacy were met by providing care for their babies (Fig. 10–4). Another inhibiting factor for some couples concerns territoriality and the mother's breasts when she is nursing: She may feel that her breasts are "off limits" to her husband as long as she is lactating. Finally, fear of pregnancy may also be an inhibiting factor.

Some of the tasks with which the new mother must cope include acceptance of her infant, integrating a changed body into her

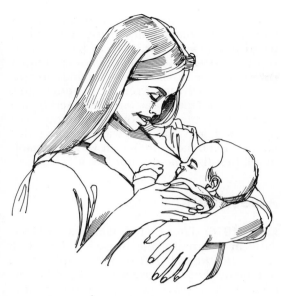

FIGURE 10–4. Women's needs for touch and intimacy are sometimes met by providing care for their babies.

self-concept, and accepting the responsibility of parenthood (Carlson, 1976). Rubin (1983) has provided a framework describing the importance of the woman's assessment of her own and her infant's intactness and the role this plays in the *binding-in* process. This process encompasses *identification* of herself as mother and of the infant as a person, *claiming* the infant as her own, and *polarization*, or separation of the infant from herself. Rubin notes that at about 3 or 4 weeks there is a healthy revolt against total absorption with these processes, which she terms "*bursting out*" (Rubin, 1983, p 253). At this time the woman is ready to reenter the wider adult world. Guilt after this event promotes mothering behaviors but with reinforced awareness of the baby's separateness from herself.

Fathers, too, have issues to resolve, including integration of their new image of their wife as mother and of the awesome capabilities of her body (Bing and Colman, 1977). Additionally, they must define their role vis-à-vis their child and determine for themselves what it means to be a good father (Newton, 1983). Other common concerns include the expense of the child and of the wife's lost income, interference with life style, and their wives' decreased interest in sex.

LeMasters' (1965) classic study of the impact of parenthood on 48 couples confirmed that the adjustment to the birth of the first child constitutes a developmental crisis. Thirty-eight of the couples reported extensive or severe crisis, even though the group as a whole was well adjusted, 35 of the couples desired and planned their pregnancies, and 34 of the couples and their friends rated their marriages as good or better. Although the group was well educated and middle class, LeMasters was surprised to find that the couples had almost completely romanticized parenthood. There had been little preparation for its realities. The crisis was most severe in couples in which the wives were highly educated professionals who quit working after birth. Despite the difficulty of the transition, the parents felt the experience was worth it.

The implications for professionals in contact with couples contemplating parenthood, pregnant couples, and new parents are great. Concerns of parents regarding the addition of their second or later child to the family include economic pressures, anxiety about how the older siblings will react to the intruder, further demands on the time available to the couple for themselves and each other, and the issue of being a good parent to the new arrival as well as to older siblings. There may be external social or family pressures to enlarge or *not* to enlarge the family, and the timing of the later birth, or its occurrence at all, may or may not be desirable to the couple. Health professionals must not assume that experienced parents have resolved issues around childbearing and parenting once and for all. The nurse who is involved in childbirth education is in a position to help expectant or new parents articulate their concerns. They can be reassured that this is a time of tremendous upheaval and that they are not alone in their reactions. She can act as a catalyst in identifying problems and in helping couples to devise strategies for dealing with them.

NURSING PROCESS

Many of the implications of the issues described in the previous sections may be apparent to the reader. Anxiety usually occurs when individuals are confronted with novel situations, and knowledge can serve to alleviate anxiety. Providing information to couples on these topics, at appropriate times and in amounts and terms that they can handle, can go a long way toward reassuring couples that they are not abnormal in their feelings or questions.

Nurses, with their background in both the biological and behavioral sciences, are in an ideal position to provide initial counseling in the area of human sexuality. The professional maternity or family care nurse has experience with expanding families; increasingly, a family-centered approach is being adopted. Pregnancy and postpartum are natural times for consideration of issues related to sexuality: It was sexuality that led to the couple's current state. There are also many times throughout the maternity cycle that the couple, or at least the woman, has contact with nurses: during prenatal clinic or home visits, in birth preparation classes, on the maternity unit, and during postpartum and well-baby clinic or home visits.

Most nurses are not sex therapists. However, nurses working with expanding families can identify actual or potential problems in self-concept, role transition, and/or sexual activity; collect data; interpret findings; formulate a nursing diagnosis; and intervene directly or refer the couple to other more specialized resources.

Nurses must first examine their own attitudes and prejudices about issues related to sex during pregnancy and the post partum, premarital and extramarital sex, and noncoital forms of sexual expression such as masturbation, fellatio, and cunnilingus (Zalar, 1976). Objectivity about their own biases will facilitate receptiveness to intimate information shared by clients. The nurse should generally speak in professional terms that are at a level comprehensible to the client; sometimes, however, it may be fruitful to adopt sexual jargon with which the clients most comfortably express themselves. Insensitive responses to clients' terms may damage their self-esteem and block further communication between client and nurse.

Permission-giving is the term Jack Annon (1974) used to describe the establishment of a secure environment in which the couple can freely share their intimate concerns. Privacy and confidentiality are essential. As part of permission-giving, the nurse, viewed as an authority, can give the couple reassurance that specific feelings or sexual practices are neither harmful nor abnormal. For example, if sexual intercourse undertaken by the woman in a supine position becomes uncomfortable as pregnancy advances, the nurse can reassure her that this is a common problem and that many couples use this time to try different positions, such as female superior (Fig. 10–5). Likewise, the nurse can give the couple permission *not* to engage in specific sexual activities if one or the other does not want to. One client was distressed by her husband's preference for cunnilingus. The nurse told her that this was a feeling that many women have and that it was reasonable to tell him that she did not like it.

Assessment

Zalar (1976) states that by taking a *sex history* early in pregnancy the nurse validates that sex is an integral part of the couple's total well-being. Four general areas should be covered: *Attitudes about sexuality* include attitudes about specific sexual practices, what the partners were taught about sexuality in childhood, and how each partner's ideas may differ.

Sexual self-concept constitutes how a man and a woman see themselves as sexual beings and how the pregnancy and changes associated with it might alter their feelings about themselves and each other. Nurses also need to explore the quality of the *relationship* as perceived by each partner. They may get a good assessment of this by asking questions regarding the couple's feelings about the pregnancy, whether it was planned or desired, how they see the pregnancy and birth changing their lives, and how they have spent time with each other in the past.

Physical status includes the reproductive history of the mother, the history of the current pregnancy, the general health of both partners, and the presence of any chronic diseases or disabilities in themselves or their families.

In addition to areas suggested by Zalar, the nurse should determine the couple's usual *coping strategies* when faced by life stressors and their general and present effectiveness.

When there is a particular sexual problem, Annon (1974) has recommended the following approach to a sexual history: the nurse should assess the couple's description of their problem, its onset and course, their perceptions of why the problem began and why it is persisting, what they have done about it and the result of this, and their current expectations and goals in seeking help.

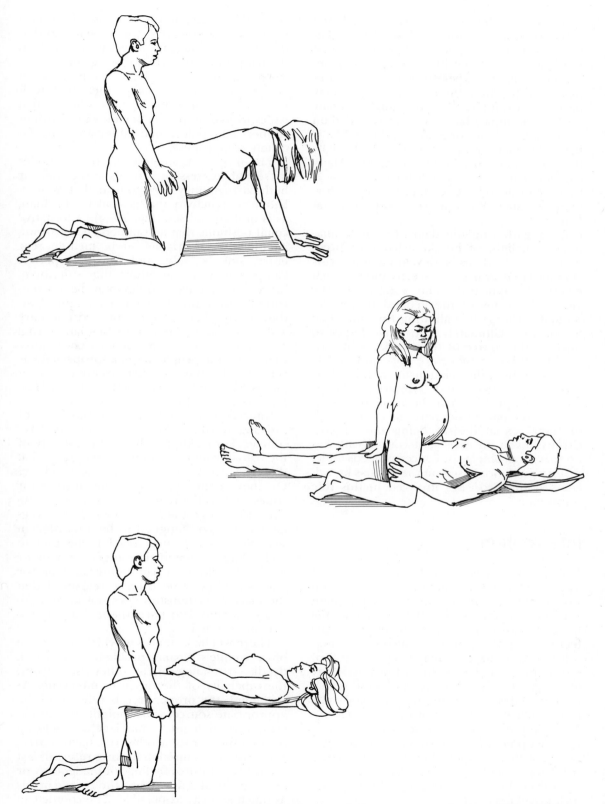

FIGURE 10–5. If the supine position is uncomfortable for the woman during pregnancy, couples can try different positions.

As a rule, the couple will be less threatened if the nurse directs the discussion from general questions to specific ones, from least sensitive to most sensitive topics, and from comments about experiences that *many* couples have to questions that *this* couple may have. For example, the nurse might initially ask, "What impact has this pregnancy had on your lives?" A later question might be, "How has your relationship changed?" And finally the nurse may specifically comment, "Many couples fear that they will hurt the baby if they continue to have sexual intercourse during pregnancy. What are some concerns that you have had?"

After gathering the data, the nurse analyzes it in light of her knowledge of pregnancy and birth as a developmental crisis characterized by many concerns and by much emotional upheaval. The couple can be viewed in terms of the general trends described earlier, while allowing for individual differences. Ultimately, the nurse hopes to uncover the source of the couple's concerns or difficulties, if there are any, and clearly convey to them the relationship among their feelings, conflicts, and symptoms (Mims, 1975). The problem may be a lack of knowledge on the part of the partners or the result of their sexual desires being out of synchrony. Even an expectant couple who has no specific problems or concerns needs anticipatory guidance based on the nurse's knowledge of the processes involved in this role transition.

Intervention

Nursing strategies depend on the nature of the problem and the client's goals. Education will be a major intervention with pregnant and postpartum couples. This may take the form of reassurance that many other people feel the way they do and that their feelings will pass in time; or it may take the form of specific information, such as the physiology of pregnancy and how it may alter sexual responsiveness. For example, hormonal shifts in the first trimester often result in nausea. This can put a damper on sexual expression. If developmental issues are named and discussed with a couple, they may experience relief that what they feel is a known entity; this will enable them to examine their feelings with greater security.

The nurse is also in a position to provide accurate information when misconceptions exist. For example, they might be afraid that the man's penis actually comes in contact with the baby and can harm it during coitus.

The nurse may facilitate communication between the partners about their true feelings and sexual wants. Simply raising such issues with an impartial person who provides support may relieve marital tensions and facilitate compromise.

The nurse can suggest alternative modes of sexual expression. For example, one or both partners may need to hear that masturbation is an activity that is available to them, as is oral-genital sex (Fig. 10–6). Alternative coital positions that accommodate a growing abdomen or a friable cervix include rear entry, side by side, and female superior. Couples may devise others that suit them. More conservative couples may be uncomfortable with novel sexual techniques, but they need to know that options exist and are widely adopted. There are Christian marital sex manuals, found in religious bookshops, to which some people might appropriately be referred. Another excellent resource for couples is Bing and Colman's (1977) book, *Making Love During Pregnancy*.

Intervention might also take the form of assisting a couple in identifying their resources. For example, who could take care of the baby for an afternoon or evening so that they can get away to spend time together? Or, they might be able to problem solve for issues such as the reallocation of tasks or the need to change their schedules if the pregnant wife is too fatigued to be interested in sex. New parents may need to be told to make dates to spend time together daily or weekly for attentive communication or for enjoyment. They need to be reassured that the marital relationship does not have to be totally sacrificed to parenthood, although it may be strained.

There will be instances in which the source of a couple's sexual problem is medical, dyadic, psychological, or otherwise beyond the capability of the nurse to intervene. At this point, the proper step is referral to the appropriate source, which might be a physician, a psychologist, a marriage counselor, a sex therapist, or some other reliable resource. Sensitivity is required in making referrals lest the nurse reinforce feelings of inadequacy or abnormality at a time when the couple needs as much security as possible. The couple can be reassured that many people seek such

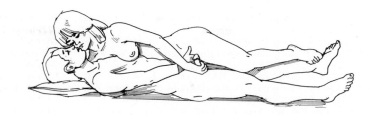

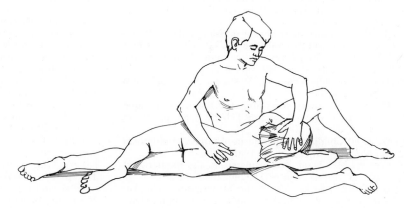

FIGURE 10–6. Masturbation and oral-genital sex are alternative forms of sexual expression during pregnancy.

help, that birth represents such a tremendous transition that normal abilities to cope may be taxed, and that they will not be negatively judged because of it. Referral need not represent the end of the nurse's relationship with the couple if she is in a position to follow up and meet other more common needs that they will have.

As can be seen from the issues raised in this chapter, the dynamics occurring during the maternity cycle may significantly alter a couple's pattern of sexual activity. Informed health professionals are in a good position to help parents experience this transition as a positive one, in which mutual growth occurs and through which their relationship can deepen.

REFERENCES

Alcott WA: Physiology of Marriage. Reprint of 1866 ed. New York, Arno Press & NY Times, 1972.

Annon JS: Brief therapy. In Annon JS (ed): The Behavioral Treatment of Sexual Problems, Vol 1. Honolulu, Enabling Systems, 1974.

Antle K: Psychologic involvement in pregnancy by expectant fathers. JOGN Nurs 4:40–42, 1975.

Aronson ME, Nelson PK: Fatal air embolism in pregnancy resulting from an unusual sex act. Obstet Gynecol 30:127–130, 1967.

Ballou JW: The Psychology of Pregnancy. Lexington, Lexington Books, 1978.

Benjamin H: Case of fatal air embolism through an unusual sexual act. J Clin Psychopathol 7:815–820, 1946.

Bennett EA: Coping in the puerperium: The reported experience of new mothers. J Psychosom Res 25:13–21, 1981.

Bing E, Colman L: Making Love During Pregnancy. New York, Plenum, 1977.

Boston Women's Health Collective: New Bodies, Ourselves. New York, Simon & Schuster, 1985.

Bram S: Voluntarily childless women: Traditional or nontraditional? Sex Roles 10:3–4, 1984.

Briggs E: Transition to parenthood. Matern Child Nurs J 8:69–83, 1979.

Campbell FL, Townes BD, Beach LR: Motivational basis of childbearing decisions. In Fox GL (ed): The Childbearing Decision: Fertility Attitudes and Behavior. Beverly Hills, Sage, 1982, pp 145–159.

Caplan G: Psychological aspects of maternity care. Am J Public Health 47:25–31, 1957.

Carlson SE: The irreality of postpartum: Observations on the subjective experience. JOGN Nurs 5:28–30, 1976.

Clark AL, Hale RW: Sex during and after pregnancy. Am J Nurs 74:1430–1431, 1974.

Colman AD, Colman LL: Pregnancy: The Psychological Experience. New York, Herder & Herder, 1971.

Colman LL: Psychology of pregnancy. In Sonstegard L, Kowalski K, Jennings B (eds): Women's Health. Vol. 2. New York, Grune & Stratton, 1983.

Comfort A: The Joy of Sex. New York, Simon & Schuster, 1972.

Debrovner CH, Winikoff B: Trends in postpartum contraceptive choice. Obstet Gynecol 63:65–70, 1984.

Deutsch H: The Psychology of Women: A Psychoanalytic Interpretation. New York, Grune & Stratton, 1944.

Duvall EM: Marriage and Family Development. 5th ed. Philadelphia, JB Lippincott, 1977.

Ellis DJ: Sexual needs and concerns of expectant parents. JOGN Nurs 9:306–308, 1980.

Erikson EH: Childhood and Society. 2nd ed. New York, WW Norton, 1963.

Falicov CJ: Sexual adjustment during first pregnancy

and postpartum. Am J Obstet Gynecol 117:991–1000, 1973.

Family Planning Perspectives 14:213–214, 1982.

Fawcett J: Body image and the pregnant couple. MCN 3:227–233, 1978.

Fischman SH, Rankin EA, Soeken KL, Lenz ER: Changes in sexual relationships in postpartum couples. JOGN Nurs 15:58–63, 1986.

Fox GS, Fox BR, Frohardt-Lane KA: Fertility socialization: The development of fertility attitudes and behavior. In Fox GL (ed): The Childbearing Decision: Fertility Attitudes and Behavior. Beverly Hills, Sage, 1982, pp 19–47.

Frank DI, Scanzoni J: Sexual decision-making: Its development and dynamics. In Fox GL (ed): The Childbearing Decision: Fertility Attitudes and Behavior. Beverly Hills, Sage 1982, pp 51–72.

Friedan B: The Feminine Mystique. New York, WW Norton, 1963.

Friedan B: Twenty years after the feminine mystique. New York Times Magazine Feb 27, 1983, pp 35–36, 42, 54–57.

Gabel H: Childbirth experiences of unprepared fathers. J Nurse Midwife 27:2–9, 1982.

Giminez ME: Feminism, pronatalism, and motherhood. Int J Women's Stud 3:215–240, 1980.

Goodlin RC, Keller DW, Raffin M: Orgasm during late pregnancy: Possible deleterious effects. Obstet Gynecol 38:916–920, 1971.

Goodlin R, Schmidt W, Greevy DC: Uterine tension and fetal heart rate during maternal orgasm. Obstet Gynecol 39:125–127, 1972.

Gough K: The origin of the family. In Freeman J (ed): Women: A Feminist Perspective. 2nd ed. Palo Alto, Mayfield, 1979.

Grudzinskas JG, Atkinson L: Sexual function during the puerperium. Arch Sex Behav 13:85–91, 1984.

Grudzinskas JG, Watson C, Chard T: Does sexual intercourse cause foetal distress? Lancet; 11:692, 1979.

Hangsleben KL: Transition to fatherhood: An exploratory study. JOGN Nurs 12:265–270, 1983.

Hetherington SE: Common postpartum sexual problems: A management guide. The Female Patient 13:43, 47–48, 50–51, 53, 1988.

Hollender MH, McGehee JB: The wish to be held during pregnancy. J Psychosom Res 18:193–197, 1974.

Howells JG: Childbirth is a family experience. In Howells JG (ed): Modern Perspectives in Psycho-Obstetrics. New York, Brunner/Mazel, 1972.

Kumar R, Brant HA, Robson KM: Childbearing and maternal sexuality: A prospective study of 119 primiparae. J Psychosom Res 25:373–383, 1981.

Lee G: Relationship of self-concept during late pregnancy to neonatal perception and parenting profile. JOGN Nurs 11:186–190, 1982.

LeMasters EE: Parenthood as crisis. In Parad HJ (ed): Crisis Intervention: Selected Readings. New York, Family Service Association of America, 1965.

Levinson DJ: The Seasons of a Man's Life. New York, Ballantine, 1978.

Lidz T: The Person. 2nd ed. New York, Basic Books, 1976.

Liebenberg B: Expectant fathers. Child Fam 8:264–267, 1969.

MacLaughlin SM, Taubenheim AM: A comparison of prepared and unprepared first-time fathers' needs during the childbirth experience. J Nurse Midwife 28:9–16, 1983.

Masters WH, Johnson VE: Human Sexual Response. Boston, Little, Brown Co, 1966.

McBride AB: Living with Contradictions: A Married Feminist. New York, Harper Colophon, 1976.

McGinnis DG: Anxiety about Coitus During Pregnancy and Its Effect on Sexual Activity. Thesis, University of Delaware College of Nursing, Newark, Delaware, 1982.

Mims FH: Sexual health education and counselling. Nurs Clin North Am 10:519–528, 1975.

Morris N: Stress in labor. In Zichella L, Pancheri P (eds): Psychoneuroendocrinology in Reproduction. Amsterdam, Elsevier/North Holland, 1979.

Naeye RL: Coitus and associated amniotic fluid infections. N Engl J Med 301:1198–1200, 1979.

Newton LD: Fourth trimester. In Sonstegard L, Kowalski K, Jennings B (eds): Women's Health. Vol 2. New York, Grune & Stratton, 1983.

Newton N: Interrelationships between sexual responsiveness, birth and breast feeding. In Zubin J, Money J (eds): Contemporary Sexual Behavior: Critical Issues in the 1970s. Baltimore, Johns Hopkins University Press, 1973.

Newton N: Trebly sensuous woman. Psychol Today 5:68–71m, 98–99, 1971.

Phillips CR, Anzalone JT: Fathering: Participation in Labor and Birth. St. Louis, CV Mosby, 1978.

Porter LS, Demeuth BR: The impact of marital adjustment on pregnancy acceptance. Matern Child Nurs J 8:103–113, 1979.

Pritchard JA, MacDonald PC (eds): Williams Obstetrics. 16th ed. Norwalk, Appleton-Century-Crofts, 1980.

Pugh WE, Fernandez FL: Coitus in late pregnancy. Obstet Gynecol 2:636–642, 1953.

Richardson AC et al: Decreasing post-partum sexual abstinence time. Am J Obstet Gynecol 126:416, 1976.

Richardson P: Approach and avoidance behaviors by women in labor toward others. Mater Child Nurs J 8:1–21, 1979.

Rosen RH, Benson T: The male role in family-planning decisions. In Fox GL (ed): The Childbearing Decision: Fertility Attitudes and Behavior. Beverly Hills, Sage, 1982.

Rossi A: Transition to parenthood. J Marriage Fam 30:26–39, 1968.

Rubin R: Attainment of the maternal role, 1, processes. Nurs Res 16:237–245, 1967.

Rubin R: Basic maternal behavior. Nurs Outlook 9:683–686, 1961.

Rubin R: Two psychological aspects of the postpartum period. In Sonstegard L, Kowalski K, Jennings B (eds): Women's Health. Vol 2. New York, Grune & Stratton, 1983.

Scott-Palmer J, Skevington SM: Pain during childbirth and menstruation: A study of locus of control. J Psychosom Res 25:151–155, 1981.

Semmens JP: Female sexuality and life situations: An etiologic psycho-socio-sexual profile of weight gain and nausea and vomiting in pregnancy. Obstet Gynecol 38:555–563, 1971.

Solberg DA, Butler J, Wagner NN: Sexual behavior in pregnancy. In LoPiccolo J, LoPiccolo L (eds): Handbook of Sex Therapy. New York, Plenum, 1978.

Spielberger CD, Jacobs GA: Maternal emotions, life stress and obstetric complications. In Zichella L, Pancheri P (eds): Psychoneuroendocrinology in Reproduction. Amsterdam, Elsevier/North Holland, 1979.

Steinhorn AI, Weiss HW: Speaking out on lesbian mothers, on gay fathers. SIECUS Report 12:7–8, 1984.

Stichler JF, Bowden MS, Reimer ED: Pregnancy: A shared emotional experience. MCN 3:153–157, 1978.

Tolor A, DiGrazia PV: Sexual attitudes and behavior patterns during and following pregnancy. Arch Sex Behav 5:539–551, 1976.

U.S. Department of Commerce. Bureau of the Census. Statistical Abstract of the United States 1985, 105th ed. Washington, DC, US Government Printing Office, 1984.

Vellay P: Anxiety and maternity. In Zichella L, Pancheri P (eds): Psychoneuroendocrinology in Reproduction. Amsterdam, Elsevier/North Holland, 1979.

Weinberg JS: Body image disturbance as a factor in the crisis situation of pregnancy. JOGN Nurs 7:18–21, 1978.

Woods NF: Human Sexuality in Health and Illness. 2nd ed. St. Louis, CV Mosby, 1979.

Zalar MK: Sexual counseling for pregnant couples. MCN 1:176–181, 1976.

Zelnic M, Kantner JF, Ford K: Sex and Pregnancy in Adolescence. Beverly Hills, Sage, 1981.

11: Contraception and Sexuality

Susan H. Kalma
Diane Lauver

Sexuality, or the expression of oneself as a sexual being, is important to individual development. Expressing oneself sexually involves a dynamic interaction of one's physiological being, self-concept, and perceived social roles. Psychotherapist Carl Jung well described the importance of sexuality:

Normal sex life, as a shared experience with apparently similar aims, further strengthens the feeling of unity and identity. This state is described as one of complete harmony, and is extolled as a great happiness ("one heart and one soul")—not without reason, since the return to that original condition of unconscious oneness is like a return to childhood. (Jung, 1953, p 105)

Sexual intercourse can be an integrating, healthy part of relationships and does not necessarily coincide with the desire to reproduce. The benefits of using contraception to delay childbearing, space children, or limit the number of children have been amply demonstrated for women, children, families, and societies (Maine, 1982). A challenge to sexually active couples is to be sexually expressive and prevent unplanned conceptions.

Although couples frequently wish to avoid or delay pregnancy, unintentional pregnancies continue to occur. Many couples are not

The authors gratefully acknowledge the assistance of Dennis Kalma, Percy James, and Wendy Williams, RN in the preparation of this chapter.

adequately protected from pregnancy at first intercourse. They may continue to risk pregnancy for some time if, as is often the case, they use contraception only irregularly. The length of this risk-taking interval varies. Surveys conducted in the United States indicate as many as 95 per cent of married women favor trying to limit pregnancy (Forrest and Henshaw, 1983). Only about 6 per cent of U.S. women aged 15 to 44 (3.1 million women) report being sexually active without use of birth control (Forrest and Henshaw, 1983). About 37 per cent of births among women aged 15 to 44 years were unplanned in the United States in 1982 (Jones et al, 1988). The discrepancies among these figures point to a significant challenge for clinicians: how can one best help clients to achieve their own goals with regard to number and spacing of pregnancies?

In order for effective contraceptive behavior to occur, the following conditions may be important: (1) motivation to use the method, (2) acceptance of and satisfaction with the method, (3) accurate knowledge base of reproduction and the contraceptive method of choice, (5) partner support, and (6) ready availability and accessibility of the method. Also, trust in clinicians at a contraceptive clinic may be especially important to adolescent clients (Silber, Addlestone, and Ragsdale, 1982). It is a challenge to the clinician to enhance these conditions and to understand the factors that influence contraceptive behavior.

FACTORS INFLUENCING CONTRACEPTION

Sexual and contraceptive choices reflect multiple factors: social, cultural, psychological, and developmental. For example, effectiveness of contraceptive use is positively associated with age and family income (Schirm et al, 1982); age may reflect a developmental phase and income a sociocultural context. Sociocultural factors may influence not only motivation but also continuation of contraception. For example, clients who are poor, black, or young are relatively more apt to stop using contraception for reasons other than a change of method or desire for pregnancy. Childlessness, Catholic religion, and lack of high school education are associated with, but are not necessarily causes of, discontinuation of contraception (Hammerslough, 1984).

An individual's beliefs, attitudes, and values may influence the choice and use of contraceptive more than the reported efficacy of the method. For example, ambivalence about pregnancy is well recognized as a factor influencing contraceptive use. Denial of the possibility of pregnancy ("It won't happen to *me*.") appears to be associated with nonuse of contraception. In one study, college women who consistently used effective contraception viewed themselves as "significantly more susceptible and vulnerable to pregnancy" than did inadequate users of contraception (Hester and Macrina, 1985, p 248). Clients who perceive their contraceptive method as highly reliable and satisfactory may be more likely to use it consistently and thus be less likely to conceive. One study of 172 college women found fewer pregnancies among women reporting their method as reliable and satisfactory than among those perceiving the method as unreliable or unsatisfactory (Bachmann, 1981). Paradoxically, there is a relatively high discontinuation rate of one of the most effective methods, the pill, and a low discontinuation rate of a relatively ineffective one, the rhythm method. Discontinuation rates may indicate client doubts about the method (for example, concerns about side effects) or about the person's role in using birth control.

Misperceptions may affect contraception decisions; sometimes clients overestimate the risk of contraceptive use and underestimate other risks, such as the risk of having intercourse without contraception. Table 11–1 is useful for putting the risk of death associated with contraceptives into perspective. For example, sexual activity without birth control involves more risk than does the use of any reversible contraceptive, unless the woman is taking birth control pills *and* is a smoker (Hatcher et al, 1988).

Sexual expression and contraception are issues relevant to nursing practice. In promoting health, nurses often act to facilitate clients' development and adaptation in sexual and contraceptive domains. Using a biopsychosocial model in their practice, nurses examine the psychosocial dimensions of their clients' health, including self-concept, social functioning, and interdependence (Roy, 1980; Table 11–2). By assessing each of these dimensions, or modes, of functioning, nurses may more comprehensively intervene to promote adaptation for the client along a health-illness continuum.

To clarify the many factors that influence clients seeking or using contraceptives, the following section first addresses psychological considerations in relation to contraceptive behavior. This discussion is followed by general physiological considerations in relation to contraceptive behavior, emphasizing the assessment phase of the nursing process. The remainder of the chapter addresses physiological and psychosocial issues for each spe-

TABLE 11–1. Risk of Contraceptive Use Compared with Other Activities

Activity	Chance of Death (in 1 Year, U.S.)
Motorcycling	1 in 1000
Smoking	1 in 200
Driving a car	1 in 6000
Playing football	1 in 25,000
Canoeing	1 in 100,000
Barrier methods	None
IUD	1 in 100,000
OCs (nonsmoker)	1 in 63,000
OCs (smoker)	1 in 16,000
Vasectomy	None
Laparoscopic tubal ligation	1 in 20,000
Pregnancy, continuing	1 in 10,000
Pregnancy, legal abortion, 9–12 weeks	1 in 100,000
Abortion, before 9 weeks	1 in 400,000

Adapted from Hatcher RA et al: Contraceptive Technology 1988–1989. New York, Irvington, 1986.

TABLE 11–2. Psychosocial Considerations for Nursing

Self-concept: how and what client believes about the self
  Physically: body image
  Personally: self-esteem, expectations of self, beliefs and attitudes about one's self-image, moral self, and evaluation of self in relation to value system; coping abilities
Social functioning: definition of self in relation to others
  Role mastery: primary present roles and specific developmental tasks
Interdependence mode: developing social integrity, being and acting in meaningful way, achieving a balance between feeling loved and supported, and achieving a balance between dependent and independent support systems

Adapted from Roy C: The Roy adaptation model. In Riehl JP, Roy C (eds): Conceptual Models for Nursing Practice. 2nd ed. Norwalk, Appleton-Century-Crofts, 1980.

cific method of birth control, with an emphasis on the implications for clients' sexuality and nursing interventions, especially client education. Throughout, we point out special considerations for the care of adolescents and the handicapped.

PSYCHOSOCIAL FACTORS, CONTRACEPTION, AND SEXUALITY

Self-concept

A person's self-concept incorporates beliefs about physical image, self-worth, and moral self (Roy, 1980). It is important for the nurse to be alert to many aspects of a client's self-concept that may influence contraceptive choice and behavior. For effective contraception, a woman needs to incorporate into her self-concept the image of herself as a physical and sexual being as well as a potential parent (Pollock, 1972).

Obtaining contraception may reflect an altered self-concept that includes one's first acknowledgment of sexual activity. As such, it may be a more significant step than would appear. A 19-year-old client getting a diaphragm confided, "I feel like I'm becoming a *woman* now." The first contraceptive visit may reflect a maturing self-concept.

Fisher et al (1979) studied sexual attitudes among university women. They assessed erotophobia (negative emotional orientation to sexuality) and erotophilia (positive emotional orientation to sexuality) and found a positive correlation between erotophilia and consistency of contraceptive use. Further analysis supports the idea of an indirect effect; erotophilia or erotophobia may be associated with attitudes that are facilitators of or barriers to contraceptive behavior. Individuals with high erotophobia scores seem to be less likely to engage in behavior associated with effective contraception; perhaps they may have difficulty in learning what they need to know about conception and contraception, they may not accurately predict future intercourse, they may be reluctant to engage in public behaviors to acquire contraception (purchasing condoms or going to a clinic), and they may hold relatively negative attitudes about discussion of sexuality and birth control (Fisher et al, 1983). These findings reinforce the importance of personal attitudes about sexuality and contraceptive behavior.

Failure to use contraception may result from women's conflicting feelings about their own sexuality and pregnancy. Ambivalence about pregnancy and parenthood may result in not using contraception (Cassell, 1984). "Failure" to make a decision may actually be a decision to risk pregnancy. Other psychological factors that have been associated with the failure to use contraception and are related to self-concept include (1) denial of realistic consequences of sexual behavior, (2) unrealistic fear of complications, (3) confusion between fertility and sexuality, (4) anxiety associated with affirming one's sexual behavior, (5) fear that contraceptives will be discovered, and (6) apathy (Sandberg and Jacobs, 1971). Perceptions of the seriousness of unintended pregnancy and the costs (material and psychosocial) of using contraception can influence decision-making (Herold, 1983).

Adolescents may experience conflicts in developing sexual and contraceptive roles. Despite changing mores, many parents provide little information on sex but do convey expectations about sexual behavior. Adolescents may react to this by concealing their practices or by elevating their belief in the value of spontaneity in intercourse (Needle, 1977). An adolescent who conceals her contraceptive is probably most concerned with hiding her sexual activity. She may fear immediate disapproval if her use of contraception is discovered more than she fears the distant possibility of pregnancy (Dembo and

Lundell, 1979). This may lead to her deciding not to use contraception.

During adolescence, one's level of cognitive development changes. An adolescent's failure to "take in" information on sexuality may be due to denial, a coping technique that is more common before the development of formal (abstract) thinking. After moving from the level of concrete operational to formal operational thinking, one is better able to anticipate the future and its consequences (Dembo and Lundell, 1979). This is of prime importance in contraceptive behavior. Even so, the taboos, conflicts, and anxiety associated in our society with sexual behavior may continue to make it difficult for the adolescent to plan ahead (Dembo and Lundell, 1979). Thus, the adolescent may have difficulty sustaining a self-image with high value on responsibility.

Role Function

Roles refer to positions people hold in society. Examples include lover, spouse, and parent (Roy, 1980). Role mastery is related to mastery of developmental tasks. Adolescents face the tasks of achieving autonomy, then intimacy (Erikson, 1963). Gilligan (1982), who stresses that psychological development in girls differs from that described by Erikson (1963), states that girls are faced with the two tasks simultaneously. Adults of all ages also have developmental tasks; for example, generativity, the bestowing of something of oneself on the next generation. Some adults express their generativity through nurturing others, whether or not they have children of their own.

Roles may be influenced by sociocultural expectations. Societal norms and values about sexuality and procreation appear prominent. Sexual and contraceptive behavior may reflect one's role in a given sociocultural milieu. Woodhouse (1982, p 2) posits that sex is "more than a physical interaction, it is a social interaction, informed and molded by cultural prescription, occurring within a vastly complex matrix of social expectations, gender roles and patriarchal control."

Societal messages about roles can be confusing. In some cultures, spontaneous sex without evident provision for contraception has a positive value, and at the same time pregnancy, outside of marriage, has a negative value. Unmarried couples who are sexually active may perceive or experience difficulties in obtaining contraception. In the United States, for example, conventional morality holds that marriage should occur before intercourse. Peer pressure frequently counters this. Johnston (1974) studied unmarried university students and found that both women and men felt pressured to have intercourse to live up to the expectations of friends and roommates. In many cultures, individuals can find little reliable factual information on which to base sexual and contraceptive decision-making. Also, adolescents may be making their first major decision on their own when they decide whether or not to have intercourse ("Counseling," 1987).

Regarding social role expectations, clients may base their behavior on beliefs that their partners, parents, or caregivers want (or do not want) them to use birth control (Fisher et al, 1979; Nathanson and Becker, 1985). In the 1960s, oral contraceptives (OCs) were hailed as a "great sexual liberator" for women. Since then, women have re-examined "free love," and Woodhouse (1982) suggests that the nonuse of oral contraceptives enables some young women who feel unsure about their sexuality to decline a partner's request for intercourse.

In addition, there is a double standard in the United States, as in many countries, about premarital sexual activity. Such activity is more acceptable among males than among females (Rosenfield, 1981). Women are thus more likely to feel that their behavior is wrong, and they may deny or conceal it. The net effect is that they are less likely to use a reliable method of contraception or to use one consistently. If a woman cannot talk with her partner about contraception and if she fears he may reject her for using it, she will be at risk for pregnancy if she chooses to have unprotected intercourse.

Regarding gender roles, it is usually the woman who goes to a health professional for reliable contraception because of social pressures and the traditional belief that contraception is a woman's concern. This belief is often reinforced by educational programs (Needle, 1977). In contrast, societal expectations focus on men as primary decision-makers in other areas. Young couples may especially need to clarify who *is* responsible for contraception.

It is not surprising that sexually active young women may find it difficult to take responsibility for consistent use of contraception. For example, among a sample of single young women seeking abortions, some had become pregnant by proceeding with intercourse after their partners stopped using condoms. Their partners had substituted "promises of being careful and assurances that everything would be alright [*sic*]" (Woodhouse, 1982, p 8). If women accept the man's role as decision-maker, they are particularly at risk for pregnancy if he views pregnancy as a "female" problem (Woodhouse, 1982). Thus, one major interactional factor affecting contraception is the assignment of responsibility for contraception.

Although men have unmet needs regarding contraception, they tend to feel that the "family planning world [is] structured for women" (Swanson, 1980, p 51). Concerns of men interviewed at the Men's Reproductive Health Clinic in San Francisco included (1) a changing social milieu, with the women's and ecological movements raising questions about the use of chemicals; (2) feeling that they are invisible to the providers of contraceptive services, since advertisements and female receptionists may reinforce the idea that women are the usual clients; (3) relative discomfort in the clinic as they imagine the clinic to be or as they experience it; and (4) relative inaccessibility of contraceptive information and services. Men do not have an annual regimen of a Pap smear or the traditions of health care associated with childbearing. Frequently, they disguise their chief concern (contraception) with an "acceptable" medical problem, or they may use their partner's problem to legitimize gaining access to the caregiver (Swanson, 1980).

Interdependence

Interdependence relates to the giving and receiving of support and affection. It is "the comfortable balance between dependence and independence in relationship with others" (McIntier, 1976, p 291). Adaptation in a role mastery mode overlaps with that in an interdependence mode. Interdependence issues of mutuality of respect, love, and support are relevant to sexual and contraceptive behavior.

Couples in relatively stable, exclusive, long-term relationships use contraception more reliably and visit a contraceptive clinic more consistently than those engaged in casual sex. This may be because the former have achieved a level of intimacy that renders discussion of contraception more acceptable. It also may be that intercourse becomes more predictable, so there may be a greater opportunity to obtain contraception (Fisher et al, 1979). Teenage girls who date "more seriously and regularly" are more likely to use birth control than others (Peacock, 1982).

Some therapists maintain that couples are not ready to begin having intercourse until they have discussed and provided for birth control. Unfortunately, this is frequently not the case. Woodhouse (1982) found the greatest lack of birth control discussions among couples with irregular or no contraceptive use.

Maladaptive patterns related to issues of developing interdependence include risk-taking "to demonstrate love," hostility (or desire to punish partner), use of possible pregnancy as leverage, and fear of loss of control in sexual encounters (Sandberg and Jacobs, 1971). Some men and women associate oral contraceptive use with promiscuity, since pill users are protected with *any* partner.

Although primarily of importance to the male-female relationship, interdependence issues may relate to a client's relationship with the caregiver. Studies of hundreds of adolescent clients at a contraceptive clinic showed phases in their relationship to the clinic: first developing trust, then learning, and finally working through a contraceptive decision (Silber, Addlestone, and Ragsdale, 1982). This finding underlines the importance of the nurse's role in facilitating the client's choice of contraception.

A new study raises questions about the effect of a nondirective approach with teenage clients. Researchers interviewed unmarried women under age 20 during their first contraceptive visit to county health department family planning clinics. Of the 2900 women surveyed, nearly 75 per cent expected the clinic nurse to tell them what contraceptive to choose. (By contrast, only 34 per cent of the clinic nurses stated that they take such a directive approach.) Based on follow-up telephone calls 6 and 12 months after the initial visit, the highest contraceptive continuation rates were found in clinics in which clients had expected, and nurses often gave, authoritative guidance regarding contraceptive choice (Nathanson and Becker, 1985). There was an inverse relationship between age and clients' desire for direction; younger women wanted more direction, i.e., dependence. It is important for nurses to consider these results when choosing how to interact with their younger clients. The effect of interaction styles may vary among populations of various ages and developmental states and may have an impact on the immediate- and long-term consequences of independence with self-care measures such as contraception.

Nursing Process for the Contraceptive Client

In working with a contraceptive client, the nurse follows these steps: assessment (data collection), diagnosis (data interpretation), plan (goal setting), implementation of plan (intervention), and reassessment (evaluation) of interventions and health status. A logical pattern of critical thinking, the nursing process is flexible rather than rigid. Thus, the nurse does not start and complete all assessment before any data interpretation or nursing intervention. Rather, the steps in the process serve as general guides during an encounter, with more assessment at the beginning of the encounter and more intervention at the end.

ASSESSMENT

The nurse is sensitive to and assesses the previously discussed psychosocial factors throughout the client's visit. These factors provide data about the context in which the client's sexual and contraceptive behavior occurs. The nurse and client use this information in conjunction with physiological data to create an individualized plan. The following discussion focuses on the physiological assessment component of a contraceptive visit.

Subjective Data. Subjective data, according to the problem-oriented record system, is historical information reported by the client to the clinician. There are many questions to ask the contraceptive client; some clients may perceive this as personal or threatening. Others, like the majority of the young women studied by Nathanson and Becker (1985), expect clinic staff to ask them personal questions. It is essential to affirm the confidentiality of the client's records, especially for adolescents.

A self-administered questionnaire (for example, Fig. 11–1) introduces the client to some areas of concern. It can greatly increase clinician efficiency. Note that the questionnaire does not replace the oral history. Rather, it is a supplement, providing a starting point that can be developed as appropriate. The questionnaire illustrated addresses chiefly physiological aspects of sexuality for young adults. The nurse may supplement it, as necessary, with questions about childbearing, menopausal or premenopausal symptoms, and the like.

Subjective data gathering includes collecting information to help determine physiological compatability of a contraceptive. For example, women with some serious chronic illnesses are at risk for complications if they take hormonal preparations. Allergies to spermicides or rubber could be contraindications to barrier methods. A woman inquiring about sterilization needs to discuss whether she has finished childbearing.

The nurse also assesses the client's competence and psychological readiness to use a given method. Asking about ability to plan ahead, delay gratification, or maintain a daily habit (such as taking vitamins) gives the nurse lifestyle data that may indicate how consistently a client will use a contraceptive. If a client has a mental illness, the nurse assesses mental stability, rationality, emotional state, and knowledge base before proceeding.

Taking a careful sexual history is essential to the assessment process. Asking questions in a matter-of-fact, yet sensitive, way will help put the client at ease. The skillful nurse is nonjudgmental and conveys permission to the client to address any concerns. The nurse may deliberately mention certain common concerns in order to show that these are "permissible" topics. The nurse may offer information that in turn facilitates the client's sharing further information. People in our society have difficulty admitting that they have questions or concerns about their sexuality. The sensitive nurse lets the client "save face" by acknowledging common questions and offering information. The clinician uses language that is clear and specific; repetition and open-ended questions may be useful techniques (Grimes, 1984).

For every client, and particularly for those who are disabled, it is helpful to identify and respond to individual needs and preferences in the following areas: learning skills (affected by mental, hearing, or visual disability); manipulative skills (affected by paralysis, amputation, arthritis); social skills (affected if the client's social life has been restricted);

Please answer these questions as completely as you can.

( ) If you are here for an annual exam, please check here and answer sections A and B.
( ) If you wish to discuss birth control methods, please check here and answer section A.
( ) If you wish to obtain birth control pills for the first time, please check here and answer sections A, B, and C.
( ) If you are here because of vaginal discomfort, itching, burning, or discharge, please check here and answer sections A and E.
( ) If you wish to renew your prescription for birth control pills, please check here and answer sections A and D.
( ) If you are here to get a diaphragm or to have yours checked, please check here and answer sections A and B.
( ) Other. Please specify. (You may indicate "personal.") Please answer sections A and B. _____

SECTION A
My last menstrual period began _____. Normal? _____
I have had sexual intercourse without birth control since my last period. ( ) No ( ) Yes
I have been instructed in breast self-examination. ( ) No ( ) Yes
I do breast self-examination monthly. ( ) Never ( ) Sometimes ( ) Usually ( ) Always
I have had a full gynecologic examination. ( ) Never ( ) Within year (date) _____
( ) Other (specify) _____
This examination was ( ) Normal ( ) Not normal; please explain _____

I have determined that my mother did not use DES while pregnant with me. ( ) No ( ) Yes ( ) Need more information on DES
I have had toxic shock syndrome. ( ) No ( ) Yes (date) _____
I am having some difficulties that I would like to discuss. ( ) No ( ) Yes

SECTION B
I began having menstrual periods around age _____
My periods are generally ( ) regular ( ) irregular
(If irregular, please describe) _____
My periods usually come about every _____ days.
My periods usually last _____ days.
Heaviest flow _____ ( ) pads ( ) tampons/day
I have severe cramps during my period. ( ) Never ( ) Sometimes ( ) Always
Remedies used, if any _____
I have bleeding between periods. ( ) No ( ) Yes
I currently use a method of birth control. ( ) No ( ) Yes (please specify) _____
Other past methods used _____

FIGURE 11–1. Self-administered health history form for contraceptive clients (Kalma, 1985).

access to people and community services (affected if there are architectural barriers or a negative self-image); and expression of sexuality (potentially an important factor in determining well-being and ability to cope with life) (Leavesley and Porter, 1982).

Objective Data. Objective assessment of the family planning client begins with attention to body language and affect. How clients reveal information about themselves, partners, and their sexual practices can provide valuable clues to effective nursing intervention. For example, the extremely anxious client may have difficulty inserting and fitting a diaphragm or may even suffer a vasovagal reaction during a pelvic examination.

The annual examination includes measurement of blood pressure and a general head-to-toe checkup (Fig. 11–2). The nurse documents carefully any deviations from normal and obtains consultation as needed. It is im-portant to conduct the examination sensitively for all clients, particularly adolescents ("Adolescent Gynecology," 1979).

NURSING DIAGNOSIS

Nursing diagnoses refer to health problems that are manageable within the domain of nursing practice. Each diagnosis represents a statement of a person's response or behavior that is causing the person difficulty (Campbell, 1984). Nursing diagnoses pertaining to contraception are usually classified under health maintenance or problems in psychosocial adaptation. Examples of nursing diagnoses include unknowledgeable about contraception, potential for pregnancy due to unprotected intercourse, and inability to use contraceptive sponge correctly due to insufficient instruction. A second diagnosis may

SECTION C   Please check as applicable
I have or have had the following:
   Condition   No   Yes   ?   Interviewer Comment
   High blood pressure
   Diabetes
   Kidney problems
   Liver problems
   Cancer
   Blood clots in legs
   Seizures (epilepsy)
I take medications regularly. (   ) No   (   ) Yes (please list) _____
I smoke _____ packs a day; I have for _____ years.

SECTION D   Please check as applicable
While using oral contraceptives I have had the following:
   Condition   No   Yes   ?   Interviewer Comment
   Abdominal pains (severe)
   Chest pain or shortness of breath
   Headaches (severe)
   Eye problems
   Emotional changes
   Severe leg pains
Any inconvenient side effects? (please list)
   Caregiver use only:
   (   ) Informed consent and release form on file
BP _____
Rx _____
Follow-up (   ) prn   (   ) other _____

SECTION E
   I have a vaginal discharge which is unusual for me. (   ) No   (   ) Yes, for _____ days
   I have pain/discomfort during intercourse. (   ) No   (   ) Yes   (   ) Not Applicable
   I have burning or itching around the (   ) vagina   (   ) external genitals for _____ days.
      Remedies tried _____
   I have had similar infection(s) before. (   ) No   (   ) Yes (dates) _____
      Treatment: _____
   I am allergic to (   ) sulfa   (   ) ampicillin or penicillin   (   ) other (please specify) _____
   I have recently been taking antibiotics. (   ) No   (   ) Yes (specify) _____

FIGURE 11–1 Continued

be risk of acquiring sexually transmitted disease.

PLAN

A comprehensive plan for the client may include further assessment (for example, physical examination or laboratory studies); therapeutic measures (for example, a prescription); client education; advice and/or counseling; and provision for follow-up. Teaching, a vital part of all nursing, is essential. The nurse provides full factual information on each method, then is available to counsel or advise the client as she weighs her options. (Informed consent is required in some settings.) Clear communications that promote confidence in the method and in the caregiver are important (Gillmor-Kahn, Oakley, and Hatcher, 1982). If the client's choice of contraceptive would be physiologically unsafe, the clinician explains this and

discusses alternatives, providing a referral to other sources of contraceptives that cannot be comfortably supplied.

A Gallup poll showed that women consistently underestimate the efficacy of all contraceptive methods ("Americans Misinformed," 1985). The nurse needs to know how to explain contraceptive effectiveness to the client. It is important to distinguish between two rates. *Theoretical* effectiveness is the pregnancy prevention rate of a contraceptive method when it is used ideally, that is, without error for every act of intercourse. *User* effectiveness is the pregnancy prevention rate of a contraceptive method when averaged for many different users, some using it consistently and perfectly and some using it inconsistently and/or with error. Contraceptive "failures" (pregnancies) may be due to inadequacy of a method, faulty user technique, nonuse, or other factors. An excellent discussion of some complicated variables that

Annual Exam   First ( )   Date _____
Objective
BP _____ Wt. _____
Urine Color _____, pH _____, pro _____, glu _____, ket _____, blood _____, UCG _____
Neck
   Thyroid wnl ( ) Other _____
   Cervical nodes ( ) wnl Other _____
Breasts
   Skin clear ( ) Other _____
   Supraclavicular nodes not enlarged ( ) Other _____
   Indentations/protrusions on maneuvers ( ) No   Other _____
   Abnormalities
     Left ( ) No Other _____
     Right ( ) No Other _____
   Discharge ( ) No Other _____
Lungs ( ) Clear Other _____
Heart ( ) No murmur or ES Other _____
Abdomen ( ) wnl Other _____
Pelvic
   External genitals ( ) Free of lesions   Other _____
   Vagina ( ) wnl Other _____
   Cervix ( ) wnl   ( ) Eversion
     ( ) Nontender Other _____
     ( ) Viewed by client   ( ) Client declined 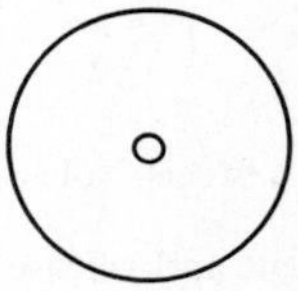
   Uterus
     Size ( ) wnl Other _____
     Position ( ) Ant ( ) Mid ( ) Post
     Tenderness ( ) No ( ) Yes
   Adnexae
     Right ( ) wnl ( ) Mass ( ) Tenderness
     Left ( ) wnl ( ) Mass ( ) Tenderness
   Rectovaginal ( ) Confirms above ( ) Not done
   Stool guaiac ( ) Neg ( ) Pos ( ) No stool present ( ) Not done
Assessment
Plan
   ( ) Pap done ( ) Pap to be done _____
   ( ) Other lab _____
   ( ) BSE taught ( ) BSE pamphlet given
   ( ) BC methods discussed
( ) Rx OC _____ x _____ mo.
   Informed consent and release signed ( ) No ( ) Yes
   Info sheet given ( ) No ( ) Yes
( ) Rx diaphragm _____ _____ mm
   Teaching done ( ) No ( ) Yes Info sheet given ( ) No ( ) Yes
   Inserted correctly by patient ( ) No ( ) Yes
   Comments
     Urged to return for check ( ) No ( ) Yes
( ) Other Rx _____
( ) Follow-up
   ( ) PRN ( ) Annual exam ( ) 6 mo ( ) 3 mo Other _____

Vaginal Discharge
Objective
   External genitals ( ) wnl ( ) Inflamed ( ) Swollen ( ) Lesions
   Discharge ( ) Vaginal ( ) Cervical
     ( ) Curds   ( ) Mucoid   ( ) Filmy
     ( ) Trich   ( ) Hyphae   ( ) Clue cells
     ( ) White   ( ) Yellow   ( ) Frothy
     ( ) Copious   ( ) Scant   Other _____
Cervix
     ( ) Eroded   ( ) Nonfriable   ( ) Friable
     ( ) Other _____
Assessment
Plan
   ( ) Culture done _____
   ( ) Rx
   ( ) Hygiene ( ) Info sheet given
   ( ) Follow-up
   ( ) PRN Other _____

Caregiver _____

FIGURE 11–2. Contraceptive health care data sheet (Kalma, 1985).

influence failure rates is found in Chapter 16 of *Contraceptive Technology 1988–1989* (Hatcher et al, 1988). Most sources agree on theoretical effectiveness rates. Because averaging methods and study populations vary, so too do the user effectiveness rates found by different investigators. A client may ask for clarification of discrepancies. In this text, efforts have been made to present consistently the widest range of user effectiveness rates reported in the literature, without bias toward any method.

There is *no* contraceptive method that is both entirely psychologically pleasing and 100 per cent effective. In counseling about any method, the nurse determines the comfort level associated with its risk. It may be useful to ask a possibly offensive question: "What would you do if this method failed and you became pregnant?" Discussion of options in unplanned pregnancy may motivate the client to select a more effective method of contraception. Of course, not all unplanned pregnancies are unwanted. In any case, discussion of pregnancy options at this point may help the couple to adapt with less difficulty if the need arises later. Therapeutic abortion remains one of the options for women who conceive despite, or in the absence of, contraception. The U.S. and Canadian Supreme Courts have upheld the individual client's right to choose abortion in consultation with her physician. If a caregiver opposes abortion, the client may be referred to another caregiver.

Client decisions reflect their values about effectiveness, chemical use, spontaneity, low cost, convenience, and degree of female/male control over use of the method. Some couples tolerate a relatively high risk of pregnancy; others want to minimize this risk. Some clients may come to the nurse with their minds made up about a contraceptive choice. Others may come already using a nonprescription contraceptive, such as a sponge, that they obtained without benefit of caregiver instruction.

The rhythm method, coitus interruptus, and condoms are especially popular in the early stages of a relationship. Individuals having intercourse several times a week may prefer to use oral contraceptives. The diaphragm may be commonly chosen by those who generally have sex less frequently. The IUD is rarely recommended for young women who have not completed childbearing. On the other hand, it may be a choice for the monogamous woman who has completed childbearing but who wants to maintain her options for a few more years. Sterilization has been the choice of older couples who have completed childbearing; it is increasingly the choice of young couples who consider their families complete with one, two, or no children of their own.

The nurse provides education that is appropriate to the individual client, informing about the contraceptive of choice and a back-up method, reinforcing the client's correct knowledge, and clarifying incorrect information. It is useful to ask, "Please tell me what is your understanding of how you will use _____ for birth control." This enables assessment of the client's knowledge and motivation. It can also help uncover myths and erroneous notions. Asking for a return demonstration is useful. Clients appreciate handouts, written material that they may peruse leisurely or when questions arise at home. Such material reinforces the teaching done with the client and may serve as outreach if the client shares it. A valuable factual reference for clients is *My Body, My Health* (Stewart et al, 1981).

Although there is some correlation between level of information and contraceptive use (Needle, 1977), information alone rarely changes behavior (Dembo and Lundell, 1979). Sex information programs (strictly factual) differ from personalized sex education that "attempts to integrate factual information with a person's existing knowledge, attitudes, and perceptions about sexuality" (Dembo and Lundell, 1979, p 661). Personalized education is congruent with nursing's biopsychosocial emphasis and is appropriate in one-to-one encounters as well as clinic or public health outreach programs.

Promoting positive attitudes toward contraception may be more important than promoting specific methods (Hester and Macrina, 1985). If clients do not accept sexuality as a normal and natural part of life or themselves as sexual beings, they may not use factual information about contraception because they may not see it as relevant (Reichelt, 1977; Winter, 1988). Long-term correct and consistent use of contraception is most likely to result if the individual, fully aware of the problems of pregnancy and the facts about her method, makes her own decisions (Gillmor-Kahn, Oakley, and Hatcher, 1982).

A contraceptive visit can help to promote open dialogue and a caring relationship. We encourage clients to discuss contraceptive options with their partners; the partner's understanding and acceptance of the method can enhance cooperation and psychological support. Client couples may need to clarify roles; for example, who will pay for pills, purchase the condoms, or be sure the diaphragm is on hand when needed?

Handicapped clients deserve special attention. Mentally disabled individuals profit most from material that is concrete and realistic, used repeatedly over a period of time, adapted to the individual's real-life situation, and presented with patience and understanding. Be sure that any visually impaired client can identify her oral contraceptives by touch (Leavesley and Porter, 1982; see this reference for resources).

The nurse needs to ensure that every client leaves the clinic able to use *two* methods of birth control—the first choice and a back-up. The couple uses the back-up method at the start of contraceptive use (for example, condoms or foam or abstinence for the first 1 to 3 months of oral contraceptives or until sterile after a vasectomy), for particularly fertile times (condoms in addition to diaphragm with spermicide midcycle), or if they discontinue use of the first choice (foam and condoms if oral contraceptives are stopped because of side effects or because of desire for pregnancy after a pill-free interval). Careful teaching and a demonstration of client comprehension are as important here as with the method of first choice. It is crucial that the nurse support the client's choice and use of her chosen method (Cupit, 1984).

The final step in the plan regards follow-up. Ensuring that adolescent clients are satisfied with the contraceptive method they have chosen may enhance their attendance at follow-up appointments ("Teenage FP Clients," 1985). Follow-up visits also are a predictor of consistency of contraceptive use: Around 70 per cent of adolescent clients who did not return for their first follow-up visit revealed (in telephone interviews) that they were using their method inconsistently ("Teenage FP Clients," 1985). In public clinic settings, discontinuation rates of clinic attendance or contraceptive method tend to be around 50 per cent (Dryfoos, 1982). Teaching about back-up methods and offering the client written materials to take home are useful strategies, as they may facilitate continued use of contraception even if the client chooses not to return.

Other Nursing Considerations in Contraception

Nurses may also intervene to prevent unwanted pregnancy on a community level. Educational programs about the facts and myths of conception and contraception are needed. Teenagers state that they want more information on birth control; involving them in the planning and execution of programs can enhance the appropriateness and usefulness of content and format. It may be important to clarify that research reveals that sex education programs have *not* led to increased teen sexual activity (Reichelt, 1977). A study of nearly 500 15- to 16-year-olds indicates that sex education programs in schools are associated with *reduction* in the level of sexual activity (Furstenberg, Moore, and Peterson, 1985). Nurses may be involved in the training of outreach workers, such as educators in school settings or community health workers in specially targeted areas, e.g., developing countries. A recent publication describes useful training methods and includes a counseling guide for the nonprofessional ("Counseling," 1987; "Why Counseling," 1987).

Contraceptive services must be available and accessible to all who need them; nurses can be advocates for such services. At especially high risk for lack of contraceptive services are teenagers, low-income women, and those in underserved areas. They need services available at low cost, in accessible locations, and at convenient hours. Some clinics render themselves effectively inaccessible to teenagers by requiring parental consent or notification as a condition of service for younger patients. In 1981 this was true for about 20 per cent of family planning facilities for patients 15 years or younger; at 10 per cent of facilities it also affected patients under age 16 or 17. There have been continued efforts to impose such policies on clinics that receive Federal funds. Surveys of young people currently attending clinics show that if such policies were imposed, about 25 per cent would stop coming to the clinic—but only 2 per cent would stop having intercourse; they would switch to the less reliable nonprescription methods or go without birth control ("Family Planning and Teens," 1981). It is important for nurses to safeguard the accessibility of contraceptive services for all clients. The Committee on Maternal Health Care and Family Planning, Maternal and Child Health Section of the American Public Health Association recommended that adolescents have access, without a parental consent requirement, to education about sex and family life, contraceptive counseling and services, pregnancy testing, and abortion (Barnes, 1978).

Men's need for information on birth control may manifest itself in a variety of clinical settings. A thorough nursing history for men includes questions about sexual functioning and contraception. It is important to acknowledge a male's concerns about sexuality or contraception regardless of the setting in which they arise. Clarifying information may be given along with a referral to an appropriate professional if the concern arises in a setting poorly equipped to offer the requested service. However, greater efforts must be made to make men feel welcome at contraceptive clinics.

Some clients may seek information on how a contraceptive will affect their sexual expression. Unfortunately, relatively little is known about the effects of contraceptives on sexuality. Reading, Cox, and Sledmere (1982) point out methodological problems: (1) research methods, such as diaries, urine tests, or questionnaires, may be unacceptable to subjects; (2) information may be inaccurate if, for convenience, it is gathered at intervals rather than daily; (3) it is difficult to quantify and compare subjective, culture-related values attached to changes in sexual functioning. Also, subtle value differences appear to influence contraceptive research. It is generally accepted that contraceptives for men must be effective in suppressing spermatogenesis, reversible, nontoxic, and without detrimental effects on male sexuality. On the other hand, women's contraceptives have been assessed for their effectiveness, reversibility, and lack of toxicity, but effects on female sexuality, e.g., libido, remain inadequately addressed (Reading, Cox, and Sledmere, 1982). We have summarized available information on contraceptive safety and effects on sexuality in the sections on specific methods in this chapter.

Learning about one's sexuality is a life-long process. For their own personal growth, nurses may wish to try attitude and values clarification exercises, which are also useful in client groups (see Morrison and Price, 1974). Recognizing personal conflicts and

feelings may help the nurse to avoid imposing them on others (Gillmor-Kahn, Oakley, and Hatcher, 1982). Reichelt (1977) cautions that adult educators need to stand outside their personal value systems to promote full discussion of all points of view, so that clients can work through their own feelings about sexuality.

In the remainder of the chapter, we shall discuss specific methods of contraception, including their implementation, implications for client education, advantages, disadvantages, and effects on sexuality. We introduce first the reversible methods, from most to least effective, followed by the irreversible methods.

ORAL CONTRACEPTIVES: THE PILL

In this book, the term oral contraceptives (OCs), or the pill, refers to combinations of synthetic estrogen and progesterone that when taken consistently inhibit ovulation. Oral contraceptives have been used by as many as 55 to 56 million women around the world, 10 million of them in the United States (Hatcher et al, 1986). Oral contraceptives were the first reversible contraceptive that was both under the woman's control and used independent of coitus.

Development of the pill depended on basic research that was started in the 1930s. Margaret Sanger, a public health nurse, and Katherine McCormick, a wealthy supporter of the birth control movement, believed in the need for a contraceptive that could be utilized independently by women. Sanger and McCormick approached Gregory Pincus, a researcher at the Worcester Foundation for Experimental Biology, who facilitated the development of the first OCs. In 1960, the U.S. Food and Drug Administration approved OCs for use. Scrimshaw (1981) describes how the development of OCs has significantly and positively altered female sexuality, male-female relations, family choices, and women's career development.

The most popular reversible contraceptive, the OC is theoretically and, in actual practice, the most effective. User effectiveness rates range from 90 to 99.5 per cent. Failures generally reflect incorrect use due to the client's inadequate understanding of OCs or simultaneous use of certain other medications.

Oral contraceptives prevent conception via several mechanisms, including the following:

1. Inhibition of ovulation. During the normal menstrual cycle, changes in estrogen and progesterone levels in the blood result in release of follicle-stimulating hormone (FSH) and luteinizing hormone (LH) from the anterior pituitary. Certain levels of these hormones trigger ovulation. Oral contraceptives provide a carefully calculated, constant level of estrogen and progestin, so the hypothalamus and pituitary are prevented from stimulating ovulation.

2. Alteration of cervical mucus. An increased level of progesterone renders cervical mucus hostile to sperm penetration.

3. Alteration in tubal transport. The action of progesterone on the fallopian tubes inhibits movement of the ovum to the uterus. Although estrogen has an acceleratory effect, it is probably not sufficient to affect conception.

4. Inhibition of implantation. High doses of estrogen and progesterone, if given before ovulation, cause changes in the endometrium, making implantation less likely (Morris, 1973; Fogel, 1981; Hatcher et al, 1986).

CLIENT EDUCATION

Because of the wide variety of OCs (with different packaging and schedules), the numerous misconceptions and fears about them, and the possible troublesome side effects and serious complications, client teaching is of prime importance. Details on how to take oral contraceptives, side effects, symptoms of serious dangers, and follow-up care are important. To assess future compliance with the one-tablet-a-day regimen, the nurse assesses the client's understanding of how OC use will affect her physically and psychologically.

Clients may be overwhelmed by the amount of information presented. Giving them a reference sheet with the most important instructions and cautions can help alleviate anxiety and reinforce correct learning. It is important to present information clearly, fairly, and comprehensively. The nurse engages the client in deciding how much information beyond that necessary for safe use she would like to receive and discuss. This shows respect for client autonomy. The nurse clarifies facts and myths about physical effects of OCs, possibly anticipating some unvoiced concerns. It may be useful to compare risks

of pill use with risks of certain daily activities (see Table 11–1); this helps some clients to put OC risk into perspective.

All women using oral contraceptives need to know of possible adverse consequences. Approximately 40 per cent of users will experience side effects of some kind. When discussing these with the client or couple, allow adequate time for the client to ask questions and voice concerns. Anticipate the probability of breakthrough bleeding (BTB) and reassure the client about this in advance. It is important to discuss this in detail to avoid the client's concluding, "The pill isn't working right; I may get pregnant," if she later experiences BTB.

Be sure that instructions are clear and complete, especially to teenagers. Although the pill is the most popular reversible contraceptive for teenagers, clients in this age group show the highest incidence of OC misuse and method failure of any age group (Tyrer, 1984). The caregiver may wish to follow adolescent clients at frequent intervals to assess for pill-related side effects that may affect usage and to reinforce consistent and correct pill use.

INSTRUCTIONS TO THE USER OF ORAL CONTRACEPTIVES

For maximum contraceptive effectiveness, instruct the client to follow these steps (Fogel, 1981):

1. Start your first pack of pills when recommended. This may be the fifth day after your period starts, the Sunday after your period begins, the day your period begins, the day of an abortion, or 4 weeks after childbirth. Your clinician may advise you to take your first pill the day of your clinic visit if there is no possibility of pregnancy (Hatcher et al, 1988). Following the calendar on the package, take one pill every day until the pack is finished. With the 21-day pack, wait 1 week before resuming pills. Start the next pack on the same day of the week as before. With the 28-day pack, you take a pill every day, beginning a new pack the day after you finish the first one. The 28-day pack has seven inert reminder pills, so the daily pill-taking habit is continuous.

2. Take the pill at the same time each day to ensure the proper level of hormones in the blood. You may find it helpful to associate pill-taking with an established daily habit such as tooth brushing.

3. Use an additional contraceptive during the first month of pill use for best protection. The contraceptive sponge or foam plus a condom provides reliable back-up.

4. If you miss *one* pill, take it as soon as you remember and use a back-up method. Take the next day's pill on schedule. If you miss *two* pills, take both pills as soon as you remember. Some spotting may occur. Use an additional contraceptive for the remainder of the cycle. If you miss *three or more* pills, stop the pill, *and* use another method of contraception. Spotting or bleeding will probably occur. Start a new package the Sunday after discontinuing the old pack (even if bleeding is still present), *and* use a back-up method of birth control for the time you are not taking pills and the first month of the new pack.

5. You may miss some periods while using the pill. If you skip a period and have not missed any pills, pregnancy is unlikely. If you miss one pill or more and then do not get your period, you may be pregnant. If you miss two periods, even if you did not skip any pills, have a pregnancy test performed right away.

6. If you wish to stop taking oral contraceptives, it is best to do so at the end of a pack to avoid irregular bleeding. To prevent pregnancy, start using another method of birth control immediately.

7. Remember that the pill is a medication. Whenever you see health professionals, tell them that you are using oral contraceptives. The brand name of pill you are taking is _____.

8. There are some symptoms that may be serious. They are summarized in the list at the bottom of the page using the mnemonic ACHES.

Do not ignore these symptoms or wait to see whether they will go away; if any of them appear, contact your health professional right away. Call for information or an ap-

pointment if you are worried about any other symptoms or if you feel you want to stop taking pills. *Any* symptoms that last for more than three cycles need to be checked.

9. If you are considering a change to another method, weigh the benefits of taking oral contraceptives against the hazards, including the risk of becoming pregnant. Using the pill confers long-term protection against certain serious illnesses.

10. Follow-up is essential after two to three cycles of pills. If there are no apparent problems or side effects, you may return annually (for example, on the anniversary of your Pap smear) (Fogel, 1981; Hatcher et al, 1986).

ADVANTAGES

The outstanding physiological benefits of the OC are its effectiveness and reversibility. The average user effectiveness rate is 98 per cent in the first year of use (Hatcher et al, 1986). Most women can use OCs safely without interruption until age 35 ("Using OCs Safer," 1985). In fact, it has been argued that some women (i.e., nonsmokers and those without diabetes and without a family history of myocardial infarction prior to age 50) may continue to use OCs safely until age 50 or menopause (Hatcher, 1988; Tyrer, 1988).

Recent research has elucidated several noncontraceptive health benefits of OCs (Table 11–3), including decreased incidence of (1) benign breast diseases, (2) ovarian cysts, (3) endometrial cancer, and (4) ovarian cancer. It is interesting to note that the decreased incidence of both endometrial and ovarian cancer among ever-users persists for several years after discontinuation of OCs (Ory, 1982; "Oral Contraceptives in the 1980s," 1982). Also, the protective effect of OCs against ovarian cancer has been observed among women who had used them for as little as 3 to 6 months and regardless of the specific OC formulation ("Cancer and Steroid

Symptom	*Possible Problem*
Abdominal pain (severe)	Gallbladder disease, hepatic adenoma, blood clot, or pancreatitis
Chest pain (severe) or shortness of breath	Pulmonary embolism or myocardial infarction
Headache (severe)	Stroke, hypertension, or migraine
Eye problems (blurred vision, flashing lights, blindness)	Stroke, hypertension, or temporary vascular problem
Severe leg pain (calf or thigh)	Thrombophlebitis

TABLE 11–3. Noncontraceptive Health Benefits of Oral Contraceptives*

Disease	Rate of Hospitalizations Prevented per 100,000 Pill Users	Number of Hospitalizations Prevented	Number of Deaths Averted
Benign breast disease	235	20,000	—
Ovarian retention cysts	35	3000	—
Iron-deficiency anemia*	320	27,000	—
Pelvic inflammatory disease			
Total episodes*	600	51,000	100
Hospitalizations	156	13,300	—
Ectopic pregnancy	117	9900	10
Endometrial cancer†	5	2000	100
Ovarian cancer†	4	1700	1000

Rate of hospitalizations prevented and deaths averted annually by use of oral contraceptives, per 100,000 pill users, and estimated number of hospitalizations and deaths prevented annually, by specific disease, in the United States; except where noted, figures refer to hospitalizations prevented among the estimated 8.5 million current users of oral contraceptives in the United States.

*Episodes prevented regardless of whether hospitalization occurred.

†Based on an estimated 39 million U.S. women who have ever used oral contraceptives.

Reproduced by permission of Hatcher RA et al: Contraceptive Technology 1988–1989. New York, Irvington, 1988.

Hormone Study," 1987). In the United States, annual OC-related deaths number 200 to 300; about 1210 deaths due to ovarian and endometrial cancer, pelvic inflammatory disease (PID), and ectopic pregnancy have been prevented annually by OC use (Hatcher et al, 1986). The use of OCs may diminish the symptoms of rheumatoid arthritis and thus prevent hospitalizations, but there is no evidence that they actually reduce the incidence of rheumatoid arthritis ("New Study," 1985).

New cases of PID among OC users are decreased, presumably because (1) thicker cervical mucus impedes bacterial movement, (2) decreased menstrual flow provides less growth medium for bacteria, (3) decreased uterine contractions limit the movement of bacteria into the fallopian tubes, (4) progesterone inhibits the growth of gonococcus, and (5) fewer pregnancies and abortions decrease the number of opportunities for infection ("Oral Contraceptives in the 1980s," 1982). Some of these factors may explain the fact that OC users may be less at risk for toxic shock syndrome (TSS) than nonusers. Ectopic pregnancies are decreased because the incidence of PID is decreased and because ovulation is inhibited.

Dysmenorrhea is decreased for many OC users; in fact, some women use OCs for this reason alone. Menstrual blood loss is decreased by half in OC users when compared to non-users ("Oral contraceptives in the 1980s," 1982), and the incidence of anemia is decreased among OC users. Some clinicians treat endometriosis with OCs (Hatcher et al, 1986). The hormones in some OCs decrease sebum production, thus decreasing the severity of acne.

Oral contraceptives interact with some commonly prescribed drugs (Table 11–4). Drugs may reduce the efficacy of OCs, potentiate the adverse effects of OCs, or have their action modified by OCs. We recommend careful counseling, based on the information in Table 11–4. Women who use antibiotics (e.g., tetracycline, penicillin) are advised to use an additional means of contraception because of possible decreased contraceptive effect. Women who use anticonvulsants and desire to use OCs may need to use 50 mcg of ethinyl estradiol because of lowered plasma estrogen levels with anticonvulsants (Hatcher et al, 1988).

Oral contraceptive use affects the serum levels of several vitamins and minerals (Prosad et al, 1977; Roe, 1976 and 1977). However, Hatcher et al (1986) do not recommend routine vitamin supplementation. Most clinicians agree that even in developing countries, women have not been adversely affected nutritionally by OCs. Undernourished women have less body fat and may not retain a full dosage of the hormones in OCs. Thus, malnourished women may not be effectively protected with the lowest dose OCs ("Oral Contraceptives in the 1980s," 1982). Research has continued to document noncontraceptive benefits of OCs, particularly for women over 35. For example, OCs are associated with a diminution of perimenopausal symptoms

TABLE 11–4. Interactions of Oral Contraceptives with Other Medications

Drugs That May Reduce the Efficacy of Oral Contraceptives

Therapeutic Agent	*Mode of Action*

Anticonvulsants
  Phenobarbital
  Carbamazepine
  Ethosuximide
  Phenytoin
  Primidone
	Reduced efficacy of OCs occurs primarily due to induction of hepatic microsomal enzymes causing reduced circulating levels of contraceptive steroids. Also, increased levels of sex-hormone–binding globulin (SHBG) results in decreased free-circulating hormones.

Antibiotics
  Ampicillin
  Penicillin
	Altered intestinal flora and "intestinal hurry" (resulting in reduced enterohepatic circulation) have been implicated in reduced OC efficacy.

Griseofulvin	Stimulation of hepatic metabolism of contraceptive steroids may occur.
Chloramphenicol Metronidazole Neomycin Nitrofurantoin Sulfonamides Tetracycline	Induction of hepatic microsomal enzymes; also disturbance of enterohepatic circulation.
Rifampicin	Increased metabolism of progestogens; suspected acceleration of estrogen metabolism.

Sedatives and hypnotics,
tranquilizers
  Benzodiazepines
  Barbiturates
  Chloral hydrate
  Glutethimide
  Meprobamate
	Induction of hepatic microsomal enzymes.

Antacids	Decreased intestinal absorption of progestogens.

Other Drugs
  Phenylbutazone
  Antihistamines
  Analgesics
  Antimigraine products
	Reduced OC efficacy has been reported; remains to be confirmed.

Drugs Whose Action May Be Modified by Oral Contraceptives

Therapeutic Agent	*Mode of Action*
Aminocaproic acid (inhibitor of fibrinolysis)	Theoretically, a hypercoagulable state may occur because OCs augment clotting factors; should not be given with OCs.
Anticoagulants	Because the estrogen component augments coagulation factors, increased dosages of anticoagulants may be required. Paradoxically, OCs potentiate the action of anticoagulants in some patients.
Anticonvulsants	Fluid retention may precipitate seizures in epileptics. OCs may also enhance the activity of anticonvulsants.
Antihypertensive Guanethidine	Antihypertensive effect is reduced.
Methyldopa	Estrogens cause sodium retention.
Beta blockers	Increased drug effect owing to decreased metabolism.
Betamimetic drugs Isoproterenol	Estrogens cause decreased response to these drugs.
Corticosteroids	Estrogens enhance anti-inflammatory activity. This may retard the metabolism of cortisol. Excessive corticosteroid effects should be watched for.
Cholesterol-lowering agents Clofibrate	The action of these agents may be antagonized by OCs.

Table continued on following page

TABLE 11–4. Interactions of Oral Contraceptives with Other Medications *Continued*

Drugs Whose Action May Be Modified by Oral Contraceptives *Continued*

Therapeutic Agent	Mode of Action
Meperidine	Possible increased analgesia and CNS depression due to decreased metabolism of meperidine. Use combination with caution.
Oral hypoglycemics, insulin	OCs may decrease glucose tolerance and increase blood glucose. Increased dosage of hypoglycemic medication may be required.

Tranquilizers
  Phenothiazines
  Reserpine
	Estrogens potentiate the hyperprolactinemic effect of these drugs, which may cause mammary hypertrophy and galactorrhea. Also, potentiation of the ataractic effect of promazine has been reported, possibly due to enzyme induction.

Chlordiazepoxide Diazepam Lorazepam Oxazepam	Increased effects of these drugs may occur owing to decreased metabolism.
Alcohol	Increased blood levels of ethanol or acetaldehyde have been reported.
Folic acid and vitamin B_{12}	OCs have been reported to impair metabolism and reduce serum levels of vitamin B_{12}.

Drugs That May Potentiate the Adverse Effects of Oral Contraceptives

Therapeutic Agent	Mode of Action
ASA Allopurinol Chloramphenicol Disulfiram Isoniazid Methylphenidate MAO inhibitors PAS Phenothiazines	These drugs all may cause hepatic enzyme inhibition, which may potentiate the action of OCs by delaying their metabolism. This may increase the incidence or severity of adverse effects of OCs.

Reproduced by permission of Health and Welfare Canada: Report on Oral Contraceptives, 1985 by the Special Advisory Committee on Reproductive Physiology to the Health Protection Branch, Health and Welfare Canada. Minister of Supplies and Services Canada, 1985.

and decreased loss of bone mass after menopause (Hatcher, 1988).

DISADVANTAGES

There are some major physiological risks to OC use, especially for women who smoke, are over age 35 to 40, or who are already predisposed to the conditions for which the OC may pose higher risk, for example, diabetes or vascular disease. It is appropriate to tell the nonsmoking, healthy client under 35 years of age that the risk of serious complications is small but measurable.

The concept of relative risk is useful here, for it enables comparison of incidence rates of morbidity and mortality in fertile users of OCs, of other methods, and of no method of contraception (see Table 11–1). Relative risk (RR) is a ratio of the rate of one condition, for example, disease or death, in a population exposed to a possible risk factor divided by the rate in those not exposed to that risk factor. A relative risk of one implies no association between the risk factor and the condition studied. A relative risk of less than one implies a negative (or protective) effect, between one and two implies a weak positive association, and greater than four indicates a strong positive association of the risk factor with the condition studied (Kanell, 1984). Oral contraceptive package inserts show relative risks. Diagramming relative risks as follows may help in your explanation to the client.

If RR = 0   1   2   3   4   >

the association between risk factor A and increase in condition X

is   —   0   +   ++   strongly +

The increased risks largely reflect threats to the cardiovascular system (Table 11–5). Assessment of this is complicated because of the contributory role of other factors, most notably smoking. Oral contraceptive use increases the relative risk of hypertension, first episodes of venous thromboembolism, ischemic heart disease, cardiovascular accidents, myocardial infarctions, and deaths due to a cardiovascular cause, especially for smokers and women over age 35. The relative risk of circulatory mortality in nonsmoking OC users ranges from 2.5 to 4.6 in different studies (Kanell, 1984; Pettiti, 1986).

There are inconsistent reports about an association between OCs and myocardial infarction. However, the apparent risk of OCs in contributing to myocardial infarction may be because of other critical factors such as smoking, lipid levels, hypertension, diabetes, arteriosclerosis, and family history of heart disease or diabetes (Dickey, 1987; Knopp, 1986; Layde, Ory, and Schlesselman, 1982). There are also inconsistent reports about the effect of OCs on cardiovascular disease among former users of OCs (Dickey, 1987; Mishell and Davajan, 1986). Most of the studies on OCs and cardiovascular risks are based on higher dose preparations than those currently used. Whether the currently used low-dose preparations are associated with similar cardiovascular risks as previously documented is not known (Hatcher et al, 1988).

Smoking increases the risk of death for OC users of all ages (Fig. 11–3). There are interactive (synergistic) effects of smoking and OC use on risk of cardiovascular diseases. "Adverse effects are increased in all women who smoke in excess of 15 cigarettes per day, especially in those who are over 35 years of age" ("Health and Welfare Canada," 1985,

p 7). Women could decrease the deaths associated with OCs by half if they did not smoke (Layde, Ory, and Schlesselman, 1982; Pettiti, 1986). Presentation of such information may give some clients the motivation they need to quit smoking. Figure 11–4 may be useful as a client handout.

Women with certain health conditions should not use OCs. Table 11–6 lists absolute, strong relative, and other possible relative contraindications to OC use. In considering OC prescription, the health professional assesses whether the client shows any of these contraindications and weighs the overall risks and benefits. For example, impaired liver function is an absolute contraindication because OCs are metabolized in the liver. On the other hand, benefits of OC use may outweigh risks for a healthy client with a strong family history of diabetes, particularly if she will cooperate in regular follow-up.

It is important to understand the physiological effects of both estrogen and progesterone. Estrogen is believed to be responsible for certain cardiovascular side effects of OCs (Hatcher et al, 1988) as well as for problems secondary to retention of sodium and water. Estrogen contributes to cardiovascular disease in OC users by increasing platelet aggregation and fibrin accumulation, which may promote thromboembolic disease. Progestin compounds contribute to cardiovascular disease by increasing triglyceride levels and/or decreasing high density lipoprotein levels, thereby promoting atherogenic changes in OC users (Kanell, 1984; Knopp, 1986). Progesterone causes side effects similar to those seen in pregnancy. Table 11–7 elucidates the relationship of OC side effects to estrogen and progestin.

TABLE 11–5. Major Cardiovascular Risks Associated with Oral Contraceptive Use*

Condition	Relative Risk	Factors Affecting Risk				
		Duration of Use	Dose		Past Use	Other Risk Factors
			Estrogen	Progestin		
Hypertension	1–3	Yes ?	?	Yes	No	Age, race
Venous thromboembolism (first episode)	2–4	No	Yes	No	No	ABO blood type, smoking?
Ischemic heart disease	2–6	Yes ?	Yes	Yes ?	?	Age, smoking, hypertension, high cholesterol, diabetes
Stroke, thrombotic	9†	?	?	?	?	Hypertension
Stroke, hemorrhagic	1.5–4	Yes ?	No ?	Yes	Yes ?	Smoking, hypertension, race

*Summary of cohort and case-control studies of white women in the United Kingdom and United States.
†Relative risk ranges from 3 for users with normal blood pressure to 14 for users with severe hypertension.
Adapted from Oral contraceptives in the 1980s. Popul Rep 10:A189-A222, 1982.

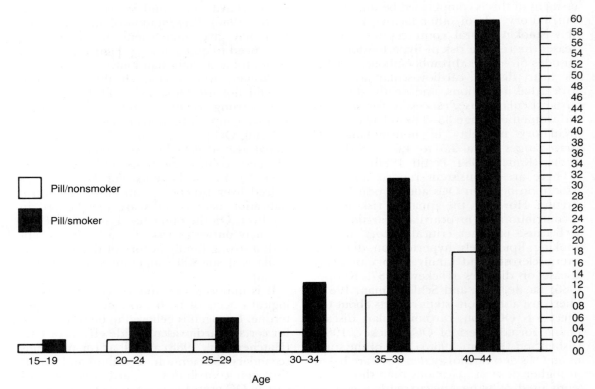

FIGURE 11–3. Smoking and the birth control pill: Age is the key. Can a heavy smoker safely be given the pill? Maybe, say experts, although smoking is not really healthy for anyone. Popular belief has been that a smoker should not take the pill. However, the real key to the increased risk of heart attack, stroke, or death in women who both smoke heavily and use the pill is age. A woman under 30 years years of age can take the pill with little risk, even if she smokes heavily. But a women over 30 may be taking some big risks if she both smokes and takes the pill. The main causes of death associated with pill use are stroke (subarachnoid hemorrhage) and heart attack (mycocardial infarction). Smoking by itself also is a risk factor for heart attack and stroke. Age underscores every risk. Looking at age alone, the risk of heart attack in women between the ages of 15 and 45 years more than doubles with every decade of life. In pill users under 30 years of age, the risk of death is only slightly higher in smokers than in nonsmokers. In pill users over 30, however, the risk soars to three or four times higher in smokers than in nonsmokers. Moreover, women over 40 have more of a chance of dying of the effects of both smoking and taking the pill than of the effects of childbirth. (Reproduced by permission of Hatcher RA, et al: Contraceptive Technology 1982–1983. 11th ed. New York, Irvington, 1982.)

OTHER PHYSIOLOGICAL CONSIDERATIONS ABOUT ORAL CONTRACEPTIVES AND HEALTH STATUS

Clients are often concerned about major OC side effects, especially cancer. Ruling out the possibility that a new drug may cause cancer is difficult, since cancer takes many forms, some of which have a long latency period. Numerous studies have failed to show an overall association between OCs and breast cancer (Rubin and Peterson, 1985; Hennekens et al, 1984; Rosenberg et al, 1984; Schlesselman et al, 1988). Experts agree that two studies purporting to show associations

between OC use and breast or cervical neoplasia are methodologically weak (Speroff, 1984; Rubin et al, 1984). Actually, OCs appear to be protective against endometrial and ovarian cancer. The issue of OC use and its role in cervical cancer is controversial; the FDA has been concerned "that there may be an increased risk of cervical carcinoma among OC users" ("Oral Contraceptives and Cancer," 1984, p 2). However, the association between OCs and cervical cancer may be confounded by frequency of health care visits and Pap smears, exposure to sexually transmitted diseases, and number of sexual partners. In a careful study, researchers failed to find any association between OCs and cervical

1. Should you take the pill if you are a smoker?

If you	*Then*
Are under 30 years Smoke heavily Want the pill	OK to use pill if no contraindications Cut down or stop smoking
Are 30 to 39 years Smoke heavily Want the pill	Consider another contraceptive method, especially if you are in your late 30s or have any of the following: diabetes, obesity, hypertension, or high cholesterol Cut down or stop smoking
Are 40 years or older Smoke heavily Want the pill	Stop taking the pill Cut down or stop smoking

2. What are the most common causes of death linked to pill use and smoking?

   The common causes of death from either smoking or taking the pill are stroke and heart attack. The risk of heart attack or stroke if you both smoke heavily and take the pill is far greater than just adding the risk of each together—they are synergistic.

3. What is your chance of having a stroke?

   You are nearly *six times* more likely to have a stroke if you smoke than if you do not.
   You are nearly *six times* more likely to have a stroke if you take the pill than if you do not; *but*
   You are *22 times* more likely to have a stroke if you both smoke and take the pill than if you do neither.

4. What is your chance of having a heart attack?

   You are *20 times* more likely to have a heart attack if you smoke heavily than if you do not.
   You are *four times* more likely to have a heart attack if you take the pill than if you do not; *but*
   You are *40 times* more likely to have a heart attack if you both smoke and take the pill than if you do neither.

5. What is your chance of dying?

   You are *two times* more likely to die of smoking-related causes, such as the above, if you smoke than if you do not.
   You are *five times* more likely to die of pill-related causes, such as the above, if you take the pill than if you do not; *but*
   You are *14 times* more likely to die of pill- and smoking-related causes if you both smoke and take the pill than if you do neither.

6. How does your age affect your chances of dying?

   If you are a pill user under 30, your risk of dying is only *slightly increased* if you smoke than if you do not; however,
   If you are a pill user over 30 who smokes, your risk of dying is *three to four times* greater if you smoke than if you do not; *but*
   If you are a pill user over 40 who smokes, your risk of dying is *two to ten times* that of a younger woman who does the same.

7. Can you kick the smoking habit?

   Of course you can, if you want to.
   Seventy per cent of smokers say they would attempt to stop smoking if urged to do so by their physicians. Ninety-five per cent of ex-smokers have quit on their own; only 2 per cent have used formal programs.

FIGURE 11–4. Smoking and the birth control pill: seven questions. (Reproduced by permission of Hatcher RA, et al: Contraceptive Technology 1982–1983. 11th ed. New York, Irvington, 1982.)

cancer; in fact, there was a tendency for OCs to have a protective effect *against* such cancer (Celentano et al, 1987).

Increased risk of skin cancer (malignant melanoma) in OC users has been suggested by some data, but this has not been further substantiated (Rubin and Peterson, 1985). A benign liver tumor, hepatocellular adenoma, is associated with OC use. Such tumors may rupture, causing blood loss and shock ("Oral Contraceptives in the 1980s," 1982). Although the risk of developing a hepatocellular adenoma is 100 times greater among OC users than nonusers (Swenson, 1981), the actual incidence is only 1.2 per 100,000 OC users. There is no strong evidence of a relationship between OC use and liver cancer (Rubin and Peterson, 1985). We need more

TABLE 11–6. Contraindications to Oral Contraceptive Use*

Absolute contraindications
1. Thromboembolic disorder (or history of)[a]
2. Cerebrovascular accident (or history of)
3. Ischemic heart disease or coronary artery disease (or history of)
4. Known or suspected carcinoma of the breast (or history of)
5. Known or suspected estrogen-dependent neoplasia (or history of)
6. Pregnancy, known or suspected
7. Benign or malignant liver tumor (or history of)
8. Undiagnosed abnormal genital bleeding[b]

Strong relative contraindications
9. Severe headaches, particularly vascular or migraine
10. Hypertension with resting diastolic BP of 90 or higher, a resting systolic BP of 140 or higher on three or more separate visits, or an accurate measurement of 110 diastolic or more on a single visit[c]
11. Diabetes[d]
12. Active gallbladder disease
13. Mononucleosis, acute phase
14. Sickle cell disease (SS) or sickle C disease (SC)
15. Elective major surgery planned in next 4 weeks or major surgery requiring immobilization
16. Long-leg cast or major injury to lower leg
17. Age of 40 years or older, accompanied by a second risk factor for the development of cardiovascular disease*
18. Age of 35 years or older and currently a heavy smoker (15 or more cigarettes a day)†

Other possible relative contraindications
May contraindicate initiation of OCs:
19. Prediabetes or a strong family history of diabetes
20. Previous cholestasis during pregnancy, congenital hyperbilirubinemia (Gilbert's disease)
21. Known impaired liver function at present time[e]
22. Impaired liver function within past year
23. Age of 45 years or older†
24. Completion of term pregnancy within past 10 to 14 days†
25. Weight gain of 10 pounds or more while on OC†
26. Failure to have established regular menstrual cycles[f]
27. Cardiac or renal disease (or history of)†
28. Conditions likely to make patient unreliable at following OCs instructions (mental retardation, major psychiatric illness, alcoholism or other chemical abuse, history of repeatedly taking oral contraceptives or other medication incorrectly)
29. Lactation†
30. Use of rifampin unless the woman is willing to use a backup contraceptive
May initiate OCs for women with these problems and observe carefully for worsening *or improvement* of the problem:
31. Family history of death of a parent or sibling due to myocardial infarction before age 50. Myocardial infarction in a mother or sister is especially significant and indicates a "coronary risk" lipid evaluation.
32. Family history of hyperlipidemia (check 14-hour fast lipids first)
33. Depression†
34. Chloasma or hair loss related to pregnancy (or history of)†
35. Asthma†
36. Epilepsy†
37. Varicose veins†

See footnote on opposite page

definitive studies on OC use and its relationship to cancer.

Some researchers associate higher incidences of bacteriuria and urinary tract infection with OC use. These problems are also associated with increased frequency of intercourse, a variable that has not been taken into account thus far in most studies.

EFFECTS ON SEXUALITY

For many, use of a contraceptive unrelated to intercourse enhances sexual spontaneity. The extremely high effectiveness rate of OCs means that couples need have little or no fear of pregnancy. This knowledge may contribute toward making their sex life more enjoyable. Some women prefer to be in charge of contraception; OCs make this possible. If, on the other hand, they value shared responsibility, the man can help his partner remember to take the pill, accompany her on clinic visits, or contribute toward the cost of OC purchase. Some partners may object to a systemic, daily contraceptive on the grounds that it may harm the woman or that she is protected if she has intercourse with *any* partner. The nurse may invite the client to bring her partner to the clinic so they can discuss these concerns together.

Clients may have concerns regarding the effects of OCs on the reproductive system, such as questions about future fertility, birth defects, and sexual desire. Although fertility is decreased significantly in the first 3 months after OC cessation, fertility rates for users and nonusers are the same after 30 months have elapsed ("Oral Contraceptives in the 1980s," 1982). Researchers do not agree on the extent and seriousness of postpill amenorrhea. Although Romney (1981) found persistence of postpill amenorrhea in 2 to 3 per cent of clients at 6 months, a comprehensive report cites the incidence of amenorrhea that lasts more than 3 months after discontinuing OCs as 1 per cent or less ("Health and Welfare Canada," 1985). Such amenorrhea is similar to physiological anovulatory amenorrhea occurring in nonusers ("Oral Contraceptives in the 1980s," 1982). Some clinicians prefer not to prescribe OCs to women with a history of marked menstrual irregularities, especially if these clients are very young and have ovulated infrequently (Burkman, 1986). Women who take OCs can postpone a period by taking extra pills, for example, during a vacation (Siemens and Brandzel, 1982).

There is no conclusive evidence to support a causal link between OCs and birth defects or miscarriage (if OCs are taken inadvertently in early pregnancy) or in infant status (if OCs are taken during breast-feeding) ("Oral Contraceptives in the 1980s," 1982). Conservative advice recommends that women wait a few months after discontinuing OCs (or any medication) before attempting to conceive in order to minimize any possible risk of birth defects. It is desirable that a woman wait at least 1 month after stopping OCs before trying to conceive; this enables more accurate dating of the pregnancy. Since estrogen may reduce milk production, some clinicians have tended to discourage breast-feeding mothers from pill use (Gillmor-Kahn, Oakley, and Hatcher, 1982). However, starting low dosage OCs 4 to 6 weeks after parturition does not appear to interfere with lactation (Health and Welfare Canada, 1985).

Nursing interventions include providing time and encouragement for the client to express her feelings about sexual desire and her sexuality. The nurse provides *p*ermission for her to raise this topic, *i*nformation as needed, and *e*mpathy, according to the PIE model for sex counseling (Martin et al, 1979).

The reliability and spontaneity afforded by OC use generally produce a positive or neu-

---

*When considering use of OCs for women with strong relative contraindications, it is extremely important to weigh the risks and benefits of OCs and to consider carefully alternatives to their use. In some settings, the contraceptive options available to a woman are limited. When a wide range of choices is not available, then OCs may become a more attractive choice. Patient concerns regarding an unplanned pregnancy due to use of a less effective contraceptive may be a factor in the woman's decision to use OCs. It is strongly suggested that you not consider the relative contraindications as categorical prohibitions against a specific method for a specific patient.

†Refers to a contraindication to combined OCs which *may not* be a contraindication to progestin-only OCs or may be *less* of a contraindication to progestin-only OCs than to combined OCs.

[a]Some clinicians do not consider thromboembolic events related to known trauma or an intravenous needle a contraindication to OCs.

[b]Several clinicians strongly feel that this should be listed as an absolute contraindication to OC use. It remains here, since we cannot in a simple, straightforward manner define "abnormal." If you, the clinician, feel that the specific patient's bleeding pattern is "abnormal" and that the cause is unknown, do not provide her with OCs.

[c]Some clinicians consider three diastolic pressure readings higher than 90 an absolute contraindication to combination OCs.

[d]Some clinicians do not consider diabetes, OC prediabetes, or a family history of diabetes a contraindication to combined OCs and are willing to initiate OCs and observe carefully. Other clinicians require that the patient's primary care physician, the endocrinologist, or whoever cares for her diabetes participate in the decision to provide OCs. The evaluation and decision to provide OCs is a shared responsibility, and the primary care physician must renew his or her approval annually.

[e]There are places in the world where endemic infections alter liver function tests for a high percentage of the population. In those areas few women would be started on OCs were this used as an absolute contraindication.

[f]In the past, the following has been given as a possible relative contraindication to OC use: "Patient with profile suggestive of anovulation and infertility problems; late onset of menses or very irregular, painless menses." Some clinicians now specifically choose OCs as the method of choice for women with irregular menses suggestive of anovulatory cycles. There is no convincing evidence that prolonged oral contraceptive use increases a woman's difficulty in becoming pregnant due to anovulation above her risk of having this problem had she never taken OCs. The woman with a profile suggestive of a problem prior to taking OCs will have greater difficulty becoming pregnant than the woman with very regular menses prior to taking OCs.

Reproduced by permission of Hatcher, RA et al: Contraceptive Technology 1988–1989. New York, Irvington, 1988, pp 209–210.

TABLE 11–7. Hormonal Side Effects of Oral Contraceptives

Estrogen Excess*
Vascular system and liver enzyme effects:
1. Vascular headache
2. Hypertension
3. Thromboembolic disease
4. Increase in serum proteins and lipids
5. Telangiectasia
Reproductive system effects:
1. Mucorrhea
2. Uterine enlargement
3. Fibroid growth
4. Cervical extrophy
5. Cystic breast changes
6. Increase in breast size (ductal and fatty tissue)
7. Hypermenorrhea, menorrhagia, dysmenorrhea
Fluid retention effects:
1. Nausea and vomiting
2. Epigastric distress
3. Dizziness, syncope
4. Edema, leg cramps
5. Irritability
6. Bloating, cyclic weight gain
7. Visual changes
8. Nonvascular headaches
Estrogen Deficiency†
1. Spotting and bleeding (day 1 to 14)
2. Decreased flow (hypomenorrhea)
3. No withdrawal period
4. Pelvic relaxation
5. Nervousness
6. Vascular symptoms
7. Atrophic vaginitis

Progestin Excess‡
Progestational effects:
1. Tiredness
2. Feeling weak
3. Depression
4. Breast tenderness
5. Increase in breast tissue (alveolar)
6. Decreased libido
7. Dilated leg veins
8. Pelvic congestion syndrome
9. Decreased days of flow
10. Moniliasis
11. Anovulation following discontinuation
12. Noncyclic weight gain
13. Increased appetite
Androgenic and anabolic effects:
1. Increased libido
2. Oily skin and scalp
3. Acne
4. Hirsutism
5. Rash
6. Pruritus
7. Cholestatic jaundice
Progestin Deficiency§
1. Late spotting or breakthrough bleeding (day 15 to 21)
2. Heavy flow and clots
3. Dysmenorrhea
4. Delayed withdrawal bleeding

*Symptoms tend to decrease in severity in a few months time.
†Symptoms get worse with time and may not appear until months or years of use.
‡Symptoms get worse with time.
§Symptoms may improve in 3 to 4 months time.
Reproduced by permission from Fogel CI: Fertility control. In Fogel CI, Woods NF (eds): Health Care of Women: A Nursing Perspective. St. Louis, 1981, The CV Mosby Co.)

tral effect on sexual desire, but the effect may be negative in a small percentage of women (Glick and Bennett, 1981). There are several possible causes of decreased desire, so it is important to take a careful history and suggest measures that may be helpful. Decreased desire may be due to dyspareunia, which may in turn be due to a vaginal infection. The incidence of monilial vaginitis is increased in OC users, so it may be helpful to suggest preventive hygiene measures. For example, wiping the perineal area from front to back only, avoiding douches or other chemicals, wearing white cotton underwear, and avoiding prolonged use of sanitary napkins are measures that may help prevent vaginitis.

Another factor contributing to decreased desire may be a reduction in natural lubrication, resulting in vaginal dryness. This may be a direct result of excessive progestational effects or lack of estrogen (Dickey, 1984). Skilled nursing intervention can put the client at ease for discussing this problem. Many clients need "permission" to try a personal lubricant or saliva to enhance their sexual pleasure.

Sexual desire depends in part on the level of effective testosterone in the blood. Decreased desire may result either if the progestin and estrogen from OCs suppress the hypothalamus to the extent that it suppresses ovarian testosterone production or if the estrogen in the pill causes an increase in sex hormone binding globulin (SHBG). SHBG normally keeps most of the serum testosterone inactive in women. A change in prescription to an OC with lower estrogen and progestin activity or to one with greater androgen activity may be necessary (Dickey, 1987).

CONTENT OF THE VISIT

Each check-up of a client taking OCs should include the following (Martin, 1978; Fogel, 1981):

1. Assessment
   a. Subjective data: review of how the client takes her pills, pattern of withdrawal bleeding, and whether she is satisfied with this contraceptive; review of symptoms, specifically any abdominal or chest pain or shortness of breath; headaches; eye problems, such as blurred vision; emotional changes, such as depression; severe leg pains; irregular bleeding; or any other side effects.
   b. Objective data: physical examination and laboratory tests, as outlined in Figure 11–2.
2. Nursing diagnosis: assessment of suitability of OCs for individual client.
3. Plan
   a. Provision for any additional data gathering required.
   b. Interventions: therapeutic measures, e.g., prescription; client education, including discussion of concerns and questions, review of the mnemonic ACHES for symptoms of serious complications and what to do should they occur, verification of the client's ability to use an alternate contraceptive method, knowledge of the most common side effects (nausea, BTB, and missed menses), and other items as appropriate; and follow-up plans.

CLINICAL RATIONALE FOR ORAL CONTRACEPTIVE SELECTION

Regardless of the OC chosen, a 3- to 4-month period is necessary to evaluate fully the match of the OC to an individual. An OC that is well-matched to a given client inhibits ovulation, permits cyclic bleeding, and is associated with no BTB or other bothersome side effects. New biphasic and triphasic OC formulations produce hormone levels that more closely correspond to natural fluctuations. It is noted that the estrogen dose *per cycle* with a triphasic may be greater than with Ovcon-35 or Modicon (Hatcher, 1988). Theoretically, these OCs should be associated with fewer menstrual irregularities, such as BTB ("Three Triphasic," 1985) and amenorrhea. Oral contraceptives and their composition are listed in Table 11–8. Some guidelines for OC selection include the following:

For anticipated long-term use, choose an OC containing 35 mcg or less of ethinyl estradiol (Dickey, 1987). If necessary for therapeutic reasons, the estrogen dosage may be increased temporarily. Clinicians generally believe the lower the estrogen dose, the safer the pill. Modicon, Brevicon, Demulen 1/35, Norinyl 1/35, Ortho-Novum 1/35, and Ovcon-35 are examples of 35 mcg pills. Because there are some concerns about mestranol, pills containing this form of estrogen should be avoided (Hatcher, 1988).

Progestins are rated in terms of both estrogenic and androgenic potency. From least to most potent in terms of androgenic effects are (1) norethynodrel, (2) norethindrone, (3) norethindrone acetate, (4) ethynodiol diacetate, and (5) norgestrel. Different progestins used in combination with ethinyl estradiol will affect endometrial activity differently. Many clinicians choose to start OC clients on triphasic OCs, such as Ortho-Novum 7/7/7, Tri-Norinyl, and Triphasil or on Brevicon, Modicon, Norinyl 1/35, Ortho-Novum 1/35, or Ovcon-35. Especially for women over 35, it is wise to choose an OC with a progestin that is not likely to alter high density lipoproteins or increase risk of arteriosclerotic heart disease (e.g., norethindrone rather than norgestrel) (Burkman, 1986; Knopp, 1986).

In general, OCs with low endometrial activity are best suited for women with light flow and minimal cramping. Underweight women do best on OCs with low estrogen and progestin. Women with a heavy flow for 6 to 7 days with cramps may do best with 50 mcg estrogen and 1.0 mg progestin. Women who are overweight may initially need OCs with higher endometrial activity than women who are not overweight. (Dickey, 1987).

Follow-up for OC users entails careful assessment of how the woman is adapting, physiologically and psychologically, to pill use. Adverse side effects have been so publicized and are so feared that the nurse expects to hear of "pill problems." When clients complain of OC "side effects," the nurse gathers detailed data to aid in determining whether OCs are indeed the cause. Every complaint deserves serious attention. For example, headaches, common in the general population, are rarely due to life-threatening causes. In the OC user, headaches could signal thromboemboli, so careful assessment is indicated. Hawkins and Higgins (1982) have compiled guidelines for nursing management of common OC side effects (see Table 11–9). If any side effects such as those listed in Table 11–9 develop, the nurse elicits an exact description of the problem and its

TABLE 11–8. Composition and Identification of Oral Contraceptives

Name	Progestin	mg	Estrogen	mcg	Manufacturer	Color[2]
Brevicon	Norethindrone	0.5	Ethinyl estradiol	35	Syntex	Bl/O
Demulen	Ethynodiol diacetate	1.0	Ethinyl estradiol	50	Searle	W/P
Demulen 1/35	Ethynodiol diacetate	1.0	Ethinyl estradiol	35	Searle	W/Bl
Enovid E	Norethynodrel	2.5	Mestranol	100	Searle	P
Enovid 5	Norethynodrel	5.0	Mestranol	75	Searle	P
Enovid 10	Norethynodrel	9.85	Mestranol	150	Searle	P
Loestrin 1.5/30	Norethindrone acetate	1.5	Ethinyl estradiol	30	Parke-Davis	G/Br[3]
Loestrin 1/20	Norethindrone acetate	1.0	Ethinyl estradiol	20	Parke-Davis	W/Br[3]
Lo/Ovral	Norgestrel	0.3	Ethinyl estradiol	30	Wyeth	W/P
Micronor	Norethindrone	0.35	None	—	Ortho	G
Modicon	Norethindrone	0.5	Ethinyl estradiol	35	Ortho	W/G
Nordette	Levonorgestrel	0.15	Ethinyl estradiol	30	Wyeth	Pe/P
Norinyl 1 + 35	Norethindrone	1.0	Ethinyl estradiol	35	Syntex	G/O
Norinyl 1 + 50	Norethindrone	1.0	Mestranol	50	Syntex	W/O
Norinyl 1 + 80	Norethindrone	1.0	Mestranol	80	Syntex	Y/O
Norinyl 2	Norethindrone	2.0	Mestranol	100	Syntex	W
Norlestrin 1/50	Norethindrone acetate	1.0	Ethinyl estradiol	50	Parke-Davis	Y/W (Br)[3]
Norlestrin 2.5/50	Norethindrone acetate	2.5	Ethinyl estradiol	50	Parke-Davis	P/Br[3]
Nor-Q.D.	Norethindrone	0.35	None	—	Syntex	Y
Ortho-Novum 1/35	Norethindrone	1.0	Ethinyl estradiol	35	Ortho	O/G
Ortho-Novum 1/50	Norethindrone	1.0	Ethinyl estradiol	50	Ortho	Y/G
Ortho-Novum 1/80	Norethindrone	1.0	Mestranol	80	Ortho	W/G
Ortho-Novum 2	Norethindrone	2.0	Mestranol	100	Ortho	W
Ortho-Novum 10/11[1]	Norethindrone (10)	0.5	Ethinyl estradiol (10)	35	Ortho	W/Pe/G
	Norethindrone (11)	1.0	Ethinyl estradiol (11)	35		
Ovcon-35	Norethindrone	0.4	Ethinyl estradiol	35	Mead-Johnson	Pe/G
Ovcon-50	Norethindrone	1.0	Ethinyl estradiol	50	Mead-Johnson	Y/G
Ovral	Norgestrel	0.5	Ethinyl estradiol	50	Wyeth	W/P
Ovrette	Norgestrel	0.75	None	—	Wyeth	Y
Ovulen	Ethynodiol diacetate	1.0	Mestranol	100	Searle	W/P
Ortho-Novum 7/7/7[4]	Norethindrone (7)	0.5	Ethinyl estradiol (7)	35	Ortho	W
	Norethindrone (7)	0.75	Ethinyl estradiol (7)	35		Light Pe
	Norethindrone (7)	1	Ethinyl estradiol (7)	35		Pe/G
Triphasil[1]	Levonorgestrel (6)	0.050	Ethinyl estradiol (6)	30	Wyeth	Br
	Levonorgestrel (5)	0.075	Ethinyl estradiol (5)	40		W
	Levonorgestrel (10)	0.175	Ethinyl estradiol (10)	30		Light Y Light G
Tri-Norinyl[1]	Norethindrone (7)	0.5	Ethinyl estradiol (6)	35	Syntex	Bl
	Norethindrone (9)	1.0	Ethinyl estradiol (5)	35		G
	Norethindrone (5)	0.5	Ethinyl estradiol (10)	35		Bl/O

[1]Multiphasic product; number in parenthesis equals days of each phase.
[2]Color abbreviations: Bl, blue; Br, brown; G, green; O, orange; P, pink; Pe, peach or light orange; W, white; Y, yellow; slash (/) indicates colors of 21 active/7 inactive tablets.
[3]Brown tablets contain 75 mg ferrous fumarate.
Reproduced by permission of Dickey R: Managing Contraceptive Pill Patients. Durant, Creative Informatics, 1984.

timing during the cycle. Sometimes a change in pill prescription is advisable. In adjusting pills, consider *relative* as well as *absolute* amounts of hormone. Dosage modifications to decrease side effects of OCs are discussed by Fogel (1981), Dickey (1987), and Hatcher and associates (1988). We urge careful attention to Table 11–9, as we shall discuss here only those side effects for which supplementary explanation is needed.

Spotting and breakthrough bleeding are among the most common concerns of new pill users. Starting OCs on schedule and

taking them at exactly the same time each day will usually minimize spotting. Spotting is a potential problem with all pills containing less than 50 mcg of estrogen; it may be necessary to switch to higher estrogen content to eliminate spotting that occurs during use of the first half of the package of pills. Spotting in the second half of the cycle may indicate the need for a more potent progestin. Breakthrough bleeding is the most common reason women give for discontinuing OCs and is a common cause of anxiety about contraceptive efficacy. The nurse intervenes

TABLE 11–9. Management Considerations of Common Side Effects in Oral Contraceptive Users

Side Effect Presenting Concern	Inquire about Possible/Probable Causes	Management Considerations
Nausea, abdominal pains	High-estrogen pill	Change to lower estrogen pill; change type of estrogen
	Taking pills on empty stomach	Take with meal or snack
	GI virus or reaction to food	Rule out other causes and treat
Headaches	Estrogen	Low-estrogen pill
	Severe migraine (present before starting OCs?)	Discontinue; physician consultation
	Histamine reaction between pill packets	Higher-estrogen pill
	Occur before pill due to school or work pressure, tension, economic or social problems, lack of sleep	History to sort out cause
	Too much TV, poor light for TV or reading	Referral for eye check
	Premenstrual tension	
	Vision problems	Monitor BP carefully
	Hypertension	Lower salt use
	Anemia	Check hematocrit
Weight gain	Increased appetite	Change to estrogen-dominant pill; low-androgen pill, low-estrogen pill
	Poor diet	Elicit diet history, diet counseling and teaching
	Hypertension and edema	Monitor, physician consultation, may need to change method
	Emotional	Counseling
	Physical release from pregnancy	Observe for 3 to 6 months
Weight loss	Poor appetite	Query cause
	No time to eat	Schedule, priorities, social life
	Emotional or social problems	Counseling, referral as needed
	Medical problems: anemia, tuberculosis, hyperthyroid	Careful history and physical, physician referral
	With nausea or vomiting	Low estrogen with high progesterone, consider anorexia nervosa in young client
	Fear of OC effects	Explore comfort with method, fears
	Imagination	Compare weight records, history, progestin-dominant pills
Fatigue	Anemia	Hematocrit, hemoglobin, diet history, teaching
	Infection	Careful history and physical, physician referral
	Overwork, lack of sleep, insomnia	Careful history, help set priorities
	Poor diet habits	Referral for counseling—social and academic as needed
Spotting, bleeding	Improper taking of pills; delay of more than 7 days between packs, mix-up of 28-day packets, takes only before or after coitus, never stops taking OC with 20- or 21-day packet	History of use—any missed, time of day, reassurance of normalcy when first on OC
	Vaginitis, cervical ectropion	Pelvic exam, smears, cultures as indicated; Pap smear yearly
	Gynecological pathology—polyps, cysts, tumors, DES exposure	Check history of DES exposure
	OC	Early cycle (pill 1–14)—higher estrogen; late cycle (pill 15–21)—higher progesterone pill
Amenorrhea	Taking 20 or 21 pills without 1 week break	Check use of OC
	Pregnancy	Pregnancy test, pelvic exam
	Prolonged use of OC	Switch to higher estrogen for few months, another method for few months, endocrine work-up
Milk in breast	Pill use	
	Pregnancy	Pelvic exam, pregnancy test
	Sucking on breasts, foreplay, squeezing nipples, especially after pregnancy, abortion	Other forms of sexual stimulation until milk disappears

Table continued on following page

TABLE 11–9. Management Considerations of Common Side Effects in Oral Contraceptive Users
Continued

Side Effect Presenting Concern	Inquire about Possible/Probable Causes	Management Considerations
	Pituitary disorder	Physician consultation
	Use of other drugs: tranquilizers, heroin, morphine	Query as to drug use, physician consultation
	Breast pathology	SBE, exam by practitioner, referral mammogram as needed
Chloasma	Estrogen excess	Low-estrogen pill
	Pregnancy	Pregnancy test, pelvic exam
	Other pathology—endocrine, lupus	Careful history, physical, referral
Scant menses	Long use of OC, especially high-androgen pill	Estrogen-dominant pill, nonandrogen progestin
	Pregnancy	History of pill use, pregnancy test, pelvic exam
Skin rash	If related to starting OC, due to pill	Physician consultation, try another brand of OC
	Localized, unrelated to OC use	Physician consultation, rule out infection, communicable diseases, syphilis
Fluid retention	Renal, vascular, cardiac pathology	Physician consultation, careful history and physical
	Cyclical pedal edema—OC	Low-estrogen pill, consider another method
Loss of hair	Hair products, curling irons, ironing hair, dyes, straighteners, wig use	Careful history
	Postpartum	Assure patient, cycles of hair in different stages—temporary
	Progestin-dominant androgenic OC	Change to estrogen-dominant pill
	Pathology—endocrine, malignancy	Physician referral
Loss of libido	Excess progestin	Lower progestin, estrogen-dominant pill
	Scant estrogen—premenopausal women	Physician consultation
	Marital, sexual, social problems	History, counseling referral
	No orgasm, relationship stressors	Knowledge of anatomy and physiology, sexual responsiveness, need for foreplay
Excessive bleeding	High-estrogen OC	Change to low-estrogen, high-progestin pill
	PID, vaginitis, myomata, pelvic pathology, DES exposure	Pap smear, smears and cultures, pregnancy test, history, pelvic exam, physician referral
Dyspareunia	Pelvic, vaginal, cervical pathology, PID, STD	Pelvic exam, physician referral
	Scant lubrication, irritations due to clothing, soaps, deodorants, douching	Education on sexual arousal, foreplay, avoidance of irritants
	Severe retroversion or retroflexion of uterus	Position for coitus
Vaginal discharge	High-estrogen pill	Switch to low-estrogen pill
	Vaginitis, irritants, cervicitis, PID, STD	Pelvic exam, smears, cultures, physician consult
Hirsutism	High-progestin, androgenic pill	Low-progestin, nonandrogenic, estrogen-dominant pill
	Endocrine causes, Stein-Leventhal syndrome	History, physical, physician consultation
Oily scalp, skin, acne	Androgenic, high-progestin pill	Low-progestin, nonandrogenic, estrogen-dominant pill
	Hygiene	Health teaching
Depression, labile moods	High-estrogen, high progestin pill	Low-estrogen, low-progestin, may need to discontinue OC
	Social problems, school, peers, marriage, job	History, counseling, referral

Reproduced by permission of Hawkins J, Higgins L: Health Care of Women: A Gynecological Assessment. Monterey, Wadsworth, 1982.

by listening and providing information that will reassure the client. If the client is using an OC with at least 35 mcg of estrogen daily, has started the pills on the correct day, and has not missed a pill, the probability of pregnancy is very small. Still, according to Dickey (1984, 1987), clients should use additional contraception on any day of BTB.

Many clients express concern that they will gain weight while taking the pill. It is realistic to assure them that most pill users do not experience weight changes. Note that pill-associated weight gain may occur in either of two ways. If the client associates pill use with increased appetite, change to a lower androgen drug or one lower in anabolic effects. If the weight gain is caused by fluid retention, stress dietary salt reduction and change to OCs containing less than 50 mcg of estrogen.

If follow-up examinations show a mild increase in blood pressure, switch to an OC with less progestin for 3 months. If blood pressure elevation continues, switch to a mini-pill or discontinue OCs altogether. Estrogen-containing OCs should not be used if diastolic pressure is consistently above 90 mm Hg (Hatcher et al, 1988).

The role of OCs in the etiology or exacerbation of depression is controversial. It is difficult to separate genetic and psychosocial variables from the physiological and pharmacological ones. A nurse can help by listening empathically and gathering data about symptoms occurring before and during OC use. Tiredness and weakness (as in mid and late pregnancy) attributed to OC use may be due to progestin excess; however, thyroid and blood glucose problems should be considered before switching pills (Dickey, 1987). A check for anemia is also indicated.

It can be challenging to find the right OC for a given client. Most clinicians urge a woman to continue with the OC prescribed for 3 months before concluding that she needs to change formulations. Anticipatory guidance about common side effects is critical; women forewarned about such side effects may be less likely to discontinue pill use. Nurses can help clients by listening carefully to their concerns and questions and reassessing or reassuring them as appropriate. Most women can use OCs without problems; it is a source of satisfaction to facilitate a woman's adjustment to the prescription that best suits her.

OTHER HORMONAL METHODS OF CONTRACEPTION

Hormonal preparations other than the daily combined OC may be used to prevent conception. These include the mini-pill and long-acting progestins.

Mini-pills

The term mini-pill refers to progestin-only compounds, not to sub–50-mcg combination oral contraceptives. Examples of mini-pills are Nor-Q.D. and Micronor (35 mg of norethindrone) and Ovrette (0.075 mg of norgestrel).

Mini-pills do not inhibit ovulation. Progestin modifies cervical mucus, impeding the passage of sperm. Also, progestin inhibits implantation through mechanisms previously discussed, such as delay in tubal transport and alteration of the endometrial lining. Because ovulation may occur, the theoretical and user effectiveness rates of the mini-pill are slightly less than those of combination OCs. Mini-pills are most effective in preventing pregnancy if they are begun directly after a combination OC and after 6 months of use.

Instructions to the User of Mini-pills. The nurse should communicate the following important directions to the client: (1) Take one pill every day without a break. If you miss one, take it as soon as you remember it, even if this means taking two on the same day. (2) For best protection against pregnancy, use a back-up method of contraception during the first 3 to 6 months and at midcycle in a regular 28- to 30-day menstrual cycle. (3) If you have no period for 45 days, seek a health professional's advice to rule out possible pregnancy. (4) Possible undesirable side effects include depression, irritability, and decreased sexual desire. Contact your health professional if these arise.

ADVANTAGES

Theoretically, mini-pills are much safer than OCs because of the lack of estrogen compounds, which have been associated with cardiovascular risks. The mini-pill is generally most useful for women who have experienced serious estrogen-related side effects with combination OCs. Women who are over

40 years old, or who have had migraine headaches or leg pain with combination OCs may be good candidates for mini-pill use. Mini-pills contain less progestin than combination OCs, so they may be useful to try in women who develop hypertension while taking combination OCs. Mini-pills do not interfere with milk production and are preferred over combination OCs for breast-feeding women. As with combination OC use, the client can experience spontaneous lovemaking with a high level of contraceptive efficacy. Some users enjoy alleviation of dysmenorrhea.

DISADVANTAGES

Because they include no estrogen and do not consistently inhibit ovulation, mini-pills are associated with irregular menses. About 40 per cent of women using mini-pills consistently have ovulatory cycles, and another 20 per cent have intermittent ovulatory and anovulatory cycles (Hatcher et al, 1986). Both spotting and amenorrhea are frequent. A client with abnormal vaginal bleeding needs a thorough history and examination before starting the mini-pill. The long-term cardiovascular risks of mini-pill use are not known. Progestins negatively affect the ratio of high to low density lipoproteins and thus may contribute to atherosclerosis. Discourage the choice of progestin-only pills if a client's history is positive for diabetes, acute mononucleosis, irregular menses, or ectopic pregnancy.

Long-acting Progestins

Injectable progestins, such as Depo-Provera (medroxyprogesterone acetate), are contraceptives effective for 3 to 6 months. Studies based on over 40,000 woman-years of observation, including follow-up of some women for up to 13 years, showed no evidence of increased risk of breast, uterine, or ovarian cancer ("Depo-Provera," 1983). The U.S. Food and Drug Administration continues to label Depo-Provera unsafe for contraception (Gold, 1983), even though it is being used in over 80 other countries.

Norplant, a set of six silicone rubber capsules 34-mm long each containing 36 mg of levonorgestrel, is being used now in several countries outside the United States. Inserted subdermally (usually under the skin of the inner upper arm) by a trained clinician, the implant releases progesterone slowly, providing continuous contraceptive protection and some noncontraceptive benefits for 5 years. The clinician can remove the implants if the client so desires.

CLIENT EDUCATION

Teach the client how to care for the implant site as the incision heals and explain possible side effects (see the following) and what to do about them.

ADVANTAGES

Depo-Provera, 150 mg injected every 3 months, is associated with a pregnancy rate of 1 to 2 per cent (Gold, 1983; "Hormonal Contraception," 1987). Not having to take any contraceptive precautions for 3 months at a time makes it a great convenience. It is safe to breast-feed an infant while using Depo-Provera. Studies on Norplant have shown a user effectiveness rate of 99.3 per cent through 5 years of use ("Hormonal Contraception," 1987; "Norplant," 1982). Client continuation rates are high: 90 per cent at 12 months and 75 per cent at 24 months, indicating high satisfaction with the implants (Lopez et al, 1986). MacLachlan and Peppin (1986), in an excellent article on contraception for the developmentally handicapped, note that a method such as Depo-Provera requires less compliance and education for efficacy. Also, when it is associated with amenorrhea, it lessens the difficulties of menstrual hygiene for the mentally handicapped (Elkins et al, 1986).

DISADVANTAGES

Long-acting progestins have some drawbacks. Irregular bleeding, either in the form of BTB or oligomenorrhea, is common. In fact, clients can expect amenorrhea 9 to 12 months after starting Depo-Provera. Because Depo-Provera is long-acting, infertility may occur for 6 to 12 months after cessation of its use. There remains controversy about the effect of Depo-Provera use on tumors (benign and malignant) of the breast and endometrium. The concern about a possible association between Depo-Provera and cancer explains why the drug has not been approved for contraceptive use in the United States ("Hormonal Contraception," 1987).

Other side effects associated with progestin use include: depression, headaches, weight gain, and decreased sexual desire. Norplant may lead to disturbances of the menstrual cycle; these tend to become less marked after the first 6 months (Lopez et al, 1986). The insertion and removal of an implant are minor surgical procedures; the latter may be more difficult ("Hormonal Contraception," 1987).

POSTCOITAL CONTRACEPTION

Hatcher and associates state that morning-after birth control is needed "as long as condoms break, inclination and opportunity unexpectedly converge, men rape women, diaphragms and cervical caps are dislodged, people are so uncomfortable about sex that they need to feel 'swept away,' IUDs are expelled and Pills are lost or forgotten" (Hatcher et al, 1988, p 374). Morning-after methods prevent pregnancy after unprotected intercourse by inhibiting implantation of sperm. The individual client must weigh risks and benefits, considering that the chance of pregnancy from any unprotected midcycle intercourse is estimated to be 20 to 30 per cent each time. Postcoital preparations are useful in times of crisis, not as routine contraception. Be sure the client has and understands how to use a reliable contraceptive method before again having intercourse.

Postcoital insertion of an intrauterine device (IUD) is effective and practical if the client desires ongoing contraception. The device is inserted within 5 days of unprotected intercourse. This practice is highly effective: Only one of 1300 reported postcoital IUD insertions failed to prevent pregnancy (Johnson, 1984). Nonetheless, due to side effects (e.g., pain and heavy menses) as well as availability factors discussed in the following section, postcoital IUD insertion may be relatively infrequent in the United States.

Ovral, an oral contraceptive containing 0.50 mcg ethinyl estradiol and 0.5 mg norgestrel in each tablet, may be used as a postcoital agent. The regimen consist of two tablets within 72 hours of unprotected intercourse and two tablets 12 hours after the first dose. This treatment is 96.5 to 100 per cent effective in preventing pregnancy (Johnson, 1984). Nausea may be a side effect, and if the woman vomits within an hour, the clinician may prescribe additional Ovral and an antiemetic. Oral contraceptive complications are unlikely from such short-term use, but the client should be instructed to watch for side effects suggested by the mnemonic device ACHES, as described earlier. Clients may expect menses within 2 to 3 weeks. In one study, 50 per cent of morning-after pill users had periods when they would have expected them (Johnson, 1984). The bleeding may be somewhat different from that accompanying their usual period. If no period has begun in 3 weeks, a pregnancy test is indicated. Diethylstilbestrol (DES), previously used as a morning-after preparation, is no longer available for such use in the United States. Troublesome short- and long-term effects resulted from the high dosage of estrogen in DES treatments.

Despite the effectiveness and proven safety of Ovral and IUDs as postcoital contraceptives, they are not universally popular. Some women think of the morning-after pill as a treatment for rape victims only. Morning-after pills are marketed in England and are readily available on an emergency basis in Canada and Western Europe. It is unlikely that U.S. pharmaceutical companies will press for FDA approval, since it is reasonable to expect a relatively small market and some opposition from anti-abortion factions (Johnson, 1984). Nonetheless, it is legal to prescribe Ovral as a postcoital contraceptive. It may be necessary for the nurse to reassure clients that morning-after pills are highly safe and effective in preventing pregnancy.

Clinical trials with antiprogesterone drugs, such as RU 486 (Mifepristone) are now under way. RU 486 is a synthetic steroid that interrupts pregnancy, especially if given in the first 5 weeks after the last normal menstrual period (Elia, 1986). Judging from results to date, in terms of efficacy and safety RU 486 may prove useful as a postcoital contraceptive.

INTRAUTERINE DEVICE

The intrauterine device (IUD) is a 22- to 36-mm plastic or metal object that once inserted in the uterus by a clinician prevents implantation of a fertilized egg (see Fig. 11–5). Because of high efficacy, relatively low cost, and lack of OC side effects, the IUD has achieved great popularity in family planning

INTRAUTERINE DEVICES

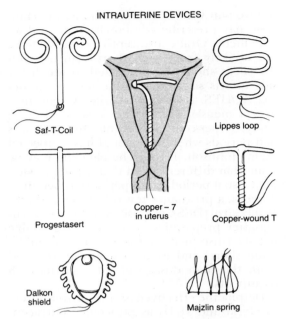

FIGURE 11–5. Types of intrauterine devices. Some IUDs have been associated with serious complications and should not be used, e.g., Dalkon Shield. Be familiar with current recommendations. (From Luckmann J, Sorensen KC: Medical-Surgical Nursing. 3rd ed. Philadelphia, WB Saunders, 1988.)

programs. About 70 million women in the world use IUDs (Hatcher et al, 1986). Concerns about IUD-related side effects decreased the availability of IUDs to women in the United States in the mid 1980s; worldwide usage rates may decrease because of this trend in the United States.

Although there has been much publicity about serious side effects of IUD use, the method offers many advantages to carefully selected clients. In the mid 1980s, U.S. manufacturers made only the Progestasert IUD, citing economic reasons. The Paragard model T380A, a copper-containing device, has been released in 1988. U.S. women who can afford to go to Canada or Europe have obtained IUDs there. Because of the high number of women who already have IUDs and because IUDs may again become more available in the United States, we include here a full discussion of this contraceptive.

The association between a foreign object in the uterus and a decreased pregnancy rate appears as early as the writings of Hippocrates (Fogel, 1981). Experimentation with IUDs in the nineteenth and early twentieth centuries was limited because of the frequency of IUD-related infections and expulsions.

The first modern study on the use of an intrauterine device to prevent pregnancy was done by Dr. Richard Richter, who in 1909 reported the use of dried silkworm gut. Dr. Ernst Graefenberg is more widely recognized. In 1929 he reported the use of an intrauterine ring of silver wire (Thomsen, 1982). In the early 1960s the Margulies Spiral (Gynekoil), Lippes Loop, and Saf-T-Coil first came into use. The Dalkon Shield was used from 1971 to 1974, until research associated it with septic abortions and deaths. Its multifilament string may have facilitated passage of bacteria into the uterus ("Intrauterine Devices," 1982). Since the 1970s, copper-wrapped and progestogen-releasing IUDs have become popular, largely because of their higher contraceptive efficacy (up to 99 per cent) and lower expulsion rate.

It has been believed that IUDs do not prevent conception but rather prevent pregnancy by inhibiting implantation of a fertilized egg. Four mechanisms of action may account for this effect. First, the IUD stimulates a local inflammatory process in the endometrium, making the environment hostile to implantation; second, it stimulates tubal movement and ovum transport, which inhibit implantation; third, it causes increased production of prostaglandins, which prevent implantation; and fourth, it may cause mechanical dislodging of the blastocyst. In contrast, a recent study concludes that IUDs may prevent conception by interfering with release and transport of ova from the ovaries to the tubes (Alvarez et al, 1988). Of note, the newly marketed Paragard IUD may also inhibit fertilization by altering the number or viability of sperm. The progesterone found in certain IUDs alters the maturation of the endometrial lining, thereby inhibiting implantation. Copper found in some IUDs may alter mineral and estrogen metabolism in cells of the endometrium. The contraceptive effectiveness of most IUDs is 97 to 99 per cent theoretically and about 94 per cent in the first year of actual use (Hatcher et al, 1988). Sometimes pregnancies occur with an IUD in place. Other times, failures occur when the client has expelled the IUD without realizing it.

The variety in shapes of IUDs shown in Figure 11–5 reflects a history of research on safer and more effective devices. A clinician in the United States is most apt to find that clients have one of the IUDs listed in Table 11–10. The efficacy of the inert IUD correlates with the size and shape of the device:

TABLE 11–10. Characteristics of IUDs

IUD Type	Strings Number	Strings Color	Need to Change	Pregnancy Rate (%)	Expulsion Rate (%)
Cu-7	1	Black, light blue	Every 3 years	1.5	3.3
Cu-T	2	Blue		1.5	5.3
Paragard T 380 A	2	White	Every 4 years	<1.0	3.3 ± 0.7
Lippes					
Loop A	1 or 2	Blue		8.0	6.9
Loop B	1 or 2	Black		5.8	6.5
Loop C	1 or 2	Yellow	prn	4.1	5.3
Loop D	1 or 2	White		3.6	3.6
Progestasert-T	2	Translucent	Yearly	2.5*	7.5*
				1.9†	3.1†
Saf-T-Coil	2	Green		0.1*	10.0*
Saf-T-Coil†	2	Green	prn	1.3†	11.4†

*For nulliparous women
†For multiparous women
(Sources: Compiled from Cole et al, 1985; Hatcher et al, 1984; Hatcher et al, 1986.)

These parameters determine the amount of contact with the endometrium (Keith, Hughey, and Berger, 1978). The larger the IUD, however, the greater the likelihood of pain and increased bleeding. The plastic Lippes Loop comes in four sizes; it can be left in place indefinitely in the asymptomatic woman (Bernstein et al, 1978). High fundal placement enhances efficacy (Perlmutter, 1978).

The presence of copper or slow-releasing progesterone in the IUD also enhances efficacy. The Cu-7 is small; it has been preferred for use with nulliparous women. Relatively lower perforation and expulsion rates as well as less blood loss are its advantages (Gromko, 1980). Because the copper is slowly absorbed by the body, the Cu-7 must be replaced every 3 years. Another copper-wrapped IUD, the Copper-T, has been commonly used in the United States and elsewhere. The newest model (380A) is the most effective IUD to date: "well under one pregnancy per 100 women after the first year" ("Highly Effective," 1985). It may be left in place for 4 years. The Progestasert-T, which contains progesterone, may be preferred for women with heavier and more painful periods. It must be replaced yearly (Bernstein et al, 1978; Gromko, 1980).

Most IUDs include one or two inert "tails" or "strings." These enable the wearer to verify that the IUD is still in her body, and they may facilitate removal by a clinician. The IUD comes prepackaged in a sterile barrel with a plunger. After it is inserted, it regains its shape because of the "memory" feature of its composition. IUD insertion is somewhat uncomfortable for many individuals. For a small percentage, it may cause severe cramping. The client may be anxious because she is unable to see what is happening during the insertion; anxiety may make the insertion more difficult. It is important to promote the woman's sense of control through anticipatory guidance and by giving her permission to request that the procedure be halted at any point.

CLIENT EDUCATION

Anticipatory guidance can help the client to feel more at ease and more in control during insertion. A diagram depicting IUD placement is a helpful adjunct to the nurse's anticipatory guidance. Each client needs to know exactly what kind of IUD she has and the facts about it: effectiveness, possible side effects, and warning signs of complications. It is now common practice to obtain written informed consent for IUD use after full discussion and before IUD insertion.

Describe procedures and sensations before they occur, including the following: (1) The clinician will perform a pelvic exam, inserting a speculum. (2) The speculum may feel cold. (3) The clinician applies an antiseptic solution, which may feel cool, to the cervix, then (4) uses a tenaculum to straighten the uterus; this may feel like pinching. (5) The clinician may use a metal sound (instrument) to determine the size of the uterus; this may cause pressure or cramping. (6) Insertion may feel much like sounding. After insertion, cramping may persist for minutes to hours. (7) A few women experience a fainting sensation during manipulation or dilation of the cervix. The client needs to know that someone may remain with her and that she is safest lying flat. A nurse is responsible for observing vital signs before and after IUD insertion or removal to assess for a vasovagal reaction, which may occur during cervical dilation. With a vasovagal reaction, the nurse assists the client with positional changes and may provide ammonia capsules or, upon a physician's order, atropine sulfate (0.6 mg intravenously) (Gromko, 1980).

For the first week after IUD insertion, the woman may be told to insert nothing in the vagina to prevent infection. Each client should be able to demonstrate a successful string check and perform this at least monthly. All IUD users need a back-up method during the first month of IUD use, in case of IUD expulsion, and during midcycle if greater protection is desired. Each client should receive and be encouraged to record a menstrual calendar. The nurse should stress awareness of dietary iron sources and, for at least 2 to 3 days of each week, iron supplementation (Hatcher et al, 1988). Instruct the client to contact her caregiver immediately if she experiences fever, chills, pain, foul-smelling discharge, excessive bleeding, or any other untoward symptoms or if she suspects pregnancy. If she wishes to have her IUD removed, she will need to return to her caregiver. Otherwise, an annual examination and Pap smear should be sufficient.

ADVANTAGES

The IUD has been used in large-scale family planning programs because it is comparatively inexpensive, effective, and easy to use. Its presence does not interfere with sexual intercourse; it permits spontaneity. Barring complications, plain plastic IUDs may be left in place indefinitely. Client continuation rates are high. The "ideal" IUD client appears to be a woman who has only one partner and who has completed her family, because of concerns about infection and infertility.

DISADVANTAGES

Not every woman can safely use an IUD. Absolute contraindications to IUD use include active pelvic infection and known or suspected pregnancy. Nulliparous women who wish some day to have children are advised not to use an IUD, as are women who have more than one sexual partner or partners who are at high risk for sexually transmitted diseases (Cramer et al, 1985). Relative contraindications to IUD use include (1) history of one pelvic infection if client desires future pregnancy, (2) purulent cervicitis, (3) history of repeated pelvic infections, (4) history of an ectopic pregnancy, (5) abnormal Pap smear or suspected malignancy, (6) altered response to infection (for example, in diabetes), (7) altered response to coagulation, (8) severe dysmenorrhea, (9) severe menorrhagia, and (10) unusual shape of uterine cavity (e.g., less than 4.5 cm or presence of fibroids) (Bernstein et al, 1978; Hatcher et al, 1986). Other contraindications may include certain chronic health problems, such as anemia or valvular heart disease; concern and desire for future fertility, especially if the client has a past history of gonorrhea; normal variants or abnormalities of the reproductive system that might make IUD use difficult, such as cervical stenosis, a small uterus, endometriosis, or fibroids; and an inability to check IUD strings or to report danger signs.

All side effects of IUD use deserve careful evaluation because some may be symptoms of serious complications. IUD use is associated with pelvic inflammatory disease (PID), which may damage the fallopian tubes. Such damage is associated with infertility. Although clinicians employ sterile technique during IUD insertions, bacteria may enter the normally sterile uterine cavity. They may also ascend along the IUD tail. The risk of developing primary tubal infertility escalates rapidly during the first few months of IUD use and then rises more gradually (10 to 15 per cent per year) (Cramer et al, 1985). Nulliparous women with more than one sexual partner have twice the risk of tubal infertility if they use the IUD instead of another contraceptive (Cramer et al, 1985). The relative risk of primary tubal infertility, studied in 54 women who had used only one type of IUD, varied from 1.3 with copper-containing IUDs to 11.3 with the Dalkon Shield (Daling et al, 1985).

The symptoms of PID vary and may be subtle. They include purulent or foul-smelling discharge, vaginal bleeding or spotting, discomfort or pain in lower pelvis or back, and generalized flulike symptoms. In an IUD user, a persistent foul-smelling discharge should be considered PID until proved otherwise. If an IUD user experiences a sudden onset of flulike symptoms (fever, chills, myalagia, and headache), sepsis must be presumed until proved otherwise (Hatcher et al, 1986). Once PID is diagnosed, IUD removal will minimize morbidity and mortality ("Another Look at IUDs," 1980). Vigorous antibiotic therapy, sometimes given intravenously, begins immediately; some clinicians begin antibiotics prior to IUD removal. A woman who has had IUD-associated PID and who desires future pregnancy is best advised not to use the IUD again. If she has no plans for pregnancy and desires another IUD, it is safest to wait 3 months before insertion (Hatcher et al, 1986).

Another IUD side effect may be menorrhagia (increased cyclic bleeding), which may in turn lead to iron-deficiency anemia. IUD users commonly experience longer menstrual periods, heavier flow, and more intermenstrual bleeding than nonusers. The exact reason for this is not known. Mechanical stress on the endometrium could trigger changes in the clotting mechanism, and menstrual bleeding may occur earlier in the cycle than in women without IUDs ("Intrauterine Devices," 1982). A woman using the Lippes Loop or Saf-T-Coil may lose twice as much menstrual blood as a woman not using an IUD. Blood loss may be less with medicated devices because they are usually smaller and cause less distortion of the uterine cavity (Fogel, 1981). Because menorrhagia may be due to factors unrelated to the IUD, a thorough assessment is advisable.

Bleeding between periods may be due to a local endometrial response to the IUD, infection, expulsion, or causes unrelated to the IUD (e.g., hormonal imbalances or benign or malignant tumors). The clinician cannot afford to miss partial expulsion of the IUD. Hatcher and associates (1986) recommend removal of the IUD if increased bleeding is associated with partial expulsion, endometritis, a hematocrit of 30 to 32 per cent or lower, or a hematocrit drop of five points. If the client desires removal of her IUD, the nurse can facilitate this and prepare the client.

Another serious side effect can be pelvic pain, most commonly experienced with menses or with insertion or removal of the IUD. When an IUD user experiences pelvic pain, the clinician must first, without delay, rule out ectopic pregnancy. Ectopic pregnancies are more common in women using contraceptives who have a past history of PID or who are present IUD users. The incidence of ectopic pregnancy is 5 to 10 per cent among IUD users, twice the rate found in women using any other means of contraception (Gromko, 1980).

Painful uterine contractions may also occur if the uterus expels the IUD, although this can also happen painlessly. From 1 to 24 per cent of users expel their IUD during the first year (Gromko, 1980). IUDs may perforate through or embed into the uterus. Estimated frequencies of perforation are 1 per 2500 insertions for all types (Hatcher et al, 1986), and 1 per 3000 for the Cu-7 (Gromko, 1980). Lack of clinician skill or experience is correlated with perforations. The clinician may locate a "lost" IUD by uterine sound, IUD remover hook, ultrasound, x-rays, or hysterosalpingogram.

A common problem for IUD users is inability to feel the string(s). Women who cannot feel their IUD strings may become anxious if they fear they have lost the IUD. Often the IUD strings are present, but the client may need assistance in verifying their presence. Occasionally, the string extends only as far as the os, so that just its tip protrudes. Or, the string may be long and soft enough to adhere to and curve around the ectocervix. Alternatively, the strings may be coiled in the cervical os, where a clinician may reach them with a sterile cotton-tipped applicator or narrow forceps.

IUD "failures" include intrauterine as well as ectopic pregnancies. Pregnancy occurs in 0.5 to 5.0 per cent of IUD users in the first year ("Intrauterine Devices," 1982). This figure includes those users who had not realized they had expelled their IUDs and thus were not protected against pregnancy. The likelihood of a normal pregnancy outcome after conception with an IUD in place is usually enhanced by *removal* of the IUD. When the IUD is left in place, 50 per cent of pregnancies may result in spontaneous abortions. When the IUD is removed, 30 per cent of pregnancies may result in spontaneous abortions. The risk of infection with an IUD in place during pregnancy is great (Perlmutter, 1978).

EFFECTS ON SEXUALITY

The high efficacy of the IUD is its primary advantage; freedom from fear of pregnancy produces positive attitudes. The IUD user does not have to prepare for intercourse, so lovemaking can be spontaneous. It is important to check for the strings at the os, but this does not need to be done at the time of intercourse. Since the IUD is worn by the woman, the male partner may feel diminished responsibility for contraception. This may make it more or less appealing to some couples.

Sarrel and Sarrel (1979) list three possible adverse effects of the IUD on sexual expression: (1) postcoital bleeding, which may be frightening; (2) uterine cramping at orgasm (less of a problem with newer IUDs); (3) association with unpleasant vaginal odor. One proposed mechanism of action of the IUD concerns some couples and may lead them to choose another method. For some individuals or couples, interrupting the development of a blastocyst is morally less acceptable than preventing conception.

BARRIER METHODS

Barrier methods, including condoms, the diaphragm, the vaginal contraceptive sponge, the cervical cap, and spermicides, can be very effective contraceptives (Table 11–11) and pose relatively low risks. Certain barrier methods are associated with decreased risk of sexually transmitted infections and tubal infertility (Cramer et al, 1987). Many couples enjoy sharing responsibility for their use. One of the few disadvantages is that using barrier methods requires a certain amount of manual dexterity. It is important to assess whether a client with quadriplegia, multiple sclerosis, upper limb amputation, or the like can correctly position a condom, diaphragm, or spermicide. If the partner is more able-bodied and is involved in contraception, he or she can assist (Leavesley and Porter, 1982).

Diaphragm

The precursor to the diaphragm and spermicidal jelly was a lemon half partially carved out with the acidic pulp and juice serving as a spermicide. Diaphragms were first popularized early in this century in the United States by a nurse, Margaret Sanger. Concerned after having seen women die from undesired pregnancies and illegal abortions, she went to Holland to learn more about contraception. After opening a clinic to offer contraceptive services, including the diaphragm, Margaret Sanger was thrown in jail in 1916. Sanger's belief in women's right to control reproduction threatened societal values on many levels. Only after several years of political organizing were contraceptive services legally available to New York women (Sharpe, 1978).

A diaphragm is a rubber dome-shaped cup with a flexible rim 55 to 100 mm in diameter. In the United States there are three rim types: coil, arcing, and flat (Fig. 11–6). A diaphragm, properly inserted, covers the cervix (Fig. 11–7), holding a spermicidal cream or jelly against it (Martin, 1978). It is the spermicide that provides primary contraceptive protection.

Muscle tone and pelvic anatomy influence the size and type of diaphragm that best fits an individual (see "Careful Choice," 1988). An experienced professional incorporates client teaching by fitting with actual diaphragms rather than fitting rings. A well-fitted diaphragm meets the following criteria, which are also the guidelines whereby a woman and her partner will know that the diaphragm is in the right place: (1) There is less than a finger breadth of space between the posterior aspect of the symphysis pubis

TABLE 11–11. Comparative Effectiveness Rates of Barrier and Spermicidal Methods

Method	Theoretical Effectiveness (%) (Used Correctly and Consistently)	Average User Effectiveness (%)	Reference
Condoms alone	96.4–99.6	90–97	Hatcher et al, 1984; Fogel, 1981
Condoms and foam	99	95	Fogel, 1981
Diaphragm with spermicide	97–98	81–98	Hatcher et al, 1984
Cervical cap with spermicide	98	87–91.6	"High Rates," 1981; Koch, 1982
Spermicidal agents alone (suppositories, cream, foam, or jelly)	95–97	64–98.5	Adasczik, 1981a Hatcher et al, 1984
Contraceptive sponge	~96	72–86	Hatcher et al, 1988

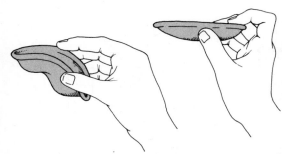

FIGURE 11–6. Arcing diaphragm (left); coil spring or flat diaphragm (right).

and the anterior rim of the diaphragm. (When a woman is sexually excited, her vaginal vault expands, creating more space; hence, the need for the largest comfortable diaphragm.) (2) The diaphragm is fully unfolded. (3) The diaphragm covers the cervix. (4) The woman does not feel pressure from the diaphragm on her rectum or bladder. She is comfortable walking around with the diaphragm in place. The largest diaphragm that meets these criteria is prescribed for the client.

The theoretical effectiveness rate of the diaphragm with spermicide is 97 to 98 per cent. The user effectiveness rate is 81 to 98 per cent (Table 11–11). A National Center for Health Statistics survey yielded an extended use effectiveness rate of 84.1 per cent for large groups of women who used it for long periods of time, either correctly or incorrectly (Connell, 1979). Effectiveness is enhanced by using the diaphragm correctly for every act of intercourse. Lane, Arces, and Sobrero (1976) found a user effectiveness rate of 98 per cent among 2175 women who were mostly young, unmarried, and of lower socioeconomic status. Higher than usual effectiveness may have been due to careful instruction, practice, and client confidence in the method. In this and a second study, diaphragm users had high continuation rates: 80 per cent, compared with 58 to 67 per cent for users of other contraceptives (Lane, Arces, and Sobrero, 1976; Gorosh, 1982).

CLIENT EDUCATION

Both members of a couple may wish to participate in the diaphragm fitting and teaching visit. Teach the client, in simple terms, how the diaphragm is fitted so she understands how to use it herself. Teach her to feel her cervix, first uncovered, then covered by the diaphragm. If she feels pain or pressure it will usually be because the diaphragm is mispositioned. Each client deserves private practice time with a diaphragm. Check her insertion and removal techniques during the visit and on a return visit if desired. Stress the advisability of a follow-up diaphragm check. In one study conducted in a university health service, approximately 10 per cent of the new diaphragm users returned for a follow-up check with the diaphragm *incorrectly* positioned (Sarrel and Sarrel, 1979).

Arranging an appointment for a diaphragm fitting can be an affirmation of one's sexuality and responsibility. A professional can use the diaphragm fitting visit to reinforce these positive attitudes and to provide further information. Permission giving is another important component of the intervention. Some women are uncomfortable and/or inexperienced with touching their genitals. Virgins and women who have not used tampons may be hesitant in their first attempts to insert a diaphragm; the clinician's sensitivity, understanding, and encouragement are important. Occasionally, a woman will be frustrated by diaphragm insertion and opt for another method of contraception. A sensitive professional will allow for expression of feelings such as frustration or anger.

Several aspects of recommended diaphragm use have not been validated by research. Craig and Hepburn (1982) challenge the usually recommended 6- to 8-hour minimum retention time. It is not known whether a diaphragm might be safely removed within fewer hours, e.g., within 3 hours of coitus. Some retention time is necessary because of changing pH levels in the vagina with intercourse. However, only during sexual excitement do cervical secretions and vaginal transudate neutralize the pH to 7. After sexual excitement wanes, the pH returns to 5, a condition hostile to sperm. Other aspects of diaphragm use also need further study. Putting spermicide around the rim of the diaphragm, as recommended, might make displacement of the diaphragm during intercourse more likely. It has been common practice to recommend that women have diaphragms rechecked if they gain or lose 10 to 15 pounds or have a baby. However, Fiscella (1982) studied 80 diaphragm users and found *no* relationship between weight change and change in recommended diaphragm size. This finding indicates that clinicians should encourage and support related research.

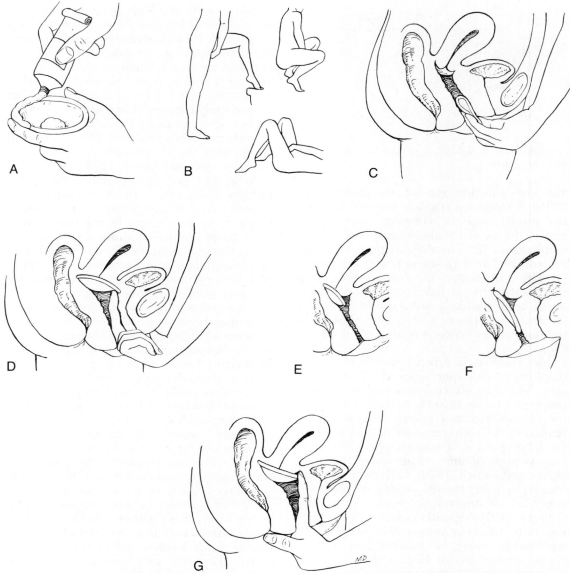

FIGURE 11–7. Use of a diaphragm. A, Application of gel. B, Positions for insertion. C, Folding to insert. D, Pushing diaphragm up above pubis. Correct fit. E, Diaphragm too small. F, Diaphragm too large. G, Diaphragm removed. (From Luckmann J, Sorensen KC: Medical-Surgical Nursing. 3rd ed. Philadelphia, WB Saunders, 1988.)

INSTRUCTIONS FOR THE DIAPHRAGM USER

Instruct the women to follow these directions to use and care for the diaphragm properly:

1. Be sure the diaphragm is in place before each and every act of intercourse.

2. Use 1 tablespoonful of contraceptive cream or jelly inside the cup, with some of it spread around the rim. If intercourse will first occur 2 hours or more after diaphragm insertion or if a subsequent act of intercourse is to occur, first insert additional spermicide into the vagina, without dislodging the diaphragm.

3. Check for proper placement of the diaphragm.

4. Leave it in place for 6 to 8 hours after the last act of intercourse.

5. Carefully wash it with mild soap and water, dry it with a soft towel, and, optionally, powder it, preferably with cornstarch.

6. Check for holes by holding it to the light.

7. Return it to its case for storage away from direct heat. Do not douche after re-

moving the diaphragm (Gunning, 1981). When the expiration date on the spermicide draws near, get another package to have on hand so that you are never using outdated cream or jelly. Replace your diaphragm when the rubber begins to feel dry or look cracked.

ADVANTAGES

Possible attitudinal advantages include (1) confidence in the physiological safety and lack of any systemic pharmacological effects, (2) fostering a positive body image and self-concept regarding female sexuality through learning about and touching one's body, (3) use limited to times of sexual activity, and (4) ease of use for most people. Physical advantages include the small relative protective effects against certain sexually transmitted diseases, cervical dysplasia, and carcinoma in situ. Nonoxynol-9, a commonly used spermicide, has also been shown to be toxic to the human immunodeficiency virus in vitro and may offer some protection against the virus (Peterman and Curran, 1986; Rietmeijer et al, 1988). Some women appreciate the fact that the diaphragm may be used to hold menstrual flow. (Due to the risk of toxic shock syndrome, explained in the following paragraph, it is prudent to remove and clean the diaphragm at least daily).

DISADVANTAGES

Disadvantages of diaphragm use include the following:

1. The user effectiveness rate, 81 to 98 per cent, is lower than that for OCs, the IUD, and sterilization.

2. There is some evidence that diaphragm users experience a higher rate of cystitis and urethritis than users of other methods (Hatcher et al, 1986). Foxman and Frerichs (1985) suggest that the diaphragm may cause decreased sensitivity to the need to void or decreased circulation to areas on which the diaphragm exerts pressure. They calculate that 34 per cent of the first urinary tract infections and 15 per cent of secondary ones in their college student population could have been prevented by use of an alternative contraceptive.

3. Some women or their partners may be allergic to rubber, latex, or spermicides.

4. Some women have difficulty learning insertion and checking placement.

5. Toxic shock syndrome (TSS) can occur in women who have left the diaphragm in the vagina for 30 hours or more, whether or not they are menstruating. TSS is a relatively rare, sometimes fatal condition caused by *Staphylococcus aureus,* and it occurs most frequently in young women who are using absorbent tampons. If a woman who has had TSS elects to use a diaphragm, she should be aware of the risk of TSS recurrence.

6. Privacy and soap and water are necessary for aesthetic use (Hatcher et al, 1984).

7. Women with lax muscle tone or some anatomical abnormalities cannot use the diaphragm.

8. Pelvic discomfort, especially with a larger diaphragm, and infrequently, vaginal infections or cramping may occur (Pyle, 1984).

Certain attitudes may limit consistent and effective diaphragm use. Some women who are not comfortable with their body may have difficulty using and checking the diaphragm. Some women who may not have fully incorporated their sexual practices and need for birth control into their self-concept and role perceptions may not feel sexually comfortable with their partners and may not take time to insert the diaphragm. Some couples may object to inserting the diaphragm just before coitus, or they may find it inconvenient to use the diaphragm every time if they have intercourse frequently. Some couples do not plan ahead, for example, to ensure that they will have the diaphragm along if intercourse occurs away from home.

EFFECTS ON SEXUALITY

In clinical practice it is observed that the adolescent women who choose the diaphragm do so primarily to avoid systemic side effects. Even when presented with the documented safety of OCs, they are generally motivated to learn diaphragm use. Those who have intercourse infrequently or who anticipate a long abstinent interval are particularly apt to choose the diaphragm.

Some couples complain that use of this method interferes with the spontaneity of intercourse. They may take chances by omitting the diaphragm on days when they think it is safe to do so. Or, they may elect another method. For other couples, diaphragm use is a shared responsibility and an enjoyable part of foreplay. It is suggested that partners alternate the responsibility for preparing, inserting, and checking the diaphragm. The professional's own attitude toward such experimentation and toward foreplay may influence client attitudes and practices. Shared responsibility in contraception may encourage or signal interdependence in other areas of the couple's relationship.

Some women or their partners may feel the diaphragm during intercourse. Occasionally, a diaphragm becomes dislodged during intercourse, most frequently when the couple uses the woman superior position. Advise clients to recheck the diaphragm after penile insertion. The disagreeable taste of most spermicides used with the diaphragm may be an impediment to oral-genital sex. This is minimized by careful cleansing of the external genitals after diaphragm insertion or by insertion of the diaphragm after oral-genital sex but before insertion of the penis into the vagina. Some manufacturers advertise a neutrally or even pleasantly flavored spermicidal cream or jelly. Diaphragm cream or jelly may make the vagina too slippery for the enjoyment of some couples (Sarrel and Sarrel, 1979). Some women are especially sensitive at the Grafenberg spot (G-spot), an area in the anterior wall of the vagina. A diaphragm may fit in such a way that it interferes with stimulation of this spot (Barbach, 1983).

Cervical Cap

The cervical cap is a thimble-shaped device that fits closely over the cervix. It has a long history. In ancient Sumatra, women molded opium into a cuplike device to cover the cervix. In Europe, women molded beeswax into cervical caps. Caps have been made of firm materials, for example, resin, ivory, lucite, or a variety of metals; and, for about 140 years, of soft rubber. Wax impressions of the cervix, allowing for custom-made cervical caps, were used by Dr. Wilde in Germany in 1923 (King, 1981); this idea has only recently been reintroduced in the United States. King (1981) attributes the lack of popularity of the cervical cap in the United States to the reluctance of physicians to master its fitting, devote extra time to client education, increase client contacts, and prescribe a contraceptive not promoted by pharmaceutical companies. The cap has been, and still is, quite popular in Europe. There are presently several ongoing studies of the cervical cap in the United States.

Cervical caps are of several types (Fig. 11–8). The most popular cap in the United States today is the Prentif Cavity Rim Cap, which comes in four standard sizes, ranging from 22 to 31 mm in diameter. Current research focuses on the design and use of custom-made caps, including those with one-way valves to allow for permanent wear (Gilbirds and Jonas, 1982). Guidelines for fitting the cervical cap are discussed by Brokaw, Baker, and Haney (1988).

The cervical cap protects against pregnancy by blocking the entrance to the uterus. Spermicidal jelly may not be theoretically necessary but is used to maximize protection. Thus, the primary contraceptive mechanism of the cap works as a mechanical barrier. Average user effectiveness rates range from 87 to 91.6 per cent (Table 11–11).

CLIENT EDUCATION

The client fills the cap about one-third full of spermicide before inserting it in the vagina and placing it on the cervix (Johnson, 1985). It is best to insert it at least one-half hour before intercourse (King, 1981). Insertion is easiest before sexual excitement; with excitation the uterus and cervix rise in the pelvic cavity and may be harder to reach. Either partner can check its position by running a finger around the cap. It is left in place for a minimum of 6 to 12 hours postcoitally. Some authors state that it may be left in place for a maximum of 3 to 7 days (Canavan and Lewis, 1981). Many clinicians recommend that caps not be worn more than 3 days (Johnson, 1985), as cervicitis, odor, and TSS are concerns.

Some professionals recommend filling the cap with spermicide if it is to be left in place more than 12 hours (Koch, 1982). Others suggest that too much spermicide may increase the chances of the cap becoming dislodged during coitus (Craig and Hepburn, 1982). Research on this question and on the most effective form of spermicide is needed. Most sources do not specify a need to insert additional spermicide before repeated acts of intercourse. After removal, the cap is washed and dried (like the diaphragm) and, optionally, powdered with cornstarch.

ADVANTAGES

Clients cite advantages such as those associated with the diaphragm. Specific advantages of the cervical cap include (1) convenience, especially if it is left in place for 2 or more

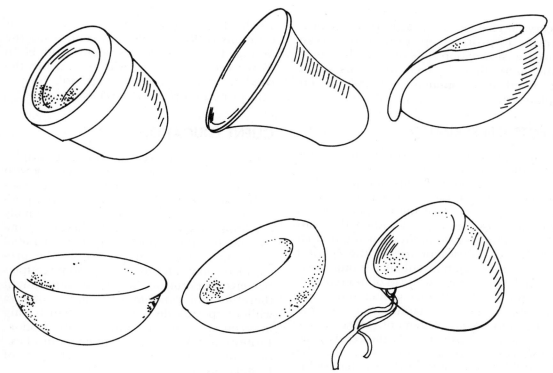

FIGURE 11–8. Types of cervical caps.

days; (2) for some women, relative ease of insertion (since the cap is smaller than the diaphragm); (3) economy and decreased discharge due to the relatively small amount of spermicide required; (4) perception of efficacy, based on the moderate degree of suction experienced with removal ("like breaking a seal"); (5) decreased sensation of pelvic pressure after intercourse as compared with the diaphragm; and (6) less cystitis in women who are prone to it with the diaphragm. Cagen (1986) found that 80 per cent of the women in his sample continued using the cervical cap after 1 year; they cited convenience and comfort as major positive features in their decision.

DISADVANTAGES

The cap has not been manufactured in the United States, and its distribution in this country was limited to research clinics until May of 1988, when the FDA approved the Prentif Cavity Rim Cap for contraceptive use. Given such approval, the manufacture and availability of the cap in the United States may increase. Health care professionals in the United States have had relatively little information about the cervical cap (Canavan

and Lewis, 1981). Some women cannot be fitted with currently available cervical caps if their cervix deviates from usual shape; for example, if it is very short, has an irregular shape due to laceration suffered during childbirth, or points toward the spine. Nabothian cysts or venereal warts are a contraindication if, by their location on the cervix, they interfere with suction (King, 1981). Some women have difficulty finding their cervix and thus have difficulty inserting or removing the cap. Inserting the cervical cap is often more difficult than inserting the diaphragm and may require longer fingers. Coitus and/or bowel movements may dislodge the cap, increasing the risk of pregnancy. Because the diameter of the cervix may vary during the menstrual cycle, the degree to which the cap fits may vary, thus exposing some women to greater risk of pregnancy. The cervical cap cannot be used during menses, as suction would be lost.

Health problems may be associated with use of the cervical cap. Cervical mucus cannot drain away when the cap is in place, so long-term usage may lead to cervicitis. There is also at least a theoretical possibility that the use of a cervical cap may predispose a woman to endometriosis. The role of the cervical cap in cervical changes is unclear. It seems prudent not to provide caps to women with an active transformation zone of reddish-orange tissue more than ½ inch in radius or, if prescribed, to recommend that they be left in place only 6 hours (King, 1981).

EFFECTS ON SEXUALITY

In our experience, many women are enthusiastic about the cervical cap. These women appear to have positive self-concepts and to be comfortable with their sexual and contraceptive roles. They are highly motivated to obtain and use the cap, providing they can be fitted. This level of motivation augurs well for effective, consistent use of the cervical cap. Use of the cap may enhance spontaneity, as it can be inserted well ahead of intercourse. The cap is rarely felt during intercourse and is less likely than the diaphragm to become dislodged in sexual excitement. The cap may create increased pressure on the cervix during intercourse; for some women this may be pleasurable. Also, more of the vaginal wall is exposed to penile stimulation than with the diaphragm, and this may enhance the sexual response (King, 1981).

Condoms

Condoms, also called rubbers or prophylactics, are penile sheaths worn during intercourse to contain the ejaculate so that sperm cannot enter the vagina (Fig. 11–9). Men used such sheaths for decoration in Egypt as far back as 1350 B.C. In the sixteenth century, linen sheaths and penile coverings made from animal intestines were available. In the eighteenth century, Casanova popularized condom use for protection against both infection and pregnancy. In the nineteenth century, rubber became available for condoms. Today many condoms are lubricated for increased comfort. Some incorporate spermicides that at least theoretically protect against failure from a slow leak or spilling during withdrawal (Free, 1985). Latex condoms with nonoxynol-9 are also promoted for physical and chemical protection against the human immunodeficiency virus (Reitmeijer et al, 1988).

Condoms offer men a contraceptive option. Of reversible methods used in the United States, they are second in popularity after oral contraceptives (Hatcher et al,

1986). Theoretical method effectiveness of condoms is 96.4 to 99.6 per cent, while the average user effectiveness ranges from 90 to 97 per cent. Used along with spermicide, the condom may offer an average user 95 per cent protection (Fogel, 1981).

CLIENT EDUCATION

Clinicians usually recommend that couples use a vaginal spermicide simultaneously with a condom. Some recommend putting spermicide on the tip of the penis before application of the condom because occasionally condoms burst or tear and also because some couples put the condom on after an initial penetration; sperm, if present in the pre-ejaculate, may enter the vagina. Some couples perceive spermicides as messy and might therefore limit condom use. Using a condom without spermicide is far safer than having intercourse without other contraception. Professionals who encourage condom placement by the woman as an enjoyable part of foreplay help to encourage condom use.

INSTRUCTIONS FOR THE USER OF CONDOMS

Effective use of the condom involves the following steps:

1. Buy individually sealed condoms.

2. Unwrap the condom carefully and set it in a convenient place before starting foreplay.

3. Unroll the entire condom onto the erect penis before penetration.

4. Use a condom with a reserve space at the tip or leave about ½ inch of condom beyond the tip of the penis to serve as a reservoir. It is important to squeeze the reservoir end with fingers to keep air out while unrolling. Many couples prefer lubricated condoms and find they are less apt to tear. If other lubrication is desired, use a personal lubricant that will not harm the rubber. (Petroleum jelly may cause deterioration.)

5. After intercourse and before erection fades, hold the condom against the base of the penis carefully while withdrawing to avoid spilling any semen on the woman's genitals.

6. Use a new condom for each and every act of coitus.

7. Store condoms where they will not get too hot or get punctured. Discard any that

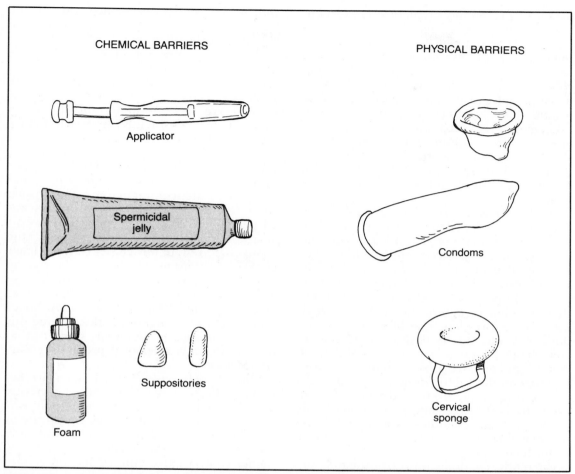

FIGURE 11–9. Nonprescription contraceptives that use physical and chemical barriers. Spermicidal jelly and foam are inserted intravaginally with a tamponlike applicator. Suppositories are inserted with a finger. (From Luckmann J, Sorensen KC: Medical-Surgical Nursing. *3rd ed. Philadelphia, WB Saunders, 1988.)*

are over 2 years old as well as any that have passed the manufacturer's expiration date.

ADVANTAGES

Practical advantages of the condom include (1) availability without prescription, (2) relative protection against sexually transmitted diseases, (3) physiological safety (no systemic effects), and (4) possible prevention of cancer of the cervix. The cost of condoms varies from a few cents apiece (bought in bulk) to several dollars apiece for special, usually imported, types.

DISADVANTAGES

A few people are allergic to rubber in condoms. Some men feel sexual pleasure is significantly reduced with condom use. If this

inhibits erectile function, condoms are contraindicated. Condom use necessitates interruption of sexual activity. This may be unacceptable to couples who highly value spontaneity. A few couples may feel that "nice people" do not use condoms (Arnold, 1975).

EFFECTS ON SEXUALITY

Use of any contraceptive can enhance sexual pleasure if it alleviates fears of unwanted pregnancy. Condoms are no exception, and they can also decrease the chances of acquiring sexually transmitted diseases. In fact, condoms are commonly recommended by sex counselors and sex therapists. The fact that the condom may diminish the amount of stimulation experienced by the male is a drawback for some couples. For others, it is useful in preventing premature ejaculation, a sexual dysfunction that may be very distressing. It is defined as ejaculation before the couple would like to have this occur; it is more common in younger couples. Using condoms may enable some couples to slow down the pace of their lovemaking, prolonging the man's preorgasmic period of sexual excitement. If a man cannot maintain his erection after putting on a condom, he should rely on other birth control (Hatcher et al, 1988). If insufficient lubrication in the female is a problem, lubricated condoms can help.

While discussing condom use, the nurse may acknowledge that sexual practices are many and varied by mentioning that the penis should be protected by a condom before rectal penetration and the condom removed prior to further genital contact to prevent infections. Such a statement shows that the nurse recognizes that there is variety in sexual expression. Use of different condoms can add variety to sex life. Condoms come in a wide range of colors, textures, and quality. Some have ribs or other textured patterns on the rubber designed to stimulate the woman. Some are named and packaged suggestively. Couples may enjoy using some of the "special" condoms as a change from traditional condoms or from other methods of birth control.

Currently, condoms represent the only reversible contraceptive for which a male may, if he chooses, take full responsibility. If they are used concomitantly with a vaginal spermicide, partners may share responsibility. Giving the male a concrete role in preventing conception is important to many couples. Also, some couples feel safer if both partners are taking precautions.

Vaginal Contraceptive Sponge

In 1983 the spermicidally treated sponge Today (see Fig. 11–9) was introduced in the United States. It is a disc of polyurethane foam about 2 inches in diameter with an indentation in the center. A polyester tape, which forms a loop through the sponge, facilitates removal. Open cells in the spongy polymer contain the spermicide nonoxynol-9 and release it over 24 hours. Two other features contribute to the efficacy of the sponge. If correctly positioned, the sponge blocks sperm from the cervix. Also, the sponge absorbs some sperm.

User effectiveness rates for the contraceptive sponge vary widely from 72 to 86 per cent, depending on the user (Hatcher et al, 1988; see Table 11–11). New users of any method are less apt to be able to use it correctly and consistently; first year failure rates may be 17 to 25 per cent. After the second year of correct and consistent sponge use, effectiveness may rise to about 96 per cent. In some studies, sponge users were compared with diaphragm users. In one such study, the failure rate for both groups was 14 per 100 nulliparous women users over 1 year; however, for parous women, the sponge failure rate was 28 per cent (Hatcher et al, 1986). This may be because the sponge does not fit parous women as well or because parous women desire to space rather than to avoid pregnancy (Hatcher et al, 1988). About 50 per cent of sponge users discontinue this method during the first year, some due to discomfort and/or removal problems ("Barrier Methods," 1984).

Clinical trials in the United States are beginning on the Benzaltex sponge, currently available only abroad. This is a polyvinyl sponge containing benzalkonium chloride as the spermicide, and it is packaged already moist. Greater convenience and possibly higher contraceptive efficacy and fewer side effects make this a promising new development ("Canadian-made," 1986).

INSTRUCTIONS FOR THE USER OF THE CONTRACEPTIVE SPONGE

To use the sponge correctly, follow these steps:

1. With clean hands, hold the sponge with the indentation up.

2. Wet the sponge with clean tap water (about 2 tablespoons), then squeeze gently to remove excess water.

3. Fold the sides of the sponge upward.

4. Slide the sponge through the vaginal opening and push it along as far as you can reach. When you let go, it will unfold.

5. Check to be sure the cervix is covered by feeling around the edge of the sponge. (The sponge may not remain in this position during intercourse, but it will still be effective as long as it is in the vagina because it continues to give off spermicide.) The sponge can be inserted up to 24 hours before inter-

course and can be used repeatedly within 24 hours of its insertion.

6. Leave the sponge in place at least 6 hours after the last act of intercourse before pulling the sponge out by hooking a finger around the ribbon loop.

7. Never use the contraceptive sponge during your menstrual period or if you have ever had toxic shock syndrome; use an alternative contraceptive, such as condoms. If you choose to douche, wait until after removing the sponge.

ADVANTAGES

User effectiveness of the contraceptive sponge alone averages about 72 to 86 per cent. Couples can increase their contraceptive protection by also using condoms. This is particularly important in the first 3 months of use, when, as with any new contraceptive method, failures are most frequent (Lemberg, 1984). It is convenient and economical to use a single sponge repeatedly for 24 hours. Contraceptive sponges cost about a dollar each in packages of three; on sale or in larger packages, they may cost less.

DISADVANTAGES

Some women experience difficulty in inserting the sponge, particularly if they have not used a diaphragm. With careful coaching by the clinician, most can learn its use. Sometimes after intercourse the sponge is high in the vaginal vault. Women with short fingers may have difficulty reaching the tape loop to remove the sponge. About 2 to 4 per cent of users may be allergic to sponge components (Lemberg, 1984). Manifestations of allergy include itching, burning, or rash in either partner. Women who are irritated by the sponge may produce a discharge. These effects are reversible, disappearing after sponge use ceases. The sponge is not to be used during menstruation. There have been some reports of TSS occurring in sponge users, even though the spermicide to some extent inhibits the growth of TSS-causing bacteria.

EFFECTS ON SEXUALITY

Ease of purchase (no prescription needed, one size fits all, relatively low cost) and efficacy over a 24-hour period are major advantages that can increase peace of mind and thereby enhance sexual enjoyment. There is no need to wait (as with suppositories) after insertion before having intercourse. Spontaneity is easier to achieve with this method than with the other vaginal barrier and/or spermicidal methods, with the exception of the cervical cap. There are no worries about systemic side effects or long-term threats to fertility. With the sponge in place, there is little or no postcoital discharge, an aesthetic consideration that is important to some couples. The spermicide may offer some protection against gonorrhea, AIDS, and other sexually transmitted diseases. The sponge is very soft, like normal vaginal tissue. If a man feels it during intercourse, it is usually not objectionable ("Vaginal Contraceptive Sponge," 1983). He may participate in contraception by inserting and/or removing the sponge.

New Female Barrier Methods

Additional female barrier methods are being produced and tested. One is a vaginal spermicidal barrier (VSB), informally called a disposable diaphragm. It is a flat, oval, plastic disc coated with nonoxynol-9. The mechanism of action is both chemical, by killing sperm, and mechanical, by blocking the cervix. The VSB is proposed to offer effective contraception for 24 hours, to be inserted like a diaphragm, to be removed 2 hours postcoitally, and to allow one size to fit all women (Sondheimer, personal communication).

Another barrier method under study is a woman's condom. It is a disposable polyurethane sheath with two rings: one fits over the cervix, somewhat like a diaphragm, and one fits over the labia. It is to be inserted like a tampon. Designers of the device claim that it is as effective as a male condom for contraception, that the polyurethane is 40 per cent stronger than latex used with male condoms, and that the female condom offers relative protection against the human immunodeficiency virus (Wolinsky, 1988).

Spermicides: Contraceptive Foams, Jelly, Creams, and Suppositories

Spermicides are substances used vaginally to kill sperm and inhibit fertilization (see Fig.

11–9). Even before the role of sperm in conception was understood, women used a variety of acidic or alkaline solutions to prevent pregnancy. Solutions were made with oils or honey and sodium carbonate in the times of Aristotle and Cleopatra. Salt, quinine, lactic acid, and boric acid solutions were popular in the nineteenth century (Seamon, 1977).

Today, contraceptive spermicidal preparations contain two substances. A vehicle ingredient keeps the active ingredient in place around the cervix. Usually, the active ingredient is nonoxynol-9, a surfactant that disrupts the sperm membrane (Christakos, 1983). Vaginal foam creates both a mechanical barrier and a spermicidal environment. Other vehicles for spermicides are creams, jellies, gels, and effervescent "foaming" tablets or suppositories (see Fig. 11–9). The user effectiveness rate of foam, when used alone, ranges from 71 to 98.5 per cent, according to studies done between 1961 and 1971 (Hatcher et al, 1984). The effectiveness of contraceptive jelly or cream alone ranges from 64 to 96 per cent (Adasczik, 1981a). The effectiveness of the spermicide depends chiefly on consistent and correct use. If used alone, foam is preferred over jelly or cream because of its superior ability to cover the cervix.

CLIENT EDUCATION

In the sections that follow, we list current guidelines for spermicide use. Craig and Hepburn (1982) call for more research on the most effective use of spermicides, including specific amounts needed, timing, and duration of effectiveness. Clinicians need to keep informed about new findings and modify their client instructions accordingly.

INSTRUCTIONS FOR THE USER OF VAGINAL FOAM

For maximum contraceptive effectiveness, remember that contraceptive foam is effective for only 30 minutes. Some foam comes in preloaded applicators.

1. For aerosol foam, shake the can thoroughly, at least 20 times, to create bubbles and mix the ingredients.

2. Fill the applicator either by direct pressure applied to the top of the container (for example, with Emko or Koromex) or by tilt-ing the applicator against the top of the container (Delfen).

3. Use one applicator full of Emko, Because, or Dalkon foam *or* two applicators full of Delfen or Koromex foam.

4. Insert the filled applicator as far back in the vagina as possible and push the plunger. Hold the plunger pushed in as you remove it.

5. Repeat this application before each act of intercourse.

6. Use only foam that has not passed the manufacturer's expiration date on the package.

7. Keep a spare can at all times, as you will not be able to see when the foam will run out.

INSTRUCTIONS FOR THE USER OF SPERMICIDAL SUPPOSITORIES

For maximum contraceptive effectiveness, follow these steps:

1. Plan to insert the suppository (for example, Encare, Semicid, Intercept) into the vagina 10 to 30 minutes before intercourse so it will have time to "foam up," or effervesce.

2. Note the time intervals provided by the manufacturer of the spermicide you are using.

3. With clean hands, remove suppository from wrapper.

4. Insert it as far back in the vagina and as close to the cervix as possible.

5. Repeat application for each act of intercourse *or* if intercourse is delayed.

6. Avoid douching, which might facilitate sperm passage through the cervix. (Routine douching is never advisable but particularly within 8 hours of intercourse with a spermicidal contraceptive.)

ADVANTAGES

Spermicides are readily available without a prescription, are used only when needed, offer some protection against transmission of AIDS, and rarely have any systemic effects. They are practical as a back-up for contraception with OCs, IUDs, and natural contraceptive methods. They are especially effective in conjunction with a barrier method, since combining two contraceptives theoretically maximizes the effectiveness rate.

DISADVANTAGES

The physiological side effects of spermicides are few. Occasionally, a man or woman is allergic to the spermicide or its vehicle. Disadvantages of spermicides include a potentially low efficacy rate (depending on accuracy and consistency of use) and rare occurrence of a local allergic response in either partner. Some persons may view sperm as life forms and object to "killing" them.

There appears to be no significant association between birth defects and foam use (Hatcher et al, 1988), although controversy remains about such an association. Health professionals may need to clarify this issue for clients. Although some experts believe that spermicides should carry a warning about this possibility, others believe there is insufficient evidence to justify this measure ("Despite Court Ruling," 1985). More research is needed in this area.

EFFECTS ON SEXUALITY

Spermicidal preparations produce little or no systemic effect. They offer a high degree of physiological safety, even for women with complicated health problems. They do not cause stillbirths (Porter et al, 1986) or affect future fertility. Spermicides may somewhat decrease the spread of gonorrhea, trichomonas, herpes, and chlamydia and the likelihood of pelvic inflammatory disease (Hatcher et al, 1988). Most spermicides, at least in the laboratory, inhibit the growth of *Candida albicans* (Keith, Berger, and Jackson, 1985). Since *Candida* causes yeast vaginitis, which is often associated with dyspareunia, spermicide use may enhance sexual functioning.

Spermicidal preparations are easy to use for most couples. A male partner can help with placing the contraceptive. This can enhance a couple's sense of mutual caring and responsibility. Contraceptive foams, jellies, gels, and creams provide lubrication in the vagina. This may enhance enjoyment for both partners.

If a couple integrates spermicide application into foreplay, they will not have to interrupt their lovemaking to insert spermicide. Some couples find spermicidal preparations messy to use. Others may object to the taste during cunnilingus. Cleansing of the external genitals after spermicide insertion can help

in overcoming this, and flavored preparations are available. A sensitive professional anticipates these objections and encourages the couple to find ways of dealing with them.

EXPERIMENTAL CONTRACEPTIVES

Vaginal Long-acting Progestins

Progestins reversibly alter the fallopian tubes, endometrium, and/or cervical mucus, interfering with sperm travel and implantation. Research is under way on long-acting progestin contraceptive devices, including a progestin-releasing vaginal ring. Slightly smaller in diameter than a diaphragm, it is worn after menses each month for 21 days. The user removes it temporarily for intercourse (Hatcher et al, 1986). World Health Organization researchers are studying a similar ring that can be left in place for 3 months; this ring releases about 20 μg of levonorgestrel a day. In a study of 1000 women over a period of 1 year, there were 25 pregnancies with the ring ("Hormonal Contraception," 1987).

Research is proceeding on progestin-releasing IUDs that might be effective for more than 1 year (Hatcher et al, 1988). This would be more convenient than the Progestasert IUD, which is replaced annually.

Male Pill

There has been interest in gossypol, a cottonseed derivative, as a male contraceptive. Men who had ingested gossypol were found to be infertile. The Chinese have experimented with 20 mg daily doses and 150 to 220 mg monthly doses for temporary infertility (Lawrence, 1981). Gossypol has been taken orally, rubbed on the skin, or used as a vaginal spermicide. Enthusiasm about gossypol has waned since some toxic effects have emerged. The major side effect is hypokalemia; enteritis, edema, and neuritis are found in men who overdose (Lawrence, 1981). There have been reports of fertility not returning after use of gossypol (Fortney, 1983). More research is needed on reversible methods of male contraception.

FERTILITY AWARENESS METHODS

An especially thorough understanding of the menstrual cycle and reproductive physiology is necessary for effective use of fertility awareness methods. Studies show wide variability in effectiveness rates (Table 11–12). However, artificially low failure rates result if the investigator disregards the lengthy learning period or excludes users judged to be unreliable (Schirm et al, 1982) or desirous of pregnancy. Fewer than 5 per cent of married couples in developed countries choose these methods (Sapire, 1986). The most effective fertility awareness methods involve combining two or more techniques of fertility estimation. Each of the fertility awareness approaches is discussed in the following sections.

Calendar Method (Rhythm)

Although the interval between menses is variable among women, the interval between ovulation and menses is fairly constant. Women ovulate about 14 days before their menses regardless of the interval between menses. After ovulation, the ovarian follicle changes into a corpus luteum. The corpus luteum continues to function, secreting progesterone, for only 14 ± 1 to 2 days (Martin, 1978). When it ceases functioning, menses begin. The calendar method must be individualized for each couple. Ideally, a client records her menstrual cycles for 12 months to establish a baseline before relying on the rhythm method.

To calculate the fertile period, one assumes that ovulation occurs 14 ± 1 to 2 days before menses, that an ovum can remain fertilizable up to 1 day, and that sperm are active for 2 to 3 days (Martin, 1978). A fertile period would exist from days 18 to 11 prior to menses: 14 + 2 + 2 = 18; 14 − 2 − 1 = 11. Assuming every cycle is exactly 28 days, the calculation would be as in the chart below:

From the date of predicted menstrual onset (M), count back 14 days for the predicted date of ovulation. Abstain (A) 2 days on either side of this date for ovulation. Abstain for 1 extra day after the last date for ovulation because the egg may remain fertilizable. Abstain for 2 days before ovulation in case sperm are present before ovulation. Thus, the fertile period begins 18 days before and ends 11 days before menses start. *If* every cycle were precisely the same length, one would abstain from intercourse from 18 through 11 days before the next period was due. *Because cycles vary and cannot be precisely predicted in advance,* one must subtract 18 from the shortest cycle length and 11 from the longest cycle length to calculate the recommended abstinent period (Britt, 1977).

Two examples illustrate how to do these calculations. One woman has 21 to 25 day cycles recorded over 10 months. Counting the first day of menses as day 1, days 3 to 14 of her menstrual cycle would constitute her fertile period (21 − 18 = 3 and 25 − 11 = 14). Another woman has 30 to 36 day cycles recorded over 12 months and calculates her fertile period as follows: 30 − 18 = 12 and 36 − 11 = 25. Days 12 to 25 are her fertile days, very unlike those of the first woman. One must abstain from intercourse on all fertile days to prevent pregnancy by this method. The calendar method is theoretically 80 to 90 per cent effective, but the user effectiveness rate is only 60 to 85.6 per cent (Martin, 1978; Hatcher et al, 1984). Travel and emotional stress are among the factors that can cause alteration in the timing of ovulation (Gillmor-Kahn, Oakley, and Hatcher, 1982), making precise calculations impossible.

```
day
1  2  3  4  5  6  7  8  9  10 11 12 13 14 15 16 17 18 19 20 21 22 23 24 25 26 27 28
                                                                             M

predicted ovulation:                      A
variation in ovulation:          A  A     A  A
egg fertilizable:                               A  A
sperm active:                 (A) A  A
total abstinence
  (= fertile period):         A  A  A  A  A  A  A  A
```

**TABLE 11–12. User Effectiveness Rates of Fertility Awareness Methods,
Coitus Interruptus, and Abstinence**

Method	User Effectiveness Rates (%)	Reference
Calendar (rhythm)	60–85.6	Martin, 1978; Hatcher et al, 1986
Thermal (BBT)	93.4	"Natural Family Planning," 1983
Cervical mucus	72–85	"Natural Family Planning," 1983
Thermal + mucus	78–88.8	Hatcher et al, 1986
		Marshall, 1976
Symptothermal (BBT, mucus, calendar, and symptoms)	85–94	"Natural Family Planning," 1983
Coitus interruptus	75–84	Adasczik, 1981a; Hatcher et al, 1986
Abstinence	100	

1. Purchase a special thermometer calibrated in tenths of degrees between 96 and 100° F.
2. Place the thermometer under the tongue for at least a full 3 minutes (preferably 5 minutes) after waking in the morning and before *any* activity (e.g., lifting your head off the pillow, shaking thermometer down, intercourse, or urinating).
3. If you forget to take your temperature and have already gotten up, *do not take it*. Write *missed* on that day.
4. Take your temperature in the same manner about the same time each day.
5. Carefully record the reading on the graph by placing a dot at the proper location. Start this chart on the first day of your period.
6. Insert the month and day in the space provided.
7. The first day of menstrual flow is considered to be the start of a cycle (day 1). Each day of flow should be indicated with an M on the graph, starting at extreme left under number 1 day of cycle.
8. Record any obvious reason for temperature variation such as a cold, flu, or infection on the graph above the reading for that day.
9. If you are placed on medication, please indicate it in the space labeled medications on the days you take it.
10. If you feel you have menstrually related symptoms, such as breast tenderness or cramping, note these also.
11. If intercourse has taken place during the previous 24 hours, mark it with an (X).

Calendar for Thermal Method of Fertility Awareness

Day of Cycle: 1 2 3 4 5 6 7 8 9 10 11 12 13 14 15 16 17 18 19 20 21 22 23 24 25 26 27 28 29 30 31

Temperature
99.0
98.8
98.6
98.4
98.2
98.0
97.8
97.6
97.4
97.2
97.0

Menses (M):
Intercourse (X):

Mucus
  Color
  Consistency
  Amount

Other factors
  Medications
  Breast tenderness
  Cramps

FIGURE 11–10. Instructions for keeping symptothermal record.

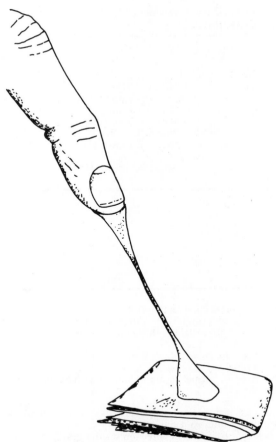

FIGURE 11–11. Spinnbarkeit of midcycle cervical mucus. Midcycle cervical mucus, collected on a tissue, can be stretched into a thread up to 20 cm long. This property is called spinnbarkeit.

Thermal Method

Basal body temperatures (BBTs) cannot be used to predict ovulation. Rather, they are used to validate the luteal, or postovulatory, phase of the menstrual cycle. The basal body temperature, the lowest waking temperature, decreases slightly before ovulation. One to three days after this drop, ovulation occurs, and the BBT rises an average of 0.7 to 1.0°F, owing to the thermogenic effect of progesterone (Gaines, 1981). After the temperature remains elevated for 3 consecutive days, a *relatively* safe period exists for about the next 18 days, *if* the woman has a perfectly regular 28-day cycle.

CLIENT EDUCATION

The client must obtain accurate temperature readings in order to detect subtle variations.

Refer to Figure 11–10 for complete directions and a chart for the client. Instruct the client to establish a baseline of 3 to 6 months of daily BBTs before relying on only this method of contraception. The client uses this baseline to predict ovulation and abstains from unprotected intercourse from the fifth day prior to the earliest expected ovulation (based on the number of days from the onset of menses to the rise of temperature in past cycles) through the third day after, as determined from temperature graph changes (Adasczik, 1981a).

Cervical Mucus Method

Mucus, secreted by exocrine glands lining the cervical canal, changes during the menstrual cycle in response to hormone levels. In the course of a normal menstrual cycle, a woman experiences menses, then progresses through a series of stages: a few days of a dry sensation, early mucus (milky white, translucent, yellow, or clear, sometimes tinged with old or new blood, sticky at first, then smooth), ovulatory mucus (lubricative, clear, stretchable), postovulatory mucus (sticky or pasty), dryness, and finally menses again. Mucus production decreases about 3 days after ovulation, and the woman is relatively "dry" until menstruation.

Ovulatory mucus is clear and slippery like eggwhite and has a high degree of stretchability (spinnbarkeit); it can be stretched up to 5 to 20 cm (Mastroianni, 1981; Fig. 11–11). Around the time of ovulation, the arrangement of the component mucin strands facilitates sperm transport (Fig. 11–12). The clinician can recognize a characteristic ferning pattern in ovulatory mucus that has been dried on a glass slide (Fig. 11–13). In contrast, luteal mucus is more thick, viscid, and white because of the hormonal influence of progesterone. It is usually described as pasty or tacky in consistency. Ferning does not occur with luteal mucus.

CLIENT EDUCATION

Clients can learn to distinguish ovulatory mucus with practice. Nofziger (1979) provides readable instructions and helpful diagrams. Teach the client about other variables that may affect what she feels when checking mucus. For example, arousal and coitus result in increased transudate and possible ejac-

FIGURE 11–12. Structural characteristics of cervical mucus. Schematic three-dimensional views of type E (estrogenic, ovulatory) mucus and type G (gestagenic, luteal) mucus. In both drawings the macromolecular cores (consisting of several long molecules side by side) are shown in black, with the surrounding hydration cells in white. These drawings show a sperm moving in the cervical plasma in the ovulatory mucus and a sperm blocked from passage by the luteal mucus. (Reproduced by permission of Odeblad E: Biophysical techniques of assessing cervical mucus and microstructure of cervical epithelium. In Elstein M, Moghissi KS, Barth KS (eds): Cervical Mucus in Human Reproduction. Geneva, World Health Organization, 1973, p 62.)

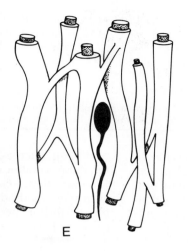
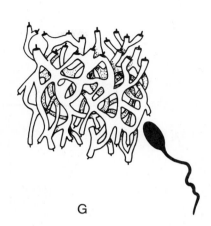

E   G

ulate in the vagina. Vaginal infections may increase the amount and alter the character of discharge.

INSTRUCTIONS FOR THE USER OF THE CERVICAL MUCUS METHOD

Check cervical mucus in the following manner, starting optimally on the day after your period is over:

1. Use three sheets of toilet tissue over your hand and wipe the perineum from front to back, observing whether the sensation is dry, smooth, or very slippery (wet). Dry days, usually just after menstruation and again just before the next period starts, are days on which no discharge is felt. A smooth sensation is due to early mucus, a sign that ovulation is approaching (Nofziger, 1979). Lubri-

cation, a very wet sensation, is a sign of ovulation.

2. Look at the material on the tissue to observe the color (clear, white, or yellow).

3. Dip your fingertip into the secretion and lift. Observe whether the mucus is stretchy and determine its consistency (like eggwhite or pasty). Clear, eggwhitelike, stretchy mucus is characteristic around the time of ovulation.

4. Do not rely solely on cervical mucus observations during the dry (preovulatory) days (Marshall, 1976) just after your period.

5. Avoid intercourse prior to ovulation, i.e., when the discharge is smooth and of varied color.

6. Abstain from unprotected intercourse from at least 5 days before through 3 days after ovulation, based on the number of days from the onset of menses to the appearance of ovulatory mucus in past cycles.

7. You may need to keep careful records and practice this method for up to 1 year before becoming proficient enough to use it as your sole means of contraception. Note that the example on page 256 is meant as a general guide only; women differ significantly in their patterns.

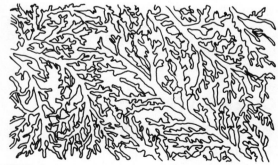

FIGURE 11–13. Ovulatory cervical mucus fern pattern. Due to its salt content, midcycle mucus produces a fernlike pattern when allowed to dry on a glass slide. This is best observed without a coverslip under low or medium power magnification. (Reproduced by permission from Fogel CI: Nursing practice with women. In Fogel CI, Woods NF (eds): Health Care of Women: A Nursing Perspective. St. Louis, 1981, CV Mosby Co.)

Symptothermal Method

Couples who use this method observe basal body temperatures, cervical mucus, and various symptoms associated with phases in the menstrual cycle. Mittelschmerz, a brief grabbing pain, and spotting sometimes occur with ovulation. Some couples can detect changes in the cervix at different phases in the men-

day:	1	2	3	4	5	6	7	8	9	10	11	12	13	14	15	16	17	18	19	20	21	22	23	24	25	26	27	28	1	2
observe:	B	B	B	B	B	d	d	d	m	m	m	m	m	m	m	m	m	m	d	d	d	d	d	d	d	d	d	d	B	B
texture:									p	p	p	s	s	l	l	p	p	p												
color:									o	o	o	o	o	c	c	o	o	o												
stretch:														+	+															
abstain:									A	A	A	A	A	A	A	A	A	A												

Key: B = bleeding; d = dry; m = mucus present; s = smooth; l = lubricative; p = pasty; o = opaque; c = clear; A = abstain from unprotected intercourse.

strual cycle. Some women experience breast tenderness and bloating in the luteal phase. Observations such as these supplement mucus examination, BBTs, and calendar calculations and may enable more accurate prediction of the days on which intercourse is least likely to lead to pregnancy.

Even so, user effectiveness for this combination of methods is in the range of only 85 to 94 per cent ("Natural Family Planning," 1983). Perhaps the complexity of so many steps in determining when to have intercourse accounts for some of the failures. Fertility awareness methods are not effective or convenient enough to be the first choice of sexually active couples for whom pregnancy would be unacceptable.

ADVANTAGES

Advantages of fertility awareness methods include (1) physiological safety, (2) low cost, (3) increased awareness of normal female body processes and fertility, and (4) compatibility with most religious beliefs. Some couples prefer a method for which they share responsibility, and they may wish to avoid chemicals, devices, or surgery. In some groups, fertility awareness methods may be the only contraceptives acceptable because they are known and understood; other methods may be considered foreign and unreliable.

DISADVANTAGES

The chief disadvantage of fertility awareness methods is low user effectiveness (see Table 11–12). Some couples may have difficulty in documenting a fertile period, and women with irregular cycles may have difficulty observing a pattern. Periodic abstinence is difficult for many couples. Temporary abstinence may be perceived as unnatural and not consistent with marriage or with either partner's role. Another possible problem is that if conception occurs, it may involve an

"old" egg, increasing the theoretical risk of fetal abnormalities (Hatcher et al, 1984).

Some clients cannot reliably use fertility awareness methods because of time, commitment, and/or necessity for handling one's genitals. It is not an appropriate method just after menarche or during the perimenopausal period, when cycles are irregular (Bernstein, 1983). It is particularly unreliable if a woman has just discontinued OCs (Nofziger, 1979). Women who work varying shifts cannot obtain reliable BBTs on which to base calculations. If either partner is away from home during a nonfertile period, it may be more difficult to practice abstinence when the couple is reunited. Mentally disabled people may find it difficult to keep accurate records and differentiate types of cervical mucus. Disabilities involving the upper extremities can also render fertility awareness methods too difficult or unreliable, although a partner's help may overcome this (Leavesley and Porter, 1982).

EFFECTS ON SEXUALITY

Spontaneity may be sacrificed with fertility awareness methods of family planning. For some couples, a high degree of mutual cooperation and responsibility may not be feasible. On the other hand, Klaus argues that fertility awareness "prevents routine and boredom and appears to add interest to the marriage" (Klaus, 1984, p 67).

OTHER REVERSIBLE CONTRACEPTIVE METHODS

Abstinence

Refraining from intercourse is a totally effective means of contraception. Couples rarely use it for prolonged periods, but it may be useful along with fertility awareness methods or before obtaining another contraceptive. Prolonged abstinence from any sexual activity may be very difficult for one or both partners; it may interfere with resumption or initiation of sexual intercourse. Gemme (1980) suggests that orgasmic noncoital sex, practiced by many but rarely discussed, should be legitimized as a contraceptive. Regardless of personal feelings about abstinence or noncoital sexual expression, the health care professional should show respect for a client's choice of these as a contraceptive method.

Coitus Interruptus (Withdrawal)

Coitus interruptus is of historical and contemporary significance. The Bible mentions its use, and it was largely responsible for falling population growth rates in nineteenth century Europe (Djerassi, 1981). However, in a 1976 U.S. study, only 2 per cent of currently married women aged 15 to 44 reported using this method (Potts, 1985). It may still be used more commonly than has been reported, since some users may not identify it as a method of birth control when questioned. Its use is important among adolescents (Withington, Grimes, and Hatcher, 1983).

To use this method, a man removes his penis from the vagina before ejaculation, so that he ejaculates away from the vagina and external genitalia (Gillmor-Kahn, Oakley, and Hatcher, 1982). A couple using this method with every act of intercourse should theoretically experience an effectiveness rate of 85 per cent (Gillmor-Kahn, Oakley, and Hatcher, 1982). Actual user effectiveness rates are lower (see Table 11–12). Advantages of this method include its constant availability at no cost and its lack of medical side effects.

Lack of success with this method may be due to the presence of sperm in the preejaculate, which is emitted without the man's being aware of it. It is frequently difficult for some men to predict when they will ejaculate, and some ejaculate soon after insertion. Cooperation and effective communication are important; these may be obstacles, especially for adolescents (Withington, Grimes, and Hatcher, 1983). Sometimes, sexual dysfunctions begin when a couple use coitus interruptus. Some women are unable to achieve orgasm because of their fear that they will become pregnant if their partner's timing is not perfect. It may be frustrating to interrupt lovemaking, and women as well as men may experience decreased desire or lack of full enjoyment. It is a challenge to the professional to teach clients about other, more reliable options while at the same time supporting them for their use of coitus interruptus.

Lactation

Some women rely on lactation to prevent pregnancy. The hormone prolactin inhibits luteinizing hormone, which is a major factor responsible for ovulatory menses. Postpartum amenorrhea lasts 4 to 24 months in breast-feeding mothers and only 2 to 3 months in non–breast-feeding mothers. Pregnancy rates are lower among lactating women whose children receive no other food supplement than among those who supplementally bottle feed their babies. There is the greatest likelihood of a contraceptive effect if sucking is vigorous and if feedings occur every 2 to 4 hours. After menses resume, the risk of pregnancy is the same in breast-feeding and non–breast-feeding women. Because ovulation normally precedes menses, couples who wish to prevent pregnancy cannot reliably do so by using lactation as a method. From 3 to 7 per cent of breast-feeding women conceive before their first postpartum menses (Hatcher et al, 1986). The significance of lactation as a contraceptive practice is apparent only in large-scale international studies.

STERILIZATION

Sterilization, the surgical interruption of the pathway for sperm or ova, is the most common form of contraception for married women in the United States (Hatcher et al, 1988). There are at least 137 million sterilized adults in the world, 16.6 million of them in the United States. By 1984, the worldwide number of voluntary sterilizations had increased seven times over that in 1970 (Hatcher et al 1988; "Sterilizations not Declining," 1986). In the United States, about one-half million women elect sterilization every year ("Research Continues," 1988). Of U.S. women aged 15 to 44 and married, about 20 per cent rely on sterilization, about half on tubal ligation and half on spouse's vasectomy (Moore, 1980; Lageson and Griffith, 1982).

General Concerns

DECISION-MAKING

Elective sterilization involves the issue of client autonomy. Caregivers are challenged to respect the opinions of any individual over 18 years of age who is rational and intellectually competent. If one respects the autonomy of an adult, one would not try to dissuade a rational and competent individual over 18 years of age who clearly understands the advantages and disadvantages of sterilization. To do so would be to deny the essential autonomy of that individual. To persuade or coerce an adult is to act paternalistically, as if the professional knows what is best for the client.

Historically, physicians have acted paternalistically toward women regarding sterilization. The American College of Obstetrics and Gynecology recommended restriction of sterilization to women whose age, multiplied by the number of living children, was 120 or greater. Thus, sterilization was available to a 40-year-old woman with three children or to a 24-year-old woman with five. Unless the woman had borne "sufficient" children, sterilization was denied. On the other hand, two physicians in South Carolina refused prenatal care to Medicaid recipients who had two or more children unless they agreed to postpartum sterilization—an example of the opposite kind of discrimination (McNall, 1980).

Regulations govern sterilization whenever federal funds are used. Regulations prevent federal reimbursement for sterilization for individuals who (1) are less than 21 years of age, (2) are mentally incompetent, or (3) do not sign a standard federal consent form *at least 30 days before* the procedure (McNall, 1980). These are federal rules; states may apply these or other regulations when state funds are to be used. Such regulations protect the retarded against involuntary sterilization and make it less likely that they will undergo voluntary sterilization.

Complete client preparation requires that the nurse address all of the issues in the

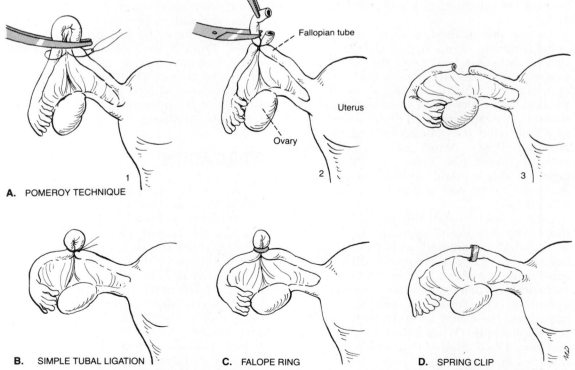

A. POMEROY TECHNIQUE

B. SIMPLE TUBAL LIGATION **C.** FALOPE RING **D.** SPRING CLIP

FIGURE 11–14. Tubal ligation techniques. The Pomeroy technique is the most common. (From Luckmann J, Sorensen KC: Medical-Surgical Nursing. 3rd ed. Philadelphia, WB Saunders, 1988.)

following mnemonic, *braided:* *b*enefits, *r*isks, *a*lternatives, *i*nquiries, *d*ecision to change, *ex*-planation, and *d*ocumentation (Hatcher et al, 1986). Be sure to provide clients with an opportunity to read carefully and discuss the informed consent release before they sign. The nurse may need to ensure special pro-visions for mentally handicapped clients. There is no ethical or legal support for re-quiring partner or spouse consent before sterilization. Today, The American College of Obstetrics and Gynecology recommends that clients seek a second opinion if sterili-zation is recommended for a medical reason and if it is not a couple's contraceptive choice (Adasczik, 1981b).

ADVANTAGES

Sterilization is extremely effective as a con-traceptive. For vasectomy, the failure rate is 0.15 per cent; for tubal ligation the failure rate is 0.04 per cent. Couples who use steri-lization for contraception enjoy high contra-ceptive efficacy, convenience, freedom from systemic side effects, and spontaneity of in-tercourse.

DISADVANTAGES

Sterilization must be considered permanent. The fact that sterilization is not easily revers-ible is an advantage to its use as a contracep-tive but a disadvantage to clients who change their mind about parenting. Reversibility de-pends on the type of procedure that was done originally as well as on the reversal technique. The reversibility rate ranges from 5 to 90 per cent for vasectomy and from 10 to 90 per cent for tubal ligation (Hatcher et al, 1986). In women, the clip method may be most reversible because it interferes least with blood supply. As a rule, the shorter the fallopian tube postsurgically, the smaller the chance of reversibility and pregnancy (Fogel, 1981). Microsurgical restoration after tubal occlusion by ligation or mechanical process may be successful in 50 to 70 per cent of clients (Hatcher et al, 1986). The relatively high one-time expense of sterilization may deter some potential clients, although the procedure is covered by major health insur-ance policies.

EFFECTS ON SEXUALITY

The greater freedom from fear of pregnancy brings relief and reduced anxiety and often healthier, more spontaneous sexual relations for both partners. Valuing a safe and non-invasive method, some couples may choose sterilization in order to avoid the risks asso-ciated with other methods. Some individuals choose sterilization out of a concern for fu-ture generations; they take responsibility for not conceiving unwanted children.

Tubal Ligation

Bilateral tubal ligation (BTL) is a procedure in which the fallopian tubes are ligated and cut, clipped, plugged, or cauterized to pre-vent ova from traveling into the uterus (Fig. 11–14). The fallopian tubes may be ap-proached via the abdomen, either by lapa-roscopy or minilaparotomy, or via the vagina. Laparoscopy is usually done under general anesthesia, utilizes gas in the peritoneal cavity for visibility, leaves a small scar, and cannot be done right after delivery. Minilaparotomy requires only local anesthesia and leaves a small scar. For either, the client is cleansed, draped, and incised. The tubes are identified carefully and then occluded by resection, clips, bands, or cauterization. The clinician then sutures up the incision. With either abdominal approach there are low rates of significant complications (0.9 to 1.5 per cent in international studies; Pritchard, Mc-Donald, and Gant, 1985). The vaginal ap-proach is equally effective and does not in-volve a visible scar but yields up to twice the rate of complications, such as infection and hemorrhage. The reader may wish to refer to Adasczik's (1981b) comparison of 19 vari-ations of tubal ligation.

CLIENT EDUCATION

Requirements for federally reimbursed ster-ilization affect the client and dictate certain nursing interventions. The client must have signed her consent 30 days *beforehand* if she wishes a BTL while under care for a delivery or abortion. This is designed to protect women from making a decision for a BTL around the time of labor and delivery or pregnancy termination. However, it means that some women go without sterilization because of not having met the 30-day re-quirement. Nurses, as client advocates, must inform their clients well ahead of time (U.S. Department of HEW, 1978). Stress the need for contraception postpartally until the operation.

There was no relationship between sterilization and altered menstrual pattern in one investigation (Bhiwandiwala, Mumford, and Feldblum, 1982) when prior contraceptive use and prior menstrual history were both considered. Women who are discontinuing use of OCs or an IUD following BTL need information on how their menses may change, since their previous contraceptive may have altered their menses.

INSTRUCTIONS FOR THE CLIENT WHO CHOOSES BTL

Provide the client with the following directions:

1. Bathe thoroughly before the procedure.
2. Arrange to have a companion drive you home.
3. Understand that pain at the incision site, in the pelvis, or in the shoulder or chest is likely but not usually severe.
4. After your operation, rest for 2 days; avoid strenuous lifting for a week; use aspirin or acetaminophen to reduce discomfort; return for follow-up in 1 month or sooner if fever (> 100°F), fainting, severe abdominal pain, or bleeding from the incision develops; and avoid intercourse until it is comfortable, usually in about 7 days. You do not need birth control *if* you can be sure you did not ovulate within 48 hours of the procedure (Hatcher et al, 1988).

ADVANTAGES

Female sterilization can usually be done at the time of some other abdominal surgeries, cesarean section, or vaginal delivery, which can be a convenience. Given correct timing, it is effective immediately. Once the procedure has been done, there is virtually no risk of reanastomosis of the fallopian tubes, so the woman and her partner can enjoy freedom from any concern about pregnancy.

DISADVANTAGES

BTL by minilaparotomy or laparoscopy very rarely results in serious complications such as tears of the mesosalpinx, burns on the bowel, perforation of the uterus, hemorrhage, and infection (Fogel, 1981; Hatcher et al, 1986). Some women experience alterations in ovulation, menorrhagia, or cyst formation after BTL (Pritchard, McDonald, and Gant, 1985). This is believed to be due to alteration in blood supply to the adnexae and ovaries. Some women experience increased menstrual pain after BTL; this may be due to resumption of ovulatory cycles if the woman had previously used OCs.

Vasectomy

Vasectomy is a procedure in which each vas deferens is ligated in two places, then cut between the ties so sperm cannot mingle with the ejaculate (Fig. 11–15). Vasectomy is associated with lower morbidity, mortality, and cost and greater possibility of reversal than BTL.

Socioeconomic variables appear to influence the popularity of sterilization. The 968,000 Americans sterilized in 1982 represented a 15 per cent drop from 1981. The number of reported vasectomies decreased by about 30 per cent (from roughly 425,000 to 300,000) from 1981 to 1982. One explanation for this is media coverage of a controversy over long-term side effects of vasectomy. Another factor may have been the rise in unemployment. At the time when men lost their jobs they also lost their health insurance benefits, which may have covered vasectomy costs ("Sterilizations Off," 1984). Also, the pool of men who could consider sterilization each year is decreased by the number who have already been sterilized. Vasectomy rates may be on the rise again, perhaps because fears of adverse side effects have been laid to rest by reliable research. The number of men choosing vasectomy rose to over 450,000 in 1983 (Hatcher et al, 1988).

INSTRUCTIONS FOR THE CLIENT WHO CHOOSES VASECTOMY

Provide the following directions to the client before the procedure:

1. Trim the pubic hair with scissors.
2. Bathe thoroughly.
3. Arrange for someone to drive you home.
4. You may expect to be cleansed and draped, injected with a local anesthetic, and incised in the scrotum. The physician will identify, cut, and tie or coagulate the vas deferens on each side. This procedure takes about 10 to 15 minutes. Absorbable sutures are usually used. Following the procedure,

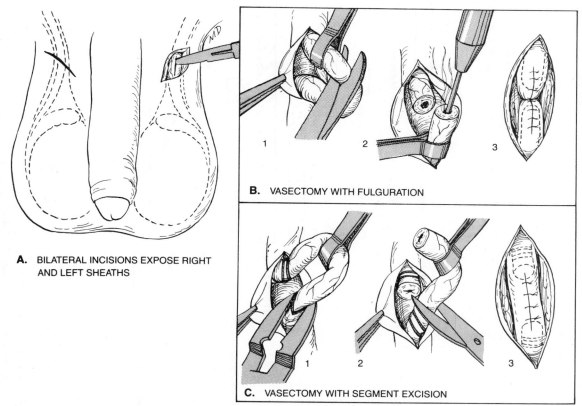

A. BILATERAL INCISIONS EXPOSE RIGHT AND LEFT SHEATHS

B. VASECTOMY WITH FULGURATION

C. VASECTOMY WITH SEGMENT EXCISION

FIGURE 11–15. Vasectomy. (From Luckmann J, Sorensen KC: Medical-Surgical Nursing. *3rd ed. Philadelphia, WB Saunders, 1988.)*

you will be observed at the clinic for 15 to 30 minutes. A man is not sterile until about 4 to 6 weeks or 6 to 36 ejaculations after the vasectomy. Negative sperm counts at follow-up demonstrate sterility and at 6 to 12 months rule out recanalization (Olds, London, and Ladewig, 1984).

5. Plan to rest for 2 days after the procedure and avoid strenuous exercise for 1 week. Protected intercourse may be resumed after 2 or 3 days if comfortable.

6. You may experience some swelling, bleeding, and discomfort. To reduce swelling and pain, use a scrotal support, ice packs to the areas, and aspirin. Sitz baths also promote healing.

7. Return for a follow-up appointment in 1 to 6 weeks to verify healing. See your caregiver without delay if you experience fever (> 100.4°F), bleeding from the incision, excessive pain or swelling (Hatcher et al, 1988), or pus or redness at the incision sites.

ADVANTAGES

Vasectomy permits a man to take responsibility for contraception and costs about one fifth as much as female sterilization. Evidence presented at meetings of the American Public Health Association confirmed the safety of vasectomy. Researchers studied the incidence of 50 diseases in 10,000 vasectomized men and matched controls. Most of the subjects had had their vasectomy 8 to 10 years earlier. They found vasectomized men had an increased incidence of only one condition: localized inflammation around the incision site, experienced by 4 per cent of men in the first year after the procedure. They found no increase in the incidence of immunopathological conditions (asthma, multiple sclerosis, arthritis), cardiovascular diseases, cancer, gout, hepatitis, erectile dysfunction, and hypothyroidism ("Study of Some," 1984).

DISADVANTAGES

For some couples, it is a disadvantage to have to continue with other birth control until all the sperm stored in the reproductive tract have been expelled. This usually takes 4 to 6 weeks but may take several months (Pritchard, McDonald, and Gant, 1985). Physically,

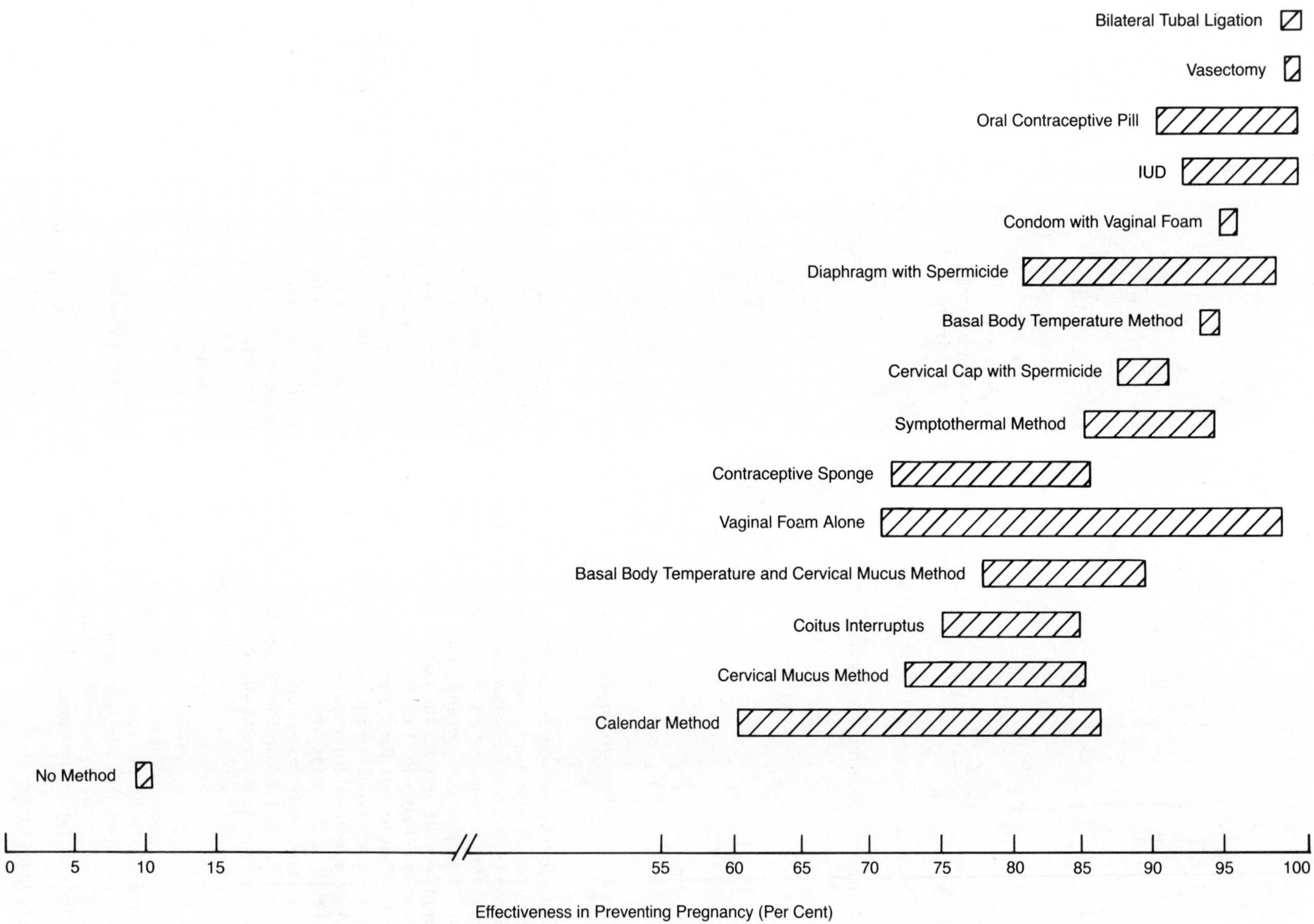

Bilateral Tubal Ligation
Vasectomy
Oral Contraceptive Pill
IUD
Condom with Vaginal Foam
Diaphragm with Spermicide
Basal Body Temperature Method
Cervical Cap with Spermicide
Symptothermal Method
Contraceptive Sponge
Vaginal Foam Alone
Basal Body Temperature and Cervical Mucus Method
Coitus Interruptus
Cervical Mucus Method
Calendar Method
No Method
0
5
10
15
55
60
65
70
75
80
85
90
95
100
Effectiveness in Preventing Pregnancy (Per Cent)

FIGURE 11–16. A comparison of effectiveness rates of birth control methods.

TABLE 11–13. Summary of Comparative Efficacy Rates of Major Contraceptive Methods

Method	Average User Effectiveness (%)
Reversible Methods	
Oral contraceptives	90–99.5
Intrauterine device	92–99.9
Barrier methods	
Diaphragm with spermicide	81–98
Cervical cap with spermicide	87–91.6
Condom with vaginal foam	95.0
Vaginal foam alone	71–98.5
Contraceptive sponge	72–86
Fertility awareness methods	
Symptothermal	85–94
Basal body temperature	93.4
Basal body temperature and cervical mucus	78–88.8
Cervical mucus	72–85
Calendar (rhythm)	60–85.6
Coitus interruptus	75–84
Irreversible Methods	
Sterilization	
Bilateral tubal ligation	99.96
Vasectomy	99.85
Chance (No Method Used)	10

the primary disadvantages are associated with the surgical procedure itself. Mild tenderness immediately after the surgery is common. Some clients experience infection (1.5 per cent), hematoma (1.6 per cent), epididymitis (1.4 per cent), or granuloma (0.3 per cent) (Hatcher et al, 1986). Some men may be apprehensive about systemic side effects, although there is no scientific basis for this. The sensitive nurse is aware that her client's partner may have questions and concerns about the procedure and will arrange for her to have an opportunity to discuss this also.

SUMMARY

Effective contraception hinges on the acceptance of oneself as a person who is valuable and worthy of respect, as a sexual being, and as a potential parent. In contraceptive interventions, the nurse can reinforce or introduce these ideas. This chapter began with an overview of the nursing process as it applies to contraceptive clients. The nurse can use these guidelines for subjective and objective assessment, diagnosis, planning, and intervention. We organized contraceptive concerns around Roy's (1980) adaptation model, stressing self-concept, role function, and the interdependence aspects of contraception de-

cision-making. Nursing goals include more than simply preventing unwanted pregnancy. The perceptive nurse fosters a positive self-concept, positive expressions of the client's sexuality, and positive relationships with others.

Although we have discussed currently available contraceptive methods as well as some not yet approved in the United States, none is perfect; all have some drawbacks as well as advantages. Table 11–13 summarizes efficacy rates, and Figure 11–16 presents effectiveness in a chart form, which the nurse can share with clients. It is a challenge to the nurse to provide up-to-date contraceptive information fairly and to assist the client in deciding on the best method for her situation. Because contraceptive methods and usage are not ideal, legal abortion remains essential as a back-up method for the prevention of unwanted births.

Choice and use or nonuse of a contraceptive has much to do with a person's concept of body and sexuality. Contraceptive decisions frequently mark a turning point in the degree of commitment in a relationship and/or an epoch of growth in maturing and role mastery. Many professionals enjoy the challenge of facilitating this growth.

REFERENCES

Adasczik JP: Contraceptive methods. In Smith ED (ed): Women's Health Care. Norwalk, Appleton-Century-Crofts, 1981a.

Adasczik JP: Sterilization by tubal ligation. In Smith ED (ed): Women's Health Care. Norwalk, Appleton-Century-Crofts, 1981b.

Adolescent gynecology: The initial pelvic examination. NAACOG Tech Bull No. 5. Nov 1979.

Alvarez F, Brache V, Fernandez E, et al: New insights on the mode of action of intrauterine contraceptive devices in women. Fertil Steril 49:768–773, 1988.

Americans misinformed about contraception, survey reveals. Contracept Technol Update 6:69–72, 1985.

Another look at IUDs. Med Lett 22:86, 1980.

Arnold CB: Proper use of the condom. Med Aspects Human Sexual 9:147–148, 1975.

Bachmann GA: Women who trust their method have fewer pregnancies. Fam Plann Perspect 13:149, 1981.

Barbach L: For Each Other: Sharing Sexual Intimacy. New York, Anchor, 1983.

Barnes FEF (ed): Ambulatory Maternal Health Care and Family Planning Services. Washington, DC, American Public Health Association, 1978.

Barrier methods. Popul Rep 12:H157–H190, 1984.

Berggren H, Zagornik AD: Teaching nursing process to beginning students. Nurs Outlook 16:32, 1968.

Bernstein G et al: When avoiding pregnancy is the issue. Patient Care Sept 15:2, 1978.

Bernstein IC: Terminating contraception when menopause nears: A psychiatric review. Med Aspects Human Sexual 17:32A, 1983.

Bhiwandiwala PP, Mumford SD, Feldblum PJ: Menstrual pattern changes following laparoscopic sterilization: A comparative study of electrocoagulation and the tubal ring in 1,025 cases. J Repro Med 27:249–255, 1982.

Britt SS: Fertility awareness: Four methods of natural family planning. JOGN Nurs 6:2, 9–18, 1977.

Brokaw AK, Baker NM, Haney SL: Fitting the cervical cap. Nurse Pract 13:49–55, 1988.

Burkman R: Selection criteria for oral contraceptive use: Current concepts. J Reprod Med 31:929–933, 1986.

Cagen R: The cervical cap as a barrier contraceptive. Contraception 33:487–497, 1986.

Campbell C: Nursing Diagnosis and Intervention in Nursing Practice. 2nd ed. JP Wiley & Sons, 1984.

Canadian-made contraceptive sponge now undergoing U.S. clinical trials. Contracept Technol Update 7:124, 1986.

Canavan PA, Lewis CA: The cervical cap: An alternative contraceptive. JOGN Nurs 10:271–273, 1981.

Cancer and Steroid Hormone Study of the Centers for Disease Control and The National Institute of Child Health and Human Development: The reduction in risk of ovarian cancer associated with oral contraceptive use. N Engl J Med 360:650–655, 1987.

Careful choice of vaginal methods ensures maximum safety, efficacy. Contracept Technol Update 9:18–20, 1988.

Cassell C: Swept Away: Why Women Fear Their Own Sexuality. New York, Simon & Schuster, 1984.

Celentano DD, Klassen AC, Weisman CS, Rosenstein, NB: The role of contraceptive use in cervical cancer: The Maryland cervical cancer case-control study. Am J Epidemiol 126:592–604, 1987.

Christakos AC: Vaginal spermicidal agents. Med Aspects Human Sexual 17:129–132, 1983.

Cole LP et al: An evaluation of the TCu 380Ag and the Multiload Cu375. Fertil Steril 43:214–217, 1985.

Connell EB: Barrier methods of contraception: A reappraisal. Int J Gynaecol Obstet 16:479–481, 1979.

Counseling makes a difference. Popul Rep 15:1–32, 1987.

Craig S, Hepburn S: The effectiveness of barrier methods of contraception with and without spermicide. Contraception 26:347–359, 1982.

Cramer DW et al: Tubal infertility and the intrauterine device. N Engl J Med 312:941–947, 1985.

Cramer DW, Goldman MB, Schiff I, et al: The relationship of tubal infertility to barrier method and oral contraceptive use. JAMA 257:2446–2450, 1987.

Cupit LG: Contraception: Helping patients choose. JOGNN 13(Mar/Apr Supplement):23–295, 1984.

Daling JR et al: Primary tubal infertility in relation to the use of an intrauterine device. N Engl J Med 312:937–940, 1985.

Dembo MH, Lundell B: Factors affecting adolescent contraception practices: Implications for sex education. Adolescence 14:657–663, 1979.

Depo-Provera controversy still brewing at FDA. Contracept Technol Update 4:85–87, 1983.

Despite court ruling, experts insist spermicides are safe. Contracept Technol Update 6:37–39, 1985.

Dickey RP: Manging Contraceptive Pill Patients. 4th ed. Durant, Creative Informatics, 1984.

Dickey, RP: Managing Contraceptive Pill Patients. 5th ed. Creative Informatics, Durant, 1987.

Djerassi C: The Politics of Contraception: Birth Control in the Year 2001. San Francisco, WH Freeman, 1981.

Dryfoos JG: Contraceptive use, pregnancy intentions and pregnancy outcomes among U.S. women. Fam Plann Perspect 14:81–94, 1982.

Elia D: Uses of RU 486: A clinical update. IPPF Med Bull 20:1–4, 1986.

Elkins TE et al: A model clinic approach to the reproductive health concerns of the mentally handicapped. Obstet Gynecol 68:185–188, 1986.

Erikson EH: Childhood and Society. 2nd ed. New York, WW Norton, 1963.

Family planning and teens: Confidentiality (Public Policy). Issues in Brief 1:1–2, 1981.

Fiscella K: Relationship of weight change to required size of vaginal diaphragm. Nurse Pract 7:21, 1982.

Fisher WA, Byrne D, White LA: Emotional barriers to contraception. In Byrne D, Fisher WA (eds): Adolescents, Sex, and Contraception. Hillsdale, Erlbaum, 1983.

Fisher WA et al: Psychological and situation-specific correlates of contraceptive behavior among university women. J Sex Research 15:38–55, 1979.

Fogel CI: Fertility control. In Fogel CI, Woods NF (eds): Health Care of Women: A Nursing Perspective. St. Louis, CV Mosby, 1981.

Forrest JD, Henshaw SK: What U.S. women think and do about contraception. Fam Plann Perspect 15:157–166, 1983.

Fortney J: Personal communication. Fam Health Int July 15, 1983.

Foxman B, Frerichs RR: Epidemiology of urinary tract infection: I. Diaphragm use and sexual intercourse. Am J Public Health 75:1308–1313, 1985.

Free MJ: Condoms: The rubber remedy. In Corson SL, Derman RJ, Tyrer LB (eds): Fertility Control. Boston, Little, Brown & Co., 1985.

Furstenberg FF, Moore KA, Peterson JL: Sex education and sexual experience among adolescents. Am J Public Health 75:1331–1332, 1985.

Gaines F: Secondary amenorrhea: Assessment plans. Nurse Pract 6:14, 1981.

Gemme R: Some sexological aspects of contraception. J Sex Educ Ther 6:20–21, 1980.

Gilbirds W, Jonas H: The cervical cap: An alternative barrier contraceptive method. Mo Med 79:216, 1982.

Gilligan C: In a Different Voice. Cambridge, Harvard University Press, 1982.

Gillmor-Kahn M, Oakley MM, Hatcher RA: Nurses in Family Planning. New York, Irvington, 1982.

Glick ID, Bennett SE: Psychiatric complications of progesterone and oral contraceptives. J Clin Psychopharmacol 1:350–367, 1981.

Gold RB: Depo-Provera: The jury still out. Fam Plann Perspect 15:78, 1983.

Gorosh M: Patterns of contraceptive use among female adolescents: Method consistency in a clinic setting. J Adol Health Care 3:96–102, 1982.

Grimes DA: Common mistakes patients make regarding contraception. Med Aspects Human Sexual 18:154, 1984.

Gromko L: Intrauterine devices. Nurse Pract 5:17, 1980.

Gunning JE: Common errors in use of the diaphragm. Med Aspects Human Sexual 15:43, 1981.

Hammerslough CR: Characteristics of women who stop using contraceptives. Fam Plann Persp 16:14–18, 1984.

Hatcher RA: Contraception: Future risks and responsibilities. May 28, 1988, American College Health Association Annual Meeting, Denver, CO.

Hatcher RA et al: Contraceptive Technology 1982–1983. 11th rev ed. New York, Irvington, 1982.

Hatcher RA et al: Contraceptive Technology 1984–1985. 12th rev ed. New York, Irvington, 1984.

Hatcher RA et al: Contraceptive Technology 1986–1987. 13th rev ed. New York, Irvington, 1986.

Hatcher RA et al: Contraceptive Technology 1988–1989. 14th rev ed. New York, Irvington, 1988.

Hawkins JW, Higgins LP: Health Care of Women: A Gynecological Assessment. Monterey, Wadsworth, 1982.

Health and Welfare Canada: Report on Oral Contraceptives, 1985 by the Special Advisory Committee on Reproductive Physiology to the Health Protection Branch, Health and Welfare Canada. Minister of Supplies and Services Canada, 1985.

Hendershot GE: Coitus-related cervical cancer risk factors: Trends and differentials in racial and religious groups. Am J Publ Health 73:299–301, 1983.

Hennekens CH et al: A case-control study of oral contraceptive use and breast cancer. J NCI 72:39–42, 1984.

Herold ES: The health belief model: Can it help us to understand contraceptive use among adolescents? J School Health 53:19–21, 1983.

Hester NR, Macrina DM: The health belief model and the contraceptive behavior of college women: Implications for health education. J Am Coll Health 33:245–252, 1985.

High rates of pregnancy and dissatisfaction mark first cervical cap trial. Fam Plann Perspect 14:48, 1981.

Highly effective Copper-T 380A IUD earns FDA approval. Contracept Technol Update 6:25–27, 1985.

Hormonal contraception: New long-acting methods. Popul Rep 15:K57–K87, 1987.

Intrauterine devices. Popul Rep 10:B101–B135, 1982.

Johnson JH: Contraception—The morning after. Fam Plann Perspect 16:266–270, 1984.

Johnson M: The cervical cap as a contraceptive alternative. Nurse Pract 10:37–45, 1985.

Johnston CD: Sexuality and birth control: Impact of outreach programming. Personnel Guid J 52:406–411, 1974.

Jones EF, Forrest GD, Henshon SK, et al: Unintended pregnancy, contraceptive practice and family planning services in developed countries. Fam Plann Perspect 20:53–57, 1988.

Jung CJ: Psychological Reflections: A New Anthology of His Writings, 1905–1961. Princeton, Princeton University Press, 1953.

Kafka D, Gold RB: Food and Drug Administration approves vaginal sponge. Fam Plann Perspect 15:146, 1983.

Kanell RG: Oral contraceptives: The risks in perspective. Nurse Pract 9:25–29, 62, 1984.

Keith LG, Berger GS, Jackson MA: Foams, creams, and suppositories. In Corson SL, Derman RJ, Tyrer LB (eds): Fertility Control. Boston, Little, Brown & Co., 1985.

Keith L, Hughey M, Berger G: Experience with modern inert IUDs to date: A review and comments. J Repro Med 20:125, 1978.

King L: The Cervical Cap Handbook for Users and Fitters. Iowa City, Emma Goldman Clinic, 1981.

Klaus H: Natural family planning. Med Aspects Human Sexual 18:59, 1984.

Knopp R: Arteriosclerosis risk: The roles of oral contraceptives and postmenopausal estrogens. J Repro Med 31:913–921, 1986.

Koch J: The Prentif contraceptive cervical cap: A con-temporary study of its clinical safety and effectiveness. Contraception 25:135, 1982.

Lageson J, Griffith R: Masters thesis. University of North Carolina, 1982.

Lane ME, Arceo R, Sobrero AJ: Successful use of the diaphragm and jelly by a young population: Report of a clinical study. Fam Plann Perspect 8:81–86, 1976.

Lawrence S: Gossypol: A potential male contraceptive? Am Pharm 21:57, 1981.

Layde PM, Beral V, Kay C: Further analyses of mortality in oral contraceptive users. Lancet I:541–546, 1981.

Layde PM, Ory HW, Schlesselman JJ: The risk of myocardial infarction in former users of oral contraceptives. Fam Plann Perspect 14:78–80, 1982.

Leavesley G, Porter J: Sexuality, fertility and contraception in disability. Contraception 26:417–441, 1982.

Lemberg E: The vaginal contraceptive sponge: A new non-prescription barrier contraceptive. Nurse Pract 9:24–37, 1984.

Lopez G et al: Two-year prospective study in Colombia of Norplant implants. Obstet Gynecol 68:204–208, 1986.

MacLachlan R, Peppin P: Sexuality and contraception for developmentally handicapped persons. Can Fam Physician 32:1631–1637, 1986.

Maine D: Family Planning: Its Impact on the Health of Women and Children. Columbia University, Center for Population and Family Health, 1982.

Marshall J: Cervical mucus and basal body temperature method of regulating births. Lancet II:282, 1976.

Martin JD et al: Good sex is as easy as pie: The role of permission, information, and empathy in brief sex therapy. J Sex Educ Ther 1:25–28, 1979.

Martin L: Health Care of Women. Philadelphia, JB Lippincott, 1978.

Mastroianni L: Reproductive physiology. In Romney SL et al (eds): Gynecology and Obstetrics: Health Care of Women. 2nd ed. New York, McGraw-Hill, 1981.

McIntier TM: Theory of interdependence. In Roy C (ed): Introduction to Nursing: An Adaptation Model. Englewood Cliffs, Prentice-Hall, 1976.

McNall LK: Contemporary Obstetric and Gynecologic Nursing. St. Louis, CV Mosby, 1980.

Miller MA, Brooten D: The Childbearing Family: A Nursing Perspective. Boston, Little, Brown & Co., 1983.

Mishell DR, Davajan V: Infertility, Contraception & Reproductive Endocrinology. Oradell, Medical Economics Books, 1986.

Moore E: Women and health. Public Health Rep Sept–Oct Suppl, 1980.

Morris JM: Mechanisms involved in progesterone contraception and estrogen interception. Am J Obstet Gynecol 117:167, 1973.

Morrison ES, Price MU: Values in Sexuality: A New Approach to Sex Education. Denver, Hart, 1974.

Nathanson CA, Becker MH: The influence of client-provider relationships on teenage women's subsequent use of contraception. Am J Public Health 75:33–38, 1985.

Natural family planning. NAACOG OGN Nursing Practice Resource No. 9. Nurses Association of the American College of Obstetricians and Gynecologists. Dec, 1983.

Needle RH: Factors affecting contraceptive practices of high school and college-age students. J School Health 47:340–345, 1977.

New study shows OCs don't reduce rheumatoid arthritis risk. Contracept Technol Update 6:12–13, 1985.

Nofziger M: A Cooperative Method of Natural Birth Control. 3rd ed. Summertown, The Book Pub Co, 1978.

Norplant TM: Instructions for clinicians. Program for the Introduction and Adaptation of Contraceptive Technology, 1982.

North Carolina Memorial Hospital: Department of Obstetrics and Gynecology Patient Education Materials, 1982.

Odeblad E: Biophysical techniques of assessing cervical mucus and microstructure of cervical epithelium. In Elstein M, Moghissi KS, Barth KS (eds): Cervical Mucus in Human Reproduction. Scriptor, 1973 (World Health Organization).

Olds SB et al: Obstetric Nursing. Boston, Addison-Wesley, 1980.

Olds SB, London ML, Ladewig PA: Maternal-newborn Nursing: A Family-centered Approach. 2nd ed. Boston, Addison-Wesley, 1984.

Oral contraceptives and cancer. U.S. Food and Drug Administration Drug Bulletin 14:2–3, 1984.

Oral contraceptives in the 1980s. Popul Rep 10:A189–A222, 1982.

Ory H: The noncontraceptive health benefits from oral contraceptive use. Fam Plann Perspect 14:82, 1982.

Peacock N: Contraceptive decision-making among adolescent girls. J Sex Educ Ther 8:31–34, 1982.

Perlmutter J: Pregnancy and the IUD. J Repro Med 20:133, 1978.

Peterman TA, Curran JW: Sexual transmission of human immunodeficiency virus. JAMA 256:2222–2226, 1986.

Pettiti DB: Epidemiologic assessment of the risks of oral contraception. J Reprod Med 31:887–891, 1986.

Pollock GH: Psychoanalytic considerations of fertility and sexuality in contraception. Israel Ann Psychiatr Related Disciplines 10:203–229, 1972.

Porter JB et al: Drugs and stillbirth. Am J Public Health 76:1428–1431, 1986.

Potts M: Coitus interruptus. In Corson SL, Derman RJ, Tyrer LB (eds): Fertility Control. Boston, Little, Brown & Co, 1985.

Pritchard JA, McDonald PC, Gant NF: Williams Obstetrics. 17th ed. Norwalk, Appleton-Century-Crofts, 1985.

Prosad AS et al: Effect of oral contraceptives on micronutrients and changes in trace elements due to pregnancy. In Moghissi KS, Evans TN (eds): Nutritional Impacts on Women. New York, Harper & Row, 1977.

Pyle CJ: Nursing protocol for diaphragm contraception. Nurse Pract 9:35, 1984.

Reading AE, Cox DN, Sledmere CM: Psychological issues arising from the development of new male contraceptives. Bull Br Psychol Soc 35:369–371, 1982.

Reichelt PA: The desirability of involving adolescents in sex education planning. J School Health 47:99–103, 1977.

Reitmeijer CA, Krebs JW, Reorino PM, Judson RN: Condoms as physical and chemical barriers against human imunodeficiency virus. JAMA 259:1851–1853, 1988.

Research continues to focus on sterilization side effects. Contracept Technol Update 9:37–39, 1988.

Roe DA: Nutritional effects of oral contraceptives. In Roe DA (ed): Drug Induced Nutritional Deficiencies. New York, AVI, 1976.

Roe DA: Nutrition and the contraceptive pill. In Winick M (ed): Nutritional Disorders of American Women. New York, AVI, 1977.

Romney SL et al: Gynecology and Obstetrics: The Health Care of Women. 2nd ed. New York, McGraw-Hill, 1981.

Rosenberg L et al: Breast cancer and oral contraceptive use. Am J Epidemiol 2:167–176, 1984.

Rosenfield A: The adolescent and contraception: Issues and controversies. Int J Gynaecol Obstet 19:57–64, 1981.

Roy C: The Roy adaptation model. In Riehl JP, Roy C (eds): Conceptual Models for Nursing Practice. 2nd ed. Norwalk, Appleton-Century-Crofts, 1980.

Rubin GL, Peterson HB: Researchers can now investigate long-term effects of OCs on cancer. Contracept Technol Update 6:7–12, 1985.

Rubin G, Layde PM, Peterson HB: Is this study valid? A closer look at the OC-breast Ca data. Contemp Obstet Gynecol 24:171–176, 1984.

Sandberg EC, Jacobs RI: Psychology of the misuse and rejection of contraception. Am J Obstet Gynecol 110:227–239, 1971.

Sapire KE: Contraception and Sexuality in Health and Disease. New York, McGraw-Hill, 1986.

Sarrel LJ, Sarrel PM: Sexual Unfolding: Sexual Development and Sex Therapies in Late Adolescence. Boston, Little, Brown & Co., 1979.

Schirm AL et al: Contraceptive failure in the United States: The impact of social, economic and demographic factors. Fam Plann Perspect 14:68–75, 1982.

Scrimshaw S: Women and the pill: From panacea to catalyst. Fam Plann Perspect 13:254–262, 1981.

Seamon B: Back to foam? Ms Aug:16, 1977.

Sharpe J: The birth controllers. In Dreifus C (ed): Seizing Our Bodies: The Politics of Women's Health. New York, Random House, 1978.

Siemens S, Brandzel RC: Sexuality: Nursing Assessment and Intervention. Philadelphia, JB Lippincott, 1982.

Silber TJ, Addlestone I, Ragsdale R: A birth control clinic within an adolescent medicine program at a children's hospital. J Sex Educ Ther 8:29–31, 1982.

Sondheimer S: Personal communication about the investigation of the vaginal spermicidal barrier. University of Pennsylvania, Department of OB/GYN, Family Planning Services Division, June 1988.

Speroff L: Safety of oral contraception: A quarrel with the recent literature. Contemp Obstet Gynecol 23:17–22, 1984.

Stewart F et al: My Body, My Health: The Concerned Woman's Book of Gynecology. New York, Bantam, 1981.

Sterilizations not declining, AVSC survey results show. Contracept Technol Update 7:139, 1986.

Sterilizations off sharply in 1982; drop due mostly to vasectomy decline. Fam Plann Perspect 16:40–41, 1984.

Study of some 20,000 men finds no evidence vasectomy has any adverse health consequences. Fam Plann Perspect 16:35–36, 1984.

Swanson JM: Knowledge, knowledge, who's got the knowledge? The male contraceptive career. J Sex Educ Ther 6:51–57, 1980.

Swenson I: Oral contraceptives. Presentation at North Carolina Nurses' Association meeting, District 11. April 9, 1981.

Teenage FP clients respond to strong direction about their choice of method from clinic staff. Fam Plann Perspect 17:223–224, 1985.

Thomsen RJ: Atlas of Intrauterine Contraception. Washington, DC, Hemisphere, 1982.

Three triphasic oral contraceptives now available in U.S. Contracept Technol Update 6:1–2, 1985.

Tietze C, Bongaarts J, Schearer B: Mortality associated with control of fertility. Fam Plann Perspect 8:6, 1976.

Tyrer LB: Oral contraception for the adolescent. J Reprod Med 29(Suppl):551–559, 1984.

Tyrer L: Contraceptive update. Presentation for 12th Annual Postgraduate Seminar for Nurse Practitioners in Family Planning, Sponsored by Planned Parenthood Federation of America and others, Philadelphia, PA, Feb 18, 1988.

U.S. Department of Health, Education, and Welfare: Information for women: Your sterilization operation. Department of Health, Education, and Welfare Publication No. (os) 79–50061, Washington, DC, U.S. Government Printing Office, 1978.

Using OCs safer for younger women than having child, CDC expert says. Contracept Technol Update 6:4–6, 1985.

Vaginal contraceptive sponge. Planned Parenthood Federation of America, 1983.

Why counseling counts! Popul Rep 15:J1–J28, 1987.

Winter L: The role of sexual self-concept in use of contraception. Fam Plann Perspect 20:123–127, 1988.

Withington AM, Grimes DA, Hatcher RA: Teenage Sexual Health. New York, Irvington, 1983.

Wolinsky, H: A woman's condom. Amer Health June:10, 1988.

Woodhouse A: Sexuality, femininity and fertility control. Women's Stud Int Forum 5:1–15, 1982.

12: Multidimensional Aspects of Caring for the Abortion Client

Colleen Keenan

The topic of induced abortion remains controversial in the United States and elsewhere despite its widespread and historical practice in most geographical areas. Political, ethical, religious, and economic factors contribute to the complexity of the abortion issue, making abortion much more than merely a routine medical or surgical procedure. Women with an unintentional and unwanted pregnancy who opt for termination have correspondingly complex health care needs. The termination or loss of a pregnancy before the fetus is capable of surviving separately from the mother, at approximately 24 to 26 weeks of gestation, is called *abortion*. More specifically, spontaneous abortion and miscarriage are terms used for loss as a result of fetal or maternal abnormality that precludes continued gestational development, whereas induced abortion refers to the deliberate termination of a pregnancy through surgical or chemical intervention.

In this chapter the historical background, the ethical and legal perspectives, and the incidence of abortion are presented. Following sections are devoted to the process of decision-making and the psychological, developmental, and sociocultural factors that

combine to make pregnancy termination a critical life event for many women. Finally, the nursing role in the assessment, counseling, preparation, and care of the client during and after the abortion procedure are discussed.

ABORTION AND SEXUALITY

Abortion and sexuality are closely interwoven when viewed from a personal and political context. On the personal level, whether or not sexual activity leads to an unwanted pregnancy and, subsequently, to an abortion depends on many individualized factors, such as the use of contraceptives and their effectiveness as well as the availability and quality of internal and external resources, that is, the means to meet the demands of the current situation. On the political level, prevailing social and cultural mores influence not only the sexual behavior of individual women and men but also social regulation of these behaviors, including abortion, through social action, public policy decisions, and legislation.

Both abortion and sexuality are linked to women's self-determination and control over their bodies. However, sexuality is more than a form of pleasurable self-expression and

The author expresses appreciation to David Gandell, MD, for comments on an earlier draft of this chapter.

individual assertion; abortion is more than a private choice. Varying perspectives on sexuality and abortion lead to different formulations of the relationship between the two concepts. From a feminist perspective, the ease of access to both birth control and legal abortion reflects women's power and social status, while restrictions in these practices coincide with limitations on the social and sexual autonomy of women (Petchesky, 1985). Therefore, the degree of access to abortion and contraception is seen as an important indicator of women's self-determination and ability to make reproductive choices. From a highly conservative and traditional perspective, sexuality outside of marriage is something to be discouraged, and contraception and abortion are viewed as providing license for and as facilitative of "irresponsible" sexual behavior. From a family planning and epidemiological perspective, changes in social mores during the early seventies have been associated with increased sexual activity outside of marriage, corresponding with increased use of contraception (Zelnick and Kantner, 1977) and legal abortion. However, trends toward the use of less effective contraceptives (Gerrard, 1982) are likely to lead to a higher incidence of unintentional pregnancies and, as a result, to have an impact on the health status of women. The diverse social and political viewpoints held by various groups arise from specific interests and concerns. All are strong forces within our society. The contrasts highlighted by these and other perspectives discussed in this chapter underscore some of the fundamental issues many women face when they have an unintentional or unwanted pregnancy. Women with an unintentional pregnancy may experience conflict in response to these divergent social attitudes.

HISTORICAL BACKGROUND

Historical Practices

Surgical techniques of abortion have been documented since the time of Hippocrates. Among his writings is included a full description of graduated cervical dilators similar to those introduced by Hegar in the late 1800s. Archaeological excavations of ancient Rome have revealed a full range of surgical equipment needed to perform an abortion, such as several forms of the vaginal speculum and syringes for the purpose of irrigating the uterus. Cervical dilation was accomplished using techniques similar to present methods, such as laminaria made of asparagus steeped in alcohol, dried slippery elm, and compressed seaweed. However, the high incidence of infection discouraged their use until the relatively recent availability of methods for sterilization of the laminaria. In the late eighteenth and early nineteenth centuries, abortion was commonly performed by flushing the uterus with caustic substances or by inserting sticks of silver nitrate into the cervix. The associated problems of bleeding and infection with such past methods were diminished after curettage, or scraping the uterine lining, was introduced in the latter part of the nineteenth century (Potts, Diggory, and Peel, 1977).

Various home remedies and herbal folk medicines were also used by women themselves to bring on a missed period or to actually abort an established pregnancy. In the nineteenth century, gunpowder solutions, quinine, oil of juniper, pennyroyal, and ergot were used with varying (and most likely low) levels of success as abortifacients (Potts, Diggory and Peel, 1977).

Illegal Abortions

It is clear from historical documentation that despite legal prohibitions beginning in the early 1800s induced abortions persisted as a common practice. Typical methods commonly implemented by illegal abortionists of the nineteenth and early twentieth centuries included the recommendation to ingest abortifacient chemicals such as lead and phosphorus, introduction of foreign bodies into the cervical canal and the uterine cavity, intrauterine injection of liquid solutions such as soapy water, and illegal dilation and curettage procedures.

These common practices persisted into the twentieth century until abortion was legalized. An estimated 1 million women died each year from illegal and unsafe abortion attempts in Europe alone before the recent abortion law reforms (Potts, Diggory, and Peel, 1977). After legalized abortion, the incidence of spontaneous abortions decreased in the United States, suggesting that many of the abortions formerly reported as "spontaneous" were in fact illegal. In a review of the public health effects of legal abortion, Tietze

(1984) notes that mortality associated with all types of abortion (legal, illegal, and spontaneous) has declined markedly and can be attributed to several factors, including the increased use of more reliable contraceptive methods and the improved management and prevention of serious complications of abortion such as hemorrhage and uterine perforation. However, the shift from illegal and frequently unsafe abortions to legal procedures by competent physicians is the most important factor in abortion mortality reduction. The practice of legal abortions has also contributed to the reduction in pregnancy-related mortality and morbidity during the past decade through the termination of a larger proportion of medically and psychosocially high-risk pregnancies and the circumvention of the higher rate of pregnancy complications associated with illegally attempted abortions (Tietze, 1984). In addition, access to legal abortions has increased the numbers of abortions being performed early in pregnancy when the procedure is inherently safer. Undoubtedly, the higher mortality and morbidity rates would recur if women were again restricted from access to legal abortion by qualified health care providers.

Legal Reform of Abortion Laws

A wave of social change related to women's rights in the 1960s and early 1970s culminated in the U.S. Supreme Court's 1973 decision in *Roe* v. *Wade*. This ruling (*Roe* v. *Wade*, 1973) determined that the states could not interfere with a woman's right to privacy, including the right to decide whether or not to bear children, and that antiabortion laws did, in fact, violate this right. The court did not recognize the fetus as a full person and in effect concluded that the constitution and the protection of persons did not extend to fetuses. In summary, the *Roe* v. *Wade* decision included the following: (1) During the first trimester of pregnancy, the woman and her physician may alone decide about pregnancy termination. (2) During the second trimester of pregnancy, the woman is still free to decide to have an abortion, but the state is permitted to regulate abortion procedures to the extent that they are reasonably related to maternal health. (3) After fetal viability, in the third trimester, the state has the right to limit abortions to situations in which preservation of life or health of the pregnant woman is jeopardized.

The Supreme Court has also ruled on the access to abortion services for minors. Individual states may require an unmarried minor to notify or obtain consent of parents; if the minor does not wish to comply, she must be able to obtain permission from a judge. Donovan (1983) cites several problems with this judicial bypass mechanism. Since most minors who do not want to consult with parents regarding an abortion have either poor family relationships or believe their parents would prevent them from obtaining an abortion, the process of standing before a judge may be unnecessarily traumatic. In addition, no constructive benefit for the minor in terms of improved family communication or contributions to informed consent are apparent. In states in which this additional barrier to abortion access for minors is operational, it is likely that some young women decide to continue a pregnancy that they otherwise would have terminated (Clary, 1982).

Legal debate also surrounds the access of poor women to federal funds for an abortion. The Hyde Amendment (1976) allows the restriction of federal Medicaid funds for abortion except in cases in which the woman's life is in danger. Subsequent legislation regarding federal funding of abortion had slightly more lenient restrictions, adding the exceptions of reported rape or incest or if two physicians certify that the health of the woman would be permanently damaged if the pregnancy were not terminated (Smith, 1982). In 1979, the Supreme Court supported the constitutionality of the power of individual states to deny funding for elective abortions. The degree of flexibility with which these laws are interpreted varies according to each state. The ultimate outcome, however, is that actual access to elective abortion is not guaranteed for indigent women in the same manner that it is available to women with greater economic resources.

Another area of controversy has been the issue of informed consent. Informed consent implies that individuals can act autonomously in their own behalf to make decisions regarding their care, based on information provided by the health care professional (Kirby, 1983). Informed consent, based on the principle of individual autonomy, is an attempt to avoid inappropriate and paternalistic interventions that are not in the recipient's own best interests. The identification of specific informational content necessary for informed consent in a given situation must be tailored to the needs of the individual. Although women have the right to be informed of the risks and benefits of an abortion just as in any other surgical procedure, legislation mandating specific descriptions of fetal development and lengthy lists of physical and emotional implications of abortion were ruled unconstitutional in *City of Akron* v. *Akron Center for Reproductive Health* (1983).

An unresolved controversy is reflected by The Human Rights Amendment previously proposed by Jesse Helms and groups such as the Moral Majority and Right to Life. The proposal would protect the life of the fetus in all situations. Those opposed to such an amendment take the stance that it would interfere with the woman's individual freedom to choose for herself how to resolve an unintended pregnancy.

The abortion controversy is a dilemma for which no simple legal or moral solution is readily apparent. Politically active groups from both sides of the controversy, such as Right to Life and National Abortion Rights Action League (NARAL), are strong lobbying forces in both state and federal legislatures. Professionals practicing in women's health care should be informed regarding current state and national legislative issues. Professionals need to be aware of the legal rights of women related to privacy, the right to choose to either continue or terminate a pregnancy in consultation with a health care professional, and the right to informed consent in the same nonjudgmental manner as for any other surgical procedure, should the woman choose abortion. In addition, health care professionals must examine their own personal set of beliefs and values. If moral or religious beliefs prevent a professional, such as a nurse, from participating in the care of the woman requesting an abortion, she or he can refer the woman to another professional for the full range of services indicated, including counseling, screening, and the abortion itself.

ETHICAL CONSIDERATIONS

The ethical question of abortion is complicated by the real and potential conflicts between the pregnant woman and the fetus. There is no clear-cut answer to the question: Is abortion right or wrong? Arguments range from the very liberal to the very conservative. The issues germane to the ethical dilemma of abortion will be briefly summarized.

Personhood

Rights and responsibilities are associated with persons. The definition of personhood is a critical focus regarding the morality of abortion. There is no commonly accepted point between fertilization of the ovum and adulthood at which personhood begins. In contrast to a specific point in development, other criteria have also been suggested as definitive of personhood in addition to being living and being human, such as self-awareness and the capacity to reason (English, 1981). Many authors refer to the *process* of developing personhood as continuous. Therefore, personhood is not able to be clearly established from an ethical or legal perspective as occurring at any particular point in time, such as conception, at quickening, at birth, or even at adulthood.

Conflict of Rights

When discussing the concept of personhood, a conflict arises over the rights of the fetus versus the rights of the woman with an unwanted pregnancy; one directly opposes the other. Smith (1984) summarizes three positions related to the rights conflict issue: one position suggests that the fetus is a person and has a right to life that supersedes the right of a pregnant woman to exert autonomy or to make decisions about what happens to her body. In contrast, another position suggests that a fetus is not a person with fully developed rights and responsibilities; therefore, a woman's right to choose is the foremost concern. Finally, a third position suggests that even if a fetus is a person and has a right to life, a woman has no moral duty to sustain that life simply because it relies on her bodily resources; this is an argument proposed by Thomson (1971).

Third-trimester Abortions

Under very special circumstances, when the life or health of the mother is in jeopardy, third-trimester abortions (at or beyond 28 weeks' gestation) may be performed. Chervenak and associates (1984) have argued that this exception should be extended to cases in which reliable prenatal diagnostics can determine either that the fetus cannot survive postnatally or that cognitive function would be absent. Such is the case with anencephaly, a condition in which profound fetal defects include absence of the cranium and all or part of the brain. These authors argue that the benefit to parents in terms of reducing the time the woman must carry a fetus with a hopeless prognosis is not counterbalanced by any benefit to the fetus in prolonging life with usual or heroic measures.

Summary

Arguments can be made both in defense and against the morality of abortion. Positions can be taken concerning the rightness or wrongness of abortion in the diversity of contexts in which abortion occurs. However, the principles of individual autonomy, counterbalanced with personal rights and responsibilities, will continue to influence legislation and the thinking of clients and professionals alike. Health care professionals must be aware of the interplay among these factors and evaluate their own moral position on abortion in order to provide nonjudgmental care to individuals facing this decision.

INCIDENCE OF ABORTION

Most authors agree that despite adequate knowledge and the availability of effective contraception, unintentional pregnancies constitute approximately one half of all pregnancies (Dryfoos, 1982; Hilliard, Shank, and Redman, 1982; Klein, 1985). In the United States in 1983, 1,268,987 abortions were performed; this was a decrease over the number performed in 1982. Abortions account for about one third of all pregnancy outcomes; the remaining pregnancies end in live births, stillbirths, and miscarriages (Ellerbrock et al, 1987). An unintentional pregnancy may not necessarily be unwanted but rather mistimed, and the woman may choose childbearing as the outcome of the pregnancy. Conversely, another woman may terminate a planned pregnancy because of physical or psychoso-

cial health risks or because of severe fetal genetic abnormalities.

Although there is no stereotypical pattern, women who obtain abortions often tend to be young, white, unmarried, contraceptively inexperienced, and of low parity (O'Reilly, Dorfman, and Cates, 1982). A contrasting pattern of married, contraceptively experienced older women who have completed their families is not unusual, however. Although statistics provide important aggregate information about women seeking abortions, it is also useful to think about the contextual factors that influence the situation of an individual woman. If followed over the entire course of their reproductive lives, a large proportion of women now in their childbearing years will likely choose to continue one pregnancy at one given time and choose to abort a different pregnancy at another time (Murphy, Symington, and Jacobson, 1983). The decision to terminate a pregnancy is strongly influenced by a complex combination of psychological, developmental, and sociocultural factors. These factors are discussed in the following sections.

ABORTION AS A CRITICAL LIFE EVENT

Although abortion may not be experienced as a crisis per se, that is, with associated emotional dysfunction and disorganization of resources or means used to deal with a difficult situation, many women certainly identify abortion as a critical life event. Frequently, this decision is the first significant moral dilemma the woman has ever faced. Conflict between previously held beliefs regarding abortion and the personal exigencies of the situation is a common occurrence. Ambivalent feelings are a common pregnancy experience in the first trimester. Pregnancy also represents important psychological aspects of the woman as a sexual being, an adult, and a female. Socially, significant persons in the woman's life, such as parents, lover, or husband, may also have strong feelings about the pregnancy, playing an important role in the support of the woman and in some instances even contributing to a sense of crisis. Potential new social roles, such as mother and transition to full adult status, may be received with varying levels of comfort. In this section, the developmental, psychological, and sociocultural factors contributing to the experience of women electing to terminate a pregnancy are reviewed.

Developmental Factors

The outcome of a particular pregnancy may depend in part on developmental issues that color the woman's experience. Certain common characteristics of adolescent and adult development are likely to influence the way a woman experiences her pregnancy. In addition, the process of decision-making and self-evaluation provides a challenging opportunity for significant personal growth.

ADOLESCENCE

The establishment of intimate relationships outside of the family is a hallmark task of adolescence. When the need for intimacy is expressed sexually, the adolescent is frequently unprepared for the practice of contraception, if pregnancy is not desired. Many adolescents feel that contraception takes away from the spontaneity of sex, that it is not "natural," or that it connotes a planned sexual encounter. Peers take on an increasingly important role in the adolescent's life, and pressure to engage in sexual activity may be very strong within certain groups.

Independence from parents is a particularly acute issue during adolescence and can be initiated by sexual behavior departing from family norms and values. Pregnancy is also seen by many adolescents as a desirable sign of adulthood and independence. However, the development of autonomy and personal responsibility is a gradual process and many, particularly younger, adolescents may need assistance in assuming an appropriate level of responsibility for their pregnancy decision. For example, some adolescents may avoid active participation in the decision-making process and allow parents or significant others to make the decision for them (Brown, 1983). This compliance does not necessarily remove conflict, however, and feeling forced into a particular decision by external influences such as parents may lead to a negative emotional outcome regarding the pregnancy (Lewis, 1980).

Finally, the physical-sexual development during early adolescence and the necessary adjustment to a new female body image is followed closely by additional adjustments of body image changes related to pregnancy. These signs of sexuality and adult status can be perceived negatively by some adolescents, while for others the experience may be positive.

YOUNG ADULTHOOD

Issues arising in young adulthood concerning autonomy and intimacy are associated with questions about long-term commitment to one's partner, the suitability of the partner, and the couple's perceived readiness for parenting. Many young adults plan to begin their families at some point in the future rather than at the time of the unintentional pregnancy. Young adulthood is a time when career training and development are paramount goals for many individuals. Women in particular may feel conflict concerning career and family. However, when compared with adolescents, young adults generally tend to be better prepared to cope with complex problems such as pregnancy decisions and to use external resources such as friends, social workers, or financial counselors, more effectively (Olson, 1981).

MIDDLE ADULTHOOD

In the early years of middle adulthood, the transition to the thirties and beyond is frequently a "now or never" situation as the woman realizes that for her the traditional childbearing years are drawing to a close. This time squeeze may be accentuated by the typical life assessment common in the thirties. Major events leading to psychosocial changes are evident for many women in this age group (Reinke, Holmes, and Harris, 1985). An unintentional pregnancy and subsequent abortion is an example of such an event. Middle adulthood may increase the underlying ambivalence the woman may feel about pregnancy; this is particularly true for the primigravida. This situation may also be compounded by the woman's awareness that fertility gradually declines in the third decade and that another pregnancy at a later time may not be as easy to achieve.

In the latter part of middle adulthood, perimenopausal pregnancies (occurring in the late forties and early fifties) frequently present an unexpected dilemma. Women in this age group commonly have completed their family several years ago, and a major consideration is whether to begin the process of childbearing again. Perhaps even more importantly, the risk of genetic defects increases with advanced maternal age. A genetic amniocentesis can be performed at approximately 16 weeks of pregnancy; this provides additional information about the fetus and can be used as a basis for a pregnancy decision. For some women, however, there is no advantage to obtaining the amniocentesis because they would not terminate a pregnancy in any case beyond the first trimester. With first-trimester chorionic villus biopsy more widely implemented, this conflict may be resolved through earlier diagnosis of fetal genetic defects (Hogge, Hogge, and Golbus, 1986).

Psychological Factors

EMOTION AND COGNITION

These elements contribute to the psychological experience of abortion in several ways and intertwine to create the personal and individual aspects of the abortion experience. For example, on the affective level, strong emotions may interfere with a realistic perception of the situation at hand and may impede decision-making. The rational, cognitive processing of the alternatives available in an unintentional pregnancy may be mediated by varying affective tones of pleasure and sadness about this irrevocable situation. The subjective meaning of fertility and pregnancy, the established and newly tried coping patterns, and potential experiences of loss and ambivalence are all important aspects of the abortion experience.

SUBJECTIVE MEANING OF FERTILITY

The ability to become pregnant and to impregnate may have important significance for a couple. The associated feelings of fertility, adult status and its attendant rights and responsibilities, and the potential losses and gains connected with pregnancy are factors resulting from the individual meanings the person attaches to pregnancy. If one carefully examines the concepts of fertility, pregnancy, and parenthood, it is apparent that while they are linked and dependent upon one another, they are experienced as quite separate and unique. For example, while a woman may have barely considered whether she desires parenthood and its responsibilities, feelings of fertility and the potential for becoming pregnant may enhance her sense of self-worth as a woman and also serve to represent in a tangible way her valued relationship with her partner.

Major, Mueller, and Hildebrandt (1985) found that those women who attached strong meaning to the terminated pregnancy coped less well following the abortion, experiencing more physical complaints, and anticipating more negative consequences from the abortion. However, other important factors such as coping abilities and perceived social support are likely to mediate this potential effect.

COPING WITH UNINTENTIONAL PREGNANCY

Using the framework of Lazarus and Folkman (1985), coping is defined as the dynamic process of handling, through behavioral and cognitive strategies, either internal or external demands that are appraised as exceeding personal resources. The strategies called forth to cope with a critical life event such as abortion vary according to the specific nature of the situation as well as the woman's personal characteristics and resources. Appraisal of the situation is a cognitive process incorporating the assessment of personal and environmental resources. The potential appraisals resulting from this evaluation are benign-positive, threat, harm/loss, and challenge. Because of the complexity and changing nature of stressful life events as they unfold, these appraisals are often mixed.

When a person confronts a stressful situation such as an unintentional pregnancy, the potential threats to well-being may lead to an appraisal of harm or loss. Such threats might include disruption of one's future life goals, the more immediate fears of undergoing a surgical procedure, the loss of a potential child (regardless of the pragmatics of actually having and raising the child), and conflicts between one's idealized vision of what one would do based purely on moral/ethical grounds versus the actual situational demands of the present dilemma. Alternately, a woman's appraisal of unintentional pregnancy as a challenge may predominate or coexist with another appraisal in a given abortion situation. She may, for example, perceive this critical life event as an opportunity for self-evaluation and clarification of goals related to reproduction and parenting. Finally, benign appraisals certainly may occur in the situation of abortion, although the likelihood is diminished because of the complexity of the problem and the wider sociocultural and political context in which abortion is practiced.

Several techniques of coping have been described by Lazarus and Folkman (1985) and have been broadly categorized as (1) problem-focused and (2) emotion-focused coping. These two categories of coping refer to separate processes, in which attempts are made to manage or alter the stressful problem in the former, while attempts are made to regulate emotional responses to the problem in the latter (Lazarus and Folkman, 1985). In the situation of an unplanned pregnancy, an example of problem-focused coping would be the thorough examination of each of the available alternatives (abortion, adoption, and motherhood). Although this form of coping does not alter the pregnancy, it is likely to be helpful to the woman in her management and resolution of the problem. Problem-focused techniques can be based on established patterns of dealing with stressful problems as well as new approaches that augment the woman's coping repertoire. Emotion-focused coping can be seen in diverse ways, sometimes directed at lessening the emotions associated with the situation and sometimes at changing the meaning of the event. For example, minimization, distancing, and selective attention may be used to lessen negative emotional feelings. In some cases, negative feelings may result from self-blaming mechanisms. Self-blame is characterized by a person's assumption of responsibility for an uncontrollable (or unchangeable) event in an effort to feel better by enhancing a sense of control over the situation (Wortman, 1983). The woman may also use other techniques, such as positive comparison (e.g., "At least I don't have to have a saline abortion like my friend Mary."). In addition to the cognitive coping techniques mentioned previously, behavioral attempts such as seeking social support and activities to divert attention or alleviate stress (e.g., physical exercise, shopping, meditation, drinking alcohol, or use of prescription or illicit drugs) are also examples of coping techniques.

Another conceptualization useful in understanding the process of coping is an approach-avoidance dimension. Behaviors and cognitions included within this framework are designed to focus attention either directly toward or away from the stressful situation.

The degree to which the individual is disposed to confront or repress threat or stress determines, in part, the success of coping maneuvers within a given situation. For example, in the case of a woman with a suspicious breast lump of 2 months' duration, avoidant techniques such as trying to keep her mind off a biopsy (a potentially stressful medical procedure) scheduled for the following day may improve coping by allowing her to attend to matters at hand. Ignoring the suspicious breast lump may temporarily relieve her anxiety yet may make long-range coping more difficult. Similarly, approach techniques such as making sure her schedule is cleared for the following day's biopsy appointment and ventilating feelings about her fears are more likely to yield success in reducing stress than reading detailed medical textbooks on the surgical treatment of advanced cancer. It is important to note that both approach and avoidance are potentially useful techniques in dealing with stressful situations; however, the extreme use of either may lead to less successful coping outcomes. Figure 12–1 summarizes the various dimensions of coping strategies.

Specific studies examining coping with abortion-related stress are beginning to appear in the literature. Whereas earlier studies tended to focus on how and why abortion decisions were made and on the measurement of negative emotional sequelae of abortion, more recent studies have examined the process of coping and positive emotional outcomes.

In general, confidence in one's ability to cope appears to enhance positive psychological outcomes for abortion clients (Major, Mueller, and Hildebrandt, 1985). In another study of coping behaviors related to abortion, Cohen and Roth (1984) found that clients using coping strategies that were aimed at approaching rather than avoiding the situation fared better over time than those clients who did not use such strategies. Approach strategies enabled them to determine consciously actions appropriate to the situation and to ventilate feelings; avoidant strategies (in this study equated only with denial) may have temporarily circumvented the experience of negative emotions but did not facilitate the woman's sense of mastery and active participation in the situation. However, had these researchers used a broader definition of avoidance, they might have found a cor-

Problem Focused ——————————————————— Emotion Focused

Approach ·————————————————————· Avoidance

Behavioral ·—————————————·Cognitive

FIGURE 12–1. Dimensions of coping strategies.

respondingly broader range of positive outcomes with this coping dimension.

LOSS

The experience of loss is integral to most women's perceptions about abortion—the loss of a part of oneself and the loss of what might have been. A pregnancy may have important meaning as an expression of a couple's closeness. A first pregnancy, in particular, may also have a special meaning to the woman. The finality of the termination of a pregnancy and any sense of associated loss must be recognized and dealt with if the woman is to integrate this experience successfully. Indeed, this finality can bring immense relief for many women, who feel they can now move on to a new phase in their life.

PSYCHOLOGICAL SEQUELAE

In the early 1970s, when legal abortions were starting to be widely practiced, researchers began to study extensively the psychological impact of abortion. They were primarily interested in identifying groups at risk for negative emotional reactions such as depression following an abortion. Several studies noted the association between negative psychological sequelae and at least one of the following risk factors: (1) ambivalence about the abortion, (2) preexisting psychiatric problems, and (3) lack of support from significant others (Bracken et al, 1974; Shusterman, 1979; Ashton, 1980; Schmidt and Priest, 1981; Moseley et al, 1981). In addition, Donnai, Charles, and Harris (1981) reported that women undergoing abortion for genetic reasons were also more likely to experience adverse psychological and social reactions following pregnancy termination.

In general, however, long-term negative psychological sequelae of abortion appear to be minimal or nonexistent in most women (Robbins, 1979; Shusterman, 1979). This finding holds true for both early and second trimester procedures (Brewer, 1978; Athanasiou et al, 1973). In terms of the impact of a previous abortion on psychological functioning during subsequent pregnancies, Bradley (1984) found no differences in levels of anxiety, labor and delivery, and postpartum maternal function when she compared women who had not previously aborted a pregnancy with those who had. Indeed, it is likely that in many cases, rather than contributing negatively to a woman's psychological health, the availability of abortion contributes positively to a woman's well-being in terms of enhancing self-determination, the ability to follow through with career or school goals, and allowing for planned pregnancies. Other positive effects experienced by many women are an enhanced awareness of their own coping capacities and confidence in their ability to deal with problems (Howe, Kaplan, and English, 1979).

Ambivalence, the emotional conflict resulting from a difficult decision when no option seems viable, is an important predictor of negative emotional sequelae to abortion (Ashton, 1980). Although the majority of women do not experience strong negative emotions following abortion, Bracken (1978) found that the women in his study who were ambivalent about their decision (approximately 15 per cent of the sample) had a higher incidence of anxiety both before and after the procedure as well as depression following the abortion. Guilt and unresolved loss are the most likely sources of this depression. Although it is impossible to predict whether post-decisional regret would have occurred had the woman continued her pregnancy, it is likely that the depression stems from the quality of the decision-making process rather than the actual decision outcome (Bracken, Hachamovitch, and Grossman, 1974; Shusterman, 1979).

Delays in seeking and obtaining abortion

are often, but not always, the result of ambivalence. Conflict about the pregnancy may impede the decision-making process and therefore prolong the period of time between when the woman suspects pregnancy and when she actually reaches a decision. In some cases, the delay may be so long that the advanced gestational age precludes termination and the woman must continue the pregnancy. Other factors contributing to delay in seeking abortion are denial of the pregnancy, fear of parental disapproval in the case of minors, and health care system failures, such as inadequate referral mechanisms (Bracken and Kasl, 1975).

REPEAT ABORTION

There are strong negative sanctions in our culture against using abortion as a primary method of contraception. Women who repeatedly seek abortions are frequently characterized as being irresponsible and immature, lacking motivation to use contraception, and failing to learn from their mistakes. Indeed, the slight increase in emotional distress experienced by repeat versus first-abortion clients found by Freeman and associates (1980) may be a result of concerns about evidence of disapproval from significant others. However, many studies have demonstrated that following the first abortion, increased contraception use is the overwhelming norm (Howe, Kaplan, and English, 1979; Cvejic et al, 1977; Abrams, DiBose, and Sturgis, 1979). Howe, Kaplan, and English (1979) proposed that, rather than being irresponsible, most clients seeking repeat abortions had a higher probability of becoming pregnant because of increased frequency of sexual activity, the imperfection of available contraceptive methods, and deficits in the structure of health institutions that provide barriers to access to care.

Sociocultural Factors

The social context in which the decision to terminate a pregnancy occurs may exert a powerful influence. Significant others, such as parents, boyfriend, siblings, spouse, and close female friends, are important sources of support, may participate in values clarification, and are frequently confidants as the woman makes a decision. External resources that affect the financial, material, and inter-

personal qualities of the woman's life may also be important contributing factors, because many women hesitate to bring a child into the world unless they can provide a good environment. Of course, the woman's or couple's perceived ideal circumstances for child-rearing are to a large extent culturally and socially determined and therefore differ from individual to individual.

SOCIAL SUPPORT

The impact of social support on stressful situations has been widely studied. While the influence of a network of significant persons generally provides a reservoir of helpful resources upon which a stressed person can rely, social networks can also exact a toll on individuals when they can least afford it. Frequently, women identify within their social networks those persons they want to include or eliminate from their confidence in making pregnancy decisions based on anticipated support. For example, a young woman may choose not to tell her parents of her decision to have an abortion because she is afraid of a disappointed or angry response. In another situation, a woman might delay telling her partner about her decision until after the abortion because she fears that he would pressure her into continuing the pregnancy.

Several studies have identified the critical importance of the woman's support network in enhancing positive emotional outcomes following abortion (Shusterman, 1979; Bracken et al, 1974; Moseley et al, 1981). For adolescents, parental support appears to be the most powerful predictor of a positive outcome; for adult women, the support of their partner serves a similar function (Bracken et al, 1974). Adolescent and adult women also differ somewhat in terms of whom they seek out for advice regarding their decision, with adults more likely to feel comfortable in consulting a professional in addition to significant others (Lewis, 1980). For both groups, however, if the partner is involved and supportive throughout the abortion experience, he is likely to provide a unique kind of emotional support no one else can provide because of his direct sharing of responsibility for the pregnancy (Robbins and DeLamater, 1985).

Little is known about the impact of cultural differences on the use of support networks by women seeking an abortion. Shusterman

(1979) found that in general the degree of intimacy with the partner was positively associated with whether or not he knew of the pregnancy and whether he supported the woman's decision. In this study, cultural factors were found to be associated with the degree of partner intimacy reported by women, with Asian women most likely to inform the partner and claim the highest degree of intimacy. The black women in this group were least likely to tell their partner of the pregnancy and also received the least amount of support from their partners (Shusterman, 1979). Much additional research is needed in this area before assertions about cultural differences can be made confidently, however.

Summary

Complex developmental, psychological, and sociocultural factors contribute to the experience of abortion as a critical life event. Much of the research exploring these factors has focused on the psychological impact of abortion. From the extensive literature reviewed, it is clear that although negative emotional sequelae resulting from abortion are rare, the abortion experience can be stressful as well as potentially growth promoting. Many different factors may mediate this process. Particular factors may be more or less salient at different points in a woman's life and in the context of different life situations. The decision-making process discussed in the following section can be viewed to a large extent as a function of these factors.

UNINTENTIONAL PREGNANCY CHOICES AND THE PROCESS OF DECISION-MAKING

A theoretical perspective on reproductive decisions is useful in guiding the nurse in facilitating the decision-making process in unintended pregnancy. Janis (1984) examined client health care decisions in stressful, problematic situations in which conflict may precipitate a crisis and proposed a progression of stages of decision-making in which the individual attempts to identify and utilize the best or most appropriate strategies to solve the problem. The stages are summarized in Table 12–1.

TABLE 12–1. Stages of Decision-Making

Appraisal of challenge
Appraisal of alternatives
Choosing the best available alternative
Commitment
Adherence

Adapted from Janis I: The patient as decision maker. In Gentry W (ed): Handbook of Behavioral Medicine. New York, Guilford Press, 1984.

The first stage is *appraisal of challenge*. The term challenge as used by Janis refers to "events or communications that convey threats or opportunities" (Janis, 1984, p 335). The person begins to assess whether the event is important enough to warrant an active decision to meet the challenge. In the case of the woman with an unintentional pregnancy, this situation may pose a distinct impact on immediate and future goals; her sense of identity, body image, current social roles; and the general status quo. An unintended pregnancy may also bring with it perceived opportunities for improved self-image and fantasies of solidification of a marriage or partnership. Many women and their partners are ambivalent when faced with an unexpected pregnancy. It is during this phase that the woman must determine whether she will act to meet the opportunity or threat or rather, for the time being, will ignore the situation.

The second stage, *appraisal of alternatives*, is initiated when the person begins to seek out and examine information about available alternatives. Evaluation of information is based on identifying which choice is most likely to avert potential losses. It is in this phase that the potential choices seen as too dangerous or incompatible with life style, resources, or values are excluded. For example, since the advent of legalized abortion, the vast majority of women eliminate pregnancy continuation and adoption as a pregnancy choice because of the high emotional costs of carrying a pregnancy to term and then giving up an infant. For other women, moral beliefs prevent them from considering abortion as an option, and they exclude this choice from serious consideration.

The third stage, *choosing the best available alternative*, is a refinement of stage two, in which the decision maker weighs each alternative in terms of salient personal criteria for maximizing positive and minimizing negative outcomes. At this stage, the decision is often private, although the decision maker usually considers the impact of the various choices on significant others. Unintentional pregnancy, similar to many other health care situations, poses a conflict because both losses and benefits are usually associated with any choice the woman may make. The decision is rarely conflict free, and the stakes are high. The use of a balance sheet during the client-professional encounter may help to clarify the decision-making process by sorting out the pros and cons for each of the alternatives. This hypothetical exercise may be particularly useful in cognitively representing a situation that is characteristically charged with emotion (Janis and Rodin 1979).

In the fourth stage, *commitment*, the person tests out the tentative decision by revealing it to others. Particularly in such controversial matters as pregnancy options, the individual can anticipate disapproval from important people in their lives and initially, at least, will often choose not to confide in those persons who may not support the decision. However, there are usually persons important in the woman's life who will offer support. As more and more support is garnered, commitment is strengthened.

The fifth and final stage, *adherence*, occurs when in the face of conflicting new information or negative response from a significant person, resolve remains firm to adhere to the decision. A hypothetical situation that exemplifies this stage is one in which a woman avoids informing her partner of an unintentional pregnancy until she has decided to terminate. Despite his desire for her to continue the pregnancy, she adheres to her abortion decision. Another example is the situation of a woman seeking pregnancy termination who believes she is only "a few weeks" pregnant yet finds out at her appointment that her pregnancy is already into the second trimester. Moving into the fifth stage requires that the woman integrate this new information (which may conflict with currently held values and beliefs) while still adhering to her decision to terminate the pregnancy.

Janis' perspective on decision-making is useful to clinicians in understanding decision-making behavior and in guiding counseling interventions that facilitate well-thought out choices. The focus is on process over time .and decribes, in general terms, how many people might solve a difficult problem. In addition, this framework includes the important aspect of emotion and its contribution to the process of decision-making. The affective component has not been considered in many other purely cognitive theoretical models of decision-making. Therefore, while this framework gives little guidance in understanding those clients who deviate from the stepwise process, it does provide a useful theoretical perspective for understanding the general sequence of stages many women go through in making a pregnancy decision.

Unintentional pregnancy decisions can be conceptualized from other vantage points as well. For example, Smetana (1981) has analyzed the reasoning process in women choosing abortion or pregnancy continuation in terms of "domains" of cognition—the moral and the personal. She found that women reason within distinct realms in order to reach a workable solution to the problem of an unintentional pregnancy. Reasoning in the moral domain, women in Smetana's (1981) study considered the fetus to possess enough genetic and spiritual potential to qualify it as a human life and therefore focused on abortion as the taking of a life. Another group, reasoners in the personal domain, attended to the needs for autonomy and self-regulation of the woman as most salient. The fetus was seen as an extension of the pregnant woman, since birth represented the point at which a fetus attained a separate status independent of the woman. Therefore, for the personal reasoners, the judgments about abortion focus on choices and needs of the woman.

Coordination between the two domains occurs for some women and is determined by gestational duration, so that even women who initially draw upon personal reasoning will shift to moral reasoning at some point in the pregnancy, such as the second trimester and, for virtually all, at the third trimester (Smetana, 1981). This finding has been supported by Luker, who describes the moral reasoning process of pro-choice women as contextual and *gradualist*, in that "a fetus may not be fully a person until it is viable, but it does have potential rights at all times, and these rights increase in moral weight as the pregnancy continues" (Luker, 1984, p 108).

The view of human reproductive behavior as a series of conscious, reflective, and rational decisions is only partially based in reality. While it is true that individuals with an unintentional pregnancy are confronted with a situation that demands an immediate choice, many of the preceding choices related to sexuality (such as whether or not to initiate a sexual relationship) and contraception frequently are influenced by a multiplicity of interacting psychosocial and cultural factors. Decisions about problems (as in the choice between continuing or terminating a pregnancy) or goals to be attained (as in contraception or the decision to conceive) result, to some degree, in an active behavioral outcome. On the other hand, no-decision situations, or when no conscious decision is made but frequently results in an outcome, are characterized by passive client behaviors. The latter may be as instructive as the active decision-making process in providing information regarding how individuals determine the directions of the reproductive aspects of their lives.

Although the process of decision-making will vary from woman to woman and even from situation to situation for a given individual, generally an unintentional pregnancy presents itself as a complicated and stressful life event. In order for the health care professional to be of maximal assistance to the woman and her significant others facing the demands and potential conflicts of making a decision, clinical interventions should be guided by theories of decision-making available in the literature. The emphasis on decision-making has been selected because it represents the client as an active (to a greater or lesser extent) individual initiating behaviors on her own behalf. For many women, a particular pregnancy decision is one among several in the course of her reproductive career (Murphy, Symington, and Jacobsen, 1983; Bracken et al, 1978), and each must be considered as unique.

Major decision points in a woman's reproductive life occur under diverse circumstances and with varying levels of conflict, deliberation, and ambivalence. The decision to initiate sexual activity, prevent pregnancy, plan children, and identify the best possible outcome of an unintended pregnancy are all examples of the decisions women encounter during their potential childbearing years. In addition to *types* of reproductive decisions, the *process* also varies considerably. For example, the decision to initiate a particular method of contraception such as the contraceptive pill may occur for one couple only after lengthy consideration of the pros and cons of this method, while for another individual, the choice of the pill as a contraceptive method may be based solely on the fact that female friends and relatives have had problems with other methods. Reproductive decision processes may be categorized generally as life style choices and as critical event decisions; these are summarized in Table 12–2.

Physiological Factors and Abortion

In addition to the psychodynamic and sociocultural aspects of the woman's experience in undergoing an abortion, clinical factors contribute to her complex set of needs. Abortion procedures vary according to the gestational age of the fetus, the skills of the physician, community standards, and the health status of the woman. In this section, the various types of abortion procedures and the implications for nursing practice will be presented. The nurse's role in providing clinical care for the woman seeking an abortion includes counseling, assessment of health and psychological status, and client education related to the abortion procedure and contraception. In addition, the nurse may be called upon to assist with the procedure itself or handle the products of conception.

Several abortion techniques are currently implemented and are summarized in Table 12–3. The advent of legalized abortion has

TABLE 12–2. Reproductive Choices

Life style reproductive decisions
  These are continuous, dependent on the preceding choices reflective of an individual's life style characteristics, such as future versus immediate orientation and problem-solving skills.
  Developmental issues determine in part the goals, motivations, and resources associated with the particular decisions at a given point in time.
  Much of the work of decision-making may occur in "latent" periods in which no particular action is required. Maintenance and adherence factors ensure continuity of experience.

Critical event reproductive decisions
  Critical decision events require mobilization of resources such as social supports and new coping mechanisms.
  Adaptations are situation specific, calling for a unique assessment of contributing factors that are specific to the particular situation and are facilitated by deliberate, conscious sorting through of relevant issues.
  Moral and ethical judgments are often indicated (e.g., abortion, use of IUD, infertility treatments such as artificial insemination, and in vitro fertilization).

TABLE 12–3. Summary of Abortion Techniques

Type of Procedure	Technique	Lami-naria	Pain Management	Complications	Setting	Expense	Psychological Impact	
							Woman	Staff
First Trimester (up to 12 Weeks of Pregnancy)								
Menstrual extraction (up to 6 weeks)	Suction curettage	No	Paracervical block with optional IV/oral sedation	Incomplete AB, cervical laceration, perforation; infection, undetected tubal pregnancy	Outpatient	Low; few or no lost work days	Low	Low
Dilation and suction (up to 12 weeks)	Cervical dilation and suction curettage	Yes	Paracervical block and IV sedation, oral analgesia as required	Uterine perforation, bleeding, infection, incomplete AB	Outpatient	Low; Laminaria requires additional visit day before procedure	Low to moderate	Low
Second Trimester (13 to 24 Weeks of Pregnancy)								
Dilation and evacuation (13 to 24 weeks)	Cervical dilation and suction curettage, sharp curettage/instrumental removal of fetus and placenta	Yes	Paracervical block and IV sedation or general anesthesia	Uterine perforation and increased bleeding with gestational age, ?cervical incompetence	Generally inpatient	Moderate; may require overnight hospitalization	Low to moderate	Physician high
Intra-amniotic saline instillation (16 to 24 weeks)	Injection of 20% saline; amount varies with gestation; labor and delivery of fetus		Local anesthetic at injection site; limited amounts of analgesia during labor	Hypernatremia, coagulopathy, bleeding, uterine rupture, incomplete AB	Inpatient	High; unpredictable length of hospital stay	Moderate to high	Nurse high
Prostaglandin in instillation (13 to 24 weeks)	Intra-amniotic injection or vaginal suppositories most common route; labor and delivery of fetus		Local anesthetic if intraamniotic; limited amounts of analgesia during labor	Retained placenta, frequent GI side effects, nausea, vomiting, diarrhea (medications can be given prophylactically)	Inpatient	High; unpredictable length of hospital stay	Moderate to high	Nurse high

AB = abortion.
(Reproduced by permission of Keenan C: Unintentional pregnancy: Education choice. In Littlefield V (ed): Health Education for Women: A Guide for Nurses and Other Professionals. Norwalk, Appleton-Century-Crofts, 1986.)

resulted in the growth of technical skills of medical professionals (Tietze, 1984), counseling, and client education programs as well as abortions earlier in gestation, all of which contribute to the generally low risks associated with pregnancy termination by surgical curettage. The earlier the procedure is performed, the lower the risks of morbidity and mortality (O'Reilly, Dorfman, and Cates, 1982). Surgical abortions in the second trimester, while associated with greater risks than those performed in the first trimester, are still safer than the medical induction methods of saline and/or prostaglandin instillation (Grimes, 1984).

Several studies have examined the impact of induced abortion on future fertility or its possible association with complications of subsequent pregnancies. Hogue, Cates, and Tietze (1982) in an extensive review of previous studies, found no evidence for secondary infertility following multiple induced abortions. This finding was corroborated by Stubblefield and associates (1984), who further noted that in women with three or more induced abortions, pregnancy rates were actually higher, perhaps suggesting a higher fertility rate in these women. Additionally, while earlier studies claimed that induced abortions were associated with subsequent complications in later pregnancies, such as low birth weight, premature delivery, and spontaneous abortions, later studies have not supported these findings (Linn et al, 1983; Hogue, Cates, and Tietze, 1983; Stubblefield et al, 1984).

FIRST-TRIMESTER ABORTION

Termination of pregnancy during the first 12 weeks is done via a surgical procedure, *dilation and suction (D&S)*, in which the cervix is dilated (if necessary) and the products of conception removed from the uterus by means of vacuum aspiration. In many cases, a paracervical block provides local anesthesia and greatly reduces the pain of cervical dilation. Frequently, laminaria are also used to provide a gradual and gentle cervical dilation up to 24 hours preceding the D&S procedure. Laminaria are dried, sterile rods of compressed seaweed stems that are inserted into the cervical os and, during the day before surgery, absorb moisture and increase in diameter, thereby dilating the cervix. Synthetic laminaria of various materials are also available. The advantages of using laminaria

before the D&S procedure are decreased likelihood of cervical and uterine trauma and diminished pain during the surgery through the rapid dilation of a firm, tightly closed cervix. Disadvantages of using laminaria include an additional visit to the health care professional preceding the surgery and, occasionally, uterine cramping requiring mild analgesia. Additionally, the risk of uterine infection may be slightly increased.

On the day of the procedure, a mild preoperative sedative such as diazepam or perioperative analgesia such as an antiprostaglandin may be given. The woman is requested to fast for 6 to 8 hours before the procedure. The laminaria, if used, are removed, and the cervix and vagina are cleansed with an antiseptic solution. After anesthetizing the anterior lip of the cervix, a tenaculum is applied to stabilize the cervix, and local anesthesia is injected into the paracervical area. The cervix is then dilated as necessary, depending on the gestational length of the pregnancy. After adequate dilation is obtained, a flexible plastic curette attached to suction tubing is inserted into the uterine cavity, and suction is applied. The curette is gently rotated, and the products of conception are removed. The uterine cavity is then explored with a small metal curette to ensure that all tissue has been extracted. The entire procedure lasts about 10 to 20 minutes.

The major risks of this procedure are uterine perforation, infection, and hemorrhage from incomplete removal of tissue. As mentioned earlier, the risks of cervical and uterine trauma are lessened with the use of laminaria.

Menstrual extraction (ME) is essentially identical to the D&S procedure except that ME refers to very early pregnancy terminations (usually up to 6 weeks' and not exceeding 8 weeks' gestation). Cervical dilation is usually not required, and laminaria are rarely used. Following a paracervical block, a small-lumen catheter is inserted into the uterus, and the products of conception are removed with suction, following the same techniques as that in the D&S.

When serum tests detecting very early pregnancies were unavailable, the major disadvantage of the ME was that some women underwent the procedure when in fact they were not pregnant. With the availability of improved serum and urine assays for human chorionic gonadotropin (HCG), which are sensitive at or before the first missed menses, a positive pregnancy test is now indicated before a pregnancy termination is undertaken. However, even if the pregnancy is documented, another disadvantage of the ME is the possibility of missing the pregnancy or incomplete removal of the pregnancy, necessitating a second procedure. Generally, even though a positive pregnancy can be documented much earlier, surgical pregnancy termination is usually deferred until 6 weeks after the last menstrual period (4 weeks after conception).

SECOND-TRIMESTER ABORTION

Dilation and evacuation (D&E) is the surgical method of pregnancy termination in the second trimester (13 to 24 weeks' gestation). The D&E and D&S procedures are similar. The cervix is initially dilated with multiple laminaria inserted the day before surgery and further dilated immediately preceding surgery with metal Hegar or Pratt dilators. A larger bore suction curette is required because of the increased volume of tissue. Extraction instruments called ring forceps are also used to remove the products of conception. General anesthesia may be used, especially beyond 16 weeks' gestation because of the increased complexity and time associated with this more advanced surgical procedure.

The complications associated with any surgical pregnancy termination, particularly uterine perforation due to the increased softness and thinning of the uterine wall as the pregnancy progresses, are more common during the second trimester. In a relative sense, however, the complication rates are still lower than those associated with other abortion techniques used in the second trimester, i.e., saline and/or prostaglandin instillation (Grimes and Cates, 1981).

Saline abortion is a medical technique for pregnancy termination in which a hypertonic solution of saline is infused into the amniotic sac, causing rapid death of the fetus. This procedure is generally performed between 16 and 24 weeks' gestation; attempts to puncture the amniotic sac before this time are usually unsuccessful. The gestational time at which this procedure must be performed can be a major disadvantage for the woman in the early midtrimester who must then wait up to 3 weeks between her decision to terminate and the time of the actual procedure.

The 24-week cutoff is the commonly accepted standard beyond which elective abortions are no longer performed; fetal survival outside of the womb beyond this gestational age is possible. Community standards vary, however, and many physicians may elect to use an earlier gestational criterion for the maximal date.

The procedure for saline abortion includes cleansing the abdomen, injecting a local anesthetic and inserting a large-gauge needle transabdominally into the amniotic sac. Approximately 100 to 250 ml of amniotic fluid is withdrawn and replaced with 150 to 250 ml of a hypertonic saline solution. Labor usually begins within several hours, and the abortion is generally complete within 24 to 36 hours (Kerenyi, 1981).

Several major complications are associated with saline abortion. Hypernatremia is the result of injecting the salt solution directly into the maternal vascular system. Coagulation defects may also result from fibrin depletion following hemorrhage or large placental clot formation. In addition, uterine rupture and cervical laceration following a rapid progression of labor are potential complications (Kerenyi, 1981). Incomplete abortion is not uncommon, and the client may require suction completion to remove the placenta.

Prostaglandin abortion is another method of medically inducing pregnancy termination that has in recent years been used with increasing frequency in midtrimester because of the lower associated risks. Prostaglandins stimulate uterine contractions, and labor is usually complete within 24 hours (Neubardt and Schulman, 1977). Commonly used routes are intra-amniotic injection and vaginal suppositories. Vaginal administration is associated with a higher incidence of gastrointestinal side effects, such as nausea, vomiting, and diarrhea.

The major complication of prostaglandin induction is incomplete abortion, with retention of the placenta or placental fragments and missed abortion. Infection and bleeding may also occur. In addition, with advanced midtrimester procedures, the delivery of a living but nonviable fetus is possible. This problem creates ethical concerns for care of the fetus and stressful experiences for the nursing staff. For this reason, the saline and prostaglandin methods may be combined in order to avert this situation.

Nursing Process and The Client Seeking Abortion

Assessment of health and psychological status, counseling, and client education are roles the nurse assumes before, during, and after the abortion procedure. The role of the nurse may vary depending on the type of practice setting. For example, in some instances, the nurse may be the primary health professional, who after initial pregnancy diagnosis and counseling, refers the client to a physician or agency for pregnancy termination. In other settings, the nurse may provide more of the direct client education and supportive care during the abortion procedure. In any case, the nurse must draw upon diverse skills in assessing and providing for the complex psychosocial, educational, and physical needs of these clients as well as in ensuring that continuity of care is maintained.

The nurse has an important role as client advocate and, even more important, as a facilitator of health-promoting and -enhancing behaviors. A nursing goal is to maximize client control over events that will yield the best possible health outcomes and to enhance client coping and adaptation in situations in which they may often have diminished control. The current nursing literature reflects the profession's orientation toward client self-determination and self-actualization (Lenz, 1984; Cox, 1982). Individual client control is particularly relevant in reproductive matters in which choice-related behaviors often have marked and long-range impact.

HEALTH CARE PROFESSIONAL ATTITUDES

The attitudes of health care professionals may have a significant impact on the woman's abortion experience. A nonjudgmental attitude toward counseling for the purposes of exploring available options can facilitate a growth-producing exchange leading to further client self-awareness and coping abilities and a positive outcome. A negative experience could result if the professional's own feelings about abortion, if not examined and clarified, are communicated and impede this important process. In an early study of the effects of nurses' attitudes toward abortion, Harper, Marcom, and Wall (1972) found that when the caregivers' attitudes were less fa-

vorable regarding abortion, clients perceived their care as less satisfactory in terms of factors such as staff interest, helpfulness and respect.

In addition to the impact on the client, abortion attitudes also affect the health care professional on a personal level. In a study of the effects of second-trimester abortion on clients and professionals, Kaltreider et al (1979) found that the degree of involvement with the abortion contributed to the emotional impact on the professional. Therefore, nursing staff reported more emotional difficulty with saline and prostaglandin abortions because of their extensive role in client care, while physicians experienced more difficulty with the surgical procedure of dilation and evacuation.

Health care professionals have diverse attitudes about abortion. The factors that determine whether the professional decides to be involved in the care of the abortion client are complex. For example, moral and religious beliefs and attitudes about sexuality and contraception as well as more pragmatic issues such as level of financial reimbursement all may affect this decision. The reader is referred to Smith (1982) for a thorough review of these factors. Of utmost importance both for professionals and ultimately for clients is that professionals be aware of their own attitudes and values concerning abortion and that they actively decide the level of care they are comfortable providing.

ASSESSMENT*

Physiological Factors. The health history yields important information regarding health status, risk factors, pregnancy dating, and previous health behaviors. The following are critical elements in the history of the woman seeking a pregnancy termination:

1. Current history: Pregnancy symptoms (fatigue, nausea, skipped menses, breast tenderness, urinary frequency, and quickening), patterns of sexual activity, and use (regular or irregular) or nonuse of contraceptives.

2. Last menstrual period: Was it normal or abnormal? Was the previous menstrual

---

*Portions of the Assessment and Interventions sections appear in Keenan C: Unintentional pregnancy: Education for choice. In Littlefield V (ed): Health Education for Women: A Guide for Nurses and Other Professionals. Norwalk, Appleton-Century-Crofts, 1986, and are included here with permission of the publisher.

period normal or abnormal? Were oral contraceptives used in the past 3 months?

3. Menstrual history: Age of onset of menses, frequency and duration of periods, amount of flow, and premenstrual or menstrual symptoms.

4. Obstetrical history: Number of full-term births, premature births, spontaneous or induced abortions, and number of living children; pregnancy complications of previous abortions and full-term pregnancies, labor, deliveries, or the postpartum period; and prior cesarean sections.

5. Gynecological history: Previous gynecological surgery, past history of infertility, sexually transmitted infections (salpingitis), abnormal Pap smear, other gynecological illnesses, previous contraceptive use (note dates, duration, and any problems experienced), and breast disorders.

6. Past medical history: Any serious medical illnesses (past or present), surgery, or hospitalizations; previous or current psychiatric illness; current medications; allergies or drug sensitivities (specifically to antibiotics, analgesics, iodine, and previous adverse effects of local or general anesthesia); history of thrombophlebitis; and Rh blood type.

7. Family history: Diabetes, cardiovascular disease, and cancer and hereditary diseases.

8. Health habits: Usual sleep patterns; bowel and bladder habits; last Pap smear and health checkup; regularity of breast self-examination; use of caffeine (contained in coffee, tea, chocolate, and cola), tobacco, and alcohol; use of marijuana and/or other illicit drugs.

The health history can provide a useful base for an initial, thorough evaluation of health risks and behaviors that might have a direct impact on a woman's pregnancy decision and on subsequent health care. For example, a preexisting medical illness such as diabetes, asthma, or cardiac or renal disease may preclude an outpatient procedure. If the woman has a significant cardiac murmur, prophylactic antibiotics may be prescribed. Additionally, if the woman's blood type is Rh negative, there is a risk of her becoming sensitized when Rh-positive fetal blood cells enter the maternal circulation at the time of the abortion. For this reason, Rh_o (D) immune globulin (300 μg RhoGAM for 12 weeks' gestation and above and 60 μg MICRhoGAM for under 12 weeks' gestation) is administered to all Rh-negative women at the time of the pregnancy termination.

A complete physical examination should include a thorough pelvic examination and careful estimation of uterine size. Laboratory data complete the health assessment and routinely include blood pressure, hematocrit, Rh blood type, pregnancy test, syphilis screen, Pap smear, if not done in the previous year, and cervical culture. In addition, the pregnancy dating information along with physical examination findings combine to determine the exact gestational age and appropriate type of abortion procedure. On occasion, an ultrasonogram may be indicated if there is a discrepancy in the pregnancy dating criteria, or if the client is near the gestational age limit for obtaining the procedure.

Psychosocial Factors. As discussed previously, any pregnancy has the potential to create stress in a woman's life, and the unintentional pregnancy is no exception. Psychosocial assessment includes evaluation of actual and potential stressors, adequacy of coping strategies (including use of social supports), decision-making status, and developmental issues. After an initial and often intense response consisting of shock, anger, pleasure, sadness, or fear, the woman begins to mobilize internal and external resources to cope with and adapt to her new situation. The following content areas should be covered for a thorough psychosocial evaluation, which forms the basis for nursing interventions:

1. Actual and potential stressors: What are the woman's perceptions regarding the unintentional pregnancy? Are there associated factors that also affect her response to the pregnancy? What are her appraisals of this event?

2. Adequacy of coping strategies: What are the woman's usual patterns of coping? Does her range of strategies include both problem-focused and emotion-focused coping? Are they adequate to meet the current demands?

3. Decision-making status: Has the woman thoroughly considered all the alternatives available to her (abortion, adoption, and motherhood)? Has she included significant others in her decision if this is appropriate? Who are her sources of support? Is there opposition from significant others? If she is ambivalent, to what extent?

4. Developmental issues: At which point in the developmental life cycle does the unintentional pregnancy occur? What are the

specific developmental issues relevant to the woman at this time?

INTERVENTIONS

Pregnancy Counseling. Each woman must ultimately make her own decision concerning the outcome of her pregnancy. Health care professionals are available as consultants in the decision, providing information, clarification, and assistance in mobilizing resources necessary to carry out her intentions. In the process of helping the woman to make her decision, it is essential that health care professionals examine and resolve personal biases concerning pregnancy options. Many pregnancy choices carry strong negative sanctions and may be totally unacceptable in certain segments of our society. Abortion for other than medical reasons and single adolescent motherhood are examples of socially controversial reproductive decisions that nevertheless should not be eliminated or minimized as a pregnancy alternative if the woman herself is considering it. Nonjudgmental counseling is mandatory if the woman is to consider fully all available options and to choose from the greatest number of feasible alternatives. If the health care professional has a strong bias against a particular option, it is then appropriate to refer the client to another professional who can provide comprehensive counseling.

Counseling Goals. Nurses may be involved in counseling the woman at many different stages in decision-making regarding her pregnancy. In many cases, counseling occurs at the time the woman receives the result of her pregnancy test. In other instances the woman may be referred for counseling. When the woman decides to terminate her pregnancy, there are frequently counselors available as part of the abortion service. Regardless of the initial setting for counseling, however, the purposes are to (1) facilitate deliberate decision-making and personal growth, (2) ensure informed choice, and (3) identify high-risk individuals and initiate intervention.

Counseling Strategies. An initial strategy is the exploration of the problem as the woman perceives it and the possible alternatives she has identified. The pros and cons of each choice are examined even if the woman has previously excluded a particular option. This process is often facilitated by writing down the choices in columns and listing the positive and negative aspects of each to determine more objectively the factors that enter into the decision (Janis, 1984). The roles of each member of the support network and their potential for providing real or tangible support for a particular decision option are reviewed. If possible, it is also beneficial to retrace the woman's history of decisions regarding sexuality, beginning with initial choices about sexual activity and contraception, and to examine the underlying rationales for these choices. Issues of contraception may also be raised at this time, if appropriate. During this initial phase of counseling, information exchange and reality validation are crucial elements in the decision-making process.

Another focus is on the decision itself. Many woman have difficulty making a choice because previous values may conflict with the present set of circumstances in her life. In this situation it is helpful to emphasize the best possible choice given all the factors she must consider. The resolution of conflict regarding such important issues is very difficult; this fact should be acknowledged by the nurse.

Resolution in decision-making is fostered by engaging the woman in playing an active role. The insights that are gained by the woman can then be more easily incorporated into future coping and health behaviors. The role of the counselor includes information gathering and assessment, reflection on the content and process of the interview, and the use of summary and appropriate validation of the knowledge and insights of the woman.

In counseling the woman with an unintentional pregnancy, psychological risk factors should be screened and assessed, and referrals should be made when appropriate. Women with great ambivalence may be at risk for regretting their decision and experiencing more physical and emotional distress. Both the very young teenager and the woman nearing the end of her reproductive years may also be at risk because of developmental issues. In addition, women with previous psychological difficulties may experience an increased sense of crisis and not be able to cope effectively with the demands of making a difficult decision (Shusterman, 1979). Women who choose abortion after a diagnostic amniocentesis may also be at risk for experiencing additional stress. These women may have a more difficult abortion experience as a result of having wanted the pregnancy and perhaps having felt fetal movement. Generally speaking, however, most women, once they have worked through the decision-making process, are satisfied with their choice. When a woman does regret her choice after a reasonable length of time and psychological functioning is affected, referral for more intensive counseling is indicated.

Client Education. Client-centered education for the woman electing to terminate a pregnancy is directed toward the following goals:

1. Provide information and anticipatory guidance.

2. Promote well-being before, during, and after the procedure, minimizing complications and emotional difficulties.

3. Enhance client independence in self-care activities.

The reader is referred to additional sources for examples of client education plans for women seeking pregnancy termination (Keenan, 1986; Smith, 1981).

Because the process of client education is interactive, the woman participates in the evaluation of her own learning needs. However, the professional must be aware of several factors that influence the process of client education and the success of teaching interventions. Examples of these factors are the client's emotional status, her learning style, and the level of content required to meet the preceding goals.

The emotional status of the woman may be affected by feelings of loss, anxiety about possible pain associated with the abortion itself, and uncertainty. This must be recognized and care taken not to overload the woman unnecessarily with voluminous information in brief periods of time. In addition, terminology such as "the baby" and "father of the baby" are inappropriate and should be avoided. Terms such as "fetus," "pregnancy," and "partner" are less psychologically loaded and adequately convey the meanings.

Learning style is another factor to consider in developing a plan for client education. Many women prefer to learn in a one-to-one situation with their health care professional, particularly in the situation of a pregnancy

---

What to Expect

You may feel tired for the next few weeks, but you may resume full activities as soon as you wish. You may have heavy bleeding like a period starting a few days after the surgery. It may be heavier than usual and you may pass clots and small pieces of tissue. These come from the thickened lining of the uterus (womb).
You may expect to experience the following:

1. Bleeding for as long as 2 weeks.
2. Mild lower abdominal cramps.
3. Breast firmness and tenderness starting about the third postoperative day and lasting for several days. There may be some secretion from the nipples.
4. First *normal* period will occur 4 to 8 weeks after surgery. It may be lighter or heavier than usual.

Self-Care

You may shower or take a bath. But it is very important that you *do not* douche. You may resume sexual relations in 2 weeks if you feel ready. Tampons may be used if your flow is relatively heavy but use minipads for lighter flow. If you have not done so already, please contact us in the next few days to make a follow-up appointment in about 1 month.

Birth Control

It is very important that you use a method of birth control as soon as you resume sexual relations because there is no "safe" period after an abortion. If you have decided to use the birth control pill, you will be starting on the Sunday following surgery. If you have decided to use another method, such as the diaphragm or IUD, you will need to use a condom (prophylactic, rubber) and birth control foam until your postoperative checkup. Please do not rely on douching, withdrawal, or foaming vaginal tablets. You have shown yourself to be fertile, and these methods have a higher failure (pregnancy) rate.

Emotional Changes

After pregnancy termination, most women feel relieved but may also feel sad or tearful. If you find that you are feeling down for longer than a few days and would like some help, we will see you or suggest others who may help you.

Notify Us If You Experience Any of the Following

1. Fever of over 100°F.
2. Moderately severe abdominal or back pain.
3. Bleeding much heavier than your normal period.
4. Foul vaginal discharge.

Health Care Provider _____

Telephone Number _____

FIGURE 12–2. Example of postoperative instructions.

CASE STUDY

Mary Ann is a 17-year-old primigravida who presents to her health care provider requesting an abortion. Her last menstrual period occurred approximately 4 months ago, but since her cycles tended to be somewhat irregular, she did not begin to feel concerned until the time of her third missed period. Although her boyfriend, Steve, had earlier expressed concern about a possible pregnancy, Mary Ann felt quite confident that she would get her period and in fact was reassured by her transient menstrual cramps and breast tenderness. She was very angry when her mother, noting that her supply of tampons had not been used in several months, asked Mary Ann if she were pregnant.

Mary Ann and Steve had been going out with each other for 1 year and had started having intercourse about 8 months ago. They did not view themselves as "sexually active," since they had sex only about once a week. Neither had used contraception, although they had discussed it a few times. They did practice withdrawal occasionally. At the time of her third skipped period, Mary Ann brought up the topic of birth control, and they decided that the pill would be the most convenient method for them. It was at the time of her first visit to a family planning center that she was told of her pregnancy. She heard this news with mixed feelings of excitement, fear of how her parents would react, and anger at herself that she had "let this happen, because I knew better."

Both are seniors in high school and plan on attending a local college after graduation. They have discussed marriage, but neither feels ready to settle down. Adoption was raised as an alternative by the counselor and rejected by Mary Ann because she could not "go through a pregnancy all that time and just give away my baby." They have discussed the abortion with their parents, who are supportive of their decision. Concerns were raised by Mary Ann and her parents about her future fertility after having an abortion.

STUDY QUESTIONS

1. What are the coping mechanisms attempted by Mary Ann and Steve? How effective are they?
2. Trace the decision-making process for this couple.
3. Identify some of the common misconceptions held by this couple and state the approaches and information you would use to clarify them.
4. Describe the counseling strategies you would implement with this young woman, her boyfriend, and her parents.
5. How would you respond to the question regarding fertility after an abortion?
6. What are the critical elements of client education for this couple?

termination, in which confidentiality and privacy may be highly desirable. In other instances, however, the woman may request that a significant other be present for part or all of the session. In the case of young adolescents, whose parent or other responsible adult must sign the consent form for termination in compliance with the regulations of selected states, this is particularly true. In every case, however, the woman should be given the opportunity for some time alone with the health care professional to discuss any topics she may not feel comfortable raising in the presence of others.

The woman's own preference for information must be taken into account as well as her needs for anticipatory guidance in order to enhance coping. Some women come prepared with a list of extensive questions about the abortion, its risks, anesthesia, and post-abortion contraception. Others prefer to be told only what the professional thinks is necessary. In either case, the woman should be encouraged to ask questions, think about the information given to her, and then follow up by telephone with any further questions. Written information regarding the procedure, self-care measures following the procedure, and contraception should be provided for the woman.

Obviously, the *level of content* depends to a certain extent on the woman's age, intelligence, and her own goals for self-care. Minimally, however, she must have enough information to prevent complications and to participate in her care. The level of language should be tailored individually, and technical terminology should be limited. Additionally, graphic details of the surgical procedures are not indicated unless the woman herself requests information; they may contribute unnecessarily to feelings of anxiety or guilt.

Postabortion Contraception. Selection of an appropriate method of contraception and adequate understanding of its implementation are also important aspects of client education. Oral contraceptives are usually started within several days after the abortion, whereas the diaphragm and IUD are usually obtained at the postoperative checkup. The reader is referred to Chapter 11 for a discussion of the methods of contraception.

Postabortion Care. An example of postoperative instructions for the abortion client is provided in Figure 12–2. Written instructions augment the verbal information given to the client at the time of the abortion, so that the woman can refer to them after the abortion. Written instructions should always include the health care professional's telephone number and method of contact should a problem arise. Specific information concerning the usual physical symptoms the client is likely to expect following an abortion, self-care measures, contraception, and abnormal symptoms (fever, heavy bleeding, moderate or severe pain, and abnormal vaginal discharge) should also be included.

SUMMARY

Historical, legal, and ethical factors as well as the woman's unique psychological and sociocultural constitution make the decision to terminate an unintentional pregnancy a challenge to the woman, her significant others, and the counselors who attempt to facilitate her decision. From the clinical perspective of providing direct care to the woman seeking pregnancy termination, a thorough assessment of health status, risks, and practices in both the physical and psychosocial realms is necessary. Client education relates to the individualized evaluation of needs and implementation of a plan that will facilitate the client's self-care knowledge, informed consent to surgical procedures, and partnership with her health care professionals. The case study appearing on page 288 is intended to stimulate the reader to apply the concepts presented in this chapter to the care of clients choosing abortion.

REFERENCES

Abrams M, DiBase V, Sturgis S: Post-abortion attitudes and patterns of birth control. J Fam Pract 9:593–599, 1979.

Athanasiou R, Oppel W, Michelson L, et al: Psychiatric sequelae to term birth and induced early and late abortion: A longitudinal study. Fam Plan Perspect 5:227–231, 1973.

Ashton J: The psychosocial outcome of induced abortion. Br J Obstet Gynaecol 87:1115–1122, 1980.

Blumenfield M: Psychological factors involved in the request for elective abortion. J Clin Psychiatry 39:17–25, 1978.

Bracken M: A causal model of psychosomatic reactions to vacuum aspiration abortion. Soc Psychiatry 13:135–145, 1978.

Bracken M, Hachamovitch M, Grossman G: The decision to abort and psychological sequelae. J Nerv Ment Dis 158:154–162, 1981.

Bracken M, Klerman L, Bracken M: Coping with pregnancy resolution among never-married women. Am J Orthopsychiatry 48:320–334, 1978.

Bracken MB, Kase DV: Delay in seeking induced abortion: A review and theoretical analysis. Am J Obstet Gynecol 121:1008–1019, 1975.

Bradley C: Abortion and subsequent pregnancy. Can J Psychiatry 29:494–498, 1984.

Brewer C: Induced abortion after feeling fetal movements: Its causes and emotional consequences. J Biosoc Sci 10:203–208, 1978.

Brown M: Adolescents and abortion: A theoretical framework for decision making. J Obstet Gynecol Neonatal Nurs 12:241–247, 1983.

Chervenak F, Farley M, Walters L, et al: When is termination of pregnancy during the third trimester morally justifiable? N Engl J Med 310:501–504, 1984.

City of Akron v. Akron Center for Reproductive Health, 462 U.S. 416, (1983).

Clary F: Minor women obtaining abortions: A study of parental notification in a metropolitan area. Am J Pub Health 72:283–285, 1982.

Cohen L, Roth S: Coping with abortion. J Human Stress 4:140–145, 1984.

Cox C: An interaction model for client health behavior: Theoretical prescription for nursing. Adv Nurs Sci 5:41–56, 1982.

Cvejic H, Lipper I, Kinch R, Benjamin P: Follow-up of 50 adolescent girls 2 years after abortion. Can Med Assoc J 8:44–46, 1977.

Donnai P, Charles N, Harris R: Attitudes of patients after "genetic" termination of pregnancy. Br Med J 282:621–622, 1981.

Donovan P: Judging teenagers: How minors fare when they seek court-authorized abortions. Fam Plann Perspect 15:259–267, 1983.

Dryfoos J: Contraceptive use, pregnancy intentions and pregnancy outcomes. Fam Plann Perspect 14:81–94, 1982.

Ellerbrock TV, Atrash HK, Rhodenhiser EP, et al: Abortion surveillance, 1982–1983. MMWR 36:11–42SS, 1987.

English J: Abortion and the concept of a person. In M. Vetterling-Braggin, Ellston F, English J (eds): Feminism and Philosophy. Totowa, Littlefield, Adams & Co, 1981, pp 417–428.

Freeman E, Rickels K, Huggins G, et al: Emotional distress patterns among women having first or repeat abortions. Obstet Gynecol 55:630–636, 1980.

Gerrard M: Sex, sex guilt and contraceptive use. J Pers Soc Psychol 42:153–158, 1982.

Grimes D: Second trimester abortions in the United States. Fam Plann Perspect 16:260–266, 1984.

Grimes D, Cates W: Dilation and evacuation. In Burger G, Brenner W, Keith L (eds): Second Trimester Abortion: Perspectives After a Decade of Experience. Boston, John Wright, 1981.

Harper M, Marcom B, Wall V: Abortion: Do attitudes of nursing personnel affect the patient's perception of care? Nurs Res 21:327–330, 1972.

Henshaw S, Forrest J, Sullivan E, Tietze C: Abortion services in the United States. Fam Plann Perspect 14:5–14, 1982.

Hilliard D, Shank C, Redman R: Unplanned pregnancies in a midwestern community. J Fam Pract 15:259–263, 1982.

Hogge J, Hogge W, Golbus M: Chorionic villus sampling. J Obstet Gynecol Neonatal Nurs 15:24–27, 1986.

Hogue C, Cates W, Tietze C: The effects of induced abortion on subsequent reproduction. Epidemiol Rev 4:66–94, 1982.

Hogue C, Cates W, Tietze C: Impact of vacuum aspiration abortion on future childbearing: A review. Fam Plann Perspect 15:119–126, 1983.

Howe B, Kaplan H, English C: Repeat abortions: Blaming the victims. Am J Public Health 69:1242–1246, 1979.

Janis I: The patient as decision-maker. In Gentry W (ed): Handbook of Behavioral Medicine. New York, Guilford Press, 1984, pp 326–370.

Janis I, Rodin J: Attribution, control and decision making: Social psychology and health care. In Stone G, Cohen F, Adler N (eds): Health Psychology. San Francisco, Jossey-Bass, 1979, pp 487–521.

Kaltreider NB, Goldsmith S, Margolis AJ: The impact of midtrimester abortion techniques on patients and staff. Am J Obstet Gynecol 135:235–238, 1979.

Keenan C: Unintentional pregnancy: Education for choice. In Littlefield V (ed): Health Education for Women: A Guide for Nurses and Other Professionals. Norwalk, Appleton-Century-Crofts, 1986.

Kerenyi T: Hypertonic saline instillation. In Burger G, Brenner W, Keith L (eds): Second Trimester Abortion: Perspectives After a Decade of Experience. Boston, John Wright, 1981.

Kirby M: Informed consent: What does it mean? J Med Ethics 9:69–75, 1983.

Klein L: To have or not to have a pregnancy. Obstet Gynecol 65:1–4, 1985.

Lazarus R, Folkman S: Stress, Appraisal and Coping. New York, Springer Publishing, 1985.

Lenz E: Information seeking: A component of client decisions and health behavior. Adv Nurs Sci 7:59–72, 1984.

Lewis C: A comparison of minors' and adults' pregnancy decisions. Am J Orthopsychiatry 50:446–453, 1980.

Linn S, Schoenbaum S, Monson R, et al: The relationship between induced abortion and subsequent pregnancies. Am J Obstet Gynecol 146:136–140, 1983.

Luker K: The war between the women. Fam Plann Perspect 16:105–110, 1984.

Major B, Mueller P, Hildebrandt K: Attributions, expectations and coping with abortion. J Pers Soc Psychol 48:585–589, 1985.

Moseley D, Follingstad D, Harley H, Heckel R: Psychological factors that predict reaction to abortion. J Clin Psychol 37:276–279, 1981.

Murphy J, Symington B, Jacobson S: Pregnancy-resolution decisions: What if abortions were banned? J Reprod Med 28:789–797, 1983.

Neubardt S, Schulman H: Techniques of Abortion. Boston, Little, Brown & Co, 1977.

Olson L: Social and psychological correlates of pregnancy resolution among adolescent women: A review. Am J Orthopsychiatry 50:432–445, 1981.

O'Reilly K, Dorfman S, Cates W: The epidemiology of abortion services. Fam Community Health, 5:29–39, 1982.

Osofsky J, Osofsky H: The psychological reactions of patients to legalized abortion. Am J Orthopsychiatry 426:48–60, 1972.

Petchesky R: Abortion and Woman's Choice. Boston, Northeastern University Press, 1985.

Potts M, Diggory P, Peel J: Abortion. Cambridge, Cambridge University Press, 1977.

Reinke B, Holmes D, Harris B: The timing of psychosocial changes in women's lives: The years 25 to 45. J Pers Soc Psychol 48:1353–1364, 1985.

Robbins J: Objective versus subjective responses to abortion. J Consult Clin Psychol 5:994–995, 1979.

Robbins J, DeLamater J: Support from significant others and loneliness following induced abortion. Soc Psychiatry 20:92–99, 1985.

Roe v. Wade 93 S. Ct. 705, 1973.

Schmidt R, Priest R: The effects of termination of pregnancy: A follow-up study of psychiatric referrals. Br J Med Psychol 54:267–276, 1981.

Shusterman L: Predicting the psychological consequences of abortion. Soc Sci Med 13A:683–689, 1979.

Smetana J: Reasonings in the personal and moral domain: Adolescent and young adult women's decision-making regarding abortion. J Appl Develop Psychol 2:211–226, 1981.

Smith E: Abortion. In Smith E (ed): Women's Health Care: A Guide for Patient Education. Norwalk, Appleton-Century-Crofts, 1981, pp 90–105.

Smith E: Abortion: Health Care Perspectives. Norwalk, Appleton-Century-Crofts, 1982.

Smith J: Rights-conflict, pregnancy and abortion. In Gould C (ed): Beyond Domination: New Perspectives on Women and Philosophy. Totowa, Rowman and Allenheld, 1984.

Stubblefield P, Monson R, Schoenbaum S, et al: Fertility after induced abortion: A prospective follow-up study. Obstet Gynecol 62:186–193, 1984.

Thomson J: A defense of abortion. Philosophy and Public Policy 1:47–66, 1971.

Tietze C: The public health effects of legal abortion in the United States. Fam Plann Perspect 16:26–28, 1984.

Woods N, Luke C: Sexuality and abortion. In Woods N (ed): Human Sexuality in Health and Illness. St. Louis, CV Mosby, 1979.

Wortman C: Coping with victimization: Conclusions and implications for future research. J Soc Issues 39:195–221, 1983.

Zelnick M, Kantner J: Sexual and contraceptive experience of young, unmarried women in the United States, 1976 and 1971. Fam Plann Perspect 9:55–71, 1977.

13: Infertility and Sexuality

Barbara Derwinski-Robinson

For many Americans, development in adult life includes both marriage and childbearing, but for between 10 and 15 per cent of couples, the problem of infertility occurs and requires special adjustment (Shane, Schiff, and Wilson, 1976; Speroff, Glass, and Kase, 1983; Hatcher et al, 1982; Woods, 1984). The purpose of this chapter is to discuss infertility, including its cause, diagnostic measures, biomedical treatments, and psychosocial interventions.

The World Health Organization has developed internationally accepted definitions of infertility:

Primary infertility: The woman has never conceived despite cohabitation, exposure to the possibility of pregnancy, and the wish to become pregnant for at least 12 months.
Secondary infertility: The woman has previously conceived but is subsequently unable to conceive despite cohabitation, exposure to the possibility of pregnancy, and the wish to become pregnant for at least 12 months.
Pregnancy wastage: The woman is able to conceive but unable to produce a live birth.
Clinical subfertility (subfecundity): The difficulty experienced by some couples, both members of whom may have reduced fertility, to conceive jointly. (Hatcher et al, 1982, pp 214–215)

It is important to note that infertility and sterility are not synonymous. Sterility is the permanent inability to conceive a child.

Hatcher and associates (1982) have described the following time frame during which 100 couples having intercourse without contraception might expect to become pregnant. Twenty-five of 100 couples will conceive in the first month of unprotected intercourse, 35 of 100 in the second through sixth month, 20 of 100 in the seventh through seventeenth month, and 10 of 100 in the eighteenth through twenty-fourth month. The time of conception for 10 of 100 couples is unknown.

There are multiple factors that contribute to infertility. To be sensitive to and to correct common misperceptions, health professionals must be aware of the commonly held myths about infertility as well as the documented causes. The following list contrasts commonly held beliefs with facts about infertility.

1. "*Infertility is a female problem.*" In 40 to 50 per cent of cases, males are wholly or partly responsible for infertility.

2. "*Infertility is caused by psychological factors.*" There is a discernible, physiological explanation in 80 to 90 per cent of all cases of infertility. No etiology is found for the remaining 10 to 20 per cent.

3. "*Adoption increases the chance of conceiving.*" A study by Rock and associates (1965) found no significant increase in conception among 113 couples who had adopted and 249 couples who had not adopted.

4. "*Infertility is incurable.*" Over 50 per cent of couples who seek assistance of qualified health care professionals become pregnant (Speroff, Glass, and Kase, 1983).

5. "*Infertility is a sexual disorder.*" For most couples, infertility is not related to their ability to perform sexual intercourse.

6. "*It is immoral to want to bear children and to work at it.*" For those who wish to have children, infertility is an involuntary obstacle to their choice of biological parenthood. Cou-

291

ples should not be made to feel guilty because they wish to become biological parents in a world in which some people are concerned with the increasing world population.

7. *"Having a dilation and curettage (D&C) enhances fertility."* This operation subjects a woman to the risks and expense of anesthesia and does not provide information that cannot be found in less invasive procedures. Also, the dilation of the cervical canal does not necessarily improve fertility (Speroff, Glass, and Kase, 1983).

8. *"The benefits of taking unneeded clomiphene (Clomid) outweigh the risks."* Clomiphene is a drug used to stimulate ovulation when a lack of ovulation has been documented as a cause of the infertility (e.g., polycystic ovarian disease). Some infertile patients demand clomiphene, which is sometimes perceived as the "fertility pill." Some physicians prescribe it so they can "do something" for their patients. There is no evidence that unneeded clomiphene improves fertility. Although a relatively safe drug, clomiphene is not without risks. Its use exposes the woman to the risks of multiple births and ovarian cysts and the low risk of unrecognized hazards (Sheridan, Patterson, and Gustafson, 1982). During studies of in vitro fertilization of human ovum, Trounson and associates (1980) found that many cases of unexplained infertility are caused by failure of the sperm to penetrate the ovum. This finding confirms that unneeded pharmacological intervention with clomiphene is inappropriate and gives very little promise of enhancing fertility. With this review of myths and facts about infertility as an introduction, the biophysical factors contributing to infertility are addressed. Subsequently, nursing interventions for the infertile couple are addressed.

BIOPHYSICAL FACTORS AND INFERTILITY: ETIOLOGY

The biophysical etiology of infertility is diverse. After reviewing conditions necessary for fertilization, it seems remarkable that pregnancy occurs. There is some disagreement about what percentage of infertility is attributed to each partner. Hatcher and associates (1982) estimate that male and female factors each account for 40 per cent of the problem with factors from both partners responsible for the remaining 20 per cent.

Shane, Schiff, and Wilson (1976) have attributed 40 per cent of infertility to male factors, 15 per cent to cervical factors, 10 per cent to uterine factors, 30 per cent to tubal and peritoneal factors, 20 per cent to ovarian factors, and 5 per cent to miscellaneous factors. The percentages equal more than 100 per cent because 35 per cent of couples have multiple causes (Table 13–1).

Of the 30 per cent of female infertility related to tubal or peritoneal factors, a number of causes are implicated, including infection, occlusion, fimbrial damage, and pelvic adhesions. *Neisseria gonorrhoeae*, once believed to be the leading cause of pelvic inflammatory disease and its sequelae, has been surpassed by *Chlamydia trachomatis* (Hatcher et al., 1982). The Centers for Disease Control have reported that chlamydial infection is now the most prevalent of sexually transmitted diseases (Droegemueller, 1984). Hatcher and associates (1986) state that sexually transmitted diseases are the cause of 20 to 40 per cent of cases of infertility in the United States. Infertility results because of pregnancy wastage, neonatal death, and damage to male or female reproductive capacities. Another cause of tubal damage is endometriosis. It is no longer believed that only nulliparous, white women over 30 years of age are affected by endometriosis. If a woman complains of dysmenorrhea and dyspareunia as well as infertility, endometriosis should be suspected (Garner and Webster, 1985).

Ovarian, cervical, and uterine factors that influence infertility are listed in Table 13–1. Disorders of the ovary may inhibit ovulation, while those of the cervix may inhibit the passage of sperm. Diethylstilbestrol (DES) exposure and cervical abnormalities may interfere with implantation.

The etiology of the other female causes of infertility include age or nutritional status (starvation or obesity); extreme age or nutritional deficiency may inhibit ovulation. Immunological incompatibility between sperm and cervical mucus may also be a cause.

Approximately 40 per cent of infertility has a male-related etiology. Male infertility is often attributed to alterations in semen production. Abnormalities in semen, which may or may not be associated with documented testicular abnormality, include inadequate volume, failure of semen to liquefy, and decreased sperm concentration or motility. Oligospermia means abnormally low sperm

TABLE 13–1. Summary of Biophysical Causes of Infertility

Tubal or Peritoneal (30%)*	Ovarian (20%)	Women Cervical (15%)	Uterine (10%)	Other (5%)
Infection	Anovulation	Cervicitis	Uterine fibromyomas	Age
Occlusion	Severe oligo-ovulation	Inadequate or poor	Congenital	Drugs
Fimbrial damage	Inadequate luteal	quality cervical	malformations	Nutritional deficiency
Pelvic adhesions	phase	mucus	Intrauterine adhesions	Immunological
Endometriosis	Polycystic ovarian	Diethylstilbestrol	Endometrial	incompatibility
	syndrome	(DES) exposure	abnormalities	Excessive alcohol
				consumption

Seminal	Genetic	Men (40%) Transport	Testicular	Other
Failure of semen to	Klinefelter's syndrome	Hypospadias	Severe oligospermia	Age
liquefy	Reinfenstein's	Retrograde ejaculation	Azoospermia	Drugs
Inadequate volume	syndrome	Epididymitis	Cryptorchidism	Excessive alcohol
Low sperm		Impotence	Testicular agenesis	consumption
concentration		Ductal occlusion	Severe febrile episodes	Cigarette smoking
Decreased sperm		Ductal adhesions		Pollution
motility				Poor nutrition
Poor forward				Immunological
motility				incompatibility
Sperm				Scrotal exposure to
dysmorphology				heat
Varicocele				

Endocrine (men and women)

Panhypopituitarism
Hypothyroidism
Adrenal insufficiency
Congenital adrenal hyperplasia
Cushing's disease
Cirrhosis of liver

*Percentages are according to Shane, Schiff, and Wilson, 1976. They equal more than 100 per cent because of multiple causation.

production; azoospermia, no sperm production.

Some causes of seminal abnormalities are correctable. A slight increase in scrotal temperature can decrease spermatogenesis. Wearing jockey shorts and excessive exposure to heat (saunas, steam baths, hot tubs, or occupations requiring long periods of sitting) may diminish fertility. Excessive use of alcohol and/or cigarettes may also decrease fertility. By making life style changes, these causes can be corrected. Varicoceles are varicose veins of the scrotum or lower abdomen that may interfere with circulation and sperm production. It is noteworthy that 25 per cent of infertile males will have a varicocele. Ligation of a varicocele is associated with a 50 per cent pregnancy rate (Speroff, Glass, and Kase, 1983).

Febrile episodes from hepatitis, mononucleosis, and epidemic parotitis (mumps) can cause decreased sperm production. Febrile episodes can result in permanently decreased sperm count and motility. Although orchitis and resulting decreased or absent fertility are believed to be a major cause of infertility, Shane, Schiff, and Wilson (1976) have found that this condition complicates only 25 per cent of all cases of postpubertal male epidemic parotitis. Usually, cases that result in infertility or sterility are those in which the male's temperature remains over 103°F for 3 or more days.

Cryptorchidism (undescended testicle) or testicular agenesis (incomplete testicular development) are testicular causes associated with permanently inadequate sperm production. Alterations in the transportation of sperm include hypospadias, erectile dysfunction, and retrograde ejaculation. Also, inflammatory or infectious processes (e.g., epididymitis or gonorrhea) may result in occlusions or adhesions of the seminal transport system. Klinefelter's syndrome and Reifenstein's syndrome are two genetic factors that contribute to male infertility. Klinefelter's syndrome is seen in phenotypic males with an XXY chromosome pattern. Males with Klinefelter's syndrome have androgen deficiency, increased development of the breasts (gynecomastia), excessively long legs, and small testes (Rosenthal, 1970; Shane, Schiff, and Wilson, 1976). Reifenstein's syndrome is seen in phenotypic males with an abnormal chromosome pattern and is characterized by decreased testosterone production, increased development of the breasts, and hypospadias (opening of the male urethra upon the undersurface of the penis) (Shane, Schiff, and Wilson, 1976).

Other male factors influencing infertility include increasing age, excessive alcohol consumption, cigarette smoking, toxic exposure (pesticides, radiation), nutritional status (i.e., starvation or obesity), and drug use (e.g., nitrofurantoin, sulfasalazine, chemotherapeutic agents, marijuana, and antihypertensives, such as guanethidine and methyldopa).

Endocrine disorders that contribute to male and female infertility are Kallman's syndrome (hypogonadotropic hypogonadism), panhypopituitarism, hypothyroidism, adrenal insufficiency, congenital adrenal hyperplasia, Cushing's disease, and cirrhosis of the liver.

The assessment of infertility, obviously, assumes that penile-vaginal intercourse is occurring on a regular basis. Occasionally, there is anatomic evidence that vaginal intromission has never taken place. A thorough yet sensitive sexual history is necessary prior to assuming that a couple is infertile (see Chapter 2 on the components of a sexual history).

A detailed discussion of the coital habits of the couple is necessary because the frequency of intercourse, position in which intercourse occurs, use of lubricants (which may be spermicidal or interfere with sperm migration), immediate arising of the female after intercourse, and postcoital douching may all contribute to infertility. The contributions of these sexual factors become more important when the couple has marginal fertility.

A sensitive approach to the sexual history is essential because the private and personal act of intercourse is evaluated for clinical diagnosis. Few people eagerly share the frequency, feelings, and positions used during intercourse. Even in the more sexually liberated culture of today, many clients may be uncomfortable, anxious, or silent during such discussions. Before being able to deal comfortably with a client's sexuality, health professionals must be comfortable with their own sexuality. They need to resolve their sexual identity; have current factual knowledge about human sexual practices; develop a positive self-concept; be able to accept the orientation, preferences, and activities of others without being judgmental; acquire skill in interviewing and in therapeutic use of the self; develop sensitivity to the nonverbal cues of others; and be knowledgeable of sociocultural and religious tenets. If comfortable with their own sexuality, health professionals can assist the client in understanding why the couple's patterns of intercourse need to be clarified and may prevent misperceptions from developing by clarifying the reasoning behind certain questions.

EFFECTS OF INFERTILITY ON PSYCHOSOCIAL ADAPTATION

Regardless of the cause, the psychological impact of infertility on couples may be similar. According to Roy (1980), the following three psychosocial modes of adaptation may be affected. First, an individual's self-concept, one's view of oneself and one's worth, may be taxed. A person may be challenged to maintain a positive self-image when feeling unable to conceive; self-image may have always included being a parent. A second mode of adaptation that may be affected is role function. Roles are persons' expectations or duties based on their given position within society. Society often expects a married couple eventually to become parents. Motherhood and fatherhood are seen, by society, as the ultimate fulfillment of the adult gender role. Third, interactions with others may be taxed. Interdependence involves an individual's ways of seeking help, attention, and affection.

If individuals feel negatively about their self or role function, they might be hesitant to seek out another for help. This may result in feelings of loneliness and alienation. As a self-protective mechanism, couples may distance themselves from each other, changing their customary means of obtaining affection and attention; however, coping strategies such as distancing may not ultimately facilitate positive outcomes. Common responses to threats to self-esteem, social roles, and interdependent functioning will be discussed next.

Psychological Factors and Infertility

From a study of 48 women (26 private and 22 clinic clients) between the ages of 21 and 45, Sandelowski and Pollock (1986) identified three constituent elements of the women's experiences of infertility. These three dominant themes were ambiguity, temporality, and otherness.

Ambiguity was the prevalent theme of both private and clinic clients' descriptions of their infertility experience. Some variants of the ambiguity theme included uncertainty about the etiology of infertility, fumbling in life pursuits, and ambivalence (both loving and hating) toward physicians. For some private clients, the relentless pursuit of fertility became like a career. Some women suspended professional or career goals for the sole purpose of conceiving a child. The ambiguity of infertility itself served to make it virtually impossible for some women to discontinue their pursuit. As long as there were no definite answers, some women refused to stop trying to become a biological parent. Conversely, few clinic clients believed that giving birth to a child was interfering with some other desired life goal. The influence of the feeling of ambiguity was "directly related to the continued hope that pregnancy would be achieved and carried to term" (Sandelowski and Pollock, 1986, p 143).

Temporality was defined as the "heightened consciousness of chronological and biological time" (Sandelowski and Pollock, 1986, p 143). Half of the private-practice clients delayed childbearing until the most opportune time was reached. Having been very goal oriented and accustomed to accomplishing goals within a specific time frame, the inability to become a biological mother caused these women to review past decisions and to extend the time limits to continue the pursuit of biological motherhood. In contrast, the clinic clients waited longer to request medical assistance to determine why they were unable to have children.

Otherness was demonstrated by the making of social comparisons between themselves and women who had become biological parents, feelings of being unfairly singled out, and feelings of not fitting in and being left out. Again, the feelings of "otherness" were experienced more frequently by private

clients than by clinic clients (Sandelowski and Pollock, 1986).

It is interesting to note that these feelings were described by both university-clinic clients and by private-physician clients, although the private client saw her life goals as more disrupted and her "differentness" as being more profound. This may be because real differences occur between private and clinic clients or because the private client is more articulate. Regardless of etiology, health professionals must note that women respond differently to the inability to become biological mothers. Thorough assessment and individualization of care is essential to provide appropriate care for a client experiencing infertility.

The frequently described psychological responses to the threat of infertility are schematically represented in Table 13–2. It is important to note that not all persons or all couples necessarily experience each response and that not all individuals experience responses to the same degree or in the stated sequence. Table 13–2 is a suggested framework for assessment of how couples respond to infertility. It is a description of recurring themes in the literature, not a prescription for normal or ideal coping.

The responses and feelings of denial, self-blame, guilt, anger, depression, and loss have been voiced by infertile individuals. The feelings of loss may include both loss of control over one's body and life plans and loss of the ability to choose or not choose biological parenthood. More specifically, these commonly described responses often represent the threats to one's self-concept stimulated by infertility. Many couples have difficulty with their feelings of anger. An individual may be angry with himself because he cannot father a child or with his partner because she cannot conceive or bear his child. If the source of anger is not acknowledged and worked through, i.e., in relation to one's own self-concept, it may lead to depression, withdrawal, aggression, or disrupted relationships.

Role Function

Throughout life, an individual's role is constantly changing. Roles are defined as "a cluster of related meanings and values that guide and direct an individual's behavior in

TABLE 13–2. Possible Responses to Diagnosis of Infertility

Surprise and Denial	Depression	Anger	Isolation	Acceptance
Denial of reality of infertility and its related issues	Loss of wish fulfillment	Bitterness	Communication gap between partners	Cope with reality of losses of control and choice
	Loss of control over one's life	Feelings of inadequacy	Withdrawal of self from others and spouse (e.g., with feelings of depression)	Deal with feelings of loss and worthlessness
	Loss of ability to choose or not choose parenthood	Self-blame or guilt from past behaviors (masturbation, premarital sex, abortion)		Reevaluate societal value of parenthood and deal with life tasks other than parenthood
	Loss of control over one's body	Anger or blame expressed toward environment or others	Confrontation with others or spouse (e.g., with feelings of anger)	
	Feelings of worthlessness and bodily defectiveness	Depression		
	Loss of sexual attractiveness			
	Feelings of failure to live up to expectations of self and society			

Sources: Hertz, 1982; Rosenfeld and Mitchell, 1980; Williams and Powers, 1977.

a given social setting" (Riehl and Roy, 1980, p 43). Some roles are innate, others are acquired. Everyone is born into the role of a baby and to an assigned role of a specific gender. Upon marriage, the acquired role of parent is often socially expected.

When discussing the psychological impact of infertility, one must consider the social meaning of parenthood and nonparenthood. Veevers (1973) described representative themes of the dominant American cultural definition of parenthood. Although dated, these themes may reflect subtle undercurrents in today's society, especially in more traditional cultures. According to Veevers (1973), nonparenthood may be perceived socioculturally as an avoidance of responsibility, as unnatural, a rejection of gender role, a hindrance to marital adjustment, a sign of immaturity, or emotional maladjustment. If an individual accepts this concept, it is understandable why he or she might have difficulty in accepting infertility and in discussing it with a professional.

An infertile couple's inability to become parents changes their expected versus actual role function. The degree of loss felt by infertile couples is related, in part, to the value they place on the role of parent. Many view the inability to parent as a loss of status. Loss of status may result in anxiety and tension unless appropriate adaptive responses are found.

Interdependence

The varied psychological responses to infertility may tax the functioning of a couple. Often, this interferes with the giving and receiving of physical and sexual closeness. If self-concept is threatened and the person no longer feels positively about him- or herself because of infertility, it follows that sexual interactions can be affected. In addition, the proscriptions and prescriptions for achieving conception—frequency and timing of intercourse and use of certain positions—may contribute tension to a couple's sexual relationship. It is not surprising that couples often complain of decreased desire for intercourse, orgasmic dysfunction, or midcycle erectile dysfunction. A once spontaneous act of loving has become a highly emphasized mechanical act for procreation. Debrovner and Shubin-Stein (1975) asked women who were attempting to conceive to describe their sexual relationships. The sexual problems most frequently identified were changes in desire and enjoyment, achievement of orgasm, initiation of sexual activity, and frequency of intercourse. Those women who were keeping basal body temperature (BBT) charts found it hard to make love because temperatures or a calendar indicated that it was the right time.

For some women studied, coitus became a

distressing reminder of the all-encompassing wish to become pregnant. Some women described a decline in the frequency of orgasm. This sometimes contributed to an already low self-concept. For about half the women, their role changed from passive recipient to active initiator, which sometimes led to the feeling of being a "task master" rather than an initiator of a pleasurable activity. For some women an interesting pattern of intercourse arose: There was a frenzy of sexual activity around the time of ovulation and a sharp decline, to the point of abstinence, after the fertile period. For other women, their sexual activity after the fertile period was similar to that prior to attempting to conceive.

For men, infertility may interfere not only with feelings of virility but also with sexual behavior. Whereas a woman can conceive with a minimum of pleasure and sexual excitement, a man must achieve enough excitation to attain orgasm and ejaculation for conception. The need for "sex on demand" could interfere with male sexual desire or erectile ability.

Infertility As a Crisis

When a couple finds that they are infertile, a state of crisis may often ensue. This is a time when their usual adaptive mechanisms are taxed. In defining crisis, Aguilera and Messick identify Caplan's definition of a crisis. A crisis occurs

when a person faces an obstacle to important life goals that is, for a time, insurmountable through utilization of customary methods of problem solving. A period of disorganization ensues, a period of upset, during which many abortive attempts at solutions are made. (Aguilera and Messick, 1982, p 5)

Four phases of a crisis may be described as the following: (1) An initial rise in tension begins when the usual problem-solving techniques are tried to maintain a state of equilibrium. (2) Increased discomfort is felt as the stress continues with lack of success in coping. (3) A further increase in tension acts as a powerful stimulus, mobilizing emergency problem-solving mechanisms. At this stage, the problem may be redefined or resignation may occur. (4) If the problem continues without either solution or avoidance, tension increases, and major disorganization results (Aguilera and Messick, 1982). Each couple's

response will vary depending on the presence or absence of balancing factors. For example, when Mary and David Simpson (see case study at end of the chapter) did not conceive a child during a year of unprotected intercourse, their equilibrium was disturbed. They felt the need to restore equilibrium. Two pathways are available to such couples. If couples perceive their infertility in a realistic manner, receive adequate situational support, and adapt to nonbiological parenthood or nonparenthood, the problem may be resolved. On the other hand, if their infertility is seen as a personal threat to one or both of them and if they are unable to communicate their feelings and concerns, isolation may occur with resultant feelings of helplessness and hopelessness. For some individuals, the day-to-day sense of failure becomes an ongoing, unresolvable emotional stress.

Usually, nurses do not have contact with infertile couples during the first phases of crisis coping. At this time some couples are in a state of denial and do not seek outside help. Denial, which involves pretending the problem does not exist, demands a tremendous amount of energy. Over time this energy expenditure leads to further discomfort.

As the discomfort rises in the second phase, couples may tentatively examine available resources. Frequently, this occurs by sharing "the secret" of infertility with a friend or relative. They may try the treatments suggested by friends or may discuss whether or not to seek assistance from a health care professional.

If resolution does not occur in phase two, the mounting tension mobilizes emergency problem-solving mechanisms. If the couple's self-esteem is low or if the situation is perceived as especially threatening, the couple seeks situational supports, i.e., those persons who are perceived as facilitators in problem solving.

It is in this phase that health professionals can have the greatest impact. The couple's need for correct and current knowledge is surpassed only by their need for compassionate and empathetic support. Couples need to be given time to ask the many questions they may have. These questions represent a range of concerns: "What did I do?" "Why did this happen?" "Will an endometrial biopsy hurt?" and "Just how do you know when to inseminate me?" In a busy office, it is easy to lose sight of a couple's psychosocial needs. Health professionals, particularly nurses or social workers, can see that sufficient time is scheduled for appointments as well as for providing a time for a couple to discuss physiological and psychological concerns. Anticipating and intervening to meet concerns provide holistic care. If these opportunities are not provided, couples may make frequent phone calls requesting specific, minute information about the plan of care or go without their concerns addressed. It is also recommended that the couple be referred to self-help organizations such as RESOLVE, which is one group that makes possible mutual support and education.

The fourth phase of the crisis in infertility can be reached in two ways—resolution or disequilibrium. Resolution of the crisis can occur by birth of a baby, adoption of a baby, or acceptance of the reality of nonparenthood. Disequilibrium occurs when a couple cannot accept the reality of nonparenthood or use appropriate coping mechanisms to deal with their distress.

Table 13–3 summarizes the common responses of infertile couples related to role concerns, interdependence concerns, and personal expectations. Personal expectations color responses to any perceived threat to a life goal. Successful coping with the threat of infertility would be described as having some degree of resolution about feelings and decisions about parenthood. Successful resolution does not imply either becoming a parent

or living without some feelings of loss. Rather, adaptation implies that the problem of infertility is no longer threatening to a person's usual means of coping or causing a state of crisis.

Health professionals, especially nurses, may facilitate successful coping with and adaptation to the threat of infertility by recognizing that couples vary in their responses to a perceived threat. Therefore, it is important to assess each person and couple to provide the best possible individualized assistance with adaptation to infertility. Two assessment tools may assist health professionals in meeting the needs of infertile individuals. One, an infertility questionnaire, was developed by Bernstein, Potts, and Mattox (1985). This measures specific effects of infertility on self-esteem, blame/guilt, and sexuality. A second tool, developed by Sherrod (1988) assists in evaluating an individual's stage of grief. Individuals and couples may be assisted in their ability to adapt to the reality of infertility if health professionals initially explore alternative courses of action, show concern, allow for discussion of feelings, and are nonjudgmental, empathetic listeners (see Table 13–3). In order to provide correct and current information, health professionals must have a sound knowledge of evaluations and treatments for infertility. Common recommended evaluation procedures and treatment modalities are discussed next.

TABLE 13–3. Common Responses, Nursing Interventions, and Factors Influencing Adaptation to Infertility

Common Responses of Infertile Individuals
  Denial of issues, feelings of loss of control, loss of self-esteem
  Anger (blaming self or others)
  Depression
  Isolation
  Resolution (acceptance or disequilibrium/crisis)

Nursing Interventions To Facilitate Adaptation
  Genuine concern
  Nonjudgmental empathetic listening
  Exploration of feelings
  Exploration of alternative courses of action
  Exploration of life style alternatives
  Emphasis on individual couples' strengths
  Identify social supports and resources
  Identification of new resources (e.g., self-help groups)
  Provision of correct and current information

Factors Influencing Infertile Individual's Adaptation to Infertility
  Personal expectations
  Support of others

ASSESSMENT OF INFERTILITY

Rates of infertility cures are estimated to be between 40 and 65 per cent. Kilmann (1984) reported that 40 per cent of the couples who seek medical help for infertility discover the etiology, correct the cause, and conceive; 40 per cent discover an uncorrectable cause; and 20 per cent neither determine a cause nor conceive. Kilmann studied couples who sought assistance from any health professional, i.e., nurse clinician, general practitioner, and a "generalist" practitioner of obstetrics and gynecology. Speroff, Glass, and Kase (1983) stated that 50 per cent of women attending an infertility clinic will become pregnant; they studied women who specifically sought the assistance of an infertility specialist. For the remaining 50 per cent, diagnoses are found for approximately 90 per cent, but not all of these conditions are correctable. Despite knowing the etiology, approximately 40 per cent of these individuals still will be unable to conceive. For 10 per cent of the individuals seeking assistance from infertility specialists, no known cause of their infertility is found. Rousseau and associates (1983) investigated 1500 women who sought care at an infertility clinic in Canada. After undergoing complete infertility investigations according to the World Health Organization criteria, 47 couples received a prognosis of unexplained infertility. According to Rousseau and associates (1983), the cumulative pregnancy rate, without treatment, was 65 per cent. Despite the absence of demonstrable pathology, couples with 4 or more years of infertility have a poor conception prognosis. For these couples alternatives need to be discussed in greater detail.

Considerations During Assessment and Treatment of Infertility

During the period of evaluation of infertility, the health professional can play a major role in providing relevant information—explaining what procedures are performed, when they are done, and the rationale for the tests and timing. Table 13–4 provides a summary of frequently performed infertility tests. For the sake of clarity a 28-day menstrual cycle is used in the table.

Health professionals, particularly nurses, are in an ideal role to provide sensory information about such tests. According to McHugh,

Christman, and Johnson (1982, p 780), sensory information is "information about our environment that is acquired by way of our sensory modalities—sight, hearing, touch, taste and smell." Health professionals can obtain the commonly used descriptions about tests, in sensory terms, from interviews with current clients and can share the most frequently occurring and neutral descriptions with future clients. Providing preparatory information may assist clients to form an image of what an experience will include and thus help to make those experiences more tolerable and less distressing. In the following paragraphs, the specific client implications of infertility tests are addressed. This is done so that health professionals can be better prepared to provide preparatory information about such tests and to offer emotional support throughout such procedures.

A woman having a hysterosalpingogram can be told that the procedure will be done in a radiology department. A hysterosalpingogram tests for tubal obstruction, which may be corrected using microsurgical techniques. A woman having a hysterosalpingogram should bring a friend to drive her home. The woman is placed in the lithotomy position, a vaginal speculum is inserted, and forceps are used to grasp the cervix. A stick may be felt by some women. A small catheter is inserted in the uterus and a radiopaque dye is injected into the uterus. A woman may experience uterine cramping, burning, and a warm sensation from the dye. If the dye spills into the fallopian tubes, as expected, these three sensations may be felt along her sides. If the dye spills into the peritoneal cavity, referred shoulder pain may be experienced. During the procedure, many radiologists permit the

TABLE 13–4. Timing and Rationale for Frequent Infertility Tests

Days	Test	Rationale
1–4	Hysterosalpingogram, tubal insufflation (Rubin's test)	Late follicular, early proliferative phase will not disrupt a fertilized ovum; may open fallopian tubes before time of ovulation
5–9	Postcoital (Sims-Huhner test) check of cervical mucus	Ovulatory late proliferative phase; cervical mucus should have low viscosity, high spinnbarkeit
14–19	—	—
20–25	Plasma progesterone	Midluteal midsecretory phase—check adequacy of corpus luteal production of progesterone
26–27	Endometrial biopsy	Late luteal, late secretory phase—check endometrial response to progesterone and adequacy of luteal phase
28	—	—

Adapted from Shane JM, Schiff J, Wilson EA: The infertile couple—evaluation and treatment. Clin Symposia 28:14–26, 1976.

woman to observe the passage of dye on the monitor. The woman is given a perineal pad to protect her clothing from the dye. The procedure usually takes 1 hour. Afterward, some women experience uterine cramping and may be instructed to take a warm bath or use a heating pad. Some women require antiprostaglandins or mild analgesics for pain relief.

Tubal insufflation tests are performed to check for tubal patency. Most tubal insufflations are done in physicians' offices. The woman is placed in the lithotomy position, a vaginal speculum is inserted, and forceps are used to grasp the cervix. A small cannula is inserted into the cervix and carbon dioxide is passed through the cervix. Some women experience slight uterine cramping. If the carbon dioxide passes through the fallopian tubes, the woman may experience referred shoulder pain. The woman is given a perineal pad to protect her clothing from the spotting sometimes experienced. The test takes about 15 to 20 minutes. Sometimes after hysterosalpingography or tubal insufflation, fallopian tubes may become more patent and conception occurs.

A couple is instructed to have intercourse approximately 8 hours before a postcoital, or Sims-Huhner test. The woman then comes to the physician's office and is placed in the lithotomy position. A vaginal speculum is inserted, with warm water as a lubricant, so the viscosity of cervical mucus is not changed. Mucus is removed with forceps from the cervical os. Slight cramping may be experienced. The mucus is examined for abundance, clarity, spinnbarkeit (stretchability), and ferning (an ovulatory mucus pattern seen by microscopy). The specimen is also examined for the presence of living, motile sperm with progressive forward motility. Sometimes inadequate cervical mucus can be treated with hormones. If the cervical mucus is inhospitable, artificial insemination with the husband's sperm may be tried. Some couples experience difficulty having sex on demand and this test may need to be rescheduled.

When a couple shares their feelings about the lack of spontaneity of coitus, the health professional can listen. Many physicians limit the period of infertility investigation to help alleviate this problem. The less time a basal body temperature (BBT) must be taken, the less time cervical mucus must be checked, and the shorter the diagnostic period, the less the disruption of a couple's sexual life style.

A nurse can try to schedule appointments for postcoital examinations at the most convenient time for the couple. If a woman is to have artificial insemination with her husband's sperm, the health professional can take the woman to an examining room soon after her arrival. The woman will be less likely to feel as if everyone in the waiting room knows she is carrying a pouch of semen in her bra, which is the usual method of transporting semen to the office.

For an endometrial biopsy, a woman comes to a physician's office. While in the lithotomy position, a small catheter is inserted into the uterus, and a small amount of endometrial tissue is withdrawn from the uterus. The endometrium is examined to determine whether it is proliferative or secretory. Lack of secretory endometrium may imply anovulation or inadequate production of progesterone by the corpus luteum. Anovulation may be treated with clomiphene or bromocriptine (Parlodel). An inadequate luteal phase may be treated with progesterone. Women frequently experience uterine cramping after an endometrial biopsy. Because bleeding may occur after a biopsy, the woman is given a perineal pad to protect her clothing.

Case Study

The following case study on page 301 illustrates some of the psychological and sexual concerns of an infertile couple and serves to synthesize issues presented in this chapter.

ASSESSMENT

Mary and David had married and decided they wished to become parents. They began having unprotected intercourse in their middle thirties (fertility is believed to peak around age 25). Their coital habits are compatible with those recommended for conception. Mary's not arising immediately after coitus might facilitate sperm migration to the fallopian tubes. Her newly acquired difficulty in achieving orgasm may be a response to a perceived threat to her self-concept.

CASE STUDY

Mary and David Simpson have sought care from an infertility specialist. Mary is a 35-year-old, 5-foot 6-inch, 130-pound teacher who married David, a 37-year-old, 6-foot, 160-pound accountant, 2 years ago. They have not been using contraception for 1 year.

SUBJECTIVE DATA

Couple

Coital history revealed a coital frequency of three to four times a week. Intercourse usually took place before bedtime. Mary did not arise after coitus to void or douche. In the past 2 months, Mary has had difficulty achieving orgasm. She reported, "I feel so inadequate, so much less than a normal woman. I was a virgin when I married David. Not being able to conceive a child seems like such an unfair burden. What did I do wrong?" David said little.

Mary

By appearance Mary was in good general health. She was not taking any medications, did not smoke, and drank only occasional alcohol. Gynecological history revealed that menarche occurred at age 12. Her menses were 26 to 28 days in frequency, with a 3- to 5-day duration. Her last menstrual period was February 22, with a previous menstrual period on January 25. Mary experienced mittelschmerz, an abundant stretchy vaginal discharge at midcycle, and had no history of pelvic inflammatory disease, peritonitis, or venereal disease. She had never been pregnant.

David

By appearance David was in good general health. He had no history of mumps, diabetes, or tuberculosis. David had experienced no injury to his scrotum, no hernias, and no history of venereal disease. He had not been exposed to unnecessary x-rays, lead, or chemicals; was not taking any medications; did not smoke; and drank one or two drinks two to four times a month. He wore jockey shorts and enjoyed taking long hot showers and sitting in a sauna after his biweekly racquetball games.

OBJECTIVE DATA

Mary

Her thyroid was nonpalpable. Breasts contained no masses and were without galactorrhea. Examinations of heart, lungs, and abdomen were within normal limits. Pelvic examination revealed a female escutcheon, normal-sized clitoris, and clear cervical mucus. Bimanual examination revealed a pink vagina and a nonparous pink cervix. Uterus was pear shaped, 6 cm long, 3.5 cm wide, 2 cm thick, moveable, anteverted, and slightly antiflexed. Ovaries were smooth, firm, and ovoid; tubes were nonpalpable. Rectovaginal examination confirmed pelvic findings.

Mary's complete blood count and urinalysis were within normal limits. Her serology was nonreactive, gonorrhea culture was negative, and the rubella titer was positive (greater than 1:16).

David

His general physical examination revealed a well-developed male, without signs of feminization or obvious endocrine disease. Urological examination revealed a male escutcheon, circumcised penis, and a central location of the urethral meatus. His testes were ovoid, each measuring 4 cm long by 3 cm wide and 2 cm thick, with epididymis and vas deferens within normal limits. No varicocele was noted. David's prostate was conical, symmetrical, and moveable, with a rubbery consistency. Microscopic examination of prostatic fluid revealed no leukocytes.

David's complete blood count and urinalysis were within normal limits. His serology was nonreactive, and gonorrhea smear was negative.

David had a semen analysis done after 48 hours of abstinence. The results were as follows: volume = 3 ml (normal, 1 to 7 ml); sperm count = 15,000,000 per ml ("good" is 20,000,000 or greater); motility = 50 per cent ("good" is 60 per cent or greater); progressive motility = 50 per cent ("good" is 50 per cent or greater); and normal morphology = 50 per cent ("good" is 60 per cent or greater). (Normal values from Speroff, Glass, and Kase, 1983, pp 508–509.)

Mary's feelings of inadequacy and her searching for blame are common psychological responses. That David volunteered few verbal statements may not be surprising. Perhaps he views infertility as a threat to his manhood. He may be concerned about letting his wife down. Further assessment is indicated.

Mary's menstrual history places her cycles within normal range. Her midcycle symptoms suggest an ovulatory response. Physically neither Mary nor David has any major health problems. Neither takes any medications or smokes. Both drink alcohol only occasionally. Neither has a significant past medical history. No deviations from normal were found after their physical examinations. Mary's and David's complete blood counts, urinalyses, serologies, and gonorrhea cultures were normal.

David has some bathing and recreational practices that might contribute to subfertility. He wears jockey shorts instead of boxer shorts, plays frequent racquetball, and enjoys long hot showers and sitting in a sauna. These practices may increase scrotal temperature and may diminish fertility by decreasing sperm count.

David's semen analysis showed one source of their infertility problem. The volume of seminal plasma was within the normal range of 1 to 7 ml, the sperm count was low (20,000,000 is seen as good), the overall motility was equivocal (60 per cent is seen as good), the progressive motility is within normal limits, and there is an equivocal percentage of sperm with normal morphology (60 per cent is seen as good).

INTERVENTIONS

Some adaptations of activities of daily living may be suggested. David and Mary should be given a rationale for the suggested changes.

The health professional can see that sufficient time is scheduled for appointments to give Mary and David time to ask questions of and share feelings with their health care professional, who can assist the couple's understanding of why the private act of intercourse needs to be discussed openly for professional analysis.

The interventions suggested in Table 13–3 may assist the health professional in providing care for this couple. Realistic nursing goals might include the maintenance of good communication between Mary and David, assistance with achieving and maintaining a satisfactory sexual relationship, and support in adapting to this developmental crisis.

Also, Mary and David should be taught about fertility awareness. This might include taking basal body temperature (BBT) and monitoring cervical mucus to determine if an ovulatory pattern exists. For taking BBTs, Mary would be instructed to purchase a thermometer calibrated in tenths and would be given graph paper on which to record basal

body temperature, coitus, and condition of cervical mucus. She would be instructed to shake the mercury into the tip of the thermometer before retiring for the night. Upon awakening and before any activity, including getting out of bed, voiding, or eating, she would take her oral, vaginal, or rectal (always by the same route) temperature and record it on graph paper. David could be involved in this by reading and recording the temperature. Ovulation may also be detected by use of such home urine tests as Ovu Stick, Quest, or First Response. Since the frequency of ovulation may decrease with age, one or two monophasic BBTs over 3 months should not result in panic. If further infertility tests are planned, the couple can be given additional information to facilitate understanding and adaptation.

It should be suggested that David try to wear boxer shorts, decrease the length and/or temperature of his showers, and limit his time in saunas. Since it takes 74 days for an undifferentiated spermatogonium to become a mature spermatozoa, changes in semen analysis will not be expected for at least 2½ to 3 months. Coital frequency can remain the same.

Information about common causes of infertility and prognosis rates should be discussed. Mary and David need to know that their infertility may or may not be resolved.

If infertility is not resolved by increasing fertility awareness, changing coital techniques, or altering life habits, the possibility of ovulation induction, artificial insemination, in vitro fertilization and embryo transfer, and surrogate motherhood should be discussed. Ovulation induction refers to inducing ovulation with drugs such as clomiphene, bromocriptine, or gonadotropin-releasing hormone (Smith, 1985). Artificial insemination is done by placing semen, from the husband or an anonymous donor, around the cervical os, just inside the cervical canal, or directly into the uterus (Olshansky and Sammons, 1985). Couples must be made aware that acquired immunodeficiency syndrome (AIDS) may be transmitted through donor semen. The American Fertility Society has proposed that fresh semen not be used for donor insemination. Rather, donor semen should be frozen and quarantined for 180 days until the donor is tested for human immunodeficiency virus and found to be seronegative ("Revised New Guidelines," 1988).

In vitro fertilization involves fertilizing a

woman's ovum with the husband's or a donor's semen in a special culture medium. Usually, at the four-cell stage the embryo is placed into the client's uterus via a catheter inserted through the cervical canal. Pace-Owens (1985) states that the procedure costs from $3000 to $6000 per treatment cycle and has a success rate of only one in ten. Surrogate motherhood can be achieved by a number of methods. A woman may be inseminated with semen from the infertile woman's husband, carry the baby to delivery, and have the baby formally adopted by the infertile couple. A newer method is to retrieve an ovum from the infertile woman, fertilize it with the husband's sperm, and place it in the uterus of the surrogate mother-to-be.

Two major ethical problems arise from artificial insemination. These are donor selection and record keeping. Donor selection may result in eugenic decisions being made for clients. Inadequate record keeping may prevent tracing of potential birth defects and may not allow tracing of fathers. Therefore, it would be possible for one donor to father several children, two of whom would be half siblings who might one day meet and marry. The result would be an intermarriage with its increased genetic risks. Two major issues surround human in vitro fertilization with resultant embryo transfer: "Do human beings have the right to interfere so drastically in natural reproduction?" and "Is it permissible to deliberately destroy blastocysts before transfer to the woman's uterus if they are found to be defective?" (Fromer, 1983, p 274). The main ethical issue revolving around surrogate motherhood is to whom the child belongs (Fromer, 1983).

It should be remembered that individuals grieving about infertility do not receive the social support provided individuals grieving other losses. Menning (1977) suggests five reasons why this may be so. One, there is no perceived loss. The couple may not consciously acknowledge being infertile as a loss. In addition, family and friends may be unaware that infertility exists. Therefore, they are unlikely to provide support for the couple. Second, because of the social and sexual overtones, infertility may be seen as a loss that is not socially acceptable, i.e., a loss that is not to be discussed with others. Third, there may be a sense of uncertainty about the loss. Many people do not see possible loss as the same as actual loss. After a definitive diagnosis of infertility is made, some couples choose permanent sterilization to alleviate the uncertainty of the remote possibility of conception occurring some time in the future. Fourth, there may be social negation of the loss. Fifth, there may be a lack of a support system.

Health professionals can help infertile couples become aware that they have experienced a loss of sizable magnitude and that grief is normal. Also, they can assure clients that grief runs a predictable course.

Referral for psychological counseling may be necessary if serious depression appears. Sharing information about RESOLVE, an organization designed to help people with infertility problems, or other infertility networks should be done. RESOLVE's national headquarters is P.O. Box 474, Belmont, Massachusetts 02178. Books about infertility have been written for the public. Two recommended books are Menning's *Infertility: A Guide for Childless Couples* and Silber's *How to Get Pregnant*.

In summary, for health professionals to assist a couple to adapt to and live with their infertility, they must be knowledgeable about the etiology of infertility and the usual psychological, social, and sexual responses to infertility. With knowledge and sensitivity, health professionals can then intervene more effectively. While everyone cannot have a baby, everyone can work toward achieving and maintaining a satisfying interpersonal and sexual relationship.

REFERENCES

Aguilera DC, Messick JM: Crisis Intervention—Theory and Methodology. St. Louis, CV Mosby, 1982.

Bernstein J, Potts N, Mattox JH: Assessment of psychological dysfunction associated with infertility. JOGNN 14:63S–66S, 1985.

Debrovner CH, Shubin-Stein R: Sexual problems in the infertile couple. Med Aspects Human Sexuality 9:140–150, 1975.

Droegemueller W: Pelvic inflammatory disease. Drug Therapy 14:31–34, 1984.

Fromer MJ: Ethical Issues in Sexuality and Reproduction. St. Louis, CV Mosby, 1983.

Garner CH, Webster BW: Endometriosis. J Obstet Gynecol Neonatal Nurs 14:10S–20S, 1985.

Hatcher RA, Guest S, Stewart S, et al: Contraceptive Technology 1986–1987. 13th ed. New York, Irvington, 1986.

Hatcher RA, Stewart GK, Stewart F, et al: Contraceptive Technology 1982–1983. 11th ed. New York, Irvington, 1982.

Hertz DG: Infertility and the physician-patient relationship: A biopsychosocial challenge. Gen Hosp Psychiatry 4:95–101, 1982.

Kilmann PR: Human Sexuality in Contemporary Life. Boston, Allyn and Bacon, 1984.

McHugh NG, Christman NJ, Johnson JE: Preparatory information: What helps and why. Am J Nurs 82:780–782, 1982.

Menning BE: Infertility: A Guide for the Childless Couple. Englewood Cliffs, Prentice-Hall, 1977.

Olshansky EF, Sammons LN: Artificial insemination: An overview. J Obstet Gynecol Neonatal Nurs 14:49S–54S, 1985.

Pace-Owens S: In vitro fertilization and embryo transfer. J Obstet Gynecol Neonatal Nurs 14:44S–48S, 1985.

Revised new guidelines for the use of semen-donor insemination. Fertil Steril 49:211, 1988.

Riehl JP, Roy C: Conceptual Models for Nursing Practice. 2nd ed. Norwalk, Appleton-Century-Crofts, 1980.

Rock J, Tietze C, McLaughlin HB: Effects of adoption on infertility. Fertil Steril 16:305–312, 1965.

Rosenfeld D, Mitchell E: Childless—not by choice. Sex Med Today 4:14–17, 1980.

Rosenthal D: Genetic Theory and Abnormal Behavior. New York, McGraw-Hill, 1970.

Rousseau S, Lord J, Lepage Y, Campenhout JV: The expectancy of pregnancy for "normal" infertile couples. Fertil Steril 40:768–772, 1983.

Roy SC: The Roy adaptation model. In Riehl JP, Roy C (eds): Conceptual Models for Nursing Practice. 2nd ed. Norwalk, Appleton-Century-Crofts, 1980.

Sandelowski M, Pollock C: Women's experiences of infertility. Image: Journal of Nursing Scholarship. 18:140–144, 1986.

Shane JM, Schiff I, Wilson EA: The infertile couple—evaluation and treatment. Clin Symposia 28:1–40, 1976.

Sheridan E, Patterson HR, Gustafson EA: Falconer's the Drug, the Nurse, the Patient. 7th ed. Philadelphia, WB Saunders, 1982.

Sherrod R: Coping with infertility: A personal perspective turned professional. MCN 13:191–194, 1988.

Silber SJ: How to Get Pregnant. New York, Charles Scribner's Sons, 1980.

Smith PM: Ovulation induction. J Obstet Gynecol Neonatal Nurs 14:37S–43S, 1985.

Speroff L, Glass RH, Kase NG: Clinical Gynecologic Endocrinology and Infertility. 3rd ed. Baltimore, Williams & Wilkins, 1983.

Trounson AO, Leeton JF, Wood C, et al: The investigation of idiopathic infertility by in vitro fertilization. Fertil Steril 34:431–438, 1980.

Veevers JE: The social meaning of parenthood. Psychiatry 36:291–309, 1973.

Williams LS, Power PW: The emotional impact of infertility in single women: Some implications for counseling. J Am Med Women's Assoc 32:327–333, 1977.

Woods NF: Human Sexuality in Health and Illness. 3rd ed. St. Louis, CV Mosby, 1984.

PART FOUR:

DISTURBANCES IN SEXUALITY

14: Illness, Chronic Disease, and Sexuality

Michael Carter

The experience of illness can lead to changes in sexuality and sexual functioning. These changes are different, depending on whether the illness is short-term and acute or will be present for the rest of the client's life. The purpose of this chapter is to assist health care professionals in understanding how these changes in health affect the client, the sexual partner, and the family. The conceptual differences between acute illnesses and chronic diseases, with three prototypes of chronic illnesses, are covered, and selected psychobiological and psychosocial aspects of illnesses and their relationship to sexuality are highlighted. By understanding these aspects of chronic illness, health care professionals will be better able to assess and treat clients in relation to their sexuality and sexual functioning.

ACUTE VERSUS CHRONIC ILLNESS

The most obvious distinction between acute and chronic illness is the duration of time that illness is expected to be present. There are no clearly defined time limits, however, that would allow one form of illness to be separated from another. Acute illnesses are short-term but can last from a few hours to a few months; chronic illnesses exist for the rest of the client's life. The aspect of time duration is important; in acute illness there is believed to be a finite period of illness followed by recovery. This expected remission of most or all symptoms allows the client and the health professional to postpone making decisions concerning long-term behavioral changes. Sexual functioning can be postponed, for example, during an acute upper respiratory tract infection, since the person only expects to be ill for a few days. Chronic illnesses, on the other hand, require dramatic alterations in the way clients go about all aspects of their daily living, since no recovery is expected.

A second major distinction between acute and chronic illnesses is the role of health professionals. Major professional roles during acute illness are those of diagnosis and prescription of therapy. An important aspect is providing a name to the cluster of signs and symptoms the client is experiencing. This act of assessment or diagnosis legitimates the problem for the client, who is now "really" sick, and the illness has a name. Therapy is prescribed in order to make the client well again or to cure the illness that has been named. A new treatment may be ordered if the illness is not cured within a specified time frame. For example, an adult who receives a diagnosis of diarrhea may be prescribed a diet of clear liquids. The expectation is that the diarrhea will stop within a relatively short period of time. If the diarrhea is still present beyond these few days, a new prescription will be provided by the health professional and may include medications to slow or stop bowel mobility. The role of the health professional in acute illness is to diagnose and to prescribe a cure for the problem.

The role of the health professional in chronic illness takes on added dimensions. There is still the responsibility for assessment and legitimating the illness. This aspect may be more psychologically difficult, since the diagnosis generally means that the client will have to make lifelong changes. The diagnosis of a chronic illness also means that there is no cure. There is an ongoing responsibility for the health professional to reconfirm that the illness is chronic throughout the treatment process. Continuous assessment is also performed to determine improvement or worsening of the illness.

The prescription of therapy for chronic illness is not intended to cure the illness, as is the case in acute illness. Instead, therapy is designed to manage symptoms or to prevent complications in most instances. Therapy continues for the duration of the illness, and this is usually for the rest of the client's life. The health professional takes on the added responsibility of consultant to the client and family: Advice and opinions are offered concerning appropriate therapy and alterations in daily living, but the client and the family must ultimately decide which alterations are acceptable and which are unacceptable. Clients can be labeled as "noncompliant" when they do not understand or choose not to follow the suggestions of their health professional.

A third distinction that exists between acute and chronic illness is the effect of the type of illness on the family. Acute illnesses usually require only temporary alterations in family functioning, since recovery of the sick member is expected. Various family members assume some of the responsibilities of the sick member with the expectation that these new activities will be given up shortly. A familiar situation occurs when a parent who usually prepares meals is hospitalized. Someone else must now take on the family cooking responsibilities. This is done with the understanding that the parent will become well soon and will resume cooking.

Recovery is not expected from chronic illness, so changes in roles within the family are much more complex. Some chronic illnesses become progressively worse over time, and this requires the family to redefine their roles almost constantly. Sexual functioning can be temporarily suspended during acute illness, but the lifelong nature of chronic illness means that temporary suspension is not an option. New definitions of sexuality and new forms of sexual functioning may be necessary for persons with chronic illness. In fact, research indicates that sexual behavior is positively related to overall adjustment to chronic illness or disability (Berkman, Katz, and Weissman, 1982; Berkman, Weissman, and Friedlid, 1978; Conine and Evans, 1982; Sadoughi, Lesher, and Fine, 1971).

FORMS OF CHRONIC ILLNESSES

There are a number of ways to categorize chronic illnesses. One method is to consider the trajectory of the illness (Glaser and Strauss, 1967; Strauss et al, 1975). From this perspective there are at least three forms of chronic illnesses. One form is a permanent illness or disability that is stable and does not progress over time. Examples include a traumatic amputation of a limb and hypertension. The client and the family are usually re quired to develop new patterns of living only one time in response to the problem. Health professionals attempt to develop an appropriate rehabilitation program to return the client as much as possible to previous levels of functioning. Persons with permanent-stable illnesses or disabilities are usually able to make the necessary life adjustments without too much difficulty.

A second form of chronic illness is permanent and at the same time progressive. The client with this form of illness is not expected to recover and is expected to get progressively worse. Examples include arteriosclerotic heart disease and osteoarthritis. As the illness worsens, the client and the family have to undergo progressive changes in their patterns of daily living. What initially worked in an earlier stage no longer does so.

A third form of chronic illness is characterized by repeated episodes of exacerbations and remissions. There is usually a progression, so that each exacerbation can make the client a little sicker than the previous episode. Examples include rheumatoid arthritis, ulcerative colitis, and multiple sclerosis. Exacerbations of these illnesses are often unpredictable, leading to a great deal of anxiety on the part of the client and the family. In addition, remissions that last for fairly long periods of time cause the client to question whether the illness is real or just imagined.

These three forms of chronic illness are not mutually exclusive. Some clients with rheumatoid arthritis may develop a remission that can last for the rest of their lives (Carter, 1986). These clients would move from an exacerbation and remission form of illness to a permanent-stable illness. Some clients with permanent-stable hypertension can develop progression of their illness with kidney and heart damage.

EFFECTS OF CHRONIC DISEASE SYMPTOMS ON SEXUAL FUNCTION

Three psychobiological factors commonly seen in illness are pain, fatigue, and depression. These factors can affect the sexuality and sexual functioning of acutely or chronically ill persons. In recent years new findings in research have led to a much better understanding of the biological mechanisms that underpin these concepts and allow for much improved assessment and interventions.

Pain

One of the most common psychobiological conditions seen in both acute and chronic illness is pain. The presence of pain can have a profound effect on the sexuality and sexual functioning of clients by altering desire or by disrupting the sexual response cycle.

Pain is very difficult to define for two reasons: (1) We all know what pain is because we have experienced pain in a number of different forms, and (2) the experience of pain is different for each of us. Pain is an unpleasant sensation referred to the body that represents the suffering induced by the psychic perception of real, threatened, or fantasized injury (McCaffery, 1979).

Pain is a subjective and unique experience for each person. Influences upon pain perception include previous experiences, the cultural background and expectation of the person, and the person's unique biology. The perception of pain proceeds through three phases. In the first, or physical, phase, the stimulus is brought into contact with the pain sense organ. Research has not definitely identified what is the primary sense organ for pain. The most common opinion is that cellular or tissue damage activates specific pain receptors through either direct action or by a release of biochemical mediators (Bonica, Lindblom, and Iggo, 1981).

During the second, or physiological, phase of pain perception, the message is transmitted from the initial sense organ to the brain. Melzack and Wall (1970) proposed the "gate control theory" to explain this phase of pain perception. They indicate that there are three spinal cord systems that transmit nerve impulses that are produced in the skin: (1) the cells of the substantia gelatinosa of the doral horn, (2) the dorsal column of fibers, and (3) the T cells of the dorsal horn. These cells are interrelated in modulating the types of stimuli reaching the brain and thereby the perception of pain (Melzack, 1982).

Exciting research has been reported that has changed our understanding of pain perception. New biochemical mediators and endogenous opiate-like peptides (endorphins) have been discovered throughout the body. Endorphins are almost identical to opiates in their analgesic properties and are found in the peripherally circulating blood as well as within the brain. Evidence of nonopiate endogenous pain modulatory systems has also been found (Watkins and Mayer, 1982; Terman et al, 1984).

The psychological phase is the final phase of pain perception (Shikora-Wachter, 1981). In this stage the person assigns meanings to the stimuli received by the brain. These meanings are often context dependent, can be learned through conditioning, can be altered by cultural background, or can be modified by differences in brain biochemistry. These influences on pain perception can account for why some persons report pain for an experience while others report sexual arousal. For example, firm pressure on the nipple during the excitement phase of the sexual response cycle is perceived as stimulating. The same amount of pressure at another time would be perceived as painful.

Pain can have a number of effects on sexual functioning. Chronic pain and pain control drugs may decrease desire (Kolodny et al, 1979). Acute pain experienced during sexual activity can disrupt the response cycle. New findings concerning pain perception will lead to better understanding of the relationships that exist among pain, sexuality, and sexual functioning.

Fatigue

The fatigue that is frequently seen in a wide range of illnesses can cause a marked decrease in sexual functioning. Persons with fatigue will feel depleted and exhausted and may also experience weakness. Fatigued persons will have difficulty beginning and remaining in an activity that requires more than simple attention. There are no valid, objective measures of fatigue in clients (Potema et al, 1986). The best measure is the person's description (Pigg, Driscoll, and Caniff, 1985).

Physiological changes occur in fatigue, including a depletion of the glycogen stores along with build up of lactic acid and other metabolites in the muscle. These changes lead to a decrease in the ability of the muscle to contract and an increase in the time the muscle must spend in recovery (Andreoli et al, 1986).

Fatigue can be a result of the disease process and its effects on various body organs and may be an adverse effect of the drugs or other therapy used to treat the illness.

Fatigue can also result from some of the psychosocial processes seen in illnesses, particularly in chronic illness. Accepting a diagnosis of a chronic illness and working through the acceptance of the permanent nature of the illness can lead to fatigue that is overwhelming at times. There is little emotional gratification in working through these processes. Substantial emotional conflict arises at this time. The fatigue seen in this situation goes away rather quickly when the conflicts have been resolved.

Clients who have fatigue will not be able to develop their sexuality fully or to engage in their ususal sexual activities because the initiation of the sexual response requires conscious focusing, and sexual activity usually requires the use of a large number of muscle groups. Assessment of fatigue may show areas in which fatigue can be decreased in order to increase sexual functioning. Alteration of drug therapy may relieve some fatigue. An example would be replacing lost potassium in a patient taking diuretics. Decreasing the energy requirements of sexual activity may also be helpful. This includes recommending different positions for sexual activity that are less demanding (usually supine) and resting prior to the initiation of sexual activity.

Counseling and emotional assistance to help work through the conflicts of acceptance of a chronic illness can diminish psychological fatigue. This form of intervention does not require a specialist but can be done by nurses and other health professionals in general practice. For example, questioning the client and allowing expression of feelings of anger and loss can be of great assistance.

Depression

Depression is frequently seen in illness. Clients with chronic illnesses are particularly at risk for the development of depression (Miller, 1983). Depression can lead to a marked decrease in desire and disruption of usual sexual functioning. Depression presents an inability to engage to the full extent in usual role responsibilities and can lead to increased focus on somatic complaints as well as to fatigue. Persons who are depressed frequently stop their usual sexual activity. The biochemical nature of depression is currently being investigated.

While there are psychotic depressive illnesses, these are different from the type of depression that accompanies chronic illness. The most common form of depression seen is reactive depression and is an expected behavioral state for people with a chronic illness. Reactive depression is brought on by the reaction to the nature and magnitude of the losses caused by the chronic illness. People with reactive depression will report that they feel discontented, tired, or anxious. They do not enjoy doing things that were previously enjoyable. When questioned closely, depressed clients will give a history of low feelings of self-worth, inferiority, or guilt (Andreoli et al, 1986).

The treatment of reactive depression generally involves assisting clients in working through their feelings of loss associated with their illness. As clients work through these losses, their feelings of depression lift. Antidepressant and anxiolytic drugs are not very effective in the treatment of reactive depression and may, in fact, prolong the problem. The supportive interpersonal relationships that clients have with their primary caregivers are generally useful in the self-limited response to loss. The resumption of the usual pattern of sexual functioning is an indicator that reactive depression is resolving.

EFFECTS OF CHRONIC DISEASE ON PSYCHOSOCIAL ADAPTATION

There are a number of psychosocial concepts that are helpful in understanding the client's response to illness. These concepts are body image, self-concept, sick role, and adaptive tasks. The theoretical formulation and research of these concepts has been done primarily by psychologists, sociologists, and social psychologists, but these concepts are frequently utilized by nurses and other health professionals.

Self-Concept

A great deal has been written about self-concept, but most of this literature is conceptual and not research based, and thus there is a lack of agreement among scientists concerning the meaning of self-concept.

Self-concept is usually used to refer to the qualities that people attribute to themselves (Kinch, 1963) and is made up of the psychosocial components and processes that people use to form a view of themselves. One component of self-concept is the view of the self as an object and consists of the attitudes and feelings that people have about themselves. The other component of self-concept is the psychological processes that people use to govern their behavior; this is referred to as the self-process component (Hall and Lindzey, 1970).

People learn to view themselves as objects through their many experiences with others. Newborns do not consider themselves as objects. Rather, the development of the view of the self as an object evolves through interactions with others who treat the person as an object, such as the self as an object of sexual attention. This view is developed through sexual experiences and evolves across the life span.

Persons with acute illness and those in the first phases of a chronic illness frequently do not view themselves as desirable objects for sexual activity. (The reader is referred to Chapter 25, Body Image Concerns, Surgical Conditions, and Sexuality, for a complete discussion of the impact of body image on sexuality.) This view of the self is present because their major task at this point is to return to health. Sexual activity is a part of wellness behavior, not illness behavior. As the acute illness resolves, normal sexual activity can resume. There can be problems for persons with chronic illnesses, however. There is a tendency for chronically ill persons to see themselves as well and as an appropriate object of sexual attention, while others view them as ill and not appropriate objects for sexual activity.

Chronically ill persons constantly revise their self-concept in response to the reactions of others. These revisions will require new views of the self as a sexual object as well as new value systems that support sexual functioning if the person is to continue to develop a satisfying sexuality. Guidance and counseling may be required for sexual partners of chronically ill persons to allow for resumption of sexual activity. For example, sexual partners of persons with rheumatoid arthritis will need to know that sexual activity will not do damage and can enhance feelings of normalcy. Careful explanations of the illness and its limited effects on sexual functioning can help the partner.

Body Image

Body image refers to the way people organize the complex set of sensations and spatial relationships of the body. The framework for our current understanding of body image was developed by providing a psychoanalytic symbolism framework for how people relate to their physical body (Ritchie, 1973).

McDaniel (1976) proposes that body image develops from the combination of postural and tactile impressions, visual sensations, and the spatial relationships persons have with their bodies. Body image is made up of the meanings and values that people give to these sensations and relationships. Body image is strongly influenced by how people interact with their environment. The exact relationship between body image and sexuality is not known, but the assumption is generally made that a positive body image enhances sexuality. Actual research findings to support this assumption are very limited.

Illness brings about changes in body image. For example, illnesses that cause deformity or disfigurement mean that the person cannot move or interact with others as was done before the illness. Acute illness usually only brings temporary changes, but chronic illnesses can lead to dramatic changes in body image. The ways in which alterations in body image influence the person's response to chronic illness are poorly understood. The relationship of "distortions," or changes, in body image to alterations in sexuality or sexual functioning is not known. Logically, persons who view their bodies negatively will likely have disrupted sexuality.

Role Function

The concept of sick role is a common part of everyday practice and is used to explain the behavior of people who are ill. Talcott Parsons (1951, 1958) developed this concept to focus on the behavior of people in Western societies. There are four important assumptions of the sick role:

1. People do not choose illnesses; therefore, they are not held responsible for developing them.

2. Illnesses exempt people from normal obligations.

3. People are obligated to attempt to overcome their illnesses, since being ill is undesirable.

4. If people cannot get well by themselves, they are expected to seek competent help for their illness and to cooperate with attempts to get them well.

Important in these assumptions is the view that being well is the normal state, and illness is an unintentional and abnormal state. Also, people are not held responsible for being sick even when their illness resulted from their own actions or irresponsibility.

Parsons' sick role model seems to fit acute illnesses but does not account for chronic illness in the same manner. Recovery is not expected from chronic illness and exemption from normal role obligations could not be expected to last forever. In addition, some people with chronic illnesses may be held responsible for their illnesses, as in the case of people who have chronic obstructive lung disease and are also smokers.

Stopping sexual activity may be viewed as a way to increase the likelihood of getting well. An example is the man who has a myocardial infarction and believes he should conserve all his strength to get well. This view may be held by the client as well as any sexual partners. Again, for the person with an acute illness this is a time-limiting situation, but for chronically ill persons and their sexual partners this view may lead to stopping all sexual activity permanently. Guidance from a health professional can be helpful in maintaining sexual functioning. Open, frank, and frequent questioning concerning sexual activity is beneficial. Concerns or problems can then be discussed.

Adaptive Tasks

People who are ill will go through a number of psychosocial adaptive tasks as they progress through their illness. The assumptions concerning the sick role apply to the tasks for the acutely ill person. In general, acutely ill persons have to give up their normal role responsibilities and focus all of their activities on getting well. This is not quite the case for chronically ill persons, who must first obtain and accept a diagnosis. This is no small task when one considers that several chronic illnesses present themselves initially with a few diverse signs or symptoms. People with hypertension, for example, may go for years without an appropriate diagnosis. Frequently, the chronically ill person will have to spend time convincing the health professional that something is wrong. For example, women in the very early stages of rheumatoid arthritis may have only transient symptoms. There may be no visible signs of the disease, and all laboratory work can be negative. The health professional may diagnose the woman as having depression. Chronically ill persons can sometimes refuse to agree that there is anything the matter with them. They can become convinced that some type of error was made in assessment and can go to a number of different health professionals for different opinions.

Once the diagnosis is made and agreed on by both the client and the health professional, the next task is to accept that the condition is permanent and that complete recovery cannot be expected. This is a very difficult task and can be accompanied by periods of denial and bargaining. The client may say that the illness will be cured if he or she follows all aspects of the diagnosis and treatment plan. Completing this task can be further compounded if the illness is characterized by periods of exacerbations and remissions. The person in remission can become convinced that an error was made in the diagnosis and that the condition is not permanent after all.

The third task is to learn how to deal with the health care team in order to have the chronic illness treated in an acceptable manner. When the illness progresses, clients learn that health professionals can become angry with them for not getting well and can accuse them of not following therapeutic orders. In addition, most chronic illnesses require treatment from a surprisingly large number of different specialists, who usually do not interact with each other. The only common point is the client. Clients learn whom to ask what, which provider will prescribe what is needed, and how to please their providers in order to continue the long-term relationship necessary for the management of the illness.

There are different effects on sexuality with each adaptive task. During the first task, there may be a great deal of anxiety for both the person and any sexual partners. This anxiety may reduce normal sexual functioning. While the client completes the second task, sexuality may vary from decreased to normal to increased. This will depend on how easily the person and the usual sexual partners accept the permanent nature of the illness. Sexuality usually returns to normal as the client learns how to deal with the health care team.

All ill persons do not either fit the sick role or go through the adaptive tasks of chronic illness. There may be family or cultural sanctions that direct them to respond to their illnesses in other ways. For example, some families may strongly believe that all ill members should only follow the directions of their physician, that there should not be any client-initiated changes in the treatment, and that there should be no "normal" role function as long as the person is ill. This would mean that rehabilitation of long-term illness would be very difficult. Understanding these concepts will help in a number of situations and will allow for planning interventions that foster sexuality and sexual functioning.

NURSING PROCESS

Assessment

Health professionals can facilitate the sexuality and sexual functioning of clients with chronic illness by first making a complete assessment of factors that impede the client's sexual functioning. These can include the nature and course of the illness, the types of medications used in the treatment, the perceptions of the client about the illness, the appropriate role in sexual functioning while ill, and any physical limitations imposed by the illness that could prevent the client from expressing sexuality in the usual way.

Intervention

Open and frank discussion of problems or potential problems in sexual functioning is very helpful. Any misconceptions concerning limitations imposed by the illness need to be corrected. The sexual partner of a client with an amputation may believe that sexual intercourse would cause pain. Discussion can be focused on sexual positions and alternative forms of sexual expression that better fit the client's situation. Male clients with spinal cord injuries and their partners will need assistance in attaining and maintaining erection for intercourse. Tactile sexual stimulation above the site of the cord lesion will be more satisfying than genital stimulation. (The reader is referred to Chapter 20, Spinal Cord Conditions and Sexuality, for a complete discussion of this topic.) Clients who are chronically ill or who have handicaps may need assistance in locating suitable sexual partners and in discussing the fear of rejection because of their condition. Support groups such as arthritis clubs can be very helpful.

The sexual functioning of the chronically ill person is the primary focus of assistance, since persons with acute illnesses usually return quickly to their previous level of sexual functioning. An encouraging note, however, is that most chronically ill clients can and do develop new forms of sexual activity. Clients who have a history of satisfying sexual relationships prior to the development of their illness are most likely to make these changes with the most ease. A more concerted effort may be required for clients who are just developing sexual relationships, such as young adults, and for clients who have to develop new partners, such as those who are divorced or widowed.

REFERENCES

Andreoli TE et al: Cecil Essentials of Medicine. Philadelphia, WB Saunders, 1986.

Berkman AH, Katz LA, Weissman R: Sexuality and lifestyle of home dialysis patients. Arch Phys Med Rehab 63:272–275, 1982.

Berkman AH, Weissman R, Friedlid MH: Sexual adjustment of spinal cord injured veterans living in the community. Arch Phys Med Rehab 59:22–23, 1978.

Bonica JJ, Lindblom U, Iggo A: Advances in Pain Research and Therapy: Proceedings of the Third World Congress on Pain. New York, Raven Press, 1981.

Carter, MA: Rheumatoid arthritis. In Price SA, Wilson LM (eds): Pathophysiology: Clinical Concepts of Disease Processes. 3rd ed. New York, McGraw-Hill, 1986, pp 967–973.

Conine TA, Evans JH: Sexual reactivation of chronically ill and disabled adults. J Allied Health 11:261–270, 1982.

Emanuel E: We are all chronic patients. J Chronic Dis 35:501–502, 1982.

Feldman D: Chronic disabling illness: A holistic view. J Chronic Dis 27:287–291, 1974.

Glaser BG, Strauss A: The Discovery of Grounded Theory. Chicago, Aldine Press, 1967.

Hall CA, Lindzey G: Theories of Personality. New York, John Wiley & Sons, 1970.

Kinch JW: A formalized theory of self-concept. Am J Soc 68:481–486, 1963.

Kolodny RC et al: Textbook of Human Sexuality for Nurses. Boston, Little, Brown & Co, 1979.

McCaffery M: Nursing Management of the Patient with Pain. Philadelphia, JB Lippincott, 1979.

McDaniel J: Physical Disability and Human Behavior. 2nd ed. New York, Pergamon, 1976.

Melzack R: Recent concepts of pain. J Psychosom Res 19:319–324, 1982.

Melzack R, Wall P: Psychophysiology of pain. Int Anesthesiol Clin 8:3, 1970.

Miller JF: Coping with Chronic Illness: Overcoming Powerlessness. Philadelphia, FA Davis, 1983.

Parsons T: The Social System. New York, Free Press, 1951.

Parsons T: Definitions of health and illness in the light of American values and social structure. In Jaco EG (ed): Patients, Physicians, and Illness. New York, Free Press, 1958.

Pigg JS, Driscoll PW, Caniff R: Fatigue. In Pigg JS et al (eds): Rheumatology Nursing: A Problem-Oriented Approach. New York, John Wiley & Sons, 1985.

Potema K et al: Chronic fatigue. Image 18:165–169, 1986.

Ritchie J: Schilder's theory of the sociology of the body image. Matern Child Nurs J 2:143–153, 1973.

Sadoughi W, Lesher M, Fine HL: Sexual adjustment in chronically ill and disabled population: A pilot study. Arch Phys Med Rehab 52:311–317, 1971.

Sakalys JA: The meaning of health and illness. In Mitchell PH (ed): Concepts Basic to Nursing. 2nd ed. New York, McGraw-Hill, 1977.

Shikora-Wachter NL: Pain theories and their relevance to the pediatric population. Issues Compr Pediatr Nurs 5:321–326, 1986.

Strauss A et al: Chronic Illness and the Quality of Life. St. Louis, CV Mosby, 1975.

Strauss A et al: Social Organization of Medical Work. Chicago, University of Chicago Press, 1985.

Terman GW et al: Intrinsic mechanisms of pain inhibition: Activation by stress. Science 226:1270–1277, 1984.

Watkins L, Mayer D: Organization of endogenous opiate and nonopiate pain control systems. Science 216:1185–1192, 1982.

15: Cancer and Sexuality

Rebecca Ingle

The topic of sexuality and cancer has long been shrouded in mystery. It is an area that health professionals have been reluctant and afraid to deal with, sometimes treating it as a nonentity. Sexuality has been arbitrarily designated as a low priority need for cancer patients, even when quality of life is considered, because we are more concerned with psychological adjustment than with psychosexual adjustment (Schain, 1981). However, sexuality for the cancer patient often means being human and being alive (Woods and Lamb, 1981). Therefore, since sexual dysfunction can occur in up to 100 per cent of patients (Derogatis and Kourlesis, 1981; Gunby, 1981), the message to caregivers is that this area cannot be ignored.

Cancer and its therapies may affect sexuality in many ways. The purposes of this chapter are to explore these effects and to discuss implications for nursing. Because Chapter 25, Body Image, Surgical Conditions, and Sexuality, addresses the effects of many surgeries associated with cancer, only a few selected surgical procedures will be discussed here. (Chapter 22, Gynecological Conditions and Sexuality, addresses the unique concerns of women having a vulvectomy for cancer.)

EFFECTS OF CANCER-RELATED SYMPTOMS ON SEXUAL FUNCTION

Fatigue

Fatigue and general malaise are common effects of the cancer disease process and are due to increased tumor nutrient utilization (Woods and Lamb, 1981). Fatigue is usually progressive during the day and is often associated with decreased sexual desire and decreased ability to express sexual feelings physically. Sexual activity is most easily tolerated after a nap or in the morning. The patient should be encouraged to experiment with positions requiring the least physical exertion and should plan for rest after intercourse. A heavy meal or alcohol should be avoided prior to sex (Woods and Lamb, 1981).

Dyspnea

Dyspnea in the cancer patient may be caused by lung cancer, anemia, infectious lung processes, ascites, lymphangitic spread of tumor, or a pleural effusion. Since the oxygen requirement for intercourse is roughly equivalent to the oxygen requirement for climbing one flight of stairs (Fedak, 1981), the patient's ability to perform this activity should be evaluated. Positions of least exertion should be suggested, and alternatives for sexual expression should be explored with the patient and partner. The use of oxygen or bronchodilators prior to sex can enhance the enjoyment of sexual activity (Fedak, 1981).

Pain

When pain is experienced, pain stimuli compete with sexual stimuli, resulting in decreased sexual desire (Woods and Lamb,

1981). Pain medication should be taken 1 hour prior to sexual activity, although narcotic pain medications may decrease sexual desire or interfere with erection (Greenberg, 1984; Silberfarb, 1984). Other suggestions for maximizing comfort include use of relaxation techniques, a warm bath or hot soak to the affected area prior to intercourse, and the use of pillows or a waterbed (Fedak, 1981). Again, alternatives to intercourse can be suggested, and use of different positions should be encouraged.

Tumor Invasion

Organ, nerve, and vascular damage from tumor invasion can have devastating effects on sexuality. Lesions and ulcerations of the genitals due to vascular impairment may cause body image and sexual intimacy disturbances (Jusenius, 1981). Cancers of the reproductive and genitourinary systems may cause erectile dysfunction, sterility, or infertility due to interference with sympathetic or parasympathetic innervation. Spinal cord compression from tumor invasion not only can block perception of sexual sensations but also can interfere with reflex mechanisms for erection or ejaculation (Woods and Lamb, 1981).

EFFECTS OF CANCER-RELATED SURGERY ON MALE SEXUALITY

Erection is a function of the parasympathetic nervous system, and ejaculation is a function of the sympathetic nervous system (Shipes and Lehr, 1982). Disruptions in erection or ejaculatory function can occur after surgical interventions for both testicular and prostate cancers.

The treatment for testicular cancer often begins with unilateral orchiectomy and retroperitoneal lymphadenectomy. With unilateral orchiectomy alone, sexual function and fertility are preserved (Gorzynski and Holland, 1979); an artificial gel-filled testicle may be implanted when there is no evidence of disease (Hubbard and Jenkins, 1983). Retroperitoneal lymphadenectomy, on the other hand, often results in loss of the lumbar sympathetic ganglia or severance of the hypogastric plexus along the celiac vessels (Greenberg, 1984), causing retrograde ejaculation of semen into the bladder. In a study of 101 patients between 1969 and 1982, Nijman (1987) reported that 89 of those patients had "dry ejaculation" after bilateral retroperitoneal lymph node dissection for testicular cancer. This may be due to incomplete closure of the bladder neck (Howard-Ruben, 1983) and should be explained to the patient. Nijman suggests that a modified or unilateral retroperitoneal lymph node dissection may help preserve antegrade ejaculation. In an earlier study, Nijman and associates (1982) reported that 10 out of 14 patients resumed antegrade ejaculation after receiving 25 mg of imipramine (Tofranil) twice a day. Five of the patients' partners became pregnant after treatment with imipramine was instituted. Even though ejaculation after retroperitoneal lymphadenectomy is retrograde, the basic ejaculatory and erectile functions are preserved.

Radical prostatectomy causes impotence in 85 to 90 per cent of patients because of the severance of the sympathetic and parasympathetic nerves (Fisher, 1983), although nerve-sparing radical prostatectomy, with preservation of potency, is now an option in some medical centers for men with prostate cancer (Schover, 1987). When erectile dysfunction is a potential outcome of surgery, preoperative counseling is imperative. Orgasmic function is not affected by radical prostatectomy, although ejaculation is "dry" owing to removal of the prostate gland and seminal vesicles.

Although a penile prosthesis is an option for men with no genitourinary, metastatic, or recurrent disease (Hammond and Middleton, 1984). It is not appropriate for everyone (Hammond and Middleton, 1984). The reader is referred to Chapter 21, Genitourinary Conditions and Sexuality, for an in-depth discussion of this option.

EFFECTS OF CHEMOTHERAPY ON SEXUALITY

Treatment with chemotherapeutic agents can produce both general, systemic side effects that interfere with sexual expression and specific effects on potency and fertility in both men and women. General systemic effects are numerous; one of the most common is fatigue, which is usually most pronounced the first few days after a chemotherapy treatment. While fatigue may cause decreased desire, often the patient has sexual desire but is physically incapable of an active sex life. Nausea and vomiting from chemotherapy certainly inhibit sexual expression. Bone marrow suppression can cause increased susceptibility to infection; yeast infections are common. The patient should be instructed in excellent perineal hygiene and may use Povidone-iodine (Betadine) douches after intercourse. When the patient is thrombocytopenic, bruising or bleeding can occur, particularly with vigorous sexual activity. Water soluble lubricating jelly should be recommended to prevent friction-induced ecchymosis.

Some chemotherapy drugs can affect sexuality by interfering with organ function. Bleomycin can cause pulmonary fibrosis with resulting dyspnea. Doxorubicin in high cumulative doses can cause cardiomyopathy, limiting tolerance of physical activity. Vincristine and vinblastine are neurotoxic and can cause erectile dysfunction in men (Nevidjon, 1984).

Hair loss (alopecia), acne, skin changes, weight loss, urticaria, and dry skin cause changes in body image that are very difficult for patients to accept (Hogan, 1980). A hypothermia cap used to prevent or delay alopecia should be offered to the patient unless contraindicated, and reassurance should be given that hair will grow back after chemotherapy is completed. Moisturizing creams or lotions are helpful for dry skin; petrolatum should not be used because it removes moisture from the skin.

Effects on intestinal, oral, and genital mucosa can occur after treatment with some types of chemotherapy. Painful lesions at these sites and decreased vaginal lubrication may inhibit sexual expression. Antiestrogen therapy (tamoxifen) for breast cancer is associated with menopausal symptoms in about 25 per cent of patients (Flynn and Durivage, 1982), including hot flushes, sweating, nausea, irritability, and vaginal bleeding or spotting (Greenberg, 1984). Chapman (1982) reports that oral clonidine or diphenhydramine hydrochloride may be helpful in reducing the severity of hot flushes.

In addition to chemotherapy, antiemetics and analgesics are also frequently prescribed for cancer patients. The phenothiazine antiemetics can decrease libido and ejaculatory ability (Fedak, 1981; Silberfarb, 1984), and narcotics may suppress erectile function, slow ejaculation, and decrease sexual desire (Fedak, 1981; Greenberg, 1984).

Fertility and Men

Since one goal of cancer chemotherapy is cure, we must learn more about the effects of therapy on fertility for those who wish to bear children. Many chemotherapy drugs, especially the alkylating agents, have documented depressant effects on spermatogenesis, including oligospermia and azoospermia (Thachil, Jewett, and Rider, 1981, Table 15–1). The effect on spermatogenesis is abrupt, not progressive, and dose related (Kaempfer, Hoffman, and Wiley, 1983). Testicular damage results in atrophy of the seminiferous tubular epithelium, where spermatogenesis occurs. Leydig cell function remains intact with continued testosterone production.

Spermatogenesis often recovers after single-agent treatment but is less likely to recover after intensive combination chemotherapy (Johnson et al, 1984). Patients with testicular cancer and Hodgkin's disease have been the most-studied groups regarding infertility. Of note is that prechemotherapy sperm counts in these patients have been reported to be subfertile in nearly 50 per cent of cases (Johnson et al, 1984; Kaempfer et al, 1983). The reason for this is unknown but may be related to the disease process itself. The antiandrogen flutamide, in combination with medical or surgical castration for the treatment of prostate cancer, has been associated with decreased libido and inability to maintain an erection in up to 70 per cent of men receiving the drug (Rousseau et al, 1988).

One chemotherapy regimen that illustrates the general effects of chemotherapy on sexuality is the CHOP protocol (cyclophosphamide, doxorubicin, vincristine, and prednisone). Twenty-three lymphoma patients treated with CHOP were interviewed 24 to 78 months after discontinuing therapy. Twelve of twenty patients who were previously sexually active described sexual dysfunction related to their treatment, including (1) decreased sexual desire, (2) decreased ability to maintain an erection, (3) decreased ability to engage in sexual activity due to doxorubicin-associated congestive heart failure, and (4) paresthesias that interfered with sexual pleasure (Armitage, 1984).

Several other chemotherapy protocols have been studied regarding their effects on fertility. The MOPP, or MVPP (mechlorethamine, Oncovin (vincristine)/procarbazine,

TABLE 15–1. Chemotherapeutic Agents and Regimens Associated with Testicular and Ovarian Damage in Humans

Agent/Regimen	Ovarian Damage (Reference)	Testicular Damage (Reference)
Agents		
Mechlorethamine		Chapman, 1982
Cyclophosphamide	Warne et al, 1973; Koyama et al, 1977	Miller, 1971; Fairley et al, 1972
Chlorambucil	Ezdinili and Stutzman, 1965	Richter et al, 1970; Miller, 1971
Busulfan	Galton et al, 1958	Chapman, 1982
Alkeran	Fisher et al, 1979; Sherman et al, 1978	
Procarbazine		Sieber et al, 1978
Hydroxyurea		LUCC, 1979
Vinblastine	Sobrinho et al, 1971	Vilar, 1974
Cisplatin		Yarbro and Perry, 1985
Methotrexate		Shamberger et al, 1981
Cytosine arabinoside		Chapman, 1982
5-Fluorouracil		Chapman, 1982
Doxorubicin		LUCC, 1979; Decunha et al, 1979
Regimens		
MOPP/MVPP	Chapman et al, 1979	Whitehead et al, 1982
ABVD		Yarbro and Perry, 1985
CMF vincristine	Rose and Davis, 1977	
Doxorubicin, cyclophosphamide, methotrexate	Shamberger et al, 1981	

prednisone), regimens for Hodgkin's disease have been associated with azoospermia after 1 to 2 courses of therapy that persists up to 8 years or longer after chemotherapy is completed (Johnson et al, 1984). The vinblastine, cisplatin, and bleomycin (VPB) regimen for testicular cancer has also been associated with azoospermia, but 50 per cent of men have recovery of spermatogenesis 24 to 36 months after completion of treatment (Drasga et al, 1982). Evidence of any spermatogenesis at testicular biopsy after completion of chemotherapy is a favorable prognostic sign for return of reproductive function (Kaempfer, 1981). Clearly, pretreatment counseling regarding potential infertility, artificial insemination, and adoption is indicated for men receiving intensive combination chemotherapy.

Cryopreservation of semen (sperm banking) is an option for some men who will receive combination chemotherapy. The goal of sperm banking is to store the patient's own sperm prior to chemotherapy for future use via artificial insemination. While sperm banking should be offered as an option, there are several problems associated with the procedure. First, as mentioned before, some men have subfertile sperm counts at the time of diagnosis, so that the semen is unacceptable for cryopreservation. Second, three to six ejaculates collected 2 to 4 days apart are required, which can cause an unacceptable delay of treatment in many cases. The danger of mutagenicity exists if semen is collected after treatment begins. Cryopreservation is also expensive, since it is not reimbursed by insurance companies (Kaempfer et al, 1983). All patients considering sperm banking must be advised about collection and storage procedures, costs, and artificial insemination.

Fertility and Women

Chemotherapy in women may cause irregular menses, amenorrhea, and premature menopause. The ovarian dysfunction is due to ovarian fibrosis with a decrease in the number of ova. Unlike the effects of chemotherapy on spermatogenesis, ovarian dysfunction is progressive rather than abrupt; the duration and reversibility appear to be dose related (Kaempfer, 1981).

Ovarian dysfunction has been associated with several drugs (see Table 15–1), including cyclophosphamide, chlorambucil, busulfan, melphalan, and vinblastine (Johnson et al, 1984). With cyclophosphamide, ovarian failure appears to be dose and age related: Women receiving higher doses and older women experience earlier dysfunction (Johnson et al, 1984).

A study of women with Hodgkin's disease receiving the MVPP protocol showed that 88 per cent had amenorrhea or irregular menses 3 years after treatment. Many of the women experienced menopausal symptoms and reported decreased sexual desire. The divorce rate for these women was also significantly higher than for women in the general population (Chapman, Sutcliffe, and Malpas, 1979). In an attempt to preserve ovarian function in women receiving MVPP, Chapman and Sutcliffe (1981) used oral contraceptives to arrest follicular activity. The women treated had more primordial follicles and fewer "failing ovary" hormonal findings after chemotherapy treatment was completed.

Adjuvant chemotherapy treatment for breast cancer and soft tissue sarcoma has also been associated with a high incidence of ovarian dysfunction, with variable recovery (Johnson et al, 1984). Women receiving chemotherapy treatment must be advised regarding potential ovarian dysfunction, noting that it appears to be more common and more severe in women over 35 years old (Yarbro and Perry, 1985).

FUTURE FERTILITY OF CHILDREN

Because of the advances made in cancer treatment over the past decade, many children with cancer are now being cured. It becomes increasingly important, therefore, to investigate the long-term effects that chemotherapy may have on these children. Effects on fertility is certainly an area worthy of study. In boys, it appears that the prepubertal testes may be relatively resistant to the adverse effects of MVPP specifically and combination chemotherapy in general (Johnson et al, 1984). The germinal epithelial injury is dose related, and the threshold for injury appears greater than that with the adult testes (Schilsky et al, 1980). In adolescent males treated with chemotherapy there has been evidence of decreased sperm count and of Leydig cell failure with decreased testosterone levels. Function may return after treatment (Kaempfer et al, 1983).

Little is known about the late effects of chemotherapy in girls, although prepubertal girls have fewer adverse effects than prepubertal boys or than adults of either sex (Ruccione and Fergusson, 1984). Because there are few data at present, childhood cancer survivors should be advised not to assume sterility, and they should be given birth control information.

Teratogenicity and Mutagenicity

Teratogenicity and mutagenicity are also possible effects of chemotherapy. Teratogenesis is the production of fetal abnormalities or death through drug effects exerted in utero. Based on theoretical and animal studies it is probable that (1) chemotherapy is highly teratogenic during the first trimester, with a higher spontaneous abortion rate; (2) alkylating agents and antimetabolites are likely to cause fetal abnormalities, while antimitotic agents (vinblastine, vincristine) are less teratogenic; and (3) little is known regarding the effects of combination chemotherapy during pregnancy (Kaempfer, 1981).

If a woman is pregnant at the time of diagnosis, either chemotherapy should be delayed or the option of therapeutic abortion discussed. Breastfeeding is contraindicated for women receiving chemotherapy, since the drugs are excreted in the breast milk.

Mutagenesis is genetic damage to sperm or ova prior to conception. Fetal abnormalities in women who became pregnant after completion of chemotherapy have occurred but have been infrequent. Many normal pregnancies in women previously treated with chemotherapy, and in wives of men treated with chemotherapy, have been reported (Johnson et al, 1984).

The incidence of cancer in the offspring of patients treated with chemotherapy has been slightly higher than in the general population. It is unknown whether exposure to chemotherapy in utero can cause changes in germ cells that will present in later generations (Kaempfer, 1981).

EFFECTS OF RADIATION THERAPY ON SEXUALITY

As with chemotherapy, extreme fatigue is a common effect of radiation therapy. It is usually related to the length of treatment, dose, and other concurrent side effects. Radiation fatigue may last 1 to 2 months after completion of treatment. The most common result of fatigue is decreased sexual desire; the partner needs to know that fatigue is not a sign of rejection (Fedak, 1981; Nevidjon, 1984). The patient may have more energy for sexual activity early in the week after having a weekend break from radiation treatment. The nurse should encourage touching and cuddling rather than strenuous sexual activity. Since depression is sometimes associated with extreme fatigue, the patient should be encouraged to get up, dress, and get out of the house. Reassurance should be given that fatigue will diminish after treatment completion, and it is not a sign of disease progression (Nevidjon, 1984).

Depending on the site irradiated, nausea and vomiting, diarrhea, oral ulceration, and sore throat may occur, all of which may inhibit sexual expression. Thrombocytopenia and leukopenia increase the risk of vaginitis or oral, vaginal, or rectal bleeding. Alopecia due to radiation therapy is often permanent, causing a dramatic change in body image.

Although skin changes are not as common now, skin erythema, dry or moist desquamation, and severe skin reactions with slow healing due to blood vessel destruction can occur (Hogan, 1980; Nevidjon, 1984). The patient should be advised to avoid irritation or friction to irradiated areas, which may discourage sexual activity. Because patients are usually advised not to use soaps, deodorants, perfumes, or lotions on the treated area, they may fear that their body odor will be repulsive (Nevidjon, 1984).

Effects on Men

Radiation therapy has been shown to affect spermatogenesis in men. Even with testicular shielding, doses as low as 15 rad to the gonadal area can produce oligospermia lasting 12 to 18 months (Thachil et al, 1981; Hubbard and Jenkins, 1983). Recovery of spermatogenesis is unpredictable with doses greater than 400 rad. Low-dose radiation to the testes can also produce genetically transmittable abnormalities in the sperm (Kaempfer et al, 1983). Schover, Gonzales, and Von Eschenbach (1986) reported in their study of 84 men who had received radiation therapy for seminoma that 30 per cent were concerned about the possibility of infertility.

Erectile dysfunction is another radiation-associated abnormality. In men with prostate cancer, radiation therapy causes erectile dysfunction in 22 to 84 per cent of patients due to vascular damage to penile arteries (Herr, 1979; Thachil et al, 1981; Bergman et al, 1984; Goldstein et al, 1984), although Schover (1987) reports that many men have erectile dysfunction before radiation therapy,

illustrating the need for prospective research in this area. If the patient is cured, he is eligible for a penile prosthesis. Herr (1979) studied the implantation of ^{125}I with bilateral pelvic lymphadenectomy as an alternative to radical prostatectomy or radiation therapy for treatment of localized prostate cancer. No patient treated with ^{125}I developed erectile dysfunction. Others report erectile difficulty for approximately 13 per cent of patients treated with ^{125}I or [198]Au (Andersen, 1985).

In boys treated with radiation, the severity of testicular damage is directly related to the radiation dose. Testosterone production is not affected.

Effects on Women

In women, doses of 600 to 1000 rad to the pelvic area can affect oogenesis and may induce menopause in women over age 40 (Fedak, 1981). A study of prepubertal girls receiving radiation therapy to the abdomen showed ovarian failure in 68 per cent when both ovaries were in the radiation field, in 14 per cent when the ovaries were at the edge of the field, and in 0 per cent when the ovaries were outside the field (Stillman et al, 1981). Therefore, ovariopexy—a surgical technique that positions ovaries outside of the radiation field—is often done during the staging laparotomy for women with Hodgkin's disease (Ruccione and Fergusson, 1984).

Pelvic irradiation in women has been associated with multiple problems, including vaginal stenosis, dyspareunia, decreased lubrication, vault necrosis, fistulas, ileitis, cystitis, bladder ulcers, and shortening of the vagina (Seibel, Freeman, and Graves, 1980; Fedak, 1981; Jusenius, 1981). Seibel, Freeman, and Graves (1982) studied 100 women with cervical cancer, comparing the effects of radiation with those of surgical treatment. Women who received radiation had significantly greater changes in sexual function and enjoyment not correlated with vaginal stenosis or loss of self-image; many experienced decreased desire.

Suggestions for women receiving pelvic irradiation may include using water-soluble jelly for lubrication (not petrolatum-based products); intercourse three times per week to help keep the vagina open; and use of a dilator with lubrication to help recover adequate vaginal dimensions (Jusenius, 1981).

Rehabilitation programs are often helpful and can provide education, opportunities to share feelings and concerns with other women, and individual counseling.

EFFECTS OF CANCER ON PSYCHOSOCIAL ADAPTATION

Psychological Function

The psychological effects of cancer on sexuality extend throughout the course of the disease and its treatment. Cancer terminology is stressful in itself; the words malignancy, cancer, terminally ill, sick, and patient can affect the behavior of the ill person and significant others (Leviton, 1978). For many persons, the word cancer means death, and death evokes many unpleasant emotions. Therefore, we must be specific in defining what cancer words mean. A diagnosis of cancer may evoke fears not only of death but also of abandonment, treatment toxicity, recurrence, loss of functional ability, and loss of social value and self-esteem; it threatens a sense of worthiness and competence (Schain, 1980).

Often, cancer is experienced as a punishment for something, especially specific sexual "transgressions" (extramarital affairs, abortions, early masturbation, prior venereal diseases), and the patient experiences guilt and shame (Cantor, 1980). An example of this is cervical cancer in women, which has been related to sex at an early age and multiple sex partners (Hogan, 1980). Another major psychological threat is fear of abandonment; the actual risk for this is usually related to the nature of the relationship prior to diagnosis (Fisher, 1983). The fears of isolation and rejection may cause more anxiety than fears of pain and death and are sometimes related to the belief that cancer is contagious. For people who believe this, sexual intimacy is frightening.

Changes in self-concept and body image may also impact on sexual functioning. The ability to give and receive pleasure is very closely bound to self-esteem; this ability affects how we feel about ourselves—whether we are worthy to live and enjoy life (Cantor, 1980). Cancer threatens this sense of worthiness, and the patient may withdraw from sexual activity (Wood and Tombrink, 1983). Also, after surgery, the patient may generalize a sense of devaluation to the whole body, feeling that general health has been impaired, and may experience malaise and fatigue (Hogan, 1980; Schain, 1980).

The patient may also have feelings of hopelessness and inadequacy due to the loss of ability to bear children. This may occur even when the *desire* to parent is not strong (Fisher, 1983; Silberfarb, 1984).

Illness with cancer may bring many losses that can cause depression and anger: loss of health, beauty, job, life, activity, youth, and independence. Depression often causes a greater loss of sexual desire than the biological effects of cancer. The patient may also experience depression or anger regarding inability to have sexual intercourse. If satisfying alternatives cannot be established, emotional crisis may result (Fisher, 1983). Anger is often directed at a loved one, resulting in inhibition of sexual expression. The dependency that often accompanies cancer may be an assault on the individual who equates masculinity/femininity with self-care and independence.

The health professional must recognize psychological reactions of the sexual partner as well as the cancer patient. Often the partner is afraid of hurting the loved one, especially when there is risk of infection or bleeding. The concerned partner or family member may go so far in protecting the sick individual that he or she completely shields the patient from sex and intimacy, or the well partner may feel guilty for thinking about sex (Woods and Lamb, 1981). Sometimes a diagnosis of cancer may actually enhance sexuality because the partners re-evaluate the relationship and what is important to them about living.

Sociocultural Factors

There are many general sociocultural factors that affect sexual adjustment: race, religion, education, socioeconomic class, emotional satisfaction from sexual aspects of life, and attitudes toward cancer. All of these factors are a reflection of who we are and the cultural environment in which we live. In addition, there are other societal factors that may affect the cancer patient's sexual adjustment; one of these is myths. Unfortunately, myths about cancer are prevalent in our society and include (1) cancer is a punishment, (2) cancer is contagious, (3) abstinence from sex will prevent a recurrence, (4) cancer is dirty and unclean, and (5) a diagnosis of cancer means the patient will have no interest in sexual expression. Myths only contribute to a patient's isolation from emotionally important persons, resulting in despair and depression (Fisher, 1983).

Cancer may also necessitate a change in sexual roles within a family, especially with long-term treatment or progressive illness. The patient may be denied employment due to employer fears about the cancer patient's ability to be productive. The partner or family member may be ill-prepared to assume financial responsibilities and the huge expenses for cancer; anxiety about paying the bills may block out other parts of the relationship. Anger that the ill person is creating a hardship may also affect a relationship (Hogan, 1980). The patient is often forced by the illness to be in a dependent role; the spouse may then assume a nurturing role, resulting in negative effects on sexual expression.

Because the masculine role in society is equated with productivity and activity, chronic illness often threatens masculinity. Many cancers occur in men during midlife, which is a vulnerable time when men realize they may never reach the goals they set when younger (Shipes and Lehr, 1982).

It is interesting to note the relationship between some sexual practices and cancer incidence. Cancer of the penis is virtually unknown in circumcised men, a fact that is probably related to better hygiene (Hogan, 1980). Cervical cancer has several sociocultural risk factors; the most important is sexual intercourse prior to age 18. There is evidence that the cervix of teenagers is more susceptible to carcinogenic agents. Since 60 to 80 per cent of the population engages in intercourse before age 20, the nurse must counsel young women regarding this increased risk and the need for regular Pap smears (Krantz, Magrina, and Capen, 1984).

Another risk factor for cervical cancer is multiple sex partners. One hypothesis is that cancer of the cervix is caused by a virus transmitted during sexual intercourse, so that a woman's risk may depend not only on her own sexual behavior but also on that of her partner, if he has had many partners (Skegg et al, 1982). There appears to be a lower incidence of cervical cancer in women with circumcised partners, and women with genital herpes may be at high risk for cervical cancer (Krantz, Magrina, and Capen, 1984).

THE TERMINALLY ILL AND SEXUAL FUNCTION

Although persons with life-limiting cancer may be physically and psychosocially debilitated, they may retain a fundamental need for sexual closeness. In a study of patients receiving chemotherapy for advanced cancer, the patients reported decreased desire for sexual intercourse and increased desire for physical closeness, such as embracing, kissing, or holding hands (Leiber et al, 1976). This finding suggests that comforting reassurances are needed more than sexual stimulation.

Death and intimacy are entwined; many theorists view intimacy as crucial in achieving the ultimate integrity that comes with accepting the inevitability of death. Lack of intimate relationships can be very stressful, and the terminally ill are at high risk for this kind of stress. Health professionals must be willing to offer education and counseling to relieve intimacy and sexual deprivation among these especially vulnerable people (Leviton, 1978).

There are many factors that interfere with sexual expression of the terminally ill patient (Mims and Swenson, 1980). Often, patients use all of their energy just to cope with the crisis of being terminally ill and may be confused by all of the feelings involved, such as love, anger, hate, hopelessness, selfishness, and selflessness. The ill person and/or the healthy partner may feel that it is inappropriate to give or receive pleasure at such a time, and either person may feel guilty about having sexual interest. There is very little opportunity for privacy in hospitals and nursing homes, and the predominant attitude in most institutions is that terminally ill patients are not interested in sex. The healthy partner may undergo an emotional separation upon anticipation of the loss of the loved one, and sexual expression may be inhibited.

The nurse should promote the idea that sex is good and should educate other health professionals about sexuality and the terminally ill. Privacy in the hospital room should be allowed, with posting of a "Do not disturb" sign if necessary. The well partner should be encouraged to express affection and caring, which may require reassurance from the nurse that death is not contagious. In general, tenderness and intimacy in the hospital environment should be reinforced (Mims and Swenson, 1980).

NURSING PROCESS

Although some specific nursing interventions have been suggested throughout this chapter, I would like to address the more general recommendations for nursing practice. If we are to be effective in dealing with the sexuality of our patients, we must first deal with our own sexuality: our sexual identity, our biases, fears, morals, and attitudes toward cancer (Fisher, 1979). The health professional who is straightforward, kind, and interested will open the door for communication of sexual concerns.

Before initiating discussion, the health professional should understand the effects of different types of cancer on sexuality and how cancer treatments may be sexually disabling. Discussion should be initiated at all stages of the illness and treatment; an initial interview only is not sufficient in determining the sexual concerns of the patient throughout the course of the illness.

Assessment

The nursing assessment of sexual concerns and sexual function should be initiated early to establish its appropriateness in the nurse/client relationship (Woods and Lamb, 1981). A study by Bullard and associates (1980) indicated that women with cervical cancer wanted more information about sexuality than they were receiving from the nurse or physician, and they expected the health professional to bring up the topic first.

In assessing the patient the nurse should plan for an uninterrupted period of time; the patient is rarely comfortable discussing sexual concerns if the nurse is busy with another task. Privacy and confidentiality should be assured. The assessment should begin with exploration of the patient's knowledge of the diagnosis, the disease, and the effects of treatment. The patient should be questioned specifically about the meaning given to the diagnosis of cancer and the organ involved and the effects of the disease and treatment on self-esteem and sexual functioning. Pretreatment sexual attitudes

and responsiveness should be assessed, including (1) frequency of sexual activities, (2) quality of performance, (3) history of sexual dysfunction, (4) personal and family attitudes toward sexuality, and (5) usual coping strategies (Derogatis and Kourlesis, 1981; Schain, 1981). These questions can give the nurse clues regarding the patient's motivation for professional intervention.

It is helpful to both the patient and the nurse to progress from less sensitive to more sensitive areas. Questions should be prefaced with statements that legitimize any response the patient might make. For example, the nurse might state, "Many women with breast cancer have fears or concerns about how the loss of a breast will affect their sexual relationships. What concerns do you have?" The nurse must recognize the role of culture, familial beliefs, and religious convictions, allowing for many interpretations of correct sexual behavior (Fedak, 1981).

Idle questioning is not appropriate; a systematic approach is most effective, and nurses should always know why they are asking a particular question. Other assessment techniques include soliciting questions about specific sexual concerns, using language that is understandable to the patient, and including the partner in the interview (Fedak, 1981).

Intervention

The goal of nursing interventions should be rehabilitation of the patient to the highest level of sexual function possible. The nurse must be flexible in terms of goal setting and changing by the patient and his/her partner (Hogan, 1980).

Several major nursing interventions are important in facilitating the cancer patient's adjustment to disturbances of sexuality. The first is acting in a supportive/facilitative role. Often just talking with the patient helps to validate normalcy and gives reassurance that behaviors, feelings, fantasies, and concerns are accepted (Woods and Lamb, 1981). Just as important is facilitating or encouraging open, honest communication between the patient and partner. The nurse can help the patient shift the emphasis from the body defect to positive attributes, such as intelligence, general strength, job, and loving relationships (Fedak, 1981).

The supportive role includes helping the

patient explore and use defense mechanisms that have helped in dealing with previous stresses. Enlist the aid of the sexual partner in preventing social isolation and affection deprivation (Hogan, 1980). The social worker can be consulted for financial problems, and if indicated, the patient can be referred for psychotherapy or sex therapy.

The second major nursing intervention is anticipatory guidance. Give accurate information about what to expect from treatment and surgery; this allows for more effective coping.

The third area of intervention relevant to nursing practice is education and counseling about sexuality and alternate means of sexual expression. In teaching alternate ways of expressing physical love the nurse must first explore the values and attitudes of the couple. What is acceptable to one may not be to another, and the subject should be approached with sensitivity. Often we as a society stereotype penile/vaginal intercourse as the only means for expressing physical love. Genital intercourse is only one way; manual, digital, and oral stimulation are others. Intrathigh and intramammary intercourse are alternatives if vaginal penetration is not possible (Woods and Lamb, 1981). When fatigue and decreased sexual desire are problems, foreplay techniques such as hugging, fondling, kissing, and caressing can produce satisfaction and a sense of well-being. The use of a vibrator can be suggested.

Autoerotic activities such as masturbation, mutual masturbation, and sexual fantasizing can be explored, and variations in intercourse positions can be suggested. Nurses should emphasize that pleasure can be received from physical closeness with or without orgasm; they should encourage the couple to explore different methods but must recognize when there are no acceptable alternatives in a relationship (Woods and Lamb, 1981).

Evaluation

Evaluation of the effectiveness of nursing interventions can sometimes be difficult when those interventions are aimed at promoting psychological adjustment to changes in sexuality. However, if the nurse has established goals with the client and sexual partner on an ongoing basis, then outcome criteria can be established as a means for evaluation (Hogan, 1985). Outcome criteria may include the following: (1) The client and sexual partner can describe expected side effects of treatment that may affect their sexuality and sexual expression. (2) The client and sexual partner report sharing their feelings about the potential changes in sexuality. (3) The client and sexual partner describe alternate means of sexual expression that are compatible with the client's physical limitations.

The best approach to evaluation is to ask the client and the partner specific questions about their adaptation (Kirchner, 1984). This approach also continues to give the client permission to discuss any new concerns that may have arisen.

CONCLUSION

The nurse who is knowledgeable about sexuality and sexual function can serve as a consultant for other health professionals. However, nurses should not feel that they have to be experts before initiating discussion with a patient. It is important to remember that problems and concerns that are beyond the scope of the nurse's expertise can always be referred.

Matters of sexuality are very important to cancer patients. No nurse or patient should ever feel forced to discuss these matters, but it is an area that clearly should not be ignored. Perhaps a nurse or a sex therapist should be a part of every oncology team, so that patients are immediately allowed to begin expressing their sexual concerns. The knowledgeable nurse can be a tremendous asset to any health team and is in a unique position to explore the issue of sexuality with patients because of the frequent day-to-day contact that nurses often have with their patients. Only when sexuality is included in the care of cancer patients will they be cared for in a holistic manner.

REFERENCES

Andersen BL: Sexual functioning morbidity among cancer survivors. Current status and future research directions. Cancer 55:1835–1842, 1985.

Armitage JD: Long-term remission durability and functional status of patients treated for diffuse histiocytic lymphoma with the CHOP regimen. J Clin Oncol 2:898–902, 1984.

Bergman B, Damber JE, Littbrand B, et al: Sexual function in prostatic cancer patients treated with radiotherapy, orchiectomy, or aestrogens. Br J Urol 56:64–69, 1984.

Bullard DG, Causey GG, Newman AB, et al: Sexual

health care and cancer: A needs assessment. Front Radiat Ther Oncol 14:55–58, 1980.

Cantor RC: Self-esteem, sexuality, and cancer-related stress. Front Radiat Ther Oncol 14:51–54, 1980.

Chapman RM: Effect of cytotoxic therapy on sexuality and gonadal function. Semin Oncol 9:84–91, 1982.

Chapman RM, Sutcliffe SB: Protection of ovarian function by oral contraceptives in women receiving chemotherapy for Hodgkin's disease. Blood 58:849–851, 1981.

Chapman RM, Sutcliffe SB, Malpas JS: Cytotoxic-induced ovarian failure in Hodgkin's disease: Effects on sexual function. JAMA 242:1882–1884, 1979.

DeCunha MF, Meistrich ML, Reed HL, Powell ML: Effect of chemotherapy on human sperm production. Proc ASCO/AACR 20:100, 1979.

Derogatis LR, Kourlesis SM: An approach to evaluation of sexual problems in the cancer patient. CA 31:46–50, 1981.

Drasga RE, Williams SD, Stevens EE, et al: Gonadal function after platinum, vinblastine, bleomycin (PVB) and adriamycin (A) in testicular cancer. Proc ASCO/AACR 1:105, 1982.

Ezdinili EZ, Stutzman L: Chlorambucil therapy for lymphomas and chronic lymphocytic leukemia. JAMA 191:444–450, 1965.

Fairley KF, Barrie JU, Johnson W: Sterility and testicular atrophy related to cyclophosphamide therapy. Lancet 1:568–569, 1972.

Fedak MK: Teaching the patient about sexuality. In Donovan MJ (ed): Cancer Care: A Guide for Patient Education. Norwalk, Appleton-Century-Crofts, 1981, pp 257–288.

Fisher B, Sherman B, Rockette H, et al: L-phenylalanine mustard (L-PAM) in the management of pre-menopausal patients with primary breast cancer. Lack of association of disease free survival with depression of ovarian function. Cancer 44:847–857, 1979.

Fisher SG: Psychosexual adjustment following total pelvic exenteration. Cancer Nurs 2:219–225, 1979.

Fisher SG: The psychosexual effects of cancer and cancer treatment. Oncology Nurs Forum 10:63–68, 1983.

Flynn KT, Durivage HJ: Anti-estrogen therapy for breast cancer: Focus on tamoxifen. Oncology Nurs Forum 9:21–25, 1982.

Galton DAG, Till M, Wilshaw E: Busulfan: Summary of clinical results. Ann NY Acad Sci 68:967–973, 1958.

Goldstein I, Feldman MI, Deckers PJ, et al: Radiation associated impotence. JAMA 251:903–910, 1984.

Gorzynski JG, Holland JC: Psychological aspects of testicular cancer. Semin Oncol 6:125–129, 1979.

Greenberg DB: The measurement of sexual dysfunction in cancer patients. Cancer 53:2281–2285, 1984.

Gunby P: Dealing with sexual problems of cancer patients. JAMA 245:1902–1903, 1981.

Hammond DC, Middleton RG: Penile prostheses. Med Aspects Human Sex 18:204–208, 1984.

Herr HW: Preservation of sexual potency in prostatic cancer patients after ¹²⁵I implantation. J Am Geriatr Soc 27:17–19, 1979.

Hogan R: Human Sexuality: A Nursing Perspective. Norwalk, Appleton-Century-Crofts, 1980.

Hogan R: Human Sexuality: A Nursing Perspective. Norwalk, Appleton-Century-Crofts, 1985.

Howard-Ruben J: Restoring antegrade ejaculation after retroperitoneal lymph node dissection. Oncol Nurs Forum 10:79, 1983.

Hubbard SM, Jenkins J: An overview of current concepts in the management of patients with testicular tumors of germ cell origin—Part II: Treatment strategies by histology and stage. Cancer Nurs 6:125–139, 1983.

Johnson DH, Hainsworth JD, Linde RB, Greco FA: Gonadal function following combination chemotherapy with cis-platin, vinblastine, and bleomycin. Med Pediatr Oncol 12:233–238, 1984.

Jusenius K: Sexuality and gynecologic cancer. Cancer Nurs 4:479–484, 1981.

Kaempfer SH: The effects of cancer chemotherapy on reproduction: A review of the literature. Oncol Nurs Forum 8:11–17, 1981.

Kaempfer SH, Hoffman DJ, Wiley FM: Sperm banking: A reproductive option in cancer therapy. Cancer Nurs 6:31–38, 1983.

Kirchner CW: Sexuality and selected cancer therapies. In Woods NF (ed): Human Sexuality in Health and Illness. St. Louis, CV Mosby, 1984.

Koyama H, Wada T, Nishaziwa Y, et al: Cyclophosphamide induced ovarian failure and its therapeutic significance in patients with breast cancer. Cancer 39:1403–1409, 1977.

Krantz KE, Magrina JF, Capen CV: Sexual risk factors for developing cervical cancer. Med Aspects Human Sex 18:144–153, 1984.

Leiber L, Plumb MM, Gerstenzang ML, Holland J: The communication of affection between cancer patients and their spouses. Psychosom Med 38:379–389, 1976.

Leviton D: The intimacy/sexual needs of the terminally ill and the widowed. Death Ed 2:261–280, 1978.

LUCC, Meistrich ML: Cytotoxic effects of chemotherapeutic drugs on mouse testis cells. Cancer Res 39:3575–3582, 1979.

Miller DG: Alkylating agents in human spermatogenesis. JAMA 217:1662–1665, 1971.

Mims FH, Swenson M: Sexuality: A Nursing Perspective. New York, McGraw-Hill, 1980.

Nevidjon BM: Sexuality. In McIntire SN, Cioppa AL (eds): Cancer Nursing: A Developmental Approach. New York, John Wiley & Sons, 1984.

Nijman JM: Sexual function after bilateral retroperitoneal lymph node dissection for nonseminomatous testicular cancer. Arch Androl 18:255–267, 1987.

Nijman J, Jager S, Boer P, et al: The treatment of ejaculation disorders after retroperitoneal lymph node dissection. Cancer 50:2967–2971, 1982.

Richter P, Calamera JC, Morgenfeld MC, et al: Effect of chlorambucil on spermatogenesis in the human with malignant lymphoma. Cancer 25:1026–1030, 1970.

Rose DP, Davis TE: Ovarian function in patients receiving adjuvant chemotherapy for breast cancer. Lancet 1:1174–1176, 1977.

Rousseau L, Dupont A, Labrie F, Couture M: Sexuality changes in prostate cancer patients receiving antihormonal therapy combining the antiandrogen flutamide with medical (LHRH agonist) or surgical castration. Arch Sex Behav 17:87–98, 1988.

Ruccione K, Fergusson J: Late effects of childhood cancer and its treatment. Oncol Nurs Forum 11:54–64, 1984.

Schain WS: Sexual functioning, self-esteem and cancer care. Front Radiat Ther Oncol 14:12–19, 1980.

Schain WS: Role of the sex therapist in the care of the cancer patient. Front Radiat Ther Oncol 15:168–183, 1981.

Schilsky RL, Lewis BJ, Sherins RJ, Young RC: Gonadal dysfunction in patients receiving chemotherapy for cancer. Ann Inter Med 93:109–114, 1980.

Schover LR: Sexuality and fertility in urologic cancer patients. Cancer 60(3 Suppl):553–558, 1987.

Schover LR, Gonzales M, Von Eschenbach AC: Sexual and marital relationships after radiotherapy for seminoma. Urology 27:117–123, 1986.

Seibel MM, Freeman MG, Graves WL: Carcinoma of the cervix and sexual function. Obstet Gynecol 55:484–487, 1980.

Seibel M, Freeman MG, Graves WL: Sexual function after surgical and radiation therapy for cervical carcinoma. South Med J 75:1195–1197, 1982.

Shamberger RC, Rosenberg SA, Seipp CA, et al: Effects of high-dose methotrexate and vincristine on ovarian and testicular functions in patients undergoing postoperative adjuvant treatment of osteosarcoma. Cancer Treat Rep 65:739–746, 1981.

Shamberger RC, Sherins RJ, Ziegler JL, et al: Effects of postoperative adjuvant chemotherapy and radiotherapy on ovarian function in women undergoing treatment for soft tissue sarcoma. JNCI 67:1213–1218, 1981.

Sherman BM, Fisher B, Rockette H, et al: The endocrine consequences of adjuvant chemotherapy in women with breast cancer. Clin Res 26:446A, 1978.

Shipes E, Lehr S: Sexuality and the male cancer patient. Cancer Nurs 5:375–381, 1982.

Sieber SM, Correa P, Dalgard DW, Adamson RH: Carcinogenic and other adverse effects of procarbazine in nonhuman primates. Cancer Res 38:2125–2134, 1978.

Silberfarb PM: Psychosexual impact of gynecologic cancer. Med Aspects Human Sex 18:212–226, 1984.

Skegg DCG, Corwin PA, Paul C, Doll R: Importance of the male factor in cancer of the cervix. Lancet 2:581–583, 1982.

Sobrinho L, Levine R, DeConti R: Amenorrhea in patients with Hodgkin's disease treated with antineoplastic agents. Am J Obstet Gynecol 109:135–139, 1971.

Stillman RJ, Schinfeld JS, Schiff J, et al: Ovarian failure in long-term survivors of childhood malignancy. Am J Obstet Gynecol 139:62–66, 1981.

Thachil JV, Jewett MAS, Rider WD: The effects of cancer and cancer therapy on male fertility. J Urol 126:141–145, 1981.

Vilar O: The effect of cytostatic drugs on human testicular function. In Macini RE, Martini L (eds): Male Fertility and Sterility. New York, Academic Press, 1974, pp 423–440.

Warne GL, Farley KF, Hobbs JB, et al: Cyclophosphamide induced ovarian failure. N Engl J Med 289:1159–1162, 1973.

Whitehead E, Shalet SM, Blackledge G, et al: The effects of Hodgkin's disease and combination chemotherapy on gonadal function in the adult male. Cancer 49:418–422, 1982.

Wood JD, Tombrink J: Impact of cancer on sexuality and self-image: A group program for patients and partners. Soc Work Health Care 8:45–54, 1983.

Woods NF, Lamb MA: Sexuality and the cancer patient. Cancer Nurs 4:137–144, 1981.

Yarbro CH, Perry MC: The effect of cancer therapy on gonadal function. Semin Oncol Nurs 1:3–8, 1985.

16: Chronic Musculoskeletal Symptoms and Sexuality

Joanne Dalton

Individuals with chronic musculoskeletal symptoms, including pain, weakness, stiffness, and/or swelling, constitute a large segment of the population of the United States. Although the pathophysiological causes of these symptoms include a variety of diseases, this chapter focuses on causes of symptoms in the greatest proportion of those affected—connective tissue disorders such as arthritis and lupus, and neuromuscular disorders such as the muscular dystrophies. Because of the changes associated with musculoskeletal symptoms, affected individuals are continually involved in adapting their physiological and psychological responses, including sexual responses, to their environment. The degree to which individuals are able to adapt positively is influenced by their knowledge, attitudes, and previous behavior; adaptability is also influenced by the knowledge and skills of health professionals.

The etiology, pathology, and progression of disease processes that cause common musculoskeletal symptoms will be briefly described. The effects of these symptoms (pain, stiffness, fatigue, weakness), drugs, decreased self-concept, anxiety, altered body image, change in role function, and social isolation on sexual functioning are then discussed using Roy's model of adaptation (Roy and Roberts, 1981). Important aspects of nursing assessment and intervention with persons experiencing chronic musculoskeletal symptoms are presented.

The goal of the chapter is to assist health professionals to increase their knowledge of the problems that individuals with musculoskeletal symptoms may experience and interventions that will aid in altering those problems. With this background, health professionals will be better able to assist persons with musculoskeletal symptoms to achieve adaptation in sexual functioning and to communicate that the presence of musculoskeletal symptoms should not be a deterent to satisfying sexual function.

CONNECTIVE TISSUE DISORDERS

Rheumatoid Arthritis

Rheumatoid arthritis is a chronic inflammatory disease of the connective tissue that most typically affects the synovial membrane, especially in the proximal interphalangeal, metacarpophalangeal, metatarsophalangeal, wrist, elbow, shoulder, hip, knee, and ankle joints. Hypertrophy of the synovial membrane, accompanied by increased synovial fluid and the development of a layer of pannus (granulation tissue covering the surface of the cartilage), eventually erodes the articular cartilage, causing pain and stiffness. Extra-articular problems such as rheumatoid nodules, vasculitis, pericarditis, and lung disease, although less common, can also be symptomatic.

Although the etiology of rheumatoid arthritis is unknown, a variety of causative factors have been implicated, including viruses, immunodeficiency, and stress. The disease occurs more frequently in women (4:1) in midlife. Its onset is frequently characterized by complaints of morning joint stiffness without pain, fatigue, anorexia, and weight loss. Individual occurrence of these symptoms is followed by an insidious progression of joint swelling, pain, and limitation of motion; muscle weakness and atrophy of the pectoral and quadricep muscles may also be present. Most individuals experience progressive symptoms, which usually are more severe in the morning, although fatigue may cause exacerbation of symptoms at any time of day. Joint deformity may be limited or extensive, causing varying degrees of restriction of activity and/or affecting the individual's self image.

Juvenile Rheumatoid Arthritis

Juvenile rheumatoid arthritis occurs most frequently in children less than 5 years of age, although the differential diagnosis is appropriate for youths up to 16 years of age. It may be characterized by complete or partial remissions throughout the developmental years, and in the older youth its onset should be differentiated from adult rheumatoid arthritis. Symptomatically, individuals with juvenile rheumatoid arthritis complain of the frequent incidence of single-joint involvement, rash, and persistent high fever. Highly individualized progression and/or exacerbation of symptoms may include polyarticular joint swelling, limitation of motion, contractures, and muscle atrophy.

Osteoarthritis

Osteoarthritis is a degenerative joint disease of uncertain etiology more commonly found in older individuals. It is characterized by joint pain, stiffness, and a crackling sensation that is sometimes perceived with movement. Most commonly, the disease affects only a few joints, primarily the distal interphalangeal, proximal interphalangeal, metatarsophalangeal, hip, and knee joints or the spine. Attempts by the body to repair changes in the cartilage result in proliferation of the cartilage and bone and the formation of spurs in many individuals, although degenerative changes of the spine may result in narrowing of the disc and/or nerve root compression.

While the etiology of osteoarthritis is uncertain, individual enzymatic and biomechanical stresses have been investigated. In contrast to the symptoms of rheumatoid arthritis, the stiffness of degenerative arthritis often lasts less than 15 minutes, and pain occurs when an activity is initiated after prolonged immobility. As the disease progresses, the individual's complaint of pain commonly occurs at the end of the day. In individuals with advanced disease, synovitis may be responsible for additional pain; joint enlargement and subluxation also become more distinct.

Ankylosing Spondylitis

Ankylosing spondylitis, or Marie-Strümpell disease, is a chronic inflammatory disease of the spine with pathological changes similar to those found in individuals with rheumatoid arthritis. It most commonly affects the joints and paravertebral ligaments, where synovitis and joint adhesions are responsible for the individual's complaint of pain and stiffness of the back. While calcification with fibrous and bony ankylosis produces the characteristic "bamboo" spine, the erosive and deforming joint changes found in rheumatoid arthritis usually are not present.

The etiology of ankylosing spondylitis is unknown. It occurs more frequently in men (9:1) during their thirties and frequently goes into remission in midlife. Although the most common complaint may be lack of lumbar flexion, the shoulder, hip, costovertebral, manubriosternal, and symphysis pubic joints may be involved, with the insidious onset of symptoms occurring after prolonged sleep or rest. Fatigue, anorexia, weight loss, and low-grade fever may be present.

Lupus Erythematosus

Lupus erythematosus is a chronic connective tissue disorder also of unknown etiology that most commonly affects the joints, skin, and kidneys. Anti-DNA antibodies have been implicated in the development of symptoms such as joint swelling and tenderness, fever, malaise, anorexia, and weight loss. Muscle pain sometimes occurs, although individual complaint of morning stiffness is uncommon. Arthritic symptoms often are accompanied by the more troublesome individual complaint of facial erythema (butterfly rash) and a rapid loss of scalp hair. Lupus erythematosus occurs more frequently in females, especially black females, during the sometimes more sexually active second and third decade. Its clinical course is highly individualized and is characterized by repeat exacerbations and remissions.

NEUROMUSCULAR DISORDERS

Muscular Dystrophies

The muscular dystrophies are a group of neuromuscular disorders characterized by individual complaints of progressive weakness and wasting of the skeletal muscles, particularly those in the proximal limb girdles. Duchenne type (pseudohypertrophic) muscular dystrophy is perhaps the most devastating form of these disorders because of its rapid progression of weakness, leading to early disability and death. Individuals with myotonic dystrophy, a disorder that is less common and more variable in progression, sometimes also develop cataracts, diabetes mellitus, and frontal baldness. The individual's sexuality may be affected by atrophy of the testes, testosterone deficiency, and impaired spermatogenesis (Harper et al, 1972). Characteristically, muscle weakness is complicated by the development of contractures that occur because of the difficulty in relaxing muscles.

As in the aforementioned joint disorders, the etiology of the muscular dystrophies is unknown. The maladaptive symptoms appear to be inherited as a sex-linked recessive trait and an autosomal dominant trait for individuals with pseudohypertrophic and myotonic dystrophy, respectively. Pseudohypertrophic dystrophy is associated with difficulty in locomotion until late in the disease, when problems with small motor movements become evident. In myotonic dystrophy, muscle weakness more often involves the face, jaw, and distal limb muscles.

EFFECTS OF SYMPTOMS ASSOCIATED WITH MUSCULOSKELETAL DISORDERS ON SEXUAL FUNCTION

Pain

Pain often is the primary deterrent to continuation of sexual activity by men and women with changes in musculoskeletal integrity (Blake et al, 1987). Pain may be localized to the joints of the hand, the hips, or the back, or it may be related to a more generalized stiffness occurring systemically or in association with flexion contractures. Localized pain in the metacarpophalangeal and proximal interphalangeal joints is responsible for a variety of problems, such as making it difficult or impossible to touch and/or caress a partner's or one's own body. Pain may prevent or diminish the individual's ability to participate in foreplay and/or masturbation; it may also affect sexual functioning because it limits or prevents the individual from supporting his or her own body or the body of a partner.

Pain in the hips, knees, and/or back often prevents or decreases the individual's ability to continue previously utilized sexual positions. Pain associated with abduction and external rotations of the hip joints interferes with the common female supine position for females with rheumatoid arthritis. Pain in the lower back area sometimes prevents the male with ankylosing spondylitis from assuming the male superior position. Pain often is the cause of decreased frequency of genital intromission.

The following case description illustrates how pain may alter and interfere with sexual expression and activity:

Ben, a 32-year-old white male with bilateral sacroiliitis, probable ankylosing spondylitis, reports that when he was 13 years old, he fell off a grapevine and subsequently developed lower back symptoms. The symptoms were resolved with weight lifting. He has experienced constant lower back pain and stiffness since age 20 that is worse in the morning and for the past 2 years has been worse in the winter. Recently, he has noted difficulty putting on his shoes and, in general, trouble bending forward.

Ben's sexual relationship with his sexual

partner has been affected physiologically by his need to always assume the supine position. He also finds that he usually needs to get up and walk around for a few minutes immediately following coitus. He expresses this need to his sexual partner and she is understanding, although she wishes that he could remain in bed during the time that she has a heightened desire to be close to and to be held by him.

The pain of rheumatoid arthritis may be complicated by balanitis, painful disfiguring lesions of the penis, or ulcerative lesions of the genitalia (Behçet's syndrome) that result in dyspareunia. Sjögren's syndrome, also associated with arthritis, is characterized by a decrease or absence of vaginal secretions, resulting in atrophic vaginitis and dyspareunia.

In addition to the physiological problems caused by pain, adaptive problems in sexuality are also associated with the fear of pain. Individuals may avoid sexual activities because they are afraid that the activity will cause joint pain. Although documented by only 4 per cent of the respondents in one Japanese study (Yoshino and Uchida, 1981), avoidance also occurs because of fear that increased pain may result from the activity. Many patients find that fear of pain interferes with orgasmic response. Partners of the individual with musculoskeletal symptoms may also be more reserved in their sexual behavior because of their fear of causing pain during sexual activity.

Pain may occur that prevents a woman from inserting tampons or barrier contraceptive devices such as the diaphragm or vaginal sponge because of difficulty and pain associated with using the hand to place them in the vagina. Men may have difficulty putting on a condom.

Stiffness

Although not implicated as frequently as pain as a contributor to sexual difficulties, joint stiffness is also responsible for problems associated with sexual activity (Blake et al, 1987). Individuals with rheumatoid arthritis, osteoarthritis, and ankylosing spondylitis frequently complain of early morning stiffness; the location and the length of time that the stiffness persists varies with each disease and among individuals. Prolonged stiffness has greater implications for time of day for sex-

ual activity. Individuals with ankylosing spondylitis often find that they are awakened from sleep by stiffness, perhaps contributing to their generalized fatigue, or they have transient stiffness commonly associated with the radiological diagnosis of "poker" back. Men, because they are more commonly affected, sometimes demonstrate excessive forward carriage in their posture, contributing to decreased respiratory function, which can affect sexual activity. They also are more vunerable to fractures of the spine because of inelasticity and associated osteoporosis. These problems, as well as similar problems of the hands and hips, interfere with stroking and caressing the body in some positions.

Involvement of the hands may be responsible for problems related to self or mutual masturbation. Flexion contractures of the hips cause pain if the individual attempts to abduct or externally rotate the hips for positions of anterior penetration. Erlich (1973) suggests that surgical ankylosis of the hip to decrease pain may result in total inability to move the hips, which will also prevent anterior penetration.

Fatigue

Generalized fatigue occurs most commonly in the evening in individuals with musculoskeletal disease. As a manifestation of systemic disease it may or may not occur secondary to anemia. In either case the individual's lack of energy and/or strength may be associated with change in responsiveness, frequency, and/or satisfaction with sexual activity. As noted in one study (Elst et al, 1984), prolonged foreplay, sometimes needed by individuals coping with pain or other distractors, becomes difficult or impossible. Maintenance of sexual positions frequently utilized by couples can add further stress to the individual with musculoskeletal symptoms who already has experienced diminished strength and energy. If fatigue causes the individual with musculoskeletal symptoms to be less responsive to simple amorous gestures or to more overt sexual advances, other sexual problems such as lack of female responsiveness or erectile dysfunction may occur. Intermittent complaints of fatigue and intermittent desire for sexual activity may be confusing to the unaffected partner. Decreased sexual activity can be associated with an increase in relationship problems.

Weakness

Weakness may be associated with musculoskeletal changes accompanying connective tissue disorders and the muscular dystrophies. It may be minimal, causing few if any problems, or it may be more extensive, causing problems with immobility and/or difficulty supporting the trunk and/or extremities. Weakness may alter an individual's ability to utilize some of the more common coital positions or to maintain any position for an extended period of time. The latter may be a problem if a weakness is confined to the lower extremities, as in the dystrophies, but decrease in strength in any part of the body can affect sexual function.

EFFECTS OF DRUGS PRESCRIBED FOR MUSCULOSKELETAL DISORDERS ON SEXUAL FUNCTION

Although the pharmacological agents most commonly used in the treatment of musculoskeletal symptoms—nonsteroidal anti-inflammatory drugs—do not have known side effects contributing to sexual dysfunction, this is not true of steroids. Prolonged utilization of steroids sometimes causes an inability to achieve an erection or may cause vasculitis, which ultimately results in atrophy of the testes. One author (Erlich, 1973) suggests that steroids oppose the stimulating action of androgens on the brain and sex organs, thus causing a decrease in libido. Prolonged utilization of steroids also is responsible for the development of cushingoid symptoms, such as moon facies, the buffalo hump, purple striae, thin skin, and facial flushing. These physiological changes can be deterrents to sexual attraction and socialization, ultimately resulting in decreased opportunity for sexual activity.

EFFECTS OF CHRONIC MUSCULOSKELETAL CONDITIONS ON PSYCHOSOCIAL ADAPTATION

Psychological deficits associated with changes in musculoskeletal integrity may be the result of decreased self-concept and may occur because individuals do not accept themselves as sexually attractive, capable, or adequate or because messages of acceptance, approval, or desire are not communicated by their partners. Deficits may also occur because of previous difficulty coping with musculoskeletal symptoms, because of the partner's response, or because of fear of not meeting the expectations of the partner.

Individuals with musculoskeletal symptoms sometimes develop anxiety secondary to unmet expectations, frustrations, and conflict as well as helplessness that relates to change. Feelings of apprehension are caused by changes in the individual's ability to continue previously utilized sexual patterns or behaviors. Difficulties may occur when the present sexual relationship is viewed only in relation to past relationships. Individuals with musculoskeletal symptoms fear the loss of responses that establish and maintain sexual relationships. They are concerned that their sexual performances will be unsatisfactory as a result of pain, stiffness, and limitation of motion. The situation becomes even more problematic if affected individuals fear loss of their partner due to decreased ability to continue previously satisfactory sexual practices. Depression can occur if individuals feel unable to cope with change and/or loss in the sexual relationship or if their expectations for future relationships appear to be unsatisfactory.

Threats to the physical self can contribute to an individual's negative attitude toward the psychological self. The image of individuals with musculoskeletal symptoms is influenced by the degree of physical deformity present and their ability to cope with physical changes. Joint or muscle changes vary from individual to individual, as do reactions or responses to change. For example, an individual with minimal involvement of the metacarpophalangeal joints may have a more negative body image than another individual with extensive multiple joint involvement. A young adult with juvenile rheumatoid arthritis who has experienced early closure of the epiphyses of one leg, so that one leg is shorter than the other, may feel severely deformed even though an elevated shoe can equalize his stature. The presence of a disfigured chin and/or disfigured hands can cause an individual to hide from the public, feeling ugly and unattractive—perhaps even handicapped.

Because Western culture so frequently seems to place high value on the healthy perfect body, individuals with musculoskeletal symptoms react to messages from the environment with frustrations or denial of limitations due to their perceived inability to assume the expected sex role. Individuals may be depressed or anxious because they fear rejection or feel that they should not expect someone else to accept or cope with their physical changes and limitations. Individuals' fear of becoming a burden to their partners may contribute to feelings of decreased self-concept.

Role Functioning

Although many individuals with musculoskeletal symptoms attempt to remain self-sufficient, their physiological and psychological deficits may ultimately lead to changes in interpersonal relationships. Changes in role function occur as the individual is forced to give up positions of productivity and/or responsibility. Joint deformity and weakness may cause changes in interdependent roles that can lead to maladaptive sexual roles. Sexual desires may become sublimated or restricted by social taboos that assume that individuals with musculoskeletal symptoms should not care about sexual relationships. Hospitalization imposes physical separation but rarely allows for the privacy that may be desired for continuation of sexual activity.

Social isolation may occur when individuals with musculoskeletal symptoms are unable to participate in strenuous physical activity. Joint pain and stiffness prevent young and older adults from participating in sports, exercise, or dancing. Severe involvement of the metacarpophalangeal and proximal interphalangeal joints may even deter the individual from more sedentary activities, such as card playing or handicrafts, that not only provide companionship but also bring the individual into a social setting. Restriction or alteration of social activity may lead to devel-

opmental dysfunction that may ultimately affect sexual activity.

ADAPTATIONS TO MUSCULOSKELETAL CONDITIONS IN SEXUAL FUNCTIONING

Individuals with musculoskeletal symptoms have sexual needs that are the same or similar to those of males and females at all developmental levels. These requirements may be influenced by changes that reflect maladaptations of the individual's physiological, psychological, or social integrity (Roy and Roberts, 1981).

Physiological Functioning

Individuals with musculoskeletal symptoms experience physiological maladaptation when pain, stiffness, limitation of motion, and weakness interfere with their sexual development and/or their usual sexual functioning. Further, sexual expression is altered by difficulty using the hands and supporting and/or positioning the torso or extremities, by changes in mucosal lubrication of the vagina, and by generalized fatigue.

Psychological Functioning

Psychological maladaptations develop when the individual with pain, limited joint motion, and/or muscle weakness experiences alterations in self-concept secondary to feelings of loss, anger, anxiety, or depression. Individuals with musculoskeletal symptoms may develop a decreased self-concept secondary to decreased independence and pride. Their psychological maladaptation may be further intensified as they experience a decrease in sexual desire. Fear of an increase in physiological symptoms or fear of loss of a partner may produce anxiety and depression. Anger and resentment may surface as behaviors.

Psychological maladaptation can also occur if young adults with musculoskeletal symptoms are protected from normal developmental sexual interest and behavior by parents who feel that the individual should not have sexual feelings because of the seriousness and or limitations of the disease. The well-meaning parents of individuals with Duchenne type muscular dystrophy sometimes feel that because the individual's condition is deteriorating and because prognosis is poor sexuality should be ignored. At times the role-modeling sexual behaviors of the parents are maladaptive because the parents themselves are physically and mentally fatigued by the care of the young adult with musculoskeletal symptoms. They may also feel guilty (Kornfeld and Siegel, 1979) because of real or presumed concerns about the genetically transmitted history of the disease and may transit that guilt to the young adult.

Role Functioning

Social maladaptations result from society's failure to recognize sexual needs or to appreciate changes in role function and interdependence experienced by individuals with musculoskeletal symptoms. Perhaps the most serious social maladaptation that affects individuals with musculoskeletal symptoms is lack of or poor communication between the symptomatic partner and the spouse or partner, family, friends, or health professionals. The symptomatic partner, more often the female because of the gender prevalence of the disease, may not feel comfortable expressing her needs for adaptation in the sexual relationship. Frequently, because open discussion of sexual needs, likes, and dislikes has been missing from the relationship prior to the development of the disease, the symptomatic partner is reluctant to verbalize feelings in such a way that the partner fully understands the continued need for intimacy. The unaffected partner may feel that it is unreasonable to expect a sexual relationship because of the symptomatic partner's limitations and thus not ask how the relationship can be adapted for sexual expressions to be less painful. Difficulties intensify if individuals with musculoskeletal symptoms refuse sexual advances from their spouses or become more inhibited during periods of intimacy. If they become overly demanding because of various physiological needs resulting from the musculoskeletal symptoms, the unaffected spouse may withdraw from the relationship. The situation then becomes cyclic as the demands intensify. The situation may be more maladaptive if symptomatic partners become suspicious that their behavior is causing their partners to develop new, perhaps sexual, relationships (Buckwalter, Wernimont, and Buckwalter, 1982).

Individuals with musculoskeletal symptoms may become anxious because they feel unable to be the partner they are expected to be. Stress in the relationship may then cause disequilibrium in the family, as the sexual partners act out their frustrations in unrelated settings with other family members.

Health professionals are generally reticent to discuss sexual matters with their clients, including individuals with musculoskeletal symptoms. Too often they adopt a passive attitude and in doing so fail to initiate communication with the individual who is also reticent to ask about problems related to sexual activity. Clients with musculoskeletal symptoms want physicians to ask questions (Blake et al, 1986; Cohen, 1987). Health professionals should, but do not always, discuss with parents the impact of musculoskeletal symptoms on affected children or young adults to determine whether problems exist for the child or the parent. Maladaptations can occur when parents are unable to assist the young adult in the development of sexuality or when the severity of the young adult's symptoms have an impact on the parents' sexual relationship.

Social isolation sometimes results from the individual's decrease in strength or activity. Pain, weakness, and limitation of motion prevent the individual from participating in activities such as sports events or dancing, thus altering the opportunity for social interaction and contributing to potential maladaptation in sexual development. Some individuals with musculoskeletal symptoms feel that their sexual maladaptation is more related to the lack of available partners than it is to specific problems of intimacy (Flynn, Schwartz, and Williams, 1979). This is especially true in the older age groups, in which the female population outnumbers the male population.

ASSESSMENT

In order to assist individuals with musculoskeletal symptoms, the nurse should first identify deficits in behavior. The sexual history of the individual can be taken at any time during a nurse-client interaction. Because of the sensitivity of the subject, sexuality may be most easily approached during the initial history taking; however, it may be delayed until there has been time for a trusting relationship to develop, but like any other gathering of pertinent data, it should be continuous.

Depending on the perceived needs or problems of the individual, the sexual history may utilize an indepth questionnaire such as the one recommended by Masters and Johnson (1970). Specific items to be addressed include sexual knowledge, presenting symptoms, erotic responses, and expectations for resolving problems (Spergel, 1977). Hogan (1980) proposes that discussion of sexual functioning be preceded by discussion of differences in family functioning and anticipated changes in the perception of oneself as a man or a woman. Specific questions to be asked are shown in Figure 16–1.

Whatever form of the story is used, it should include an assessment of the sexual relationship as it existed before the onset of musculoskeletal symptoms. The assessment should identify adaptive and maladaptive behaviors that communicate messages of desire or rejection, foreplay and positions that are pleasing and uncomfortable, and alternative expressions of sexuality that are perceived as acceptable or deviant. An important area of psychological assessment is the identification of stimuli influencing sexual behavior, e.g., loss of ability to use traditional positions for sexual activity, suggestions by partner to decrease sexual activity, and previous ability to cope with pain. Anxiety that relates to sexuality may be assessed in the individual's manner, posture, voice, or in more subtle cues. The health professional taking the history should look for obscure problems in individuals who have difficulty discussing their sexual needs and should keep in mind that the presence of pain may interfere with desires that would be more fully expressed in the absence of pain. The sexual history should also take into account the effect of medications, such as steroids, which may decrease desire. The reader is referred to Chapter 2, Sexual Health Care and the Nursing Process, for an indepth discussion of sexual history and to Chapter 24, Drugs and Disturbed Sexual Functioning, for a more thorough discussion of drugs and sexuality.

Following the sexual history, the nurse should assess any physiological deficits that relate to sexual functioning. Physical assessment should include determination of flexion, abduction, and external rotation (FABER maneuver) to ascertain the extent of hip and hand involvement and to determine musculoskeletal pain and/or contractures in all joints. Inspection of the skin should note real or potential problems, such as the presence of subcutaneous nodules or cutaneous thinning caused by long-term use of steroids. Weakness of the extremities, especially the lower extremities in individuals with muscu-

---

1. In what ways, if any, has your arthritis affected your sexual relationship with your spouse/significant other?
   Physiological problems:
   Psychological problems:
   Social problems:
2. Do you and your spouse/significant other talk about your sexual relationship problem?
3. How important has your sexuality and sexual functioning been to your spouse/significant other?
4. Have you discussed any problems that may exist with your physician or a nurse?
5. What was your sexual relationship like before you had arthritis? How has that changed?
6. Have you found it difficult to explain/inform your sexual partner of your limitations?
7. What type of sexual aids have you used in the past?
   Have satisfactory adaptations been achieved?
8. Specifically, what adaptations have been helpful?
   Exercise and rest
   Increase or decrease in analgesics
   Increase or decrease in steroids
   Contraceptives
   Local lubricants
   Time of day
   Positions of comfort
   Expressions of intimacy
9. In what ways, if any, have the adaptations or lack of adaptations in your sexual relationship affected your family? Other interpersonal relationships?
10. What expectations do you have for future adaptations?

FIGURE 16–1. Sexual health assessment for chronic musculoskeletal symptoms.

lar dystropy, should be evaluated to assess problems of motion as well as locomotion.

INTERVENTION

Assisting individuals to adapt to physiological, psychological, and role changes associated with musculoskeletal symptoms requires thoughtful, continuous assessment of individual problems. Each change must be evaluated in relation to individual coping styles and desire for adaptation and in relation to realistic interventions and outcomes. Priorities are based on the severity of the maladaptation and the intensity of the threat to the individual's integrity.

Physiological Factors

Physiological deficits in the sexual activity of the individual with musculoskeletal symptoms may require change or adaptation of the therapeutic regimen in order to achieve the desired goal. Pain, the greatest deterrent to sexual activity, and stiffness can be altered through manipulation of the inflammatory response. Adjustments may compensate for decreased joint mobility, flexibility, and contractures. Medication, joint protection, and surgery are the foundations of adaptation that should be used. Systemic analgesics are the treatment of choice for musculoskeletal symptoms. While usually taken every 4 hours or upon arising and at bedtime, aspirin or its equivalent should be taken at a time when its peak action (1 hour after ingestion) will coincide with the time of sexual activity. If the individual is utilizing flexible dosage, maximal dosage should also be considered at this time. If medication other than aspirin is used, it too should be taken to provide maximal relief during the period of sexual activity. Although this adaptation may diminish spontaneous sexual activity, it may be considered preferable to a lessening in activity. Although narcotics are rarely used to treat the chronic pain of arthritis, it should be kept in mind that continuous use may be responsible for a decrease in sexual desire. Pain problems may also be altered with the use of small doses of muscle relaxants such as chlorzoxazone (Parafon Forte) or methocarbamol (Robaxin).

Choosing a time of day for sexual activity that is associated with the least amount of discomfort provides an additional mechanism of adaptation. If the time before going to sleep is commonly linked with fatigue and the time after awakening in the morning is associated with stiffness, the individual with musculoskeletal symptoms may need to experiment with alternative periods of time, such as early evening or before the evening meal. Such experimentation clearly requires the interest, cooperation, and availability of a sexual partner. It may also require planning that involves other family members, including dependent children. Experimentation with sexual activity may need to be planned while children are out of the home.

Gentle massage of painful joints provides an alternative solution to coping with painful foci. According to the gate-control theory of pain perception, massage may interfere with transmission of the pain impulse. Although the period of decreased pain may be brief, it is a good supportive therapy. Incorporating massage, with or without the use of lotions, creams, or oils, in the period of foreplay enhances it as an adaptive mechanism. Using tapes of pleasing sounds or music and/or imagery interferes with pain perception and promotes relaxation.

The following example illustrates many of these points:

> Larry, a 35-year-old white male with spondyloarthropathy, reports that he has had lower back pain for 12 years, with increased pain in his ankles and neck for the past 2 years. He notes that he has decreased motion in his neck and stiffness that is worse in the evening. However, he does work full-time evenings in a textile mill. He finds that he requires 6 to 7 hours of sleep and 8 to 9 hours of total rest every day. He has been treated in the past with gold, aspirin, and indomethacin (Indocin) but is currently taking tolmetin (Tolectin).
>
> Larry's sexual relationship with his wife of 1 month has been affected by his need for rest and relaxation prior to the period of foreplay and intercourse. He finds that foreplay requires more time and that massage is good for joint stiffness. Although he reports that he has not needed to increase his analgesics before sexual activity, he finds that pain does decrease his desire and feels that he could increase his dose of analgesics 2 to 3 hours prior to coitus. He has taken 7.5 mg of prednisone every day for 2 years but has not noted any change in his ability to achieve an erection during that time.

Small pillows may be used to support painful joints such as the knees during sexual activity. Although generally contraindicated, pillows provide comfort and increased adaptation, which enhances the individual's ability to participate in the sexual relationship, and do not jeopardize joint protection when used for short periods of time. Using a waterbed may also be helpful if the individual does not have difficulty getting on or off the bed and can afford it.

There is no uniformly effective treatment for ulcerative lesions of the genitalia, although local and/or systemic application of antibiotics and/or corticosteroids may provide some relief. Dyspareunia, associated with decreased vaginal secretions, can be altered with the use of water-soluble jelly during foreplay and intromission. Kegel excercises—contracting and relaxing the vaginal musculature—increases the ability of the vagina to grasp the penis and may enhance the responsiveness of both partners.

Selection of an appropriate and desirable method of contraception is important in adaptation of the individual with musculoskeletal symptoms. It should be based on a variety of factors, such as life style, age, past medical and obstetrical history and desire for pregnancy by the affected partner and his or her sexual partner, and cost. Understanding that pregnancy may cause remission of the disease with possible exacerbation following delivery, the female patient will need to consider current plans for or size of her family when and if pregnancy is desired. If the female patient wishes to preserve her reproductive capacity, decisions regarding the safety and effectiveness of oral contraceptives, IUDs, diaphragms, cervical cap, vaginal spermicides, and condoms should be discussed. Of particular importance are problems associated with placement of a diaphragm, cervical cap, or condom. These problems may be minimized by teaching the nonaffected sexual partner how to assist with application of the device selected or by teaching the affected female partner how to use appliances that assist in placement of the diaphragm or cervical cap. Selection of these methods also should be contingent upon the ability of the patient to remove the barrier. (For a more thorough review of contraceptive methods, see Chapter 11.) The patient with musculoskeletal symptoms who is taking steroids and considering oral contraceptives will need to evaluate the potentially compounded problem of fluid retention, while the patient who has chronic anemia should consider the risk of increased

menstrual flow sometimes associated with use of the IUD.

Closely associated with the musculoskeletal symptoms of pain is the physiological deficit of decreased joint mobility and flexibility. Adaptation for this deficit is achieved through utilization of a variety of interventions. Initially, the individual may find that taking a hot shower or applying hot compresses to the involved joints prior to sexual activity provides increased comfort as well as more active participation. The shower may be enjoyed by both the symptomatic individuals and their sex partners and can be viewed as an appealing setting for foreplay. An individualized program of range-of-motion therapy will decrease tension and promote flexibility. Perhaps the most beneficial adaptation is change in coital position. The commonly used female-inferior position requires abduction and external rotation of the hip and is often found to be difficult, if not impossible, for women with musculoskeletal symptoms. These women should experiment with alternative positions such as side lying or back to front, which allow rear entry into the vagina. Men experience the same deficits but do not require the same adaptations. With lower back involvement, the male may find that the back-lying position is preferable. If alternative positions do not provide increased comfort and/or satisfaction, the individual with musculoskeletal symptoms and his or her partner may decide to assume a more passive role. Other alternatives of adaptation include manual and oral stimulation and gratification, depending on the willingness and acceptance of both partners (Blake et al, 1987). Total hip replacement, sometimes recommended to decrease pain and improve joint mobility, also provides a mechanism for adaptation of sexual activity. However, females who have a total hip replacement should be counseled to avoid sexual positions that involve marked adduction and internal rotation of the hip to prevent dislocation of the acetabular cap.

Although not well documented, anecdotal reports have suggested that sexual activity stimulates the adrenal cortex to release increased amounts of cortisone, resulting in decreased stiffness and increased mobility (Halstead, 1977). Myotonic dystrophy may be treated symptomatically with the use of quinine.

Successful adaptation of the individual with musculoskeletal symptoms of necessity also includes counseling of the sexual partner. The nurse should encourage a high level of communication, in which both partners are not embarrassed to identify and discuss needs and problems and to experiment sexually to aid in solving problems. Consider the following case study:

Brenda, a 39-year-old married black female with two children, reports that she has had joint pain affecting the neck, shoulder, finger, knee, and foot joints intermittently for 2 to 3 years. She has experienced increasing alopecia as well as occasional joint swelling, weakness, and dizziness. She is unable to take aspirin but takes prednisone to decrease her pain. Her mother and father have a positive history of arthritis.

Brenda's sexual relationship has changed since the onset of her illness. She states that she often "doesn't want to be bothered" and that her husband understands when she is hurting. She finds that her desire for sexual activity is very unpredictable, but she believes that communication is the key to positive adaptation in her relationship with her husband.

The nurse can assist both partners to cope with guilt feelings that sometimes emerge because the sexual act cannot take place using traditional positions or simply because the healthy partner is concerned that he or she should not expect the unhealthy partner to respond. Some health professionals (Smith, 1979) suggest that the healthy individual should be counseled to try not to withdraw or discontinue sexual activity when the individual with pain or stiffness complains of pain, but they should remain sensitive to their partner's limitations and discomfort. Sexual partners sometimes need reinforcement of their knowledge that the diseases causing musculoskeletal symptoms are not contagious. Depending on the degree to which sexual maladaptations exist, and on the degree to which the involved individuals are interested in and committed to change, structured behavior modification may contribute to the re-establishment of the sexual relationship. If either the healthy or the affected partner is observed to be or reports making jokes about the sexual relationship, an effort should be made to determine the underlying maladaptation in order to treat the cause. All individuals with musculoskeletal symptoms and their partners should be free of the old taboos that suggest that sexual activity in the ill or disabled is unhealthy or perhaps even perverted.

While the problems of pain, stiffness, and decreased joint mobility may be treated symptomatically, assisting the person with musculoskeletal symptoms to cope with fatigue is also important. Fatigue associated with chronic anemia can be improved with the administration of oral iron or by increasing the intake of foods high in iron, such as liver, red meats, fortified cereals, cooked dried beans, peas, and spinach in the diet. Fatigue that has an impact on sexual activity can be decreased with thoughtful and concerned planning of daily activities. The symptomatic partner may need to omit some routine activities and/or plan additional rest periods on days that sexual activity is desired. Adaptation to fatigue requires good communication and good planning between the sexual partner.

The following case study exemplifies one person's adaptation:

Claudia, a 27-year-old black female with polyarticular arthritis secondary to lupus erythematosus, reports that for the past 8 to 10 weeks she has experienced pain, swelling, and stiffness in the joints, especially in the knees, wrists, metacarpophalangeals, proximal interphalangeals, elbows, and shoulders. She says that she has lost 10 pounds and has problems with sleep disturbance and fatigue. She used to work as a school custodian but has had to give up that job with the recent exacerbation of her symptoms. She takes 20 to 30 mg of prednisone every day when needed to decrease her symptoms.

Claudia says that the key to satisfactory adaptation in her sexual relationship with her husband is communication and planning. If she and her husband want to make love at night, she tries to rest more during the day; her husband then helps get the children to bed. After intercourse, she finds massage and application of heat to the hip important to maintain comfort and prevent soreness the following morning. Taking a shower before intercourse unfortunately makes her sleepy. Claudia feels that her husband is very understanding about her symptoms, but if he gets tense because she does not feel like having sex, he understands and chooses an alternative activity, such as working in his shop. She says that she is very determined not to let her symptoms control her life.

Psychological Adaptation

Psychological deficits affecting the sexuality of the individual with musculoskeletal symptoms may be as devastating as physiological deficits, or more so. The result of decreased self-esteem, psychological deficits sometimes need assistance that will increase the individual's value of self and help others to improve feedback that reinforces self-worth and acceptance. Nurses can provide this assistance but should first recognize that barriers to adaptation can be related to the attitude of the health professional as well as to the attitude of the individual. Nurses should be comfortable with their own sexuality and should communicate a feeling of openness in discussing sexual matters and an acceptance of varied sexual behaviors and sexual fantasies. Care should be taken not to assume that because individuals are coping with musculoskeletal symptoms they do not have concerns about their own sexuality and, indeed, are not interested in sexual activity. Nurses should be realistic when assisting individuals to plan adaptive behaviors; they need to be able to accept reasonable limitations. By understanding contributing forces, such as the sexual partners' verbal and nonverbal communication of desire and acceptance, nurses can aid individuals with musculoskeletal symptoms to change perceptions that are causing decreases in self-concept.

The nurse should help individuals with musculoskeletal symptoms causing psychological deficits to become more aware of their own feelings, to find ways of expressing feelings, and to understand and try out acceptable control of the environment. Nurses should use good communication skills to help individuals to identify areas of confusion and change, encouraging individuals to verbalize wishes while formulating realistic expectations for the sexual relationship. Individuals should be encouraged to be involved in caring for their bodies; they can maintain an attractive appearance compatible with the level of hygiene and grooming that were practiced prior to the onset of the symptoms. If the individual appears depressed, reassurance and support are needed from family and health professionals. The individual should be encouraged to make short-term goals and should be praised for progress. Some individuals may need short-term or long-term counseling that will enhance their feelings of self-worth, desirability, or adequacy.

Individuals with musculoskeletal symptoms may change their sexual behavior; they need not give up sexuality. Health professionals,

nurses in particular, can assist individuals with musculoskeletal symptomatology to maintain their sexuality. Through understanding of the concept of sexuality, health professionals promote individual adaptation and contribute to quality of life.

The pamphlet *Arthritis: Living and Loving—Information About Sex* (1982) was developed under the direction of the Arthritis Foundation in response to an identified need for information to aid individuals with musculoskeletal symptoms in adapting to sexual problems. Self-Help Arthritis Resources and Education (SHARE), 1314 Spring Street, NW, Atlanta, Georgia 30309, provides support and information, including a newsletter to patients and families.

REFERENCES

Arthritis: Living and Loving—Information about Sex. Atlanta, Arthritis Foundation, 1982.

Blake DJ, Maisiak R, Alarcon GS, et al: Sexual quality-of-life of patients with arthritis compared to arthritis-free controls. J Rheumatol 14:570–576, 1987.

Blake DJ, Maisiak R, Brown S, Koplan A: Acceptance by arthritis patients of clinical inquiry into their sexual adjustment. Psychosomatics 27:576–579, 1986.

Buckwalter T, Buckwalter JA: Musculo-skeletal conditions and sexuality. Sexual Disabil 5:Winter 1982.

Cohen M: Sexuality and the arthritic patient—how well are we doing? J Rheumatol 14:403–405, 1987.

Erlich GE: Sexual problems of the arthritic. Total Management of the Arthritic Patient. Philadelphia, JB Lippincott, 1973.

Erlich GE: Social, economic, psychologic and sexual outcomes in rheumatoid arthritis. Am J Med 75:27–34, 1983.

Elst P, Sybesma T, Van der Stadt RJ, et al: Sexual problems in rheumatoid arthritis and ankylosing spondylitis. Arthritis Rheum 27:217–220, 1984.

Flynn I, Schwetz K, Williams D: Muscular dystrophy: Comprehensive nursing care. Nurs Clin North Am 14:123–132, 1979.

Halstead LS: Aiding arthritic patients to adjust sexually. Med Asp Hum Sex 11:85–86, 1977.

Harper P, Penny R, Foley TP, et al: Gonadal function in males with myotonic dystrophy. J Clin Endocrinol Metab 38:852–856, 1972.

Hogan RM: Human Sexuality: A Nursing Perspective. Norwalk, Appleton-Century-Crofts, 1980.

Kornfeld M, Siegel I: Parenteral group therapy in the management of a fatal childhood disease. Health Soc Work 4:99–118, 1979.

Masters WH, Johnson VE: Human Sexual Inadequacy. Boston, Little, Brown & Co, 1970.

Roy SC, Roberts S: Theory Construction in Nursing: An Adaptation Model. Englewood Cliffs, Prentice Hall, 1981.

Smith LL: Helping to manage the emotional effects of arthritis. Health Soc Work 4:1340–1350, 1979.

Spergel P: Psychological aspects of joint disease. Rheumatic Diseases, Philadelphia, JB Lippincott, 1977.

Yoshino S, Uchida S: Sexual problems of women with rheumatoid arthritis. Arch Phys Med Rehabil 62:122–123, 1981.

17: Endocrine Disturbances and Sexuality

Ginger Manley

Sexual health, or integrity, is a product of the integration of multiple components into one complex, unified system. The endocrine system, through its hormonal regulators, acts with the vascular, nervous, and psychic systems as a direct influence on biological sexual integrity. The endocrine system also acts as an indirect influence on sexual integrity by its secondary effect on the psychosocial systems. In discussing sexual integrity, it is important to remember that while the components can be separated for purposes of analysis, they must be reassembled and viewed in the context of the whole person.

In this chapter the influence of endocrine regulation upon the biological, psychological, and social factors that underlie sexual integrity is examined separately in terms of sexual response, physical characteristics, reproductive capacity, psychic identity, and social relationships.

ENDOCRINE DISTURBANCES AND SEXUAL FUNCTION

Roy's adaptation model of nursing practice is used as the framework for discussing interactions with clients around the issue of endocrine disturbances and sexual health. Roy (1984) asserts that a person adapts to constantly changing environments through four modes or manners: physiological, self-concept, role function, and interdependence. A person's level of adaptation is a function of the stimuli to which the person is exposed. These stimuli may be focal, or primary, causative factors; contextual, or situational, determinants; and residual, or cultural and attitudinal, influences. An endocrine disturbance may be a focal stimulus precipitating a biological response; or, it may be a contextual or residual stimulus contributing to or coinciding with a biological, psychological, or social response.

Adaptive sexual behaviors are those responses that maintain the sexual integrity of the individual. Ineffective sexual behaviors, or sexual dysfunctions, are those behaviors that disrupt the sexual integrity of the individual. Assessments of the effectiveness or ineffectiveness of a sexual behavior may be individual or require collaboration with the person's partner.

The goal of nursing is to support and promote a person's adaptation specifically by altering stimuli to be within the person's adaptational level. In the case of sexual dysfunctions associated with endocrine disturbances, the nurse may intervene to alter stimuli that are influencing the dysfunction. Interventions include administering specific therapeutic measures, promoting normal body functioning, teaching about changes that are occurring, promoting role mastery, and promoting a positive emotional response to the therapy.

337

SEXUAL ADAPTATION, ENDOCRINE REGULATION, AND PHYSIOLOGICAL FUNCTION

Three dimensions of sexual adaptation can be identified in the physiological mode: sexual response, reproductive capacity, and physical characteristics. These categories assume that sexuality is both recreational and procreational and that sexuality can be both independent and dependent of a sexual relationship.

For the purposes of this discussion, Kaplan's (1983) triphasic model of the human sexual response cycle will be used. Kaplan (1983) describes a model consisting of a desire phase, an excitement phase, and an orgasm phase.

The desire phase is regulated by the hormonal and psychic systems. Sexual adaptation in the desire phase is observed through sexual interest. Dysfunction in the desire phase is characterized by variances in sexual desire that are out of the normal range for the individual. Hormonal disturbances as primary stimuli for desire dysfunction are rare, such as hypogonadism and low testosterone levels. Desire dysfunction is most often a product of psychic disturbances.

The excitement phase is regulated primarily by the parasympathetic component of the autonomic nervous system and secondarily by the capacity of the vascular system to respond to neural and psychic input. There is no evidence to support direct hormonal regulation as a mediator of sexual excitement. Sexual adaptation in the excitement phase is observed through intact erections in the male and intact vaginal lubrication and genital swelling in the female. Dysfunction in the excitement phase is characterized by erectile dysfunction (impotence) in the male and by vaginal dryness or inadequate lubrication in the female.

The orgasm phase is regulated by the sympathetic branch of the autonomic nervous system and, as with excitement, there is no direct endocrine influence. Sexual adaptation in the orgasm phase is observed through intact emission and ejaculation in the male and by intact orgasm in the female. Dysfunctions in the orgasm phase include premature ejaculation, inhibited ejaculation, and retrograde ejaculation in the male. Females may experience lack of orgasm (preorgasmia) or decreased intensity of orgasm.

Reproductive capacity is basic to preservation of the species. The major regulator of reproductive capacity is the endocrine system through both reproductive hormonal secretion and target organ receptivity. The reproductive hormones include those secreted by the anterior pituitary, adrenal cortex, testes, and ovaries. Reproductive sexual adaptation is observed in intact pituitary and gonadal function and in intact reproductive organs. Dysfunctional reproductive capacity is characterized by excessive or diminished reproductive hormone production and by structural and functional deficits in the reproductive organs.

Endocrine regulation of physical characteristics is maintained through hormone production and target organ receptivity. The physical characteristics associated with sexual adaptation include body stature and size, development of secondary sex characteristics, and altered appearance of physical structures. Alterations in physical characteristics may be genetic or acquired.

EFFECTS OF ENDOCRINE FUNCTION ON PHYSIOLOGICAL SEXUAL BEHAVIOR

Our understanding of the relationship between hormones and biological sexual functioning assumes that specific hormonal levels are necessary for specific functions. Alterations in physiological sexual behavior, therefore, may be the person's response to altered hormone levels, either excesses or deficits.

The role of hormones in human sexual behavior is not well understood because not enough is known and what is known is not clear. It is important to note that measures of levels of hormones in circulating plasma do not necessarily describe hormone receptor activity. Another problem is that although we have some understandings of the role of hormones in lower animals and their corresponding sexual behavioral effect, we cannot readily generalize this effect to humans. Bancroft states, "Hormones and human sexual behavior present us with a jigsaw puzzle and as yet only a few of the pieces are in place" (Bancroft, 1984, p 18).

The endocrine system acts as a regulator mechanism on a feedback loop. Specific hormone disruptions signal other hormones that attempt to intervene to restore homeostasis. Because of multiple hormonal factors, it is often difficult to demarcate clearly the effect of one discrete disruption on a person's total sexual response. Hormonal disturbances may be innate (genetic or endogenous) or may be acquired (exogenous or surgical) and frequently are part of a constellation of polyendocrine disease. In general, hormones seem to have their greatest physiological sexual effect on reproductive capacity and physical characteristics and a much lesser effect on

sexual desire and on the genital responses of excitement and orgasm.

The relationship along the hypothalamic-pituitary-gonadal axis and the corresponding changes in sexual behavior offer the clearest conceptual model for understanding endocrine-mediated sexual alterations (Fig. 17–1). Dysfunctions in this axis are frequently associated with erectile dysfunction and other impairments (Nickel, 1984). Endocrine regulation and sexual dysfunction in pregnancy and lactation are beyond the scope of this chapter and are discussed in Chapter 10, The Maternity Cycle and Sexuality. Sexual dysfunctions common to endocrine diseases are summarized in Table 17–1.

The endocrine system may be simplistically organized into the following structural and

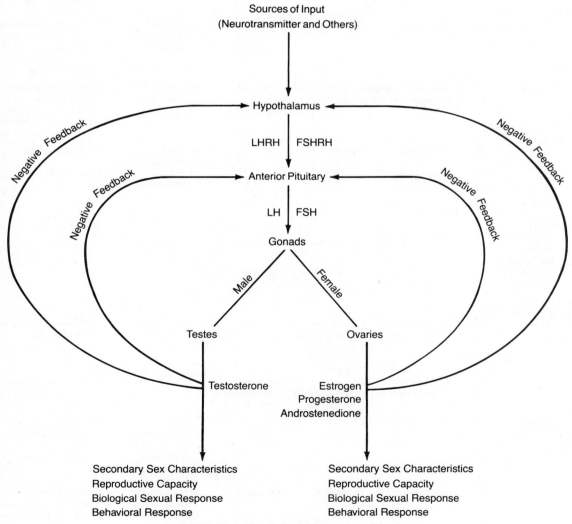

FIGURE 17–1. *Hypothalamic-pituitary-gonadal axis.*

TABLE 17–1. Physiological Sexual Dysfunctions Common to Endocrine Diseases Other Than Diabetes Mellitus

		Desire	Excitement	Orgasm	Reproductive Capacity	Selected Physical Characteristics
Disruption in Endocrine System						
1. Hypothalamus						
LHRH	M	*	*	*	Indirect	*
FSHRH	F	*	*	*	Indirect	*
2. Pituitary						
Gonadotropins						
FSH, LH	M	Indirect—associated with gonadal testosterone production			Disrupted spermatogenesis	Failure to mature
	F				Low fertility anovulation	Failure to mature
Growth hormone						
Excess	M	Decreased	Decreased	*	Altered spermatogenesis	Gigantism (childhood), acromegaly (adulthood), hypogonadism, gynecomastia, galactorrhea
	F	Decreased	Decreased	Decreased (acromegaly)	Menstrual irregularities, amenorrhea	Gigantism (childhood), acromegaly (adulthood), hypogonadism, galactorrhea
Deficit	M	Indirect—associated with gonadotropin and glucocorticoid production			Reproductive immaturity	Pituitary dwarfism (childhood) failure to mature weight gain (adults)
	F					
Prolactin						
Excess	M	Decreased	Erectile dysfunction	*	Altered spermatogenesis	Rare galactorrhea
	F	Decreased	*	*	Menstrual irregularities	Galactorrhea
Deficit	M	*	*	*	*	*
	F					
ACTH (corticotropin)		See adrenal disorders				
TSH (thyroid stimulating hormone)		See adrenal disorders				
3. Thyroid						
Thyroxine						
Excess	M	Increased or decreased	Erectile dysfunction associated with increased desire	*		Increased growth rate (childhood)
	F	Increased or decreased	Increased, decreased or no change	Increased, decreased or no change		Weight loss, sweating, overt psychological changes
Deficit	M	Decreased	Erectile dysfunction	*	Decreased spermatogenesis secondary to decreased testosterone levels	Decreased growth rate, failure to mature, sexual precocity (rare)
	F	Decreased	Decreased	Retarded	Menstrual irregularities Spontaneous abortion	Failure to mature, increased, decreased growth rate, sexual precocity (rare)

TABLE 17–1. Physiological Sexual Dysfunctions Common to Endocrine Diseases Other Than Diabetes Mellitus *Continued*

		Desire	Excitement	Orgasm	Reproductive Capacity	Selected Physical Characteristics
4. Adrenals						
Cortisol						
Excess (Cushing's disease)	M	Decreased	Erectile dysfunction	*	Decreased spermatogenesis	Acne, hirsutism, truncal obesity, atrophied testes, gynecomastia, feminization
	F	Increased or decreased	*	Decreased or retarded	Amenorrhea, oligomenorrhea	Virilization, hirsutism, clitoral hypertrophy, masculine voice
Deficit (Addison's disease)	M	Decreased	Erectile dysfunction	*	Decreased spermatogenesis and testosterone synthesis	Weight loss, hyperpigmentation of nipples and genitals
	F	Decreased	Intact	Decreased	No change	Hyperpigmentation of nipples and genitals
5. Gonads						
Testosterone						
Excess	M	Increased	Indirect, effect on ability to fantasize	*	No change	Hypertrophy of gonads
	F	No change	Indirect	*	No change	Masculinization and virilization, ovarian atrophy
Deficit	M	Decreased	Probably no change	Decreased seminal fluid volume	Decreased spermatogenesis	Atrophy of penis and testes, failure to mature, male eunuch (childhood)
	F	No change, unless both adrenalectomized and oopherectomized	No change	*	No change	Altered maturity
Estrogen						
Excess	M	Possible decrease	Erectile dysfunction	*	*	Gynecomastia, feminization
	F	No effect	*	*	Intermenstrual bleeding, postmenopausal bleeding, infertility, endometriosis	No effect
Deficit	M	*	*	*	*	No effect
	F	No effect	Secondary decreased lubrication	*	Ovarian failure	Failure to mature, breast atrophy, decreased pubic hair
Progesterone						
Excess	M, F	Possible decreased secondary to decreased androgens	*	*	*	*
Deficit	M, F	*	*	*	*	*

* = unknown

functional categories for ease of understanding its effect on sexual behaviors.

Hypothalamus

The hypothalamus is the part of the brain that controls the pituitary by nerve signals transmitted from the hypothalamus. While the hypothalamus produces several hormones, only *luteinizing hormone releasing hormone* (LHRH) and *follicle-stimulating hormone releasing hormone* (FSHRH) are considered in this chapter. LHRH is known to enhance sexual function in castrated lower animals. However, the role of LHRH in male erectile functioning has yet to be specified (Kaplan, 1983).

Pituitary Gland

The anterior pituitary produces six hormones that affect sexual behavior: the gonadotropins (1) follicle-stimulating hormone (FSH) and (2) lutenizing hormone (LH), (3) growth hormone, (4) prolactin, (5) corticotropin (ACTH), and (6) thyroid-stimulating hormone (TSH). The posterior pituitary produces two hormones: (1) antidiuretic hormone (ADH) and (2) oxytocin. Posterior pituitary hormones are not discussed in this chapter.

Some overall observations may be made about altered sexual responses and pituitary dysfunction. Briefly, pituitary disruptions from surgical or chemical mechanisms or disease processes are associated with mild to marked impairment of sexual behaviors. These may be summarized as (1) hypogonadism, (2) alterations in sexual desire, (3) inhibited orgasm, (4) menstrual irregularities, (5) difficulty with lactation and conception, (6) alterations in physical characteristics with corresponding changes in body image, and (7) debility. The specific hormone disruptions and resulting sexual behaviors will be discussed by discrete hormone entity, as follows.

The *gonadotropins* control ovarian function and the menstrual cycle in females as well as production of testosterone and spermatogenesis in males. In females, FSH stimulates ovarian function in the follicular stage and LH stimulates ovarian function in the luteal stage. In males, FSH mediates spermatogenesis, and LH mediates testosterone secretion. In relation to alterations in desire, excite-

ment, and orgasm, the role of gonadotropins appears to be indirect and associated with their influence on gonadal testosterone production.

Alterations in reproductive capacity associated with gonadotropic alterations are well known. In females, low fertility and anovulation associated with ovarian failure is almost always a function of altered LH production. Since LH levels in males are associated with production of testosterone in the testicular interstitial cells, altered LH levels can affect spermatogenesis.

Alterations in physiological characteristics associated with altered gonadotropins are generally the result of childhood rather than adult onset of the problem. These include failure to mature sexually and physically, with corresponding short stature and skeletal as well as reproductive immaturity. Prepubertal boys with LH and FSH deficiency show the same failure to mature as do males with testosterone deficits (Braunstein, 1983).

Produced by the pituitary, *growth hormone* promotes tissue growth throughout life. Excessive growth hormone production prior to puberty leads to gigantism and, if not controlled, may further lead to diabetes and/or early death. Excessive growth hormone in adulthood leads to acromegaly and may also lead to overt diabetes.

Both gigantism and acromegaly can result in hypogonadism. The diseases may be accompanied by decreased sexual desire and excitement secondary to diminished testosterone. Also, desire may be altered by associated changes in body image. Acromegaly may retard orgasm in females through its effect on neural pathways in the brain and/or cellular responses of the genitals (Kaplan, 1983).

Both gigantism and acromegaly can alter reproductive capacity. Women commonly note menstrual irregularities or amenorrhea (Kolodny, Masters, and Johnson, 1979). Alterations in physical characteristics can be generalized as excessively long limbs (gigantism) or thickened, coarse facies, hands, and feet (acromegaly). Women with acromegaly often have galactorrhea; men with either condition may have gynecomastia and galactorrhea.

Deficits in growth hormone may affect both adults and children. When a growth hormone deficit occurs in adults, it is accompanied by hypothyroidism and the corresponding behaviors of lethargy and weight gain. Additionally, glucocorticoid and gonadotropin production is compromised, leading to decreased sexual functioning. If deficits in growth hormone occur in childhood, pituitary dwarfism, with a balanced but small stature, results. Many pituitary dwarfs will also have decreased reproductive capacity secondary to partial failure to mature sexually.

Prolactin controls the establishment and maintenance of lactation in females and appears to contribute to female sexual desire. No corresponding physiological function of prolactin has been identified in males (Bancroft, 1984), but prolactin may contribute to sexual desire in males by an unexplained relationship between prolactin and testosterone (Segraves, 1983). Excesses of prolactin (hyperprolactinemia) are commonly associated with decreased desire in both males and females (Kaplan, 1983). Among men with hyperprolactinemia, erectile dysfunction occurs in 70 to 90 per cent of cases (Braunstein, 1983). One possible explanation for this is that hyperprolactinemia appears to decrease testosterone synthesis in the testes and therefore directly contributes to decreased desire, which may then lead to erectile dysfunction (Pont et al, 1979). An interesting and significant relationship has been noted among prolactin levels, testosterone levels, and marital status of men: Married men have higher prolactin levels and lower testosterone levels than unmarried men (Segraves, 1983). The explanation for this phenomenon is currently unknown.

Among women, hyperprolactinemia may be responsible for 20 per cent of reproductive dysfunctions through its interference with FSH and LH secretion and the ensuing menstrual irregularities. Hyperprolactinemia is associated with galactorrhea in females but only rarely causes galactorrhea in males (Pont et al, 1979). Hyperprolactinemia is also occasionally associated with acromegaly.

ACTH controls the secretion of adrenocortical hormones. Excesses of ACTH lead to Cushing's disease, while decreases of ACTH lead to Addison's disease. These conditions and their relation to sexual behavior are discussed in the following section.

TSH controls the rate of secretion of thyroxine by the thyroid gland. Sexual dysfunctions associated with altered thyroxine are discussed in the following section.

Thyroid Gland

Thyroid hormone (thyroxine) influences overall metabolic activity. There is a "significant association between thyroid disease and sexual problems" (Kolodny, Masters, and Johnson, 1979, p 116).

Hyperthyroidism may be a result of Graves' disease, toxic goiter, or thyrotoxicosis, all representing hyperplasia of the thyroid gland with corresponding increased hormone production. Excesses of thyroid hormone are associated with increased growth rate (in children), weight loss, excitement of mental processes, sweating, nervousness, and overt psychological changes.

Alterations in sexual response associated with hyperthyroidism may include both increased and decreased desire, especially associated with manic behaviors and with increased levels of FSH, LH, testosterone, and estradiol (Kaplan, 1983). Among hyperthyroid men, 50 to 71 per cent have decreased desire and 40 to 56 per cent have erectile difficulties (Braunstein, 1983; Cooper, 1984; Kolodny, Masters, and Johnson, 1979). In contrast, increased desire, sometimes accompanied by erectile dysfunction, has been seen in 10 to 20 per cent of men with hyperthyroidism (Kolodny, Masters, and Johnson, 1979). Aggressive sexual behavior in men associated with increased desire has been noted in cases of Hashimoto's thyroiditis and thyrotoxicosis (Kolodny, Masters, and Johnson, 1979; Leigh and Kramer, 1984).

Among women with hyperthyroidism, 70 to 80 per cent describe no change or a mild decrease in sexual responsiveness. Another 5 to 10 per cent of these women have heightened sexual arousal and orgasm response (Kolodny, Masters, and Johnson, 1979).

Hypothyroidism may result from a goiter or from antithyroid medications and may be only slight or may progress to myxedema or cretinism (in childhood). Thyroid deficiency results in somnolence, lethargy, decreased growth of hair, and increases in prolactin and free estrogen (Kaplan, 1983).

Alterations in female sexual response associated with hypothyroidism include decreases in desire, with secondary diminution of excitement (Kaplan, 1983). Kolodny, Masters, and Johnson note that "approximately 80 per cent of hypothyroid women report a decrease in libido, and about half of these women describe difficulty in becoming sexually aroused" (Kolodny, Masters, and Johnson, 1979, p 117). Hypothyroidism may also retard female orgasm (Kaplan, 1983), with approximately 37 per cent of women who have untreated hypothyroidism reporting nonorgasmia (Kolodny, Masters, and Johnson, 1979).

Among men, hypothyroidism is associated with decreased desire and erectile dysfunction in an unknown way (Braunstein, 1983). About 80 per cent of men with hypothyroidism experience decreased desire; about 40 to 50 per cent of these men also have erectile dysfunction to varying degrees (Kolodny, Masters, and Johnson, 1979).

While these alterations in sexual function may largely be a manifestation of the effect of the thyroid disease on the person, they may also be reflections of decreased synthesis of testosterone in the testes and adrenal cortex (Kolodny, Masters, and Johnson, 1979). Also, hyperprolactinemia is associated with hypothyroidism, giving an added stimulus for the decreased testosterone production and metabolism.

Reproductive capacity in thyroid disorders is altered by ovarian failure and menstrual irregularities in females and decreased sperm production in males. In addition, "pregnancies in women with untreated hypothyroidism exhibit an increased rate of spontaneous abortion" (Kolodny, Masters, and Johnson, 1979, p 118).

Changes in physiological characteristics associated with thyroid disorders include failure to mature physically, mentally, and sexually in untreated cretins. Hypothyroidism occurring prior to puberty results in general retardation of physical growth and development; if severe and untreated, it will result in failure of onset and development of secondary sex characteristics, all of which are reversible by adequate replacement of thyroid hormone. "Rarely, primary hypothyroidism may be associated with sexual precocity, including early breast development, maturation of the vaginal mucosa, vaginal bleeding, and galactorrhea in girls, and testicular and penile enlargement in boys" (Kolodny, Masters, and Johnson, 1979, p 117).

Adrenal Glands

The adrenals are composed of two layers: the medulla and the cortex. The medulla secretes the hormones epinephrine and norepinephrine; these are not directly pertinent to this chapter and are not discussed. The cortex secretes hormones known as steroids, which contribute to the synthesis of proteins, carbohydrates, and fats. Three categories of adrenal cortical steroids affect sexual behavior: (1) glucocorticoids, (2) mineralocorticoids, and (3) adrenal androgens.

Cortisol, a glucocorticoid, mediates metabolism of carbohydrates, proteins, and fats. *Aldosterone,* a mineralocorticoid, mediates fluid and electrolyte balance. *Adrenal androgens* (such as testosterone) mediate the development of sex organs in males (childhood) and the appearance of axillary and pubic hair in females. Adrenal androgens also contribute to maintenance of desire.

Cushing's disease, associated with excess adrenal cortical hormone, usually cortisol, may result in alterations in sexual response. They include changes in desire and orgasm. Either a marked increase or marked decrease in desire occurs in about 10 to 20 per cent of women with this condition (Kolodny, Masters, and Johnson, 1979). Cushing's disease may retard orgasmic response in women (Kaplan, 1984), with as many as 30 per cent of women reporting nonorgasmia "despite a previous history of normal sexual responsiveness" (Kolodny, Masters, and Johnson, 1979, p 122). Men with Cushing's disease may have diminished desire and erectile dysfunction, with incidence rates varying from 70 per cent (Braunstein, 1983) to 100 per cent (Kolodny, Masters, and Johnson, 1979).

Reproductive capacity in Cushing's disease is altered in as many as 80 per cent of women by amenorrhea or oligomenorrhea (Kolodny, Masters, and Johnson, 1979). Male fertility is decreased by disrupted spermatogenesis, with as many as 70 per cent of men having decreased sperm count (Braunstein, 1983). While some of these alterations in sexual response may result directly from corresponding alterations in adrenal androgen production or from disruptions in testicular function, others may result from the effects of coexisting diabetes mellitus or from antihypertensive drugs used to treat the symptoms of the illness.

Physiological characteristics are altered in hypercortisolism (Cushing's disease) by acne, hirsutism, truncal obesity, and weight gain, all contributing to alterations in body image. Overt personality changes in Cushing's disease are more marked than with any other endocrine disease. Men with Cushing's disease commonly experience atrophy of the testes and gynecomastia and other feminizing signs. Women experience mild to moderate "virilism, including hirsutism, clitoral hypertrophy, deepening of the voice, and, occasionally, temporal hair recession" (Kolodny, Masters, and Johnson, 1979, p 122).

Addison's disease is a result of deficits of both cortisol and aldosterone. If untreated, it can result in death in 3 to 14 days. Alterations in female sexual response associated with Addison's disease include a marked decrease in desire and a decrease or diminished orgasmic response, possibly as a result of a decreased sensory threshold to tactile stimuli, a common condition associated with Addison's disease. Usually, sexual arousal in women with Addison's disease remains intact unless another condition occurs to alter arousal and lubrication (Kolodny, Masters, and Johnson, 1979; Kaplan, 1983).

Alterations in sexual response in men with Addison's disease include decreased desire and decreased initiatory sexual behaviors (Kolodny, Masters, and Johnson, 1979). This is probably not a reflection of lowered circulating testosterone levels but is probably secondary to weight loss and debility (Braunstein, 1983). The incidence of erectile dysfunction in males with Addison's disease is approximately 35 per cent (Kolodny, Masters, and Johnson, 1979). Information on orgasm disturbances in males is not available but may be hypothesized as paralleling that of women.

Alterations in reproductive capacity in Addison's disease is usually not marked in women because the menstrual cycle is usually not altered. Males with secondary adrenal insufficiency may have marked changes in spermatogenesis and testosterone synthesis (Kolodny, Masters, and Johnson, 1979), contributing to decreased fertility.

Alterations in physical characteristics associated with Addison's disease include hyperpigmentation, especially in unexposed areas such as the genitals and nipples. Weakness, weight loss, and personality changes may all contribute to alterations in body image and role function.

Androgen-producing adrenal tumors may occur in both males and females but are more readily observed in females. Alterations in desire, excitement, orgasm, and reproductive capacity parallel those of alterations in gonadal testosterone production. Alterations in physiological characteristics of adrenal androgen-producing tumors may be recognized in male children through premature masculinization but are obviously less easily detected in adult males.

Other adrenocortical alterations include feminizing tumors in men that produce large amounts of estrogen and lead to diminished desire and erectile dysfunction. Because of suppressed testosterone production and decreased spermatogenesis, reproductive capacity is also altered. Physiological changes include feminization, gynecomastia, and atrophy of the testes (Kolodny, Masters, and Johnson, 1979).

Gonads

The testes secrete the hormone *testosterone*, and the ovaries secrete the hormones *estrogen* (estradiol), *progesterone*, and *androstenedione*, a testosterone precursor.

In the adult male, 95 per cent of the circulating testosterone is produced by the testes, and 5 per cent is contributed by the adrenal cortex. The normal range in concentration of serum plasma testosterone in males varies considerably, but it may be between 385 and 1000 mg/100 ml (Kolodny, Masters, and Johnson, 1979). Testosterone levels in males fluctuate in a diurnal variation, with peak concentrations in the morning.

In the adult female, androgen production occurs in the adrenal cortex and the ovaries, with each structure contributing about 50 per cent of the total (Bancroft et al, 1980). The principal plasma androgen in females is androstenedione, which is converted peripherally to testosterone. The normal range of testosterone in adult females is 20 to 80 ng/100 ml; in women who use oral contraceptives it is 45 to 125 ng/100 ml (Kolodny, Masters, and Johnson, 1979). Testosterone levels in females fluctuate in patterns corresponding to the menstrual period, with a "substantial increase in testosterone and other androgens . . . during the middle third of the cycle, mainly due to increased ovarian production" (Bancroft, 1984, p 17).

The absolute ranges of testosterone associated with adequate sexual function are not known (Bancroft, 1984), but it is known that testosterone production in males declines slightly with age. Comparable declines in androgen levels in women with aging have not been demonstrated. Testosterone facilitates sexual desire in both males and females, but the evidence for this is much clearer for males than for females.

In observing sexual patterns of lower animals, female animals show an estrous pattern that corresponds well with fluctuating hormone levels, including testosterone. In human females, however, there is no corresponding increase in sexual interest with a partner at peak testosterone levels. Bancroft (1984) hypothesizes that the relationship between testosterone levels and sexual behavioral changes is more indirect than direct in human females.

Bancroft (1984) has also studied the relationship of testosterone to female sexual behavior *independent* of a partner. He observed that while autosexuality in these women was androgen dependent, sexuality within a relationship was not or may even have been adversely affected by androgens. Further, he noted that while testosterone was positively related to both sexual desire levels and to role function, some "high testosterone" women may note role conflicts within a conventional relationship, which may lead to a secondary loss in desire for their partner.

Testosterone excess can result from androgen-producing tumors and from exogenous testosterone, especially from injections or oral ingestion of the hormone. There has also been "some evidence to suggest that testosterone levels tend to be higher during periods of sexual inactivity . . . or anticipation of sexual activity" (Schwartz, Kolodny, and Masters, 1980, p 363), although these data are controversial. Testosterone deficits can result from genetic absences, gonadal insult, and adrenalectomy.

Excess testosterone has been associated with increased sexual desire in some males, occasionally to a compulsive level. No corresponding evidence of excess testosterone and compulsive sexual desire exists in women.

Deficits in testosterone in hypogonadal men result in declines in sexual interest; resumption of interest occurs within 1 to 2 weeks after beginning replacement androgen therapy (Bancroft, 1984). Several studies (Bancroft et al, 1980; Dow and Hart, 1983; Matthews, Whitehead, and Kellett, 1983) have not demonstrated any benefit in administering exogenous testosterone to women with low sexual interest, and the problematic side effects of such treatment can outweigh any theoretical benefits. However, administration of testosterone (in levels higher than normal) to postmenopausal or oophorectomized women is sometimes tried to treat decreased desire (Goleman, 1988). It has been observed that oophorectomized and adrenalectomized women become sexually disinterested (Kaplan, 1983), assumingly because of loss of the testosterone-producing ovaries and adrenals.

The effects of testosterone on the excitement and orgasm phases of sexual response are indirect. Testosterone per se does not influence male erection, as is evident in the presence of penile erections with minimal testosterone levels in infants and preadolescent males (Segraves, 1983). Bancroft (1984) observed that androgens may be necessary for normal tactile sensitivity of the penis but questioned whether such penile sensitivity is *only* androgen dependent; androgens may facilitate psychic or other stimuli. Since androgens *are* necessary for erotic fantasy to result in arousal and penile erection, as has been demonstrated in studies with sex offenders, it can be assumed that the control of cognitive mechanisms leading to erection *are* androgen dependent but that the erectile response is *not directly androgen dependent* (Bancroft, 1984). One may assume that this is also true for clitoral erection, since the structures are homologous.

Testosterone affects the emission phase of male orgasm through target organ response of the prostate and seminal vesicles to androgen stimulation. When a severe testosterone deficiency is present, seminal fluid volume and spermatogenesis are diminished, thus decreasing reproductive capacity in males (Kolodny, Masters, and Johnson, 1979).

The reproductive capacity of males with severe testosterone deficiency is also diminished through decreased spermatogenesis. Male reproductive capacity is rarely affected by testosterone excess. In females, testosterone excesses and deficits are also only rare causes for alteration of reproductive capacity by interruptions in the menstrual cycle.

Physiological characteristics are altered by testosterone as the hormone acts on target organs to produce masculinization, with male distribution of body hair, deepening of the voice, increases in sizes of the penis and scrotum in the mature male, increased thickness of bones, and increased musculature and thickness of the skin. Testosterone excess in females leads to masculinization and virilization (clitoral hypertrophy and ovarian atrophy) and, in the male, to increased size of target organs.

Testosterone deficits in mature males result in atrophy of the penis and testes, decreased growth of body hair and beard, and gynecomastia (Braunstein, 1983). Prior to puberty, uncorrected testosterone deficits in the male may cause retention of juvenile physical characteristics, increased height outside of the predictable range for the individual, muscle weakness, and abnormal body hair distribution. All of the foregoing are characteristics of the male eunuch.

Estrogen, through its effect on target organs, is responsible for the development of secondary sex characteristics at puberty and for maintaining target organ integrity throughout the life of the female. Estrogen is responsible for pubertal changes that include increased size of the uterus, and external genitalia and breast and the early starting and stopping of bone growth. Throughout the fertile years, estrogen contributes to maintenance of vaginal epithelium through mucus production (contributing to lubrication) and through increasing vascularization of the vagina and the endometrium of the uterus.

Estrogen (estradiol 17-beta) levels vary during the menstrual cycle, with average serum levels of 200 pg/ml in the premenopausal female. Estrogen deficiency may be genetic or acquired, such as the premature menopause from oophorectomy or natural menopause. At midlife (in the absence of oophorectomy) estrogen levels begin to decrease, resulting in an average serum level of less than 25 pg/ml at menopause (Sarrel, 1988). The effect of this decrease is noted both in target organ responsiveness (especially vascular, neurological, genitourinary, and skeletal systems) and in changes in emotional states and behaviors. Physiological changes in target organs relative to sexual responsiveness include decreased touch perception, decreased sexual desire, decreased clitoral receptivity to stimulation, dyspareunia with or without vaginal lubrication, and increased threshold for orgasm (Frazer, 1987; Hufnagel, 1987).

Changes in emotional state and behaviors relative to estrogen deficiency include depression, alterations in body image, and the onset of sexual dysfunctions in the male partners of estrogen-deficient females. These male dysfunctions include inhibitory sexual feelings, fear of hurting the female, perform-

ance anxiety, inability to penetrate, and prolonged stimulation time (Sarrel, 1988).

The direct effect of estrogen on male sexuality is less well known. There is some evidence, however, that administering estrogens to men decreases their sexual desire, with effects similar to those associated with antiandrogens or the condition of androgen deficiency (Bancroft, 1984).

Estrogen excess may be endogenous or induced, such as from estrogen-containing drugs. Estrogen-producing tumors are rare but can produce feminization, which is obviously more noticeable in males. Increased estrogen in males, from testicular tumors or treatment with antiandrogen medications, has been noted to lead to decreased desire, erectile dysfunction, and gynecomastia (Braunstein, 1983). The physiological effects of excess estrogen on women are hypertrophy of the endometrium with intermenstrual bleeding or dysfunctional postmenopausal bleeding. Estrogen excess has also been hypothesized to mediate the development of endometriosis, which can lead to dyspareunia and infertility.

The biological effect of progesterone is to enhance conception, retention of pregnancy, and to stimulate lactation. Progesterone is often used, either alone or in conjunction with estrogen, as an oral contraceptive. Progesterone may reduce sexual desire in both males and females by reducing the levels of circulating androgens (Hogan, 1980), but as yet the role of progesterone on desire is speculative (Bancroft, 1984). More research on the effect of progesterone on sexuality is needed.

Pancreas

Insulin mediates carbohydrate metabolism by intercellular transport of glucose. Excessive insulin effect (hypoglycemia) can result from insulin-producing tumors (rare) or from excessive exogenous insulin injection or use of other hypoglycemic substances. Although many persons believe they have hypoglycemia, true endogenous hypoglycemia is extremely rare, and "present evidence does not support the general association of sexual difficulties with low blood sugar" (Kolodny, Masters, and Johnson, 1979).

Deficiencies of insulin (diabetes mellitus) may result from genetic or acquired mechanisms and may be absolute or relative. Diabetes is the endocrine disturbance about which the greatest amount of study has been done regarding its effect on sexual behavior. These effects will be discussed in the following section.

SEXUAL ADAPTATION IN DIABETES MELLITUS

The most common, as well as the most completely understood, endocrine disturbance associated with sexual dysfunction is diabetes mellitus. Diabetes can affect sexual behavior in all of Roy's four modes of adaptation (Roy, 1984). Much more is known about the effect of diabetes upon male sexual adaptation than upon female sexual adaptation. Sexual dysfunctions associated with diabetes mellitus are summarized in Table 17–2.

A number of stimuli thought to influence biological sexual adaptation in diabetes mellitus have been studied (Block, 1982; Ellenberg, 1977; Furlow, 1979; Kolodny, 1971; Krosnick and Podolsky, 1981; Pieper, 1982; Podolsky, 1982a and 1982b; Renshaw, 1978; Wabrek, 1979). Factors studied include severity and duration of the illness, degree of metabolic control, neurovascular complications, hormonal influences, relative degree of depression, and age of the person. Two distinct conclusions can be made from these studies. First, initial severe metabolic decompensation of uncontrolled diabetes is often associated with sexual dysfunction that resolves once metabolic control is achieved

(Wagner and Green, 1981). Second, with varying degrees of control over time, the only two factors that seem to be reliable predictors of biological sexual dysfunction in diabetes are age of the person and presence of autonomic neuropathy.

In general, persons with diabetes maintain levels of sexual desire comparable with those of the general population (Krosnick and Podolsky, 1981; Jensen, 1981; Jensen et al, 1979; Ellenberg, 1977 and 1979; Schiavi and Hogan, 1979). As for other clients, the major cause of diminished desire is depression. Diabetics as a group have not been found to be more depressed than the general population (Krosnick and Podolsky, 1981) or than others with chronic illness (Cassileth et al, 1984). Since depression may affect one's sexual responsiveness, if depression is present in a person with diabetes, then depression may play a role in altering sexual desire. Excitement and orgasmic phase dysfunction associated with diabetes are considered separately for males and females in the following sections.

Diabetic Males

Erectile dysfunction may be the first symptom of diabetes in men. The problem is that of attaining and maintaining effective rigidity rather than merely experiencing changes in circumference. A man may note progressive softening of his penis over a period of months or years, eventually leading to inability to perform vaginal penetration. The first

TABLE 17–2. Physiological Sexual Dysfunctions Associated with Diabetes Mellitus as Compared with General Population

	Desire	Excitement	Orgasm	Reproductive Capacity	Characteristic Changes in Appearance
Males	Unchanged, except secondary to erectile dysfunction	Erectile dysfunction (30 to 60%) with duration of illness and neuropathy	No greater risk for premature or retarded ejaculation	Slight decrease secondary to retrograde ejaculation and abnormal sperm	Uncommon (except with childhood onset)
			Retrograde ejaculation (< 5%)		
Females	Unchanged	Some decreased lubrication, especially with neuropathy or vaginal infection	Increased threshold of stimulus necessary for orgasm	Decreased capacity to sustain pregnancy to delivery of viable infant	Uncommon (except with childhood onset)

report of the association between diabetes and erectile dysfunction was in 1797 (Wabrek, 1979). While studies vary, it is generally recognized that the prevalence of erectile dysfunction among diabetic males is 30 to 60 per cent (Wabrek, 1979; Ellenberg, 1979; Tattersall, 1982).

The direct effect of decreased insulin secretion and the indirect effect of hyperglycemia do not appear to be of major importance as causes for excitement phase disorders in males with diabetes. Specifically, high blood sugar levels or the lack of glucose control do not affect erectile capacity, except perhaps at onset of the illness (Wagner and Green, 1981). While it is recognized that the presenting symptom of diabetes in some men may be erectile dysfunction, these men "have usually not been evaluated for vascular and neurological abnormalities, which may occur rapidly in some patients" (Wagner and Green, 1981, p 53). Men who have impaired insulin function have not been found to have changes in testosterone, prolactin, gonadotropins, or estrogen secretion at a rate different from the general population (Jensen et al, 1979). These hormonal states are usually not responsible for erectile dysfunction in diabetes. Based on his review of the literature, Podolsky states that "there is no evidence that deficiency of testosterone is other than a rare cause of impotence in diabetic men" (Podolsky, 1982, p 1391).

Wagner and Green (1981) describe changes in the autonomic nervous system that can be demonstrated in the majority of diabetics after 10 to 15 years of the illness. First, repeated studies (Ellenberg, 1971, 1978; Jensen, 1981; Karacan et al, 1978) have shown that peripheral neuropathy is correlated significantly with erectile dysfunction. Less is known about the effect of defects in the sympathetic nervous system on penile function of insulin-dependent males. Second, Kaplan (1983) describes laboratory studies showing a reduction in norepinephrine content in erectile tissue of men with erectile dysfunction and diabetes. Third, both Kaplan (1983) and Wagner and Green (1981) conclude that there may be a yet undescribed relationship between a defect in the sympathetic nervous system and penile dysfunction in insulin-dependent males.

It is difficult to separate vascular factors from neurological factors in diabetes (Renshaw, 1979). This is particularly true in relation to sexual function. From a vascular perspective, diabetes causes both macro- and microangiopathy that impairs circulation in the genital area. It is suspected that decreased blood flow to the genitals may interfere with ability to attain an erection, while neuropathy and/or microlesions in the veins may cause inability to maintain engorgement once erection occurs. Erectile dysfunction associated with neurovascular impairment often develops gradually over time and is usually progressive. This differs from erectile dysfunction of a psychogenic basis, which usually has a sudden onset and may be specific to a partner or place.

Much less is known about the frequency of all types of orgasmic phase disturbances in the diabetic male than about excitement phase disturbances. In a study of age-matched groups, both diabetic and nondiabetic men noted about the same frequency of ejaculatory problems (Jensen, 1981). Premature ejaculation and retarded ejaculation are usually psychological problems for either diabetic or nondiabetic males; they have not been reported to be directly caused by diabetes (Podolsky, 1982b). Retrograde ejaculation occurs in some diabetic men, although its exact incidence is not known (Wabrek, 1979). It is thought to be a result of pelvic autonomic neuropathy that inhibits the reflex closure of the sphincter of the bladder neck after emission and prior to expulsion of semen. Rather than being propelled through the urethra to the meatus, semen flows through the relaxed sphincter into the bladder. The male feels as though he has ejaculated but notes no semen to confirm this, experiencing a "dry ejaculation." The condition is usually not associated with erectile dysfunction. Its effect is to produce infertility, which may or may not be of concern to the man.

Diabetic Females

The incidence of decreased vaginal lubrication among women with diabetes is not well documented. In one study (Jensen, 1981) significantly more diabetic women (19 of 80) reported reduced vaginal lubrication than did nondiabetic women (3 of 40) in a matched sample. In another smaller study, no significant differences in vaginal lubrication, genital swelling, or use of exogenous lubricants existed between diabetic women with peripheral neuropathy and diabetic women without neuropathy (Brown, 1983). Diabetic women do report a higher rate of dryness and pain during intercourse and masturbation than do nondiabetic women; this dryness seems to be associated with duration of the illness and with neuropathy (Whitley and Berke, 1983). Rostalpil and Zrustova (1978) reported the observation of degenerative changes in nerve fibers of autopsied clitoral tissue in diabetic women but not in a control group. The significance of these findings awaits further investigation.

The paucity of studies on women in relation to diabetic control and vaginal lubrication hampers our understanding of this relationship. It is likely, however, that since hyperglycemia is often associated with vaginal infections and reduction in vaginal moisture, women may be more at risk than men in developing excitement phase disorders when diabetes is out of control.

It is difficult to understand why women with diabetes who have impairment of neurovascular function do not report excitement phase disorders similar to those experienced by men. It has been suggested that since the female excitement phase is not as dependent on complex vasocongestive changes as the male excitement phase, the female excitement phase is less affected than the male excitement phase by illness and drugs (Kaplan, 1983, citing Kolodny, 1971). Jensen explained this phenomenon by noting that disruptions in the excitement phase in men can be demonstrated both visibly and functionally. A similar physiological disruption in the female "might present either no or an easily handled problem in sexual functioning of the female" (Jensen, 1981, p 502). This comment parallels observations of women in general; that is, while it is necessary for males to maintain erections in order to have vaginal intercourse, it is not necessary for females to swell or to lubricate in order to have vaginal intercourse.

Kolodny (1971) reported that 35.2 per cent of hospitalized diabetic women noted a complete absence of orgasm compared with 6 per cent of hospitalized nondiabetic women from an age-matched group with other illnesses and concern about absence of orgasm. Ellenberg (1979), on the other hand, found no significant differences between diabetic and nondiabetic women in terms of orgasmic function. Interestingly, a third study found that orgasm with a partner and orgasm with masturbation were both unaffected by peripheral neuropathy (Brown, 1983). Whereas male sexual dysfunctions in diabetes are primarily a result of neurovascular deficits related to the excitement phase, female sexual dysfunctions in diabetes are primarily a result of an elevated stimulatory threshold before the orgasm phase that "necessitates more time and a higher level of stimulus to trigger the orgasmic reflex" (Unsain and Goodwin, 1982, p 389).

Reproductive Capacity and Physiological Characteristics

Biological factors influencing reproductive capacity in persons with diabetes include (1) relative infertility/sterility in both males and females and (2) ability to sustain a pregnancy to successful delivery of a viable infant.

Fertility in diabetic men is somewhat less than that in the general male population. Male infertility has been associated with a high incidence of abnormal sperm production and retrograde ejaculation causing a "dry" ejaculate. In the latter instance, successful artificial insemination with the male's own sperm has been achieved by collection of a fertile ejaculate after masturbation with a full bladder (Templeton and Mortimer, 1982).

Until recently, many diabetic women were discouraged from conceiving because of concerns for maternal and fetal health. With the advent of more precise technology to control diabetes, such as self-monitoring of blood-glucose levels, and continuous insulin infusions, many women with diabetes are now experiencing healthy pregnancies and delivering healthy infants (Hinnen and Hume, 1982). The decision to conceive should be made carefully and with input from the woman, her partner, and her health professionals.

Biological alterations in physical appearance secondary to diabetes are uncommon. The most notable exception to this statement is the short stature that may accompany juvenile onset of diabetes. Thickened skin and callus formation may be a problem for some diabetics, as can lipodystrophy, especially at injection sites. Acquired alterations in appearance resulting from treatment (e.g., insulin pumps) or interventions (e.g., implanted penile prostheses) are a part of the stimuli to which diabetics may be adapting.

In summary, neither males nor females with diabetes are likely to experience alterations in sexual desire at any greater rate than the general population. Diabetic males who are older are most prone to experience erectile dysfunction that is progressive and associated with neurovascular changes secondary to the illness. Diabetic females may experience varying rates of vaginal dryness associated with diabetes; this may be an organic problem associated with neurovascular changes. Though rare in comparison to erectile problems, retrograde ejaculation occurs in some diabetic males. Orgasm problems in diabetic women are not well understood but probably are of concern to many diabetic women. Reproductive capacity can be altered in both males and females with diabetes but recently has improved through better control of the diabetes. Overt alterations in physiological characteristics are not a problem for most persons with diabetes.

EFFECTS OF ENDOCRINE SYSTEM DISTURBANCES AND PSYCHOSOCIAL ADAPTATION

Hormonal disturbances are frequently associated with, and are sometimes the cause of, a number of psychiatric and behavioral alterations, which can be summarized as follows: (1) organic brain syndromes with behaviors of confusion, delirium, and dementia; (2) psychosis with behaviors of disturbed thought content, ineffective cognitive processes, and perceptual aberrations, (3) depression, both transient and prolonged; (4) mania with inappropriately elevated self-esteem and hyperactivity; (5) anxiety with apprehensiveness, irritability, and impatience; (6) personality changes with social withdrawal and self-destruction; (7) specific sexual dysfunctions; and (8) hysteria with somatization and conversion reaction (Leigh and Kramer, 1984).

All of the preceding psychosocial alterations may be either global or specific. Leigh and Kramer caution that

it is important to remember that cognitive, affective and behavioral disorders may be the first sign, the only sign, or a concomitant sign of endocrine disease . . . Specific sexual complaints

may be part of a depressive syndrome or an isolated symptom. Diminished desire and impaired arousal can occur owing to CNS depression, general debility, androgen deficiency in either sex, or an affective disorder—all due to endocrinopathy. (Leigh and Kramer, 1984, pp 414, 438)

The role of psychological factors in sexual behavior should not be underestimated even in the presence of endocrine abnormalities. Even when endocrine treatment *does* restore the capacity for an effective sexual behavior, continuing intrapsychic or interpersonal problems can prevent a person from acting on that capacity. For example, a man who has low sexual desire as a result of hyperprolactinemia may have his desire restored by appropriate therapeutic treatment, but he may have continuing marital stresses that prevent him from acting on his desire (Bancroft, 1984).

While it would be possible to describe the alterations in sexual behavior in each endocrine disorder, many disorders have common alterations. The present discussion will address psychosocial sexual behaviors subject to alteration in diabetes as a prototype for other endocrine disorders. Implications for other endocrine diseases are similar to those in diabetes.

Self-Concept

Individuals have a need for psychic integrity that allows them to know who they are and to have a sense of wholeness (Roy, 1984). Self-concept is concerned with the question, "Who am I?" It contains two major subareas: physical self and personal self. Self-concept is mediated by learning and by growth and development. Behaviors in the self-concept mode are observed through a person's verbalization of thoughts and feelings as well as through a person's actions.

Sexual adaptation in diabetes in the self-concept mode is observed in behaviors and disclosure of the following phenomena:

1. Having confidence in one's ability to function sexually, e.g., "I'm able to get wet most of the time."

2. Acknowledging that the presence of early morning erections shows the capacity for erections to occur in an erotic situation, e.g., "Since I often wake up with an erection the plumbing must still be working."

3. Having appropriate knowledge about the limitations that may result from sexual dysfunction, e.g., "I know that some men (women) have problems with sex, and I may expect to at some point, but so far so good."

4. Seeing oneself as sexual despite alterations in genital sexual responses, e.g., "I hardly ever reach climax anymore but I'm still a sexy lady."

5. Seeking information about ways to adapt to sexual limitations, e.g., "Now that I know that my problem is physical, what can be done?"

6. Being able to become erect or moist in response to erotic stimuli if organic function is intact, e.g., "I really get turned on when I see my partner naked."

7. Having appropriate level of self-esteem and sense of manhood or womanhood, e.g., "I'm every bit the woman (man) now that I was before I got diabetes and started having these problems."

8. Seeing oneself as well rather than ill or sick, e.g., "Even though I have diabetes I am able to do just about anything I could before. I don't think of myself as being sick."

9. Feeling hopeful about either a transient or chronic dysfunction, e.g., "I feel hopeful that when I have the penile implant put in I will have full erections again."

10. Using mechanical aids to enhance sexual responsiveness, e.g., "I've found that using a vibrator gives me more intense stimulus so I can go ahead and reach orgasm."

Ineffective sexual adaptation in diabetes in the self-concept mode may be exemplified by the following:

1. Having little confidence in one's ability to function sexually, e.g., "My penis is dead. I'm no good as a lover anymore."

2. Continuing to believe that erectile dysfunction is organic despite normal erectile capacity during sleep, e.g., "I don't care how many erections I have at night, there's something physically wrong with me."

3. Inappropriately generalizing about the limits on one's sexuality as a result of dysfunction in one phase of genital response, e.g., "Since I don't get hard anymore I guess I won't be able to come, either, before long."

4. Equating loss of genital response to being asexual, e.g., "I'm washed up as far as sex goes."

5. Constantly spectatoring about one's responses, e.g., "I can't relax because I'm so concerned about whether my penis will get hard."

6. Feeling guilty about dysfunction by associating it with earlier sexual practices such as masturbation, e.g., "I feel so ashamed. I know the reason I'm impotent is because I used to play with myself when I was a teenager."

7. Having no hope for improvement, e.g., "I just quit hoping when I was told nothing could be done."

8. Deliberately controlling one's responsiveness to erotic stimuli because of false beliefs about dysfunction, e.g., "I just quit putting myself in situations because I knew it wouldn't work."

9. Avoiding any activity that might enhance erection or orgasm because of feelings of guilt or immorality, e.g., "I'm a Christian, and only a pervert would use something like a vibrator."

Many ineffective sexual adaptations in the self-concept mode share common themes of loss. A person's perception of sexual loss may seem out of perspective to the health care provider, in comparison to the physical losses associated with diabetes. For example, "loss of erectile function is more threatening to many diabetic men than blindness or loss of lower extremity due to gangrene" (Podolsky, 1982a). In addition, the person experiencing the sexual dysfunction may value a restoration of the function above all other costs, e.g., "I wouldn't do without (my penile prosthesis) for $100,000 as broke as I am today" (Manley, 1981c, p 26).

Role Function

Whether one is healthy or ill, one has a role. The basic assumptions underlying role function are that roles exist only in relationship to others and that roles are filled by individuals. Underlying the role function mode is the need for social integrity. Role function is concerned with the question, "Who am I in relation to others?" There are three subareas under role function: primary, secondary, and tertiary. Primary role function consists of demographic data and developmental stage, for example, age, marital status, and gender. Secondary role function includes the behaviors associated with accomplishing the goals of the primary function, for example, wife, mother, lover, employee, or, in the case of a chronic illness, for example, being diabetic. Tertiary roles are temporary and usually chosen by the person, such as a social date, a member of a club, or a speaker at a program.

Sexual adaptation to diabetes in the role function mode can be observed in the following behaviors:

1. Acknowledging that some sexual functions decline with age in all persons and are not a function of diabetes, e.g., "I don't have the desire that an 18 year old has, but I still get horny once or twice a week."

2. Seeking information relative to the best methods for contraception, e.g., "At this point in my life, and with having diabetes for such a short time, I don't feel I'm ready to take on being a parent."

3. Maintaining active involvement in the role of lover or partner despite alterations in sexual function, e.g., "Even though I can't always get an erection I still want to make love to my partner."

4. Conserving energy so that one can have an active sex life, e.g., "I know that if I'm too tired I just can't make it, so I try not to let this happen."

5. Obtaining genetic counseling regarding the chances of producing an afflicted child, e.g., "I understand that there is some risk that I could pass on diabetes to my children, so I need some help in deciding how much of a risk this is for me."

6. Talking openly with health care professionals about questions of sexuality, e.g., "I don't wait for my doctor to bring up the subject. I just go ahead and ask her every time I see her."

7. Seeking opportunities to share experiences with others who have similar sexual limitations, e.g., "I volunteer to talk to anyone who is in the same boat because I know how hard it was for me to find somebody else who understood."

8. Giving oneself permission to act on sexual feelings, e.g., "There's no reason why having diabetes should mean I can't make love."

9. Engaging in an active dating relationship, e.g., "Even though I have diabetes I can still date and do almost everything my friends are doing."

Ineffective sexual adaptation in the role function mode may include the following:

1. Allowing "performance anxiety" to overshadow one's capacity to function if such capacity is organically intact, e.g., "I get so worried about not being able to get hard (get wet) that I just don't put myself in that situation."

2. Using intellectual defenses to prevent engaging in roles of lover or spouse, e.g., "Over half of all men with diabetes are impotent so I know that I am too."

3. Generalizing about genetic capacity to transmit diabetes to offspring to the extent of becoming impotent, e.g., "I don't want my child to have to suffer the way I have so I just won't allow myself to have erections."

4. Failing to talk with health care professionals about sexual function, e.g., "I just don't want to talk about it—it's too embarrassing."

5. Assuming that because one is past the developmental stage of procreation one should be asexual, e.g., "Since I'm 52 years old and I've raised my children, I don't need sex anymore, and anyway it wouldn't be good for me."

6. Feeling compulsive about finding the "fountain of youth," e.g., "If I can just get some of those shots I know I'll be as good as I was at 21."

7. Changing jobs, housing, or economic status as an attempt to make oneself more attractive to a partner, e.g., "Now that I'm defective because I have diabetes I'll just have to work harder and make more money so my wife will want me."

Interdependence

Behaviors in this mode, as with those in role function, involve interactions with others. Unlike in the role function mode, the underlying need in this mode is for affectional integrity which a person experiences through love, value, and respect. Functioning in this mode is particularly vulnerable to the effects of illness, whether chronic or acute. For example, a client may be unable to give nurturance but may seek more nurturance to the point that the balance in the relationship becomes dysfunctional. On the other hand, clients may try to overcompensate for being ill or having an organically mediated sexual dysfunction by increasing their nurturance of the partner to a dysfunctional level as a way of meeting their own nurturance needs.

Sexual adaptation by persons with diabetes in the interdependence mode includes the following:

1. Receiving and giving sexual satisfaction as defined by the couple, whether with intercourse or through noncoital behaviors, e.g.,

"We don't always depend on intercourse to satisfy us. There are lots of other options for us."

2. Being aware of a partner's likes and dislikes regarding sexual behavior, e.g., "I don't like for him to try to stimulate me by kissing my nipples, but I do like long foreplay to help me get aroused and reach climax." "I really need her to physically stimulate my penis with oral sex to help me get erect, but I know she doesn't like to do this."

3. Being able to establish intimacy, mutuality, and long-term commitment in a relationship despite organic sexual dysfunction, e.g., "My love for him goes far beyond his ability to have an erection. We've been together a long time and if it were just based on his sexual performance I wouldn't still be here."

4. Acceptance by the partner of the need for and the effects of having a penile prosthesis, e.g., "I know it's very important for him to have erections to feel good about himself, so I'm supportive of his decision."

5. Having a history of resolving conflicts within the relationship so that sexual dysfunctions do not represent crises that are unsurmountable, e.g., "We've been through a lot together over the years since she's had diabetes, and I know we'll get through this, too."

Ineffective sexual responses in the interdependence mode include the following:

1. Excessive need to please the partner sexually (Schiavi and Hogan, 1979), e.g., "I have to work extra hard to make it good for her or she will leave me."

2. Partner's excessive demands for sexual performance (Schiavi and Hogan, 1979), e.g., "If he can't have an erection, I just don't want to try."

3. Unwillingness to explore noncoital methods for sexual fulfillment (Shiavi and Hogan, 1979), e.g., "Intercourse is the right way to make love. I would never use a vibrator."

4. Dysfunctional relationships that are fueled by sexual dysfunction (Shiavi and Hogan, 1979), e.g., "We've never gotten along very well, and this just makes it worse."

5. Use and abuse of diabetes in the marital power balance (Shiavi and Hogan, 1979), e.g., "You can't expect me to be interested in sex when I'm always worrying about my blood sugar."

6. Blaming the other partner for the dysfunction or blaming oneself for the partner's

problem (Tattersall, 1982; Manley, 1981), e.g., "For a long time he blamed me, and I guess I thought I was to blame because I wasn't responding like he thought I should."

7. Marital separation or divorce as a result of the dysfunction (Block, 1982), e.g., "First we just started sleeping in separate bedrooms, and now he has moved out and we're seeing a lawyer."

8. Fearing that the partner is gay or lesbian or that the partner is having an extramarital affair (Block, 1982), e.g., "I worried that she was a lesbian or was seeing someone else, since I'm no good to her. I couldn't really blame her if she did."

9. Fearing that the diabetic partner will die if the couple makes love (Manley, 1981c; Renshaw, 1979), e.g., "I just worry about him all the time—am afraid I'll walk in and he'll be dead. I don't want to make matters worse by having sex."

10. Feigning low interest in sex as a way of concealing a dysfunction (Krosnick and Podolsky, 1981; Manley, 1981c; Tattersall, 1982), e.g., "I didn't want him to know how much of a problem it was for me when I don't get wet, so I just pretend like I'm never interested."

11. Ignorance of the partner's and the person's needs, both for sexual pleasure and for noncoital physical and emotional closeness (Renshaw, 1979), e.g., "I could live for a long time without having intercourse if he would just hold me and caress me like he used to, but he's just quit doing all those things now."

12. Fear that diabetes will be transmitted to the partner by sex (Renshaw, 1979), e.g., "I just can't have sex with him because that old sugar stuff will come out of his penis."

13. Fear that when the partner initiates sex, and when intercourse is not possible for the other, refusal would represent rejection or lack of love (Pieper, 1982; Shiavi and Hogan, 1979; Manley, 1981c), e.g., "If I'm no good to her as a man, she won't love me anymore."

14. Ignoring the partner's dislikes about specific sexual activities as a way of trying to compensate for sexual dysfunctions (Schiavi and Hogan, 1979), e.g., "I'm really turned off by oral sex, but he thinks this will make it better for me so he insists on doing it."

In general, it has been found that there is no correlation between the onset of a sexual problem with diabetes and the duration of the sexual relationship (Jensen, 1981). In addition, one cannot generalize the effects of a sexual dysfunction in diabetes to the relationship with a partner (Pieper, 1982). If one's self-concept or role function is stressed by diabetes, one's usual adaptive patterns are taxed. For those who adapt to such stress (i.e., through an intrapsychic mechanism of acceptance or redefining their situation or turning to others for support) marked negative affect may not be experienced. However, for those who do not adapt to the sexual limitations that may occur in their chronic illness, heightened negative affect (e.g., anxiety or depression) may be observed.

An individual's or couple's sexual behavior is shaped by the biological, psychological, spiritual, and social stimuli that influence sexuality. While "sociocultural factors such as social-class level and educational background affect sexual behaviors" (Roy, 1984, p 331), no correlation has been found between onset or severity of sexual dysfunction in persons with diabetes and profession, economy, housing, or social status (Jensen, 1981). In other words, sexually ineffective responses in diabetes cut across all strata; one would not necessarily expect certain groups of persons with diabetes to have more or less concern than others.

It has been noted that "a high level of self-esteem is necessary for a good sexual relationship, since the person needs to be comfortable seeking pleasure and asking another to help satisfy one's sexual needs" (Roy, 1984, p 331). Judgments about the effectiveness or ineffectiveness of sexual behaviors associated with diabetes are, therefore, most likely to reflect the person's level of self-concept.

NURSING PROCESS AND SEXUAL PROBLEMS OF PERSONS WITH DIABETES

The general goals for nursing intervention are to identify and reinforce adaptive behaviors and to change ineffective responses to adaptive responses. These goals may be met by first identifying with the person or couple those behaviors that are of concern and then by mutually setting specific goals.

First level assessment of sexual concerns consists of evaluating each of the four adaptive modes. Second level assessment consists of determining the focal, contextual, and

residual stimuli contributing to each behavior. The agreed-upon goal is stated in terms of the anticipated behavioral outcome. The nurse then identifies approaches that are expected to accomplish the goal. These approaches relate to removing, increasing, decreasing, or altering the focal, contextual, and residual stimuli to foster adaptation. After intervention, the adaptive or nursing behavioral goals are then evaluated, and nursing approaches are modified as necessary (Roy, 1984).

Assessment: First Level

Depending on the nurse's role and stage of professional development, the nurse may be involved in actually performing the physical assessment or may use data collected by others to assess the degree of adaptation in the physiological mode. The sexual health history is the best tool to use for assessing responses in all four modes, since the nurse can assess for cognitive, affective, and conative adaptation during the interview (Manley, 1981b). History taking should, if at all possible, involve both partners.

If a "problem of decreased sexual self-concept is identified, the goal is focused on the promotion of the person's sexual self-identity by increasing feelings of worth and value. A long-term goal is aimed at restoring the person's usual sexual role activities" (Roy, 1984, p 333) by helping the person reach the level of sexual health he or she chooses.

Assessment: Second Level

Once behaviors are identified and categorized by the nurse and the client or couple as adaptive or ineffective, the stimuli influencing them are assessed, and both short- and long-term goals are mutually agreed upon. If, for example, the dysfunction is organic, various options may be explored to relieve the accompanying distress. In sexual dysfunctions of diabetes, options may involve seeking further evaluation for potentially correctable problems (such as penile blood flow studies) or exploring options for surgical implantation of a penile prosthesis, if genital sexuality is essential to the relationship (Schiavi and Hogan, 1979). The long-term goal is for the partners or the individual to experience sexual pleasure consistent with their values and desires and with their physiological capacity.

If the partners are willing to consider alternatives (such as alternate sexual patterns or use of mechanical aids), these can be explored through open communication. Education and anticipatory guidance may be used to help the couple acknowledge and accept sexual limitations (e.g., organic dysfunctions that cannot be improved). In addition, exploration of attitudes and beliefs that are negatively influencing the outcome, for example, a belief that an individual with diabetes is not a sexual person, can be discussed and perhaps minimized (Schiavi and Hogan, 1979).

A nurse may encounter sexual problems of diabetes mellitus in many locations, including with hospitalized persons and in ambulatory settings. The nurse's role may be primary as well as transient or long-term. The nurse may be a generalist or a specialist and may be expected to interact not only with the person and partner but also with various other members of the health care team. The nurse needs to have a basis of sexual self-acceptance in order to be nonjudgmental and also needs to have basic knowledge about the relationships among the biopsychosocial modes, as the behaviors of each affect diabetes. Using this framework for the nursing process, the nurse may then intervene to promote the sexual integrity of the person or partnership.

CONCLUSIONS

In summary, endocrine disturbances can be associated with many sexual dysfunctions. Sexual desire is often altered by changes in emotional status and less commonly by changes in testosterone, by thyroid disease and, by hyperprolactinemia. Erectile dysfunction often occurs in endocrine disease through neurological and vascular changes and by secondary testosterone disruptions. Vaginal dryness can result from estrogen deficit. Premature ejaculation is not directly mediated by endocrine problems. Inhibited orgasm sometimes results from thyroid disease and less commonly from decreased testosterone. Retrograde ejaculation occurs, although rarely, in diabetes. Reproductive capacity is directly affected by hormonal disturbances, especially pituitary-gonadal function. Physical characteristics leading to altered body image and role performance are frequently the result of hormonal influences. Psychosocial behavior may be altered directly by endocrine disease or may be a secondary adaptation to the effect of the endocrine disease on the person's self-concept, role performance, or interdependence needs.

CASE STUDY

The following case study is used as a student learning activity. It is a typical situation of erectile dysfunction occurring secondary to diabetes mellitus. For a different case study, see the article by Manley (1986).

Mr. DRC is a 50-year-old man who has been known to have diabetes since age 30. He was noninsulin dependent for the first year and has been insulin dependent subsequently. He did well for the first 15 years. He then experienced diabetic ketoacidosis following an episode of gastrointestinal flu and was hospitalized at a local hospital at that time but recovered well. Approximately 3 years ago, he began to note a change in his insulin reactions that began to occur more often and without warning. When first seen, he was taking 25 units NPH insulin in the morning and 5 units of regular insulin in the evening.

His past history is significant for a hemorrhoidectomy and a hernia repair 3 years ago, a laminectomy several years prior to that, and an exploration of the parathyroid glands 10 years ago. He also had experienced prostatitis, which resolved after he took medication. Additional risk factors included one pack of cigarettes daily throughout his adult life. He uses no alcohol. The family history is significant for chemical diabetes in his mother. His social history includes having been married for 25 years. He is a ranger for the forestry department and is quite active in that work.

He has noted progressive erectile dysfunction for the past 5 to 6 years with no nocturnal or early morning erections. Physical examination showed him to be 6 feet tall and an ideal body weight of 150 pounds. Visual acuity is 20/20 in both eyes uncorrected. Blood pressure is 106/70. He was thin, wiry, and muscular. Examination of the eyes showed bilateral dot and blot hemorrhages, Class III. There were scattered exudates and AV nicking. The rest of the head, eyes, ears, nose, and throat examination was normal. The thyroid was not enlarged; the lungs were clear. Heart sounds S_1 and S_2 were clear, without murmur. The abdomen was soft; the liver was not palpable. There was a well-healed scar in each inguinal area. The femoral pulses were full. Neurological examination showed hyporeflexia except for the right triceps and biceps, which showed 2+ deep tendon reflex. There were absent knee and ankle jerks. The grasp was equal in both hands. Genital examination showed that he is uncircumcised. There were no testicular masses and no hernia. There were no rectal masses.

He was briefly hospitalized at the onset of care for evaluation of Somogyi reactions. His insulin dosage was adjusted accordingly. He was also monitored with the nocturnal penile tumescence monitor (NPTM) for three nights and showed no evidence of nocturnal tumescence.

After a consultation with the urologist and with the patient and his wife, he was advised to proceed with insertion of an inflatable prosthetic implant, a procedure that he underwent without difficulty and had an uneventful postoperative recovery. He has subsequently done well. He has had no problems with the penile prosthesis, and both he and his wife have been satisfied with it, as evidenced by the following condensation of an interview conducted 18 months after the surgery.*

Husband: We started having sex problems about 7 or 8 years ago. Couldn't keep an erection. This is one of the things that individuals don't want to talk about. You don't want to admit that you have anything wrong . . . to [your] wife . . . to the doctor. [It] was very frustrating to Lois. It was working on her as much or more as it was on me . . . which was bad on me. I would tell by the way she was acting. She wasn't Lois.

Wife: And another thing, when you started you didn't want to admit it to yourself. A man blames a woman at first. [He] blamed me that I didn't respond as he thought I should. I

*Reprinted with permission of The American Association of Diabetes Educators from "Interview with a Couple Who Has Experienced Sexual Dysfunction Secondary to Diabetes Mellitus" by Mary Virginia Manley, RN, MSN, CANP, in *The Diabetes Educator* 7:24–26, 1981.

finally felt it was better to just forget the whole deal. I was afraid I really wasn't responding as I should and he'd want to try anyway, and of course it wouldn't work, then he would get frustrated and that would upset me, and I would get frustrated, too.

Husband: It just goes from bad to worse. Without some knowledgeable person to talk to, someone that knows what you're talking about, it is really frustrating. [It's] not something you . . . talk to your best friend about. And sometimes it's hard to talk to somebody that's not your best friend.

Wife: I think doctors should explain to their male patients at the onset what might happen, and [that men who become impotent] can do something. Then [the impotence] would cause a lot fewer problems.

Husband: [When] I decided to have surgery . . . [the doctor] explained everything, how it worked, what he had to do, the mechanics of it, and I in turn went and told Lois. I didn't know exactly how to explain it to her. I think [the man and woman] need to be conferred with together, as a family, not as an individual, because after all, they're both in the same boat. There was a lot of physical discomfort the first week after surgery. It's kind of rough for about 3 weeks. When I first went home I had some swelling . . . but anyway, soon it was fine.

Wife: I guess I was afraid, even after he had his surgery, that I was going to get sexually aroused [only to be disappointed by having the same old problems] . . . and it took me a while to get over that fear. I haven't worked everything out yet, but I'm getting over it. [Author's note: Lois also reported that the implant is not painful to her and that she now achieves the same level of sexual gratification she experienced years ago.]

Husband [after being asked how he feels now]: When you're in the Sahara Desert for 10 years and then can come out and get a drink, how would you feel? There's a period of adjustment first because it's new and you don't know exactly what to expect.

Wife: [And] if the couple had too many problems between them, after the surgery it still takes time to [solve them].

Husband: [Before the surgery,] we were trying everything in the book. The hell of it is we didn't have a book—we were having to make our own book. If there's some way to get the patients and the doctors talking to each other instead of about each other, that would be one of the greatest things.

REFERENCES

Bancroft J: Hormones and human sexual behavior. J Sex Mar Ther 10:3–21, 1984.

Bancroft J, Davidson DW, Warner P, Tyrer G: Androgens and sexual behavior in women using oral contraceptives. Clin Endocrinol 12:327–340, 1980.

Block AM: Sexual dysfunction of the male with diabetes mellitus. Nurse Pract (Suppl) 7:19, 24–25, 1982.

Braunstein GD: Endocrine causes of impotence. Postgrad Med 74:207–211, 1983.

Brown ME: Factors Related to Sexual Functioning in Female Diabetics: A Preliminary Pilot Study. Thesis. Vanderbilt University School of Nursing, 1983.

Cassileth BR, Lusk EJ, Strouse TB, et al: Psychosocial status in chronic illness. A comparative analysis of six diagnostic groups. N Engl J Med 311:506–511, 1984.

Cooper AJ: Advances in the diagnosis and management of endocrine impotence. Practitioner 228:865–870, 1984.

Dow MGT, Hart DM, Forrest CA: Hormonal treatments of sexual unresponsiveness in postmenopausal women: A comparitive study. Br J Obstet Gynaecol 90:361–366, 1983.

Ellenberg M: Impotence in diabetes: The neurologic factor. Ann Int Med 75:213–216, 1971.

Ellenberg M: Sexual aspects of the female diabetic. Mt. Sinai J Med 44:495–500, 1977.

Ellenberg M: Impotence in diabetes: The neurologic factor. In LoPiccolo J, LoPiccolo L (eds): Handbook of Sex Therapy. New York, Plenum Press, 1978.

Ellenberg M: Sex and diabetes: A comparison between men and women. Diabetes Care 2:4–8, 1979.

Frazer J: The dilemma of the perimenopausal female: A sexual/physical health issue. Holistic Nurs Pract 1:67–75, 1987.

Furlow WL: Diagnosis and treatment of male erectile failure. Diabetes Care 2:18–25, 1979.

Goleman D: Chemistry of sexual desire yields its elusive secrets. New York Times Oct 18, 1988, sec C, p 1.

Hinnen DW, Hume JW: Pregnancy. In Guthrie DW, Guthrie RA (eds): Nursing Management of Diabetes Mellitus. 2nd ed. St. Louis, CV Mosby, 1982.

Hogan R: Human Sexuality. Norwalk, Appleton-Century-Crofts, 1980.

Hufnagel V: No more menopause. Monograph, 1987.

Jensen SB: Diabetic sexual dysfunction: A comparative study of 160 insulin treated diabetic men and women and an age-matched control group. Arch Sex Behav 10:493–504, 1981.

Jensen SB et al: Sexual function and pituitary axis in insulin treated diabetic men. Acta Med Scand (Suppl) 624:65–68, 1979.

Kaplan HS: The Evaluation of Sexual Disorders. New York, Bruner/Mazel, 1983.

Karacan I et al: Nocturnal penile tumescence and diagnosis in diabetic impotence. Am J Psychol 135:191–196, 1978.

Kolodny R: Sexual dysfunction in diabetic females. Diabetes 20:557–559, 1971.

Kolodny RC, Masters WH, Johnson VE: Textbook of Human Sexuality for Nurses. Boston, Little, Brown & Co, 1979.

Krosnick A, Podolsky S: Diabetes and sexual dysfunction: Restoring normal ability. Geriatrics 36:92–95, 99–100, 1981.

Leigh H, Kramer SI: The psychiatric manifestations of endocrine disease. Adv Int Med 29:413–443, 1984.

Manley MV: Erectile dysfunction in the man with diabetes. Diabetes Educ 7:19–22, 1981a.

Manley MV: Taking a sexual history. Diabetes Educ 7:22–24, 1981b.

Manley MV: Interview with a couple who have experienced sexual dysfunction secondary to diabetes mellitus. Diabetes Educ 7:24–26, 1981c.

Manley MV: Diabetes and sexual health. Diabetes Educ 12:366–369, 1986.

Masters WH, Johnson VE: Human Sexual Response. Boston, Little, Brown & Co, 1966.

Matthews A, Whitehead A, Kellett J: Psychological and hormonal factors in the treatment of female sexual dysfunction. Psychol Med 13:83–93, 1983.

Nickel JC et al: Endocrine dysfunction in impotence: Incidence, significance and cost-effective screening. J Urol 132:40–43, 1984.

Notelovitz M: Gynecologic problems of menopausal women: Part 3. Changes in extragenital tissues and sexuality. Geriatrics 33:51–53, 57–58, 1978.

O'Carroll R, Bancroft J: Testosterone therapy for low sexual interest and erectile dysfunction in men: A controlled study. Br J Psychol 145:146–151, 1984.

Pieper B: Women's perceived effect of diabetes mellitus on sexual function and relationship to spouse. J Sex Ed Ther 8:18–21, 1982.

Pieper B, Clarke PN, Caldwell MH, et al: Perceived effect of diabetes on relationship to spouse and sexual function. J Sex Ed Ther 9:46–50, 1983.

Pirke KM et al: Pituitary gonadal system function in patients with erectile impotence and premature ejaculation. Arch Sex Behav 8:41–47, 1979.

Podolsky S: Sexual dysfunction in diabetic men. Pract Diabetol 1:1, 4–5, 1982a.

Podolsky S: Diagnosis and treatment of sexual dysfunction in the male diabetic. Med Clin North Am 66:1389–1395, 1982b.

Pont A et al: Prolactin-secreting tumors in men: Surgical cure. Ann Int Med 91:211–213, 1979.

Randell B, Tedrow MP, Van Landingham J: Adaptation Nursing: The Roy Conceptual Model Applied. St. Louis, CV Mosby, 1982.

Renshaw DC: Diabetic impotence: A need for further evaluation. Med Asp Hum Sex April:19, 22, 25, 1978.

Renshaw DC: Sexual function and diabetes. Psychosom 20:54, 1979.

Rostalpil J, Zrustova M: Etiology of female sex disorders revealed. Diabetes Outlook 13, 1978.

Roy C: Introduction to Nursing: An Adaptation Model. 2nd ed. Englewood Cliffs, Prentice Hall, 1984.

Rubin A, Babbott D: Impotence and diabetes mellitus. JAMA 168:498–500, 1958.

Sarrel P: Sex and menopause. Paper presented at AASECT 21st Annual Meeting, San Francisco, April 1988.

Schiavi RC, Hogan B: Sexual problems in diabetes mellitus: Psychological aspects. Diabetes Care 2:9–17, 1979.

Schwartz MF, Kolodny RC, Masters WH: Plasma testosterone levels of sexually functional and dysfunctional men. Arch Sex Behav 9:355–364, 1980.

Segraves RT, Schoenberg HW, Ivanoff J: Serum testosterone and prolactin levels in eretile dysfunction. J Sex Marital Ther 9:19–26, 1983.

Sotile WM: The penile prosthesis and diabetic impotence: Some caveats. Diabetes Care 2:26, 1979.

Tattersall R: Sexual problems of diabetic men. Br Med J 285:911, 1982.

Templeton A, Mortimer D: Successful circumvention of retrograde ejaculation in an infertile diabetic man. Case report. Br J Obstet Gynaecol 89:1064–1065, 1982.

The sexually dysfunctional diabetic. Sex Med Today 3:8, 1979.

Unsain IC, Goodwin MH: Effects on sexual function. In Guthrie DW, Guthrie RA (eds): Nursing Management of Diabetes Mellitus. 2nd ed. St. Louis, CV Mosby, 1982.

Unsain IC, Goodwin MH, Schuster EA: Diabetes and sexual functioning. Nurs Clin North Am 17:387–393, 1982.

Wabrek AJ: Sexual dysfunction associated with diabetes mellitus. J Fam Pract 8:735–740, 1979.

Wagner G, Green R: Impotence. New York, Plenum Press, 1981.

Whitley M, Berke P: Sexual response in diabetic women. J Sex Marital Ther 9:51–56, 1983.

Whitley M, Berke P: Sexuality and diabetes. In Woods NF (ed): Human Sexuality in Health and Illness. 3rd ed. St. Louis, CV Mosby, 1984.

18: Cardiovascular Disturbances and Sexuality

Lora E. Burke

Over 63 million Americans have one or more forms of heart or blood vessel disease; almost one in every four adults has hypertension, and over 2 million have rheumatic heart disease (American Heart Association, 1988). While an acute event such as a heart attack may not directly affect a person's ability to engage in sexual relationships, it may indirectly affect sexual function. These sexual disorders may be affective or of a direct physical nature or both (Myerscough, 1980). While heart disease may be chronic, the sexual impairment, which may potentially result from an acute event, does not have to be.

Studies have shown that individuals do not resume pre-illness levels of activity because of fear and not because of physical inability (Burke, 1981). Clients may restrict or abstain from their sexual activity because of fears resulting from inadequate information concerning resumption of the activity (Mann et al, 1981; Scalzi and Dracup, 1978; Rosen and Bibring, 1966). Frequently, the effects can be overcome by supportive counseling and instruction from health care professionals (Dracup, 1985; Scalzi and Burke, 1989a, b; Kolman, 1984; Puksta, 1977; Papadopoulos, 1983). This chapter most thoroughly examines the effects of a myocardial infarction on an individual's sexual function, with a focus on the physiological, psychological, and sociological aspects. Counseling is presented as an important aspect of care for clients with cardiac disease. The cardiac effects of specific drugs are identified, while further discussion

of the effects of pharmacological agents is covered in Chapter 24, Drugs and Disturbed Sexual Functioning. In addition, the impact of hypertension, angina, and valvular heart disease on sexual activity is discussed. A conceptual framework for assessment and intervention is provided through Roy's Adaptation Model (Roy, 1980). The four modes of adaptation described in the model are physiological, self-concept, role function, and interdependence.

MYOCARDIAL INFARCTION AND SEXUAL FUNCTION

Several studies report decreased sexual activity following a myocardial infarction (MI) (Tuttle, Cook, and Fitch, 1964; Klein et al, 1965; Hellerstein and Friedman, 1969). One study showed that among males who had had an MI in the previous 1 to 9 years, two thirds experienced a decrease in intercourse and 10 per cent reported an erectile problem that had not resolved since the MI (Tuttle, Cook, and Fitch, 1964). In a subsequent study, Klein and associates (1965) found that 75 per cent of men had not resumed sexual activity at a level equal to their pre-MI level as late as 4 years after the infarct; Hellerstein and Friedman (1969) reported similar findings. When females were compared with males, a smaller percentage of females had resumed sexual activity within 7 weeks after an MI (Boogaard and Briody, 1985).

Reasons frequently cited for decreased sexual activity after an MI include fears, a change in desire, and symptoms such as angina and fatigue (Hellerstein and Friedman, 1969; Bloch, 1975; McLane et al, 1980; Trelawny-Ross and Russell, 1987). Either partner may fear that sexual activity may precipitate symptoms, another MI, or sudden death and, thus, decrease sexual activity. Fear of resuming intercourse is often based on misconceptions and lack of information regarding the cardiovascular demands of sexual activity.

Misconceptions and lack of knowledge may be partially attributed to insufficient instruction about sexual implications of cardiac disease by health professionals. In their study of 58 women with an MI or angina, Baggs and Karch (1987) found only 19 (33 per cent) had received any information prior to hospital discharge. In one study of wives of 100 MI patients, only 45 of the women reported receiving information prior to their husbands' discharge from the hospital (Papadopoulos et al, 1980). Researchers note there is marked variation in the instructions provided and that clients and spouses would like to receive more information about resuming sexual activity (Papadopoulos et al, 1980; Orzeck and Staniloff, 1987; Baggs and Karch, 1987). Stern reported a higher percentage of couples resuming sexual activity following an educational program (1978). Garcia-Barreto (1986) cited reports of improved performances and satisfaction among clients who received instruction and counseling 3 to 6 months after an MI. The literature supports the importance of instruction for a client and partner following an MI (McLane et al, 1980; Bloch et al, 1975).

An MI has immediate effects on self-esteem, outlook, and mood. The person who has just been admitted to the coronary unit is preoccupied with the threat to life. The technological atmosphere of the intensive care unit and perceived lack of control may reinforce feelings of threat. Anxiety may be high during the initial hours after an MI and may be followed by denial, anger, and depression (Thomas, 1983). After the initial experience, clients begin to focus on what the MI means to their future. They may question if they will be able to lead a fully active life again, including work and sexual activity (Andreoli and Foster, 1970; Cassem et al, 1970; Scalzi, 1973).

Having an MI affects the four modes of adaptation: physiological needs, self-concept,

role function, and interdependence (Roy, 1980). The coronary client's physiological needs for survival are, at first, primary. Later, human contact and relief of physical tension through sexual gratification may be threatened. Not maintaining usual activities may threaten the person's self-concept. During the acute and convalescent phase, client roles change significantly. There may be role reversals between spouses for the roles of provider and caretaker. The mode of interdependence or the ability to give and to receive affection may be altered markedly during the acute period. The ability to receive affection may not be altered as much as the ability to give it.

EFFECTS OF HEART DISEASE ON ADAPTATION

Physiological Function

Using data from Masters and Johnson's study of normal subjects, a brief review of physiological changes associated with sexual activity follows. During the arousal period, skin flush and a sense of warmth occur accompanied by gradual increases in respirations, heart rate, and blood pressure. With intromission, further increases occur. With orgasm, maximal respiratory, heart rate, and blood pressure occur. Within seconds after the completion of orgasm, the physiological parameters return to a resting level (Masters and Johnson, 1966).

Based on the early studies conducted by Masters and Johnson in the laboratory, the following data were reported on physiological changes: With orgasm, a normal respiratory rate of 16 may, on average, increase to 60 per minute. A resting heart rate of 60 to 70 beats per minute may rise to 170, with an average rise of 148.5. Blood pressure may increase from 120/80 to peak levels of 220/110, with an average increase of 170/100. Similar physiological responses were observed with penile-vaginal intercourse, masturbation, and same-sex sexual activity (Masters and Johnson, 1966).

In 1969, Hellerstein and Friedman reported the results of their often-cited study of physiological responses to sexual activity in middle-aged males with arteriosclerotic heart disease and in middle-aged coronary-prone males without evidence of heart damage. They monitored electrocardiographic tracings during a 24- to 48-hour period and compared physiological responses to sexual activity with those of other activities. Fourteen of the 40 postcoronary clients had sexual intercourse during the monitoring period. During the orgasmic phase, the mean maximal heart rate was 117.4 (minimum to maximum was 90 to 144). Similarly, the mean maximal heart rate during activity such as walking and climbing stairs was 120.1. Some factors that may explain the higher heart rates reported by Masters and Johnson (1966) and by Hellerstein and Freidman (1969) include a laboratory setting versus the familiar home and an unfamiliar partner versus a long-married spouse.

As can be seen in Table 18–1, data reported by Larson and associates (1980), parallel those from Hellerstein and Friedman's study (1969). During orgasm, mean heart rate among men with coronary heart disease (CHD) was 115; among normal males it was 123. Similarly, after walking and stair climbing, mean heart rate among men with CHD was 118; among normal males, it was 122. The mean systolic blood pressure during intercourse among CHD subjects was 144; among normal subjects it was 146. The mean systolic blood pressure was significantly higher with stair climbing than with sexual activity in the CHD subjects (164 versus 144), but it was the same in both activities for normal subjects (146 versus 146). The investigator suggested that the higher systolic blood pressure in the CHD subjects may be partially explained by a higher level of anxiety observed in these subjects prior to and during the stair climbing test. One conclusion that can be made from these studies is that

the physiological cost of sexual activity is modest for middle-aged, long-married men with CHD. Another conclusion that can be made is that climbing two flights of stairs following a 10-minute brisk walk is one method of assessing clients' readiness for sexual activity prior to hospital discharge.

Nemec, Mansfield, and Kennedy (1976) found no significant differences in heart rate or blood pressure responses in healthy males when they used the on-top or on-bottom positions for intercourse. Bohlen and associates (1984) found no differences in heart rate and rate pressure product (heart rate × systolic blood pressure) during orgasm between on-top and on-bottom coitus. However, Bohlen and associates (1984) did find significant differences in metabolic expenditure during stimulation and orgasm, depending on coital position. Energy expenditure for the on-bottom position was significantly less than that for the on-top position. The study results also showed large variations among individuals in physiological responses to sexual activity. These findings highlight the importance of considering individual differences in clinical conditions and sexual patterns when advising CHD patients about sexual activity.

Although the studies reported here attest to the modest energy expenditure of sexual activity, especially when the client uses the on-bottom coital position with a familiar partner, safety in resuming sexual activity remains a concern of both the health professional and the client. Also, partners have concerns about precipitating sudden death. One study showed an incidence of sudden death during sexual intercourse of 0.6 per cent based on 559,000 cases. Eighteen of the 34 deaths occurred in nonfamiliar surroundings and most in individuals with a history of serious heart disease (Ueno, 1963). One subject in a study involving 24-hour ECG recordings had intercourse with his lover and, later, with his spouse. Compared with sexual intercourse with the spouse, coitus with the lover produced a higher heart rate response (96 to 150 compared with 72 to 92) and occasional ventricular extrasystolic beats (Johnson and Fletcher, 1979). It is suggested that there may be an increased risk of sexual activity with extramarital partners or in nonfamiliar settings. However, it is concluded that sexual activity in a familiar environment is not associated with increased risk, especially among those clients with the ability to

TABLE 18–1. Heart Rate and Blood Pressure Response During Orgasm and Stair Climbing

	Orgasm	Stair Climbing
Hellerstein and Friedman, 1969		
CHD subjects		
mean maximum HR	117.4	120.1
Larson and associates, 1980		
Normal subjects		
mean maximum HR	123	122
SBP	146	146
CHD subjects		
mean maximum HR	115	118
SBP	144	164

CHD = coronary heart disease; HR = heart rate; SBP = systolic blood pressure.

walk and subsequently climb stairs without undue increase in heart rate or development of arrhythmias or cardiac symptoms.

Psychological Function

How clients interpret and react to an MI may have a significant impact on their self-concept or their view of self-worth. In turn, it may affect how they adapt to changing roles of spouse, parent, and worker. The nurse needs to consider a partner's response to the illness of the client. While the client may be experiencing certain emotional responses, the partner may feel responsible because of assuming the role of protector. Later, the partner may feel anger toward the client for having the MI and for its consequences on the family. If these feelings are not expressed, depression may result in the partner, who may express resentment, hostility, or anxiety to the staff, as it may not be acceptable to verbalize these to the client, particularly in the early phase of recovery. Resentment could ultimately affect levels of communication for the couple.

Two psychological responses to MI often cited in the literature are anxiety and depression (Cassem et al, 1970; Scalzi, 1973; Owen, 1987). Denial, anger, and aggressive sexual behavior are also possible responses. Initially, anxiety is due to the threat of death and the surroundings. As the client convalesces, anxiety may be due to a fear of symptoms that may limit usual activities. Client views may be shared by the spouse. The spouse may be over-protective, reinforcing the unfounded fears of the client. Fear of symptoms, another MI, or death are the reasons why most clients or spouses avoid or refuse to resume sexual intercourse (Bloch, 1975; Hellerstein, 1969).

People's perception of a changed body image and lowered self-esteem may contribute to anxiety. Individuals who have suffered damage to their hearts may feel less of a man or woman; this can affect the marital relationship. Clients may need frequent assurance of love and attraction at the time when their partners may be afraid to initiate such expressions. Or, clients may not be very receptive and withdraw because of depression. (Guillidge, 1976). This could lead to a vicious cycle of reinforced negative emotions and poor communications.

The multiple potential losses associated with an MI are the basis for the depression that is frequently observed while the client is still in the hospital or following discharge. Depression is often characterized by a loss of interest in self, others, and activities, including sexual activity. Decreased interest in sex may be manifested as arousal problems reinforcing feelings of inadequacy.

Guilt may also be expressed by clients. They may blame themselves for the MI; they may experience guilt for "doing this" to their partner or family. Clients may also feel guilty for continuing to engage in some behavior they identify as causing the MI, e.g., smoking, diet, or lack of exercise.

Because of the varied and changing stimuli over the post-MI course, clients and partners may continue to experience altered moods as they adjust to the MI. Clients and partners have been shown to experience anxiety associated with the acute event several months after its occurrence. Depression usually occurs during early convalescence when the client realizes what has happened (McLane et al, 1980). It may also occur later, up to 1 year after the MI. Guilt may occur at the same time. These feelings may resurface repeatedly and interfere with the client's ability to give and receive physical affection and sexual pleasure.

ASSESSMENT

Roy (1980) has described a two-level assessment process. First, a nurse assesses a client in the modes of adaptation: physiological, self-concept, role function, and interdependence. This is done incorporating subjective data from the client and objective data from the chart. For example, a nurse-client discussion of satisfaction with, attitudes about, and expectations of sexual activities is essential. Such a discussion provides data regarding psychosocial adaptation. Some examples of issues to be considered by a nurse in the process of discussion and assessment are level of sexual satisfaction in the client's present relationship(s); client's perception of the partner's level of sexual satisfaction; presence/absence of warmth, affection, and pleasure provided outside of sexual intercourse; and fears about sexual matters that partners are unable to share.

Second, a nurse assesses specific factors of stimuli that influence a client's behavior in relation to a given health concern. As defined by Roy (1980), these stimuli include *focal*, or primary, causative factors; *contextual,* or situational, determinants; and *residual,* or cultural and attitudinal, influences regarding behavior. The factors or stimuli to be considered in a second-level assessment can be applied to the cardiac client.

For a client recovering from an MI, one diagnosis may be sexual abstinence secondary to fears of "harming" oneself. Regarding such behavior, *focal* stimuli potentially causing abstinence may be specific fears of pain, injury, or death. *Contextual* factors that contribute to abstinence may be an inadequate knowledge base about the safety of intercourse or past sexual behaviors that were associated with pain and discomfort. *Residual* factors having potential impact on abstinence may include norms or attitudes that inhibit discussion of sexual matters. One study found that 66 per cent of males had been sexually dysfunctional prior to the MI (Wabrek and Burchell, 1980). Findings such as these underline the importance of gathering a sexual history when assessing cardiac clients. This includes, but is not limited to, frequency and manner of sexual expression as well as past experiences with sexual dysfunction and/or cardiac symptoms with sexual activity. For example, professionals should assess whether clients have maintained sexual activity and the range of this activity prior to the MI. For a review of the content of a thorough sexual history, refer to Chapter 2, Sexual Health Care. Specific considerations in the assessment of the four modes of adaptation follow.

Physiological Factors

Prior to instruction on activity resumption following an MI, the physical status of the client must be assessed through a review of the client's record, including a routine electrocardiogram, enzyme elevation, and clinical course. The client's response to exercise, such as a low-level treadmill or stair climbing test, prior to discharge can provide valuable subjective and objective data to guide the client's progression of sexual activity (Johnson and Fletcher, 1979; Larson, 1980; Sivarajan and Newton, 1984; Sivarajan et al, 1977). Frequency and severity of angina or dyspnea during the convalescence and the individual's pattern of physical activity prior to the MI must be considered. The client's general health status, presence of other medical con-

ditions, and current medications should also be reviewed. If there is concern about the individual's ability to engage in sexual activity, a 24-hour electrocardiogram can also be done to determine the presence of arrhythmias, heart-rate response, and ST segment changes with increased activities (Larson, 1980).

Self-concept

Subjective data provide the information for determining how the MI has disrupted the client's self-concept. Spontaneous verbalization by clients and direct questioning by a health professional may provide information about their interpretation of the event. Body language, as well as general behavior, provides clues about how clients perceive and cope with the MI. An example would be an anxious client who is restless and asks many questions concerning the cause of the MI in an attempt to handle guilt. If the MI is stimulating a high degree of emotional arousal or denial, a professional such as a nurse can assist the client in resolving these reactions before effective instruction about sexual activity can take place. The same will apply to the partner.

Another point to be addressed in assessing self-concept is the person's view of sexuality. Sexual preference (homosexual, heterosexual, or bisexual) and sexual practices (celibacy, monogamy, multiple partners) have implications for adaptation and can be assessed prior to counseling.

Role Function

A role involves the particular title one has and the behavior society expects of an individual in order to maintain that title. A temporary role reversal may be required; for example, the head of the household may have to relinquish many responsibilities to the mate. An acceptance of this is functional. Some individuals may become threatened or feel insecure, out of control, or anxious with the loss of usual duties, which may, in turn, influence their sexual role function. The professional needs to look at role changes secondary to the MI for the client and family. In assessing role function, it is important to be aware that an MI often increases an individual's awareness of aging. The individual who continues to deny the occurrence of the MI is not receptive to instruction regarding limitation of activities. Assessing the client and partner's level of adaptation is essential before planning interventions. Other points to consider are adjustments to past significant life events and effectiveness of past coping strategies.

Interdependence

Interdependence can be defined as the comfortable balance between dependence and independence in relationships (McIntier, 1976). Because of changes due to the MI, clients may have difficulty giving or receiving affection or sexual pleasure, particularly with a partner on whom they now feel dependent. Fear and anxiety often interfere with intimacy. In clinical settings, clients and partners express fears of engaging in intercourse because of the possibility of precipitating symptoms. Knowing that being physically or emotionally intimate may lead to intercourse, they may avoid any form of intimate expression. Partners have expressed a feeling of guilt surrounding thoughts of experiencing sexual gratification with the client. Partners may feel guilty about having such thoughts if they perceive that their lovers should not have demands placed on them during recovery. Anger may be felt by either client or partners and may be directed to the other. Inability to express feelings directly could lead to further guilt. Both anger and guilt can interfere with interactions in an interdependent relationship, including sexual expression.

INTERVENTION

An overall nursing goal is to facilitate coping responses to bring about positive adaptation (Roy, 1980). Nurses can intervene to meet such a goal by altering certain factors or stimuli, so that the client can better cope with these stimuli. Planning interventions for a positive sexual adaptation is based on data gathered in a thorough assessment. However, the topic of sexual activity should not be withheld until the end of a structured assessment or a hospital stay. Rather, it should be introduced naturally early in the hospitalization in discussions about disease implications.

If a nursing assessment of one client has revealed abstinence secondary to fears about sexual activity, a discussion about such fears may allow direct intervention by addressing the cause of the abstinence. A few clients may spontaneously identify fears or concerns about sexuality. Nevertheless, the nurse must be prepared to initiate a discussion on sexual issues for those who may desire such a discussion but find it difficult to initiate one. On the other hand, nurses may encounter clients who do not want to discuss sexual issues; this must also be respected. Intervening to address fears and concerns about post-MI sexual activity may be particularly helpful when done with both client and partner together. Counseling a couple may be an effective way of discussing myths the couple has about sexual activity following an MI and of providing time for questions from the couple and for accurate clarification of facts by the nurse. For some persons, counseling as a couple may not be desirable. If this is the case, nursing efforts should be made to share relevant information about sexual adaptation to the client and partner separately.

The nurse is in a key position to promote positive sexual adaptation for the cardiac client. The nurse can provide information about, and suggest alterations in, the contextual or situational factors to minimize cardiovascular stress with sexual activity. Critical information to be shared with clients and partners is highlighted in the following plan.

Teaching Plan for Cardiac Clients and Partners

1. Like any physical activity, intercourse places increased demands on the cardiovascular system. To avoid additional strain and promote success, the following suggestions are provided:
   a. Wait 2 or more hours after eating meals.
   b. Wait 2 or more hours after drinking alcohol (one drink, 4-ounce glass of wine, or one beer).
   c. Avoid an environment that is too hot or cold.
   d. Be rested and relaxed.
   e. Be aware that an unfamiliar environment or partner *may* increase cardiovascular response and work.
   f. Have nitroglycerine available.
   g. Use nitroglycerine prophylactically if intercourse usually precipitates angina symptoms.

h. If angina occurs, cease activity and place a nitroglycerine tablet under the tongue.

2. Depending on the individual case (e.g., presence or absence of heart failure or extent of MI), intercourse may be resumed 3 to 6 weeks following the MI. The client's tolerance of increased physical activity and/or performance on stair climbing or low-level treadmill tests are general parameters to help determine when the patient may resume sexual activity.

3. If sexual dysfunction occurs, such as erectile problems or inorgasmia, it may be due to fatigue, stress, anxiety or depression. This is a normal response and may occur again under similar circumstances.

4. If the following symptoms occur during or following sexual intercourse, inform your health professional:

   a. Persistent rapid heart beat or breathing (lasting more than 5 minutes after orgasm).
   b. Anginal symptoms (pain, pressure, or tightness in the chest, neck, arm).
   c. Extreme fatigue the day following intercourse.

By intervening and addressing focal and contextual factors for a cardiac patient in the preceding ways, the nurse may also successfully intervene to promote functioning in the four modes of adaptation; that is, addressing fears and encouraging the creation of an environment for safe, relaxed, and satisfying intimacy may strengthen a client's self-concept and abilities to be interdependent.

Content of Sexual Counseling

Integral to counseling about sexual adjustment is the demonstration of a positive, accepting attitude toward sexuality as a warm, natural part of a healthy life. The demonstration of a positive attitude about sexuality may help foster positive attitudes in clients themselves, thereby altering residual factors that may inhibit sexual adaptation.

A clinician such as a nurse or doctor can safely recommend the resumption of sexual activity given that the patient does not show signs of cardiac failure, e.g., angina or arrhythmias with increased physical activity. If the client does not show signs of failure

(resting tachycardia, dyspnea) and if there is an appropriate increase in heart rate and blood pressure without arrhythmias or angina during increased activity while in the hospital, the clinician can counsel the couple about gradual resumption of lovemaking. They should be encouraged to be intimate and to engage in pleasurable activities without intercourse during the early weeks following discharge. Depending on the individual case, sexual intercourse can be resumed within 3 to 6 weeks after the infarction when the client's exercise capacity safely exceeds the demands of coitus (Larson, 1980; Stein, 1979; Bohlen et al, 1984). Although the ability to walk and climb two flights of stairs may indicate general ability to be sexually active, further assessment of an individual client's abilities in specific sexual activities is encouraged during initial recovery. The client may need to be cautioned about specific coital positions that may require greater isometric exercise. In that situation, the partner may be encouraged to take a more active physical role in lovemaking. Prior sexual assessment should enable the clinician to know the sexual practices of the couple and whether the couple might need to alter these practices, at least temporarily.

The couple should be sensitively instructed about the potential for angina during lovemaking and how to respond. Activity should be ceased, and a nitroglycerine tablet should be taken. They may resume after relief is obtained, if they so desire. If the couple is advised that angina may occur and how to respond, they may be better able to cope when it develops. They should also be told to inform their health professional within 24 hours, particularly if the experience represents a change in the angina pattern, i.e., it is the first episode of angina, or angina occurs with much less effort. The health professional may prescribe long-acting nitrates or, if the client is already taking these, a beta blocker (Stein, 1979). Additional agents such as calcium channel blockers are available for use in preventing anginal episodes.

Couples should be encouraged to engage in intercourse at times when they are relaxed and well rested and feel good about it, not hostile or guilty. Many couples find early morning to be a good time for sexual activity, when they feel rested and have time to rest afterward.

Participating in sexual activity after eating a heavy meal may precipitate angina, as might any exercise at such a time. There is increased blood flow to the stomach postprandially, and the increased demands imposed by coitus may result in insufficient myocardial blood flow.

The client needs to be warned of sexual activity right after alcohol ingestion. The consumption of alcohol in an amount appropriate for a social drinker may reduce the amount of exercise that can be performed without precipitating angina. Significant ST segment depression has been shown to occur after alcohol ingestion. Alcohol may increase myocardial coronary blood flow in the absence of disease, but in coronary artery disease it seems to cause a redistribution of blood flow to nonischemic myocardium at the expense of the ischemic myocardium (Coffin, 1981; Friedman, 1981; Orlando, 1976).

Before closing the individual and joint counseling sessions, the topic of fear of coital death should be raised. The client and partner should be allowed to verbalize their fears and should also be informed about the low incidence of coital death. If indicated during a private conference with the client, considerations concerning other partners should be addressed.

MEDICATIONS

Drugs frequently prescribed for clients with coronary heart disease may have beneficial and/or adverse effects on their sexual performance. The nitrates, nitroglycerin and the long-acting preparations, may increase one's angina threshold, enabling the client to complete sexual intercourse without the development of angina. Beta-blocking agents are usually prescribed for angina that persists in the presence of long-acting nitrate therapy. They may also be used as an anti-arrhythmic drug. Propranolol has been implicated as the potential cause of erectile problems and loss of or decreased desire (Papadopoulos, 1980). It has also allowed individuals to complete coitus without angina or development of palpitations. Digitalis and clofibrate may cause gynecomastia in males. Two lipid-lowering agents, clofibrate and probucol, may cause dysfunction and loss of or decreased desire (Papadopoulos, 1980). Diuretics and antihypertensive drugs are frequently implicated for their association with erectile dysfunction. For further discussion of the cardiovascular

drugs and their specific effects, refer to Chapter 24, Drugs and Disturbed Sexual Functioning.

Assessment of the client's tolerance of drug therapy is an important part of clinical practice, especially for nurses. Drug side effects are not frequently volunteered by the client. Soliciting the information and sharing it with the client's primary physician or nurse practitioner may lead to a change in therapy and elimination of unwanted side effects. The widespread practice today of utilizing outpatient rehabilitation programs after MI or coronary bypass surgery provides an opportunity for health professionals to participate in the long-term management of clients. Developing safe exercise regimens is an important part of these programs. Continued education and counseling in the psychosocial, sexual, and occupational aspects of life are vital components of these programs. In addition to the long-term follow-up provided, there is the benefit of improved exercise tolerance. Stein (1979) showed that improved exercise tolerance positively influenced sexual activity. Hellerstein and Friedman (1969) reported that fewer cardiac symptoms were experienced during sexual activity after exercise training as compared with before training.

Clients with improved exercise tolerance also generally feel better about themselves. The partner who may be fearful about allowing the mate to engage in physical activity may be reassured by visiting a cardiac rehabilitation class and by observing the mate exercise without ill effects. This usually helps restore the partner's confidence in the client's ability to be physically active.

Through the long-term management of the client in the cardiac rehabilitation program or through other means of follow-up, evaluation of the clinical interventions should occur. Follow-up interviews with the couple or with the client or partners may provide the best information about adaptation and resumption of sexual activity without major problems.

OTHER CARDIOVASCULAR CONDITIONS
Angina

The previous discussion also generally applies to an individual with angina, who may be fearful of having an MI during intercourse. The client and partner need to be counseled alone or together, so that they can express their fears and concerns and be instructed about precautions as well as the use of prophylactic medications. They also need instruction about other medications prescribed for them and for potential side effects. The benefits of regular physical exercise and its salutary effects on sexual activity should be included. There are increasingly more client education materials available on this topic (American Heart Association, 1983). It is important that nurses provide this material to clients and also make other health professionals aware of it.

Postoperative Coronary Artery Bypass Graft Operation

Postoperatively, clients who have had a bypass may have difficulty knowing what activities they can perform. Generally, these clients can progressively assume activities faster than clients who have had an MI, because myocardial healing from an infarct is not an issue. Otherwise, the previous discussion of the effects of MI also applies because the client has CHD. Initially, the client may be fearful that angina will recur and may confuse the sternal incisional pain with ischemic pain (Marshall, 1985).

Prior to discharge the client should be counseled about having realistic expectations during the recovery period and about preventing fatigue. Clients and partners should be instructed that resumption of sexual activity is permissible when the client is able to engage comfortably in sexual activity. Incisional discomfort may be the prohibitive factor, which may occur for 1 to 2 weeks after discharge. If the client had a complication, such as an intraoperative MI or heart failure, the time for resumption of sexual activity is determined, as for all clients, on an individual basis. If the client had severe, limiting angina prior to revascularization, the couple may need guidance and reassurance about resuming sexual activity. The client may have previously abstained because of the symptoms. If a long time has passed since the couple had intercourse, both persons may need reassurance. Partners are fearful of inducing angina and sometimes, particularly husbands, are overly protective of their partners and do not initiate or ask for sexual activity (Sivarajan and Newton, 1984). Physical closeness and touching can be encouraged as a way of getting the couple comfortable with each other again without the fear of angina developing. Partners need to be reassured that they will not injure the patient's sternum. Postoperative depression may occur and interfere with activity progression. It is helpful to tell the client and partner about the possible occurrence of depression.

Valvular Heart Disease

One valvular heart disease that has been associated with distress during sexual intercourse is mitral stenosis. With marked stenosis of the mitral valve, pulmonary edema may be stimulated by intercourse; this occurs more frequently in women than men. Symptoms include cough, dyspnea, and tachycardia. In severe cases, with calculated valve areas 1 sq cm or less, hemoptysis has occurred during orgasm in females (Thompson, 1978). The basis for this is the increased heart rate associated with sexual stimulation, which in turn reduces diastole (transit time from left atrium to left ventricle) and results in a sharp elevation in pulmonary, venous, and capillary pressure. The client with this disorder needs reassurance and guidance concerning continued sexual activity.

Changes in position of sexual activity may be advised. If the female is less recumbent during intercourse (e.g., in a sitting position), her cardiac workload will be reduced. Also, beta blockade may be prescribed to block the increased heart rate response. Mitral stenosis may require surgical treatment. As with other major cardiac surgery, body image may be affected and negative moods, such as depression, may occur postoperatively. Counseling should be provided postoperatively to assist the client with these issues and to reassure the client that resumption of sexual activity will not induce the symptoms experienced prior to the operation.

Another form of valvular heart disease, aortic stenosis, may result in angina with exertion. This is due to the tight aortic valve, which increases the workload on the left ventricle during systole. The resultant anginal pain may be complicated with concomitant coronary artery disease. Individuals with this disease should be counseled about positions of intercourse to minimize physical effort. Assuming a more passive role during intercourse or a position in which isometric exercise is not required would be beneficial to these clients. They should inform their physician if they are experiencing angina during intercourse. Curtailment of physical activity may be necessary until surgical correction is performed. Nitroglycerin is not used in this situation unless coronary artery disease is also present.

Congestive Heart Failure

Congestive heart failure (CHF) is the clinical syndrome that occurs when the tissue requirements for oxygen are not met by the amount of blood pumped out of the heart each minute. This condition may be caused by one of the following conditions: (1) a poorly functioning myocardium, such as a damaged left ventricle from MIs or cardiomyopathy; (2) systemic demands greater than the myocardial pump can meet, such as infection, anemia, thyrotoxicosis, or exertion; (3) mechanical disorders, such as valvular stenosis or insufficiency; and (4) ineffective pumping action caused by rhythm disturbances, such as atrial fibrillation, tachycardia, or bradycardia. The clinical picture includes dyspnea with exertion, and in worse cases, dyspnea at rest, orthopnea, palpitations, weakness, fatigue, and dependent edema. Depending on the severity of the condition and the effectiveness of the treatment, the functional capacity may range from symptoms only with exertion (functional class 1 as described by the New York Heart Association) to symptoms of cardiac insufficiency at rest (functional class 4) (Burke, 1983). The individual who is severely limited by symptoms at rest should be counseled about not engaging in coital activity, since the tachycardia will cause further decompensation. For the client who is not so severely incapacitated, positions such as semireclining or on-bottom are recommended to minimize physical effort. The precautions about the best times to engage in sexual activity suggested for post-MI clients should also be suggested for CHF clients.

Hypertension

High blood pressure afflicts an estimated 54,990,000 adults in the United States (American Heart Association, 1988). Many of those who know they have hypertension are untreated or inadequately treated. Through improved detection and follow-up, the number of controlled hypertensives is increasing, and the mortality rate is decreasing.

There are two things to consider when dealing with the hypertensive client in sexual counseling. First, there is an increase in blood pressure during sexual activity. This has implications for the individual with hypertension, particularly if the person also has ischemic heart disease. The client needs to be counseled about the importance of achieving control of the blood pressure because of the additive effect of a blood pressure rise with coital activities. If individuals smoke cigarettes or are overweight, they need to be instructed about the additive effect of these conditions on blood pressure.

The second issue to address in the hypertensive patient is the pharmacological agents used for hypertension and their effects on sexuality and sexual function. Many drugs used to treat hypertension, for example, diuretics and sympatholytic agents, have been associated with alterations in sexual function, including erectile dysfunction and decreased desire. One study of 50 male and female hypertensive clients suggested that drug therapy had more frequent and more untoward effects on men; women experienced fewer adverse effects in relation to frequency of sexual activity, ability to achieve orgasm, and their general sexual relationship (Oaks and Moyer, 1972). There are increasingly more males in their third decade with hypertension who may have difficulty complying with their medication plan because of erectile dysfunction. (Refer to Chapter 24, Drugs and Disturbed Sexual Functioning, for further discussion of antihypertensive medications and sexual implications.)

Prior to the initiation of antihypertensive drug therapy, a sexual history should be taken to determine the pretreatment pattern of sexuality. Providing confidentiality and establishing rapport with clients can promote discussion of sexual issues. Once the baseline is established, follow-up assessment can more accurately determine if difficulties develop. The development of dysfunction may be the reason the client discontinued a medication without informing the clinician (Myerscough, 1980). Clients need to be asked if problems are developing and why they stopped taking a drug.

CONCLUSION

This chapter has reviewed several cardiovascular conditions and their implications for sexual function. When individuals are afflicted with a cardiac condition, they may feel threatened, alone, and unable to perform activities as before. The need to reach out and gain closeness, warmth, and reassurance from others is an important coping mechanism during such times of increased vulnerability. Future research could better illuminate the effects of cardiac disease on sexuality, particularly among women. The expression of human sexuality in the context of cardiac disease needs to be supported by nurses and other health professionals to promote the client's recovery to a full and enjoyable life.

REFERENCES

Abramov LG: Sexual life and sexual frigidity among women developing acute myocardial infarction. Psychosom Med 38:418, 1976.

American Heart Association: 1988 Heart Facts. AHA, 1988.

American Heart Association: Sex and Heart Disease. AHA, 1983.

Andreoli K, Foster S: Behavior following acute myocardial infarction. Am J Nurs 70:2344, 1970.

Baggs JG, Karch AM: Sexual counseling of women with coronary heart disease. Heart Lung 16:154, 1987.

Bloch A: Sexual problems after myocardial infarction. Am Heart J 90:536, 1975.

Bohlen JG, et al: Heart rate, rate-pressure product, and oxygen uptake during four sexual activities. Arch Intern Med 144:1745, 1984.

Boogaard MAK, Briody ME: Comparison of the rehabilitation of men and women post-myocardial infarction. J Cardiopulmonary Rehabil 5:379, 1985.

Burke LE: Current concepts of cardiac rehabilitation. Occ Health Nurs 29:41, 1981.

Burke LE: Education and rehabilitation of the patient with heart failure. In Michaelson CR (ed): Congestive Heart Failure. St. Louis, CV Mosby, 1983.

Burke LE, Scalzi CC: Behavioral responses of patient and family: Myocardial infarction and coronary bypass surgery. In Underhill SL, Woods SL (eds): Cardiac Nursing. 2nd ed. Philadelphia, JB Lippincott, 1989.

Cassem NH, et al: Reaction of coronary patients to the CCU nurse. Am J Nurs 70:319, 1970.

Coffin CE: Cardiovascular effects of alcohol ingestion. Cardiovasc Nurs 17:19, 1981.

Dracup K: A controlled trial of couples group counsel-

ling in cardiac rehabilitation. J Cardiopulmonary Rehab 5:436, 1985.

Fletcher GF: Long-term exercise in coronary artery disease and other chronic disease states. Heart Lung 13:28, 1984.

Friedman HS: Acute effects of ethanol on myocardial blood flow in the nonischemic and ischemic heart. Am J Cardiol 47:61, 1981.

Garcia-Barreto D, et al: Sexual intercourse in patients who have had a myocardial infarction. J Cardiopulmonary Rehabil 6:324, 1986.

Guillidge AD: The psychological aftermath of a myocardial infarction. In Gentry WD, Williams RB (eds): Psychological Aspects of Myocardial Infarction and Coronary Care. Englewood Cliffs, Prentice Hall, 1976.

Hellerstein HA, Friedman EH: Sexual activity and the post-coronary patient. Med Asp Human Sex 3:70, 1969.

Johnston BL: Exercise testing for patients after myocardial infarction and coronary bypass surgery: Emphasis on predischarge phase. Heart Lung 13:18, 1984.

Johnston BL, Fletcher GF: Dynamic electrocardiographic recording during sexual activity in recent post-myocardial infarction and revascularization patients. Am Heart J 98:736, 1979.

Klein RF, et al: The physician and postmyocardial infarction invalidism. JAMA 194:123, 1965.

Kolman PBR: Sexual dysfunction and the post-myocardial infarction patient. J Cardiac Rehabil 4:334, 1984.

Larson JL, et al: Heart rate and blood pressure responses to sexual activity and a stair-climbing test. Heart Lung 9:1025, 1980.

Mann, et al: The effects of myocardial infarction on sexual activity. J Cardiol Rehabil 1:187, 1981.

Marshall JL: Rehabilitation of the coronary bypass patient. Cardiovasc Nurs 21:1341, 1985.

Masters WH, Johnson VE: Human Sexual Response. Boston, Little, Brown & Co, 1966.

McIntier RM: Theory of interdependence. In Roy C (ed): Introduction to Nursing: An Adaptation Model. Englewood Cliffs, Prentice Hall, 1976.

McLane M, et al: Psychosexual adjustment and counseling after myocardial infarction. Ann Int Med 92:514, 1980.

Myerscough PR: Sexual function in illness. Clin Obstet Gynecol 7:317, 1980.

Nemec ED, Mansfield L, Kennedy JW: Heart rate and blood pressure responses during sexual activity in normal males. Am Heart J 92:274, 1976.

Oaks WW, Moyer JH: Sex and hypertension. Med Asp Human Sex 6:128, 1972.

Orlando J, et al: Effect of ethanol on angina pectoris. Ann Int Med 84:652, 1976.

Orzeck SA, Staniloff HM: Comparison of patients' and spouses' needs during the posthospital convalescence phase of a myocardial infarction. J Cardiopulmonary Rehabil 7:59, 1987.

Owen PM: Recovery from myocardial infarction: A review of psychosocial determinants. J Cardiovasc Nurs 2:75, 1987.

Papadopoulos C: Cardiovascular drugs and sexuality. Arch Int Med 140:1341, 1980.

Papadopoulos C, et al: Myocardial infarction and sexual activity of the female patient. Arch Int Med 143:1528, 1983.

Papadopoulos C, et al: Sexual concerns and needs of

the post-coronary patient's wife. Arch Intern Med 140:38, 1980.

Puksta NS: All about sex . . . after a coronary. Am J Nurs 77:602, 1977.

Rosen I, Bibring GL: Psychological reactions of hospitalized male patients to a heart attack. Psychosom Med 28:808, 1966.

Roy C: The Roy Adaptation Model. In Riehl J, Roy C (eds): Conceptual Models for Nursing Practice. 2nd ed. Norwalk, Appleton-Century-Crofts, 1980.

Russell RO, et al: Surgical versus medical therapy for treatment of unstable angina: Changes in work status and family income. Am J Cardiol 45:134, 1980.

Scalzi CC: Nursing management of behavioral responses following an acute myocardial infarction. Heart Lung 2:62, 1973.

Scalzi CC, Burke LE: Education of the patient and family: In-hospital phase. In Underhill SL, Woods SL (eds): Cardiac Nursing. 2nd ed. Philadelphia, JB Lippincott, 1989a.

Scalzi CC, Burke LE: Sexual counseling. In Underhill SL, Woods SL (eds): Cardiac Nursing. 2nd ed. Philadelphia, JB Lippincott, 1989b.

Scalzi CC, Dracup K: Sexual counseling of practice patients. Heart Lung 7:5, 1978.

Siewicki BJ, Mansfield LN: Determining readiness to resume sexual activity. Am J Nurs 77:604, 1977.

Sivarajan ES, et al: Low-level treadmill testing of 41 patients with acute myocardial infarction prior to discharge from the hospital. Heart Lung 6:975, 1977.

Sivarajan ES, Newton KM: Exercise, education, and counseling for patients with coronary artery disease. Clin Sports Med 3:349, 1984.

Stein RA: The effect of exercise training on heart rate during coitus in the post-myocardial infarction patient. Circulation 55:738, 1979.

Stern MJ: Sexual activity after myocardial infarction. Med Asp Human Sex 12:119, 1978.

Thomas SA, et al: Denial in coronary care patients—An objective reassessment. Heart 12:74, 1983.

Thompson DR: Sexual activity following acute myocardial infarction in the male. Nurs Times 76:1965, 1980.

Thompson WP: Mitral stenosis, intercourse, and hemoptysis—Letters. JAMA 239:2446, 1978.

Trelawny-Ross C, Russell O: Social and psychological responses to myocardial infarction: Multiple determinants of outcome at six months. J Psychosom Res 31:125, 1987.

Tuttle WB, Cook WL, Fitch E: Sexual behavior in post-myocardial infarction patients. Am J Cardiol 13:140, 1964.

Ueno M: The so-called coition death. Jap Leg Med 1963.

Wabrek HA, Burchell RC: Male sexual dysfunction associated with coronary heart disease. Arch Sex Behav 9:69, 1980.

19: Respiratory Disturbances and Sexuality

Rebecca Stockdale-Woolley

Chronic respiratory diseases not only affect physiological functioning but may also have an impact on psychological, social, and sexual functioning. This chapter will address these problems as experienced by individuals with chronic respiratory diseases and will present interventions to promote sexual health for these individuals. While the disease emphasized in this chapter is chronic obstructive pulmonary disease, cystic fibrosis, tuberculosis, and lung cancer are also discussed.

RESPIRATORY DISEASES AND SEXUAL FUNCTION

Chronic Obstructive Pulmonary Disease

In 1980 over 16 million Americans reported that they had seen a physician in the previous 12 months for the diagnosis, treatment, continuing care, and/or consultation of chronic obstructive pulmonary disease (COPD) (American Lung Association, 1982). In 1986,

For editorial review, the author wishes to thank Kristen Kreamer, RN, MSN, OCN, Oncology Clinical Nurse Specialist, in private practice, and Assistant Professor, School of Nursing, University of Southern Maine, Portland, Maine, and Linda Norton, RN, MSN, doctoral candidate at the University of California, San Francisco.

the National Health Interview Survey (NHIS) in the United States estimated the prevalence of chronic bronchitis and emphysema to be 13.4 million, with an additional 6.9 million estimated to have asthma (NHIS, 1986). Chronic Obstructive Pulmonary Disease is a collective term that refers to a group of diseases characterized by increased resistance to airflow, usually resulting in a variable degree of dyspnea, easy fatigability, wheezing, and a productive cough. Specific disorders included in this group are asthma (frequently a reversible process) and chronic bronchitis and emphysema (both irreversible processes). In asthma there is increased responsiveness of the airways to various stimuli (pollens, dust, molds, danders, atmospheric pollution, cold air, infection, emotions, and exercise), resulting in bronchoconstriction, bronchospasm, and mucus hypersecretion. Chronic bronchitis is associated with prolonged exposure to nonspecific irritants and is accompanied by increased mucus secretion and a chronic or recurrent productive cough. Emphysema is characterized by destructive changes of the alveolar walls, with enlargement of the air spaces and air trapping. However, chronic bronchitis and emphysema, rarely seen as separate clinical entities, are usually found in combination.

The impact of chronic lung disease on life in general and on sexuality in particular was studied by Hanson (1982). The survey participants were 128 adults, mostly married and male, with asthma (30 per cent), emphysema

(28 per cent), and a combination of asthma, emphysema and chronic bronchitis (25 per cent). Hanson (1982) inquired about the importance of 11 areas of adjustment to lung disease. The overwhelming majority of subjects rated all areas as important. Dependency on others, life in general, and effects of symptoms were rated as important by 90 to 91 per cent of the survey participants; physical/sexual aspects of marriage were rated as important by 74 per cent. Of interest, for 40 per cent of the participants, lung disease had a positive effect on both emotional aspects of marriage and on the need to rely on others. A slower life style and closer relationships were viewed as positive effects of the disease. Thus, sexual expression was one of many adjustment concerns of individuals with chronic respiratory disease.

Clients with COPD typically report difficulty engaging in sexual intercourse. In a study of the needs and concerns of persons with COPD, difficulty with or fear of sexual activity was a commonly identified concern (Curgian, 1981). According to Petty (1978), sexual dysfunction is common in persons with COPD, often presenting as erectile dysfunction in males and anorgasmia in females. Agle and Baum (1977) found that 19 of 23 men participating in a pulmonary rehabilitation program for COPD complained of impaired erectile function and decreased sexual desire. Sexual function was more often compromised in advanced disease and was attributed to shortness of breath and easy fatigability. Fletcher and Martin (1982) studied males with COPD without major accompanying illnesses; seven out of twenty subjects had stopped sexual activity as their pulmonary symptoms worsened, six because of erectile difficulty and one because of shortness of breath. Other subjects reported decreased desire and decreased frequency of sexual activity. Overall, the more severe the respiratory symptoms were, the more severe the sexual dysfunction. In contrast, in a study of 100 clients with COPD, Kass, Updegraff, and Muffly (1972) reported that only 17 out of 100 men had erectile dysfunction. They found erectile dysfunction to be uncommon early in the disease; when present, it was related more to marital and psychic conflicts.

Clients with COPD characteristically have some degree of hypoxia, with the degree increasing with severity of disease. This hypoxia results in shortness of breath and difficulty with exercise. These patients have limited walking tolerance and often avoid climbing stairs whenever possible. Thus, they may avoid sexual activity because it involves too much physical exertion.

Clients with COPD may have physiologically grounded fears of experiencing acute breathing difficulty or increased severity of shortness of breath. Especially for asthmatics, emotional anxiety and exertion may trigger a bronchospastic episode. The fear of experiencing dyspnea with intercourse may decrease desire and interfere with maintaining sexual arousal. Such a situation can be aggravated further by performance anxiety.

Both the disease process of COPD and aspects of its treatment cause changes that affect self-concept and body image. The barrel-shaped chest and sputum production seen in COPD, along with the fat deposition and muscle wasting from steroid therapy, may make the client feel less sexually attractive.

For many COPD clients, shortness of breath and limited energy reserves force activity restriction, decreased socialization and recreation, and early retirement or disability. In a study of women with COPD, the major problems reported were shortness of breath and fatigue, loneliness and depression, and restricted activity (Sexton and Munro, 1988). Particularly for men, relinquishing the primary wage earner role and assuming a more dependent role may be seen as major role changes. These altered roles may decrease self-esteem and sexual desire.

Clients with COPD may experience changes in their marital and sexual relationships. When married women with COPD were questioned regarding the effect of the illness on their relationship with their spouse, more than a third reported that the illness had brought them closer together, whereas less than a fifth reported that the illness had caused them to drift apart. Less than half of the women (46 per cent) reported that their husbands supported them in doing whatever was needed (Sexton and Munro, 1988).

Sexton and Munro (1988) also compared women with and without a diagnosis of COPD. Whereas less than half (44.8 per cent) of married women with COPD reported being highly satisfied with the sexual relationship with their spouse, about three quarters (73.1 per cent) of an otherwise comparable group of married women without COPD reported being highly satisfied. However, fewer married women with COPD (55.2 per cent) rated sexual satisfaction as highly important than did women without COPD (84.7 per cent) (Personal communication, Munro and Sexton, 1988). Although these data are from a small sample and are limited to married women, the data suggest that women with COPD make adjustments about the importance of a satisfying sexual relationship.

Spouses of clients with COPD also report changes in their marital and sexual relationships. In a study of wives of men with COPD, Sexton and Munro (1985) found that about half (48 per cent) of the wives reported they had no desire for sexual relations. Perhaps this was due to fear of precipitating an exacerbation of their husbands' symptoms. In a study of husbands of women with COPD, Munro and Sexton (1988) found that about three quarters (72 per cent) of husbands rated the importance of a sexual relationship with their spouse as high, but only about half (56 per cent) of these husbands rated their satisfaction with their sexual relationship as high. Taken together, these data seem to suggest that female spouses of COPD clients may be more likely than male spouses of COPD clients to forgo their former sexual relationship; however, this warrants further study. Davis (1981) has suggested that if the spouse remains interested in sexual activity, the partner with COPD may feel guilty for letting the spouse down or may feel angry at the spouse for wanting sex.

The COPD population, particularly those with chronic bronchitis and emphysema is, on average, an older population, ranging from 40 to 70 years of age. For these individuals, lack of knowledge regarding normal changes that accompany aging may affect sexual functioning. With advancing age, it takes longer for the male to become erect and to experience orgasm. The intensity of the ejaculatory experience is diminished, and the refractory period (time interval after ejaculation) is extended. These normal changes, while not a barrier to sexual activity, may be misinterpreted to be the onset of erectile dysfunction. Fear associated with these misconceptions may contribute to poor sexual health (Shomaker, 1980).

Other physiological changes seen in COPD clients may affect sexual activity. A significant slowing of peripheral sensory and motor nerve conduction has been demonstrated in individuals with chronic respiratory insufficiency and severe hypoxia (Narayan and Ferranti, 1978). Such a neurological disturbance

may increase the potential for sexual dysfunction.

Certain medications may affect sexual function in selected clients with COPD. Some drugs used for asthma are related to epinephrine; these can cause tremors and decrease the ability of the male to maintain a satisfactory erection (Davis, 1981). Steroids are used to decrease bronchial inflammation in exacerbations of COPD. Although steroids may not affect sexual functioning (Davis, 1981), they have been shown to depress spermatogenesis at doses of 30 mg of prednisone per day (Kolodny, Masters, and Johnson, 1979). Cor pulmonale, a complication of advanced chronic bronchitis and emphysema, is often treated with diuretics. Diuretics such as ethacrynic acid, furosemide, and the thiazides have been associated with erectile dysfunction in 5 per cent of men using them consistently (Kolodny, Masters, and Johnson, 1979). Sedation usually depresses sexual responsiveness and desire, which may lead to greater anxiety over sexuality. However, some clients, particularly asthmatics, have been helped by antidepressants or sedatives when sexual dysfunction was due to anxiety (Straus and Dudley, 1976).

In summary, individuals with COPD may experience sexual dysfunction due to the physical effects of the disease and its treatment; to psychological effects of the disease on self-esteem, body image, and general emotional outlook; or to lack of knowledge of the effects of the disease and aging. Some individuals may respond by withdrawing from their partner. Others may deny their disease and attempt to overcompensate by increasing sexual activity (Davis, 1981).

Cystic Fibrosis

Cystic fibrosis (CF) is a recessively inherited disease that affects one in every 1500 to 2000 live Caucasian births (Thompson, 1986). It is characterized by pancreatic insufficiency (manifested as failure to thrive, diarrhea, and steatorrhea), recurrent and chronic chest infection (with cough, thick and purulent sputum, dyspnea, and finger clubbing), and elevated sweat electrolyte levels.

Advances in treatment now enable 50 per cent of CF individuals to live to 18 years of age or older (Larter, 1981). As the person ages, the symptoms of pancreatic insufficiency decrease, and pulmonary involvement dominates the picture (di Sant'Agnese and Davis, 1979). Pulmonary function testing reveals obstructive disease.

Because the primary task of adolescence is the establishment of an independent ego identity and the acceptance of one's sexuality (Evans and Conine, 1982), the self-image of the adolescent with CF may be threatened by the physical effects of the disease on sexual development. In addition to being underweight, clients with severe pulmonary involvement experience inhibition of secondary sex characteristics. In males there is an increased incidence of inguinal hernia, undescended testes, and hydrocele. Women may have little breast development and irregular menses. In the prepubertal individual, androgens may be used for weight gain; in females, estrogens may be used for development of secondary sex characteristics (Taussig, Cohen, and Sieber, 1976). The chronically ill adolescent needs a supportive family and peer group, increased responsibility for self-care, an atmosphere that fosters independence, and information about sexuality and potential as a sexual being.

Cystic fibrosis also affects the procreative aspects of sexual activity (Evans and Conine, 1982). Most men with CF are sterile because of absence or atrophy of the epididymis, vas deferens, and seminal vesicles. Women have difficulty conceiving because of thick vaginal secretions. Prevention of conception is also problematic. Alternatives to oral contraceptives should be explored, since they seem to cause deterioration of pulmonary function in clients with CF.

There are certain risks for the woman with CF considering pregnancy (Hodson, 1980). Pregnancy may increase the severity of her lung disease. Furthermore, there is a genetic as well as personal risk because any child born will, at least, be a carrier of the disease. If the partner of a CF client is a carrier, then there is a 50 per cent chance that the child will have CF. Besides the physical risk of bearing a child with CF, there is the possibility that the parent with CF will die, leaving young children. In addition, the chronicity of the disease, the potential dependency involved, and the medical costs can strain a marital relationship.

Nolan and associates (1986) found that in general adolescents with CF are poorly informed about their potential for participating in a sexual relationship and the risks involved in having children. In looking at problems

spontaneously discussed by a group of CF clients and families, Brissette and associates (1987) found that information regarding sexual activity was actively sought by clients.

Coffman and associates (1984) studied the sexual adaptation of 48 single young adults with CF and a similar group without chronic disease. They found that female subjects with CF had more developmental sexual problems than physically healthy female subjects. However, there were not significant social and sexual differences between males with CF and physically healthy males. There was also no significant relationship between severity of CF and sexual health.

A study by Levine and Stern (1982) of 30 married CF clients revealed that the majority experienced consistently good sexual functioning and derived much physical and emotional satisfaction from their sexual relationships. In this sample, the spouses were all aware before marriage of possible reproductive problems; this concern was reported to be less troublesome for the spouses than the clients. Reproductive concerns created anxiety in clients soon after marriage but were subsequently resolved. Overall, clients with adequate vital capacity (e.g., greater than 70 per cent of predicted on pulmonary function tests) did not have disease-related sexual difficulties. However, one third of couples in Levine and Stern's (1982) study reported serious sexual problems. Only half of these were attributable to CF. Some subjects experienced decreased desire due to poor pulmonary function and decreased exercise tolerance. Others suffered from decreased self-esteem and chronic depression due to symptoms associated with CF (cough, sputum, stool changes, slight build, and delayed development of secondary sex characteristics). These feelings were associated with poor health maintenance, decreased self-esteem, and a poorer relationship with the partner. Those with poorer pulmonary function may be told that satisfactory sex lives can be achieved by clients with serious disease. When sexual dysfunction is present, some problems can be corrected with treatment of the pulmonary disease, while other sexual difficulties may necessitate treatment of marital problems.

Tuberculosis

Tuberculosis (TB) is an infection caused by the organism *Mycobacterium tuberculosis* or *My-*

cobacterium bovis. With the development of specific chemotherapy for TB, the mortality rate in the United States has decreased dramatically. The morbidity rate, however, has not declined as rapidly. The number of new active cases in the United States in 1978 was 13.1 per 100,000 or 28,251 cases (Guenter and Welch, 1982).

The client with pulmonary TB experiences anorexia, weight loss, fatigue, shortness of breath on exertion, fever, cough, and sputum production. Clients are treated medically and are asked to restrict social contact to family members until the infection is no longer transmissible. Family members should also be treated chemoprophylactically. The client is usually not infectious after 1 to 2 weeks of effective therapy (medications to which the tubercle bacillus is sensitive) (Karus, 1983). At this time, there is no longer the risk of the partner developing TB as a result of close contact during sexual activity (Feldman, 1977).

Both men and women with pulmonary TB may experience decreased sexual desire. The decrease in desire may be due to the physical symptoms of fatigue and shortness of breath on exertion. Feelings of shame, inferiority, and social ostracism have, in the past, been reported with TB and may affect desire. A lack of desire may also contribute to feelings of sexual inferiority and anxiety regarding sexual performance. Increased sexual impairment has been noted with more severe disease states. Of important note, there is an excellent chance of returning to the prior level of sexual functioning after treatment (Feldman, 1977). The patient may be reassured that the drugs used to treat TB have no effect on sexual function.

The effects of TB on sexual function are more permanent if the tubercle bacillus enters the blood stream. Genitourinary TB may develop, affecting the kidneys and reproductive organs. In women, genital TB may invade the fallopian tubes, resulting in sterility, pelvic pain aggravated by sexual activity, menstrual disturbances, and general debility. In men with genital TB, the prostate and seminal vesicles are infected; often the epididymis is also involved. Sterility results because of decreased semen volume or obstruction of the ductus deferens or ejaculatory ducts. Untreated men with genital TB rarely transmit the disease to a sexual partner. However, there is evidence of small children developing a positive reaction to tuberculi, perhaps due to exposure to material soiled with infected urine (Feldman, 1977). Thus, TB may be spread via fomites.

Lung Cancer

The estimated incidence of lung cancer for 1988 was 152,000 new cases, of which only 13 per cent live 5 or more years after diagnosis (American Cancer Society, 1988). A diagnosis of lung cancer may affect family relationships. In a study of persons with lung cancer and their spouses, Cooper (1984) found most subjects perceived either no change or an increase in closeness between husband and wife. The majority of subjects also reported no change in expression of affection or in need for affection expression. However, most spouses did not share concerns or fears with the clients. There also was a discrepancy between how the partners saw communication. The clients perceived the couple as talking more often than did the spouse.

Both lung cancer and its treatment have physical and psychological effects that may have an impact on sexual functioning (Hogan, 1985). The client commonly experiences weakness, a general sense of malaise, fatigue, and pain. This state contributes to a decrease in exercise tolerance, sexual responsiveness, and desire. In itself, the diagnosis of cancer has a great emotional impact, sometimes resulting in negative moods, such as anger, depression, guilt, anxiety, and fear of death, especially in the weeks following diagnosis. These feelings may decrease self-esteem and desire. In addition, the disease state produces psychological concerns, social role changes, life style changes, and financial burdens that can affect body image and decrease self-esteem. Treatments for cancer can also alter body image and self-esteem.

Clients may not maintain their former sexual role with their present sick role. However, cancer clients often experience an increased desire for physical closeness with a decreased interest in coitus (Leiber et al, 1976). This decreased interest in intercourse may be accepted by both the client and the partner. In some cases, the client may feel angry that the partner could continue to be interested in sex.

The partner, too, operates under the strain of dealing with the client's diagnosis and prognosis and the resultant role changes.

Such stress may result in diminished desire and sexual dysfunction; fatigue from assuming a caregiver role may also be a factor. If the partner continues to be interested in sex, feeling guilty about wanting sex or feeling hesitant to initiate such activity with one who is not well may further exacerbate the problem (Lamb and Woods, 1981).

The treatment of lung cancer can also affect one's sexuality through physiological and psychological effects (Fisher, 1983; Shipes and Lehr, 1982). Some chemotherapy affects the reproductive system and fertility; surgery, radiation therapy, and chemotherapy all contribute to decreased energy and poor exercise tolerance. Radiation therapy and some types of chemotherapy may cause pulmonary fibrosis, leading to a decrease in vital capacity and an increase in shortness of breath (Foote, Sexton, and Pawlik, 1986; Hogan, 1985). For some clients, the side effects of nausea and vomiting from chemotherapy and radiation therapy further contribute to a sense of malaise. Changes in appearance, such as alopecia from chemotherapy and skin changes from radiation therapy, can alter body image. Surgery may interfere with a person's sense of wholeness. Thus, physical debilitation, decreased exercise tolerance, and alterations in body image and self-esteem may all contribute to decreased desire and decreased ability to function sexually for the person with lung cancer.

EFFECTS OF RESPIRATORY DISEASE ON ADAPTATION

There are distinct and interrelated ways in which respiratory diseases affect sexual function. The disease may affect physiological function, self-concept, role function, and interdependence (Roy, 1980).

Physiological Function

There are a number of physiological problems that are present in clients with respiratory disease and that may contribute to sexual dysfunction. Many of the alterations in sexual activity are related to the physiology of exercise. In healthy individuals, sexual activity alters respiratory rate and depth as well as increases oxygen consumption and cardiovascular work; there are increases in heart rate, blood pressure, and respiratory rate.

The most marked changes occur with orgasm, after which these physiological parameters quickly return to baseline. The work of sexual activity has been compared to the cardiovascular cost of walking briskly or climbing one or two flights of stairs (Hellerstein and Friedman, 1969). In those with respiratory disease, impaired gas exchange (due to bronchoconstriction and bronchospasm, air trapping, mucus plugging, and/or infection) creates an oxygen deficit that results in decreased exercise tolerance and activity limitations. Increased cough and sputum production, associated with asthma, chronic bronchitis, cystic fibrosis, and tuberculosis, contribute to an oxygen deficit, interfere with activity, and promote a general feeling of malaise. A significant slowing of nerve conduction in clients with chronic respiratory insufficiency and severe hypoxia increases the potential for sexual difficulties.

Other medical problems in addition to the respiratory disease may affect sexual function (Woods, 1984). For example, poorly controlled diabetes results in difficulty with erections and ejaculation because of the effects on the autonomic nerves. Cardiac disease may also result in activity limitations, depression and anxiety, and fear of engaging in sexual activity. Nutritional deficiencies and anemias contribute to a poor sense of well-being and decreased exercise tolerance.

Treatments for medical problems can also contribute to sexual dysfunction. Although bronchodilators and tuberculosis chemotherapy do not affect sexual function, diuretics and epinephrine-related drugs may affect erectile abilities. Therapeutic interventions for cancer may have an effect because of the resultant general malaise and changes in body image. Medications for nonpulmonary problems, such as antihypertensives and antidepressants, may also decrease desire and affect erectile function in males (Davis, 1981).

Psychological Factors

A critical area in which respiratory disease affects sexual function is self-concept. Self-concept (Buck, 1984) is the composite of what one believes and how one feels about oneself. It is defined by both physical self (physical feelings and body image) and personal self (personality traits, expectations, and moral beliefs) and is formed largely from perceptions of others' reactions.

Physical and psychological effects of disease and treatment can alter one's body image. Respiratory symptoms such as dyspnea, cough, and sputum production, the delayed development of secondary sex characteristics in CF patients, and alopecia and skin changes from chemotherapy and radiation may make the client feel less sexually attractive. Surgery for lung cancer or the sterility associated with CF and genitourinary TB may make a person feel less whole. Embarrassment about shortness of breath with sexual activity may lead to reluctance to engage in sex. In addition, the reactions of others to symptoms and physical appearance may affect self-concept. Social isolation and ostracism because of others' misconceptions as well as self-enforced withdrawal because of lack of energy may also contribute to decreased feelings of self-worth.

Other negative feelings may affect self-concept. In our society sex has been associated with youth, physical attractiveness, and procreation. Although studies have shown that sex drive and activity are markedly consistent throughout the life span, an older person may feel guilty over continued interest in sexual activity and too embarrassed to express concern about changes in sexual function (Anderson, 1975; Steinke and Bergen, 1986).

Some clients feel inferior, become physically or sexually inhibited, and withdraw from others and from sexual activity. Others try to overcompensate to prove they are still sexually adequate and attractive. Some clients are able to work through their feelings, perceive their illness as a challenge, and cope well. Defense mechanisms commonly used to deal with the changes and losses associated with respiratory diseases include denial and testing of limits, anger at and resentment of others, projection of blame on others, intellectualization, and regression (Abram, 1972). Finally, the emotional impact for those who have a terminal respiratory illness can seriously threaten a person's sense of self-worth.

Role Function

The chronicity of respiratory illness and the activity limitations that it imposes have a profound effect on role function. The individual with COPD must often retire prematurely. The client with CF may be physically incapable of maintaining a job. Decreased energy necessitates a decrease in socialization and recreation. These physiological changes affect the person's ability to maintain social and societal roles. Recurrent exacerbations and hospitalizations may promote the assumption of the sick role.

A person's role as a sexual being is affected. For the CF client, there may be delay in and interference with the normal stages of developing childhood and adolescent intimacy, which may affect assumption of adult roles. With respiratory diseases, desire and frequency of sexual activity are often decreased, and sexual dysfunction may occur, thus threatening the client's role as a sexual partner.

Parenting role expectations may be altered. Men with CF are sterile, and women have difficulty conceiving. In addition, the person with CF is faced with a shortened life expectancy. Clients with genitourinary TB are sterile. In turn, the loss of meaningful social roles may threaten their self-concept.

Interdependence

Interdependence is defined as the close relationships of people and refers to the giving and receiving of love and respect and the valuing of others (Tedrow, 1984). Changes in physical self, self-concept, and roles influence how a person relates interdependently with others. Healthy interdependence involves achieving a balance of dependence and independence as well as giving and receiving love. With respiratory limitations, there may be threats to these balances between a patient and significant other.

Chronic illness may necessitate a gradual increase in physical dependence. Recurrent exacerbations and hospitalizations associated with respiratory disease may increase dependency. The adolescent with CF struggles for independence at a time when the disease, the parents, and health professionals are setting limits. Antagonism may develop and contribute to the deterioration of important family and provider relationships. In addition, the overprotective parent can adversely affect the child's growth and development.

Sometimes clients suffer from loneliness and alienation because of myths and misconceptions about their disease, its cause, and its treatment and because of physical limitations imposed by respiratory insufficiency. Clients with shortness of breath must set priorities

Sexual History of Individual with a Respiratory Disturbance*

A. General
  1. Has anything interfered with your being a partner, mother/father?
  2. Has anything changed the way you feel about yourself as a partner, mother/father?
  3. Are there any problems with your sexual activity?
  4. Are you satisfied with your sexual activity?
  5. Has your respiratory disease affected your sexual activity? If so, how?
B. Specific
  1. When you engage in sexual activity, do you have problems with shortness of breath?
  2. How does the shortness of breath affect your ability to engage in sexual activity?
  3. For each symptom ask questions to help define the problem:
    —What is the shortness of breath like?
    —When does it start?
    —How long does it last?
    —How severe is it (i.e., on a scale of 1–10)?
    —What makes it better? Worse?
    —What other changes do you notice besides shortness of breath?
  4. Inquire similarly about the following symptoms: coughing, wheezing, sputum, mouth odor, orthopnea/ lying down, chest pain/pressure, palpitations, anxiety, other.
C. Management
  1. What preparation(s) do you take before engaging in sexual activity? (Medications, nebulizer, metered dose inhaler, extension device, oxygen, breathing exercises, postural drainage, relaxation exercises, time, setting, positioning).
  2. After sexual activity what do you do to help your shortness of breath?

FIGURE 19–1. Sexual history of individual with a respiratory disturbance. This outline may be used in conjunction with the other aspects of a comprehensive health history (demographic; history of present illness; past medical history; management regimen; family history; occupational history; nutrition, alcohol, and smoking history; psychosocial history; and review of systems). In addition, questions related to the specific respiratory disturbance may be added.

on expenditure of energy. They may limit themselves to relationships within the family. With progressive disease, couples face balancing the client's physical need to take on a more passive role during sexual activity and both persons' desire for sexual relations. This balancing may be a source of growth for the couple.

Hanson's (1982) survey documented that lung disease had a negative impact on physical sexual aspects of marriage for 67 per cent of the respondents, on emotional aspects of marriage for 57 per cent, and on dependency on others for 38 per cent. However, lung disease was reported as having a positive impact in these same areas for 29 per cent of the respondents in physical-sexual areas and for 40 per cent in emotional and dependency issues. Some participants reported that greater dependency on others was associated with feelings of warmth and security.

As the respiratory disease progresses, clients may withdraw from family members as well. In withdrawing, clients cannot meet their interdependency needs for physical, emotional, or sexual intimacy.

Families, too, experience conflicts about balancing interdependence issues. Families of chronically ill individuals report feelings of helplessness and inadequacy when faced with a situation in which the client does not "get well" or the client withdraws or refuses assistance. The chronicity and progressive deterioration, as in CF, emphysema, and chronic bronchitis, can be very discouraging. The demand of providing care to a client over a long period of time may result in caregiver fatigue. Caregiver fatigue may signal a deficit of feeling cared for and loved.

ASSESSMENT

A sexual history (Fig. 19–1) should be part of the assessment of the total person and should be as much a part of the history as any other bodily function. It is the responsibility of the health professional to raise the subject; clients may not initiate discussion. Empathy and a matter-of-fact, problem-solving approach help to decrease anxiety and promote an open response from client and partner. Although the professional should assess the degree of the extent of sexual history needed at the time, assumptions should not be made simply on the basis of appearance. The sexual history should elicit any changes in sexual activity, the extent of their impact on sexual functioning, problems or discomforts with sexual activity, and the degree of patient and couple satisfaction (Sexton, 1981). Information related to illness severity, activity limitations, medications and treatments, and psychosocial history helps assess the effects of respiratory illness on sexual health and may be obtained during other parts of the health history. Questions may be tailored to obtain information pertaining to the four modes of adaptation (physical needs, self-concept, role function, and interdependence) and to identify factors that may be contributing to sexual dysfunction (age, lack of knowledge, other medical illnesses).

If the client admits to a breathing problem related to sexual activity, the clinician needs to assess the nature, severity, and duration of respiratory symptoms before, during, and after coitus as well as any other manifestations associated with respiratory symptoms. Particular attention should be given to the following symptoms: dyspnea, cough, wheeze, sputum, mouth odor, orthopnea, chest pain/pressure, palpitations, and anxiety. Careful clarification of what sexual activity was like prior to the disease is necessary to assess the degree of change. It may be helpful to interview the client and partner both separately and together. A couple's communications and level of knowledge regarding sexual changes can alert the nurse to possible knowledge deficits.

INTERVENTION

Education of the client and partner is an important function of a health professional such as a nurse (Table 19–1). A nurse can make suggestions that may help the respiratory client and the partner approach sexual activity more comfortably (Cooper, 1986; Stockdale-Woolley, 1983). Information may be given regarding normal sexual response as well as changes that accompany aging. It is important to communicate to the client that the respiratory disease does not directly decrease sexual ability or the capacity to enjoy sex. It is the degree of exercise intolerance associated with respiratory disease that most directly affects any limitation of sexual activity. The frequency of sexual activity is often limited, as is the frequency of other physical activities.

Treating the respiratory disease aggressively may indirectly facilitate psychosocial and sexual functioning. In addition to gen-

TABLE 19–1. Client and Partner Education

The sexual response cycle
  1. Normal response
  2. Changes with aging
  3. Limitations secondary to respiratory disease
Optimizing exercise tolerance
  1. Time of day
  2. Pacing activity
  3. Positioning
  4. Diaphragmatic and pursed lip breathing
  5. Bronchodilator therapy
  6. Low-flow oxygen
  7. Environmental control
  8. Alternative forms of sexual gratification
Optimizing related factors
  1. Regular exercise
  2. Appropriate nutrition
  3. Treatment of other medical problems
  4. Altering drug regimens
Referral
  1. Support groups
  2. Counseling, psychotherapy

eral disease management, a nurse can share specific suggestions with the client and the partner to help optimize exercise tolerance for sexual activity (Campbell, 1987; Stockdale-Woolley, 1983). The maintenance of some form of regular physical exercise tailored to the individual's ability is important for efficient cardiovascular and respiratory functioning. Clients should approach sexual activity as they do other physical activities, incorporating the same methods to ensure energy conservation. Choice of time of day is important. For some, this may be mid-morning—after a night's rest, morning medications, a breathing treatment, and raising secretions that have accumulated throughout the night. For others, the most comfortable part of the day may be the evening. Sexual activity should be paced like any other activity. It should be avoided after a heavy meal, consumption of alcohol, or an argument. The client should feel rested and relaxed, not tense or tired.

There are other modifications and adaptations a professional such as a nurse can suggest that may be helpful in engaging in sexual activity (Cooper, 1986; Davis, 1981; Haas et al, 1979). The nondyspneic partner may be encouraged to assume a more active role. The position utilized may be a consideration. Two positions are generally comfortable regardless of which person has respiratory disease: the side-lying position and the position with the male seated (on a chair or bedside) and then straddled. Pillows may be used to help position and support the patient to avoid weight on the chest and restriction of breathing. Depending on beliefs of each individual, changes in position or role may have different meanings, which may be more or less easily assimilated. Some clients find a waterbed facilitates coitus because active movement of the partner moves the client with little effort expended by the client.

Diaphragmatic breathing with exhaling through pursed lips for several minutes before engaging in sexual activity may prove helpful because it increases oxygen saturation. Exercise tolerance may be improved by using an aerosol bronchodilator before or during sexual activity. In addition to decreasing hypoxia, oxygen helps to decrease anxiety. It is suggested that the flow of oxygen be increased 1 liter during sexual activity if not contraindicated by the client's physician (Davis, 1981). Although clients may feel inhibited by the use of bronchodilators and oxygen, professionals can assist clients to accept whatever safe measures promote a fulfilling sexual relationship.

Environmental control is important, especially for the asthmatic. Allergens and other precipitants of attacks should be identified and eliminated as much as possible. Choosing familiar surroundings with a comfortable room temperature and level of humidity is helpful. The ideal room temperature is 68° F with 40 per cent humidity (Curgian and Gronkiewicz, 1988). Hygiene and cosmetic products must be considered as possible irritants. Medical precipitants of shortness of breath such as infection or cardiac disease need to be treated.

A professional such as a nurse can be instrumental in assisting the client and partner to each understand their own sexual role and the limits and possibilities of it. Since the client's adjustment will be affected by the attitudes, beliefs, and perceptions of the partner, discussion of sexuality and sexual activity should include both the respiratory client and partner. The concerns of the client and partner should be addressed on their level. It is important to dispel ignorance and correct misinformation. Such discussion helps to decrease fears and may also promote awareness of the acceptability of their conception of their own sexuality. Partners may need to be reassured that sexual activity need not be avoided, can increase the quality of life, and can contribute to both partners' feeling loved and important.

Alternative forms of sexual gratifications may be employed if mutually pleasing and acceptable to client and partner, since intercourse is only one aspect of sexual expression. Caressing, embracing, cuddling, and open communication are other forms of expression that are less fatiguing and anxiety producing and should be encouraged. An important factor in client adjustment to respiratory disease is a supportive spouse or significant other.

It is also helpful for the nurse or health professional to examine what other factors may be adversely affecting sexual function and, when possible, to minimize them (Stockdale-Woolley, 1983). This may be accomplished by optimizing nutritional status, treating other medical problems, altering drug regimens to decrease side effects, providing education regarding changes with aging and sexual potential, and promoting performance of reconditioning exercises to increase exercise and respiratory muscle endurance. If applicable, vocational rehabilitation can improve a client's sense of self-concept.

Support groups can assist both clients and families in dealing with respiratory disease. Support groups vary, depending on the degree of involvement of a health professional. The purposes of such groups generally are to provide education, skills, coping techniques, encouragement, and support. Members share helpful hints on how to deal more effectively with some of the everyday problems of living with respiratory disturbances. Clients sometimes do not realize there are others who experience the same problems. Communicating with individuals with similar experiences helps lighten the burden and often provides laughter as well. Identification with such a group can provide a sense of belonging and decrease isolation and alienation for both client and family. Information on existing support groups can be obtained by contacting the American Lung Association, the Cystic Fibrosis Foundation, and the American Cancer Society. It is an important role of the nurse to share with clients information regarding the existence of support groups and the benefits they can provide.

Counseling needs to be individualized for each client. For the client with genitourinary TB or CF, specific counseling is indicated regarding the effects of disease on sterility. In addition, clients with CF and their partners should have genetic counseling. Haas and associates (1979) recommend further psychotherapy or sexual counseling if sexual dysfunction seems to be related to either a long-standing problem or to underlying psychopathology.

SUMMARY

Respiratory disease may affect sexual function through a variety of mechanisms. Individuals can continue to enjoy sexual activity, particularly with specific modifications. Nurses may be instrumental in assisting individuals to adapt to their respiratory disease and its psychosocial and sexual effects. By discussing sexual function with individuals with respiratory disturbances, the scope of the problem can be further defined. Information gained from discussion can guide suggestions to clients and partners to maintain and promote sexual activity.

REFERENCES

Abram HS: The psychology of chronic illness. J Chronic Dis 25:659, 1972.

Agle DP, Baum GL: Psychological aspects of chronic obstructive pulmonary disease. Med Clin North Am 61:749–758, 1977.

American Cancer Society: 1988 Cancer Facts and Figures. New York, American Cancer Society, 1988.

American Lung Association: Synopsis on recent trends on chronic lung disease. Statistics from the Epidemiology and Statistics Unit. New York, American Lung Association, 1982.

Anderson CJ: Sexuality in the aged. J Gerontol Nurs 1:6–10, 1975.

Brissette S, Zinman R, Fielding M, Reidy M: Nursing care plan for adolescents and young adults with advanced cystic fibrosis. Issues Compr Pediatr Nurs 10:87–97, 1987.

Buck MH: Self-concept: Theory and development. In Roy SC (ed): Introduction to Nursing—An Adaptation Model. Englewood Cliffs, Prentice Hall, 1984.

Campbell ML: Sexual dysfunction in the COPD patient. DCCN/Dimen Crit Care Nurs 6:70–74, 1987.

Coffman CB, Levine SB, Althof SE, Stern RC: Sexual adaptation among single young adults with cystic fibrosis. Chest 86:412–418, 1984.

Cooper D: Sexual counseling of the patient with chronic lung disease. Focus Crit Care 13:18–20, 1986.

Cooper ET: A pilot study on the effects of the diagnosis of lung cancer on family relationships. Ca Nurse 7:301–308, 1984.

Curgian LM: Needs Assessment of the COPD Patient for Discharge. Master's thesis. Yale University School of Nursing, New Haven, CT, 1981.

Curgian LM, Gronkiewicz A: Enhancing sexual performance in COPD. Nurs Pract 13:34–38, 1988.

Davis K: Sexual counseling for the patient with chronic lung disease. Sex Med Today March:10–13, 1981.

di Sant'Agnese PA, Davis PB: Cystic fibrosis in adults. Am J Med 66:121–132, 1979.

Evans JH, Conine TA: Development of sexuality in

children with chronic obstructive pulmonary disease. Resp Care 27:687–692, 1982.

Feldman JM: Effects of tuberculosis on sexual functioning. Med Asp Human Sex 11:29–30, 1977.

Fisher SG: The psychosexual effects of cancer and cancer treatment. Oncol Nurs Forum 10:63–68, 1983.

Fletcher EC, Martin RJ: Sexual dysfunction and erectile impotence in chronic obstructive pulmonary disease. Chest 81:413–421, 1982.

Foote M, Sexton DL, Pawlik L: Dyspnea: A distressing sensation in lung cancer. Oncol Nurs Forum 13:25–31, 1986.

Guenter CA, Welch MH (eds): Pulmonary Medicine. Philadelphia, JB Lippincott, 1982.

Hanson EI: Effects of chronic lung disease on life in general and on sexuality: Perceptions of adult patients. Heart Lung 11:435–441, 1982.

Haas A, Pineda H, Haas F, Axen K: Pulmonary Therapy and Rehabilitation: Principles and Practice. Baltimore, Williams & Wilkins, 1979.

Hellerstein HK, Friedman EH: Sexual activity and the postcoronary patient. Med Asp Human Sex 3:70–96, 1969.

Hodson ME: Psychological and social aspects of cystic fibrosis. Practitioner 224:301–303, 1980.

Hogan RM: Human Sexuality: A Nursing Perspective. Norwalk, Appleton-Century-Crofts, 1985.

Karus CA: Tuberculosis: An overview of pathogenesis and prevention. Nurs Pract 8:21–28, 1983.

Kass I, Updegraff K, Muffly RB: Sex in chronic obstructive pulmonary disease. Med Asp Human Sex 6:33–42, 1972.

Kolodny RC, Masters WH, Johnson VE: Textbook of Sexual Medicine. Boston, Little, Brown & Co, 1979.

Lamb MA, Woods NF: Sexuality and the cancer patient. Ca Nurs 4:137–144, 1981.

Larter N: Cystic fibrosis. Am J Nurs 81:527–532, 1981.

Leiber L, Plumb MM, Gerstenzang ML, Holland J: The communication of affection between cancer patients and their spouses. Psychosom Med 38:379–389, 1976.

Levine SB, Stern RC: Sexual function in cystic fibrosis. Chest 81:422–428, 1982.

Munro BH, Sexton DL: Personal communication. May 1988.

Narayan M, Ferranti R: Nerve conduction impairment in patients with respiratory insufficiency and severe chronic hypoxemia. Arch Phys Med Rehabil 59:188–192, 1978.

National Center for Health Statistics: National Health Interview Survey, U.S. Series 10, No. 164, 1986.

Nolan T, Desmond K, Herlich R, Hardy S: Knowledge of cystic fibrosis in patients and their parents. Pediatrics 77:229–235, 1986.

Petty TL (ed): Chronic Obstructive Pulmonary Disease. New York, Marcel Dekker, 1978.

Roy C: The Roy Adaptation Model. In Riehl JP, Roy C (eds): Conceptual Models for Nursing Practice. 2nd ed. Norwalk, Appleton-Century-Crofts, 1980.

Sexton DL: Chronic Obstructive Pulmonary Disease—Care of the Child and Adult. St. Louis, CV Mosby, 1981.

Sexton DL, Munro BH: Impact of a husband's chronic illness (COPD) on the spouse's life. Res Nurs Health 8:83–90, 1985.

Sexton DL, Munro BH: Living with a chronic illness: The experience of women with chronic obstructive pulmonary disease. West J Nurs Res 10:26–44, 1988.

Shipes E, Lehr S: Sexuality and the male cancer patient. Ca Nurs 5:375–381, 1982.

Shomaker DM: Integration of physiological and socio-cultural factors as a basis for sex education to the elderly. J Gerontol Nurs 6:311–318, 1980.

Steinke EE, Bergen MB: Sexuality and aging. J Gerontol Nurs 12:6–10, 1986.

Stockdale-Woolley R: Sexual dysfunction and COPD: Problems and management. Nurse Pract 8:16–20, 1983.

Straus S, Dudley DL: Sexual activity for asthmatics—A psychiatric perspective. Med Asp Human Sex 10:63–64, 1976.

Taussig LM, Cohen M, Sieber OF: Psychosexual and psychosocial aspects of cystic fibrosis. Med Asp Human Sex 10:101–102, 1976.

Tedrow MP: Interdependence: Theory and development. In Roy SC (ed): Introduction to Nursing—An Adaptation Model. Englewood Cliffs, Prentice Hall, 1984.

Thompson JM: Respiratory system. In Thompson JM, McFarland GK, Hirsch JE, et al (eds): Clinical Nursing. St. Louis, CV Mosby, 1986.

Woods NF: Human Sexuality in Health and Illness. St. Louis, CV Mosby, 1984.

20: Spinal Cord Conditions and Sexuality

Carol Sackett

The spinal cord and the autonomic nervous system can be affected by trauma, disease, and congenital anomalies. Because the nervous system is the "electrical" network that stimulates our bodies to function, interference anywhere in its central or peripheral tracts can cause "short circuits" that lead to malfunction of the nerves distal to the anomaly present. The majority of the nerves associated with sexual functioning are located in the sacral region of the spinal cord, the most distal portion, so *any* dysfunction of the spinal cord or autonomic system has the potential for affecting some aspect of the sexual response.

The care involved with persons who have anomalies involving the spinal cord is complex and comprehensive and involves not only the physical aspects but also cognitive, emotional, and psychological ones. Because sexuality and sexual functioning are basic to our daily lives, nurses must include these in the care and education of the client with an anomaly of the spinal cord.

Spinal cord injuries (SCI) and meningomyelocele have been selected as examples of acquired and congenital interferences in spinal cord function. The individual who is rendered paraplegic by disease or injury usually is at least a young adult who already has experienced physical, intellectual, psychological, and emotional stages of growth and development prior to the disability. However, the child with a congenital disability begins, as a neonate, the long process of growth and development with the added burdens associated with the disability. The child begins a process of habilitation, while the adult is faced with rehabilitation. While both may have many physical manifestations in common, different approaches for nursing care are indicated for each.

MENINGOMYELOCELE

Spina bifida is a defect in the embryological development of the vertebral bodies of the spinal column and/or the spinal cord itself. There is no known cause for this congenital defect. Approximately 40 per cent of the population is born with spina bifida *occulta,* which is a failure of one or more of the vertebral bodies to fuse; no dysfunction occurs as a result of this, and the defect is not evident externally. In one of every 1000 live births an infant is born with spina bifida *cystica,* evident by the presence of a fluid-filled sac, usually on the lower back because the lumbosacral area of the spine is the most common site for this defect. Four per cent of these infants have a meningocele. In this instance the vertebral bodies at the site of the sac have not fused, but the spinal cord has developed normally; however, the sac may contain nerve roots. This results in varying degrees of muscle weakness in the lower extremities and, frequently, bowel and bladder dysfunction.

Ninety-six per cent of infants born with

spina bifida cystica have a meningomyelocele, which can have severe neurological manifestations. The vertebral bodies do not fuse in the area of the sac, the neural plate does not form a normal spinal cord, and the defective portion of the cord is contained within the sac. The neurological deficits include muscle weakness below the defect, sensory losses below the defect, bowel and bladder incontinence, and hydrocephalus in 70 per cent of the cases.

It is important to note that health professionals today are faced with the habilitation of children with more severe manifestations of the meningomyelocele than 25 years ago. Prior to the 1960s no treatment was available for hydrocephalus, and the management of bladder dysfunction was not so successful. Thus, children with severe hydrocephalus and/or renal failure resulting from dysfunctional bladders frequently died, often before reaching adolescence. The first implantable mechanical shunts for the drainage and reabsorption of the excess cerebral spinal fluid were introduced in the early 1960s, so more children born since then have reached adolescence and adulthood. The introduction in the 1970s of intermittent catheterization for the management of neuropathic bladders has diminished the potential for renal failure, which in the past had resulted from chronic urinary tract infections and/or from chronic obstruction of the kidneys by a bladder that would not empty spontaneously. The children, adolescents, and adults with meningomyelocele today are survivors who have more profound physical disabilities, so the process of habilitation is much more complex.

The meningomyelocele forms within 30 days after conception, perhaps before the mother even knows she is pregnant. Any pregnant woman can have a serum alpha-fetoprotein (AFP) level drawn between the fifteenth and seventeenth weeks of pregnancy. The maternal serum AFP procedure is a screening tool and is *not* diagnostic; an elevation in the serum AFP is an indication that further screening may be necessary, and frequently it is repeated. If the level is still elevated, an abdominal ultrasonogram and/or amniocentesis are often recommended for the diagnosis of a specific congenital defect. If the amniotic AFP level is high, it can be an indication of the presence of an open defect of the spinal cord. The ultrasonogram can detect the presence of the sac on the back and/or hydrocephalus, if present, in a fetus with spina bifida. Unless these studies have been performed prenatally and a diagnosis of congenital defect has been made, the prospective parents await the birth of their child with excited anticipation of its being perfect. When the child is born with a defect such as meningomyelocele, the parents must begin the process of mourning the loss of their perfect child. Eventually, they will need to accept that this infant is a child first, who happens to be handicapped. Acceptance is a serious, emotionally draining process that takes much time and effort to accomplish. Health professionals often spend days, weeks, months, perhaps years helping the nuclear and extended families see their child as a child with many abilities, who happens also to have complex disabilities.

Meningomyelocele and Sexual Function

Table 20–1 shows the physical manifestations of the neurological deficits of meningomyelocele and has implications for psychosexual development and subsequent sexual functioning. The degree of each manifestation differs with each child and depends on the location of the defect on the spinal cord and the severity of nerve damage. These manifestations can range from mild to severe in each child. For instance, a child with sacral level meningomyelocele may have incontinence of bowel and bladder only, while one with a thoracolumbar defect may exhibit the full range of manifestations as outlined in the Table 20–1. The goals of the health care team include (1) the provision of emotional and psychological support to the family as they incorporate the child into their family life; (2) helping the child to attain his highest level of physical, intellectual, emotional, psychosocial, and psychological functioning; (3) the promotion of self-care and independence to include as many activities of daily life as possible; and (4) the promotion of the psychosexual development of the child. The health care team should be multidisciplinary and include nurses, physical therapist, occupational therapist, social worker, psychologist, pediatrician, orthopedic surgeon, urologist, and neurosurgeon. Because most of the children with meningomyelocele do not live near the medical center at which they receive their specialized care, local health

TABLE 20–1. Manifestations of Meningomyelocele

Manifestation	Assessment and Treatment	Outcome
Hydrocephalus	Ventriculoperitoneal shunt, periodic replacements of shunt.	Normal IQ to varying degrees of retardation.
	Parent education to monitor for signs of increased intracranial pressure and/or shunt malfunction.	Potential for (minimal) brain damage secondary to hydrocephalus, meningitis, or shunt infections. Deficits manifest as learning disabilities (e.g., spatial-perceptual reasoning, visual-perceptual problems, visual-sequencing memory).
	Periodic ultrasound or CT scans of head to assess ventricular size.	
	Periodic neurological assessment for symptoms of tethered cord.	
	Periodic ophthalmological evaluations. Squint (crossed eyes) and optic atrophy can result from untreated hydrocephalus (e.g., in utero).	Correction of ophthalmological dysfunction by eyeglasses or surgery, if indicated.
Sensory deficits (lower trunk and lower extremities)	Parent/child education to teach concepts related to sensory loss of lower extremities and potential for skin breakdown and assessment of legs on regular basis for areas of trauma (e.g., bath water), friction, and/or pressure (e.g., shoes, braces, sitting).	Preventive measures and surveillance will diminish chances for skin breakdown.
	Management of skin irritation and/or breakdown.	
Motor deficits (lower trunk, and lower extremities)	Promotion of mobility by prevention of obesity; passive and active exercise of hips, knees, ankles to prevent contractures and to strengthen muscles; bracing to support weak muscles and prevent contractures.	Protection and support of musculoskeletal system. Prevention of muscle contractures. Upright mobility, which also promotes physical, psychological, and psychosocial development.
	Surgery to correct spinal deformities due to inequities of muscle strength.	Prevention of osteoporosis.
	Wheelchair mobility might be necessary by midteens for child with high lumbar or thoracic lesions, when mobility more difficult and limiting with braces.	
Neuropathic bladder	Surveillance of urinary tract by periodic assessment of urine and radiographic evaluation of kidneys and bladder.	Prevention of urinary tract infections and renal complications secondary to neuropathic bladder.
	Urodynamic evaluation to assess neurological status of bladder.	Continence of urine.
	Clean intermittent catheterization.	
	Anticholinergic medication to prevent bladder spasms and decrease bladder pressures.	
Neuropathic bowel	Surveillance of bowel function to prevent constipation.	Prevention of constipation. Promotion of continence.
	Education concerning diet and fluid intake.	Decreased incidence of bladder infections.
	Promotion of regular evacuation of rectum by diet and medication.	

care personnel are relied on to promote parenting skills, foster normal growth and development, and complement the care provided by the multidisciplinary team at the medical center.

Effects of Meningomyelocele on Adaptation

PHYSIOLOGICAL

The earliest "survivors" of aggressive, comprehensive neonatal care are just reaching adolescence and young adulthood. As yet, no one really knows the range of physiological sexual capabilities of these young adults, who have reached this stage of life with more severe neurological deficits than any person ever before. There are no published studies that discuss the neurological effects of meningomyelocele on sexual functioning per se. Cass, Bloom, and Luxemberg interviewed 47 young adults with meningomyelocele who were over 16 years old to ascertain their sexual functioning. They identified functional motor levels and the sexual activities practiced by those at each level, associated with methods of urinary control, and concluded that "most . . . had satisfactory sexual function" (Cass, Bloom, and Luxemberg, 1986, p 426). Even though sexual activity was related to the functional level of those interviewed, neither physical assessment to determine the clients' *potential* for function nor psychosocial variables were considered. Because of the asymmetry of the neurological deficits, it would be difficult to predict function or dysfunction in the male adolescent. However, history of erections and/or nocturnal emissions as well as a neurological examination could indicate whether a male child will be able to engage in penovaginal intercourse, and a semen analysis would ascertain his fertility. A controlled prospective study of male adolescents is needed. Regarding female adolescents, it is thought that like females with traumatic paraplegia pregnancy and childbirth are possible; most have very limited sensation in the areas of the labia, perineum, and rectum, so clitoral stimulation may not be rewarding. However, erogenous zones in other parts of the body can be identified. The effects of meningomyelocele would make a woman a high-risk obstetrical client, for example, with increased risk for urinary tract infections; however, with comprehensive medical supervision, the capability for pregnancy and vaginal delivery is present.

PSYCHOLOGICAL

The neonate with meningomyelocele usually receives intensive treatment in the hospital, often having to be transferred to a medical center from a local hospital within hours after birth. During this initial admission, the back lesion is closed. Frequently, the neonate must lie in a prescribed position in an isolette for weeks during the postoperative period to avoid stress on the suture line. This initial hospitalization often lasts from 4 to 8 weeks, during which time the family may not even be able to hold their baby normally, much less cuddle him or her. The bonding process, which is the first step in the development of sexuality, is inevitably delayed. Family members are grieving; they feel angry, hurt, resentful, and guilty and often look for a cause for the defect. They wish to affix blame on someone within the family or on some event that occurred prior to or during the pregnancy. At a time when solidarity is crucial, the family is stressed severely.

The health professional needs to support family members through the grieving process and to help them come to understand that no one knows what causes meningomyelocele and that there was no way to prevent it. Initial counseling should focus on the interactions between the parents and the child during the neonatal period, promoting bonding, despite the physical constraints, by encouraging touching, talking to, and feeding the infant.

Throughout the formative years, the child and family are seen frequently as outpatients for physical and occupational therapy as well as for orthopedic, neurosurgical, and urological evaluations and treatments. Readmissions to the hospital for elective orthopedic procedures and shunt revisions are common, so the various members of the team have many opportunities to become well acquainted with the child and some members of the family. During the early months, counseling should focus on interactions of the child within the family, as these are the bases from which sexuality develops within the young child. This is extremely difficult for the parents because in addition to any stresses present within the family prior to the birth of the child they are accepting their handicapped child. They are being taught how to carry out many physical treatments with their child while being told to incorporate the child as a functional member of the family—to treat the child as normally as possible.

Assuming that the milestones discussed previously have been achieved, the child with meningomyelocele must experience adolescence, that emotional merry-go-round of hormonal and physical upheaval. The adolescent years are tumultuous ones for all pubescent youngsters and for their families. The child with meningomyelocele has the added burden of looking different from his peers because of his braces, as well as of having to cope with bowel and bladder management and problems with mobility. The child with meningomyelocele develops secondary sex characteristics within the same time frame as the nonhandicapped child. Although not borne out by statistics, clinical experience suggests that this development appears earlier in children who have shunts for hydrocephalus; some girls begin their menstrual periods as early as 9 or 10 years of age (Passo, 1978; Parsons, 1972). This is the time when a second dichotomy appears: The child has "blossomed" physically, yet *many* parents still have not acknowledged that their child is pubescent and continue to treat the child as a youngster, thwarting the potential for independence. Health professionals may unconsciously support this behavior by continuing to address the parents during a clinic visit, rather than focusing attention on the child. Frequently, this has been the pattern within the family for so long that it is difficult to draw such children into a conversation because they literally look to the parents to respond to any questions directed at them.

Intervention

The parents of a child with meningomyelocele must be encouraged to develop the child's abilities to the fullest, and this encouragement must begin in the neonatal period. It is difficult for families to avoid preoccupation with treatments because exercises, braces, and the management of the bowels and bladder are ongoing and time consuming. However, parents must be encouraged to identify and focus on the child's abilities

and to foster normal growth and development. Because of physical limitations and possible visual perceptual problems, developmental milestones might be *delayed,* but they are attainable. If, because of continued infantilization and/or overprotection, children are delayed unnecessarily from passing through the physical, emotional, intellectual, psychosocial, and psychological stages of development, their potential sexuality will be affected significantly, as the various aspects of sexuality are progressive and cumulative from infancy. The utilization of specific instruction from the therapists and available booklets on growth and development can assist parents to integrate developmental activities into daily activities, including periods of specific treatments. Mobility is imperative for growth and development, as is the enhancement of the senses of touch, taste, and smell. The Spina Bifida Association of America (SBAA) has published *Straight Talk . . . Parent to Parent,* which gives specific suggestions to parents concerning "games" to use for the stimulation of the senses (Pieper, 1977).

As toddlers become mobile, albeit with braces and cruches or a walker for assistance, they should become involved with their own care. All parents fall into the trap of performing the care themselves because it is easier (and faster), even more so when the child's daily care requires so much time. Nurses must attempt to alter this behavior before it becomes habitual. It takes more time when *any* children attempt to do things for themselves, but it is to the detriment of the children if they are not encouraged to do whatever they can for themselves. The nurse might have to provide some specific suggestions to the parents. For instance, if children cannot put *on* coats without assistance, let them take them *off;* a parent might start the process of zipping a jacket and let the child complete the task; the child can be taught the parts of the body while learning to bathe in the bathtub. A toddler can be taught to set the table for a meal: A basket for a tricycle can be attached to a walker; the child can then place items in the basket and carry them to the table. These small achievements give the child positive feelings of confidence and self-worth and promote the development of a positive self-concept and self-esteem, the building blocks of sexuality and future independence.

The health professional must assess the

effects of siblings and the extended family on the growth and development of the child. Frequently, siblings, grandparents, and others undermine the best laid plans of the parents perhaps because they feel sorry for the child. Unfortunately, social stereotypes of disabilities permeate all relationships within and outside the family. The child frequently is seen as crippled and is subject to different considerations from the rest of the family and by others in the community as well. As with nondisabled children, disabled children must be taught behavioral skills, and they must learn to accept the consequences of their behavior. The family must not have a different set of rules for the disabled child.

If children are prevented from achieving developmental milestones, which include socialization, their "rehearsal for life" will be impeded and their potential for independence severely diminished. Despite the best efforts of health professionals, many handicapped persons *continue* to be subjected to parental control of activities, feelings, and thoughts. The family may expect little of the children, allowing them to manipulate the family and to behave in ways that would be unacceptable outside the home. Social skills have a direct effect on sexuality as well as on the ability of children to form meaningful interpersonal relationships as they mature.

The child's ability to develop interpersonal relationships may be hampered and limited because opportunities for interactions with people outside the family are limited. Interpersonal relationships are another milestone in the development of a positive self-image. Unless interactions outside the home are encouraged, the child may learn only those social skills required within the family. Parents should be encouraged to seek and promote experiences for their child with nondisabled children to foster the development of interpersonal relationships. In the preschool years, educational day care programs, church activities, and play opportunities with neighborhood children should be encouraged. Educational day care experiences, e.g., Head Start programs, can provide much needed stimulation for the growth and development of the child who is handicapped. Young, nondisabled children are not judgmental and are more accepting of children with differences, thus creating a positive experience in socialization for the child with a handicap as well as for the nonhandicapped child.

Public Law 94–142, which was implemented in 1976, provided the mechanism for the education of handicapped children in classrooms with their nonhandicapped peers. Prior to this, children with physical disabilities either were improperly placed in classrooms, for example, with severely mentally retarded youngsters, or were not in school at all. The enactment of this law has done much to increase the skills of independence and to promote the development and maturation of handicapped children. Without these opportunities the child would lack self-esteem, self-confidence, and the psychosocial and psychosexual skills that adolescents need. Because of the potential for learning disabilities, which frequently go unrecognized in the school setting, preschool testing for cognitive abilities and organic dysfunction by a psychologist is recommended, so that any disabilities can be identified; the psychologist can communicate findings to the school so the child can receive individualized assistance to achieve the highest potential despite the disability. If the learning needs are not met appropriately, the child may perform very poorly in school, which would contribute significantly to the undermining of self-confidence and self-image.

BLADDER AND BOWEL MANAGEMENT

Prior to the advent of intermittent catheterization for bladder management and specific protocols for bowel management, children and adults with meningomyelocele wore diapers (or condom-type external catheters for boys), utilized indwelling catheters, or had their urine diverted surgically through an ostomy. These children and adults had chronic urinary tract infections, they were wet, and they smelled of urine-soaked diapers or clothing and/or incontinent stool. Earlier studies revealed that this aspect of disability frequently is more distressing than any other. Incontinence of urine and stool is one of the greatest detriments to habilitation or rehabilitation. Incontinence—or fear of it—causes feelings of misery and is a major contributing factor to social isolation. Who can have positive feelings about themselves or about their potential as a sexual being or be comfortable with sexual activity if they are incontinent (Kolin et al, 1971; Dorner, 1977a; Gartley, 1985)?

The advent of clean, intermittent self-catheterization has had a revolutionary effect on the habilitation of those with meningomyelocele. By the age of 4 or 5, at least, all children are free of diapers and managed by intermittent catheterization. Some medical centers institute this protocol routinely when the children are between 12 and 24 months of age. Others wait until the children are 4 or 5 years old, unless medically indicated earlier; those following this protocol feel that promotion of mobility and attainment of growth and developmental milestones should take precedence during the toddler years and that instituting intermittent catheterization adds another responsibility to the parents' daily routine. Catheterization is just one more thing that the parents, since they have been doing it themselves, are reluctant to delegate to the child when it is appropriate. By age 5 children are excited about wearing normal underclothing and, in many cases, are capable of being independent with self-catheterization, requiring little supervision. While all of the boys can do self-catheterization at this age, many of the girls cannot pass their own catheters because of the limitations of bracing and/or problems with eye-hand coordination. Even though clean, intermittent self-catheterization has been utilized for more than 10 years, many physicians and nurses are unfamiliar with the protocol and its concepts, so it is imperative that information about this protocol be communicated to the local health professional, and that specific arrangements be made with the child's school. Some states do not have school nurses, so school personnel must, by law, provide for the catheterization of the child at school.

Although initially all of the children are excited about being dry and out of diapers, during adolescence many of the youngsters enter a stage of noncompliance when they do not seem to care whether they miss catheterizations and get wet; this has become a significant issue in many families. It appears to be a manifestation of adolescent rebellion; it is incongruous because it appears at a time when the children are most conscious of how they appear to others, so this behavior could also be a reflection of low self-esteem and/or anger (Hayden, 1979).

Historically, incontinence of stool has been a shameful experience (Hayden, 1979). While the bowels of some children can be trained by fluid, diet, and regular toileting habits, most children need medication such as bisacodyl enemas or suppositories for a more complete and predictable evacuation of the rectum. There is a correlation between incomplete evacuation and increased incidence of bladder infections. A few children have minimal or no rectal tone, which makes control of incontinence very difficult. In any case, each child presents a unique set of problems, and each must be assessed and managed according to the specific problems.

The health professional must take the initiative when it comes to discussion of sexuality in the adolescent. It must be a conscious effort because professionals get so involved with their particular focus, such as problems with the braces or the catheterization protocol, that important aspects of sexuality and sex education are often forgotten. Adolescent sexuality is a Pandora's box for all teenagers, but the child with meningomyelocele has even more needs in relation to his appearance, socialization with peers, and mobility. Because socialization might be affected by geographical and mobility issues, for instance, the professional must assist the teenager and family to overcome these by providing the teenager with opportunities to be with peers (Sherman, Berling, and Oppenheimer, 1985). Social isolation from peers has been identified as a major factor in adolescent adjustment and frequently results in an overriding depression (Castree and Walker, 1981; Dorner, 1975, 1976, 1977a). Encouraging adolescents to invite friends to visit them at home and to utilize the phone to communicate with peers are two examples of socialization without much physical effort, which may need to be communicated specifically. Encouraging families to install hand-controls on the family car will facilitate mobility. Although this suggestion should come from the drivers' education personnel in the schools, frequently parents must advocate for this specifically, or the teenager is apt to be overlooked by the school.

Privacy is an important issue for everyone. Because all youngsters with meningomyelocele continue to need some physical assistance, the need for privacy must be addressed as a specific issue. The SBAA has published a booklet for teenagers (*By, For, and With Young Adults with Spina Bifida*) that discusses typical adolescent issues, such as privacy, acceptance, and popularity; it also offers suggestions about how teenagers can explain their disabilities to peers (Pieper, 1979). This and other publications are available from the SBAA, 1700 Rockville Pike, Suite 540, Rockville, MD 20852, for minimal costs and are recommended reading for health professionals and teenagers and their families.

During adolescence, attention should be paid to the child's potential for employment and/or continued education. Exploration of goals for a vocational future should be addressed with the adolescent, and intellectual and/or aptitude testing should be considered, so that realistic expectations for employment can be pursued (Parsons, 1972). The current literature describes low rates of employment and/or job dissatisfaction for those with meningomyelocele, both of which have been associated with poor quality and quantity of assessment and guidance concerning employment opportunities as well as with problems associated with independence and mobility (Dorner, 1977b; Castree and Walker, 1981).

Unfortunately, few members of the health care team feel like experts when it comes to sexual counseling; specific courses on sexuality have been neglected in the curricula of medical and nursing schools as well as in the course work of students of occupational and physical therapy (Cole, 1975a). Myths and misconceptions about sexuality and the sexual functioning of the physically handicapped still exist. Adolescents (and their parents) *do* contemplate their potential for sexual functioning, marriage, and the parenting of children, despite a continued exhibition of behaviors that foster dependence and an appearance of asexuality (Dorner, 1976, 1977b; Castree and Walker, 1981). However, unless these subjects are introduced by the health professional, they may not be broached by the teenager or the parents.

Sexual counseling of the adolescent with meningomyelocele must include discussion concerning birth control as well as specific suggestions for positions for penovaginal intercourse if the lower extremities are involved severely. (To avoid repetition, the reader is referred to the section on paraplegia for some specific suggestions.) Genetic counseling prior to a planned pregnancy is mandatory; there is a risk that a client with meningomyelocele (male or female) will parent a child with a spinal cord defect. Alpha-fetoprotein levels, with subsequent ultrasonography, would be recommended at the appropriate times in the pregnancy. At the present time abortion is an option if the client does not wish to have a child with meningomyelocele, so the screening evaluations must be done by the sixteenth or seventeenth week if abortion is a consideration.

SPINAL CORD INJURIES

Having presented the unique needs of the child with congenital disabilities, the focus now turns to those associated with acquired lesions of the spinal cord. In contrast to children who were born with congenital disabilities and clients who have gradual onset of sensory and motor paralysis due to a disease process,* individuals who sustain a spinal cord injury (SCI) experience instantaneously the most profound and complex insults to their total being. Suddenly, they are changed from active, independent individuals to immobile and dependent ones. An injury to the spinal cord alters every aspect of daily living: physical, psychological, occupational, personal, and recreational. Nursing plays a pivotal role in the care, counsel, and education of clients with SCI, utilizing the nursing process to its fullest. In addition, frequently it is the nurses' responsibility to coordinate the other members of a multidisciplinary team who are involved with the care of these clients.

Although specific disease processes such as multiple sclerosis can affect the spinal cord or peripheral nerves, causing paralysis, trauma is the major cause. Motor vehicular accidents are the leading cause, followed by falls, diving accidents, job-related accidents, gunshot wounds, and sports-related accidents. Considerably more males than females sustain paralytic cord injuries, and those injured most often are between the ages of 15 and 29. Approximately 30 per cent of spinal cord injuries are at the cervical level, most often due to diving accidents; of the remaining 70 per cent, more injuries are sustained in the lumbar area of the cord because the spine does not have the added stability afforded by the ribs (Larrabee, 1977; Eyster, 1986).

Definition

Injuries of the cervical portion of the spinal cord cause quadriplegia, in which motor and

---

*The reader should remember that any illness that affects the spinal cord or peripheral nerves, such as diabetes or multiple sclerosis, can also affect sexuality and sexual functioning. Although neurological deficits might not be as evident or as severe as in an SCI, these clients have definite needs for evaluation and counsel.

TABLE 20–2. Functional Potential of Client with Spinal Cord Injuries

Level	Shoulder	Elbow	Wrist	Hand	Hip	Knee	Ankle	Foot	Self-care	Wheelchair Management	Transfers	Gait
C₁–C₃ (no sensation below neck)	Paralysis of diaphragm and respiratory muscles; requires respirator.											
									Has No Trunk Support			
C₄ (no sensation below clavicle)									Using mouth-stick: type, turn pages, use telephone.	Electrical wheelchair required.		
C₅ (no sensation below clavicle)	Min	Min							Type, feed self with assistance device, if food placed.	Hand projections on wheels, manipulate brakes, push on flat surface.		
C₆ (most common cervical injury; no sensation below clavicle)	Part	Part	Min						Drink, wash face, shave, brush hair, dress upper torso, sit up/lie down in bed, write with hand splints.	Hand projections on wheels, remove armrests and footplates, push on sloped surface, turn chair.	Chair↔bed Chair↔car ? Needs use of sliding board	
C₇	Comp	Comp	Part	Min					Turn in bed, dress self, perform skin care.	Pick up objects from floor, move over uneven surface, "bounce" over small elevation.	Chair↔toilet Chair↔chair ? Chair↔bath	Fully braced can stand in parallel bars.
C₈	Comp	Comp	Comp	Part					Bladder and bowel care	Negotiate curbs and ramps	Chair↔bath	Fully braced can swing-to in bars.
									Partial Trunk Support			
T₁–T₇ (no sensation below diaphragm)	Comp	Comp	Comp	Comp					Independent	Independent, "wheelies," put wheelchair in car.	Independent, chair↔floor	Braced to pelvis, can swing-to in bars.

Level							Full Trunk Support			
T₈–T₁₂	Comp	Comp	Comp	Comp			Independent	Independent, wheelchair sports, uses wheelchair primarily.	Independent	Braced to pelvis, can swing-to on crutches; household ambulator
L₁–L₃ (sensation to hips and knees)	Comp	Comp	Comp	Part	Min		Independent	Independent, uses wheelchair only part-time.	Independent	Independent with lower leg braces and forearm crutches; can use public transport during off-hours.
L₄ (sensation to hips and knees)	Comp	Comp	Comp	Part	Part	Part	Independent	Not needed		Short leg braces; occasionally needs cane.
L₅ (no sensation of sex organs deficit noticed)	Comp	Comp	Comp	Comp	Part	Part	Independent	Not needed		No orthotics.
S₁ (no sensation of sex organs deficit noticed)	Comp	Comp	Comp	Comp	Comp	Comp	Independent	Not needed		No orthotics.

Comp = complete function; Min = minimal function; Part = partial function
(Adapted from Bromley, 1981; Weinberg, 1982; Wittman, 1986)

sensory deficits occur from the neck and shoulder downward. Injuries to the cord below the cervical level cause paraplegia, with motor and sensory deficits from the midtorso down, depending on the level at which the cord has been traumatized. Injuries of the cauda equina do not cause paraplegia but affect the motor and sensory innervation of the sacral nerves, which are involved with bowel, bladder, and sexual function. Complete transection of the spinal cord is the exception rather than the rule, so there can be an unequal residual distribution of motor and sensory levels for all SCI clients; however, this inequity rarely improves the functional level of the client. (Note: Levels of SCI mentioned in this text refer to the levels of the spinal cord, *not* to the vertebral levels of the spinal column, e.g., the cord ends and the cauda equina begin at the L_1 vertebral level.)

Effects of Spinal Cord Injury on Adaptation

PHYSIOLOGICAL

For a minimum of 8 weeks after the trauma, the client is neurologically in a state of "spinal shock" during which all nerves below the level of the SCI are without response due to the effects of the trauma. The permanent neurological status of the client cannot be determined until the "spinal shock" has resolved completely, which can take up to 2 years. Therefore, a client's full potential cannot be realized until that time; the exception to this occurs when the spinal cord is transected. In this instance the residual strengths and deficits are predictable. To help the reader grasp the impact and significance of an SCI, Table 20–2 shows the functional potential of clients with injuries to various levels of the spinal cord. Rehabilitation of a client with such losses includes physical, psychological, social, spiritual, and sexual issues—a reworking of a lifelong accumulation of experiences.

The sexual response is the synergistic, coordinated stimulation of the cerebral cortex, spinal cord, peripheral pathways, and the reflex centers; spinal cord trauma affects all but the cerebral cortex, so all SCI clients experience some degree of sexual dysfunction. In a noninjured male or female the sexual response is a synergistic event involving both psychogenic and physiological stimuli and responses. In the client with an SCI there has been trauma to the nerves that provide the physiological responses, so this synergism may no longer exist. Because the majority of SCIs do not involve a complete transection of the cord, some afferent and efferent responses below the lesion level are intact; the degree of neurophysiological damage depends on (1) the location of the trauma on the cord and (2) the degree of trauma to the cord. In general, if the trauma to the cord is at T_{10} or above, reflex activity will be present following resolution of spinal shock. Because all clients with an SCI have different locations and degrees of trauma, the information in Tables 20–2 to 20–4 can be used *only* as guidelines for health professionals working with clients with SCIs.

Clients with an SCI above the level of T_4 can experience symptoms of autonomic dysreflexia, which is an exaggerated response of the autonomic system by stimuli that cannot be inhibited by the brain (Weinberg, 1982) and which can be a life-threatening emergency. Symptoms of autonomic dysreflexia are extreme hypertension, a pounding headache, bradycardia, and nausea.

Any spinal cord injury has a deleterious effect on the sexual response and functioning of the male client (see Table 20–4). Initially, all male clients will be unable to attain any kind of erection because of the effects of spinal shock, and this must be explained to each client. As the shock resolves, reflex erections may become evident within 6 to 8 weeks after the trauma, but until the shock resolves completely, the quality of the erection cannot be ascertained. The level and completeness of his injury and the result of the digital rectal examination combined with the client's exploration of his own body will demonstrate the ultimate ability of the client to have a functional erection. Because of sensory deficits, he may not be aware that an erection is present unless he looks or feels it with his hands.

A certain percentage of clients are able to ejaculate. Some can ejaculate during penovaginal intercourse, while others must rely on oral stimulation or the use of a vibrator. With some clients who ejaculate, the seminal fluid is propelled retrograde into the bladder, rather than antegrade through the urethra. Neurological dysfunction resulting from the cord trauma accounts for ejaculatory dysfunction.

TABLE 20–3. Outcome of Genital Examination of Male Clients with Spinal Cord Injuries

Lesion Classification	Sensation	Voluntary Control of Rectal Sphincter	Rectal Sphincter Tone	Bulbocavernous Reflex
Complete lesion (transection) with reflex activity	None	No	Yes	Yes
Incomplete lesion with reflex activity	Light	No	Yes	Yes
Complete lesion without reflex activity	None	No	No	No
Incomplete lesion without reflex activity	Partial	No	No	No

Adapted from Comarr and Gunderson, 1975

Orgasm as an isolated entity is not common with male clients (Comarr and Gunderson, 1975). However, both researchers and clients have reported a variety of experiences that they have classified as orgasms in male and female clients (Griffith, Tomko, and Timms, 1973). A sudden increase of lower extremity spasticity is most frequently described, followed by a protracted period of relaxation of these same muscles.

Information regarding the extent to which women have specific neurophysiological interruptions of sexual response is lacking. As with male clients, the incompleteness of most lesions permits individual variations of the sexual response. Reflex activity upon digital examination probably indicates that she will lubricate during the excitement phase of the sexual response. The extent to which female clients have orgasmic difficulties is not known.

It is not uncommon for menses to cease temporarily following an SCI, which probably is related to the physical and emotional stresses associated with the trauma. In most cases menses resume within 6 months. The ability to conceive, to carry a fetus to term, and to deliver vaginally is consistent with the client's preinjury state, unless pelvic trauma sustained with the original injury precludes vaginal delivery.

Although studies that have assessed the sexual functioning of males with SCI have been published, many of them neither adequately define nor control for many of the relevant variables, such as level of injury or the time lapse since injury (Griffith, Tomko, and Timms, 1973; Weinberg, 1982). Because

TABLE 20–4. Potential for Sexual Functioning in Male Clients with Spinal Cord Injuries

Lesion Classification	Erectile Ability	Coitus	Ejaculation	Orgasm
Complete lesion (cord transection) with reflex* activity	Reflexic, spontaneous, and/or by external stimulation of penis; may be unpredictable and/or of short duration, thus not capable of intromission.	70% of those who can achieve erection are able to achieve intromission.	Rare	Rare
Incomplete lesion with reflex* activity	Reflexic, spontaneous, and/or by external stimulation of penis; may be unpredictable and/or of short duration, thus not capable of intromission; if neurological deficits minimal, psychogenic erections possible.	80% of those who can achieve erections are able to achieve intromission.	Depends on extent of neurological deficits.	Rare
Complete lesion with no reflex† activity	Only 25% can attain any kind of erection; erections often very brief and/or of poor quality.	Few can achieve intromission because erections are not firm enough.	Few	Rare
Incomplete lesion with no reflex† activity	83% can achieve psychogenic erections.	90% of those who can achieve erections.	50 to 70% of those who can achieve intromission.	10% of those who can ejaculate.

*Reflex activity indicates lesion level above T_{12} of spinal cord (upper motor neuron).
†Absence of reflex activity indicates lesion level below T_{12} (lower motor neuron).
(Adapted from Comarr and Gunderson, 1975)

the number of women with SCI is so low, it is difficult to study this population. Of those studies that have been done, however, attention has focused only on the reproductive aspects of sexual functioning, with little to no recognition even of the potential for problems with sexuality (Griffith and Trieschmann, 1975; Cole, 1975; Zwerner, 1982). Based on the assumption that the female is a passive partner in a sexual encounter, investigators have assumed that no particular problems exist for the female (Thornton, 1981). Although females *may* have been passive sexual partners in the past, this no longer can or should be assumed. Clearly, controlled studies of male and female clients with SCI need to be done.

SELF-CONCEPT

An examination of Table 20–2 will show the health professional why the self-concept and body image of the client are jeopardized so severely. Body image, the way we see ourselves, is an integral part of our daily lives and is a reflection of the relationships and experiences we have had since infancy. This cumulative image does not change rapidly or easily after an SCI, particularly since the client's body still is intact and does not look any different. Denial is a major operative factor present in the weeks and months following an SCI. Many clients believe they will recover completely and, therefore, are not diligent with their therapy regimens. At the same time, denial is a major coping mechanism for clients, allowing them to deal more slowly with all the losses that eventually must be incorporated into a new body image (Weinberg, 1982). The health professional must support this denial until clients have come to terms with the losses and have identified their residual strengths. Individuals must grieve and accept the loss of parts of their former selves before they can develop a new image. Grieving does not begin until the client realizes that recovery is not possible, that pre-existing concepts of "normal" no longer are viable. Adjustment to an altered body and acceptance of a new self-concept takes time—time during which first the individual must experience denial, realization, anger, and despair (Larrabee, 1977a). All clients must learn to cope with bowel and bladder management, the loss of muscle mass of the affected areas of the body, and the loss of mobility as once known and, in many cases, to adjust to life viewed from a wheelchair. In addition, they may also have to cope with spasticity of the hips and lower extremities.

While the child with a congenital disability grows up with a body image associated with the underdeveloped musculature of his lower extremities, braces, crutches, and wheelchair, all of this is sudden and new to the client with an SCI. The male client may have placed a high value on physical activity as a measure of his manhood. Ever sensitive to the portrayal of the "body beautiful" by the media, clients can be devastated as they compare their paralyzed bodies with the popular image. Though typically in the late teens and twenties at the time of injury, the client with an SCI may not have experienced some of the developmental maturational tasks; this challenge and the temporary regression associated with this new dependency mean that the client will have to re-experience some of these tasks to achieve social and emotional maturity. Acceptance takes *time* and is demonstrated when clients see themselves as worthwhile individuals who have some control over their lives, despite handicaps. Out of this acceptance a new self-concept will emerge.

While the female client may have no dysfunction associated with the reproductive aspects of sexuality and sexual functioning, there are specific issues she must resolve. Like the male client, she, too, will have to grieve the loss of her former body image and build a new concept of herself as a healthy individual who has many assets, despite her handicaps. She will need reassurance that she continues to be a sexual being.

Assessment

A sexual assessment should be included with the initial assessment of the client, during which information is obtained for the formulation with the client of short- and long-term plans of care. Information is obtained about the client's educational level, vocational and recreational interests and practices, and interpersonal support systems; also assessed are wheelchair and transfer abilities, skills for self-care, skin integrity, and bowel and bladder management. Many clients will *not* take the initiative to voice their concerns about sexuality and their potential for sexual functioning. By assessing the client's needs for sex education and counseling at the time physical and interpersonal factors are examined, the health professional is giving the client permission to express these concerns as well as the assurance that these issues will be addressed with physical ones. The health professional should be a sensitive and nonjudgmental listener.

The sexual assessment should include (1) the client's knowledge and understanding of the human sexual response, including basic anatomy and physiology; (2) attitudes and feelings about sexuality and sexual functioning; (3) a history of pretrauma sexual experiences, including pre-existing erectile or orgasmic difficulties experienced by the client and/or partner; (4) the client's awareness of sexual feelings, erections, ejaculation, and orgasm since injury; and (5) sexual activities attempted since trauma. The clients' knowledge of their current abilities may be inaccurate because of a lack of knowledge of the normal sexual response and/or because they have not yet explored their own potential. Frequently, so much physical and emotional energy has been used in the struggle to acknowledge their new selves, they may not have focused on sexual capabilities, particularly if the health professional is working with the client within the first 12 months after the trauma. It is advisable to include in the assessment, education, and counseling the client's spouse or partner, who needs to learn more about the associated disabilities. Inclusion of the partner can serve to stimulate communication between the couple, to allow for discussion of fears and problems, and to enhance the physical and emotional support given by the partner, leading to a more positive outcome—the partner must also adapt to the disability.

Once a sexual history has been obtained, it is appropriate for the health professional to assess objectively the erectile potential of the male client. Based on extensive evaluations of a large number of clients with SCI, Comarr (1979) reports that the sexual ability of male clients can be predicted on the basis of several simple examinations: reflex contractions of the anal sphincter, conscious control of the anal sphincter, and the presence or absence of sensation of the penis, scrotum, and perianal dermatomes. The presence or absence of reflex contractions of the anal sphincter will determine whether the man with SCI can experience reflex erections. Reflex erections are attained by visceral or direct stimulation and not by psychogenic means, such as imagery or fantasy. This can be assessed by a digital examination of the rectum by (1) merely inserting a gloved finger into the rectum, (2) moving the examining finger back and forth within the rectum, (3) tapping the client's suprapubic area while feeling for the reflex contraction with the examining finger in the rectum, and/or (4) eliciting the bulbocavernosus reflex (squeezing the glans penis briefly several times to see if a contraction is stimulated). If *any* of these examinations is positive, reflex erectile activity is possible. Performing a similar digital examination on a female will determine the presence or absence of reflex activity and indicate whether lubrication during sexual excitement is possible.

To determine whether the SCI is a complete transection of the cord or an incomplete lesion, the examiner ascertains whether the client has conscious control of the anal sphincter and/or whether sensation is present in the genital area. Conscious control of the anal sphincter is determined by a digital rectal examination, during which the examining finger in the rectum is *not* moved (to avoid reflex contractions). The client is instructed to contract and relax the sphincter several times without using other muscles to do so. Control will be absent, weak, normal, or hyperactive. Evaluation of sensation is made by a *bilateral* pinprick examination of the penis (clitoris), scrotum (labia), and perianal areas. The presence of any degree of voluntary contraction of the anal sphincter and/or any degree of sensation present indicates that the cord lesion is incomplete, and the male client has the potential for psychogenically induced erections. Table 20–3 provides the outcome of these examinations associated with complete and incomplete, reflexic, and areflexic types of lesions. Table 20–4 depicts these lesions and the potential for male clients to have erections, intromission, ejaculation, and orgasm (Comarr and Gunderson, 1975).

Intervention

SEXUALITY AND SEXUAL FUNCTIONING

In the acute care setting the focus of rehabilitation is on the promotion of independent self-care and wheelchair mobility. Every waking hour is involved with the teaching-learning of these activities, which include wheelchair activities, strengthening of the upper extremities, transfers, skin care, bathing, dressing, and bowel and bladder management. Because much of the neurophysiological aspects of bowel, bladder, and sexual function occur through the sacral nerves of the cauda equina, virtually all clients with spinal cord trauma have dysfunction in these three areas. Bowel and bladder management are addressed routinely as part of the acute care of the client with SCI. Unfortunately, health professionals who work with SCI clients rarely address the effects of the SCI on sexuality and sexual functioning. Team members tend to assume someone else will accept this responsibility, if they even think consciously of it at all. If a client overtly or covertly refers to something sexual in nature, health professionals frequently "dismiss" the client by the very nature of their responses. This dismissal merely accentuates clients' feelings of isolation, dependence, and worthlessness and can make them feel as if indeed they will not be able to function sexually ("Paraplegics Discuss," 1972; Zwerner, 1982; Cole, Chilgren, Rosenberg, 1973; Diamond, 1974; Anderson and Cole, 1975; Cole, 1975b; Hanion, 1975; Hohmann, 1975; Chipouras et al, 1979; Weinberg, 1982).

Several factors contribute to the noninvolvement by health professionals in discussing sexuality with SCI clients. Myths about the sexual interests and abilities of clients with SCI abound, e.g., the client with an SCI no longer is interested in sex, or the client with an SCI can no longer perform sexually (Chipouras et al, 1978). Very few health professionals feel prepared to discuss sexual issues. Courses in human sexuality usually are not a required part of the curricula of schools of medicine, nursing, physical and occupational therapy, or social work; therefore, health professionals feel neither competent nor confident in their abilities to address these issues.

Sexuality must be an integral part of an individualized plan for the rehabilitation of the client with an SCI, who still maintains an interest in and desire for sex, despite the spinal cord injury. Sexuality is vital to self-concept, self-esteem, sense of fulfillment, and love of life. Male and female clients are interested in their abilities to function sexually, although this may not be expressed overtly. Sexual adjustment is as crucial to

rehabilitation as the other activities of daily living (Berkman, Weissman, Frielich, 1978). Despite ongoing reports of the paucity of attention given to sexual assessment and rehabilitation, several specific organized programs for sexual counseling of clients with spinal cord injuries have been described in the literature. Both Rancho Los Amigos and the University of Minnesota have described their programs (Cole, Chilgren, Rosenberg, 1973; Anderson and Cole, 1975; Held et al, 1975; Comarr and Vigue, 1978; Melnyk, Montgomery, and Over, 1979). One Canadian hospital has a sexual health care clinician on the staff who assesses and treats the sexual dysfunction of disabled clients (Miller, Szasz, Anderson, 1981).

Acceptance of clients as sexual beings is crucial to rehabilitation. Health professionals in any setting can become involved with sex education and counseling to the degree to which they are prepared. The issues surrounding a client's sexuality should never be ignored. The major requirements for counseling are concern about the sexuality of the client and knowledge of the human sexual response, the neurophysiological changes caused by the SCI, and the resources available to both the professional and the client. Health professionals must also examine their own feelings, attitudes, beliefs, and values concerning sexuality and related sexual issues and must consciously prevent them from interfering with the perspectives held by client or with the suggestions for alternatives for sexual functioning that might be necessary for a particular client. Attitudes of the health professional can enhance or inhibit the growth and development of realistic attitudes, beliefs, and practices of the client with SCI.

SEX EDUCATION AND COUNSELING

Once the initial assessment has been made, the health professional and client can determine goals for sex education and counseling. Remembering that aspects of sexuality affect individuals 24 hours a day and that sexual function is but a small, albeit significant, part of total sexuality, counseling about sexual *functioning* should not obscure related issues that are a major part of *sexuality*. Counseling by the health professional should center on the broad spectrum of sexuality, from attitudes, feelings, and beliefs to appearance, behavior, and sexual functioning. No matter what the outcome of the examination, the health professional can and should assure the client and the partner that a satisfactory sex life is possible (Berkman, Weissman, Frielich, 1978). In fact, despite a general lack of sexual counseling, many clients with SCI have achieved active sex lives despite their handicaps and despite the avoidance of issues by health professionals, although sexuality and sexual activities would have been enhanced by sex education and counseling (Cole, Chilgren, and Rosenberg, 1973; Berkman, Weissman, Frielich, 1978; Melnyk, Montgomery, and Over, 1979; Zwerner, 1982). Marriage and divorce statistics for those with spinal cord injuries have been found not to be different from those of the general population (Griffith and Trieschmann, 1975; Teal and Athelstan, 1975).

Having assessed the client's knowledge and understanding of the sexual response and examined the male client to determine his sexual potential, it is important for the health professional to encourage clients to explore their bodies to ascertain areas of increased and decreased sensation and to determine areas that are sexually stimulating. Frequently, dermatomes just above the level of sensory paralysis are particularly sensitive to stimulation; this can include parts of the body that may not have been sensitive prior to the injury. Exploration of the genitals and perianal areas is to be encouraged as well. While the term masturbation may be repugnant to some for personal, religious, or cultural reasons, introducing the concept of body exploration for the identification of capabilities for sexual activities, rather than as a sexual act in and of itself, frequently is acceptable. Introducing this practice with a phrase such as, "Some people report that ..." can help to assure the client and partner that the practice is acceptable; in addition, this gives them permission to experiment. The health professional can encourage the client and partner to explore the body in different ways, to include kisses, fondling, massage, and the use of a vibrator to determine what is most satisfying to the client and partner. Imagery and fantasy, coupled with touch, are encouraged for sexual stimulation. Many clients enhance sexual stimulation and pleasure with digital stimulation, oral-genital stimulation, and/or use of a vibrator. The health professional can inform the client that these options have been utilized successfully by male and female clients and that any practice that is agreeable to the client and partner is acceptable. What the client and partner agree to try in private is *their* business. The client must be instructed to communicate with the partner what forms of touch stimulate or hurt and to assure the partner that attempts at pleasure will not cause damage. In addition, the client must communicate assets and physical limitations to the partner. Including the partner in these early stages of exploration and experimentation is very useful and helpful to the enhancement of the self-esteem and sex life of a client.

A fulfilling sex life is to be anticipated for all clients with an SCI; however, sexual functioning cannot be a spontaneous occurrence as it might have been prior to the SCI. The health professional must help the client to anticipate and prepare for the many factors that must be considered so that the client feels more in control in social and sexual situations. If the client does not have a regular sexual partner who has been involved with the rehabilitation process, the problems of meeting potential partners, coupled with fears of rejection—social or sexual—are very real. The client still may be coming to grips with a new body image in addition to coping with a wheelchair and the ever present architectural barriers. Frequently, there is a reluctance for nondisabled persons to associate with the disabled. Assertiveness training by the health professional would be beneficial to clients to enable them to become more communicative and to project a more positive image, thus encouraging the nondisabled to see beyond the wheelchair and braces.

Mobility and spasms of the hips and lower extremities must be considered in relation to sexual activity, and current physical limitations must be related to previous modes for sexual expression by the client and partner. The health professional should assist the client with the identification of alternative practices to accommodate limitations, such as the use of pillows, or to try different positions, such as the client prone or supine, or side lying or rear entry, to ascertain which is more conducive to optimal sexual functioning. Books such as *The Joy of Sex* (Comfort, 1975) and *Sexual Options for Paraplegics* (Mooney, Cole, and Chilgren, 1975) can be helpful to the client and partner for various positions for sexual activity as well as suggestions for the stimulation of each partner. Spasticity of the hips and lower extremities enhances performance for some clients, while it is extremely inhibiting to others. If spasticity interferes with enjoyment and performance, some clients will want to inquire about the use of muscle relaxants to decrease the intensity of the spasms.

Clients with SCI above the level of T_4 can experience symptoms of autonomic dysreflexia, which is an exaggerated response of the autonomic system by stimuli that cannot be inhibited by the brain (Weinberg, 1982) and that can be a life-threatening emergency. Symptoms of autonomic dysreflexia are extreme hypertension, a pounding headache, bradycardia, and nausea. These symptoms must be avoided, so Comarr (1978) suggests that sexual activity take place with the client in a sitting position or with the head of the bed elevated. If this does not work, local anesthetic agents can be introduced into the bladder and rectum, or oral alpha adrenergic medications might be taken orally prior to sexual activity.

MANAGING INCONTINENCE

Fears of bowel and/or bladder incontinence can hamper any feelings of sexuality as well as sexual functioning. A specific protocol for bowel management usually is a necessity for clients with SCI to prevent stool incontinence. (Recurrent bladder infections have been associated with retention of stool, so a good bowel protocol is recommended for this reason as well.) Some clients will evacuate the rectum daily or every other day by digital stimulation. Others will utilize stool softeners and laxatives, which adds to the unpredictability of evacuation. The constipated stool, frequently described as dry "marbles" or "golf balls," is usually a symptom of incomplete evacuation, particularly if the client's fluid intake is sufficient (2 quarts per day). The daily or every-other-day use of bisacodyl suppositories (Dulcolax) or bisacodyl enemas (Fleet) immediately after a meal stimulates a complete and predictable evacuation of the rectum. Implementation of this protocol after the same meal each time actually "trains" the rectum to respond to this stimulus, and accidents are rare. Once the bowels respond to the regular use of bisacodyl, the fear of incontinence can be eased.

Bladder management is achieved in a variety of ways. Ideally, both male and female clients manage their bladders with the protocol for clean intermittent self-catheterization, with adjunctive anticholinergic medications if bladder spasms are associated with the neurogenic bladder. If the client drains the bladder every 3 to 4 hours and does not consume more than 2 quarts of fluid each day, wetness and recurrent bladder infections can be avoided. Infections irritate the bladder and can cause episodes of incontinence between catheterizations. Both male and female clients with SCI have been successful with this protocol. To avoid having to navigate a wheelchair into a restroom or having to transfer out of the chair for self-catheterization, the protocol can be adapted to the individual needs of each client, so catheterization can be done on time with minimal maneuvering. Unfortunately, self-catheterization frequently is not possible for quadriplegic clients because it is difficult to eradicate their bladder spasms pharmacologically and the client continues to be incontinent between catheterizations and because the client may not have enough upper extremity function to do self-catheterization. However, if pharmacological manipulation is successful in eliminating the bladder spasms, the person assisting the client with other activities of daily living could also perform the catheterizations. Since self-catheterization can be done as often as necessary, it is recommended that clients always drain their bladder prior to the initiation of sexual activity.

Indwelling catheters can be an esthetic problem, particularly if the partner also assists with care of the catheter. Any client with an indwelling catheter should drink a minimum of 3 quarts of fluid a day to flush the bladder and to keep the urine dilute. A *suprapubic* catheter in the male client should not present any particular problems during sexual activities if it is secured to the abdomen and attached to a bedside drainage bag that is placed out of sight below the level of the bladder. The presence of a *urethral* catheter does not preclude coitus. Obviously, scrupulous perineal cleansing is recommended prior to sexual encounters. Some clients are taught to remove their catheters prior to coitus, which then are replaced afterwards. Because bladder capacity diminishes to very small volumes when indwelling catheters are used and because the bladder is irritated from the catheter, involuntary urination probably would occur during sexual activity, so precautions should be taken to protect the bed linens. The male client can bend his catheter down the length of his erect penis, apply a condom over the penis and catheter, and use a water-soluble lubricant on the condom if intromission is uncomfortable to his partner. The female client can bring her catheter up to her abdomen, apply a piece of tape to secure it, and place the drainage bag lower than her bladder on the side of the bed.

The man who utilizes an *external,* condom-type *catheter* to prevent incontinence must remove the device prior to intromission. Since his bladder drains as a result of bladder spasms, urinary incontinence should be anticipated during sexual activity and the bed linens protected. He might also refrain from drinking fluids for about 3 hours prior to sexual activity to decrease the amount of urinary incontinence.

Unfortunately, women with urinary incontinence do not have many alternatives for bladder management and are limited to intermittent catheterization, an indwelling urethral catheter, or waterproof panties with diapers or liners. External appliances are not an alternative at the present time. Several publications are available that describe the availability of the various products. These materials are readily available at surgical supply houses as well as through the Sears Home Care Catalogue, but they are expensive. While third party payers, such as Medicaid, cover the costs of catheters, they rarely cover these items. Skin care is crucial if external products are utilized; to avoid constant wetness against the skin, the author recommends the utilization of a product that has a liner next to the skin, through which the urine passes into a central layer containing a polymer that turns gelatinous as it absorbs the urine.

Clients who have continuing problems with urinary incontinence, despite diligent attempts to achieve continence with intermittent catheterization, might be candidates for a surgical procedure to achieve continence. Several relatively new surgical procedures are being utilized in medical centers throughout the country to create a continent vesicostomy, or a Kock pouch. This is a major surgical procedure, and all clients would have to undergo a thorough urological evaluation prior to consideration. Briefly, either the bladder itself or a segment of bowel is utilized as a reservoir for urine; a nipple valve is created between the reservoir and the abdomen, which creates a continent stoma through which the reservoir is catheterized

by the client about every 3 to 4 hours per day (Brogna and Lakaszawski, 1986).

SEXUAL ACTIVITY: PREPARATIONS AND TECHNIQUES

The health professional can assist clients with a "rehearsal" for a sexual encounter, so they can anticipate the preparations that must be made, e.g., protection of bed linens, additional pillows, perineal-catheter care, and bowel evacuation. The client might want to consider how to make the environment alluring, e.g., soft lights, music, wine. The health professional can assist clients to determine how they will explain the extent of deficits to the partner and communicate preferences. It is most important that the client is prepared and rested prior to a sexual encounter, so physical, emotional, psychological, and cognitive skills are at an optimal level. It is natural for a client to feel clumsy and nervous in anticipation of a sexual encounter. For clients who have been sexually active prior to the SCI, it is helpful to remind them that they probably experienced these same feelings during those initial attempts at sexual activities. Above all, the health professional should remind their clients that sexual function is not a performance but the natural expression of feelings for their partner.

Unfortunately in our society, maleness frequently is associated with the penis, erectile ability, and penovaginal intercourse. The male client must adapt to his altered body image, and the health professional must help him to recognize that he, indeed, is masculine, despite the alterations in his erectile ability. The client who has relied on his physical appearance and sexual prowess as the indication of his sexuality must learn that a relationship with a partner encompasses much more than penovaginal intercourse and that care and concern about the partner, companionship, effective communication with the partner, tenderness, and the physical components of holding, kissing, and caressing are essential components of a positive sexual relationship. If the quality of his erections is not suitable for penovaginal penetration, the health professional can assist the client to broaden his sexual behaviors by reviewing with him past behaviors that were satisfying but did not include intercourse. Learning to be concerned about his partner's satisfaction primarily might be a new experience for the male client; the health professional can assure him that this concern will enhance his own sexual experience.

In addition to exploration of the body for the identification of erogenous areas, the male client who experiences reflex erections should be encouraged to masturbate to achieve a reflex erection. If he has a spouse or partner, mutual exploration is to be encouraged as well as attempts at intercourse. If the client who demonstrates the potential for reflex erections on examination cannot attain a functional erection by masturbation, he should be encouraged to try using a vibrator on the penis as a stimulus and/or oral stimulation by his partner (if this practice is agreeable to them). "Stuffing" is a technique employed successfully by many clients who cannot attain a functional erection. The flaccid or semirigid penis is "stuffed" into the partner's vagina, and she then "grips" it by contractions of her pubococcygeus muscle. Although this will not stimulate an erection of the flaccid penis, female partners report reaching orgasm, and clients report feelings of great pleasure at being able to satisfy their partners. Many couples prefer oral-genital sex to their mutual satisfaction. Clients with incomplete lesions and no reflex activity can learn to use imagery and fantasies to attain a psychogenic erection. This type of erection occurs as a result of a reflex within the brain and can be stimulated with imagery and fantasy as well as by visual, auditory, olfactory, and perceptual stimuli. Frequently, the sexual stimulation of the partner will intensify the client's own stimulation. The use of imagery and fantasy may be a new experience to many male clients and, if this is an option for a particular client, the health professional should encourage him to utilize this stimulus.

The University of Minnesota sponsored a 2-day program in human sexuality for SCI clients, their spouses or friends, and health professionals who work with the disabled. Through discussion it was revealed that oral-genital sex was a very important part of the sexual behavior of the SCI clients, probably because penovaginal intercourse is time consuming, if not difficult or impossible to achieve. Also revealed during the program was the strong use of fantasy, using the partner's sensory responses as a stimulus for the fantasy as well as the substitution of the partner's sexual satisfaction for the client's own satisfaction (Cole, Chilgren, and Rosenberg, 1973).

The inability to attain a functional erection is devastating and demoralizing to any man, but even more so to the man who has suffered the additional losses associated with the SCI. Emotionally, he may feel as if he were castrated and suffer from overwhelming feelings of hopelessness and depression, increasing the problems associated with body image and self-concept. Over time the nurse, along with the partner, friends, and family can help the client recognize that he is masculine, despite his physical losses; physical, emotional, cognitive, and psychological strengths must be identified to assist the man to gain a new concept of himself as a man.

A penile prosthesis is an option for men who are unable to attain and/or maintain an erection. However, this procedure and device is not appropriate for everyone. The patient and partner should be assessed to determine their motivation for wanting the device, their expectations, and their fears. The advantages and disadvantages and expected function of the prosthesis should be explained; the man and his partner must know that the prosthesis is not a panacea for all sexual disturbances. The reader is referred to Chapter 21, Genitourinary Conditions and Sexuality, for a complete discussion of this option.

Because of the genital sensory paralysis associated with the SCI, the potential for erosion of one or both of the rods through the corpora cavernosa might go unnoticed by a client who was not scrupulous about skin care or body position. For this reason alone some urologists are hesitant to insert a penile prosthesis in clients with an SCI. Another alternative would be to teach the client to induce an erection with the injection of papavarine and phentolamine.

ARTIFICIAL INSEMINATION

It is possible for semen to be retrieved from the bladder of a client so his wife can be inseminated artificially (Heslinga, Schellen, and Verkuyl, 1974). Retrieval is not as simple as it sounds, however, because the client's urine would have to be alkalinized beforehand. His bladder is then emptied prior to ejaculation; the semen is removed from the bladder by catheter aspiration and immediately placed in his wife's cervix during the ideal time for conception to occur. A client and his spouse would have to locate a urologist and/or gynecologist sympathetic to their problem who would work closely with the couple to achieve a pregnancy. However, spermatogenesis frequently is impaired in the client with SCI. Amelar and Dubin (1984) report that this probably is secondary to lumbar denervation from the cord trauma. Perkash and his associates (1985) did a controlled study of 30 clients with SCI to evaluate their sperm and hormone levels with a control group in the same age range. Although their sample size was small, their findings indicate that decreased motility of sperm was the greatest problem. Chronic urinary tract infections can be a problem for some clients. While appropriate antibiotics treat the bladder effectively, Perkash and associates (1985) feel that low-grade infections of the ejaculatory ducts are more persistent. In addition, they report that some medications contribute to creating a poor environment for sperm maturation. Of the patients they studied, few had sperm of sufficient quality to be used for artificial insemination. If these findings are applicable to larger numbers of male clients, prevention of urinary tract infections is imperative to promote spermatogenesis and motility of sperm in the client who is considering artificial insemination.

EFFECTS ON FEMALE SEXUAL FUNCTIONING

There are many unknowns regarding the effect of an SCI on female sexual functioning. Because response is individual, the health professional should counsel the woman that if lubrication does not occur as a result of psychogenic stimulation, for example, imagery, she could attempt manual stimulation of her clitoris. If manual stimulation does not produce sufficient lubrication, water-soluble lubricants can be used. Because a significant number of nondisabled women experience orgasmic disorders, it is imperative for the health professional to assess pre- and post-trauma difficulties with orgasm. As with male clients, it is important for the health professional to encourage the female client to explore her own body alone or with a partner to identify erogenous zones. Many nondisabled women never have done this or have never even examined their external genitalia. Permission to explore the body with touch, caresses, massage, vibrator, and oral maneuvers must be given, being cognizant of the personal values and cultural and religious factors that may inhibit the client. Assuring the client that "other women with SCIs report

success ..." with various methods is a good form of encouragement.

Lonnie Barbach's book *For Yourself: The Fulfillment of Female Sexuality* (1975) is recommended reading for female clients because it teaches women how to explore their bodies to learn their own sexual responses.

It is imperative that the female with an SCI have routine gynecological examinations for the same reasons as a nondisabled female: an annual pelvic examination for the assessment of her pelvic organs and a Pap smear for detection of cancer. Female clients with SCI should also practice monthly breast self-examinations after their menstrual periods; the examiner can also do this exam as well as schedule mammograms for additional screening, if indicated. The fact that she has decreased or absent perineal sensation, frequently including also the abdominal organs, means that she may not exhibit typical signs and symptoms of gynecological problems, such as pain, or the perineal itching associated with vaginitis (Griffith and Trieschmann, 1975). She must become aware of her vaginal secretions throughout her menstrual cycle so she is cognizant of any abnormalities—this may be her only symptom of vaginitis.

BIRTH CONTROL

Because fertility is not impaired, birth control is necessary if the client is sexually active. A brief description of contraceptive options is presented here. Weinberg (1982) and Shaul and associates (1980) discuss each method of birth control and their advantages and disadvantages in relation to the client with an SCI, and the reader is referred to these sources for additional information.

Oral contraceptives are contraindicated for use because of the greater risk for thrombophlebitis; in addition, because of sensory paralysis, the client would not be aware of the usual warning signs of leg and/or abdominal pain. The *intrauterine device* is a potential method. If the client is unable to check for the presence of the strings, her partner would have to do so; however, the client would not be aware of early signs of pelvic inflammatory disease. The health professional would have to teach the client to be especially aware of other potential signs, such as changes in vaginal secretions, fever, spotting, irregular periods, and increased spasticity of her lower extremities (a potential response to any kind of infection in the body). The *diaphragm* with spermicidal jelly could be utilized by the client; however, weakness in her upper extremities or tightness/spasticity of her hips might preclude its use, unless her partner could be taught how to insert it. If the client has decreased tone in her pelvic musculature as a result of the SCI, the diaphragm could become dislodged, and thus be rendered ineffective. The use of a *condom* with spermicidal foam could be utilized, again with the assistance of her partner if the client is unable to apply the foam against her cervix. *Depo-Provera* is an injectable form of progesterone, administered intramuscularly every 3 months; statistically the pregnancy rate associated with its use is the same as that with the oral contraceptives. Its main disadvantages are a delayed return of fertility after it is discontinued and vaginal dryness, which might necessitate the use of a water-soluble lubricant during intercourse (Shaul et al, 1980). Although utilized for birth control in other countries, this medication has not been approved specifically for birth control in the United States. If the client has no intention of becoming pregnant, she could discuss the advisability of having a *tubal ligation* with a gynecologist. Each method of birth control should be discussed with the client by the health professional. Each has definite physical and/or aesthetic advantages and disadvantages. Whichever method is selected, the woman must be given detailed instruction for proper utilization; if the partner will be involved with the utilization of a particular method, he should also be involved in the instruction.

CHILDBEARING

If a client decides to have a child, several aspects should be explored with her. Are her functional abilities (activities of daily living, mobility) such that she can care for a child? Are there architectural barriers that should be removed to make her home environment more conducive to her independence in caring for a child? If she cannot care for a child independently, have she and her spouse or partner determined how this will be accomplished? The client would be considered a high-risk obstetrical patient, and she should engage the services of an obstetrician prior to becoming pregnant so that a baseline status of her general health can be ascertained. The client should be stable from a urological standpoint, i.e., her renal function should be within normal limits, and she should be compliant with appropriate protocols for bladder and bowel management. Because pregnant women in general are more susceptible to urinary tract infections, the female with an SCI should probably be seen by a urologist if she has a history of recurrent urinary tract infections prior to her pregnancy. The urologist might be able to make recommendations for better management, which would decrease her risk for infections during a pregnancy.

Because of motor and sensory deficits, the labor and delivery sequences will not be as predictable as those of a nondisabled woman. If her lesion level is below T_{10}, the client would experience the normal sensations and contractions associated with labor but have increased spasms in her hips and lower extremities if these were present prior to pregnancy. Above the T_{10} level of the cord, labor is usually painless, but contractions are within normal limits, and increased spasticity might be a problem. Clients with lesions above T_6 might be unaware of labor because they cannot sense contractions; additionally, they might be troubled with symptoms of autonomic dysreflexia. Since the stimulus (labor) cannot be removed, beta-blocking agents might have to be administered to treat this condition to prevent serious sequelae, such as a stroke. An epidural block might be utilized during labor and delivery to prevent this problem from occurring if the client has a lesion at or above this level of the spinal cord.

SUMMARY

The sexual assessment, education, and counseling of the client with an SCI is a complex endeavor. It is obvious from the literature that both male and female clients with SCIs have continued to be sexual beings, despite the paucity of attention given to them by health professionals. However, since our daily lives constantly have an impact on our sexuality and since sexuality and sexual functioning are a vital part of our feelings about ourselves and our body image, clients with an SCI deserve to be taught how to cope with such a devastating attack on life. They need to be assisted to regain self-esteem and reinforced in the knowledge and assurance that they continue to be sexual beings. With the guidance from the health professional, SCI clients should be able to pursue their interests in sexual functioning.

While in some instances one person assumes the total responsibility for the education and counsel of the client with an SCI, it is probably more realistic to involve multiple members of the health care team. It is important, however, that sexuality and sexual functioning be a conscious and conspicuous aspect of the rehabilitation of the client with an SCI. For instance, because the physical therapist works one-to-one with clients on such aspects as assessment of physical strengths and weaknesses and assists clients to transfer and position their body for activities of daily living, it would be logical for this person also to counsel the client about positioning for sexual activities. It would be difficult for one individual to address all issues. However, health professionals need to identify resources available within their institutions and/or communities from which they can glean assistance or to whom the client can be referred. Coordination for these efforts should be the responsibility of the nurse.

All members of the health care team must assist the client to feel more positive about him- or herself as a male or female and to increase strengths for the achievement of a meaningful and fulfilling life, so the client eventually can look upon the effects of the SCI as a fact of life. It is hoped that on reading this chapter health professionals will be stimulated to increase their knowledge and understanding of the needs of the client with an SCI. One of the most comprehensive resources available to the reader who does not work regularly with SCI clients is *Who Cares?*, a handbook that addresses the needs for sex education and provides a multitude of resources. This 233-page handbook can be ordered from PRO-ED, 5341 Industrial Oaks Blvd, Austin, Texas, 78735, for less than $20.

REFERENCES

Amelar R, Dubin L: Infertility in the male. In Kendal AR, Karafin L (eds): Urology. Vol 2. New York, Harper & Row, 1984.

Anderson TP, Cole TM: Sexual counseling of the physically disabled. Postgrad Med 58:117, 1975.

Barbach L: For Yourself: The Fulfillment of Female Sexuality. New York, Doubleday, 1975.

Baxter RT, Linn A: Sex counseling and the SCI patient. Nurs 8:46, 1978.

Becker EF: Sexuality and the spinal cord-injured woman: An interview. In Bullard DG, Knight SE (eds): Sexuality and Physical Disability. St. Louis, CV Mosby, 1981.

Berkman AH, Weissman R, Frielich MH: Sexual adjustment of spinal cord injured veterans living in the community. Arch Phys Med Rehabil 59:29, 1978.

Bloom JL: Sex education for handicapped adolescents. J Sch Health 39:363, 1969.

Bogle JE, Shaul SL: Body image and the woman with a disability. In Bullard DG, Knight SE (eds): Sexuality and Physical Disability. St. Louis, CV Mosby, 1981.

Brogna L, Lakaszawski M: Nursing management: The continent urostomy. J Enterstomal Ther 13:147, 1986.

Bromley I: Tetraplegia and Paraplegia: A Guide for Physiotherapists. 2nd ed. New York, Churchill Livingston, 1981.

Carlson CE: Conceptual style and life satisfaction following spinal cord injury. Arch Phys Med Rehabil 60:346, 1979.

Cass AS, Bloom BA, Luxemberg M: Sexual function in adults with myelomeningocele. J Urol 136:425, 1986.

Castree BJ, Walker JH: The young adult with spina bifida. Br Med J 283:1040, 1981.

Chipouras S et al: Who Cares? (A Handbook on Sex Education and Counseling Services for Disabled People). Washington, DC, George Washington University, 1979.

Cole TM: Reactions of the rehabilitation team to patients with sexual problems. Arch Phys Med Rehabil 56:10, 1975a.

Cole TM: Spinal cord injury patients and sexual dysfunction. Arch Phys Med Rehabil 56:11, 1975b.

Cole TM, Chilgren R, Rosenberg P: A new programme of sex education and counselling for spinal cord injured adults and health care professionals. Paraplegia 11:111, 1973.

Colgan MT: The child with spina bifida. Am J Dis Child 135:854, 1981.

Comarr AE: Urinary disorders from spinal cord injury. Comp Ther 5:37, 1979.

Comarr AE, Gunderson AB: Sexual function in traumatic paraplegia and quadriplegia. Am J Nurs 75:250, 1975.

Comarr AE, Vigue M: Sexual counseling among male and female patients with spinal cord and/or cauda equina injury (2 parts). Am J Phys Med 57:107, 215, 1978.

Comfort A: The Joy of Sex. New York, Simon & Schuster, 1975.

Diamond M: Sexuality and the handicapped. Rehabil Liter 35:34, 1974.

Dorner S: The relationship of physical handicap to stress in families with an adolescent with spina bifida. Develop Med Child Neurol 17:765, 1975.

Dorner S: Adolescents with spina bifida. Arch Dis Child 51:439, 1976.

Dorner S: Problems of teenagers. Physiotherapy 63:190, 1977a.

Dorner S: Sexual interests and activities in adolescents with spina bifida. J Child Psychol Psychiatry 18:229, 1977b.

Duff RS: Counseling families and deciding care of severely defective children: A way of coping with "medical Vietnam." Pediatrics 67:315, 1981.

Evans K, Kickman V, Carter CO: Handicap and social status of adults with spina bifida cystica. Br J Prevent Soc Med 28:85, 1974.

Eyster F: Spinal injuries are forever. Letter to Ann Landers. Durham Morning Herald June 11, 1986.

Fost N: Counseling families who have a child with a severe congenital anomaly. Pediatrics 67:321, 1981.

Gartley CB (ed): Managing Incontinence. Ottawa, Jameson Books, 1985.

Gatens C: Sexuality and disability. In Woods NF (ed): Human Sexuality in Health and Illness. St. Louis, CV Mosby, 1984.

Geiger RC: Neurophysiology of sexual response in spinal cord injury. In Bullard D, Knight S (eds): Sexuality and Physical Disability. St. Louis, CV Mosby, 1981.

Golji H: Experience with penile prostheses in spinal cord injury patients. J Urol 121:288, 1979.

Griffith ER, Trieschmann RB: Sexual functioning in women with spinal cord injury. Arch Phys Med Rehabil 56:18, 1975.

Griffith ER, Trieschmann RB: Sexual function restoration in the physically disabled: Use of a private hospital room. Arch Phys Med Rehabil 58:368, 1977.

Griffith ER, Tomko MA, Timms RJ: Sexual function in spinal cord-injured patients: A review. Arch Phys Med Rehabil 54:539, 1973.

Hanion K: Maintaining sexuality after spinal cord injury. Nurs 5:58, 1975.

Hayden PW, Davenport SLH, Campbell M: Adolescents with myelodysplasia: Impact of physical disability on emotional maturation. Pediatrics 64:53, 1979.

Held JP et al: Sexual attitude reassessment workshops: Effect on spinal cord injured adults, their partners and rehabilitation professionals. Arch Phys Med Rehabil 56:14, 1975.

Heslinga K, Schellen AMCM, Verkuyl A: Not Made of Stone. Springfield, Charles C Thomas, 1974.

Hohmann GW: Reactions of the individual with a disability complicated by a sexual problem. Arch Phys Med Rehabil 56:9, 1975.

Kolin IS et al: Studies of the school-age child with meningomyelocele: Social and emotional adaptation. J Pediatr 78:1013, 1971.

Larrabee JH: The person with a spinal cord injury: Physical care during early recovery. Am J Nurs 77:1320, 1977a.

Larrabee JH: Spinal cord injury—incidence and cost. Am J Nurs 77:1340, 1977b.

MacRae I, Henderson G: Sexuality and irreversible health limitations. Nurs Clin North Am 10:587, 1975.

Madorsky JGB, Dixon TP: Rehabilitation aspects of sexuality. West J Med 139:174, 1983.

Martini L, MacTurk RH: Issues in the enumeration of handicapping conditions in the United States. Mental Retardation 23:182, 1985.

Melnyk R, Montgomery R, Over R: Attitude changes following a sexual counseling program for spinal cord injured persons. Arch Phys Med Rehabil 60:601, 1979.

Miller S, Szasz G, Anderson L: Sexual health care clinician in an acute spinal cord injury unit. Arch Phys Med Rehabil 62:315, 1981.

Montague DK: Clinical evaluation of impotence. Urol Clin North Am 8:103, 1981.

Mooney J, Cole TM, Chilgren R: Sexual Options for Paraplegics and Quadriplegics. Boston, Little, Brown & Co, 1975.

Murray RL: Symposium on the concept of body image. Nurs Clin North Am 7:593, 1972.

Myers GJ, Cerone SB, Olson AL (eds): A Guide for Helping the Child with Spina Bifida. Springfield, Charles C Thomas, 1981.

Paraplegics discuss their sexual problems: Proceedings of the Conference of Continuing Education in the Treatment of Spinal Cord Injuries, June 28–29, 1972. Milwaukee, Wisconsin.

Parsons JG: Assessments of aptitudes in young people of school-leaving age handicapped by hydrocephalus or spina bifida cystica. Develop Med Child Neurol (Suppl 27) 14:101, 1972.

Passo S: Parents' perceptions, attitudes, and needs regarding sex education for the child with myelomeningocele. Res Nurs Health 1:53, 1978.

Payton TR, Goldstein I: Intracavernosal pharmacology. J Urolog Nurs 5:611, 1986.

Pepper GA: The person with a spinal cord injury: Psychological care. Am J Nurs 77:1330, 1977.

Perkash I et al: Reproductive Biology of Paraplegics: Results of semen collection, testicular biopsy and serum hormone evaluation. J Urol 134:284, 1985.

Pieper B: Straight Talk ... Parent to Parent. Chicago, Spina Bifida Association of America, 1977.

Pieper B: By, For and With: Young Adults with Spina Bifida. Chicago, Spina Bifida Association of America, 1979.

Riddle I: Nursing intervention to promote body image integrity in children. Nurs Clin North Am 7:651, 1972.

Santana Carlos VM: Importance of communication in counseling the spinal cord injury patient. Paraplegia 16:206, 1978–79.

Shaul S et al: Toward Intimacy: Family Planning and Sexuality Concerns of Physically Disabled Women. New York, Human Sciences Press, 1980.

Sherman RG, Berling BS, Oppenheimer S: Increasing community independence for adolescents with spina bifida. Adolescence 20:1, 1985.

Shrey DE, Kiefer JS, Anthony WA: Sexual adjustment counseling for persons with severe disabilities: A skill-based approach for rehabilitation professionals. J Rehabil 45:28, 1979.

Stewart TD: Sex, spinal cord injury, and staff rapport. Rehabil Liter 42:347, 1981.

Stewart WFR: The Sexual Side of Handicap. New York, Woodhead-Faulkner, 1979.

Swinyard CA: The Child with Spina Bifida. Chicago, Spina Bifida Association of America, 1980.

Teal JC, Athelstan GT: Sexuality and spinal cord injury: Some psychosocial considerations. Arch Phys Med Rehabil 56:264, 1975.

Tew B, Laurence KM: Mothers, brothers and sisters of patients with spina bifida. Develop Med Child Neurol (Suppl 129) 15:69, 1973.

Thornton CE: Sexuality counseling of women with spinal cord injuries. In Bullard D, Knight S (eds): Sexuality and Physical Disability. St. Louis, CV Mosby, 1981.

Trieschmann RB: Sex, sex acts and sexuality. Arch Phys Med Rehabil 56:8, 1975.

Veterans Administration: A Source Book. Rehabilitating the Person with Spinal Cord Injury. Washington, DC, US Government Printing Office, 1972.

Weinberg JS: Human sexuality and spinal cord injury. Nurs Clin North Am 17:407, 1982.

Wittman MI: LPT Department of Physical Therapy, The NC Memorial Hospital, Chapel Hill, North Carolina.

Woods NF: Sexual adaptation to traumatic paraplegia. In Woods NF (ed): Human Sexuality in Health and Illness. St. Louis, CV Mosby, 1984.

Zwerner J: Yes we have troubles but nobody's listening: Sexual issues of women with spinal cord injury. Sex Disabil 5:158, 1982.

21: Genitourinary Conditions and Sexuality

Carol Sackett

An essential component of sexuality and sexual self-image is an individual's self-concept and body image. One's self-concept is influenced by a myriad of factors—interactions with nuclear and extended families from birth onward; interactions with peers, friends, and acquaintances; and one's body concept. Body image begins to form early in life and is reinforced and altered by people and the events experienced throughout a lifetime. An alteration in one's body or bodily functions may affect body image, even in the mature, stable person. If body image is threatened, the person often feels like a misfit, at least temporarily. Any change in the functioning of the urinary tract and/or genital organs has the potential to affect body image and sexual functioning adversely.

This chapter presents the information needed to provide insightful, supportive sexual education and counseling related to potential or real sexual disturbances in clients experiencing genitourinary dysfunction. Specific clinical conditions that occur in the urinary tract are reviewed for their impact on sexuality and sexual functioning, with the focus on problems common to men and women and those unique to men. (Gynecological disorders are discussed in Chapter 27.) Interventions that can diminish or eliminate the dysfunction or assist the client with adaptation to altered functioning are discussed, and the role of the nurse is highlighted. For ease of presentation, organ systems are the organizing schema.

KIDNEY

End-Stage Renal Disease (ESRD)

Chronic renal failure is the decreased ability of the kidneys to maintain the internal physiological equilibrium of the body, while ESRD is the irreversible failure of the kidneys to function. Without treatment by medication, diet, and/or fluid restriction and by dialysis or transplantation, the client with ESRD faces an inevitable death. Causes for progressive renal failure that lead to this potentially terminal disease may be congenital, as in the case of polycystic kidneys, or acquired. Diseases such as chronic glomerulonephritis and chronic pyelonephritis attack the kidneys primarily, while severe hypertension, diabetes, and lupus erythematosus cause renal failure secondarily. ESRD is no small problem in our population; currently about 85,000 people are being treated by some form of renal dialysis.

EFFECTS OF END-STAGE RENAL DISEASE ON SEXUALITY

Physiological Function

ESRD affects every system in the body. There are skin changes such as the pruritis associated with uremia. The entire gastrointestinal tract can be involved, with the potential for

407

nausea and vomiting and inflammatory changes of any or all portions, from the mouth to the rectum. There are problems with fluid and electrolyte balance necessitating dietary and fluid restrictions. Hypertension exists as well as the potential for other cardiovascular problems. Chronic anemia and changes in the red and white blood cells also occur. ESRD produces neurological changes in the central and autonomic nervous systems. From an endocrinological standpoint children with ESRD cease to grow and have delayed sexual maturation. Decreased sexual desire is a problem for both men and women with ESRD. Women experience amenorrhea, and ovulation can diminish or cease. Men can be infertile because of a decrease in the number and motility of sperm. The inability to attain or maintain an erection frequently is a problem as well.

The impact of ESRD on sexual functioning is variable and multifactorial for the client on dialysis. Multiple studies have been conducted to measure the impact of ESRD on sexual functioning, but except for the fact that decreased sexual desire, decreased potential for orgasm, infertility, and erectile difficulties are recognized as problems, specific causal factors cannot be identified in most cases because of the many variables associated with the disease, with treatment modalities, and with the individuality of clients and their relationships with partners (Abram et al, 1975; Steele, Finkelstein, and Finkelstein, 1976; Milne, Golden, and Fibus, 1977–78). Treatment by dialysis can diminish or reverse these problems, but studies do not reflect uniform improvement, probably because of the multiplicity of other factors. For instance, if the client's ESRD was the result of severe hypertension, the male client already could have experienced erectile difficulties because of his antihypertensive medication; likewise erectile dysfunction can result from the peripheral neuropathies associated with diabetes. The constant stresses of living with ESRD, coupled with the necessary adaptations in the life of clients and their families can also affect sexuality and sexual performance. It is impossible to separate these for an objective determination of causal factors.

Psychosocial Function

In addition to the physical factors associated with ESRD, multiple psychosocial factors are also involved. The client with ESRD is faced with a chronic, potentially fatal disease; the process of accepting this fact and learning to live with the disease necessitate profound psychological adaptation, as the client mourns the loss of a healthy body and learns to adapt to a new self. The effects of living with a chronic illness have been examined thoroughly in Chapter 14, Illness, Chronic Disease, and Sexuality, to which the reader is referred. With ESRD, clients are sentenced to a life with hours of treatment by dialysis at least three times a week or continuously, if the client is on such a program with peritoneal dialysis. Their sphere of existence is narrowed significantly both by the disease itself and by the treatment. Either the disease or the treatment or both can affect the ability to be gainfully employed and to maintain roles and responsibilities in the family and community. Clients are also caught in a web of struggles with dependence/independence issues, necessitated by the limitations imposed by the disease and dialysis.

NURSING CARE

The roles for the nurse working with ESRD clients are multifaceted. Fortunately, in most treatment facilities the client and partner become part of the "family" of the treatment team. Because long-term clients will be on some form of dialysis, the team, at least initially, has the time to develop a positive, therapeutic relationship with clients and partners when they are available. Although not all clients with ESRD have sexual partners, the majority do, and thus the following discussion focuses on clients in relationships.

Several options for treatment exist; each has advantages and disadvantages, so clients, in conjunction with the treatment team, select the one that best suits individual life styles and physical problems. Hemodialysis is accomplished through an arteriovenous shunt that has been implanted surgically, usually in the forearm; hemodialysis can be performed in a treatment center, or the client and partner can be taught home dialysis. Peritoneal dialysis is accomplished through a catheter that has been placed surgically through the abdominal wall into the peritoneal cavity. Clients then decide whether they will undergo dialysis intermittently, for example, during the night, or continuously (Lancaster and Pierce, 1984).

Assessment

Assessment of sexuality and problems with sexual functioning should be included as part of the initial complete assessment; this will let the client and partner know that sexuality is an acceptable subject about which questions and problems may be pursued. Opening a discussion with a statement such as, "Some people with kidney failure tell me they don't feel much like having sex anymore," gives the client and partner permission to mention problems they might be experiencing. Because degrees of dysfunction are variable, it is not advisable to suggest that the client has—or will have—specific sexual problems. In addition, because the client's renal failure is progressive over a long period of time in most cases, it may be difficult to obtain a sexual assessment of the client and partner's previous sexual relationship.

Intervention

The nurse must assist the client and partner to move through the stages of grief to acceptance of ESRD and dialysis. It is important to be sensitive to the problems of role changes that may accompany all of the restrictions associated with ESRD and dialysis. The partner, of necessity, may have to assume many of the roles and responsibilities formerly performed by the client, and both the client and partner, therefore, may suffer from role conflicts. The nurse must help the couple work through the resulting problems of dependence/independence, encouraging clients to do all they are able to do on their own, while helping the partner to foster the client's independence rather than encouraging unnecessary dependency. All of these factors have an effect on the sexual relationship of the couple. It is important for the nurse to identify coping mechanisms that the couple used to handle stresses that occurred prior to the onset of ESRD. These serve to decrease anxiety and to give the client and partner an ability to function through this highly stressful time. Coping mechanisms, including denial, must be supported until the client and partner can cope in more productive ways.

Once the client and partner have learned about dialysis and all it entails and have established a certain daily routine, the high levels of fear and anxiety may diminish, although this process might take months. Once the client begins to feel better physically be-

cause of the dialysis, the nurse can serve as a catalyst to encourage moving on with life. Fostering communication between the client and partner concerning their feelings, needs, desires, and problems can stimulate the exploration of solutions and the means for coping with sexual difficulties. If the client has pleasurable sexual relationships prior to ESRD and dialysis, the chances for this to continue, albeit in an altered state, are good. The nurse can assist clients to explore new and energy-sparing ways for sexual pleasuring.

The client who is fortunate enough to acquire a new kidney by transplantation can look forward to the restoration of sexual desire, sexual functioning, and fertility, unless these dysfunctions preceded the onset of renal failure. The female client may begin to ovulate prior to the return of menstruation, so birth control is very important, particularly since pregnancy is discouraged for 1 to 2 years following transplantation. Oral contraceptives are not advocated because of their side effects, and the use of intrauterine devices in these immunosuppressed clients is discouraged because of heavier menstrual flow and the increased potential for infection (Lancaster and Pierce, 1984).

The nurse who works with the ESRD/dialysis client has important responsibilities. Along with other members of the treatment team, the nurse must help clients come to grips with a potentially fatal disease, teach them how to perform dialysis, and facilitate the return of the client to as normal a life as possible, despite the many limitations imposed by the disease and its treatment. To include problems with sexuality and sexual functioning in this entire process must be a conscious and concerted effort.

BLADDER

Cystitis

Bladder infections are far more common in women than men. When a man develops cystitis, it is usually secondary to another physiological problem, such as benign prostatic hypertrophy or other such conditions that can prevent the emptying of the bladder during urination. The symptoms of cystitis in men and women—frequency, urgency, and burning on urination—are acute and can be very debilitating. Treatment with appropriate antibiotics usually diminishes the symptoms within 48 hours. However, if the client fails to complete the prescribed course of antibiotics, symptoms can recur because of inadequate treatment.

CYSTITIS AND SEXUAL FUNCTION

Women are more susceptible to cystitis because of the short length of the urethra (about 2 inches) and because of the proximity of the urethra to the vagina and rectum. The length of the urethra allows for the ascension of bacteria into the bladder, which then can be compounded by the irritation and "milking" action of coital thrusting. This combination can perpetuate recurrent bladder infections in some women. Postmenopausal women have the added factors of diminished vaginal lubrication and atrophic tissue changes in the urethra and vaginal mucosa secondary to decreased estrogen production. The pain, urgency, and frequency of acute cystitis, as well as the fear of recurrent episodes, can diminish the sexual desire.

NURSING CARE

The nurse who works with women experiencing cystitis should obtain a sexual history. Frequently, there is a relationship between sexual practices and the subsequent development of cystitis; for example, after a period of little sexual activity, the woman engages in frequent and vigorous activity. The nurse can help the client identify the potential causal relationships between sexual activity and the development of cystitis.

The client should be taught normal anatomy and physiology of the lower urinary tract and its relationship to the vagina, as many women have no knowledge of their internal anatomy. The nurse should suggest that after sexual activity the client should urinate to flush the urethra, and she should drink 6 to 8 ounces of water to dilute the urine that will subsequently collect in the bladder. Postmenopausal women could be encouraged to use a water-soluble lubricant during sexual intercourse.

The nurse should suggest additional measures to diminish the chances of infection and the discomforts associated with them:

1. Drink 2 to 3 quarts of fluid each day to keep the urine dilute.
2. Urinate every 3 to 4 hours to flush the urethra.

3. Wear cotton underpants (or those with a cotton crotch) to diminish the moistness of the perineum.
4. Wear pantyhose with a cotton crotch.
5. Avoid the use of bubble bath or perfumed additives that would irritate the perineum.
6. Use white, unscented toilet paper to eliminate the potentially irritative ingredients.
7. Towel dry the perineum by patting, not rubbing, and additionally use a hair blower on the cool setting to decrease irritation.

If the client with recurrent cystitis uses a diaphragm for birth control, she might be encouraged to use an alternative method. It is thought that the ring of the diaphragm serves to alter the flow of urine from the bladder, thus diminishing the flushing effect. Urologists have been successful with preventing recurrent cystitis in many women by prescribing a low dose of an antibiotic such as trimethaprim-sulfamethoxazole at bedtime to combat bacteria in the bladder. Frequently, estrogen therapy, topical creams or oral therapy, will be prescribed to treat atrophic changes in postmenopausal women.

Urinary Incontinence

The extent of the problem in our society is unknown because it is an "unmentionable" affliction; those who are known to be incontinent represent only the tip of the iceberg. A British study in 1980 compared the number of incontinent clients already known by the various health and social agencies in two London boroughs with the number of incontinent clients identified through a survey mailed to all patients of 12 physicians in different parts of England. The agencies revealed that 1.4 per cent of males and 2.7 per cent of females had urinary incontinence that had already been identified. The mail survey revealed that 8.5 per cent of the males and 20.1 per cent of the females were incontinent at least twice a month, thus implying that urinary incontinence is more prevalent than was previously thought (Fenely, 1984). In 1982 Help for Incontinent People, Inc. (HIP) was formed by Katherine Jeter. In 1983 Dr. Jeter wrote a letter to Dear Abby introducing urinary incontinence to the public, mentioning HIP as a resource. Dr. Jeter was inundated by 35,000 letters; she continues to receive 100 to 200 letters a week from individuals or their families about personal problems with incontinence.

Urinary incontinence can be a congenital problem, such as that associated with spina bifida, or acquired, such as that accompanying multiple sclerosis or traumatic paraplegia. Unless an individual has a severe problem with incontinence, fear and shame may prevent bringing the lesser degrees of incontinence to the attention of health professionals. Conversely, health professionals may not inquire about urinary problems. The problem is compounded further by the view of some health professionals that incontinence is an affliction with no resolution. In the elderly population it may be accepted as a normal consequence of the aging process; as a result, elderly people frequently are admitted to a nursing home merely because they are incontinent.

EFFECTS OF URINARY INCONTINENCE

Physiological Function

The neurophysiology of urination is a very complex process, requiring synchronous interaction among the brain, spinal cord, and autonomic nervous system. Innervation of the bladder and urethra is complex and not fully understood. Any alteration in the nervous system by disease, trauma, or congenital defects can have a deleterious effect on urination. Incontinence is merely a *symptom* of an underlying problem.

Bladder filling and emptying are associated with pressure changes within the bladder, bladder neck, and urethra (external sphincter). During the resting-filling phase, the pressure within the normal bladder is low, allowing the bladder to fill and expand with urine. Pressures at the bladder neck and in the urethra are significantly higher than those in the bladder, thus allowing for continence. When the bladder has reached its capacity (300 to 500 ml), an afferent impulse is sent via the spinal cord to the micturition center of the brain, which then transmits efferent impulses through the thoracic and sacral levels of the spinal cord to initiate voiding. During voiding, the bladder pressure increases with contraction. Pressures in the bladder neck and urethra decrease, thus allowing the bladder to empty.

Bladder function can be demonstrated easily by comparing it to an inflated balloon that has been pinched at the opening to prevent the escape of air; the pinching illustrates the higher pressures in the urethra. By relaxing the fingers and thus decreasing the pressures in the "urethra" and "bladder neck," the higher balloon (bladder) pressure will result in the escape of the air (urine). Because the full bladder looks like a balloon on x-ray, the balloon concept can be used to teach clients about the physiology of voiding as well as to illustrate their pathophysiology (Fig. 21–1).

Psychosocial Function

Urinary incontinence—or the fear of it—can be a devastating problem for an individual. It interferes with many aspects of daily life and can threaten feelings of self-concept, body image, and sexual roles. Individuals with urinary incontinence will experience feelings of anger, depression, shame, and fear, and they may isolate themselves from family, friends, and colleagues to avoid the embarrassment of incontinence. Because bladder control is one of the first milestones of self-control in the life of an individual, incontinence makes one feel childlike and lacking in self-control. The ominous association of wetness, the ever-present fear of someone noticing it, the distressing odor, and the perineal skin breakdown can prevent persons from viewing themselves as sexual beings. It can result in avoidance of close interpersonal relationships.

ASSESSMENT AND INTERVENTION

Conditions that affect the brain, spinal cord, and/or peripheral nerves can alter the pressure gradients previously described. Table 21–1 describes four major classifications of voiding dysfunction, while Table 21–2 presents a format for the assessment of the incontinent client. Although evaluation of voiding dysfunction can be difficult, most health professionals can categorize incontinence by referring to Table 21–1.

Once the assessment is complete, the data collected can be utilized to plan appropriate interventions. All interventions should be aimed at the underlying cause of the urinary incontinence, remembering that the incontinence is a *symptom*. When the client is to be referred to a physician for additional assessment and/or treatment, the health professional should provide the physician with the results of the assessment. The client should

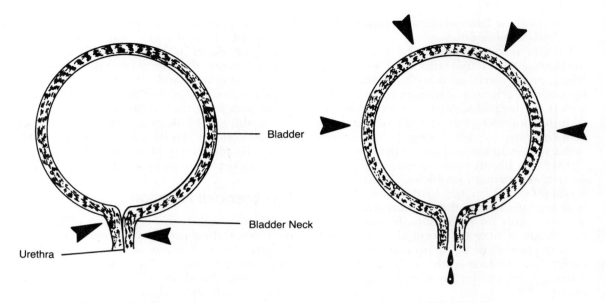

A. Resting-Filling Phase   B. Voiding Phase

FIGURE 21–1. Normal bladder. Note: Dark areas indicate areas of higher pressure. A, Resting-filling phase. B, Voiding phase.

be involved in the treatment planning so individual abilities and life style can be taken into account.

A significant number of clients can be helped just by instituting good bowel and bladder toileting habits combined with adequate fluid intake. When a client is not completely independent in his daily activities, nursing staff and families frequently perpetuate incontinence unknowingly by not encouraging the client to get out of bed, to get dressed, or to become physically active. Incontinence pads are placed in the bed and in chairs, which gives the message to the client that it is all right to be incontinent. Often in institutional settings clients are expected to notify caretakers when they need to void, whereas they may have no concept of the passage of time because they are not involved in personal daily routines. It is vitally important that the client, family members, and nursing staff (on all shifts) work together to promote continence. The client should be out of bed, dressed, and involved in this process. While total fluid intake should be 1500 to 2000 ml each day, it may need to be curtailed 3 hours before sleep. The most "normal" setting for urination should be provided, e.g., easily accessible toilet or bedside commode, if the nearest toilet is not accessible. If the client requires a bedpan, voiding and bladder emptying will be compromised. The client should be reminded every 3 to 4

hours to void, beginning upon awakening in the morning and continuing until bedtime at night. If the client takes diuretics or steroids, is diabetic, and/or is elderly, provisions should be made for nighttime urination because each of these conditions can cause nocturnal diuresis.

A number of clients will need intermittent catheterization, with or without the use of adjunctive medications. With rare exceptions, clients can be taught self-catheterization to maintain independence. Intermittent catheterization is a clean procedure, in which clients merely wash their hands then cleanse the urinary meatus with a commercial wipe or soap and water. The catheter is lubricated and passed into the bladder. After use, the catheter is washed inside and outside with soap and water, rinsed, dried, and stored in a clean manner. Children catheterize themselves every 3 hours and adults every 4 hours to replicate normal voiding patterns.

Many health professionals believe that bladder infections associated with clean, intermittent catheterization are caused by the introduction of bacteria via the catheter. In the great majority of clients, these bacteria do not cause serious hazard. By preventing overdistention of the bladder by regular catheterization, the actual incidence of infections is reduced markedly. Catheterizing less often than every 3 to 4 hours can cause overdistention, ischemia of the bladder wall, and the

TABLE 21–1. Classification of Urinary Incontinence

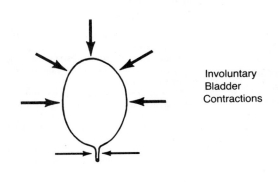

Involuntary Bladder Contractions

Bladder contracts with little or no warning.

1. *Urge* incontinence: voiding, immediately preceded by strong urge to void. (This is cause for incontinence in 50 to 75% of elderly females.) Many can remain continent unless delicate balance is tipped by illness or bed rest.
   a. Causes: CVA, diffuse changes caused by ASCVD, history of radiation therapy to pelvic area, bladder irritation from cystitis or concentrated urine.
   b. Treatment options: timed voiding every 3 to 4 hours by the clock, fluid intake of 2000 ml/day, decreased fluid intake in evening to decrease chances for incontinence during night, pharmacological manipulation with judicious use of anticholinergics to decrease bladder contractions (oxybutynin, imipramine).
2. *Reflex* incontinence: spontaneous void with no preceding desire to void.
   a. Causes: disc disease, spinal cord deficits (usually about T_{10}) such as paraplegia, multiple sclerosis, spina bifida
   b. Treatment: pharmacological use of anticholinergics, intermittent catheterization

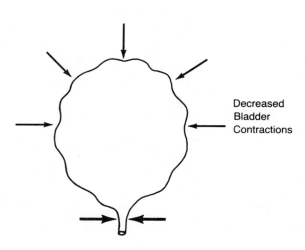

Decreased Bladder Contractions

Bladder contractions are of low pressure and inadequate to overcome urethral pressures (atonic bladder); bladder usually has capacity greater than 500 ml.

1. *Overflow* incontinence: involuntary loss of urine from grossly distended bladder, with large postvoid residual (greater than 75 ml; may have history of infrequent voiding and normal to large fluid intake; may have hesitancy initiating stream and decreased force of stream.
   a. Causes: peripheral neuropathies, e.g., diabetes, or lesions of sacral cord; medications (OTC and prescription)—cold preparations, antihypertensives, antidepressants, tranquilizers, muscle relaxants.
   b. Treatment options: discontinue offending medications; pharmacological manipulation to increase bladder contractions (bethanical chloride); or intermittent catheterization.

Table continued on following page

rapid multiplication of bacteria in the bladder. It is absolutely crucial that clients be taught these facts so that they are more likely to be compliant. Performing the catheterization *earlier* than every 4 hours is preferable to delaying or omitting a catheterization. Chronic constipation can affect bladder emptying and is associated with bladder infections in those who have voiding dysfunction. It is imperative that clients with these problems maintain a daily fluid intake of 1500 to 2000 ml, eat a high fiber diet, and, if necessary, be

put on a protocol for regular bowel evacuation. (For additional information, see Chapter 20, Spinal Cord Conditions and Sexuality.)

A small percentage of clients cannot be helped by existing medical or surgical treatments. Fortunately, improved commercial products for the inconspicuous containment of urine are available. Many of these products draw the urine away from the perineum, thus decreasing the likelihood of skin breakdown, and have an internal layer that absorbs

TABLE 21–1. Classification of Urinary Incontinence *Continued*

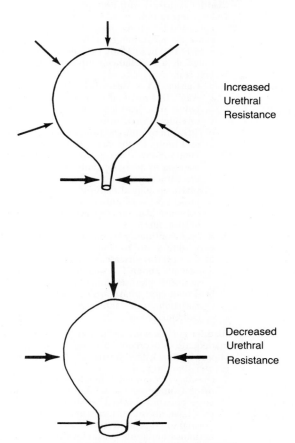

Increased
Urethral
Resistance

Decreased
Urethral
Resistance

Darker arrows indicate areas of higher pressure.

Bladder pressures not great enough to overcome higher urethral pressures/resistance.
1. *Urge* or *overflow* incontinence (described above):
   a. Causes: BPH, distended rectum, urethral strictures (male).
   b. Treatment: Remove obstruction (e.g., prostatectomy), bowel management.
2. *Reflex* incontinence: (described above):
   a. Causes: neurological deficits that cause contractions of external urethral sphincter at same time as bladder contractions (detrusor-sphincter dysynergia as seen in paraplegia, spina bifida).
   b. Treatment options: pharmacological agents to decrease urethral resistance (phenoxybenzamine) with attempted voiding trial; if voiding unsuccessful, intermittent catheterization (with anticholinergics, if indicated).

Bladder pressures higher than urethral pressures, frequently owing to anatomical malposition of female urethra because of relaxed muscles of pelvic floor.
1. *Stress* incontinence: involuntary loss of urine when intra-abdominal pressure increased (cough, sneeze); 25% also have element of *urge* incontinence.
   a. Causes: relaxed pelvic muscles because of parity, age, obesity; estrogen depletion postmenopause causes atrophic changes in mucosa of perineum, vagina, and urethra.
   b. Treatment options: weight loss; estrogen therapy to reverse changes; Kegel exercises* to strengthen pelvic musculature; surgical correction by urologist or gynecologist to suspend urethra and bladder neck to increase urethral resistance; pessary to realign/elevate urethra if other alternatives not an option.

*Client is taught to identify muscles by starting and stopping urinary stream during voiding; muscles that stop the stream are those which should voluntarily be contracted 40 to 50 times a day for 5 to 10 seconds each time. Positive results may not be seen because it takes persistent efforts for many months to achieve good tone, and many clients are not motivated to continuous exercises without continuous reinforcement.

ASCVD = arteriosclerotic cardiovascular disease; BPH = benign prostatic hypertrophy; CVA = cardiovascular accident.

urine to prevent signs of wetness on clothing. Commercial products, however, should be a *last* resort for the management of urinary incontinence. Every incontinent client should have this symptom evaluated thoroughly by a urologist, who can determine the most appropriate method of management.

There are excellent commercial devices available for male clients in the form of external condom-type catheters. As yet no one has marketed an acceptable device for females. However, there are some nonbulky, superabsorbent disposable devices on the market; a descriptive catalogue is available from HIP, PO Box 544, Union, South Car-

olina 29739. Unfortunately, all of these products are expensive, and third party payers are very inconsistent with their coverage; some will pay for condom-type devices for men but not for the kinds of products that must be used by women.

In addition to providing clients with technical information, emotional and psychosexual support is also necessary. The reader is referred to the book *Managing Incontinence* (Gartley, 1985), which was written for and by incontinent persons. It teaches the client the importance of identifying the feelings that are generated by this problem—the first step in learning to cope with it. The goals are to

TABLE 21–2. Assessment of Urinary Incontinence

I. History
  A. Current status of client
    1. Mental status: alert, lethargic, confused?
    2. Physical status: factors such as obesity, decreased mobility, lack of independence with ADLs that could affect toileting.
    3. Current medical problems.
    4. Medications client is taking or has taken recently; include both prescription and over-the-counter medications.
  B. Past medical history
    1. Abdominal or pelvic trauma, surgery, and/or radiation therapy.
    2. History of urinary tract infections. (Many clients are told by physicians that infections are "kidney infections" but client's history of symptoms indicate bladder infections, i.e., burning on urination, frequency, urgency, no fever, chills and/or flank pain.)
  C. Urination
    1. When client has urge to void, how long can client wait prior to voiding?
    2. How frequently does client urinate during the day, night?
    3. How much urine is passed at a time (drops, cup full, quart)?
    4. Does bladder feel empty after voiding?
    5. Does client have to strain to start urinary stream or to empty bladder?
    6. Any pain associated with voiding? Describe pain and its location.
  D. Incontinence
    1. How long has this been a problem?
    2. How does client manage incontinence (pads, diapers)?
    3. Is client wet all the time, wet with cough or sneeze, wet on the way to the toilet, dry with intermittent dribbling or dry with periodic gushing of urine?
  E. Fluid intake. Ask client to describe amount and kinds of fluids drunk on a typical day. Does any one kind of fluid predominate in the diet? (Notes: adults need a daily fluid intake of about 2000 ml each day for homeostasis. If this much fluid is drunk, the client should need to void every 4 to 5 hours if bladder capacity and voiding are within normal limits. A predomination of carbonated and citrus drinks make urine pH alkaline, caffeine can serve as a bladder irritant, and alcohol as a diuretic.)
  F. Assess bowel function. If neurological deficits are present that affect ability to void, bowel function frequently is abnormal.
    1. How often does client have bowel movements?
    2. Do bowels move at any particular time of day?
    3. Consistency: loose, semiformed, cigarshaped, or hard and dry like marbles or golf balls, which is indicative of chronic constipation. (Associated with difficulty in voiding, this can be a symptom of neurological dysfunction.)
    4. What does client take for constipation? How frequently?
    5. Does client have pain when passing bowel movements, which might indicate hemorrhoids or anal fissures?
  G. Additional assessment of female client
    1. Number of pregnancies and deliveries, vaginal and cesarean. Were forceps ever used in a delivery?
    2. Does she feel a "heaviness" in her perineum?
    3. Is sexual intercourse painful? Does urine seem to "scald" her perineum during voiding? (In postmenopausal women these symptoms could indicate mucosal thinning and irritation due to estrogen depletion.)
  H. Additional questions for male client
    1. Has he ever had urethritis or discharge of fluid from urethra? Has he had to wear an indwelling catheter or had other urethral instrumentation? (Positive response to these questions could have been the stimulus for urethral stricture formation, which could interfere with voiding.)
    2. Is the force and caliber of his urinary stream different from 1 or 2 years ago?
    3. Does he dribble urine after he has completed voiding?

Table continued on following page

grieve the loss of control, to find individualized and constructive ways to cope with it so the person eventually can "accept" the incontinence and get on with life as a confident individual, who recognizes the incontinence as an everpresent nuisance but who remains courageous and determined. There are chapters that teach skills for coping: management of the emotional distress, preservation of competence with a positive self-image, preservation of interpersonal relationships, and management of incontinence itself.

Sexual functioning certainly is possible when the client is incontinent, but modifications are necessary. Therefore, sexuality concerns of the client should be addressed by the health professional. The client needs specific suggestions regarding approaches to use in explaining incontinence to a potential sex partner; communication with a partner is imperative. The client should be informed that prior to sexual encounters the bladder should be emptied. Fluids, particularly alcoholic beverages or those with caffeine, should be avoided 1 to 2 hours prior to anticipated sexual activity. Hygiene is of utmost impor-

TABLE 21–2. Assessment of Urinary Incontinence *Continued*

II. Physical examination
   A. Abdominal examination by palpation for distended bladder and other masses.
   B. Depending on assessment skills, the examiner should do a bimanual exam on the female and a prostate exam of the male client (if he is over 40 years of age).
   C. Neurological examination
      1. Rectal tone is examined digitally by examiner to note whether tone is normal, weak, or absent.
      2. Bulbocavernosus reflex. Examiner inserts a finger in client's rectum, then gently squeezes the glans penis (clitoris); if the rectal sphincter contracts around examiner's finger, $S_{2,3,4}$ (the reflex arc) is intact.
         (Note: Lax rectal tone and a negative bulbocavernosus reflex should alert examiner to concomitant neurological injury to the bladder.)
   D. Female client
      1. Perineal examination
         a. Assess sensation of the perineum, labia, and perirectal area by pinprick if neurological deficits suspected.
         b. Can client voluntarily contract rectum and vagina?
         c. Look for presence of relaxed pelvic musculature, e.g., cystocele, rectocele.
      2. If symptoms and history suggest stress incontinence, evaluate this when client has a full bladder. With client in lithotomy position (or standing over disposable absorbent pads placed on the floor), ask client to bear down (Valsalva maneuver) or cough and observe for leakage of urine. If there is leakage, the examiner should insert two gloved fingers into the client's vagina pressing gently upward on either side of the urethra to support it, but not occlude it; again ask client to cough. If urinary leakage no longer is present with this maneuver to suspend the urethra, the examiner should refer her to a urologist or gynecologist for evaluation of stress incontinence.
   E. Male client. Assess urinary stream by doing a simple flow study when he has a full bladder. Using the second hand of a watch, time the client's entire voiding as he empties his bladder into a calibrated container (note also the force and caliber of his stream and whether he must strain to void). Calculate the number of ml voided per second. A calculation of 15 ml or less/second indicates poor force of the stream and indicates to the physician that assessment is needed to rule out obstruction by the prostate gland, urethral strictures, and/or poor bladder contractions.
III. Laboratory studies
   A. Urinalysis of a midstream, clean-catch urine. If possible with the female client, assist with the collection: After the client has been prepped, allow her to separate the labia using both hands while examiner collects a midportion of the urine.
   B. Urine culture. Male clients can collect a midstream clean-catch urine. To avoid contamination of the female's specimen, a sterile catheterized urine should be obtained, particularly if the urinalysis was positive for white blood cells and/or bacteria.
IV. Collect objective baseline data of intake, output, wetness, and any circumstances surrounding episodes of wetness (e.g., bedpan used instead of commode). Use a systematic flowsheet and enlist the assistance of the client and all those associated with the 24 hour care of the client. This will document the history and symptoms described by the client during his evaluation. Collect this data for 36 to 72 hours for greater accuracy.

ADLs = activities of daily living

tance and can be achieved by using clean and absorbent padding when engaging in sexual activity. The few clients who have indwelling catheters can drink copious amounts of fluid to decrease urine odor and can observe scrupulous hygiene prior to sexual encounters. Female clients can tape the catheter to the top of the thigh to prevent dislodgment; male clients can fold the catheter back alongside the penis and apply a condom over it, utilizing a water-soluble lubricant prior to penetration.

It is imperative for the physical *and* mental health of every incontinent client that health professionals pursue every avenue available to eliminate or cope with this devastating problem. Achievement of continence provides the client with a new lease on life.

Bladder Cancer

Cancer of the bladder occurs most frequently after the fifth decade of life and more frequently in men than women. The overall incidence of bladder cancer in the population over age 40 is 20 per 100,000 people (Droller, 1980a). The most common symptoms are gross, often transient, painless hematuria and/or urinary frequency and burning with urination. It is not uncommon for a client initially to ignore intermittent hematuria before consulting a physician. Because the symptoms often imitate those of cystitis, it is also not uncommon for a physician merely to treat (and retreat) the symptoms before referring the client to a urologist for further evaluation. It is imperative that every client with hematuria receive a comprehensive evaluation and that if a specific cause is not found, for example, an infection documented by a urine culture, the client be referred to a urologist for further evaluation. (The reader is referred to Chapter 15, Cancer and Sexuality, for a thorough discussion of the effect of cancer on sexuality.)

EFFECTS OF BLADDER CANCER ON ADAPTATION

The diagnosis of cancer is a severe blow to the psyche. Because in most cases the symptoms of bladder cancer are so mild and the client does not feel sick, it is even more difficult for the client to grasp the significance of the diagnosis.

The client with a diagnosis of bladder cancer will undergo a complete metastatic evaluation to determine the stage of the cancer. If the tumor is superficial, it is removed cystoscopically through the urethra; the client may subsequently be treated with a course of a topical chemotherapeutic agent, which is instilled in the bladder through a catheter on an outpatient basis. Clients with superficial tumors have periodic internal visual examinations of their bladders by their urologists as outpatients for continued surveillance. None of these examinations or treatments has more than a transient physical effect on the sexual activities of the client. Psychologically, however, the individual never can escape from the fear of recurrence, which can only be detected by periodic cystoscopic examinations. The fear itself can interfere with sexual desire and/or sexual functioning.

If the tumor has invaded the bladder muscle but not metastasized beyond, the urologist will recommend a radical cystectomy. The procedure necessitates the surgical diversion of urine through an ileal or colon conduit (ostomy) on the client's abdomen, or diversion into a continent urostomy, during which an internal reservoir is created from a piece of bowel. A continent stoma is created on the abdomen through which the client is taught to drain the reservoir every 4 to 6 hours (Brogna and Lakaszawski, 1986). Every client should also be informed of the treatment option of radiation therapy as a primary treatment, with subsequent radical surgery if this is not successful. However, surgery is more difficult when it is done on tissues that have been radiated.

Whether male or female, the optimal treatment for attaining a cure for invasive bladder cancer is extensive, with great psychological and physical effects on the client. The male will experience a temporary diminution of his sexual desire because of the effects of major surgery; he will be infertile and (perhaps) experience erectile problems, while the female will lack lubrication, engorgement, and uterine contractions during orgasm and will be infertile. Because most clients with bladder cancer are beyond their childbearing years, fertility usually is not a significant issue.

NURSING PROCESS

Nurses play a great role in the care of these clients. The nurse's first contact should be made when the initial diagnosis is made, even prior to the staging evaluation. The nursing role initially is to develop a close therapeutic relationship with the client and partner; to ascertain their strengths and weaknesses as individuals and as a couple; to learn about their family relationships, work history, and leisure time activities; and to assist with the formulation of nursing diagnoses for the development of a long-term plan of care. The relationship established between the nurse and the couple can become a deep and long-lasting one. The nurse assumes responsibility for the clarification and amplification of all explanations provided by the physician. Sketches and diagrams can be used to provide tangible illustrations of explanations, which then can be kept for review. The word cancer frequently is so devastating that little else is heard by clients initially. If the knowledge that they have cancer does not block the reception of further information, frequently the discussion of treatment options and subsequent effects will.

Assessment

During the emotional turmoil following diagnosis, the health professional must obtain a sexual history from the couple. At the same time that the male client is informed of the potential for surgically induced erectile dysfunction, he can also be told about subsequent treatment options for restoration of his erectile function. The nurse must review information pertaining to the urinary diversion that will be constructed. Frequently, the surgeon has already done this, but often clients do not have a clear understanding of what they have been told. If the client is to have a diversion that requires him to wear an ostomy appliance, it is vitally important to show him an appliance before surgery; many clients have visions of a very unsightly, bulky bag being attached to their abdomen, while others understand that the segment of bowel that serves as the conduit for the passage of urine is actually a functional new bladder.

Intervention

Client Education. The surgeon should provide extensive explanation to the client about the cancer, the options for treatment, and the statistics to support each. The male client is told that the bladder, prostate gland, seminal vesicles, urethra (in some cases), and surrounding lymph glands will be removed. He is told that he will be infertile because the vas deferens is resected and that he will potentially be unable to attain an erection because of surgical trauma to the pelvic nerve plexus during surgery. However, a modified technique for pelvic surgery is now being recommended that prevents permanent trauma to the pelvic nerve plexus and thus spares erectile ability. If sparing the nerve plexus does not compromise removal of the tumor, this technique can be utilized (Walsh and Donker, 1982).

The female client is told that her surgery includes not only removal of the bladder (and perhaps urethra), but also will include removal of her uterus, ovaries (after age 45 or menopause in some hospitals), fallopian tubes, and perhaps the anterior vaginal wall because of the anatomic proximity of these structures to the bladder and urethra. If the anterior vaginal wall is removed surgically, the posterior vaginal wall is formed into a new, shortened vagina during the surgery. However, the clitoris remains intact. It is important that all information is provided so the client can make an informed decision regarding treatment options. If indepth explanations are not provided, probably 100 per cent of the clients would elect to have radiation therapy to avoid surgery, erectile dysfunction, and an ostomy.

Interventions To Promote Adaptation. If the client elects to undergo radical surgery, the nurse serves many functions to the client and the partner: confidant, supporter, educator, caregiver. Preoperative nursing care must be extensive and include tasks such as the mechanical bowel preparation, postoperative ileus, and maintenance of the nasogastric tube to diminish the attendant fears and anxieties regarding surgery. In addition, the abdomen must be examined to select and mark the ideal site for the placement of the stoma during surgery. It is imperative that this be done by a nurse or physician who is knowledgeable with regard to stomal placement and that the site be marked during the preoperative period when the abdomen can be examined with the client in a variety of positions.

Postoperatively, the nurse cares for the ostomy and teaches the client how to care for it. By the time of discharge the client should have changed the appliance independently, should have understood all basic aspects of ostomy care, and should have been provided with all necessary supplies and literature. The client who has a continent urostomy will be discharged with an indwelling suprapubic catheter for several weeks and then return as an inpatient or outpatient to learn the technique and protocol for the intermittent catheterization of the internal reservoir. Clients can be encouraged to join a branch of the United Ostomy Association (UOA) if one is near their homes. When appropriate during the preoperative and/or postoperative periods, specially trained visitors (ostomates themselves) from the local branch of the UOA can be asked to visit with the client.

The author does not recommend routinely teaching ostomy care to the partner, so the client avoids dependence on the partner. Some clients want their partners to care for the ostomy (and many do), but the author strongly encourages independence, telling clients that after discharge, if they and their partners mutually agree that the partner will care for the ostomy, the client can teach the partner how to do it. Unlike a colostomy, when the adhesion of a urinary pouch seal loosens, the appliance must be changed immediately because one cannot "caulk" a urine leak; clients *must* be able to change their own appliances in case the partner is not at home at the time. Clients with a continent ostomy must catheterize the ostomy regularly, so they must be able to carry out this procedure independently.

Interventions To Promote Sexual Function. In order to preserve optimum feelings of sexuality and sexual functioning in the couple, open communication and physical closeness should be encouraged from the start, focusing on their strengths as individuals and as a couple; the health professional should stress that physical limitations will be negligible following the recovery from surgery. During the long hours of surgery, the nurse can focus attention on the partner, encouraging discussion of feelings and questions about the course of events. Postoperatively, physical closeness and touching should be encouraged; frequently the partner is afraid of hurting the client and hesitates to initiate touch. The nurse encourages the partner to assist with physical care, such as encouraging the client to cough and helping with ambulation. With the permission of the client, the partner is also encouraged to observe the stoma and to touch it, allowing the client to affirm that the stoma does not hurt.

The couple should be told that following recovery from surgery (6 to 8 weeks postoperatively), the client will regain sexual desire and that the sensation of orgasm will return, despite a male client's inability to ejaculate. The author has not observed any long-term deleterious effects on the overall relationship of a well-adjusted couple because of the physical changes or alterations in sexual functioning.

Until ostomates feel comfortable and competent with the care of the stoma, they (or the partner) will be afraid that intimate body contact will cause physical discomfort, leakage of urine, or even dislodgment of the appliance. Feelings of satisfaction with intimate encounters may be limited because of the everpresent consciousness of the stoma and the appliance. The nurse should assure the couple that these fears will decrease significantly as competence and confidence increase.

Alterations necessary for the physical expression of love should be discussed with the couple, stressing the importance of touching and kissing. Permission is given to explore alternative forms of sexual expression, since vaginal penetration may be impossible for clients with erectile problems. For female clients, vaginal penetration is not encouraged until the physician has determined that the vagina has healed. Once healing has occurred, the use of water-soluble lubricant during sexual intercourse is recommended because vaginal lubrication is usually not sufficient. If vaginal dilation cannot be accomplished with ease by the partner's erect penis or fingers, commercial dilators can be prescribed to enlarge the vagina slowly, over time.

The nurse can provide specific suggestions regarding the traditional conduit urostomy during sexual activity. The client is taught to examine the appliance prior to intimate encounters to be certain that it is securely adhered to the abdomen. Fluid intake can be limited an hour or so before sexual activity to decrease urine production. The appliance should be emptied immediately prior to sexual activity. Decorative covers for appliances are available commercially, or the appliance can be gently folded out of the way and covered with a piece of material used as a cumberbund. If the client utilizes a two-piece appliance, it can be positioned in any direction to prevent inconvenience.

The client with a continent urostomy should be instructed to perform catheterization prior to sexual activity to prevent pressure on the reservoir. As the abdomen is typically covered with a piece of gauze or bandage to absorb moisture from the mucosa, no other preparation is necessary.

During subsequent postoperative outpatient visits, the health professional can initiate discussions about treatment options for erectile dysfunction. Many urologists delay surgical implantation of penile prosthesis for 1 year to ensure that no additional cancer is detected. In the meantime the client can be taught to induce erections by intracavernosal injections of papaverine and phentolamine when he is physically and psychologically ready. If intercourse is infrequent, the client may elect not to have a prosthesis inserted and continue to use this method.

Because memories of the radical cancer surgery are apt to be vivid, it is important to explain the comparatively simple nature of penile prosthesis surgery. During subsequent visits, the types of prostheses are shown to the client and the partner, so eventually they can decide whether to undergo the surgery. Clients can suggest which kind of prosthesis they would rather have implanted, although the final decision rests with the surgeon who will perform the surgery.

PROSTATE

The lobes of the prostate form a "collar" around the urethra just below the neck of the bladder. Sperm are stored in the epididymis and, when combined with fluids secreted by the seminal vesicles, prostate and Cowper's glands, constitute the seminal fluid of ejaculation.

Prostatitis

Although men have few primary infections of the urinary tract, the prostate is the most common site for infections of the lower urinary tract. Symptoms of prostatitis include perineal and lower back pain and frequency and urgency of urination. Acute bacterial prostatitis can also cause fever and chills. While an acute bacterial infection is treatable with appropriate antimicrobials, chronic bacterial prostatitis (persistence of bacteria despite treatment with appropriate antibiotics) is often difficult to eradicate because of poor transmission of the medication from plasma into the prostatic tissues. In chronic prostatitis and prostatodynia (negative cultures despite presence of symptoms), the perineal and lower back pain persist, possibly decreasing sexual desire in the affected man. In addition, the continued inflammation associated with prostatitis can cause pain during the contractions that occur in the excitement and orgasmic phases of the sexual response. These problems can lead both to decreased desire and/or to avoidance of sexual activity unless the inflammation can be eradicated.

NURSING PROCESS

Nursing measures include patient education about the prostate and prostatitis. If antibiotics have been ordered, it is imperative that the client understand the diligence necessary for compliance. This particularly is important for the treatment of chronic prostatitis because the course of antibiotics may last for more than 6 weeks in an attempt to eradicate the nidus of infection; compliance is often difficult. Drinking a minimum of 2 liters of fluid a day to dilute the urine and to flush the urethra through frequent urination is also beneficial, and the client should be encouraged to do so. The use of warm sitz baths and mild analgesia can help to minimize the local symptoms. This condition is very frustrating for the client, who needs much emotional support and encouragement to persist with his treatment.

Benign Prostatic Hypertrophy

Although the cause for benign prostatic hypertrophy (BPH) is not known, the lobes of the prostate enlarge as part of the aging process, occurring in about 50 per cent of men over 50 years of age and in 75 per cent of men over 75 years of age (Lytton and Epstein, 1977). Many men fear that treatment for prostate problems will affect their sexual functioning, so they avoid seeking medical attention until the symptoms of straining to void and nocturia have progressed to the point of nocturia seven or eight times a night and/or urinary retention from urethral compression by the enlarged lobes of the prostate.

BPH is treated surgically by one of three approaches: if the hypertrophy is relatively small, the tissue will be resected through the urethra; if there is significant hypertrophy, a suprapubic incision is made, and the prostate gland is enucleated through the prostatic capsule (retropubic approach) or through the bladder (suprapubic approach) (Fig. 21–2).

BENIGN PROSTATIC HYPERTROPHY AND SEXUAL FUNCTION

Eighty to ninety per cent of men who have had prostate surgery for BPH will have irreversible retrograde ejaculation of seminal fluid into the bladder as a sequela of any of the surgical approaches because the bladder neck unavoidably is damaged during surgery; functional fertility, therefore, is lost (Kolodny, Masters, and Johnson, 1979). No erectile nerve fibers are damaged, and the vascularity of the penis is unaffected, so erectile dysfunction is not an anticipated problem. However, erectile dysfunction has been reported in 5 to 20 per cent of men following prostate surgery. It is thought that this might be of psychogenic origin due to the fears of the man and his lack of knowledge and understanding of the anatomy and physiology and of the human sexual responses (Kolodny, Masters, and Johnson, 1979).

NURSING CARE

Preoperative teaching to explain retrograde ejaculation and to dispel the fears of the man and his partner could help to prevent the occurrence of erectile dysfunction. A preop-

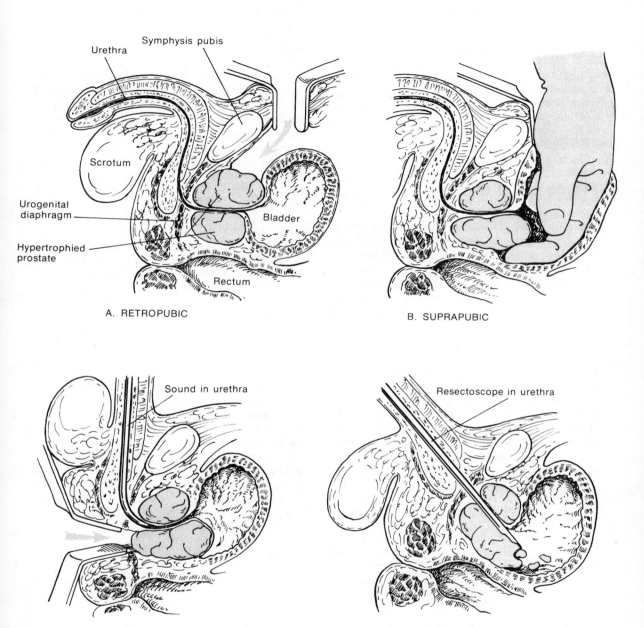

FIGURE 21–2. Surgical approaches to the prostate. A, Retropubic (extravesical) prostatectomy *is an open method in which a low abdominal incision is made between the pubic arch and the bladder.* B, Suprapubic (transvesical) prostatectomy *is an open method of treatment in which the hyperplastic prostatic tissue is enucleated through the anterior walls of the abdomen and bladder.* C, Perineal prostatectomy *is an open method involving an incision between the anus and the scrotum.* D, Transurethral resection prostatectomy (TUR) *is a closed method of treatment, i.e., no incision is made and the hyperplastic prostate tissue is removed through a resectoscope (like a cystoscope) inserted through the penis. (From Luckmann J, Sorensen KC: Medical Surgical Nursing. 3rd ed. Philadelphia, WB Saunders, 1988.)*

erative sexual assessment would be beneficial to identify pre-existing sexual difficulties of the client and/or the partner when one is present. Since most couples are beyond their childbearing years when prostate surgery occurs, the lack of fertility rarely is a problem. If the man and his partner understand that the "dry" ejaculation accompanying orgasm will not interfere with their ordinary sexual behaviors, then perhaps psychogenic erectile dysfunction could be prevented.

Prostate Cancer

While it is unusual for prostate cancer to occur in men less than 55 to 60 years of age, it is a common form of cancer. There is no known cause for prostate cancer, and the probability of acquiring it increases with age. Frequently, no symptoms are apparent until the cancer has reached an advanced stage—when supportive and palliative treatments are the only options available. More than 50 per cent of prostate cancers are found during routine digital rectal examinations, before the man has symptoms.

Table 21–3 lists stages for prostate cancer and the potential treatment modalities. The stages used here are not those recommended by the American Joint Commission on Staging but are used merely to serve as a reference point. The effects on the sexuality and/or sexual functioning of the client are influenced more by the result of the particular treatment regimen than the disease itself.

PROSTATE CANCER, TREATMENT AND PHYSIOLOGICAL FUNCTION

Radical Prostatectomy. Until the past few years, nearly all men who had radical prostatectomies for the treatment of cancer suffered permanent erectile dysfunction because of the traumatic dissection necessitated by the surgery. Both the sacral parasympathetics and the lumbar sympathetic nerves pass through the pelvis nerve plexus, branches of which are located between the rectum and urethra and innervate the corpora cavernosa. During radical pelvic surgery (prostatectomies and cystoprostatectomies), injury to this nerve plexus causes erectile dysfunction postoperatively (Walsh and Donker, 1982). By modifying surgical approaches, erectile function has been spared in a high percentage of clients. However, Walsh and Donker (1982) feel that some nerve damage is sustained temporarily as a result of surgical manipulation. A factor that appears to affect the erectile function statistics is progression of disease at time of surgery. In men in whom the cancer has progressed outside the prostatic capsule, more surgical dissection is required, causing more surgical trauma and thus increasing the chances for irreversible impotence.

Despite careful nerve dissection, some men will still experience erectile problems after radical pelvic surgery. Bahnson and Catatona (1988) studied men who experienced erectile problems following nerve-sparing radical prostatectomies and found that the vascular system involved in erection had been damaged by the surgery because vascular stimu-

TABLE 21–3. Treatment of Prostate Cancer

Stage	Treatment Options
A—entirely confined within prostate, nonpalpable. Identified in pathological examination of tissue from transurethral resection for benign prostate hypertrophy	Low-grade pathology: no treatment; follow-up surveillance by physician. High-grade pathology: radical prostatectomy or radiation therapy.
B—Confined to prostate but palpable on digital examination.	Radical prostatectomy or radiation therapy if patient prefers.
C—Tumor confined to pelvis without distant metastases.	With statistical life expectancy of 5 to 10 years: radiation therapy. With limited expected survival and client symptomatic: hormonal therapy Limited survival and no symptoms: no treatment until symptoms occur, then palliate with hormonal treatment (Grahack, 1984).
D—Distant metastases to bone, lungs, liver, and/or lymph nodes.	Hormonal manipulation: bilateral orchiectomies or oral diethlystilbesterol.

lation of erections using papaverine failed to induce erections. These men can have penile prostheses implanted surgically if the tumor has not reoccurred in 1 year. They may also elect to try intercavernosal injections (Dennis and McDougal, 1988).

When a man has had a radical retropubic prostatectomy, the vas deferens has been tied off intraoperatively, and the seminal vesicles have been removed, so the man would be infertile even after the penile prostheses were implanted. However, since the man with prostatic cancer is usually beyond the age for wanting to father a child, infertility is not a problem.

Urinary incontinence is a problem in about 10 per cent of clients who have had radical prostatectomies. Surgical excision of the prostate damages the bladder neck; depending on the extent of the cancer and the resulting surgical dissection, the external sphincter also might be damaged. If both sphincters are damaged, total incontinence might result; if only the bladder neck is damaged, the client might experience stress incontinence and have to rely on frequent emptying of the bladder to avoid wetness. The client with total incontinence following a radical prostatectomy is a candidate for the surgical implantation of an artificial sphincter, which is described in greater detail in the section on urinary incontinence.

If the client's erectile function was spared during surgery, his sexual functioning should be normal even if he experiences urinary incontinence; he will be infertile, however. The client who experiences stress incontinence should limit his fluid intake for 1 hour or more prior to sexual activity and should certainly void immediately before sexual encounters to prevent leakage of urine.

Radiation Therapy. External beam radiation therapy is a standard treatment of prostatic cancer (see Chapter 15, Cancer and Sexuality, for a general discussion of the effect of radiation on sexual function). The dosage to be delivered is extremely accurate, but it cannot be targeted to hit only the prostate, so the bladder and bowel also receive radiation. During the 6-week course of therapy, clients will usually experience diarrhea, which can last for several weeks beyond treatment. As a rule, this can be controlled by oral medication that slows transit time through the intestines. Lassitude is another problem for clients during the course of treatment. Symptoms of bladder irritation

(frequency and urgency) are common as well. Long-term effects from external beam radiation can include (1) damage to the sigmoid colon, with continued diarrhea, which usually can be controlled with oral medication; (2) chronic symptoms of bladder irritation, which may indicate the use of low doses of anticholinergics; (3) periodic bleeding from pre-existing hemorrhoids; and (4) rectal strictures, which necessitate the use of stool softeners. Erectile dysfunction has been reported, but prospective studies to assess clients before and after treatment have not been judiciously done.

Hormonal Therapy. Hormonal therapy is used for the palliation of symptoms of prostate cancer that has metastasized beyond the prostatic capsule and for which no cure exists. Because prostate tumors are hormonally fed, these therapies benefit the client by shrinking the tumor. Bilateral orchiectomies for the palliation of symptomatic stage D disease removes the major source of androgen and estrogen production. In the client who has severe bone pain resulting from bone metastases, improvement is frequently felt in the recovery room after the surgical procedure. This procedure makes the client infertile, of course, and the loss of testosterone causes a decreased sexual desire and erectile dysfunction. Research has shown, however, that some men retain erectile functioning despite hormonal manipulation; these are most probably psychogenically induced erections (Ellis and Grayhack, 1963). Despite counseling, during which the client is told the benefits of the therapy, some refuse to have the surgery because of the effects on sexuality and sexual functioning.

The oral administration of diethylstilbesterol (DES) daily is another form of hormonal therapy, which works by neutralizing the production of androgen. There are some systemic side effects from taking this medication, such as gynecomastia and the potential for fluid retention. No client with existing cardiovascular problems is a candidate for this form of treatment, so orchietomies would be the treatment of choice. Likewise, the client who would not be diligent in taking the medication daily should also be advised to undergo orchietomies. Some urologists do not advocate the use of DES and prefer orchiectomy.

NURSING CARE

As with other forms of cancer and progressive chronic diseases, the nurse should not forget that the client is a sexual being. Despite the client's having stage C or D disease at the time of diagnosis, sexuality and sexual functioning are still prominent aspects of his life. It is imperative that the nurse make an initial sexual assessment and evaluate understanding of normal sexual functioning to allow for education and to be able to clarify the effects of the diagnosis and treatment regimens on sexual functioning. The development and promotion of a close, therapeutic relationship with the client (and his partner) is also essential. Because prostatic cancer progresses slowly in most cases, the diagnosis of stage C or D disease does not mean that the client is in the terminal stages of his illness.

The shock of the diagnosis can be devastating. Because few people have any understanding of the genitourinary tract's function, the couple may abstain from any coital activity for fear that the partner will contract cancer from the client or that vigorous sexual activity will "inflame" the cancer and cause it to progress more rapidly. Neither of these fears is real, but the nurse must dispel them and teach the anatomy and physiology and pathophysiology of the cancer.

When a client begins to exhibit systemic symptoms of stage D disease, the nurse must offer supportive counsel to encourage unity and sexual closeness previously exhibited by the couple and to suggest physical measures to be utilized for symptomatic relief.

PENIS-URETHRA

Hypospadias

Any alteration or interruption of the normal embryological development of the genitalia, hypospadias is the abnormal opening of the urethral meatus anywhere on the ventral surface of the penis, from the ventral surface of the glans penis to the junction of the penis and scrotum, or the perineum (Fig. 21–3). Although hypospadias occurs in about 1 of 125 live male births, approximately half of the meatal openings are in the glans penis and thus are not a problem. Associated with this abnormality can be a ventral curvature of the penis caused by a fibrous band of tissue on the ventral surface between the urinary meatus and the glans penis called chordee (Kolodny, Masters, and Johnson, 1979). When epithelial tissue does not de-velop normally, the result is this proliferation of connective tissue.

EFFECTS OF HYPOSPADIAS, TREATMENT, AND ADAPTATION

With surgical correction to remove the chordee and to construct a new urethra extending to the glans penis, sexual functioning in adulthood will not be altered in any way. It is imperative that the neonate with hypospadias not be circumcised, as the prepuce frequently is used in the construction of the urethra. The optimal age for surgery is between 12 months and 4 years, to prevent psychological fears of castration and to correct the problem prior to school age. It is important for the surgical correction to be made before the child enters day care or experiences school socialization because, prior to the surgery, the child might have to sit to urinate if the meatal opening is proximal to the glans penis, which could be a source of embarrassment. With the advent of microsurgery, the procedure can be done when the child is between 12 and 24 months of age. Repair of hypospadias should be performed by a skilled microsurgeon because even in the most experienced hands the development of a urethral-cutaneous fistula at the anastomosis of the new urethra and the original urethra is not an uncommon postoperative complication. The development of a fistula would require additional surgery.

Parents of infants with hypospadias are often distressed at the news that their child has a defect. Parents may express feelings of guilt. The nurse can reassure the parents that no one knows the cause and that following surgical repair the child's penis will be normal both cosmetically and functionally and have no effect on his ability to function sexually.

Peyronie's Disease

A disease of men over 40 years of age, Peyronie's disease is the development of fibrous plaques on the sheaths of the corpora cavernosa, the tissue within which becomes engorged with blood during erections. These plaques usually develop on the dorsal surface of the penis and do not permit lengthening of the involved portion of the penile shaft, causing the erect penis to bend in the direction of the plaques. This results in severe

HYPOSPADIUS

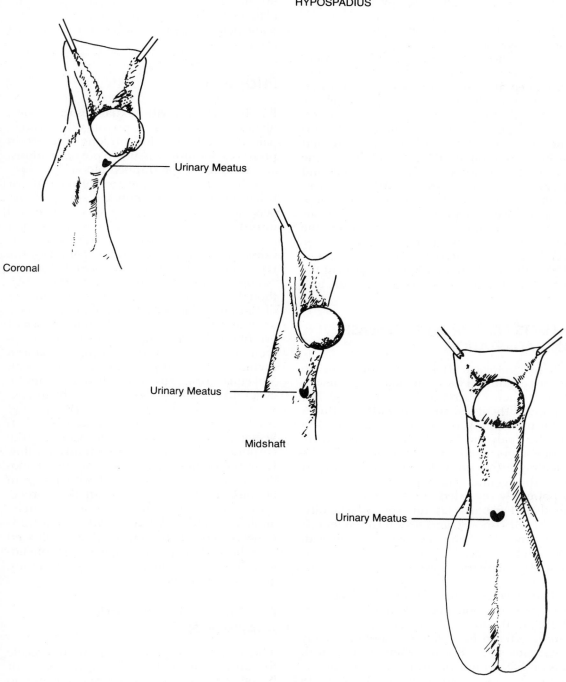

Coronal

Urinary Meatus

Midshaft

Urinary Meatus

Penoscrotal

Urinary Meatus

FIGURE 21–3. Hypospadias. A, *Coronal.* B, *Midshaft.* C, *Penoscrotal.*

angulation of the erect penis and pain associated with erections; the progression of the angulation eventually can prevent coitus. Erectile dysfunction can result from the pain with erections and from the fear associated with the symptoms.

There is no known cause for this condition, and many different treatment modalities have been attempted over the years with no consistent or favorable results. All of the treatments, ranging from oral medications, such as vitamin E, and injections of steroids into the plaques to radiation therapy and surgical excision of the plaques, have side effects that could equal the aggravation and frustration of the disease process. Treatments do not necessarily relieve the symptoms but seem to speed up the spontaneous resolution of the problem. Therefore, the self-limiting aspects of the disease must be weighed against the potential side effects of the treatment. With or without treatment the symptoms begin to resolve in 6 months to 2 years.

EFFECTS OF PEYRONIE'S DISEASE AND ADAPTATION

The psychological effects of this problem can be devastating. The client may fear he has cancer when he first feels the plaques. The erectile difficulties, coupled with the threat to his masculinity, can have a crippling effect on the body image of the affected man. Penile abnormalities can have more of a debilitating effect on male sexuality than most any other genitourinary problem. The penis is popularly regarded as the symbol of manhood and erection as the key to sexuality, sexual self-concept, and sexual fulfillment. It is no wonder, then, that any problem with the genital tract, especially the penis, is viewed with fears of castration and mutilation.

The affected man and his sexual partner need much supportive care and education: the natural course of the disease and what can be offered for treatment. Because many physicians feel helpless when dealing with this problem, most will institute some conservative therapy, such as vitamin E orally, to enhance the spontaneous remission that eventually occurs. These clients need someone who will listen to their frustrations. During the course of this disease the nurse can encourage experimentation with different positions for coitus and/or alternative forms of sexual pleasure, if necessary. Occasionally, when the angulation and pain are devastating to the man, the surgeon will excise the plaques to allow for expansion and will implant penile prostheses to restore functional erections.

Priapism

Rarely associated with sexual desire or stimulation, priapism is a prolonged, severely painful erection. This prolonged erection produces localized tissue hypoxia, acidosis, and viscosity of the trapped blood.

Although about 50 per cent of the cases of priapism have no identifiable cause, it has been associated with some specific medical disorders. Sickle cell anemia is the second major cause of priapism after idiopathic causes. During an acute sickle cell crisis, the red blood cells that have lysed form a "sludge" within the corpora cavernosa. Although it only occurs in a very small number of those with sickle cell anemia, it does have a tendency to recur, with a high incidence of erectile dysfunction because of the development of fibrosis of the corpora. Priapism occurs in about 10 per cent of patients with leukemia—primarily with chronic granulocytic leukemia, but other forms of the disease have been implicated as well (White and Nagler, 1983). Priapism associated with leukemia is caused by direct invasion of the corpora, which blocks the venous outflow from the corpora. Leukapheresis and hemodialysis have been associated with priapism because the heparin used with both procedures induces the production of antiplatelet antibodies and leukostasis, which then leads to decreased venous outflow. Also implicated have been some psychotropic drugs, phenothiazines, some antihypertensive medications, and marijuana and alcohol.

EFFECTS OF PRIAPISM AND ADAPTATION

The major sequela of priapism is erectile dysfunction or failure, which is the result of fibrotic changes in the corpora cavernosa no matter which form of treatment has been attempted to detumesce the corpora of the affected client. Treatment measures should be undertaken as soon as possible after priapism is diagnosed; conservative measures, such as hydration, sedation, and analgesia should begin at once. The chances for permanent erectile dysfunction increase dramatically once the erection has lasted 24 to 36 hours. Disease-specific treatment should also be instituted, as with clients with sickle cell disease. However, most cases of priapism must have surgical intervention to clear the corpora. Various procedures have been utilized by urologists; it appears that the most successful, as well as the quickest and easiest, is to create a temporary shunt between the corpora cavernosa and the corpora spongiosum (through which the urethra passes) to drain the accumulated "sludge" (White and Nagler, 1983). Although follow-up reports of various corrective procedures have not been reported consistently, it appears that this treatment has the greatest chance for preserving potency.

NURSING CARE

Although the overall incidence of priapism is not high, the potential for causing erectile dysfunction is alarming, and a man who suffers from this should be referred for appropriate treatment as soon as possible. The occurrence of an unexpected erection could surprise a client initially, but the prolongation of the erection and the resulting pain could make the man very frightened and anxious. Because erectile dysfunction frequently is the ultimate outcome, despite appropriate treatment, it is difficult to counsel the client until the treatment is complete. Any proposed local surgery to the penis to affect detumescence could be viewed by the client as the cause for erectile dysfunction, should it result. The psychological assessment of the client assists in determining whether the client has realistic expectations about restoration of erections. The client must be taught normal anatomy and physiology of erection and the basic pathophysiology of priapism. In addition, he must understand that if the condition is not treated, the chances for erectile dysfunction are far greater because of the fibrotic changes within the corpora cavernosa.

Penile (Urethral) Trauma

Urethral injuries result from pelvic fractures, straddle injuries, or penetrating wounds, such as those that occur from gunshot wounds or stabbings. The urethra of the male is much more susceptible to urethral trauma than that of the female because the female's urethra is protected by the symphysis pubis.

EFFECTS OF PENILE TRAUMA ON ADAPTATION

If injury occurs to the anterior (dependent) portion of the male urethra, there is usually no residual problem if appropriate care is given and if there is no neurovascular damage. Trauma to the posterior portions of the urethra usually occurs along with pelvic fractures and other internal injuries, leading to partial or complete disruption of the urethra. After the client has recovered from his multiple injuries, he might have urethral strictures, urinary incontinence, and/or erectile dysfunction. The rate of impotence from these multiple injuries is high—about 50 per cent (Webster, 1984), probably because of the neurovascular damage caused by the injury and/or the surgery necessary to correct it. Urinary incontinence, if present after complete physical recovery, usually results from injury to the bladder neck because of immediate surgery or postoperative scarring. Surgical reconstruction of the bladder neck after initial healing is complete can be done in an attempt to restore continence. These clients are not candidates for the artificial sphincter because of poor vascularity from the trauma and primary surgery (Webster, 1984).

NURSING CARE

Because of the multiple internal injuries associated with trauma to the posterior urethra, these clients are acutely ill for a long time. Nursing care revolves around physical and psychological care to allow the client time to heal. Residual damage, such as incontinence and/or erectile dysfunction, will not be known initially because the client will have his bladder managed by an indwelling catheter for a long period of time to allow for healing of the urethra and because any erectile dysfunction noted by the client could be temporary. In fact, one should not assume a client has permanent erectile dysfunction until 18 to 24 months have elapsed after the initial trauma. If erectile dysfunction is a problem at this time, a full evaluation should be made to distinguish between organic and psychogenic erectile dysfunction, and the appropriate treatment should be initiated.

Penile Cancer

This form of cancer is a quite rare entity, occurring in 1 of every 100,000 men, who are usually over age 50 (Schellhammer, 1984). It frequently presents as a painless growth or ulcer on the glans penis, but the lesion is often hidden under a tight (phimotic) foreskin. In fact, this disease is associated most often with the uncircumcised male who has a foreskin that will not retract behind the glans penis, probably having begun as irritation of the glans penis caused by the smegma trapped inside.

EFFECTS OF PENILE CANCER ON ADAPTATION

Embarrassment, fear of cancer, and fear of castration often prevent a man from seeking treatment until the disease is far advanced; it is not uncommon for the man to feel that the lesion resulted from masturbation or as punishment by God for past misdeeds. Without treatment the lesion progresses to become a fungating mass, which erodes the penile shaft, often becoming an infected and draining wound. This lesion tends to spread locally into inguinal nodes, rather than to produce distant metastases; therefore, the cancer is amenable to local treatment by penile amputation. Cure rates with amputation are high. Because lymphadenopathy can be the result of the inflammation, lymph node dissection at the time of the penile amputation is not advocated unless a node biopsy is positive; if nodes do not diminish over time, surgical removal might be necessary.

Neither orgasm nor ejaculation would be affected by penectomy. Because about one half of the penis is not visible externally, a penectomy for cancer usually necessitates removal of no more than one quarter of its actual length (Bracken, 1981), thus leaving enough length during erection for intercourse. Therefore, a majority of clients will maintain full sexual capabilities after surgery. In fact, this may be viewed as an improvement from the unsightly, foul-smelling lesion often present prior to treatment.

NURSING CARE

The impending surgery most often has a negative impact on the client's body image. The nurse must listen to the client and the partner, encouraging them to express fears and feelings; they must be helped to sustain their relationship or to renew it, particularly if sexual functioning had previously been prevented by the presence of the lesion. Postoperatively, the nurse should provide sexual counseling appropriate to the alternatives produced by surgical intervention. The psychological impact of the shortened penis may be devastating; the client may need referral for indepth psychological counseling.

Erectile Dysfunction

Erectile dysfunction is the inability of a man either to attain or to maintain an erection to permit penetration. Although the precise and complex physiological basis for penile erection still is unknown, erection does involve the synergistic interaction of the vascular, autonomic, and central nervous systems and is associated with psychogenic components as well. In the past, it was believed that most men with erectile dysfunction had psychological problems; however, as researchers have learned more about the neurophysiology of erections, this belief has been reversed.

ERECTILE DYSFUNCTION AND ADAPTATION

Erectile dysfunction can threaten a sense of manhood, a man's body image, and feelings of self-concept, as well as seriously alter a couple's relationship. In some men the insult to their body image caused by erectile dysfunction pervades all aspects of their daily lives and all interpersonal relationships by creating a reactive depression. Even though a couple may have an emotionally healthy relationship and have explored and utilized alternative forms of sexual pleasure, many men would rather engage in intercourse.

When a man seeks help for erectile dysfunction, it may seem apparent that the obvious course of treatment would be the surgical implantation of a penile prosthesis. However, the causes of erectile impotence are varied, so each client needs a detailed and systematic physical and psychological evaluation.

NURSING CARE
Assessment

A knowledgeable and compassionate health professional should (1) assess the client's sexual history beginning at puberty, (2) note his medical and surgical history, (3) perform a complete physical examination and a neurological examination pertinent to the presenting problem of erectile dysfunction, and (4) obtain a psychological evaluation by a competent psychologist or psychiatrist. The psychological assessment assists in determining whether the client has realistic expectations regarding the restoration of erections.

Nurses need to be aware of the many factors that can contribute to erectile dysfunction when providing care in a variety of settings. Clients with chronic illness can have erectile difficulties as a sequela of their diseases, such as the diabetic who has vascular insufficiencies and/or peripheral neuropathies. Fatigue and/or pain associated with chronic illness can affect sexual desire and erectile function as well. Certain endocrine disorders, for example, hypofunction of the thyroid or adrenals, can cause erectile dysfunction. Peripheral vascular disease can also affect erections. Genital disorders, such as priapism and Peyronie's disease, trauma, and iatrogenic sequelae of pelvic surgery are also causes. Neurological problems associated with the central or autonomic nervous systems, such as multiple sclerosis, spinal cord trauma, and neoplasms, frequently cause erectile dysfunction. Certain medications are a major cause of erectile dysfunction, such as antihypertensives, sedatives, and tranquilizers. The health professional should ask the client whether he has difficulties with erections and whether he is taking any of the commonly implicated medications because many clients will not bring up a sex-related issue unless asked.

Interventions

A number of treatment approaches are available to the man who experiences organic erectile disorder. Hormonal imbalances can perhaps be treated, and a different antihypertensive can be tried. Vascular insufficiencies are now being treated with greater accuracy, so that erections may return following surgery to correct the vascular insufficiency; procedures for the revascularization of the corpora cavernosa are now undergoing clinical trials. Penile prostheses are also widely available, although they are not appropriate for some clients. Unfortunately, many cases of erectile dysfunction are irreversible and

require medical and/or surgical procedures to achieve erectile competence.

A nonsurgical treatment for erectile dysfunction is the injection of a mixture of papaverine and phentolamine into a corpus cavernosum to stimulate a transitory erection. The papaverine-phentolamine combination produces tumescence by vasodilation, which when further stimulated by sexual foreplay, results in an erection capable of vaginal penetration. This treatment can be used in a carefully selected population of men who are not candidates for surgery or who do not want to undergo surgery. In our clinic, one 80-year-old man had married and wanted to be able to have penovaginal intercourse with his wife. Another man had stage D prostate cancer but was feeling well enough to have sexual intercourse periodically. Surgical implantation of prostheses seemed too radical for both of these men.

Should the client elect to utilize this method of treatment, the health professional teaches the client how to inject the medication, alternating sides of the penis each time, and provides him with a limited supply of medication and syringes, based on his frequency of intercourse. The client returns monthly for re-evaluation of his physical and psychological status before a new supply of medication and syringes is issued (Zorgniotti and Lefleur, 1985).

In our outpatient clinic the urologist and nurse clinician have taught this method to a number of clients, to the great satisfaction of the clients and their partners. Learning how to penetrate the corporal sheath to place the needle within the corpus has proved to be a challenge to the clients, and several have had local extravasation into penile tissues resulting in a transitory penile edema until they mastered the technique. This kind of injection is more difficult technically than the injection of insulin, for instance, so patient selection is crucial.

There are four types of penile prostheses (Hammond and Middleton, 1984):

1. Small-Carrion (Fig. 21–4). Semirigid silicone rods are implanted in the penis, which gives it a permanent, artificial erection (a disadvantage), but it is simple, easy to implant, less expensive than other types, and has a low risk of infection (advantages). Generally, there is high patient satisfaction.

2. Flexi-rod or Finney prosthesis (Fig. 21–5). This is a modification of the Small-Carrion but has a hinge at the level of the

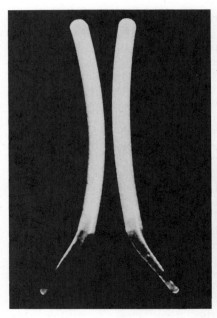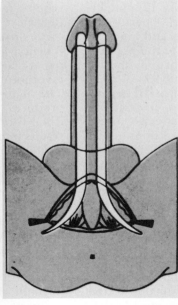

FIGURE 21–4. Small-Carrion rod prosthesis. (Reproduced by permission of Wood RY, Rose K: Penile implants for impotence. Am J Nurs 78:235, 1978.)

patient's pubis, so that it can bend out of the way. A disadvantage is that it may have too little stability during intercourse.

3. Jonas silicone-silver prosthesis (Fig. 21–6). This is similar to the Small-Carrion but has a central core of braided silver wire that holds the penis firmly in any position. It can bend out of the way easily and is more cosmetically attractive and expensive than the Small-Carrion.

4. Inflatable (Scott) penile prosthesis (Fig. 21–7). This consists of paired inflatable cylinders, a fluid reservoir, and a pump with an inflate and deflate mechanism. The biggest advantage of this device is that the erection can be controlled. However, the installation

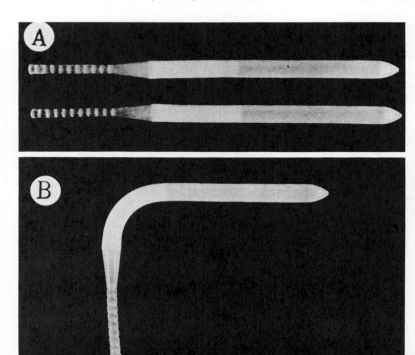

FIGURE 21–5. Finney prosthesis. (Reproduced by permission of Finney RF: New hinged silicone penile implant. J Urol 118:585, 1977.)

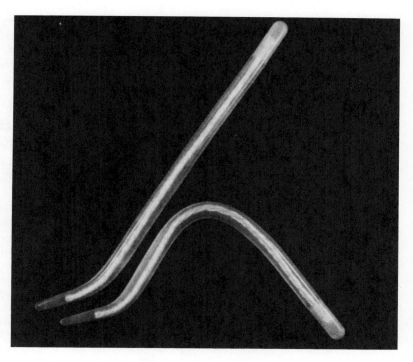

FIGURE 21–6. Jonas silicone-silver prosthesis. (Reproduced by permission of Jonas U, Jacobi GH: Silicone-silver penile prosthesis: Description, operative approach and results. J Urol 123:865, 1980. © by Williams & Wilkins, 1980.)

is more difficult and expensive and requires a longer hospital stay; mechanical failure has been reported in 10 to 35 per cent of the devices (Hammond and Middleton, 1984).

Each kind of penile prosthesis is paired, and a rod is implanted surgically within each corpus cavernosum; the surgical procedure is relatively simple and the postoperative recovery is usually benign and of short duration. The semirigid rods give the client a permanent erection that he can conceal under his clothing by wearing jockey style shorts or an athletic supporter. The flexible rods can be bent into a more normal pendulous position for concealment. Two kinds of inflatable rods are available. One requires implantation of the rods in the corpora; implantation of a fluid reservoir in the lower abdomen; and placement of a pump mechanism within the scrotal sac. Small-caliber silicone tubing connects the pump and the reservoir to the rods to make the prosthesis functional. The other inflatable device has both the pump and the reservoir contained within the rods themselves.

The physician should discuss each kind of prosthesis with the client and his partner, so they can participate in the decision regarding which should be implanted. The prosthesis selected is based on the physical condition of the client, the preference of the client, and the recommendation of the physician. For instance, the surgeon may not feel he could implant the inflatable prosthesis in a man who has undergone extensive abdominal surgery because of the technical difficulties associated with implantation of the fluid reservoir into an abdomen with scars and adhesions. Some surgeons are reluctant to implant any prosthesis, particularly the rigid or semirigid, in a paraplegic client because of the dangers of erosion and/or extrusion of the rods in a phallus that has no sensation. However, Golji (1979) found the implantation of Small-Carrion (semirigid) prostheses in 30 clients with spinal cord injuries to be no more traumatizing physically to those clients than to the nonparaplegic population. It should be noted that these clients were carefully selected and well-adjusted prior to surgery.

Beutler and his associates (1984) systematically evaluated women's satisfaction with their partners' prostheses (of all three types) using standardized measures of sexual satisfaction. The women reported high levels of satisfaction with sexual performance and that the artificial erection made little difference in their roles in sexual arousal.

TESTICLE
Testicular Cancer

Testicular tumors constitute less than 1 per cent of all malignancies in males and about

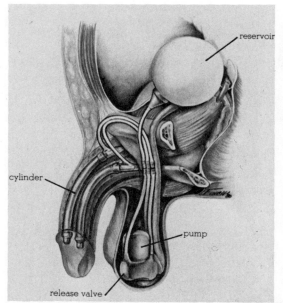

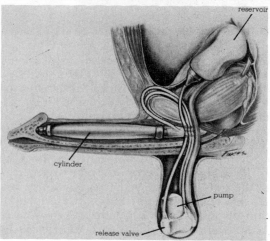

FIGURE 21–7. Inflatable penile prosthesis. When the bulb of the pump is squeezed, radiopaque fluid travels from the reservoir through tubing into the cylinders, creating an erection. When the release valve is pressed, the fluid returns to the reservoir, and erection ceases. (Reproduced by permission of Googe MCS, Mook TM: The inflatable penile prosthesis: New developments. Am J Nurs 83:1046, 1983. © by Williams & Wilkins, 1983.)

5 per cent of all genitourinary malignancies. However, except for lymphomas and leukemia, they are the most common malignancy in men between the ages of 25 and 34 (Cerny, 1984). A man with a cryptorchid (undescended) testicle has a 40 per cent chance of its becoming malignant. Surgery to bring an undescended testicle down into the scrotal sac (orchiopexy) is advocated prior to the age of 5 or 6 to preserve fertility in that testicle and to prevent malignancy from occurring

later in life. Orchiopexy does decrease the occurrence of malignancy, but statistics show that 12 per cent of testicular tumors occur in a testicle that previously had been brought into the scrotal sac surgically (Donahue, 1984).

EFFECTS OF TESTICULAR CANCER ON ADAPTATION

Testicular cancer is a disease of men in the prime of their lives—young men still pursuing an education or just beginning their careers, who may not yet have married or who may not have started a family, or men approaching their middle years, who may be married with children but who certainly have not achieved their life's goals. Cancer is a frightening disease at any stage of life, but a man at this stage does not expect such a diagnosis. He is faced with a threat to his manhood and with his own mortality at the sexual prime of his life.

Assessment

When testicular cancer is suspected, the client undergoes an extensive preoperative evaluation and is scheduled for a radical inguinal orchiectomy. The evaluation for metastases is very stressful to the client because the results of the serum and radiological examinations will affect the rest of his life. A definitive diagnosis awaits the pathologist's report following the orchiectomy.

Intervention

The client needs much emotional support, education, and clarification from the nurse. Often, so much information has been given by the physician that it is important to assess what the client has "heard" and actually understands and to clarify misinformation. The client must understand that the orchiectomy per se will not affect either his fertility or his sexual functioning in any way and that, at a later time, he could have a testicular prosthesis implanted for cosmetic purposes.

After the inguinal orchiectomy for testicular cancer, the choice of treatment depends on the type of cancer and its stage of involvement. Forty per cent of these cancers have already metastasized by the time a client sees a physician, so adjuvant therapy in the form of external beam radiation, retroperitoneal lymph node dissection, and/or chemotherapy is usually warranted. All of these treatments have effects on the sexual functioning of the client.

Forty per cent of all testicular tumors are seminomas. Because a seminoma is radiosensitive, metastatic spread to the lymph nodes is treated by external beam radiation rather than surgical lymph node dissection. Despite retraction and shielding of the remaining testicle during treatment, it receives radiation by scatter effect, which affects spermatogenesis. Recovery of sperm in the semen requires a minimum of 10 months, and maximum return of pretreatment levels may not occur for 2 to 3 years after radiation therapy. In some instances, the sperm count may never return to pretreatment levels (Bracken, 1981). Because the client with seminoma has not had the surgical trauma from a lymph node dissection (as might be done with other forms of testicular cancer), once his sperm counts have risen to levels of functional fertility he has the potential for fathering a child.

The metastases of nonseminomatous tumors, which constitute 60 per cent of testicular tumors, respond to lymph node dissection but may also require adjuvant chemotherapy for optimal treatment.

The lymphatics that drain into the testicles are located around the vena cava and aorta, between the kidneys and the bifurcation of the iliac vessels. Traditionally, a bilateral lymph node dissection was the surgical approach used when a nonseminomatous tumor was found. This extensive dissection can traumatize the lumbar sympathetic ganglia, causing permanent ejaculatory dysfunction. In a recent study of a large number of men with nonseminomatous tumors, Weissbach and Boedefeld (1987) found that many men with no evident metastases need to have only the nodes dissected on the side of the body corresponding to the cancerous testicle, thus sparing the sympathetic ganglia.

Chemotherapy, which can last for about 2 years, has an adverse effect on spermatogenesis. Although more prospective research is necessary, a few retrospective and prospective studies have been done showing that sperm counts diminish significantly during the course of therapy, but spermatogenesis returns and sperm counts return to pretreatment numbers within 2 to 3 years following completion of the chemotherapy (Drasga, 1983).

The health professional who works with the client with testicular cancer has an immense job of emotional support, education, and information clarification for the client, partner, and family and must facilitate good communication among those involved. Because the client may be roughly the same age as the medical and nursing staff, the health professional must avoid identifying too strongly with the client. If this occurs, objectivity can be lost, which can then interfere with understanding what the client himself is feeling.

As the client faces further treatment following his orchiectomy, the nurse needs to be in close communication with the primary physician to know exactly what the client and family have been told. The nurse can clarify the treatment protocols and anticipated side effects to the client as well as serve as a sounding board for the expression of fears and frustrations. In all communication with the client, the nurse must stress that his sexual desire, erections, and orgasm will not be affected permanently by any proposed treatment. However, there may be temporary effects due to the emotional and physical stresses of the treatments. Fertility will be affected permanently, and this can be a devastating event for a man at the age at which these tumors occur.

Because all adjuvant therapies interfere with fertility, the physician might suggest that the client collect several ejaculates through masturbation for preservation in a sperm bank. These could then be used for artificial insemination when children are desired. False hopes for the future must not be raised, however. The client must realize that current methods for sperm preservation are limited and that the numbers and motility of sperm are decreased by the freezing-thawing processes now utilized. In addition, the client will have a lower sperm count and/or decreased motility of his sperm at the time of collection, and these may be too low for submission to the sperm bank. Why this occurs is not known, but it has been suggested that a metabolic stress reaction to the anesthesia and surgery for orchiectomy adversely affects sperm counts and motility (Bracken, 1981). Even the inherent situational stress could affect the hypothalamus, which, in turn, affects spermatogenesis. If the client decides to store his sperm, the nurse must provide him with the instructions that will allow the semen to be collected under optimal conditions. Significant factors in the preservation of sperm are abstinence prior to masturbation, a proper container for collection of the ejaculate, the ideal temperature for storing the sperm prior to its being submitted, and how long a specimen can be collected prior to submission. The nurse should contact the sperm bank to obtain specific instructions for the client.

Communication among health professionals who work with the client in the outpatient setting, the inpatient unit, radiation therapy clinic, and the oncology unit is important to ensure that the client receives optimal care. Emotional support and physical care can be enhanced if relevant facts about the client are communicated prior to his being treated in each area. Clients must be involved with the proposed communication, and they generally appreciate the interest and concern showed by this effort. Continuity of care during the protracted time in which treatment takes place is best maintained when information about the client, his support system, and his reactions to treatments is shared. For instance, the client may not return to the outpatient setting for many months because he has been hospitalized for his initial treatment and/or has had adjuvant treatment in another setting. It is advantageous for the outpatient staff to know how the client has been responding to his treatment. With information about his emotional and physical responses, the nurse can anticipate his needs when he returns to the clinic for periodic follow-up visits. Communication will facilitate continuity of care, and the staff in the various settings will feel they are familiar with the client before he arrives for treatment.

SUMMARY

Whether congenital or acquired, many dysfunctions of the genitourinary tract affect the sexuality and/or the sexual functioning of the client. With knowledge, skill, and compassion the nurse can assess a particular dysfunction and assist the client and his family to diminish or eliminate the dysfunction or can assist the client to make adaptations to the dysfunction and/or its treatment.

REFERENCES

Abram HS et al: Sexual functioning in patients with chronic renal failure. J Nerv Ment Dis 160:220, 1975.

Bahnson RR, Catatona WJ: Papavarine testing of im-

potent patients following nerve-sparing radical prostatectomy. J Urol 139:773, 1988.

Beutler LE, et al: Women's satisfaction with partner's penile implant. Urology 24:552, 1984.

Bracken RB: Cancer of testis, penis, and urethra: The impact of therapy on sexual function. In von Eschenback AC, Rodriguez D (eds): Sexual Rehabilitation of the Urologic Cancer Patient. Boston, G.K. Hall Medical Publishers, 1981.

Brogna L, Lakaszawski M: Nursing management: The continent urostomy. J Enterostom Ther 13:139, 1986.

Brundage DJ: Nursing Management of Renal Problems. St. Louis, CV Mosby, 1980.

Cerny J: Tumors of the testis. In Kendal AR, Karafin L (eds): Urology. Vol 2. New York, Harper & Row, 1984.

Dennis RL, McDougal WS: Pharmacological treatment of erectile dysfunction after radical prostatectomy. J Urol 139:775, 1988.

Devine CJ: Surgery of the penile curvature. In Paulson DF (ed): Genitourinary Surgery. Vol. 2. New York, Churchill Livingstone, 1984.

Donahue JB: The testis. In Paulson DF (ed): Genitourinary Surgery. Vol. 2. New York, Churchill Livingstone, 1984.

Donovan MI (ed): Cancer Care: A Guide for Patient Education. Norwalk, Appleton-Century-Crofts, 1981.

Drasga RE et al: Fertility after chemotherapy for testicular cancer. J Clin Oncol 1:179, 1983.

Droller MJ: Adenocarcinoma of the prostate: An overview. Urolog Clin North Am 7:579, 1980a.

Droller MJ: Cancer of the testis: An overview. Urolog Clin North Am 7:731, 1980b.

Eccard M: Adjustments and psychosocial impact on ESRD: Nursing interventions. In Lancaster LE (ed): The Patient with End Stage Renal Disease. 2nd ed. New York, John Wiley & Sons, 1984.

Ellis WJ, Grayhack JT: Sexual function in aging males after orchiectomy and estrogen therapy. J Urol 89:895, 1963.

Fair WR: Diagnosing prostatitis. Urology (Dec Suppl) 24:6, 1984.

Fenely RCL: Incontinence clinics. In Mundy AR, Stephenson TP, Wein AJ (eds): Urodynamics. New York, Churchill Livingstone, 1984.

Finkelstein FO, Finkelstein SH, Steele TE: Assessment of marital relationships of hemodialysis patients. Am J Med Sci 271:21, 1976.

Fowler E, Goupil D: Managing an incontinence problem: Assessment, plan, and products. J Urol Nurs 4:333, 1985.

Gartley CB (ed): Managing Incontinence. New York, Jameson Books, 1985.

Glassman CN, Machlus BJ, Kelalis PP: Urethroplasty for Hypospadias: Long-term results. Urol Clin North Am 7:437, 1980.

Goldfarb M: The clinical efficacy of antibiotics in the treatment of prostatitis. Urology (Dec Suppl)24:12, 1984.

Golji H: Experience with penile prostheses in spinal cord injury patients. J Urol 121:288, 1979.

Grahack JT, Wendel EF: Carcinoma of the prostate. In Kendal AR, Kerafin L (eds): Urology. Vol. 2. New York, Harper & Row, 1984.

Gray H, Brogan D, Kutner NG: Status of life-areas: Congruence/noncongruence in ESRD patient and spouse perceptions. Soc Sci Med 20:341, 1985.

Green R: Taking a sexual history. In Green R (ed):

Human Sexuality. 2nd ed. Baltimore, Williams & Wilkins, 1979.

Hammond DC, Middleton RG: Penile prostheses. Med Aspects Hum Sex 18:204–208, 1984.

Hendry J, Geddes N: Living with a congenital anomaly: How nurses can help patients of children born with spina bifida to develop lasting patterns of creative caring. Can Nurs 74:29, 1978.

Hickman BW: All about sex . . . despite dialysis. Am J Nurs 77:606, 1977.

Hopper S, Sweeney JT, Pierce PF: The patient receiving a renal transplant. In Lancaster LE (ed): The Patient with End-Stage Renal Disease. 2nd ed. New York, John Wiley & Sons, 1984.

Kolodny RC, Masters WH, Johnson VE: Textbook of Sexual Medicine. Boston, Little, Brown & Co, 1979.

Krane RJ, Siroky MB: Neurophysiology of erection. Urolog Clin North Am 8:91, 1981.

Lancaster LE, Pierce P: Total body manifestations of end stage renal disease and related medical and nursing management. In Lancaster LE (ed): The Patient with End Stage Renal Disease. 2nd ed. New York, John Wiley & Sons, 1984.

Langemo DV: Peyronie's disease. AUAA J 3:4, 1985.

Laurence KM, Beresford A: Continence, families, marriage and children in 51 adults with spina bifida. Develop Med Child Neurol (Suppl 35)17:123, 1975.

Lepor H et al: Precise localization of the autonomic nerves from the pelvic plexus to the corpora cavernosa: A detailed anatomical study of the adult male penis. J Urol 133:207, 1985.

Lerner J, Khan Z: Manual of Urologic Nursing. St. Louis, CV Mosby, 1982.

Lytton R, Epstein F: Tumors of the urinary tract. In Thorne GW (ed): Harrison's Principles of Internal Medicine. 8th ed. New York, McGraw-Hill, 1977.

McConnell EA, Zimmerman MF. Care of Patients with Urologic Problems. Philadelphia, JB Lippincott, 1983.

Meares E: Etiology of prostatitis. Urology (Dec Suppl)24:4, 1984.

Milne JF, Golden JS, Fibus L: Sexual dysfunction in renal failure: A survey of chronic hemodialysis patients. Int J Psychiatry Med 8:335, 1977–78.

Nichols KA, Springford V: The psycho-social stressors associated with survival by dialysis. Behav Res Ther 22:563, 1984.

Oberly ET, Oberly TD: Learning to live with dialysis: A personal perspective. In Lancaster LE (ed): The Patient with End Stage Renal Disease. 2nd ed. New York, John Wiley & Sons, 1984.

Piening S: Family stress in diabetic renal failure. Health Soc Work 9:134, 1984.

Resnick NM, Rowe JW: Urinary incontinence in the elderly. In Rowe JW, Besdine RW (eds): Health and Disease in Old Age. Boston, Little, Brown & Co, 1982.

Robertson M, Walker D: Psychological factors in hypospadias repair. J Urol 113:698, 1975.

Rosenman J: ^{125}I implantation of prostate cancer. Unpublished paper, 1984.

Schaeffer AJ: Pharmokinetics of antibiotics used in the treatment of prostatitis. Urology (Dec Suppl)24:8, 1984.

Schellhammer PF, Spaulding JP: Carcinoma of the penis. In Paulson DF (ed): Genitourinary Surgery. Vol 2. New York, Churchill Livingstone, 1984.

Stecker JF: Surgical management of erectile impotence. In Paulson DF (ed): Genitourinary Surgery. Vol 2. New York, Churchill Livingstone, 1984.

Steele TE, Finkelstein SH, Finkelstein FO: Hemodialysis patients and spouses. J Nerv Ment Dis 162:225, 1976.

Subrini L: Surgical treatment of Peyronie's disease using penile implants: Survey of 69 patients. J Urol 132:47, 1984.

von Eschenbach AC, Rodriguez DB (eds): Sexual Rehabilitation of the Urologic Cancer Patient. GK Hall Medical Publishers, 1981.

Walsh PC, Donker P: Impotence following radical prostatectomy: Insight into etiology and prevention. J Urol 128:492, 1982.

Walsh PC, Mostwin JL: Radical prostatectomy and cystoprostatectomy with preservation of potency. Br J Urol 56:694, 1984.

Webster GD: The urethra. In Paulson DF (ed): Genitourinary Surgery. Vol 2. New York, Churchill Livingstone, 1984.

Weissbach L, Boedefeld GA: Localization of solitary and multiple metastases in Stage II nonseminomatous testis tumor as basis for a modified staging lymph node dissection in Stage II. J Urol 138:77, 1987.

White R, Nagler H: Priapism. In Krane RJ, Siroky MB, Goldstein I (eds): Male Sexual Dysfunction. Boston, Little, Brown & Co, 1983.

Willscher MK: Peyronie's disease. In Krane RJ, Siroky MB, Goldstein I (eds): Male Sexual Dysfunction. Boston, Little, Brown & Co, 1983.

Woods NF: Human sexual response patterns. In Woods NF (ed): Human Sexuality in Health and Illness. St. Louis, CV Mosby, 1984.

Woods NF: Restorative intervention. In Woods NF (ed): Human Sexuality in Health and Illness. St. Louis, CV Mosby, 1984.

Woods NF: Roles for professional nurses in the delivery of sexual health care. In Woods NF (ed): Human Sexuality in Health and Illness. St. Louis, CV Mosby, 1984.

Woods NF: Sexual adaptation to changed body image. In Woods NF (ed): Human Sexuality in Health and Illness. St. Louis, CV Mosby, 1984.

Woods NF, Herbert JM: Sexuality and chronic illness. In Woods NF (ed): Human Sexuality in Health and Illness. St. Louis, CV Mosby, 1984.

Zorgniotti AW, Lefleur RS: Auto-injection of the corpus cavernosum with a vasoactive drug combination for vasculogenic impotence. J Urol 133:39, 1985.

22: Gynecological Conditions and Sexuality

Linda Bernhard

Gynecological conditions are those physical entities or situations that uniquely affect women. Gynecology may be strictly defined as the study of the female reproductive system and its diseases. More broadly defined, gynecology includes the study of women's reproductive system as well as other structures, such as the clitoris, urethra, and anus, that are influenced by the reproductive system and that are involved in women's sexual activity. Although gynecology may constitute the study of the systems and structures used in sexual activity, a woman's sexuality is a total body, total life experience and is not limited to her reproductive system and its corresponding structures.

A woman's sexual system in uniquely different from a man's because, unlike a man, not all of her sexual organs also have reproductive functions. Women have one organ, the clitoris, whose sole function is related to sexuality.

Potentially *any* gynecological condition may affect a woman's sexual functioning, since each individual responds uniquely to a particular situation. What causes pleasure to one woman may cause extreme distress to another. For example, some women greatly enjoy sexual activity when they are menstruating because they associate the blood with earth, nature, and life itself. Others do not engage in sexual activity at all when they are menstruating because of cultural or other beliefs about uncleanliness or because they simply feel it is too messy.

Although the conditions included in this chapter are organized by body organs for convenience of presentation, most of the conditions are not related only to one organ but to the entire female genital and reproductive system.

CONDITIONS INVOLVING THE UTERUS

The nonparous uterus is approximately the size and shape of a small pear. The uterus has three identified functions: holding the growing fetus during pregnancy, expulsion of the fetus from the uterus, and menstruation. Although menstruation occurs during about half of nearly all women's lives, reproduction plays a part for only a few years for most women, and not at all for some.

The uterus is often perceived as the internal representation of femininity. While there are no American cultural events associated with womanhood, menstruation is viewed by many as a significant part of being a woman. The uterus is thus a valued organ, but one about which many women do not consciously formulate their feelings until its function is threatened or changed (Roeske, 1978). The major abnormal conditions associated with the uterus are alterations in menstruation and tumors.

436

Alterations in Menstruation

The primary activity of the uterus is periodic bleeding, which occurs at the beginning of each menstrual cycle when the endometrial tissue, not needed to nurture a fertilized ovum, is shed. Although this bleeding is normal and expected routinely, when menstruation is irregular or painful it can cause problems for women concerning their sexuality.

Dysmenorrhea

Dysmenorrhea, or painful menstruation, is the most common gynecological symptom complex, affecting as many as 50 per cent of postmenarchal women and representing the major cause of women's absence from work or school (Fuchs, 1982). Dysmenorrhea usually occurs a day before or with the onset of menstruation, and it improves or is resolved by the end of menstruation. Dysmenorrhea does not occur with anovulatory menstrual cycles.

Primary dysmenorrhea is an *entity* that begins at menarche or soon afterward and is not associated with any pelvic pathology. It is now believed that the cause of dysmenorrhea is related to the effects of prostaglandins released from the endometrium (Hale, 1983). However, recently when laparoscopies were performed on some adolescent women who had severe dysmenorrhea, mild endometriosis was identified (Altchek, 1985). Secondary, or acquired, dysmenorrhea occurs after a time of painless menstruation and is a *symptom* associated with organic disease in the pelvis or with the use of an intrauterine device (IUD).

EFFECTS OF DYSMENORRHEA

A study by Brown and Woods (1984) reported that while dysmenorrhea was extremely common, it produced varying amounts of psychological stress for women. Furthermore, their study suggested that neither a traditional nor a feminist sex role orientation was particularly useful in understanding dysmenorrhea. In the past the psychiatric literature promoted the belief that dysmenorrhea occurred because the woman could not accept her female role and femininity, since menstrual periods are an inherent part of being a woman. However, more recent research reveals this idea to be a myth.

The effect of dysmenorrhea on a woman's sexual health varies greatly. The sexual function of the woman with mild dysmenorrhea may not be affected, whereas women who have severe dysmenorrhea may be totally incapacitated for a day or more each month. Since primary dysmenorrhea occurs in young women, concern about when they have their menstrual periods may affect dating patterns as well as other activities, such as sports, in which they participate.

Dysmenorrhea may stimulate conflict about acceptable behavior and role functions. A woman may want to hide the fact that she is menstruating and maintain her usual roles, or she may find maintaining usual roles difficult. Her physical symptoms may keep her at home (which she must explain) or cause her to act differently than usual in a work or social setting.

Primary dysmenorrhea has been known to disappear completely after a pregnancy and childbirth (Wilson, 1984). Because of this, some young women may choose to become pregnant in order to relieve the symptoms, not thinking of the long-term consequences of having a child. On the other hand, some young women will be frustrated knowing that a pregnancy might help to relieve their symptoms, yet they do not wish to become pregnant.

ASSESSMENT

To promote adaptation in women who have primary dysmenorrhea, the nurse must assess each woman for how much of a concern it is to her health. The nurse will need to assess possible environmental forces acting on the woman that both help and hinder her adaptation to dysmenorrhea. For example, if she has heard from other women that a heating pad to her abdomen, exercise or walking, backrubs, or other self-care may relieve dysmenorrhea, she should be asked whether she has tried these measures and whether they have helped.

INTERVENTIONS

The current treatment for primary dysmenorrhea is antiprostaglandin medication. Aspirin is a mild antiprostaglandin and will relieve symptoms in some women. Antiprostaglandin drugs (e.g., ibuprofen) are now available without a prescription, but women should be cautious about using these drugs if they are allergic to aspirin. The use of oral contraceptives can relieve dysmenorrhea in some women because they become anovulatory. If a woman prefers not to use oral contraceptives for a long time, even a 3- to 6-month trial may be useful in relieving some of the dysmenorrhea.

Self-care measures such as exercise, yoga and/or meditation, heating pads, and backrubs may be suggested. The uterine contractions that can occur during orgasm may relieve the backache that often accompanies dysmenorrhea, so sexual activity may be recommended.

There is very little research related to dysmenorrhea. Existing reports consist mostly of physiological studies to determine the cause of primary dysmenorrhea. Research that would describe women's responses to dysmenorrhea and their self-care practices would aid nurses in providing care to this population. The importance of cultural differences in dysmenorrhea should also be investigated.

Hypermenorrhea

Whereas dysmenorrhea occurs with normal menses and can be expected, other types of uterine bleeding may be unexpected. Bleeding may occur between regular menstrual periods (metrorrhagia), or "regular" periods may continue longer than normal (menorrhagia). Occasionally, uterine bleeding may become nearly continuous, and some women may fear that they will bleed to death. Additionally, bleeding can recur after menopause has begun. This type of bleeding is generally related to some pathology.

The initial medical approach to problematic uterine bleeding is often a dilation and curettage (D&C). This surgical procedure, which can be threatening to some women, is performed frequently on an outpatient basis. Sequelae are rare, but the woman should not put anything—including penis, fingers, dildo, douches—in her vagina for about 2 weeks after the surgery, so that the cervical os can return to normal and infection is prevented. Other types of sexual activity are not prohibited.

ASSESSMENT

The nurse should assess whether the woman has friends or family members, such as sisters

or her mother, with whom she can discuss the problem. Some women are uncomfortable discussing bleeding problems, particularly when it is related to sexuality. If the woman does not have supportive persons with whom she can share her feelings, the nurse should be especially supportive in promoting adaptation to this condition.

Since hypermenorrhea is generally a symptom, the nurse should help the woman to see that finding the source of the problem is important. Once the woman finds out the pathology, she can decide how to deal with the underlying cause.

INTERVENTION

If hypermenorrhea is severe, the nurse should discuss its effects on the woman's life style and sexual activity. If she is too tired to engage in sex, the nurse could suggest having sex in the morning when she is rested. The woman may not even want to go out socially because she is afraid of hemorrhaging. If she has become anemic, the nurse should encourage the woman to eat foods high in iron and to begin an iron supplement, if necessary.

Menopause

Menopause is the cessation of menstruation. It is *not* an illness or a pathological condition but a normal process in a woman's life. Menopause does, however, affect women's sexual health. Myths about menopause and its effects on sexuality abound. The foundation for most myths is that there is something wrong with menopause. A lack of discussion about menopause among women helps to keep myths alive (Millette and Hawkins, 1983).

EFFECTS OF MENOPAUSE: MYTHS AND REALITIES

Perhaps the most common myth is that a woman's sexual life is automatically ended once menopause has begun. Our social values of youth and beauty, to the detriment of our experience of normal aging, are at least partly at fault for the maintenance of this myth. Since, according to the myth, only the young and beautiful may be sexual, older persons are led to believe that aging and menopause imply a decline or demise in their sexuality. When their experience proves this belief wrong, they may feel guilty and ashamed.

There are conflicting reports of both increases and decreases in women's sexual activity after menopause (Osborn, 1983). Increases may be a result of no longer having to worry about becoming pregnant, whereas decreases are often due to the presence of physical illness in the woman or her sexual partner or to the lack of a partner. Some women have heard that going through menopause will decrease sexual desire. Reports indicate that both increases and decreases in sexual desire are associated with menopause, but research has not produced any clearcut evidence to support either position.

The common occurrence of slower lubrication and possible vaginitis due to cracking and bleeding of the atrophic vaginal mucosa can make women feel that they should not be engaging in sexual activity. Regular sexual activity, by masturbation or coitus, will help to prevent these problems (Leiblum et al, 1983).

Another myth is that menopausal women become irritable, depressed, mentally disturbed, and possibly even insane. In reality it is very difficult to separate the experience of menopause from the experience of aging. Of course, the cessation of menses is an obvious sign that a woman cannot deny her aging. However, it appears that psychological symptoms of depression and irritability, if they occur in menopausal women, are more related to social and cultural events occurring in their lives than to the physiological occurrence of menopause (Semmens, 1983).

One of the symptoms of menopause that may cause difficulty for women in terms of their sexuality is hot flashes. The cause of hot flashes is unknown, but it is thought to be related to the hypothalamus. Hot flashes occur at any time and, as such, can cause difficulty and embarrassment to women. It has been suggested that hot flashes may be triggered by events or activities that alter body temperature, such as sudden emotional responses, exercise, hot weather, alcohol, caffeine, and spicy foods or by sleep (Heilman, 1980). However, one comprehensive study of women's experiences with hot flashes concluded that there is no way to predict the trigger for hot flashes (Voda, 1981). The relationship of hot flashes to specific sexual activities has not been studied.

Estrogen has been used effectively to treat hot flashes as well as to prevent vaginal degeneration. There is considerable controversy, however, regarding the use of estrogen replacement therapy (ERT) for treatment of other menopausal symptoms.

Additionally, the use of ERT has been associated with the development of endometrial cancer due to endometrial hyperplasia (Smith et al, 1975). To prevent the proliferation of endometrium, physicians are now giving progesterone with the estrogen; this is called hormone replacement therapy (HRT) (Dennerstein and Burrows, 1982). However, the progesterone results in a cyclic bleeding, which some women do not realize. They may become frightened when the bleeding starts, thinking that something is wrong. Some women would rather take the risk of developing cancer than be bleeding every month, and others find the return of menstrual bleeding causes them to feel young again.

There is very little research about menopause in general and even less about sexuality during menopause. Existing research focuses more on physiological functioning and hormonal levels than on the psychosocial or cultural experience of menopause. Lack of research is another factor that allows myths to be perpetuated.

INTERVENTION

Women must be helped to adapt physically and psychosocially to menopause. The nurse can first help women by teaching the facts about menopause and dispelling the myths that women have heard. This may be effectively done in a group situation, in which women can share with other women their feelings, concerns, and experiences (McKenzie, 1978). Women can be encouraged to talk with their mothers and older female relatives about their experiences with menopause.

If the woman is given ERT or HRT, the nurse should be sure that the woman understands the reasons for the drugs, the potential side effects, and what to observe in herself. If progesterone is given, the nurse should explain that the woman will experience bleeding if she has a uterus. The nurse should be sure that the woman knows how to perform breast self-examination and can also explain that the woman will receive some written information from the pharmacist when she has the prescription filled and that she should read the information. When the woman returns to the nurse, the nurse can clarify and help the woman to understand the medical information she has received.

If women have mild hot flashes and prefer not to have HRT, the nurse can suggest wearing layers of clothes, which can be removed when she is hot and replaced when she is cool. Clothes made of natural rather than synthetic fibers seem to be better tolerated (Morgan, 1982).

For problems with vaginal dryness, the nurse can recommend continuing regular sexual activity as well as sufficient foreplay and the use of a water-soluble lubricant such as KY Jelly, if necessary. Petroleum-base lubricants, such as Vaseline, should not be used. Women should be encouraged to find ways to enhance their sexual encounters with lighting, music, and clothing (McKenzie, 1978); this can cause them to feel more sexual and to enjoy sex more fully.

Uterine Tumors

Tumors of the uterus can be benign or malignant. In either case the most common treatment is surgical removal of the uterus, often in conjunction with the ovaries and fallopian tubes. Although women may say that a hysterectomy is the threat to their sexuality, it may actually be an oophorectomy, or loss of the ovaries.

There are innumerable myths surrounding hysterectomy that can influence how a woman will feel about the procedure. These include beliefs that hysterectomy results in weight gain, hair growth on the face and chest, and menopause; the uterus is the source of a woman's strength; menstruation purges the body of bad things (the inability to menstruate can result in a build-up of bad things in the body); and the uterus helps a woman to think. These myths result from a lack of understanding of the anatomy and physiology of the body in general and of the reproductive system specifically.

Additionally, there are also myths that are clearly specific to sexuality. These include beliefs that the uterus is the source of a woman's sexual drive, the uterus is the center of a woman's sexuality and femininity, a hysterectomy will result in a woman's being neutered or in her no longer being a "full woman," and a hysterectomy will deprive a male partner of his sexual satisfaction. If a woman believes any or all of these myths, her

sexual feelings and/or sexual expression can be greatly affected.

BENIGN TUMORS

By far the most common benign tumors of the uterus are leiomyomas or myomas, which are composed primarily of smooth muscle, not connective tissue, so that the commonly used term "fibroid" is actually a misnomer (Krieger, 1983). Myomas are present in about 20 per cent of women over the age of 35 (Hibbard, 1983), but they are two to five times more common in American black and Asian women than in white women (Krieger, 1983).

The majority of women who have myomas have no symptoms; however, symptoms that can occur include hypermenorrhea and a feeling of heaviness in the pelvis. Occasionally, very large myomas may cause symptoms as a result of pressure on other organs; there may be urinary frequency, constipation, or difficulty sitting or walking.

The most frequent treatment for myomas is hysterectomy; however, indications for hysterectomy are not clearly defined. This has resulted in the performance of many unnecessary hysterectomies. Occasionally, myomectomy (removal of the tumors only) can be performed, if pregnancy is desired. Myomas often regress after menopause, so surgery may not be needed.

Hysterectomy can be performed via an abdominal incision or vaginally; however, hysterectomy for treatment of myomas is most frequently performed abdominally because the uterus is too large to remove vaginally. Many women would prefer to have the surgery vaginally, however, because of the absence of a visible scar. Recovery from vaginal hysterectomy usually is faster than abdominal hysterectomy, but if there are complications, they are more common with vaginal hysterectomy (Rubin, 1983). Occasionally, women who have a vaginal hysterectomy may express frustration because they have no abdominal wound on which to blame their feelings of pain and loss (Moran, 1979).

EFFECTS OF HYSTERECTOMY ON SEXUAL FUNCTION: MYTHS AND REALITIES

Women who believe the myths about the negative effects of hysterectomies may be upset about the effects of surgery on their sexuality. Many women do not know before the surgery whether or not their ovaries will be removed (and some do not know after surgery) but have fears about the effect of loss of ovaries.

When women have time to prepare for a hysterectomy, they may frequently have dreams about their uterus. The dreams may concern the sexual, reproductive, and other aspects of the uterus that are significant to the woman. This is apparently a grief reaction of the woman concerning the loss. Women may be quite upset and feel guilty when they remember these dreams, but they are quite normal.

Some women worry about what will happen to the space where the uterus was. They may verbalize an expectation of feeling empty when the uterus is gone. Usually, this fear results from a lack of knowledge of the size of uterus and is relieved when they are helped to understand its actual small size.

There is a limited amount of research concerning hysterectomy and women's reactions to it. Historically, the most commonly reported reaction women have after hysterectomy is depression. This finding was reported in the classic study by Lindemann (1941), in which women who had "pelvic surgery" experienced more postoperative depression than women who had "abdominal surgery." Based on this study, the belief that depression follows hysterectomy has been perpetuated. Richards (1974) identified what he called a posthysterectomy syndrome, with women who had had hysterectomy within the previous 3 years experiencing significantly more depression than women having a variety of other surgical procedures.

Recent research is inconsistent with the idea of posthysterectomy depression. Both Moore and Tolley (1976) and Lalinec-Michaud and Englesmann (1984) found no statistically significant differences in depression before and after hysterectomy. Martin, Roberts, and Clayton (1980) reported a nonsignificant decrease in psychiatric symptoms from before to after hysterectomy. Gath, Cooper, and Day (1982) reported a statistically significant decrease in psychiatric morbidity.

Findings of a number of studies also differ concerning the effects of hysterectomy on women's sexuality. Several studies report primarily negative effects (Dennerstein, Wood, and Burrows, 1977; Drellich, Bieber, and Sutherland, 1956; Lazarov et al, 1979; Utian,

1975), which included women's reports of loss of sexual desire and orgasm, lack of sexual enjoyment, decrease in frequency of intercourse, and the presence of dyspareunia.

In contrast, several studies suggest that a woman's sexuality is not affected by hysterectomy (Coppen et al, 1981; Cosper, Fuller, and Robinson, 1978; Humphries, 1980; Martin et al, 1980). Finally, two of the most recent studies suggest that sexuality is *positively* enhanced by having a hysterectomy (Gath, Cooper, and Day, 1982; Webb and Wilson-Barnett, 1983); that is, frequency and enjoyment of sexual intercourse increased after hysterectomy. Methodological problems in these studies may partially explain the inconsistent findings, and more research is clearly needed (Bernhard, 1986).

Some authors have asserted that hysterectomy has a negative effect on a woman's *femininity* (Hollender, 1969; Wolf, 1970). Kav-Venaki and Zakham (1983) administered the Bem Sex Role Inventory to three groups of premenopausal women who 1 year earlier had had hysterectomy only, hysterectomy and bilateral oophorectomy, or cholecystectomy. Both hysterectomy groups scored lower on the femininity scale than the cholecystectomy group. The authors concluded that in this sample the "self-evident truth" that the uterus symbolizes femininity was supported (Kav-Venaki and Zakham, 1983).

However, when Budd (1977) specifically studied the effects of hysterectomy on femininity, she found the opposite of what might have been expected: Women who endorsed the homemaker role (i.e., traditional femininity) were less depressed after hysterectomy than women who did not endorse the homemaker role. The majority of women in another study (Cosper, Fuller, and Robinson, 1978) indicated that their feelings of femininity were not altered by having a hysterectomy. A small number even said they felt *more* feminine.

Williams (1972) found more similarities than differences in convalescence from hysterectomy among Mexican-American and Anglo women, although the Mexican-American women consistently reported more physical and emotional symptoms during their convalescence than did the Anglo women. Virtually no other studies have considered culture as an important variable in hysterectomy.

Apparently the male sexual partners of

women having hysterectomy are also affected sexually. Wolf (1970) reported that when husbands of women about to undergo hysterectomy were interviewed, they made comments such as, "If a woman does not have a womb, she is not a full woman, so what does that make me if I have sex with her?" Daly (1976) reports that in one study 18 per cent of the black men experienced erectile dysfunction with a woman who had had a hysterectomy but did not experience erectile dysfunction with other women.

Malignant Tumors

There are two major types of malignant tumors of the uterus—cervical and endometrial. Cervical cancer is the more prevalent of the two. The incidence of invasive cervical cancer is decreasing, but the incidence of cancer in situ is increasing (American Cancer Society, 1986). Cervical cancer is more than twice as common in black than in white women and is infrequent in Jewish women.

CERVICAL CANCER

A number of factors have been associated with increasing risk for developing cervical cancer. The most statistically significant factor is young age of initial sexual intercourse (Ramzy, 1983). Other sexual habits are also associated: having multiple sexual partners, using poor sexual hygiene, and participating in intercourse shortly after delivery. Although having multiple partners is significant, apparently frequency of intercourse is not. A male partner's multiple partners may also increase the risk for the woman (Thomas, 1984). As many as 80 per cent of lesbians have had sexual intercourse with men in the past, so they may be at risk as well (Johnson and Palermo, 1984).

Other factors such as having herpes (HSV-II) and cervical inflammation or erosion are also associated with an increased risk (Ramzy, 1983). Intrauterine exposure to diethylstilbestrol (DES) is important because of the cervical changes that occur, but this may become even more significant as women exposed to DES become older. Low socioeconomic status and living in an urban, as opposed to a rural area are also related (Ramzy, 1983).

Multiparity and a history of emotional unhappiness or divorce have also been cited as factors in the development of cervical cancer (Edlund, 1982). Although some research indicates that personality traits, stress, and inadequate coping skills are associated with the development of cervical cancer (Goodkin, Antoni, and Blaney, 1986), more research is needed.

Interventions. Treatment of cervical cancer consists of surgery, radiation therapy, or a combination of both. There are a variety of surgical procedures that can be performed, depending on the stage of the disease. Severe cervical intraepithelial neoplasia or carcinoma in situ (precancerous lesions) may be treated with lesser therapy or conization of the cervix. Advanced cervical cancer is most commonly treated with radical hysterectomy, including the uterus, both ovaries and fallopian tubes, the upper portion of the vagina, the broad ligaments, and the surrounding lymph nodes (Sharma, 1983). Pelvic exenteration is performed for cure of advanced or recurrent cancer, most commonly of the cervix but also of the endometrium, rectum, or vagina (Vera, 1981). Early stage cervical cancer may be treated by either radiation therapy or simple hysterectomy.

Radiation therapy can consist of intrauterine and intravaginal internal radiation or external beam radiation or both. Combination therapy often consists of internal radiation to shrink the tumor prior to hysterectomy.

Some research has been conducted concerning the effectiveness of treatment and the effects of treatment for cervical cancer in women. It is generally agreed that radiation and surgery have comparable effectiveness. However, the effects on women's sexuality are markedly different. (See Chapter 15, Cancer and Sexuality, for complementary information.) In the classic study of women who had stages I and II carcinoma of the cervix, the sexual outcomes of 28 women who were treated with radiation only were compared with the outcomes of 32 women who were treated with surgery only (Abitbol and Davenport, 1974). One year after treatment, in women with radiation only frequency of sexual activity was most likely to have stopped or to have been greatly reduced, whereas in women with surgery, frequency of sexual activity was most likely not to have been changed or to be improved. In addition, nearly half of the women with radiation complained of lack of desire and orgasm, and they experienced dyspareunia.

Over half were conscious of their vagina feeling shorter or narrower during coitus (Abitbol and Davenport, 1974).

Seibel, Freeman, and Graves (1980) produced virtually the same results in their study of 22 women treated with radiation for stages I, II, or III cancer of the cervix and 20 women treated with hysterectomy for cancer in situ. More than a year after treatment, the women with radiation reported statistically significant decreases in sexual enjoyment, orgasmic ability, desire, frequency of intercourse, and sexual dreams. The women treated with surgery had no significant changes in their sexual functioning.

ENDOMETRIAL CANCER

Cancer of the endometrium primarily affects women between the ages of 55 and 69, and it is twice as common in white women as it is in black women (American Cancer Society, 1986). Risk factors associated with the development of endometrial cancer include nulliparity, infertility, anovulatory cycles associated with ovarian pathology, endometrial hyperplasia, late menopause, prolonged use of estrogen (especially postmenopausal ERT), family history of endometrial cancer, obesity, diabetes, and hypertension (Edlund, 1982). Treatment is usually surgical.

Effects of Endometrial Cancer on Sexuality. The woman confronted with uterine cancer may be doubly concerned about her sexuality. Her feelings concerning reproduction and sexuality may become very intertwined. Having a diagnosis of gynecological cancer causes a woman to focus on her independence and self-image (Donahue, 1981). She is concerned about the effects of the cancer on herself, but, perhaps even more so, she is concerned about the effects on her friends and family and especially her sexual partner.

Research concerning sexuality and gynecological cancer often includes women who have several different types of cancers, including endometrial, vulvar, vaginal, cervical, ovarian, and/or tubal cancer (Cain et al, 1983; Cobliner, 1977; Harris, Good, and Pollack, 1982; Krouse and Krouse, 1982), but results suggest that sexuality and sexual functioning are significantly impaired in all groups from the time of diagnosis, before treatment (Harris et al, 1982), up to 20 months after surgery (Krouse and Krouse, 1982). Cain and associates (1983) did try to identify differences according to type and stage of cancers on

sexual relationships but found no significant differences. Thus, one might conclude that a diagnosis of any gynecological cancer is a severe threat to a woman's sexuality.

PELVIC EXENTERATION

Radical surgery for cancer of the cervix and endometrium may lead to anterior and/or posterior exenterations. The procedure involves not only a very large incision but also an ileal conduit (anterior exenteration) or a colostomy (posterior exenteration) or both (total exenteration), resulting in the need for the woman to wear pouches over the stomas. These often are not conducive to feelings of sexually desirability or attractiveness. The woman must adapt to her abdomen's being totally different after surgery. She may feel completely disfigured or mutilated. Additionally, the loss of control of normal body functions of excretion may cause her to feel repulsive.

Effects of Pelvic Exenteration on Adaptation. Several studies have been conducted about the effects of pelvic exenteration on sexuality and psychological adjustment in women (Andersen and Hacker, 1983a; Dempsey, Buchsbaum, and Morrison, 1975; Fisher, 1979; Lamont, DePetrillo, and Sargeant, 1978; Vera, 1981). These studies used very similar methodologies, and all of them concluded that sexual functioning was severely depressed in these women.

However, a feminist critique of this research suggests that the measurement of sexuality has been male oriented and has focused on intercourse as the primary means of sexual expression rather than on a more broad concept of sexuality that women themselves may endorse (Cairns and Valentich, 1986). After pelvic exenteration, the women seemed to be well-adjusted, but many of the women in these studies had completely ceased all sexual activity. They may have been unknowledgeable about sexual alternatives to traditional intercourse, unwilling to try a variety of sexual activities, or satisfied with activities not traditionally defined as sex, such as kissing or just being physically close to their partner. Body image was negatively affected, and this seemed primarily related to the presence of stomas.

Nearly all of the women who were asked whether they would have the exenteration again said they would. This may be because they are so thankful to be alive that they are able to suppress their sexual needs or because they simply express their sexuality in other ways. Donahue and Knapp (1977) emphasize that not only grief reactions but often significant *positive* feelings occur following successful treatment for gynecological cancer. Nurses and other health professionals must be careful not to impose a belief of what is normal or adequate sexuality. If they are well-adjusted and satisfied, even though sexually depressed (by traditional definitions), they may have found other methods of sexual release. A woman's feelings about her sexuality are far more important than her sexual behaviors (Millette and Hawkins, 1983).

One aspect of pelvic exenteration that has not been evaluated in research is the effect of the absence of the rectum on orgasmic ability. Many women have intense rectal contractions with orgasm but may not realize it until these sensations are not present.

NURSING PROCESS

Nursing care of women who have uterine tumors depends on many factors, including the specific pathology and the treatment selected. However, there are many commonalities when the treatment involves hysterectomy. Donahue and Knapp (1977) listed four "instruments" for the health care professional in facilitating the sexual rehabilitation of women with gynecological cancer: interest, openness, support, and the ability to provide information. These instruments are useful for nursing care to women having *any* gynecological problem.

Assessment. To combat the many myths that exist concerning hysterectomy, the nurse must first assess the woman's knowledge about gynecological and reproductive anatomy and physiology, her awareness of and beliefs about the myths, and her feelings about her uterus and ovaries. Many women (and men) are ignorant of anatomy and physiology—especially related to their sexual organs. For example, some women think that the uterus and the womb are two different organs.

The nurse should determine what myths a woman has heard and which of them she believes. By asking, "What have you heard about having a hysterectomy?" the nurse can elicit some of the myths. This can be followed with, "What good things have you heard?" or "What bad things have you heard?" The woman's answers will often suggest how

much she believes of what she has heard. They may also provide information about how she regards her uterus and how much of her sexuality and/or femininity she attributes to her uterus.

Interventions. Teaching women about their bodies, and especially about their reproductive and sexual systems, can reduce fears. The use of charts, diagrams, pictures or natural-sized anatomical models (with organs that come apart) can be helpful. Preoperatively, a teaching pelvic examination, using a mirror so that the woman can see her cervix, and explaining what it will look like when the uterus is gone, may also be useful.

Women need to understand the function of the organs, so after the organs are removed, they will know what is missing. Some women do not realize that they will be sterile or that they will not have menstrual periods after a hysterectomy. Such understanding is necessary for an informed consent to surgery.

By correcting misconceptions, the nurse may elicit further questions the woman has. Providing a realistic idea before the hysterectomy of what she can expect is very important. In Dennerstein, Wood, and Burrows' (1977) study, women's preoperative expectation that sexual functioning would be altered was significantly associated with their postoperative sexual dysfunction.

One study specifically assessed the effects of nurse counseling on sexual adjustment after hysterectomy (Krueger et al, 1979). Results showed that there was no relationship between nurse counseling and sexual adjustment 8 weeks after hysterectomy; however, the researchers concluded this was because only 11 per cent of the women identified the nurse as the person from whom they received the most valuable information. However, over half of the subjects wrote comments suggesting that nurses should provide patients with information about the effects of hysterectomy on sexuality.

Psychological Concerns. Women with cancer have special needs related to how cancer affects sexuality. It has been assumed that sexuality is of no importance to someone who has cancer because the fear of death is primary, but Derogatis (1986) claims that sexuality is *central* to women when faced with a diagnosis of gynecological cancer. Feelings about sexuality influence the delay time in seeking a diagnosis, the impact of the diagnosis, fears about the disease, and response to treatment (Derogatis, 1986).

In one study of poor white rural women who had cervical cancer, the less education a woman had and the more she enjoyed coitus, the longer she delayed in reporting inter-menstrual or postcoital bleeding to her husband or her physician. When asked about the delay in reporting the symptom, the women indicated that reporting it might mean they would have to cease engaging in coitus (Vincent et al, 1975). Thus, it is a myth that illness or cancer precludes sexuality.

Body Image Concerns. The woman who has undergone treatment for cancer may be primarily concerned with her body image and how she appears to her partner with two stomas and pouches on her abdomen and a large scar. She may feel untouchable. Once again, the nurse should help her focus on what she still has and what she can give and receive sexually. Most parts of the body can be trained to become quite erotic with time and practice.

Often, women are afraid of showing the stomas to their sexual partners for fear of rejection. If they have no partner, they may believe that they will never be an acceptable sexual partner. With careful planning of the sites for the stomas, the woman can still wear bathing suits and clothes that make her feel sexually attractive. Nevertheless, the partner may be afraid of hurting her or the stomas and may avoid sexual activities. It is important that the partner be reassured regarding this concern and encouraged to assist with physical care, such as helping the woman with ambulation. Physical closeness and touching should be encouraged. With permission of the woman, the partner can be encouraged to observe the stoma and to touch it, allowing the woman to affirm that the stoma does not hurt.

To make sexual encounters more cosmetically or esthetically pleasing, the nurse can suggest ways to cover the stomas. Fancy, appealing pouch covers can be purchased or made; or, the woman could wear a slip, negligee, or cumberbund in her or her partner's favorite color and material. Ideas are only limited by the couple's creativity.

The nurse can also suggest ways to minimize the stomas' working during sexual activity; that is, avoiding drinking before sexual activity will decrease the ileal conduit eliminating urine. If certain foods give the woman gas, she should avoid eating those before sexual activity. To minimize pouches coming off during sexual activity, they should be emptied beforehand. Also, if there will be a great deal of body contact and friction, the pouches can be taped down for security.

Resuming Sexual Roles

Postoperatively, nurses can teach specifics related to sexual activities. Two studies have documented the average time for resumption of sexual intercourse as 6 weeks after hysterectomy (Bernhard, 1986a, b; Krueger et al, 1979). This is useful information for women, so that they do not feel rushed into resuming intercourse before they are ready. It is beneficial to include the sexual partner in these discussions.

There are many reasons why the sexual partner may avoid a woman after hysterectomy. There is often a fear of hurting her; however, there may be other reasons, including the fact that the partner may subscribe to myths about hysterectomies. A male partner may not be willing to wait until the woman is healed and may find his sexual gratification elsewhere.

If the woman expects her partner to take the sexual initiative and that does not happen, she may become depressed (Hott, 1982). The partner's lack of initiative may be due to a fear of hurting the woman and not any other reason. The nurse should emphasize the importance of the couple communicating about their own needs.

Specific suggestions should be given regarding the type of sexual activities in which the woman may or may not engage; that is, nothing should be put in the vagina, and oral sex is prohibited, but masturbation is permitted. Only telling the woman "no sex" is insufficient, unclear, and assumes that sex is coitus and that coitus is the only sexual behavior in which a woman engages (Savage, 1982).

Women may be afraid to resume coitus because they are afraid it will be painful. The nurse can explain that the first time may be uncomfortable (or it may not be) but that the woman should be well-prepared for the event: adequate desire, normal energy levels, and sufficient lubrication for easy penetration. Both partners should try to be as relaxed as possible.

Depth of penetration may be decreased with radical surgery. Some couples will not be aware of any change. However, the nurse can suggest alternate positions, such as elevating the woman's hips on a pillow, the woman's cupping her hands around the penis at the introitus, or a side-lying or standing position, which the couple can use if they wish. Intrathigh or intramammary intercourse could also be suggested.

If the ovaries were removed and the woman is premenopausal, she will probably be given estrogen. No vaginal changes should occur, but the woman must understand the importance of her continuing the estrogen so that vaginal changes do not occur. In some cases in which a hysterectomy and oophorectomy were performed for an estrogen-sensitive cancerous tumor, estrogen will not be given. The premenopausal woman may experience hot flashes and other symptoms of menopause, and her vagina may gradually atrophy. In this case the nurse should recommend the use of a water-soluble lubricant to prevent the development of atrophic vaginitis.

Some women are primarily concerned with their capacity to give and receive love with their whole body (Kitzinger, 1983). The nurse should help couples to share touching and physical closeness, even when coitus is prohibited, for these feelings help the woman to affirm and have reaffirmed for her, by the partner, that she is still lovable and sexual.

Women treated with radiation therapy for cervical cancer have special sexual needs and concerns. Radiation results in fibrosis of the vagina, with shortening of the vaginal barrel and decreased elasticity and lubricability (Hubbard and Shingleton, 1985). Sexual intercourse can be continued during external radiation therapy and is beneficial in preventing vaginal fibrosis. The nurse should teach the woman and her partner about fibrosis. Sexual intercourse three times a week will keep the vagina patent; however, coitus must be engaged in very gently, using a lubricant, so that the very friable vaginal tissues do not bleed.

Alternately, the woman can use dilators (which the nurse can provide) to maintain vaginal patency. The woman should insert the well-lubricated dilator once a day, well into the vagina and hold it there for two to four minutes (Lamberti, 1979). A plain candle will also work. Sometimes it is easier for a woman to insert the dilator when she is sitting in a tub of water. If the woman has fears about masturbation, she may not be able to consider using a dilator, but she may allow a sexual partner to insert it. The nurse needs to be aware of this possibility. A woman who has no sexual partner may find vaginal dilation a painful or meaningless procedure. The nurse can encourage her to continue because she may choose to engage in sexual activity at some point in the future.

One of the side effects of radiation therapy is extreme fatigue, which can continue for 1 to 2 months after therapy has ceased. Fatigue may become progressively worse throughout the day and can lead to decreased desire, resulting in sexual difficulties. The nurse might suggest that the woman engage in sexual activity early in the morning; the partner should also be informed that her fatigue and decreased sexual interest result from the therapy and are not a rejection of the partner.

Women who have pelvic exenterations need a great deal of sexual teaching and counseling. As with any of the other situations, the woman will not know how she will feel or act sexually until she goes home from the hospital and has to deal with her sexual partner alone; with good assistance from the nurse, she can be better prepared.

The nurse can help the woman to focus on the positive aspects of her sexuality. The sexual partner's involvement in this counseling will be very useful. The importance of a warm, loving, interested, caring partner cannot be underestimated in helping a woman recover from this radical mutilating surgery.

Some concerns depend on whether a neovagina was created—or will be at a later time. In either case the neovagina will take considerable time to heal before penetration may be tried, so there will be a period during which the woman does not have or cannot use her vagina. If vaginal penetration was an important part of a couple's sexual activity, the nurse will want to help them consider alternatives, such as oral sex or intramammary or intrathigh intercourse. It may be important for the couple to consider whose needs are being met and how. If the nurse can help them to communicate their needs and feelings to each other, they may be able to try other sexual alternatives that will meet both persons' needs.

In summary, sexual health is very important to the woman who has a uterine tumor, and there is a great deal that the nurse can do to help her adapt to her condition and maintain her sexual health. Teaching about anatomy and physiology as well as providing specific suggestions concerning sexual activities after hysterectomy and other procedures will be very useful to the woman and her partner.

CONDITIONS INVOLVING THE VAGINA

Whereas the uterus is the female organ that society associates with reproduction, the vagina is the organ most associated with intercourse. The social construction of femininity as passive and submissive relates to the vagina as the receptacle for male sexuality. Many women still accept this stereotype of femininity, and even those who do not are still likely to view the vagina as extremely important to a woman's sexuality.

Infections

Vaginal and vulvovaginal infections are common in women. While each infection is an acute episode, the presence of vaginal infections often becomes chronic in individual women. There are many causes of vaginal discharge; the major causes of vaginitis are discussed in this chapter. A discussion of the assessment and intervention for sexually transmitted diseases that complements this discussion of vaginitis is found in Chapter 23, Sexually Transmitted Diseases.

The cardinal symptom of vaginitis is a vaginal discharge, the character of which varies according to the infecting agent. With minimal discharge women may be asymptomatic because there are few nerve endings for pain in the vagina. However, when the discharge is profuse or contacts the highly sensitive vulvar tissue, women may have severe symptoms (Ramzy, 1983).

The unpleasant symptoms of discharge, pruritis, foul odor and burning and/or discomfort during urination and vaginal penetration can affect a woman's sexuality and sexual health. Both the woman and her sexual partner can view her as dirty and thus not sexually appealing.

Vaginal infections can be caused simply by the transference of bacteria from the rectum to the vagina. This can result from improper hygiene, or it can result when anal intercourse or manipulation is combined with vaginal intercourse or manipulation without washing in between these activities. In lesbians, vaginal infections can be transmitted between partners by mixing vaginal discharges in any way, including direct vulva-to-vulva contact or hand-to-vulva contact. Foreign bodies, such as tampons, diaphragms, and condoms left in the vagina, can also result in vaginitis.

Women must be taught from the time they are small children to wipe themselves from front to back after elimination to prevent infection. They should also be taught the importance of remembering to remove foreign objects (such as tampons and diaphragms) from the vagina.

Some women do not feel clean unless they douche regularly. If they have a vaginal discharge or pruritis, they recognize the need for medical assistance, but in their attempt to be as clean as possible for the health care professional, and to avoid being embarrassed, they may douche before going to the doctor. Unfortunately, the douche may mask the symptoms sufficiently to prevent an accurate diagnosis and appropriate treatment.

CANDIDIASIS

Candidiasis *(Monilia)*, or yeast infection, is the most common cause of vaginitis during the reproductive years (Roy, 1983). *Candida albicans*, a part of the normal flora of the mouth, gastrointestinal tract, and vagina, is the most usual infecting agent. Classic symptoms include severe pruritus and a thick whitish cottage cheese–like discharge as well as inflammation of the vaginal tissue. Treatment usually consists of antifungal topical vaginal creams or suppositories.

Candida is often associated with diabetes, pregnancy, and the use of oral contraceptives. In these situations the glycogen content of the vagina may be increased, predisposing the woman to the development of candidiasis. The use of broad-spectrum antibiotics (e.g., those used for chronic treatment of acne or for other acute infections) may decrease lactobacilli in the vagina, altering the pH and predisposing the woman to candidiasis. Women who are taking immunosuppressive drugs may also be predisposed to the development of a *Candida* infection. Oral sex may introduce organisms, particularly *Candida*, from the mouth into the vagina, resulting in infection, and the reverse may also be true; that is, *Candida* from the vagina may infect the throat.

TRICHOMONIASIS

Trichomoniasis is the second most common type of vaginitis; it is caused by *Trichomonas vaginalis.* Trichomoniasis is classically characterized by a foul-smelling, thin, frothy discharge that may be green, yellow, gray, or white. The discharge is often worse during and after menses and is associated with pruritus and irritation of the labia from the discharge. Trichomoniasis is often asymptomatic in both men and women, leading to recurrent infections (ping-pong effect) between sexual partners.

Trichomoniasis is treated with metronidazole (Flagyl or Protostat). During treatment and for 48 hours afterwards, women should not drink alcohol, as it leads to severe nausea and dizziness. Pregnant women should not take the drug during the first trimester, and lactating women should not nurse their babies while taking the drug and for 24 hours afterwards.

Trichomonas is transmitted most frequently via direct sexual contact. Because it has been shown that the organism can survive for 24 hours in swimming pools (Ramzy, 1983), women who are infectious should not share towels, wash cloths, or soap and should avoid public pools.

BACTERIAL INFECTIONS

Gardnerella vaginalis, previously called "nonspecific vaginitis" or *Haemophilus vaginalis* is a bacteria causing vaginitis (King, 1984). Classic symptoms include a vaginal discharge that is thin, gray-white, and homogenous and may have a fishlike odor. The odor is especially noticeable after coitus, since the odor increases in an alkaline environment, which semen provides. Frequently, *Gardnerella* infection is asymptomatic, although there may be irritation rather than pruritus. *Gardnerella* is often present with other vaginal infections and is usually treated with an antibiotic such as ampicillin or with metronidazole; however, using an antibiotic can predispose to the development of candidiasis.

ATROPHIC VAGINITIS

When ovarian estrogen production decreases in women during their climacteric (menopause), the vaginal mucosa can become dry and thin. In addition, part of normal aging involves loss of elasticity of the vaginal walls and shrinking of the vaginal barrel. Friction or similar trauma to the vaginal mucosa, often resulting from coitus, can cause cracking and bleeding of the tissues. In the presence of bacteria, infection or atrophic vaginitis can occur.

The first symptom of atrophic vaginitis is often bleeding. Other symptoms may include a scanty, thin, sometimes purulent, and possibly blood-tinged discharge. There may also be dyspareunia. Older persons—both men and women—may assume that such a situation is to be expected as a part of aging, and it may lead to their decreasing frequency and perhaps termination of sexual activity (Semmens and Semmens, 1984).

Atrophic vaginitis does not occur in all women. It appears that regular sexual activity—masturbation, coitus, and oral sex—at least once or twice a week can prevent atrophic vaginitis. This may literally be the case of "If you don't use it, you lose it."

Topical estrogen creme applied to the vaginal mucosa can be very beneficial in the treatment of atrophic vaginitis. Women who are taking oral estrogen should be careful about using estrogen cream because the combined dosage may be too high for them. Although oral estrogen should help to prevent or treat atrophic vaginitis, it does not always do so. In this case, ordinary water-soluble lubricant (applied either on the penis or in the vagina) can be very useful.

OTHER INFECTIONS ASSOCIATED WITH VAGINAL DISCHARGE

Women may experience and seek evaluation for abnormal discharge secondary to infections that commonly affect the cervix rather than the vagina. These infections may be caused by *Neisseria gonorrhoeae, Chlamydia trachomatis,* and herpes simplex virus. Gonorrhea and chlamydia infections can also present with abnormal pelvic pain and often cause pelvic inflammatory disease. Herpes can also present with vulvovaginal pain and dysuria.

For an indepth discussion of the epidemiology, assessment, and intervention of gonorrhea, chlamydia infection, herpes, and pelvic inflammatory disease, see Chapter 23, Sexually Transmitted Diseases.

INTERVENTIONS

Nursing care for a woman who has vaginitis first involves helping her to achieve a psychological state in which she will be able to adapt to her situation. The nurse should evaluate her ability to cope with the treatment and should help her to respond positively to treatment. This includes explanation and teaching about the use of vaginal creams and tablets. The nurse should teach the women how to insert the medication and suggest that she lie down or rest for about 15 minutes after insertion, so that the medication will not spill out. A tampon can also be inserted to help hold the medication in the vagina.

The nurse should help the woman to understand all the ways in which infection can be acquired as well as ways to prevent spreading it. One common aspect, often unknown by many women, is that any time the anus is involved in sex play, care should be taken to wash the hands, penis, or whatever was in contact with the anus before making subsequent contact with the vagina or to avoid direct contact with the vagina.

Loose-fitting cotton clothes, especially in hot humid weather, allows air to circulate around the perineum and will be more comfortable for women when they have a vaginal infection. Sitting for long periods of time, or other activities that decrease air to the perineum may be uncomfortable, and the nurse should recommend minimizing these situations.

The safest approach for the woman with an infection is not to put anything in the vagina until she is cured. The nurse should recommend that *any* sexual activities that are uncomfortable be stopped until the infection is treated. Although vaginitis, herpes, and gonorrhea are transmitted more readily through heterosexual intercourse than through lesbian sexual activity (O'Donnell et al, 1979), lesbians must also be careful about the spread of vaginitis.

The nurse should be careful not to make assumptions about the sexual orientation of clients; they may be lesbian, bisexual, or heterosexual or have multiple partners. The nurse should be specific about recommendations; for example, vaginal touching is to be avoided, but clitoral stimulation is acceptable.

Toxic Shock Syndrome (TSS)

Toxic shock syndrome is a rare but extremely serious disease that is diagnosed primarily in young women during their menstrual periods (Wroblewski, 1981). It is believed to be caused by a toxin produced by *Staphylococcus aureus*. The initial episode is usually the most severe and is a highly acute, multisystemic illness that can result in death. TSS will recur in about 30 per cent of all cases (Borton and Oskowitz, 1983). The risk of recurrence is greatest in women who do not receive antibiotics and who continue to use tampons, although no woman is exempt. The symptoms of desquamation of the palms and soles suggest recurrence (Rosene and Eschenbach, 1983).

Women who have TSS should not use tampons because of the association of TSS with tampon use. For many women tampons are the only sanitary protection they have ever used, and sanitary napkin use may be viewed as a burden.

The effects of TSS on a fetus or the risk to a baby are unknown, and for this reason women who have TSS may delay pregnancy. However, TSS may also be associated with the use of diaphragms and the contraceptive sponge, so methods of contraception are limited.

Research on TSS has involved finding the cause and preventing the disease, but there has been no nursing research on TSS and the reactions of women and their sexual partners. It seems likely that women and partners experience a great deal of anxiety and frustration with the disease, particularly since there is no effective treatment or cure. Additionally, writings about TSS have focused only on the initial acute illness; virtually nothing is written about managing and helping women who have recurrences.

INTERVENTION

Women who have TSS, once they survive an initial episode, need information about the disease and how to prevent recurrence, so that they can adapt to the situation of having a threatening, potentially chronic illness. They need to understand the importance of avoiding the use of tampons.

If the nurse can help several women who have TSS to meet together as a group, it may be very useful for them to have the support of other women who have TSS. However, there are not many women who have been diagnosed with TSS, so forming a group may be difficult.

Vaginal Tumors

Primary vaginal cancer is rare, but it occurs in women of all ages in several different forms. Embryonal rhabdomyosarcoma occurs in infants. Clear cell adenocarcinoma has been clearly associated with in utero exposure to diethylstilbestrol (DES). About one in 700 DES daughters will develop this cancer, usually in their late teens or early twenties (Orenberg, 1981). Squamous cell carcinoma is the most common type of vaginal cancer in adult women (Gaddis, 1983).

Vaginal cancer often escapes early detection because there may be no symptoms. The first symptoms may be unexplained vaginal bleeding that may occur every day or postcoitally. Later, there may be vaginal discharge and pelvic pain (van Nagell, Powell, and Gay, 1982).

Young women who know that they are DES daughters should be closely followed so that the disease can be identified early, should it develop. It is often quite threatening to these young women to think that they could develop cancer, and their mothers may experience significant guilt. The women who do develop cancer may be sexually inexperienced, and cancer of the vagina is threatening to their concept of womanhood.

Treatment of vaginal cancer depends on the specific disease. Surgery is the treatment of choice for clear cell adenocarcinoma, but radiation is the choice for squamous cell carcinoma (Gaddis, 1983). A number of different treatments, including topical chemotherapy (fluorouracil), cryosurgery, and laser therapy, can be used. Surgical treatment may consist of anything from local excision of the tumor to total vaginectomy to pelvic exenteration (van Nagell, Powell, and Gay, 1982); there are advantages and disadvantages to each method. If the woman is young, attempts to save at least a portion of the vagina and/or ovarian function may be made. If the woman is older or a poor candidate for surgery, for any reason, radiation may be preferred.

There are no studies on sexual adjustment after vaginal cancer specifically, although some women with vaginal cancers have been included in studies of women having gynecological cancer. There have been case studies published and studies concerning the psychological effects of finding out that one is a DES daughter.

INTERVENTION

The woman who has vaginal cancer, regardless of her age, needs a great deal of support to help her deal with the feelings of loss and mutilation. Often, physicians may assume that an older woman does not need or care about her vagina, but this is a mistaken assumption. All women must be helped to maintain their sexual image if they perceive it threatened.

Nursing care definitely depends on the treatment; that is, a young woman who has a vaginectomy, partial or complete, will probably have reconstructive surgery performed, but she may feel devastated. If she has a sexual partner, it is important to involve that person in her care, so that she still feels loved and cared about but not dependent. It is important to teach the couple about what is happening and what it can mean for them. They may need to be taught about which sexual activities they can engage in until the woman heals. The woman needs to know that she is not asexual because her vagina was removed.

An older woman may need support in the use of dilators, if radiation therapy is used to treat her disease. She may be very embarrassed and unsure about the procedure. If she has a sexual partner, both she and the partner may need to know she is not radioactive and sexual activity can continue, but gentleness is required because of the fragility of the vaginal mucosa.

PELVIC RELAXATION

Pelvic relaxation is a broad term that refers to the weakening of the pelvic supportive structures for the vagina, bladder, uterus, urethra, and rectum. Although one organ may be more affected than the others, all displacements (i.e., relaxations) are varying degrees of the same anatomical process (Krantz, 1983). The more common conditions are the cystocele (herniation of the bladder into the vagina), rectocele (herniation of the rectum into the vagina), and uterine prolapse (dropping of the uterus into the vagina).

Although pelvic relaxation can be congenital and occur in young women, it most frequently occurs in postmenopausal, multiparous women. The pregnancies may have resulted in traumatic deliveries with perineal lacerations and/or large birth weight infants (Krantz, 1983).

These conditions are rarely painful; women may experience a fullness or a bearing-down sensation, particularly when in an erect position. She may describe a sensation of something "falling out," which she is able to reduce by pushing it back in. Severe uterine prolapse may prohibit vaginal penetration. Additionally, a complete prolapse that is not reducible can lead to irritation and inflammation of the uterus and the woman's inner thighs. While this is quite rare, it can happen in elderly women who do not understand their problem and are too embarrassed to seek medical assistance.

With a cystocele, one of the major symptoms is stress incontinence, the involuntary loss of urine, coincident to brief increases in intra-abdominal pressure caused by laughing, coughing, sneezing, or changing position (Nichols and Wisgirda, 1985). Stress incontinence occurs specifically when the ligaments that support the urethra are weakened (Huffman, 1983). Stress incontinence can be embarrassing and frustrating for women, which can cause them to avoid social or sexual contacts. Often, it is the embarrassment and discomfort with stress incontinence that causes the woman to decide on surgical treatment.

Treatment for the most common pelvic relaxation conditions consists of anterior colporrhaphy, posterior colporrhaphy, and vaginal hysterectomy. A particular woman may have one or more of these procedures, and it is not uncommon to have them all at once.

If surgery must be avoided in an elderly woman who has other medical problems, vaginal prolapse or cystocele can be treated medically with the use of a vaginal pessary (Huffman, 1983). It must be used with caution, however, and be removed and cleaned at least once a month, because the irritation can lead to the development of vaginal cancer.

Effect on Sexual Function

After vaginal surgery for pelvic relaxation, a woman may experience some changes sexually. Any time the vaginal wall is cut, there is a possibility of developing vaginal stenosis. If the introitus is cut, there may be entrance dyspareunia. This is more common following posterior repair than the other procedures (Amias, 1975). One study reported that the poorest sexual outcomes after vaginal hysterectomy occurred in women who also had both anterior and posterior colporrhaphy (Craig and Jackson, 1975).

Extensive vaginal repair may lead to tenderness during sexual intercourse, and certain positions may be uncomfortable. Additionally, there may be some temporary loss or dullness in vaginal sensation (Hott, 1982). Early resumption of coitus does help to prevent vaginal stenosis, but if coitus is resumed too early, it may be harmful to the repair.

One study included 71 women who had anterior and/or posterior colporrhaphies. These women experienced negative changes in their sexuality after surgery. Fewer women were orgasmic than they were preoperatively and desire for coitus dropped. In addition, more women masturbated and preferred oral sex (instead of coitus) after surgery (Chapman, 1979).

Intervention

The woman who has a pelvic relaxation problem may want to avoid surgery. If she is able to reduce the condition (by pushing the tissue back into the vagina), she may think this is sufficient. She may also have the fears common to anyone facing hysterectomy.

Huffman (1983) suggests that performing Kegel's exercises 30 times, three times a day, will "treat" stress incontinence, and strengthen the pelvic musculature enough to avoid surgery. He further suggests that the exercises must be continued without fail, however, or the stress incontinence will return. Others assert that it is better to perform the exercises 100 times only once a day.

In either case the nurse should teach the woman how to do Kegel's exercises and should help her to understand their importance. Performing Kegel's exercises involves squeezing the tissues of the perineum so that when voiding, the flow of urine is stopped. A woman will quickly learn which muscles are involved and then can perform the exercises at any time, since it is not noticeable that she is doing them. The nurse can emphasize the ease and convenience of performing Kegel's exercises, and also discuss the benefit of doing the exercises on enhancing vaginal sensation during intercourse.

After surgery, it is critical for the nurse to help the woman to understand the importance of her not placing *anything* in her vagina until the surgeon has examined her (usually 4 to 6 weeks after surgery) to be sure that healing is adequate. For some women the delay in resuming sexual activity in itself can be very stressful. The nurse should help women and their partners to understand that masturbation is not prohibited and that she can still give sexual pleasure in other ways to her partner.

When permission has been given to resume sexual intercourse, the nurse should help the couple to deal with any fears they may have about resuming sexual activity. They should know that resumption of coitus may be uncomfortable for the woman the first time, but with practice, sex should be more comfortable. The woman should also be told that she may have diminished vaginal sensation after this kind of surgery but that normal sensation should return in time.

CONDITIONS INVOLVING THE OVARY

Some persons might call the ovary the organ of womanhood and youth and may believe that once the ovaries cease to function or are removed, a woman is old. Women do value their ovaries, but they may not consciously know why. When a woman experiences problems with her ovaries or she is threatened with their removal, she may express fears of growing old, experiencing menopause, or becoming masculine. Most women do seem to understand that having only one ovary can be sufficient (so removal of one is usually not very threatening).

Although bilateral oophorectomy was performed in the late 1800s and early 1900s as a "treatment" for such conditions as insanity, epilepsy, and menstrual distress, it is almost never performed by itself today. When bilateral oophorectomy is performed, it usually is in conjunction with hysterectomy. Consequently, there are no studies regarding the physical, emotional, or sexual effects on women of oophorectomy alone.

Endometriosis

Endometriosis is characterized by the presence of endometrial tissue in a site other than the uterus. This ectopic endometrial tissue generally responds to the cyclical ovarian hormones in a way similar to that of normal endometrium (Fox and Buckley, 1984). The bleeding that occurs results in inflammation, scarring, adhesions, cysts, and pain. Endometriosis occurs most commonly in the childbearing years and apparently stabilizes or regresses when the endometrial tissue becomes atrophic after menopause (Ramzy, 1983).

Although many women are asymptomatic, the major symptom is pain (Bernhard, 1982). The pain, described as dull and crampy over the lower abdomen, tends to increase prior to or during menses. There is often dyspareunia, especially with deep penetration.

Hormonal treatment with danazol produces effective regression of the disease and relief of pain for a period of time. Danazol treatment may be associated with unpleasant side effects of weight gain, vaginal spotting or dryness, and, potentially, a decrease in sexual desire. There may also be a mild masculinizing effect that is reversible after stopping the drug. The use of intranasal luteinizing hormone releasing hormone has produced dramatic results in treating endometriosis; however, side effects of vaginal bleeding and dryness, hot flashes, and decreased sexual desire were still observed (LHRH agonist, 1984).

INTERVENTION

Nursing care for the woman who has endometriosis depends on the individual woman. If she is asymptomatic but infertile, nursing care will be much different than if she has severe pain and is facing a hysterectomy and oophorectomy. Whatever the case, the nurse should help the woman adapt to her unique situation in whatever way is best for her.

Since pain is the primary symptom, the nurse will need to assess the pain and its effects on the woman's sexual activities. If she has dyspareunia, the nurse may suggest alternate positions for coitus in which the woman has greater control, such as female superior, either lying down or sitting astride. The nurse might also recommend taking pain medication about a half hour before beginning coitus, in hopes that the drug will be maximally effective during coitus. The nurse should emphasize the importance of communication between the partners about sexual activity, so that the woman's discomfort is minimized, her partner does not feel rejected, and both can experience as much sexual pleasure as possible.

For women who are receiving hormonal therapy, the nurse should teach them about the drugs and their side effects. The nurse may counsel the women about diet to minimize possible weight gain and inform her of the potential decrease in sexual desire. For those women who experience vaginal dryness, a water-soluble lubricant can be suggested.

Polycystic Ovarian Disease

Polycystic ovarian disease (POD) is a gynecological disorder in which the ovaries are enlarged and encapsulated, with multiple cystic follicles present beneath the capsule (Kase, 1983; Ramzy, 1983). The cause is unknown. POD may present in a variety of ways, one of which is Stein-Leventhal syndrome. It was originally thought that POD was one problem (i.e., Stein-Leventhal), but it is now recognized that there are several presentations that do not all have the classic symptoms of Stein-Leventhal syndrome.

The classic symptoms of Stein-Leventhal syndrome are infertility, amenorrhea, hirsutism, and obesity (Kase, 1983). In POD there can also be virilization, menstrual irregularity, or menometrorrhagia (Ramzy, 1983). There may be PMS-like symptoms in the rare ovulatory cycles in young women with POD (Altchek, 1985). Increased production of androgens by the ovary is often the result of POD (Scommegna and Maroulis, 1983). There may also be increased production of estrone, resulting in endometrial hyperplasia. Adolescent women may be diagnosed because they have primary amenorrhea, whereas other women may have POD diagnosed when they are unable to become pregnant.

Treatment may be quite varied. Goals of treatment are usually to induce ovulation, control hirsutism, and decrease endometrial hyperplasia (Kase, 1983). If pregnancy is desired, administration of clomiphene citrate is very successful in inducing ovulation. If a woman does not want to conceive, the best treatment is oral steroid contraceptives (Droegemueller et al, 1987). Hirsutism can be controlled with the use of antiandrogens (Kirschmer, 1986). Hyperplasia can be decreased with the use of low-dose oral contraceptives. Women who do not have hirsutism but who do have endometrial hyperplasia can be given progestins (medroxyprogesterone) only (Kase, 1983).

INTERVENTION

Nursing care for women with POD is unique for each woman. The adolescent woman may be very afraid that she is a "freak," since she may already be the only one of her peers who has not menstruated. She may also feel different from her peers if she has developed hirsutism or is overweight. She needs a great deal of support (Kirschmer, 1986). The nurse can assist her with a weight-reducing diet and can explain methods of hair removal, if that is appropriate. The nurse should help the young woman to re-establish and/or strengthen her self-esteem.

The infertile woman has special concerns that may be related to her infertility or to other symptoms. The nurse should provide appropriate teaching, support, and counseling. The reader is referred to Chapter 13, Infertility and Sexuality, for specific information about infertility counseling.

Premenstrual Syndrome

Premenstrual syndrome (PMS) is defined as the regular occurrence, in at least three menstrual cycles, of distressing physical and/or psychological symptoms during the premenstruum that are not present in the postmenstruum (Dalton, 1985). The term premenstrual tension, or PMT, may be used to refer only to psychological symptoms. No specific cause for PMS has yet been determined. Until recently, the cause was thought to be psychological, or simply an inevitable part of being a woman and thus to be endured.

The onset of PMS may occur following pregnancy or the use of oral contraceptives, although it can occur at any time. PMS is most commonly a problem of women in their thirties; it rarely occurs before puberty, during pregnancy, or after menopause. In one older study of lesbians, it was found that lesbians reported significantly less premenstrual *tension* than did heterosexual controls (Kenyon, 1968).

Symptoms and severity vary greatly. Over 150 symptoms have been identified. The most common physical symptoms are breast pain, abdominal bloating, and generalized swelling. The most common psychological symptoms are tension, depression, tiredness, and irritability. Symptoms may spontaneously subside or increase (Altchek, 1985).

Women who have PMS may report an increase in sexual desire during the premenstruum (Dalton, 1982). However, many also report having no desire for sex when they are premenstrual but having great desire once the menstrual period begins. These kinds of mood changes can have a direct effect on sexual feelings and activities and could certainly present problems in a relationship, unless they are understood (Sanders, 1983). The sexual partner may be very confused by the woman's behavior.

Women who have PMS often feel ugly and nonsexual during their premenstrual time. One of the reasons for this may be the feeling of bloatedness, which causes them to feel fat—even though there are no demonstrated changes in weight. A recent study supported this idea. Two groups of women diagnosed as having PMS, one who experienced mainly psychological symptoms and one who experienced mainly somatic symptoms, were studied (Faratian et al, 1984). Both groups described a significant increase in perceived body size and the "feeling of bloatedness" without an associated change in weight or an increase in abdominal dimensions.

INTERVENTION

There is no cure for PMS. Treatment has been symptomatic and extremely varied. However, Harrison (1982) says it is the *woman* with PMS who should be treated rather than the PMS. Treatments in the same woman may be effective in one episode but not another. There seems to be a strong placebo effect with almost any kind of treatment (Gitlin and Pasnau, 1983).

One of the first treatments is a change in diet, including decreases in sugar, chocolate, caffeine, and salt. A high-protein, hypoglycemic diet has been suggested. Vitamin B_6 has also been recommended. Some women have tried oil of evening primrose, which should be taken with food to prevent gastric irritation (Harrison, 1982).

Other self-help treatments include exercise and stress management. Drug therapy has included diuretics, bromocriptine, antiprostaglandins, and both synthetic and natural progesterone. However, studies concerning the effectiveness of these therapies have not found any to be consistently or demonstrably more effective than any other.

Nursing care for women who have PMS involves primarily supportive care, that is believing them and accepting what they say. Women report that among their worst fears is the idea that they are feeling crazy and not being believed or taken seriously. The nurse should listen carefully, support them as women, and validate that their experience is real and that other women also experience it. One concrete suggestion that many women find useful is to keep a symptom diary or calendar.

The nurse should teach women as much as possible about PMS and assist them with self-care treatments that they wish to try. Stress management techniques are often helpful. The nurse must emphasize that these treatments are not offered as cures but as something that may help. Because there are so many treatments and approaches, the nurse should help the women to avoid clinics or offices that quickly appear—and disappear—for treatment of PMS; the woman should be helped to be a wise consumer, keep records of her signs and symptoms, and avoid being the victim of exploitation.

Ovarian Tumors

Ovarian tumors can be benign or malignant, with 75 to 80 per cent benign and 20 to 25 per cent malignant (Ramzy, 1983). They occur in women of all ages. However, benign tumors are more likely in premenopausal women, while malignant tumors are more common at the time of menopause or shortly after, with the peak incidence around 40 to 65 years (Weekes and Watkins, 1981). Ovarian cancer accounts for 4 per cent of the cancer in women but 5 per cent of the deaths (American Cancer Society, 1986), as it is extremely virulent. At diagnosis, 70 per cent of cases have spread beyond the ovary (Weekes and Watkins, 1981). (The reader is referred to Chapter 15, Cancer and Sexuality, which addresses the effects of cancer on sexuality and discusses implications for nursing.)

CONDITIONS INVOLVING THE VULVA

The vulva (or pudenda) refers to the female's external genitalia, including the labia and clitoris. The vulva has both a physical and a symbolic relationship with female sexuality, and as such, problems with the vulva may be disturbing to a woman and her sense of sexuality.

There are many benign and malignant conditions of the vulva, but the situation that is the most threatening to a woman's sexuality is a vulvectomy. Simple or radical vulvectomy is performed as a treatment for cancer of the vulva.

Cancer of the vulva usually occurs in older women—the average age of women who have invasive cancer of the vulva is 60 to 65 years; however, in situ cancer of the vulva is now being recognized in young women, even in their late teens and early twenties (Woodruff, 1985). There seems to be an increased frequency of vulvar carcinoma in obese women (Morrow, 1983). The primary symptom is a painless, although occasionally pruritic lesion, that may be a lump or a white patch. About 25 to 30 per cent of the lesions are asymptomatic (Woodruff, 1985). The lesion is usually located in the anterior two thirds of the labia majora but can be anywhere on the vulva (Ramzy, 1983).

Definitive treatment consists of surgical excision of the involved tissue. However, chemotherapy, cryotherapy, or immunotherapy may be preferable to a radical vulvectomy with the attendant severe scarring and potential dyspareunia in some elderly women who are sexually active (Huffman, 1983).

A more radical vulvectomy involves removal of all the fatty and connective labial tissue, the distal third of the vagina (the most sensitive part), and often the clitoris as well. Surgery can result in vaginal stenosis, particularly of the introitus, which may cause dyspareunia. There will also be less vaginal sensation than before. (Recently, vulvar reconstruction has been attempted following radical vulvectomy, but the reconstruction may be more radical than the procedure itself.) The discussion in Chapter 15, Cancer and Sexuality, in which general effects of cancer and many of its treatment modalities are discussed complements the information presented here on the effects of vulvar surgery on sexuality and sexual functioning. The interested reader is referred to that chapter.

Effect of Vulvectomy on Sexuality

Clitoridectomy may result in greatly altered sexual sensation, although some women can achieve orgasm from stimulation of the area (Moth et al, 1983). However, there has been no systematic study of orgasmic ability after clitoridectomy. Because the fatty tissue of the mons pubis is also removed, the remaining tissue may be quite sensitive. Masturbation techniques may have to be altered. The use of vibrators may be quite uncomfortable. Tribadism (mutual body rubbing) in lesbians or male superior positions for intercourse may become painful.

Some surgeons are now performing a less radical procedure, involving only a wide excision (or partial vulvectomy) of the lesion itself. This may be followed with skin grafting. DiSaia (1985) reports that in 15 women on whom he performed the wide excision with skin grafting, there was no change in sexual functioning. If this finding could be replicated, it may be a very positive change for women in terms of sexual health.

Several complications of radical vulvectomy may have an impact on a woman's sexual health. One long-term complication is the development of leg edema (Springer, 1982), which can be extreme enough to result in a change in clothes size. The loss of fat over the perineum may also make wearing fitted clothing uncomfortable, and the woman may totally change her usual pattern of dressing.

The woman may view the change in her body image as eliminating sexual activity. She may fear that she will be unable to do *anything* sexually. Especially if the woman is young, she may feel that she is sexually undesirable. Later, after she has recovered, she may wonder whether she can ever have a baby. Since radical vulvectomy has no direct effect on fertility, pregnancy may still be a possibility.

One study of 15 women (mean age 55, mean years since surgery equaled 5) who had vulvectomies reported considerable disruption in sexual behavior, with decreased sexual desire, activity, and satisfaction as well as negative body image (Andersen and Hacker, 1983b). Another study reported similar findings among 15 women who had had vulvectomies and nine of their sexual partners. Over half of the women had given up coitus—primarily because of dyspareunia and a subjective sense that the introitus was too small. The women also described an extreme lack of sexual desire and a reduced acceptance of their own bodies (Moth et al, 1983).

An earlier study also showed that women who had had radical vulvectomies had negative changes in their body image, sexual relationship, and frequency of intercourse after surgery (Sewell and Edwards, 1980). The women who had vulvectomies had less of a negative change than women who had pelvic exenterations and more of a change than women who had radical hysterectomies.

In the most recent study of women having radical vulvectomies, eight of ten of the women were said to have accomplished complete or partial sexual rehabilitation by approximately 2 years after the surgery. Specific criteria for "successful rehabilitation" were used. The investigators concluded that motivation for sexual expression and mutual affection may be more important for sexual rehabilitation than the specific results of the surgery (Schultz et al, 1986).

SUMMARY

The breadth of content in this chapter suggests the significant impact of gynecological conditions on women's sexual functioning and that of their sexual partners. Any condition that has to do with women, because they are women, can affect women's sexual health. Seemingly minor situations, such as laparoscopy, to the most radical gynecological surgery, pelvic exenteration, may affect women's sexual functioning, but in very different ways, because each woman is unique.

REFERENCES

Abitbol MM, Davenport JH: Sexual dysfunction after therapy for cervical carcinoma. Am J Obstet Gynecol 119:181–189, 1974.

Altchek A: Pediatric and adolescent gynecology. In Nichols DH, Evrard JR (eds): Ambulatory Gynecology. New York, Harper & Row, 1985, pp 20–62.

American Cancer Society. Cancer Facts and Figures. New York, American Cancer Society, 1986.

Amias AG: Sexual life after gynecological operations—II. Br Med J 2:680–681, 1975.

Andersen BL, Hacker NR: Psychosexual adjustment following pelvic exenteration. Obstet Gynecol 61:331–338, 1983a.

Andersen BL, Hacker NF: Psychosocial adjustment after vulvar surgery. Obstet Gynecol 62:457–462, 1983b.

Barber HRK: Cancer of the ovary. In van Nagell JR, Jr, Barber HRK (eds): Modern Concepts of Gynecologic Oncology. Boston, John Wright, 1982, pp 239–265.

Bernhard LA: Endometriosis. JOGN Nursing 11:300–304, 1982.

Bernhard LA: Methodological issues in studies of sexuality and hysterectomy. J Sex Res 22:108–128, 1986a.

Bernhard LA: Sexuality expectations and outcomes in women having hysterectomies. Ph.D. dissertation, University of Illinois at Chicago, 1986b.

Borton M, Oskowitz SP: Toxic shock syndrome. In Friedman EA (ed): Gynecological Decision Making. St. Louis, CV Mosby, 1983, pp 170–171.

Brown MA, Woods NF: Correlates of dysmenorrhea. JOGN Nursing 13:259–266, 1984.

Budd KW: Variations of response to hysterectomy: Bases for individualized care to women. In Lytle NA (ed): Nursing of Women in the Age of Liberation. Dubuque, Brown, 1977, pp 187–206.

Cain EN, Kohorn EI, Quinlan DM, et al: Psychosocial reactions to the diagnosis of gynecologic cancer. Obstet Gynecol 62:635–641, 1983.

Cairns KV, Valentich M: Vaginal reconstruction in gynecologic cancer: A feminist perspective. J Sex Res 22:333–346, 1986.

Chapman JD: Sexuality—The mature or childbearing years and the effect of gynecologic surgery. J Am Osteopathic Assoc 78:509–514, 1979.

Cobliner WG: Psychosocial factors in gynecological or breast malignancies. Hosp Phys 10:38–40, 1977.

Coppen A, Bishop M, Beard RJ, et al: Hysterectomy, hormones, and behaviour. Lancet 1:126–128, 1981.

Cosper B, Fuller SS, and Robinson GJ: Characteristics of posthospitalization recovery following hysterectomy. JOGN Nursing 7:7–11, 1978.

Craig GA, Jackson P: Sexual life after vaginal hysterectomy. Br Med J 3:97, 1975.

Dalton K: Diagnosis and clinical features of premenstrual syndrome. In Dawood MY, McGuire JL, Demers LM (eds): Premenstrual Syndrome and Dysmenorrhea. Baltimore, Urban & Schwarzenberg, 1985.

Dalton K: Premenstrual tension: An overview. In Friedman RC (ed): Behavior and the Menstrual Cycle. New York, Marcel Dekker, 1982, pp 217–242.

Daly MJ: Psychological impact of surgical procedures on women. In Sadock BJ, Kaplan HI, Freedman AM (eds): The Sexual Experience. Baltimore, Williams & Wilkins, 1976, pp 308–313.

Dempsey GM, Buchsbaum HJ, Morrison J: Psychosocial adjustment to pelvic exenteration. Gynecol Oncol 3:325–334, 1975.

Dennerstein L, Burrows GD: Hormone replacement therapy and sexuality in women. Clin Endocrinol Metabol 11:661–679, 1982.

Dennerstein L, Wood C, Burrows GD: Sexual response following hysterectomy and oophorectomy. Obstet Gynecol 49:92–96, 1977.

Derogatis LR: The unique impact of breast and gynecologic cancers on body image and sexual identity in women: A reassessment. In Vaeth JM (ed): Body Image, Self-esteem, and Sexuality in Cancer Patients. 2nd ed. New York, Karger, 1986, pp 1–14.

DiSaia P: Management of superficially invasive vulvar carcinoma. Clin Obstet Gynecol 28:196–203, 1985.

Donahue VC: Sexual rehabilitation of gynecologic cancer patients. In Coppleson M (ed): Gynecologic Oncology. Vol. 2. New York, Churchill Livingstone, 1981, pp 1050–1054.

Donahue VC, Knapp RC: Sexual rehabilitation of gynecologic cancer patients. Obstet Gynecol 49:118–121, 1977.

Drellich MG, Bieber I, Sutherland AM: The psychological impact of cancer and cancer surgery. VI. Adaptation to hysterectomy. Cancer 9:1120–1126, 1956.

Droegemueller W, Herbst AL, Mishell DR, Stenchever MA: Comprehensive Gynecology. St. Louis, CV Mosby, 1987.

Edlund BJ: The needs of women with gynecologic malignancies. Nurs Clin North Am 17:165–177, 1982.

Faratian B, Gaspar A, O'Brien PMS, et al: Premenstrual syndrome: Weight, abdominal swelling, and perceived body image. Am J Obstet Gynecol 150:200–204, 1984.

Fisher SG: Psychosexual adjustment following total pelvic exenteration. Cancer Nurs 2:219–225, 1979.

Fox H, Buckley CH: Current concepts of endometriosis. Clin Obstet Gynecol 11:279–287, 1984.

Fuchs F: Dysmenorrhea and dyspareunia. In Friedman RC (ed): Behavior and the Menstrual Cycle. New York, Marcel Dekker, 1982, pp 199–216.

Gaddis O, Jr: Carcinoma of the vagina. In Mishell DR Jr, Brenner PF (eds): Management of Common Problems in Obstetrics and Gynecology. Oradell, Medical Economics Books, 1983, pp 271–273.

Gath D, Cooper P, Day A: Hysterectomy and psychiatric disorder: I. Levels of psychiatric morbidity before and after hysterectomy. Br J Psychiatry 140:335–350, 1982.

Gitlin MJ, Pasnau RO: Depression in obstetric and gynecology patients. J Psychiatric Treat Eval 5:421–428, 1983.

Goodkin K, Antoni MH, Blaney PH: Stress and hopelessness in the promotion of cervical intraepithelial neoplasia to invasive squamous cell carcinoma of the cervix. J Psychosom Res 30:67–76, 1986.

Hale RW: Pediatric and adolescent gynecology. In Hale RW, Krieger JA (eds): Gynecology. New Hyde Park, Medical Examination, 1983, pp 163–177.

Harris R, Good RS, Pollack L: Sexual behavior of gynecologic cancer patients. Arch Sex Behav 11:503–510, 1982.

Harrison M: Self-help for Premenstrual Syndrome (rev ed). New York, Random House, 1982.

Heilman JR: Menopause: Myths are yielding to new scientific research. Sci Digest March 1980, pp 66–68.

Hibbard LT: Uterine myomas. In Mishell DR Jr, Brenner PF (eds): Management of Common Problems in Obstetrics and Gynecology. Oradell, Medical Economics Books, 1983, pp 241–243.

Hollender MH: Hysterectomy and feelings of femininity. Med Asp Human Sex 3:6–15, 1969.

Hott JR: Restoring sexual expression after uterine cancer. The Female Patient 7:15–18, 1982.

Hubbard JL, Shingleton HM: Sexual function of patients after cancer of the cervix treatment. Clin Obstet Gynecol 12:247–264, 1985.

Huffman JW: The diagnosis and treatment of gynecologic disorders in elderly patients. Comp Therapy 9:54–60, 1983.

Humphries PT: Sexual adjustment after a hysterectomy. Issues Health Care Women 2:1–14, 1980.

Johnson SR, Palermo JL: Gynecologic care for the lesbian. Clin Obstet Gynecol 27:724–731, 1984.

Kase NG: Anovulation. In Kase NG, Weingold AB (eds): Principles and Practice of Clinical Gynecology. New York, John P. Wiley & Sons, 1983, pp 355–367.

Kav-Venaki S, Zakham L: Psychological effects of hysterectomy in premenopausal women. J Psychosom Obstet Gynecol 2:76–80, 1983.

Kenyon FE: Physique and physical health of female homosexuals. J Neurol Neurosurg Psychiatry 31:487–489, 1968.

King J: Vaginitis. JOGN Nurs 13(Suppl 2):41S–48S, 1984.

Kirschmer MA: The PCO syndrome: Sexual and reproductive concerns. Med Aspects Human Sex 20:92–96, 1986.

Kitzinger S: Woman's Experience of Sex. New York, GP Putnam's Sons, 1983.

Krantz KE: Pelvic relaxation. In Peckham BM, Shapiro SS (eds): Signs and Symptoms in Gynecology. Philadelphia, JB Lippincott, 1983, pp 95–103.

Krieger JA: Benign lesions of the uterus. In Hale RW, Krieger JA (eds): Gynecology. New Hyde Park, Medical Examination, 1983, pp 215–230.

Krouse HJ, Krouse JH: Cancer as crisis: The critical elements of adjustment. Nurs Res 31:96–101, 1982.

Krueger JS, Hassell J, Goggins DB, et al: Relationship between nurse counselling and sexual adjustment after hysterectomy. Nurs Res 28:145–150, 1979.

Lalinec-Michaud M, Engelsmann F: Depression and hysterectomy: A prospective study. Psychosom 25:550–558, 1984.

Lamberti J: Sexual adjustment after radiation therapy for cervical carcinoma. Med Aspects Human Sex 13:87–88, 1979.

Lamont JA, DePetrillo AD, Sargeant EJ: Psychosexual rehabilitation and exenterative surgery. Gynecol Oncol 6:236–242, 1978.

Lazarov A, Jurukovski J, Adamova G, Antonovski L: Sexual response following hysterectomy. In Carenza L, Zichella L (eds): Emotion and Reproduction. Vol. 20B. New York, Academic Press, 1979, pp 1277–1281.

Leiblum S, Bachmann G, Kemmann E, et al: Vaginal atrophy in the postmenopausal woman. JAMA 249:2195–2198, 1983.

LHRH agonist reduces implants, pain. Med World News Nov 12, 1984, p 15.

Lindemann E: Observations on psychiatric sequelae to surgical operations in women. Am J Psychiatry 98:132–139, 1941.

Martin RL, Roberts WV, Clayton PJ: Psychiatric status after hysterectomy. JAMA 244:350–353, 1980.

McKenzie CAM: Sexuality and the menopausal woman. Issues Health Care Women 1:38–44, 1978.

Millette BM, Hawkins JBW: The Passage Through Menopause. Reston, Reston Pub, 1983.

Moore JT, Tolley DH: Depression following hysterectomy. Psychosom 17:86–89, 1976.

Moran S: Vaginal hysterectomy. RN 42:53–54, 1979.

Morgan S: Coping with a Hysterectomy. New York, Dial, 1982.

Morrow CP: Evaluation and management of the patient with vulvar and urethral carcinoma. In Mishell DR Jr, Brenner PF (eds): Management of Common Problems in Obstetrics and Gynecology. Oradell, Medical Economics Books, 1983, pp 268–270.

Moth I, Andreasson B, Jensen SB, Bock JE: Sexual function and somatopsychic reactions after vulvectomy. Danish Med Bull 30(Suppl 2):27–30, 1983.

Nichols DH, Wisgirda JA: Gynecological urology. In Nichols DH, Evrard JR (eds): Ambulatory Gynecology. New York, Harper & Row, 1985, pp 200–222.

O'Donnell M, Leoffler V, Pollock K, Saunders Z: Lesbian Health Matters! Santa Cruz, Santa Cruz Women's Health Center, 1979.

Orenberg CL: DES: The Complete Story. New York, St. Martin's Press, 1981.

Osborn MF: Sexual problems in obstetrics and gynaecology. Br J Hosp Med 30:264–268, 1983.

Piver MS: Ovarian carcinoma: A decade of progress. Cancer 54:2706–2715, 1984.

Ramzy I: Essentials of Gynecologic and Obstetric Pathology. Norwalk, Appleton-Century-Crofts, 1983.

Richards DH: A post-hysterectomy syndrome. Lancet 2:983–985, 1974.

Roeske NCA: Hysterectomy and other gynecological

surgeries: A psychological view. In Notman MT, Nadelson CE (eds): The Woman Patient: Medical and Psychological Interfaces. Vol. 1. New York, Plenum Press, 1978, pp 217–231.

Rosene KA, Eschenbach DA: Flulike symptoms and toxic shock. In Peckham BM, Shapiro SS (eds): Signs and Symptoms in Gynecology. Philadelphia, JB Lippincott, 1983, pp 447–454.

Roy S: Vulvovaginitis. In Mishell DR Jr, Brenner PF (eds): Management of Common Problems in Obstetrics and Gynecology. Oradell, Medical Economics Books, 1983, pp 190–195.

Rubin H: Vaginal hysterectomy. In Friedman EA (ed): Gynecological Decision Making. St. Louis, CV Mosby, 1983, pp 190–191.

Sanders D: Premenstrual tension. In McPherson A, Anderson A (eds): Women's Problems in General Practice. New York, Oxford University Press, 1983, pp 42–62.

Savage J: No sex, please, Mrs Smith. Nurs Mirror 154:28–32, 1982.

Schultz WCMW, Wijma K, Van de Wiel HBM, et al: Sexual rehabilitation of radical vulvectomy patients: A pilot study. J Psychosom Obstet Gynaecol 5:119–126, 1986.

Scommegna A, Maroulis GB: Hirsutism. In Peckham BM, Shapiro SS (eds): Signs and Symptoms in Gynecology. Philadelphia, JB Lippincott, 1983, pp 312–327.

Seibel MM, Freeman MG, and Graves WL: Carcinoma of the cervix and sexual function. Obstet Gynecol 55:484–487, 1980.

Semmens JP: Sexuality. In Buchsbaum HJ (ed): The Menopause. New York, Springer-Verlag, 1983, pp 173–180.

Semmens JP, and Semmens EC: Sexual function and the menopause. Clin Obstet Gynecol 27:717–723, 1984.

Sewell HH, Edwards DW: Pelvic genital cancer: Body image and sexuality. In Vaeth JM, Blomberg RC, Adler L (eds): Body Image, Self-esteem, and Sexuality in Cancer Patients. Vol. 14. New York, Karger, 1980, pp 35–41.

Sharma SD: Carcinoma of the cervix. In Hale RW, Krieger JA (eds): Gynecology. New Hyde Park, Medical Examination, 1983, pp 271–290.

Smith DC, Prentice R, Thompson DJ, Herrmann WL: Association of exogenous estrogen and endometrial carcinoma. N Engl J Med 293:1164–1167, 1975.

Springer M: Radical vulvectomy: Physical, psychological, social and sexual implications. Oncol Nurs Forum 9:19–21, 1982.

Thomas DB: Epidemiology of cervical cancer: The herpes virus question. In Forastiere AA (ed): Gynecologic Cancer. New York, Churchill Livingstone, 1984, pp 33–46.

Utian WH: Effect of hysterectomy, oophorectomy and estrogen therapy on libido. Int J Gynaecol Obstet 13:97–100, 1975.

van Nagell JR Jr, Powell DF, Gay EC: Cancer of the vagina. In van Nagell JR Jr, Barber HRK (eds): Modern Concepts of Gynecologic Oncology. Boston, John Wright, 1982, pp 181–212.

Vera MI: Quality of life following pelvic exenteration. Gynecol Oncol 12:355–366, 1981.

Vincent CE, Vincent B, Greiss FC, Linton EB: Some marital-sexual concomitants of carcinoma of the cervix. South Med J 68:552–558, 1975.

Voda AM: Climacteric hot flash. Maturitas 3:73–90, 1981.

Webb C, Wilson-Barnett J: Self-concept, social support and hysterectomy. Int J Nurs Stud 20:97–107, 1983.

Weekes LR, Watkins SA: Carcinoma of the ovary. J Nat Med Assoc 73:1055–1061, 1981.

Williams MA: A comparative study of postsurgical convalescence among women of two ethnic groups: Anglo and Mexican-American. In Batey MV (ed): Communicating Nursing Research. Vol. 5. Boulder, WICHE, 1972, pp 59–80.

Wilson MA: Menstrual disorders: Premenstrual syndrome, dysmenorrhea, amenorrhea. JOGN Nurs 13(Suppl 2):11S–19S, 1984.

Wolf SR: Emotional reactions to hysterectomy. Postgrad Med 47:165–169, 1970.

Woodruff JD: Noninfectious diseases of the vulva. In Nichols DH, Evrard JR (eds): Ambulatory Gynecology. New York, Harper & Row, 1985, pp 371–398.

Wroblewski SS: Toxic shock syndrome. Am J Nurs 81:82–85, 1981.

23: Sexually Transmitted Diseases

Linda Schoonover Smith

Diane Lauver

P. Allen Gray, Jr.

Sexually transmitted diseases are major public health problems because they cause severe human suffering, put heavy demands on health care facilities, and cost hundreds of millions of dollars to treat. The burden of having sexually transmissible diseases predominantly falls upon the women and children in society who are exposed to complications, which include sterility, ectopic pregnancy, fetal and infant deaths, and mental retardation. The poor who contract sexually transmissible diseases also share a greater magnitude of the burden of suffering because of greater difficulty in paying for treatment.

The purpose of this chapter is to provide a strong knowledge base for health professionals who care for clients with sexually transmitted diseases (STDs). The general nursing approach to the client with an STD is discussed first. The psychosocial issues of such clients and the prevention of STDs in the general population are emphasized. Next, STDs that are major public health problems are described in detail. The epidemiology, etiology, transmission, clinical features, medical treatment, nursing management, and client education of specific STDs are presented. Myths and misconceptions about STDs are examined, and the relation-

ship of STDs to human sexuality is discussed. A special final section focuses on acquired immunodeficiency syndrome (AIDS) because of the anxiety about and fear of the disease.

Common STDs in the United States include infections from *Neisseria gonorrhoeae* and *Chlamydia trachomatis*, herpes simplex virus 1 and 2, and syphilis. Common STDs for new immigrants and migrants, travelers to developing countries, and military personnel include chancroid, granuloma inguinale, and lymphogranuloma venereum. An increasingly prevalent and often fatal STD is AIDS. The epidemiology of each disease will be further described in detail under the appropriate section.

NURSING PROCESS WITH CLIENTS WITH AN STD

Nurses need to assess the biopsychosocial needs of clients with STDs in a holistic way. Traditionally, clients with STDs have not been treated in a biopsychosocial manner and have experienced discrimination, prejudice, and a "loftier-than-thou" attitude by health professionals. Clients with STDs need care and attention to their emotional feelings, fears, and physical comfort; they also need privacy—in consultations with their practitioners and in confidentiality of their medical records.

Nurses can be sensitive to reasons for delay in seeking care for STDs and work to minimize such delays. Clients may delay seeking treatment for STDs because they believe they may be stereotyped or suffer social stigma, embarrassment, or some degree of shame during the encounter. In some cultures, Victorian mores persist in associating sex with sin and STDs with just punishment. Other clients may delay seeking treatment because of little accessibility or availability to health care. Still other clients do not seek treatment because they may be asymptomatic, although infectious. A proportion of the population is not aware of the signs and symptoms of STDs.

Psychosocial reactions of clients with STDs vary. Anxiety and depression have been reported with a positive diagnosis (Carlton and Mayes, 1982; Leo, 1982). The theoretical literature discusses shame and guilt as secondary to stigma about STD. Although such negative effects may occur with the diagnosis of an STD, they may be different for various sociocultural subgroups, may be limited to dealing with the short-term crisis, and may actually be secondary to a changing intimate relationship rather than to a diagnosis per se.

Unfortunately, research to describe and explain individual reactions to STDs is lacking. In clinical practice with women, a wide range of reactions have been observed: acceptance ("I knew it."), hurt ("I never thought he'd been with anyone else."), disbelief ("I can't believe I've got that."), anger ("That's the end of him."), and concern ("What are the side effects of this?"). Psychosocial reactions seem to vary with the expectations and frequency of STDs within a subculture and within the client's personal experience. Although distressed at her diagnosis, one young woman stated in response to her treatment plan, "Yes, I know about these two drugs and when to take them . . . My mom told me about them." This is not to suggest that some individuals are blasé about STDs. Rather, perhaps some persons are more realistic in acknowledging the necessity of treatment. Most clients, although distressed, seem appropriately concerned about treatment and prevention of complications.

Assessment

A thorough history, medical examination, and appropriate laboratory tests are needed to diagnose STDs (Table 23–1). Clients with STDs may be anxious or embarrassed. Thus, the history is taken first, with the client dressed.

A history is elicited in a nonjudgmental manner, using open-ended questions and avoiding assumptions of sexual orientation. Refer to all partners as partners and not by gender, for example, "Did your partner have any rashes or lesions?" The history of the present concern includes a description of the data and type of sexual activity, number of contacts, symptomatology, and potential sites of infection (mouth, cervix, rectum, urethra). Pertinent medical history includes any information that will influence the treatment plan, history of allergies (especially to penicillin),

TABLE 23–1. Data Collection for the Client with an STD

History
1. The chief complaint.
2. Thorough description of the history of the present illness. (Describe major symptoms by quality, quantity, precipitating and palliative factors, radiation, associated symptoms, and chronology of events. Self-care tretments and use of prescribed or over-the-counter medicine should be noted.)
3. Major adult health problems.
4. Sexual history (type and frequency of sexual actrivity, number of contacts, past history of STDs, potential sites of infection, sexual preference).
5. Allergies.
6 General women's health (date of last menstrual period, date of last Pap smear, pattern of contraception).

Physical Examination of the Male and Female External Genitalia
1. Inspection.
2. Palpation (refer to Barbara Bates' *A Guide to Physical Assessment* for more detail).

Laboratory Tests
1. Saline wet preparation (*Trichomonas* and *Gardnerella*).
2. Whiff test (*Gardnerella*).
3. Potassium hydroxide preparation (*Candida*).
4. Urinalysis (U/A).
5. Gonorrhea culture.
6. Cervical culture.
7. Herpes cervical culture.
8. Pap smear.
9. Complete blood count.
10. Venereal Disease Research Laboratory (VDRL), fluorescent treponemal antibody absorption test (FTA-ABS).
11. Herpes simplex virus type 1 and 2 antibodies.

pregnancy, previously diagnosed conditions, and general health. The date of the last menstrual period should always be obtained to help rule out pregnancy.

At the conclusion of the history, the client is prepared for the examination. During the examination, the client's comfort, modesty, and privacy are respected. Clients are draped for privacy and warmth. For women, the speculum is warmed, and it is helpful to warm the metal stirrups of the examining table with cotton booties. Application of the general guidelines for data collection for STDs follows, with discussion of specific diseases.

Intervention

The client who has an STD needs support for seeking medical care at the earliest stage of symptoms, and sexual partners also need evaluation. Clients and partners need to know how to follow the treatment regimen adequately; specifically, whether or not abstinence may be necessary, and if so, for how long. Education is necessary for all clients so that they can respond promptly to symptoms, follow medical instructions, refer partners for treatment, return for all follow-up appointments, practice prevention, and request periodic check-ups if their life style places them at a higher risk of contracting STDs (Tables 23–2 and 23–3).

STDS ASSOCIATED WITH DISCHARGE

Neisseria Gonorrhoeae Infection

Neisseria gonorrhoeae was first isolated in 1879, although it had been recognized as early as Biblical times. Before Christ, Hippocrates made early observations of the infection. Galen is stated to be the first to use the term gonorrhea. Interestingly, street language for gonorrhea, i.e., "the clap," has its roots in the 1300s in England. At that time, the surgeon to Richard II and Henry IV used this term (Spence, 1983).

EPIDEMIOLOGY

Today gonorrhea presents a major health problem, as it infects men and women vene-

TABLE 23–2. Client Education for all STDs

What to Do
Taking Medication:
  1. How
  2. When
  3. Things to avoid.
Obtaining repeat cultures after treatment for test-of-cure:
  1. When
  2. Why
  3. What happens at the clinic.
Recheck:
  1. When
  2. Why
  3. What happens at the clinic.
Sex partners:
  1. Need for medical care
  2. Need for a period of abstinence from sexual intercourse
  3. Devise realistic health plan to include: how client is going to tell partners, where client is going to refer partners to, when partners will go, where client can reach counselor for additional help, and where counselor can reach client if needed.
Future health
  1. Respond immediately to any unusual bumps, sores, rashes, discharges.
  2. Return to the clinic occasionally—even if things appear normal.
Be Sure the Client Leaves the Clinic with *No* Unanswered Questions

really as well as infants in childbirth and children via sexual abuse. Gonorrhea invades the pseudostratified and columnar epithelium of the urogenital tract. In childbearing women, it does not affect the vagina. Only in low-estrogenized women (prepubertal or postmenopausal) may the vaginal resistance be lowered to facilitate infection. Gonorrhea may be termed *uncomplicated* to refer to limited urethral or cervical infections in symptomatic or asymptomatic clients. *Complicated* infections most commonly refer to those of salpingitis or pelvic inflammatory disease (PID) or disseminated gonococcal infection (McMaster, 1981; Spence, 1983). Gonorrhea is a health concern because of its prevalence and its short- and long-term morbidity, including acute, painful infections and preventable infertility. In addition, the asymp-

TABLE 23–3. Preventing STDs

1. Engage in sex with one mutually faithful partner.
2. Abstain from sex with a person who has lesions, rashes, or malodorous discharges from the genitals.
3. Do not have intercourse with a person whose sexual history is unknown or who is at high risk for AIDS.
4. Use condoms consistently and throughout genital contact.
5. Wash and urinate before and after sexual intercourse.

tomatic state and the emergence of a penicillin-resistant strain of gonorrhea are causes for concern.

Overall, the incidence of gonorrhea is highest among young, sexually active individuals in urban areas (Barnes and Holmes, 1984; Fiumara, 1987). The reported prevalence of gonorrhea varies among different populations. Whether this reflects different prevalence rates *or* reporting practices is unknown. Among women, 1 to 2 per cent seen in private practice and about 5 per cent seen in hospital clinics are reported to have gonorrhea (Spence, 1983). Of those women affected, 17 per cent may develop pelvic inflammatory disease, which in turn is positively associated with infertility (McMaster, 1981). The majority of males with gonorrhea are symptomatic; however, about 10 per cent may be asymptomatic. In contrast, the majority of women (75 to 80 per cent) may be asymptomatic (Fiumara, 1987). It has been found that as many as 40 to 50 per cent of the male partners of asymptomatic, but infected, females may also have positive cultures for gonorrhea (Spence, 1983). These figures reveal a high incidence of gonorrhea among unsuspecting and asymptomatic clients.

N. gonorrhoeae, a gram-negative intracellular diplococcus, is one of the many *Neisseria* species. For diagnostic purposes, it is important to note that *Neisseria* species other than *N. gonorrhoeae* are normally found in the gastrointestinal and genitourinary tract. Because there are a variety of gram-negative intracellular diplococci normally found in the genital tract, a Gram stain of cervical discharge is not specific for gonorrhea. Appropriate cultures are necessary for women and recommended for men. Menstrual blood promotes reproduction of the organism; cultures should not be omitted during menses (McMaster, 1981). Sugar fermentation tests are available to differentiate the gonococcus from other strains (*N. gonorrhoeae* only ferments glucose, not fructose or mannose) (Spence, 1983; McMaster, 1981).

Gonorrhea is spread primarily during sexual relations when the organism invades the mucous membranes of the genitourinary or gastrointestinal tract. However, it may sometimes be spread indirectly through close physical contact or the use of thermometers, that is, via fomites (Litt, Edberg, Finberg, 1974). The incubation period of gonorrhea averages 3 to 5 days but can range from 1 day to 2 weeks (Fiumara, 1983; Spence, 1983).

CLINICAL FEATURES

Primary symptoms of gonorrhea include pain or discomfort and discharge. With urethritis, dysuria and sometimes frequency occur. The dysuria is usually marked and may spontaneously resolve. With cervicitis, acute pelvic or back pain is minimal in the absence of PID. For men, the onset of symptoms 2 to 3 days after exposure is often abrupt. In over 70 per cent of cases, males present with purulent urethral discharge and dysuria (Hook and Stamm, 1983). For women, the symptoms of gonorrhea are less clearly defined (Barnes and Holmes, 1984; Fiumara, 1987).

The nature of the observed or reported discharge may vary. Gonorrhea cervicitis may be associated with or without a classic yellow-green profuse purulent discharge (Simon, 1981). However, in one study, 23 per cent of women with gonococcal PID had visually normal cervices on examination (Curran, 1979). Males with gonococcal urethritis may not have the classic discharge; a "morning drip" of a few drops of clear fluid may be reported (Spence, 1983).

Palpation of the affected area may elicit marked tenderness, for example, of Skene's or Bartholin's glands, the cervix or fallopian tubes in women, or epididymis in men. Fever, another objective sign, is more common with complicated than uncomplicated gonorrheal infections. The primary objective signs for a diagnosis of gonorrhea involve carefully performed laboratory measures.

ASSESSMENT

A microscopic slide may be prepared for documentation of gonococcal urethritis in males. Under oil immersion (100× magnification) the presence or absence of gram-negative diplococci (kidney bean shapes facing each other) inside polymorphonuclear leukocytes is assessed (Spence, 1983). This is made by rolling the swabbed discharge on a glass slide. The slide is dried with a flame. The slide is Gram stained. Finding the classic organism is diagnostic for gonococcal urethritis in males.

Although the literature is inconsistent in suggesting slide preparations of cervical discharge to rule out gonorrhea in women, the authors do not support this practice. The normal presence of gram-negative intracellular diplococci other than *N. gonorrhoeae* in the female genital tract makes this practice inaccurate (McMaster, 1981). Cultures are necessary for definitive diagnosis in women and are desirable in all clients.

Culturing is done not only to detect *N. gonorrhoeae* accurately and minimize morbidity for symptomatic or high-risk clients but also to prevent its spread to others in the general population. Culturing all exposed sites is important. Sites other than the urethra or cervix include the pharynx and rectum. Cost-effective individualized culturing of specific sites necessitates good rapport and sensitive interviewing techniques. One way to address the necessity of thorough screening is to give clients information (e.g., "Infections such as gonorrhea may grow in areas that have been involved sexually like the throat and rectum. It is important to culture all areas where gonorrhea might be.") and then to ask a simple question matter of factly (e.g., "Shall I culture your throat? Your rectum?").

Fastidious culture techniques must be followed in routine examinations to increase the diagnosis of gonorrhea. Thayer Martin plates are used. When culture techniques are correct, the sensitivity of cultures may be 85 to 90 per cent (McMaster, 1981). Culturing the pharynx and rectum increases yield. For example, in pregnant women, 15 to 35 per cent of clients have had positive pharyngeal cultures (McMaster, 1981); in women with uncomplicated gonorrhea, 44 per cent also have anorectal infection; in homosexual men, the involvement may be 45 per cent (Klein, Fischer, and Chow, 1977). When culturing the gastrointestinal tract for *N. gonorrhoeae*, sugar fermentation tests are necessary to differentiate it from other species of *Neisseria*. Correct technique necessitates using a nonlubricated speculum, swabbing the area for 30 seconds to absorb the organism, swabbing the culture medium, and placing the culture in a carbon dioxide–rich environment.

It is important to note the limitations of cultures. As symptoms subside, the organism may not be readily retrievable. This may occur in female urethritis. Also, a negative cervical culture for *N. gonorrhoeae* (or *Chlamydia trachomatis*) does not rule out the possibility of endometrial or fallopian tube involvement. A negative gonorrhea culture may not necessarily indicate an absence of infection (Hook and Stamm, 1983). Impor-

tantly, gonorrhea and chlamydia infections often occur together; 45 per cent of clients with gonorrhea have positive cultures for *C. trachomatis* (Sexually Transmitted Diseases, 1982).

INTERVENTION

A positive diagnosis of gonorrhea warrants prompt antibiotic therapy for the client and partner. Frequently, the practice of treating infections necessitates objective documentation of the infection prior to treatment. In contrast, the client with "only" a positive history of exposure to gonorrhea warrants treatment. This practice decreases the degree of complications and spread of gonorrhea. Left untreated, gonorrhea may affect body systems and parts other than the urethra and cervix, for example, the upper reproductive tract and musculoskeletal and circulatory systems.

For uncomplicated cases of gonorrhea, the following antibiotics are adequate:

1. Ceftriaxone (125 to 250 mg IM).
2. Amoxicillin (3.0 g orally) plus probenecid (1 g orally).
3. Doxycycline (100 mg orally twice a day for 7 days) or tetracycline HCL (500 mg orally four times a day for 7 days).

The ceftriaxone regimen is effective against pharyngeal and rectal gonococcal infections but not against chlamydia infections ("Treatment," 1988). See Table 23–4 for further details.

Health professionals such as nurses should clarify how to take all oral medications effectively. Concomitant therapy for candida infections may be considered for high-risk clients. Also, estrogen vaginal therapy may be desirable for pre- or postmenstruating women.

Follow-up cultures are necessary; they should be done 3 to 7 days after treatment. In women, follow-up cultures of the urethra, cervix, and rectum should be done. Encourage follow-up cultures for all individuals by saying, "I want to be able to assure you that the infection is gone and that this treatment was effective for you." Follow-up cultures are particularly important in the control of gonorrhea because of the increasing resistance of many strains to penicillin (Barnes and Holmes, 1984). Regarding sexual activity, intimate contact of any kind should be postponed until after follow-up cultures are negative for both partners.

TABLE 23–4. Recommended Regimens for Gonococcal Infections

Population	Treatment
Clients with rectal infection	Ceftriaxone (125–250 mg IM) or aqueous procaine penicillin G (4.8 million units IM) plus probenecid (1.0 g po).
Clients who are allergic to penicillins, cephalosporins, or probenecid	Tetracycline (500 mg po QID for 7 days) or doxycycline (100 mg po BID for 7 days) or spectinomycin 2 g IM (the latter does not cover chlamydia).
Pregnant women	Ceftriaxone 25–250 mg IM or amoxicillin (3.0 g or ampicillin (3.5 g po). Aqueous procaine penicillin G (4.8 million units IM) is effective but less desirable because of associated pain and toxicity.
	Ampicillin, amoxicillin, and penicillin (but not ceftriaxone) regimens are accompanied by probenecid (1 g po) plus erythromycin (500 mg) or erythromycin ethylsuccinate (800 mg po QID for 7 days).
	Pregnant women who are allergic to penicillin, cephalosporins, or probenecid should be treated with spectinomycin (2.0 g IM) plus erythromycin.
Clients with disseminated disease	Aqueous crystalline penicillin G (10 million units IV per day for at least 3 days) followed by amoxicillin or ampicillin (500 mg po QID for 7 days) *or* amoxicillin (3.0 g) or ampicillin (3.5 g) each with probenecid (1.0 g po) followed by amoxicillin or ampicillin (500 mg po QID for 7 days) *or* cefoxitin (1.0 g IV QID for 7 days) *or* cefotaxime (500 mg IV QID for 7 days) *or* ceftriaxone (1 g IV QD for 7 days).

Sources: Fiumara, 1987; "Treatment," 1988

Chlamydia trachomatis Infection

Although some infections due to chlamydia were recognized as early as 1500 BC, it was not until 1899 that the possibility of *C. trachomatis'* infecting the male genitalia was proposed; 11 years later, in 1910, it was proposed that the organism could infect the female genitalia (Hare and Thin, 1983). Not until 1976 to 1977 was *C. trachomatis* isolated from the fallopian tubes (Westrom and Mardh, 1983). For most of this century, gonorrhea has been implicated as a primary cause of urethral and cervical discharge. Today, chlamydia infection is recognized not only as more common than gonorrhea but also as one of the most prevalent STDs (Bell and Grayston, 1986).

Chlamydia infection is a health concern because of its common occurrence and because in addition to causing urethritis and cervicitis, it has been found to be associated with neonatal conjunctivitis, infantile pneumonia, endometritis, salpingitis, perihepatitis, tubal occlusion (Handsfield, Stamm, and Holmes, 1981), proctitis, epididymitis, and infertility (Felman, 1981; Fiumara, 1987; Holmes, Bell, and Berger, 1984). Greater professional and public awareness of the importance and frequency of chlamydia infection and its complications are crucial in order to reduce this public health concern (Thomp-

son and Washington, 1983; Westrom and Mardh, 1983).

EPIDEMIOLOGY

C. trachomatis is an obligate intracellular bacterial pathogen. Like a virus, it requires tissue culture for isolation and propagates intracellularly. Like a bacterium, it has both RNA and DNA and is susceptible to some antibiotics. *C. trachomatis* invades the same epithelial tissues as *N. gonorrhoeae*, specifically the columnar epithelium in the reproductive tract (Rein, 1981).

The primary mode of transmission of *C. trachomatis* among adults is sexual. The risk of developing infection from one coital exposure is not known (Hare and Thin, 1983). For newborns, transmission occurs through vaginal delivery. It has been hypothesized that infants may be reservoirs for nonvenereal transmission of *C. trachomatis* within families. Also, *C. trachomatis* is not a particularly fragile organism and may live in exudate under select conditions for some days (Thompson and Washington, 1983).

Although the incubation period is not definitely known, most sources state it as being 1 to 3 weeks (Fiumara, 1987; Thompson and Washington, 1983; Sweet, Schachter and Landers, 1983). Important to the client's understanding the effects of the infection is acknowledging the existence of a latent state of *C. trachomatis*, which has not been thoroughly described by researchers (Thompson and Washington, 1983).

C. trachomatis is associated with one third to one half of the cases of non-gonococcal urethritis (NGU) in men and with 34 to 63 per cent of mucopurulent cervicitis in women (Sweet, Schachter, and Landers, 1983). Among college-aged males, chlamydia infection may be 10 times more common than gonorrhea (Handsfield, 1982). The majority (67 to 74 per cent) of female contacts of known infected males are also infected with *C. trachomatis* and are asymptomatic (Sweet, Schachter, and Landers, 1983; Rein, 1981). In general, 3 to 5 per cent of women may carry *C. trachomatis* in their cervices (Sweet, Schachter, and Landers, 1983). Although correlations do not imply causality, chlamydia infection has been positively correlated with women using oral contraceptives, cervical ectopy, and recent changes in sexual partners (Hare and Thin, 1983; Sweet, Schachter, and Landers, 1983). Factors that may confound these associations need to be studied; for example, the degree of sexual activity may be positively correlated with both oral contraceptive use and chlamydia infection. However, using oral contraceptives may not alone contribute to infection.

A recent change in sexual partners might be associated with a primary exposure to *C. trachomatis*, but it might also be associated with an alteration in host defense environment that permits exacerbation of a latent stage (Thompson and Washington, 1983; Oriel and Ridgway, 1983). For example, gonococcal infection may reactivate latent chlamydia infection (Hare and Thin, 1983). Other potential triggers for latent disease include other infectious agents, trauma, or excessive alcohol use (Thompson and Washington, 1983).

The natural history of untreated chlamydia infection has been thoroughly explained (Thompson and Washington, 1983) and has been positively correlated with salpingitis, infertility, and cervical neoplasia in women as well as with epididymitis and infertility in men (Sweet, Schachter, and Landers, 1983; Westrom and Mardh, 1983; Oriel and Ridgway, 1983; Felman, 1981; Aria and Lindley, 1980). Cervical intraepithelial neoplasia associated with chlamydia infection warrants further explanation; there may be confounding factors, for example, degree of coital activity or the presence of other STDs, that contribute to neoplasia. In some cases the neoplasia may regress to a more benign condition with tetracycline therapy (Hare and Thin, 1983). Infertility associated with *C. trachomatis* is presumably due to tubal rather than cervical factors (Thompson and Washington, 1983).

CLINICAL FEATURES

For males and females, the primary symptoms of chlamydia infection are discharge and dysuria. Urinary frequency may occur with urethritis. Soreness or dull aching may occur in the affected areas, for example, the pelvis with salpingitis or the scrotum with epididymitis. In contrast to gonorrhea with its classical history of sudden onset (1 to 3 days) and profuse purulent discharge and marked dysuria in men, chlamydia infection is characterized by a slower progression: 6 to 14 days with a mucoid discharge that may be clear, white, or amber and of varying amounts (Fiumara, 1987; Thompson and Washington, 1983). The discomfort associated with chlamydia infection is often described as mild or aching, or it may be absent. In women with cervicitis or salpingitis, the discomfort has been described as "low degree" (Westrom and Mardh, 1983). Fifty per cent of women with chlamydia salpingitis or cervicitis may be asymptomatic.

For males, discomfort associated with epididymitis is described as a "painful, serious complication" and with urethritis as "severe" (Thompson and Washington, 1983; Oriel and Ridgway, 1983). Whether the descriptions of pain accurately reflect sex differences in the experience of chlamydia infection is an interesting question; perhaps reports are socioculturally biased. With cervical or uterine involvement, chlamydia infection may also be associated with a history of irregular bleeding (Westrom and Mardh, 1983). In summary, the symptoms of chlamydia infection may be mild and insidious.

In terms of objective findings, the discharge associated with chlamydia infection is mucoid in consistency, not necessarily profuse in amount, and clear, white, or amber in color. Systemic symptoms of infection are not usually present with cervicitis or urethritis alone; a febrile illness is uncommon. With salpingitis, fever may occur in 29 per cent of cases, while an elevated sedimentation rate may occur in about 65 per cent of cases (Westrom and Mardh, 1983).

On physical examination, a discharge (as

previously described) is often observed. Ideally, this is cultured specifically for *C. trachomatis*. Local signs of infection (i.e., redness, swelling, and tenderness) may be noted (e.g., with bartholinitis or epididymitis). Although cervicitis is difficult to define clinically, with chlamydia infection the endocervix may appear edematous, congested, and eroded (Thompson and Washington, 1983; Holmes and Stamm, 1979). The presence of lymphoid follicles has also been reported (Hare and Thin, 1983). Because *C. trachomatis* specifically infects columnar tissue, it causes cervicitis; it does not affect vaginal squamous cells to cause vaginitis. On palpation, pelvic examination findings may often be equivocal, yet laparoscopies have revealed more involved salpingitis infections than had been suggested by physical examination (Westrom and Mardh, 1983).

ASSESSMENT

One way to diagnose chlamydia infection is with a positive culture. Because it must be grown intracellularly, the organism may be difficult to culture successfully. Special tissue culture media are now available, and the cost is about $40. Thus, these cultures may not be routinely performed. However, culturing for *C. trachomatis* among high-risk groups (the young, sexually active persons, and pregnant women) is cost-effective by preventing morbidity (Handsfield, Stamm, and Holmes, 1981). In an STD clinic in Seattle, women screened for *C. trachomatis* had a positive yield of 12 per cent greater than that for *N. gonorrhoeae* (Holmes, 1982). The presence of numerous polymorphonuclear leukocytes and the absence of gram-negative intracellular diplococci are suggestive of chlamydia cervicitis. With urethritis, pyuria is frequently seen.

Because more cost-effective screening tests for *C. trachomatis* have been developed, routine screening of high-risk groups is recommended (Trachenberg, Washington, and Halldorson, 1988). *C. trachomatis* can be detected with high sensitivity, acceptable sensitivity, and at low cost (about $7) by examination of stained cervical secretions under a fluorescence microscope (Bourcier and Seidler, 1987; Stamm et al, 1984; Emmons and Courter, 1985). *C. trachomatis* can also be detected with a less specific and low cost screening test based on an enzyme immu-

noassay that uses a colorimetric reaction (Bell and Grayston, 1986).

Serological titers of chlamydia antibodies have been studied as a diagnostic tool for chlamydia infection. Significant rises (i.e., fourfold) have been positively associated with epididymitis and salpingitis (Thompson and Washington, 1983). In fact, Westrom and Mardh (1983) report positive associations between titers and infection seen on laparoscopy when evaluating salpingitis. Use of routine serology in diagnosis is limited by its cost and the need to document a rise; that is, two titers must be drawn, and the first must be lower. With past chlamydia infections, the baseline titer would not be expected to be low.

INTERVENTION

One of the nursing interventions for chlamydia infection is client education. Information about the incubation period, primary mode of transmission, usual signs and symptoms, and possible complications is shared with the client. Definitive information about transmission in the latent phase and statistical probabilities of complications have not been available. If factors relevant to the latent period were known, clients might be better able to answer the question, "How or why did I get this?" The latent stage and asymptomatic carrier state have psychosocial and sexual implications regarding monogamy or promiscuity. Simultaneous effective antibiotic treatments with tetracycline, doxycycline, or erythromycin in both the client and partner(s) are essential to minimize morbidity for individuals (e.g., advanced infections and infertility) as well as to decrease transmission to other adults and newborns. For uncomplicated chlamydia genital infections (e.g., urethritis or cervicitis), doxycycline calcium (100 mg twice a day for 7 days) or tetracycline (500 mg four times a day for 7 days) is recommended (Bell and Grayston, 1986; Trachtenberg, Washington, and Halldorson, 1988). The exact length of treatment necessary has not been well researched. For more involved infections (e.g., acute salpingitis and epididymitis), higher doses for longer duration may be necessary, such as 500 mg of tetracycline four times a day for 10 to 14 days (Sweet, Schacter, and Landers, 1983; Oriel and Ridgway, 1983; Hare and Thin, 1983); additional antibiotics and hospitalization should be considered. When treating cervical or urethral discharge, clinicians should treat for both *C. trachomatis* and *N. gonorrhoeae*. For individuals who are pregnant or allergic to tetracycline, erythromycin, 500 mg four times a day for 7 days, is recommended (Bell and Grayston, 1986; Hare and Thin, 1983).

Regardless of the regimen, clients need careful instruction to understand the rationale for antibiotic treatment. Specifically, they need to know that the specific number of pills and days prescribed is necessary in order to eradicate the infection, to prevent latent or recurrent infection, and to preserve fertility. As with other STDs, a re-evaluation is in order to document that the infection has cleared (a "test of cure"). Clients need to know that they must abstain from intercourse until both partners are fully treated. An exception may be made when the couple is being treated simultaneously. The likelihood of transmission between a couple after both taking antibiotics for 24 to 48 hours is probably quite small.

Pelvic Inflammatory Disease

Pelvic inflammatory disease (PID) is a broad term referring to infection of the female reproductive organs in the pelvis. When possible, it is more accurate to identify infection as salpingitis or endometritis or oophoritis. Unfortunately, an accurate diagnosis is not easily or frequently made, hence the general term. PID is a significant disease because of its acute and chronic morbidity, especially including infertility. Thus, salpingitis or endometritis must be differentiated from cervical infections for effective treatment. The former frequently warrant aggressive antibiotic intervention (e.g. high doses, broad-spectrum drugs, multiple antibiotics, and intravenous administration) to preserve fertility.

EPIDEMIOLOGY

The two primary causative organisms of PID are *N. gonorrhoeae* and *C. trachomatis*, but other bacteria, both aerobic and anaerobic species, and mycoplasma species may also be causes. The incidence of PID is higher among women who are sexually active, are less than 20 years old, are nulliparous, or have more than one sexual partner (Gibbs, 1983). That sexual activity is associated with PID has long

been supported, and the number of sexual partners appears to be a risk factor. However, the relationships between selected aspects of sexual behavior (e.g., frequency and timing of intercourse) and PID have not been well identified (Newton and Keith, 1985). The use of an IUD and a past history of PID may also increase the likelihood of PID; both may facilitate transmission of an infectious organism beyond the cervix. Nulliparity may be a risk factor to the extent that PID jeopardizes fertility and because the cervical tissue may be more prone to infection in adolescence prior to maturity.

CLINICAL FEATURES

The commonly reported signs and symptoms of PID are identified in Table 23–5. However, the presentation of PID may vary greatly; many women will not have high fever and marked pelvic pain and a pelvic mass.

ASSESSMENT AND INTERVENTION

The diagnosis of PID depends not only on physical findings but also on data from Gram stains of the endocervix, cervical cultures, complete blood counts, culdocentesis, laparoscopy, and ultrasonography.

The treatment of choice for acute PID is not established. No single agent is active against the entire spectrum of pathogens. Combinations of doxycycline and cefoxitin or clindamycin and gentamicin are used intravenously for hospitalized clients. Ambulatory treatment includes cefoxitin or aqueous procaine penicillin G or ceftriaxone plus probenecid. See Table 23–6 for specific regimens.

A primary nursing consideration in the care of the client with PID is the preservation of fertility. Prompt and complete antibiotic therapy is necessary, with follow-up to assure

TABLE 23–5. Signs and Symptoms of PID

Symptoms
  Lower abdominal pain
  Increased vaginal discharge
  Irregular bleeding
  Urinary symptoms
  Vomiting

Signs
  Fever (>38° C)
  Marked abdominal, uterine, adnexal, or
    cervical motion tenderness
  Palpable adnexal mass swelling
  Abnormal vaginal discharge

TABLE 23–6. Regimens for Acute PID

Population	Treatment
Hospitalized clients	*Regimen A* Doxycycline (100 mg IV BID) plus cefoxitin (2.0 g IV QID) for 4 days and at least 48 hours after client improves; then continue doxycycline (100 mg po BID) for 10 to 14 days. *Regimen B* Clindamycin (600 mg IV QID) plus gentamicin (2.0 mg/kg IV followed by 1.5 mg/kg TID) in clients with normal renal function; continue IV drugs for 4 days and at least 48 hours after patient improves, then continue clindamycin (450 mg po QID) 10 to 14 days.
Ambulatory clients	Cefoxitin (2.0 g IM) or aqueous procaine penicillin G (4.8 million units IM at 2 sites) *or* ceftriaxone (250–500 mg IM). Each of these regimens except ceftriaxone is accompanied by probenecid (1.0 g po) followed by doxycycline (100 mg po BID) for 10 to 14 days.

Sources: Fiumara, 1987; "Treatment," 1988

efficacy of treatment. Instruction in ways to prevent PID is appropriate; rates of infertility are higher among those who have had more than one episode of PID.

Other Infections Associated with Discharge

Women commonly experience and present with an abnormal vaginal discharge. In contrast to the infections previously discussed associated with cervicitis, most vaginal discharges are secondary to vaginitis. Common causes of vaginitis are *Candida vaginalis, Trichomonas vaginalis*, and *Gardnerella vaginalis*. Infections due to these organisms can be spread sexually. Although men can harbor these organisms, it is uncommon for them to present with symptoms of discharge. The assessment for these infections would follow the guidelines previously discussed in this chapter (e.g., wet preparations and cervical cultures); the presence of one STD does not preclude another. Discussions of the specific causes of vaginitis are found in Chapter 22, Gynecological Conditions and Sexuality.

STDS ASSOCIATED WITH ULCERS

Syphilis

EPIDEMIOLOGY

Syphilis ranks third among reported communicable diseases in the United States, exceeded only by chickenpox and gonorrhea.

Since 1941, the reported cases of primary and secondary syphilis and early latent syphilis have declined; primary and secondary syphilis cases have numbered about 80,000 annually. However, there has been a recent increase of syphilis in epidemic proportions, especially in urban areas ("Venereal Disease Surges," 1989). The male-to-female ratio of syphilis is about three to one (Fiumara, 1987). This trend may be due to an increasing incidence of drug use and associated prostitution.

Young adults between 20 and 24 years of age have the largest reported case rates. Primary and secondary syphilis is reported more frequently from large urban areas. Sixty-five per cent of the reported cases in 1979 came from 63 cities (only 27 per cent of the national population; CDC, 1984). Since 1941, complications caused by syphilis (e.g., blindness, congenital damage, cardiovascular damage, syphilitic psychoses, and death) have decreased. In 1979, 184 deaths were estimated to be due to syphilis, and 154 syphilitic psychotic patients were hospitalized. The hospital cost of patients with syphilitic psychoses has exceeded $62 million annually (US Dept Health Human Services, *STD Fact Sheet*).

Although free public clinics are available for the diagnosis and treatment of venereal disease, the majority of clients seek private medical care. A 1968 national survey of private physicians indicated that although they treated about three fourths of infectious syphilitic cases in the United States, they reported only 19 per cent of their cases to public health departments (Fleming, 1970). Thus, the incidence rates for syphilis are probably higher than those reported.

The causal organism of syphilis is *Treponema pallidum* and belongs to the treponeme group of spirochetes. Transmission of syphilis may be congenital or acquired. Congenital syphilis is transmitted from the mother to the unborn child through the placenta. Acquired syphilis occurs when *T. pallidum* invades the body through a mucous membrane, usually genital, or a skin abrasion. The infection is usually transmitted by sexual contact but may be transmitted by kissing or close body contact.

The *incubation period* begins when *T. pallidum* invades any moist mucosal surface and is transmitted to the host's blood stream. Within 24 hours, it spreads throughout the body. There may be no symptoms or signs of the infection for 10 to 60 days.

CLINICAL FEATURES

Primary Syphilis. This stage occurs 9 to 90 days after exposure. The chancre is a painless superficial ulcer that varies in size between 3 to 4 mm and 1 to 2 cm and has a raised, sharply demarcated border. The appearance of a chancre at the site of inoculation (e.g., labia, vagina, cervix, penis, or rectum) occurs on the average 2 to 3 weeks after exposure. Extragenital lesions on the lips, tongue, nipples, and fingers may occur. Chancres may occur at any site, are most common in the oral or anogenital regions, and often go unnoticed. Multiple chancres may occur but are less common. Regional lymph nodes may be enlarged, firm, and painless. If untreated, the chancre may persist for 2 to 6 weeks. Darkfield microscopy of discharge from a syphilitic lesion reveals spirochetes (Fiumara, 1987; Noble, 1982). The serological tests to document infection are not positive until the fourth week of infection.

Secondary Syphilis. The secondary stage of syphilis occurs 6 weeks to 6 months after the initial exposure and persists for 2 to 6 weeks in the untreated client. It is characterized by generalized lesions of the skin and mucous membrane. A bilateral, symmetrical rash occurs that may be macular, papular, follicular, papulosquamous, or pustular. Fleshy, vegetative lesions in the oral or genital areas may occur and are called condylomata lata. Mucous patches in the mouth, tongue, and cervix may also occur. The skin lesions contain spirochetes. Clients with secondary syphilis are infectious, and spirochetes may be seen on darkfield microscopy. Serological test results are now positive at this point.

Early Syphilis. The Centers for Disease Control defines early syphilis as that which occurs in first year after infection. Only syphilis cases of less than 1 year's duration are sufficiently infectious to warrant public health follow-up. During this period, if no lesions or evidence of the disease is found, it is called "early latent syphilis" to indicate that infectious lesions may recur.

Late Syphilis. Late syphilis is syphilis of more than 1 year's duration after infection. It is noninfectious, *except* to the fetus of the pregnant woman. In some cases, the serological test becomes negative even without treatment. In others, it may continue in the latent form with a persistent positive serological test for years.

Late Symptomatic Syphilis. The disease may continue to proceed to late syphilis. Approximately 50 per cent of untreated cases will develop "benign late syphilis," in which gummas or other lesions of the skin, bone, and mucous membranes occur. This form is not fatal. Among those with untreated syphilis, about 30 per cent will develop cardiovascular syphilis with aortitis and its complications of aortic insufficiency, aneurysm, or stenosis of the coronary ostia. This usually occurs 20 years or so after the initial contracting of the disease. Among those untreated, approximately 20 per cent develop neurosyphilis, which includes involvement of the central nervous system, for example, paresis, syphilis of the brain, or syphilis of the posterior columns of the spinal cord (tapes) (Noble, 1982).

Congenital Syphilis. To screen for asymptomatic syphilis, it is recommended that pregnant women have a test such as the Venereal Disease Research Laboratories (VDRL) test or the rapid plasma reagin (RPR) test performed as early as possible and again at 32 weeks' gestation. If the mother's infection is untreated, the infant may suffer (1) premature stillbirth; (2) congenital syphilis with blindness, deafness, facial abnormalities, and crippling; or (3) death (Romney, 1975). Adequate treatment of infected pregnant women is essential to prevent complications for the infant.

ASSESSMENT

The diagnosis of syphilis depends on the history of exposure and symptoms, the physical examination, and the selection of appropriate laboratory tests. The medical history should include a thorough sexual history, a history of lesions that may have been syphilitic, results of previous serological tests if known, and previous antisyphilitic treatment. A careful physical examination is done in search for signs of syphilis.

Demonstration of *T. pallidum* from a lesion (chancre, mucous patch, condylomata lata) on darkfield microscopic examination permits an absolute and immediate diagnosis of syphilis. Because lesions of primary and secondary syphilis contain many spirochetes, darkfield examination is helpful in these two stages, especially since the VDRL test may be nonreactive in early primary syphilis. In general, the shorter the duration of the lesion, the more easily it is observed on darkfield microscopy. Hence, darkfield examination of late lesions on the body surface is less useful. Failure to demonstrate the organism does not preclude syphilis, and the test should be repeated in 3 days (Neeson and Stockdale, 1981; Shofield, 1979). Darkfield microscopy should be done by professionals who are well trained and experienced in identification of the organism, since there is a great similarity between *T. pallidum* and other spirochetes found in the genitalia and in the mouth. Darkfield microscopy is not available in many primary care sites.

The VDRL antigen is a nontreponemal serological test and is dependent upon direct documentation of *T. pallidum*. It has a 75 per cent accuracy rate and because of its inexpensiveness is a standard mass screening test in the diagnosis of syphilis. It is also useful in following the response to treatment, since the test is also quantitative. Early treatment of the disease causes the VDRL titer to fall rapidly. The test does not indicate whether the syphilis is infectious, however. False-positives may be caused by pregnancy, measles, pneumococcal pneumonia, aging, drug abuse, collagen diseases, viral hepatitis, lymphogranuloma venereum, systemic lupus erythematosis, infectious mononucleosis, and rheumatoid arthritis (Romney et al, 1975; Neeson and Stockdale, 1981).

The fluorescent treponemal antibody absorption test (FTA-ABS) is the most sensitive and reliable serological test to diagnose all stages of syphilis. It is performed on all clients who have a positive VDRL test because it has greater sensitivity than the VDRL or RPR in the diagnosis of syphilis in all stages (Noble, 1982). Once this test becomes reactive it rarely ever becomes nonreactive (Fiumara, 1987). It is also slightly more expensive.

The *T. pallidum* immobilization test (TPI) is specific, expensive, and difficult to use and is limited to complex diagnostic problems only.

Cerebrospinal fluid examination is done with the VDRL and FTA-ABS tests for detection of latent disease (Neeson and Stockdale, 1981).

INTERVENTION

A thorough assessment of the client's emotional reaction and knowledge of syphilis is done first. This can be accomplished by asking the following: (1) What do you think syphilis is? (2) How do you think you got it? (3) What does this mean to you? (4) What will this mean to your loved ones? Common myths of syphilis may be revealed, for example, that syphilis confers immediate insanity and mental illness. Transmission myths also exist such as that one gets syphilis from toilet seats and bathroom faucets or that syphilis cannot be spread if either partner is orgasmic during intercourse. An immunity myth reveals the belief that one develops permanent immunity after one treatment with penicillin.

For many women, venereal disease connotes fear and shame. The diagnosis of syphilis in Western culture is associated with immorality, promiscuity, social stigma, and low social status (Fogel, 1981). As with other STDs, syphilis may negatively influence sexual relationships. Thus, a thorough assessment of the client's emotional response is made by observing nonverbal behavior and listening to verbal statements. Is the client anxious, angry, fearful, and depressed? Clients who are extremely angry can be further questioned for homocidal tendencies. If definite intention and plans exist, the client should be detained and referred for an immediate consultation with a social worker or psychiatrist, who can offer short-term crisis therapy to help the client constructively ventilate feelings and offer supportive close follow-up.

Clients should be informed about the treatment, side effects, complications of untreated disease, and need for follow-up (Table 23–7). Clients should know that syphilis is sexually acquired. When treated early, it is easily cured. Completion of medical treatment is

TABLE 23–7. Recommended Treatment for Syphilis

Stage	Treatment
Early syphilis (primary or secondary)	Benzathine penicillin G (2.4 million units IM) at a single session. Penicillin-allergic patients: tetracycline HCL (500 mg po QID) for 12 to 15 days. Tetracycline-allergic patients: erythromycin (500 mg po QID) for 12 to 15 days.
Late syphilis	Benzathine penicillin G (2.4 million units IM) once a week for 3 weeks. Penicillin-allergic patients: tetracycline HCL (500 mg po QID) for 30 days. Tetracycline-allergic patients: erythromycin (500 mg po QID) for 30 days.
Neurosyphilis	Aqueous crystalline penicillin G (12 to 24 million units IV/day in divided doses) for 10 days followed by benzathine penicillin G (2.4 million units IM weekly) for 3 doses. Or Aqueous procaine penicillin G (2.4 million units IM daily) plus probenecid (500 mg po QID) both for 10 days followed by benzathine penicillin G (2.4 million units IM weekly) for 3 doses. Penicillin-allergic patients: Tetracycline or erythromycin 500 mg po QID for 30 days. Clients should have their allergies tested and be managed by an infectious disease expert.
Syphilis in pregnancy	Penicillin should be used in dosage schedules appropriate for the stage of syphilis as recommended for the treatment of nonpregnant clients. Penicillin-allergic clients: Erythromycin in dosage schedules appropriate for the stage of syphilis as recommended for the treatment of nonpregnant patients. Tetracycline is not used in pregnancy.
Congenital syphilis	Asymptomatic or symptomatic infants with abnormal cerebrospinal fluid: aqueous crystalline penicillin G (50,000 units/kg IM or IV daily) in two divided doses for 10 days or aqueous procaine penicillin G (50,000 units/kg IM daily) for 10 days. Asymptomatic infants with normal CSF: benzathine penicillin G (50,000 units/kg IM) in a single dose.

Sources: Fiumara, 1987; "Treatment," 1988

essential to stop asymptomatic disease progression, especially if treatment consists of an alternate regimen besides one dose of IM penicillin. Partners need to be notified that they need treatment for exposure as soon as possible. Explain that contrary to some cultural beliefs, reinfection can occur and that the client must refrain from intercourse for 1 month or until follow-up test results are negative. Discuss how to examine any potential sexual partner prior to sex for signs of syphilis.

DRUG REACTIONS OF SYPHILIS TREATMENT

Penicillin reactions include skin rashes, urticaria, arthralgia, fever, and chills. Occasional fatal anaphylactoid reactions have occurred. Tetracycline and erythromycin may cause nausea, vomiting, diarrhea, and skin rashes.

Genital Herpes

Genital herpes has received much attention because of its frequency of occurrence, se-

verity of symptoms, and pattern of recurrence. Because there is not a present cure, herpes has stimulated concern as a public health problem. In addition to affecting adults, newborns who contract the infection through vaginal delivery may have serious morbidity and mortality.

EPIDEMIOLOGY

In a study of 630 clients with symptomatic genital herpes, Corey and associates (1983) found most clients to be white (96 per cent), single (64 per cent), and well educated. This is similar to other reports of herpes' occurring commonly among young, white, single, upper-middle-class people (Baker, 1983).

Herpes is a virus that affects both genital and nongenital sites. There are two types of herpes commonly recognized as affecting the genitalia, herpes simplex virus type 1 (HSV-1) and herpes simplex virus type 2 (HSV-2). HSV-1 is responsible for 75 to 90 per cent of nongenital lesions, for example, the cold sore that frequently occurs on the lip of the mouth. HSV-2 is responsible for 70 to 90 per cent of genital lesions (Fiumara, 1987; Peacock, 1982; Baker, 1983). Today, it is well recognized that either type 1 or 2 may be found with either oral or genito-urinary lesions. The prevalence of oral-genital sex is cited as a reason for this. Since the virus has a predilection for mucocutaneous tissues, it does not discriminate between "above and below the waist."

The primary mode of transmission of genital herpes is sexual contact; spread via fomites is possible but not proven. Occasional cases of nonsexually acquired genital herpes have been reported, some in children. However, clinical and epidemiological studies have shown that close, intimate contact with infected secretions and mechanical friction are needed to transmit the disease (Douglas and Corey, 1983).

The incubation period of herpes simplex virus is 2 to 20 days (Fiumara, 1987; McMaster, 1981; Baker, 1983). The average time since last sexual contact has been reported as 6 days (Corey et al, 1983). The clinical course of herpes is distinct from that of other STDs in that it invades the nerves (e.g., in genital herpes, the sacral nerve), where it may lie dormant until there is an alteration in host-environment that predisposes to recurrence. In about half of infections, the virus may reside in the nerve (Fiumara, 1982). Recurrences are more common with HSV-2 than HSV-1 (60 versus 15 per cent) and in men than in women (Baker, 1983; Corey et al, 1983). The occurrence of herpes cultured from the cervix of asymptomatic women has been reported as 1.5 to 8 per cent among those attending STD clinics (Baker, 1983; Corey et al, 1983; Raab and Lorincz, 1981) and as 0.25 to 1.5 per cent in a private practice (Corey et al, 1983).

CLINICAL FEATURES

The clinical course of primary herpes consists of initial subjective symptoms of painful lesions. The superficial, often multiple, lesions are first vesicular but later ulcerate and crust over. Ulceration may occur in 1 to 4 days, depending on the moistness of the affected area. The lesions are accompanied by dysuria (as the urine contacts the ulcerated area), dyspareunia, and sometimes rectal pain. In primary herpes, inguinal lymphadenopathy and pelvic pain are common as well as systemic symptoms of malaise, fever, and head-

ache (Table 23–8). Systemic symptoms are reported to occur more often in women than in men (68 versus 39 per cent, Corey et al, 1983). Symptoms may persist for 10 to 14 days, but the lesions may not entirely heal for 3 to 6 weeks (Corey et al, 1983; Baker, 1983). Secondary bacterial infection may occur, marked by redness surrounding the lesions and a purulent discharge.

Herpes simplex virus pharyngitis may also occur. It has been observed more commonly in primary infections than with recurrences. Symptoms include sore throat and tender cervical adenopathy. Systemic symptoms may also occur with pharyngitis (e.g., fever, malaise, myalgia, headache) (Corey et al, 1983).

ASSESSMENT

Objective measures to assess HSV are available but not inexpensive. An assessment is often made clinically. Whenever possible, viral cultures should be done to document the diagnosis. The implications of having herpes are significant. It may be especially important for clients' future peace of mind to spend the money to document the infection while it is active.

Kellum and Loucks (1982) have summarized diagnostic tests for herpes. Viral cultures are most sensitive (about 80 per cent) and also most expensive (about $40) (Baker, 1983; Kellum and Loucks, 1982). Specimens for viral culture are most reliable when obtained within 48 hours of the lesion's development. Serum viral titers may be drawn. Nurses need to note that serological testing necessitates two titers for comparison; usually a fourfold rise in antibodies is considered indicative of infection. With past exposure to herpes simplex virus, an initial and subsequent serological test may not show a significant difference (Fiumara, 1987).

Cytologic testing (i.e., a Papanicolaou's stain) may be done. With compatible clinical findings, the microscopic finding of multinucleated giant cells is suggestive of HSV (McMaster, 1981). Cytology is less sensitive for assessment—about 50 to 60 per cent as sensitive as viral cultures. Thus, there are high false-negatives with cytology as compared with cultures (Mertz and Corey, 1984).

INTERVENTION

The major reasons for interventions with herpes are (1) to promote comfort, (2) to

TABLE 23–8. Comparison of Symptoms and Signs Between Primary Genital HSV-2 and Recurrent HSV*

Symptoms and Signs	Primary Genital HSV-2		Recurrent Genital HSV	
	Male *(n = 63)*	*Female* *(n = 126)*	*Male* *(n = 218)*	*Female* *(n = 144)*
Mean day duration of prodrome before lesions (range)			1.5 (0–6)	1.2 (0–3)
Mean day duration of local pain	10.9	12.2	3.9	5.9
Mean number of lesions (range)	15.5 (3–50)	15.4 (1–60)	7.5 (1–25)	4.8 (1–15)
Mean day duration of lesions (range)	16.5	19.7	10.6 (5–25)	9.3 (4–29)
Percentage of clients with abnormal discharge	27	85	4	45
Percentage of clients with tender lymphadenopathy	80	81	23	31

*HSV = herpes simplex virus
(Adapted from Corey et al, 1983)

promote healing, (3) to prevent secondary infections, and (4) to decrease transmission of the disease.

Symptomatic measures for pain are not consistently addressed in the medical literature. Fiumara (1987) suggests the use of oral analgesics (e.g., antiprostaglandins such as indomethacin or ibuprofen) and topical corticosteroids for comfort, recognizing that such therapy will not affect the virus. Although voiding is often painful, fluids and frequent voiding are promoted. Voiding while in a tub of water or while water is poured over the genitalia may ease dysuria by diluting the urine. Sometimes topical anesthetics (e.g., lidocaine jelly) and catheterizations are also used for dysuria (Kellum and Loucks, 1982). In student health services, hospitalization may be considered for short-term supportive care. Intermittent sitz baths or warm moist compresses may be used to reduce inflammation. Careful drying should follow a sitz bath. To prevent secondary infection, the skin is kept clean and dry. Occlusive ointments (e.g., antibiotic creams) may delay healing (Raab and Lorincz, 1981).

Acyclovir is the medication used to treat primary genital herpes. Acyclovir controls the signs and symptoms of herpes but does not diminish the frequency or severity of recurrences after it is stopped. Treatment for the first clinical episode is 200 mg of acyclovir orally five times a day for 7 to 10 days, started within 6 days of the onset of the lesion. Treatment for recurrent herpes is 200 mg of acyclovir orally five times a day for 5 days started within 2 days of the onset of the lesion (Fiumara, 1987; "Treatment," 1988). The safety of systemic acyclovir for pregnant women is uncertain.

Alternative treatments with 2-deoxy-D-glucose, idoxuridine, and cytarabine are controversial (McMaster, 1981; Kellum and Loucks, 1982; Raab and Lorincz, 1981). According to Mertz and Corey (1984), the former warrants further testing; the latter two have demonstrated no change in the duration of HSV episodes.

Complications of primary HSV infections include encephalitis (manifested by headaches, behavioral changes, or seizures), aseptic meningitis (manifested by stiff neck, headache, and photophobia), and disseminated infection. Temporary neurological symptoms such as sacral anesthesia, urinary retention, and constipation have been observed (Kellum and Loucks, 1982; Corey et al, 1983; Raab and Lorincz, 1981). Genital HSV infections have been associated with the development of lesions on thighs as well as fingers, probably through autoinoculation.

Clients with a diagnosis of primary herpes need nursing interventions for both acute and chronic infections. In the acute infection, the client needs information on the treatment and spread of the disease. Clients need to know there is no cure; treatment is asymptomatic. The virus may be shed from the point of prodromal symptoms until the lesions have fully healed or re-epithelialized several days after crusting over. Thus, herpes may be spread prior to lesion formation and following crusting. Spermicides and condoms may offer some, but not absolute, protection (Peacock, 1982; Raab and Lorincz, 1981). Therefore, intimate contact must be avoided until all symptoms are absent and the skin is healed. About 60 per cent of clients with HSV-2 infections experience recurrences.

It may be helpful to prepare clients for

realistic expectations of recurrences. For example, recurrences may occur one or more times a month or year (Kellum and Loucks, 1982). Half of clients with recurrences experience a prodrome of about 1 day prior to lesion formation (Mertz and Corey, 1984). Clients may be reassured to know symptoms are often less severe and of shorter duration with recurrences. One study on coping with herpes (Manne and Sandler, 1984) reported that engaging in negative and wishful thinking, characterological self-blame (as opposed to behavioral self-blame), and repeated use of treatments for herpes were associated with psychological distress. It may be helpful to minimize such coping techniques to assist the client in dealing more effectively with herpes. Social support was associated with positive adjustment and could be encouraged. Clients may wish to know of informational sources for herpes, such as Help, PO Box 100, Palo Alto, California 94302 and HELPhiladelphia, PO Box 13193, Philadelphia, PA 19101.

Individualized assessment of a client's reaction to the diagnosis and implications of the chronic disease of herpes is necessary. Descriptive data document that anger, anxiety, fear, and guilt are responses to the diagnosis. Feelings of disbelief and uncleanliness have been reported. Affected persons report fearing and experiencing rejection from partners. Hesitations about being sexual and self-chosen abstinence, beyond the time recommended clinically, are reported by some clients (Leo, 1982). Clinician sensitivity to these potential, although not usually devastating, reactions is essential.

Research is lacking regarding the spread of herpes within a stable monogamous relationship in which one partner has had genital herpes and the other has not. Admittedly, there is some risk to the unaffected partner of asymptomatic shedding. However, the likelihood of contracting herpes is low if couples avoid intimate contact during recurrences. Prior HSV-1 infection may offer some protection against subsequent HSV-2 infection. In couples in whom both partners have had genital herpes, the likelihood of reinfection by another strain of the virus is small. "Transmission does not appear inevitable when one partner has genital herpes" (Mertz and Corey, 1984, p. 104). Clients and couples deserve empathetic understanding while adjusting to their psychosocial reaction to herpes.

Herpes raises concerns about pregnancy and cervical cancer. Of particular concern is neonatal infection. Of infants who become infected, 80 per cent have neurological sequelae (Baker, 1983). However, only a small percentage of women who have had genital HSV also have babies who acquire herpes. Transmission to the neonate is much greater with primary genital HSV (as high as 50 per cent) as compared with recurrent HSV cervicitis (about 5 per cent). Either prenatal transplacental transmission prenatally or intrapartal cervical transmission is possible; the latter is more common (Corey et al, 1983).

For pregnant women, herpes cultures may be done prior to labor (at 32, 34, and 36 weeks) to detect cervical shedding of HSV. When active lesions are present or shedding of HSV is documented, a cesarean section should be planned.

Recurrent maternal HSV infections are associated with antibodies that may protect the newborn (Raab and Lorincz, 1981; Fiumara, 1982; Baker, 1983). The degree of risk of early fetal loss or early delivery with herpes is not well known for the woman with infrequent recurrent vulvar HSV (Corey et al, 1983). "Most pregnant women with recurrent vulvar herpes deliver normal infants" (Corey et al, 1983, p 969).

Of the major viral causes of STDs, i.e., herpes, condyloma acuminatum, and cytomegalovirus, herpes has been most strongly associated with a role in carcinogenesis. Serological tests and epidemiological studies show a consistent correlation between herpes infection and cervical cancer. It appears that herpes simplex virus can, under certain conditions, transform normal cells to malignant ones (Berman et al, 1985; Rapp, 1981). Related risk factors of cervical cancer include the number of sexual partners, history of STDs, low socioeconomic status, and early age of initiation of coitus. Indeed, cervical cancer has an epidemiological profile like that of many STDs such that some call cervical cancer an STD (Roseman, Ansell, and Chapman, 1984). The clinical implication here is for careful screening and secondary prevention in high-risk women.

For women with herpes, Pap smears are recommended every 6 to 12 months. When providing client education, nurses must be sensitive to the association of herpes with cancer. The neoplasia considerations may be better discussed on a follow-up visit rather than on an initial diagnostic visit.

Of interest, the role of viral STDs in prostatic cancer is being researched. There are associations showing that past HSV infections are higher among some men with prostate cancer. Also, there are data showing positive correlations between men with prostate cancer and spouses with cervical cancer. Such associations suggest that prostatic cancer may have a venereal disease component. More research here is needed before clinical implications may be drawn (Roseman, Ansell, and Chapman, 1984).

Haemophilus ducreyi Infection (Chancroid)

EPIDEMIOLOGY

Another STD that also produces an ulcer is chancroid. While it is not as common as syphilis in the United States, it does occur in immigrants to this country. It is estimated that chancroid is several times more prevalent than syphilis in the entire world and more common than gonorrhea (Gaisin and Heaton, 1975; Marmar, 1977). Chancroid is most common in tropical developing countries and is rare in North America; there were 847 cases of chancroid reported in the United States in 1983 (Felman, 1986). In the United States it is predominantly seen among immigrants or travelers to developing countries. Chancroid affects more men than women (Karchmer, 1983).

Haemophilus ducreyi, a short gram-negative rod with round edges, is the cause of chancroid. The incubation period is 2 to 5 days. The disease is transmitted through sexual contact with either the ulcer or purulent discharge from enlarged, infected local lymph glands. As long as *H. ducreyi* is present in the purulent discharge or the ulcers, the disease is infectious. After healing, the infection is gone (Fiumara, 1987; Neeson and Stockdale, 1981).

CLINICAL FEATURES

After inoculation, a small papule forms at the site. This lesion soon converts to an irregular deep ulcer or pustule that exudes pus, bleeds easily, and is very painful and indurated. Local lymph glands enlarge (called buboes), become inflamed, and may drain pus.

Usually, only one or two ulcers develop. However, up to 10 ulcers may occur (Hart,

1977). Women are usually asymptomatic. The primary symptoms include painful genital ulcers and tender inguinal lymph nodes. On physical examination either an inflamed papule or an irregular ulcer is evident. The difference between a chancroid and a chancre is that the former is soft, very painful, and lacks induration or hardening. Bubo formation may be present. Autoinoculation can cause the transmission of lesions to the pubis, abdomen, or thighs (Fiumara, 1987; Neeson and Stockdale, 1981).

ASSESSMENT

Diagnosis is usually made clinically by the history, the appearance of the characteristic lesion on physical examination, and exclusion of other sexually transmitted diseases. The organism requires a special culture media in which to grow (Karchmer, 1983).

INTERVENTION

The treatment is erythromycin, 500 mg orally four times a day for 7 to 14 days, or ceftriaxone, 250 to 500 mg IM in a single dose. Partners are treated with the same regimen ("Sexually Transmitted Diseases," 1982; Fiumara, 1987).

Client education is similar to that for the client with syphilis. Recent partners from the past 2 to 3 weeks need to be located and treated immediately. Condoms will prevent chancoid transmission in the early stage, before bubo formation.

Granuloma Inguinale

EPIDEMIOLOGY

Granuloma inguinale (GI) is endemic in Vietnam, Indonesia, Africa, Southern New Guinea, and Southern India. It is usually found in dark-skinned individuals. Hot and humid climate, low socioeconomic status, lack of personal hygiene, and the number of sexual partners play important roles in its occurrence (Ronald, 1983). In the United States GI is rare, with fewer than 100 cases reported annually (Fiumara, 1987). Among the cases reported, GI was particularly common in gay men (Karchmer, 1983).

GI is caused by *Calymmatobacterium granulomatis*. The exact mode of transmission is not understood, but it is presumed to be transmitted sexually.

CLINICAL FEATURES

With GI, a painless papule appears at the site of inoculation after a 1- to 12-week incubation period. The papule then ulcerates and converts to a beefy-red granular lesion with rolled and elevated borders and some induration. Other painless lesions form and spread together in the genitalia. Progressive infection can become mutilating. In late stages, genital lymphedema occurs.

ASSESSMENT AND INTERVENTION

The diagnosis of GI is suggested by the history and confirmed by a biopsy and cytological examination that show Donovan bodies in the cells.

Tetracycline in a dosage of 500 mg orally four times a day for about 14 days is the treatment of choice and is continued until the lesion heals or until the Donovan bodies are no longer seen. Continued therapy for 3 to 4 weeks may be required. Lesions should heal within 6 weeks. Late follow-up examinations should exclude relapse (Karchmer, 1983). For client education, stress that if lesions are not healing, the client is to return promptly. Clients should be seen monthly until lesions are gone and yearly thereafter because the involved areas may be precancerous (Fiumara, 1987).

STDS ASSOCIATED WITH OTHER DERMATOLOGICAL CHANGES

Condyloma Acuminatum

Condylomata acuminata are most commonly known as genital or venereal warts. Venereal warts were described in ancient Greco-Roman times, but not until 1968 to 1970 was the viral agent of condyloma acuminatum identified (Meisels and Morin, 1981; Margolis, 1984).

EPIDEMIOLOGY

Condylomata acuminata are caused by a member of the human papillomavirus (HPV), of which there are several types. Only some types are responsible for genital lesions; they are different from those causing common cutaneous or plantar warts. The papillomavirus enters the cell nucleus, initiates cell division and duplication of virus particles, and produces viral particles for spread of the virus to the host and others (Margolis, 1984).

The venereal transmission of condylomata acuminata was shown in 1954. At least two thirds of clients exposed to genital warts will develop warts. The incubation period is comparatively longer than that for other STDs. A 1- to 3-month incubation is common, but a 9-month period has been reported (Margolis, 1984; Hook and Stamm, 1983). Initially, genital warts are "small, discrete, papillary growths" (Meisels and Morin, 1981, p S112). Given time, they may grow into the more classical cauliflower-like lesions. Genital warts grow where the "stratified squamous epithelium is thin, moist and warm" (Margolis, 1984, p 164). Common sites are the urinary meatus, vulva, vagina, cervix, anus; additional sites include the shaft of the penis, the scrotum, labia majora, perianal area, and any adjacent skin (Margolis, 1984).

About one half of clients with anal warts will also have lesions in the anal canal. Many women with vulvar warts will also have cervical lesions (Margolis, 1984; Deitch and Smith, 1983; Schneider, 1988). Unless colposcopy is performed, cervical lesions are often overlooked and therefore untreated. On the other hand, cervical condylomata are sometimes misdiagnosed as cervical dysplasia. Not all cervical condylomata are raised; on colposcopy many are flat and are virtually indistinguishable from cervical intraepithelial neoplasia.

CLINICAL FEATURES

The primary symptom is usually the discovery of a small lump or growth; it may be associated with some itching but not tenderness. Dyspareuria may occasionally occur. Sometimes women experience a profuse irritating vaginal discharge concurrently with condyloma acuminatum. The discharge may be secondary either to condyloma acuminatum or to another sexually transmitted disease. Being somewhat estrogen dependent, warts may hypertrophy during pregnancy and regress afterwards (Neeson and Stockdale, 1981).

Objective data include clinical observation of the suspected lesion. Condylomata acuminata are small, gray-pink fingerlike growths. They often have a pedunculated base, are soft, and occur singularly or in clusters, especially in dark moist areas of skin folds. Warts may be more firm and dry if they are in a less moist environment. A vaginal discharge and secondary vulvitis may occur. Sometimes bleeding or infection of the warts is seen (Neeson and Stockdale, 1981; Fiumara, 1983; Hatcher et al, 1982). Lymphadenopathy and fever do not occur with warts alone (Margolis, 1984).

There is an association between condylomata acuminata and cancer. Certain strains of the papillomavirus (especially types 16 and 18) are associated with cervical cancer (Meisels and Morin, 1981; Deitch and Smith, 1983; Roseman et al, 1984). In women, condylomata acuminata and cervical intraepithelial neoplasia and carcinoma in situ are seen as different points on one continuum (Reid et al, 1984). There is also an association between warts and anal cancer (Hook and Stamm, 1983; Schneider, 1988).

The mean age of women with condylomata acuminata is less than that of those with dysplasia, whereas the mean age of women with carcinoma in situ is higher (Meisels and Morin, 1981). Condylomata acuminata have been found concurrently with dysplastic and neoplastic lesions (e.g., in 25 to 50 per cent of cases) (Meisels and Morin, 1981; Schneider, 1988). Because condylomata acuminata are sometimes reversible (e.g., in about 68 per cent of the cases in one study; Meisels and Morin, 1981), having warts is not sufficient for developing malignancy; other factors are needed. Research substantiates that condyloma acuminatum may, under certain conditions, transform normal cells into a malignant state (zur Hausen, deVilliers, and Gissman, 1981; Roseman, Ansell, and Chapman, 1984; Schneider, 1988). One factor contributing to the development of malignancy is cigarette smoking.

ASSESSMENT

In a thorough assessment, data are gathered to rule out other diseases. Wet mounts are done for vaginitis, cultures for cervicitis, serology for syphilis, and a Pap smear for cervical abnormalities. The diagnosis of vulvar condyloma acuminatum is usually made clinically. Pap smears are important to rule out cervical condyloma acuminatum, which may be less noticeable on physical examination. Because of the difficulty in discriminating between condyloma acuminatum and cervical intraepithelial neoplasia, more thorough

evaluations with colposcopy and biopsy may be indicated.

INTERVENTION

Common treatments for condylomata acuminata on external lesions are trichloroacetic or podophyllin (podophyllum resin; usually a 20 to 25 per cent solution with tincture of benzoin). These are left on for a maximum of 1 to 4 hours, as tolerated (Margolis, 1984). Surrounding tissues are protected with vaseline prior to the topical application. The client then bathes the area after waiting the specified time. This is repeated weekly for 4 weeks. The treatment of warts is not always successful; the cure may be as low as 20 per cent (Margolis, 1984, "Treatment of STDs," 1984). Alternative treatment may involve topical application of 5-fluorouracil, cryotherapy, hot cautery, laser therapy, and surgical removal (Felmar, Payton, and Smietanka, 1988).

Because podophyllin may be absorbed and is toxic, authorities caution against its use for vaginal and cervical lesions. Because podophyllin may induce cellular changes that mimic dysplastic changes, thereby causing unnecessary treatments, some clinicians discourage the use of podophyllin at all. Only when small amounts are applied and the area is fully dried prior to removal of a speculum should podophyllin be used. Side effects of podophyllin poisoning include lethargy, coma, paralysis, nausea, and diarrhea (Hatcher et al, 1982). The use of podophyllin is contraindicated in pregnancy (Neeson and Stockdale, 1981; McMaster, 1981).

For cervical condyloma acuminatum documented by colposcopy and biopsy, carbon dioxide laser, cryosurgery, and cautery are used in attempts to eradicate the infection. However, there are often recurrences of condyloma, despite treatment, because the virus may remain in adjacent tissues.

Effective treatment involves prevention of reinfection from partners. Sexual contacts of those with condylomata acuminata should be examined and treated as necessary. Intimate sexual contact should be discontinued at least until all external lesions are clear. If intercourse does occur, condoms should be used.

The nursing management involves explaining the transmission, treatment, and complications of genital warts. Clients need to know of the long incubation period of 1 to 3 months (Fiumara, 1983; Neeson and

Stockdale, 1981). Abstinence (or condom use) is recommended with active external lesions to prevent spread. Clients need to know that repeated treatments may be necessary, that condylomata acuminata can regress, and that treatments may not bring immediate results.

Treating concurrent vaginitis, if present, may facilitate regression of warts. Sulfa vaginal creams have been suggested as a potentially useful adjuvant therapy (Hatcher et al, 1980; McMaster, 1981). A straightforward, nonalarming attitude and time for clarification is appropriate in discussing the need for Pap smears. Emphasizing the need to document normalcy, that is, to rule out the possibility of abnormality, or to prompt treatment, if necessary, may be helpful. Some sources suggest that treatment be postponed until Pap smear results are available to guide therapy (Margolis, 1984). Clinicians need sensitivity in addressing the association of condylomata acuminata and neoplasia with a client. This may be especially true if the client is stressed by the diagnosis of a sexually transmitted disease.

Lymphogranuloma Venereum

EPIDEMIOLOGY

Lymphogranuloma venerum (LGV) has a worldwide distribution. It is prevalent in South America, the West Indies, East and West Africa, India, and Southeast Asia (Ronald, 1983). In the United States, there are less than 400 cases of LGV annually (Fiumara, 1987). Cases occur in military personnel, travelers, immigrants, or homosexual men with anogenital syndrome.

LGV is caused by three immunotypes of *Chlamydia trachomatis*, is acquired by sexual contact, and has three phases of infection: primary lesion, lymphatic spread with systemic symptoms, and complications.

CLINICAL FEATURES

The incubation period of LGV is often 7 to 12 days, but may be 3 to 30 days (Fiumara, 1987). A primary sore appears on the site of inoculation (genitalia, mouth, rectum) and is a small painless vesicle or nonindurated papule or pustule. Next, regional painful fluctuant adenopathy occurs, with lymphatic spread. Fever, malaise, arthralgia, myalgia,

aching, diaphoresis, nausea, vomiting, and abdominal pain may occur. The adenopathy may recede or go on to form draining abscesses (Noble, 1982). Complications of untreated LGV include urethral, vaginal, or rectal strictures, nonspecific urethritis, chronic buboes, perirectal abscess, elephantiasis of the genitals, and possible increased risk of vulvar or rectal carcinoma (Fiumara, 1987; Neeson and Stockdale, 1981).

ASSESSMENT AND INTERVENTION

The infection may be diagnosed through elevated titers on a LGV complement fixation test or by a microimmunofluorescent test. While screening tests for syphilis may be positive, tests for antitreponemal antibodies are negative. LGV infections are often treated with tetracycline (500 mg orally four times a day for 14 days) or with doxycycline (100 mg orally twice a day for 14 days) (Fiumara, 1987).

ACQUIRED IMMUNODEFICIENCY SYNDROME

Acquired immunodeficiency syndrome (AIDS) is a severe loss or depression of cellular immunity caused by infection with the retrovirus known as human immunodeficiency virus (HIV). AIDS is not usually diagnosed directly but is detected from abnormal T-lymphocyte values and the presence of opportunistic diseases (Laurence, 1987). There is usually a decrease in the number (absolute cell count) of "helper" T-lymphocytes (T4) accompanied by a ratio of "helper" to "suppressor" T-lymphocytes of less than one. Common opportunistic diseases occurring in association with AIDS are cytomegalovirus infection, *Pneumocystis carinii* pneumonia, *Candida albicans* infection, and Kaposi's sarcoma, an invasive cutaneous and soft tissue malignancy. Diagnosis of an opportunistic infection or of Kaposi's sarcoma usually precedes the diagnosis of AIDS (Glover, 1984). AIDS is also manifested as AIDS dementia, a complex of neurological problems caused by HIV infection of the brain and nervous system.

Epidemiology

AIDS and HIV infection are transmitted by blood, semen, vaginal secretions, and breast milk infected with HIV. The virus has been found in other body fluids including saliva, urine, and tears, but infection has not been documented from these sources (Krim, 1987). Since HIV is blood borne, it is essential that it enter the circulatory system in order to cause infection. HIV infection most commonly results from vaginal, anal, or oral sexual intercourse or from introducing infected blood into the circulatory system (injecting infected blood with intravenous drugs or transfusing infected blood or blood products).

All persons infected with HIV are considered carriers; however, not everyone infected with HIV has AIDS. HIV infection manifests itself in four categories: (1) symptomatic infection (AIDS, usually accompanied by one or more opportunistic diseases), (2) asymptomatic infection, (3) persistent generalized lymphadenopathy (also known as AIDS-related complex, or ARC), and (4) other disease processes: specifically, constitutional, neurological, and secondary infectious diseases and secondary cancers ("Classification System," 1986).

The incidence of AIDS is increasing steadily but not at the exponential rate documented when the syndrome was first recognized. AIDS cases have been reported from all 50 states and have occurred among people of all ages and all races. As of May 1988, 60,852 cases meeting the surveillance criteria for AIDS have been reported to the Centers for Disease Control (CDC, 1988). In addition, epidemiologists estimate that 1 to 2 million people have been infected by HIV and that 250,000 to 270,000 AIDS cases meeting the surveillance criteria will be reported by 1991 ("Special AIDS Issue," 1987; Francis and Chin, 1987; Krim, 1987).

To date, AIDS has occurred primarily (about 63 per cent of all cases) among men who have sex with other men (gay or bisexual males) who have no known intravenous (IV) drug use, among heterosexual IV drug users (about 18 per cent of cases), and among homosexual or bisexual males who have used IV drugs (about 7 per cent of cases). The remainder of AIDS cases are distributed among persons with hemophilia/coagulation disorders (about 1 per cent of cases), among persons who received blood transfusions or blood products before 1985 when routine blood screening for HIV antibodies began (about 2 per cent of cases), among heterosexual sex partners of those with AIDS or of those at risk for AIDS (about 4 per cent of cases), and among those for whom a cause is unclear (about 3 per cent of cases) (Centers for Disease Control, 1988). Heterosexual spread of AIDS and HIV infection has increased rapidly, particularly among sexual partners of persons in high-risk groups. The percentage of women who were not intravenous drug users and who presumably became infected through heterosexual contact increased from 12 per cent in 1982 to 26 per cent in 1986 (Guinan and Hardy, 1987). In addition, increasing numbers of children are infected with HIV during pregnancy, by breastfeeding or by blood transfusions (Minkoff, 1986).

Groups of people who develop AIDS are also considered to be at especially high risk for acquiring HIV infection. High-risk groups include the following:

- Men who have sex with other men (gay or bisexual males).
- Users of intravenous drugs.
- Immigrants from Central Africa, which has a high incidence of HIV infection.
- Sexual partners of members of the above-named groups.
- Sexual partners of persons with AIDS or HIV infection (including both those with positive HIV antibody tests and those who are infected with the virus but have not been tested).

History of sexually transmitted disease is considered to be an additional risk factor because unsafe sexual practices leading to an STD could lead to HIV infection and because concomitant genital lesions from an STD may create portals of entry for HIV.

Clinical Features

Symptoms of HIV infection include the following:

- Unexplained increasing and persistent fatigue.
- Continued (intermittent) fever of 38° C (100.5° F) or higher for longer than 1 to 2 months associated with drenching night sweats and shaking chills that are not accompanied by a known illness.

- Weight loss (unrelated to diet or exercise) that is more than 10 to 15 pounds or more than 10 per cent of body weight within 1 to 2 months.
- Persistent palpable (> 1 cm) lymph nodes (with or without pain) in two areas of the body, excluding the inguinal nodes, for more than 3 months without other known illness to explain the finding.
- Pink to purple flat or raised patches or bumps, usually painless, occurring on or under the skin, inside the mouth, nose, eyelids, or rectum. Initially, lesions may look like bruises that do not go away; they are usually harder than the skin around them. These lesions are characteristic of Kaposi's sarcoma.
- Persistent white spots or unusual blemishes in the mouth.
- Persistent or often dry cough that is not from smoking and has lasted too long to be from a usual respiratory infection.
- Persistent diarrhea (Bennett, 1986; Selwyn, 1986c; Schietinger, 1986).

Assessment

Diagnosis of AIDS is made based on clinical presentation and laboratory findings consistent with impaired immune function. Diagnosis of HIV infection is inferred from serological testing for antibodies to HIV. The two most common HIV antibody tests are the enzyme-linked immunoassay (ELISA) and Western blot (a more specific immunoassay). The specificity of a single ELISA test is less than ideal because the inactivated HIV used as an antigen may contain components that make the specimen react falsely positive. The Western blot is confirmatory because it tests specifically for the presence of selected proteins associated with HIV. When repeated tests are carried out using both ELISA and the Western blot, the specificity rates are about 99 per cent and false-positive results are minimized (Laurence, 1987; "Update: Serologic Testing," 1988). Because the sensitivity of the ELISA and Western blot tests is extremely high (99% or greater), the likelihood of false-negative test results is extremely low, except in the earliest weeks of infection. ("Public Health Service Guidelines," 1987). Most individuals exposed to HIV develop antibodies within 6 to 12 weeks of infection ("Public Health Service Guidelines," 1987), although antibodies may appear as early as 2 to 3 weeks and as late as 9 to 12 months after infection (Laurence, 1987).

It is crucial that health professionals understand the implications of HIV antibody testing. A negative result can mean that (1) the individual has not been infected with HIV, (2) the individual has been infected with HIV and has not yet developed antibodies to the virus, (3) the individual has AIDS and is severely immunocompromised, or (4) the test results were inaccurate.

A positive antibody test indicates prior infection with HIV and an immune response to the virus. All individuals with positive antibody tests are considered to be potentially contagious HIV carriers. However, their future prognosis, that is, likelihood of developing AIDS, cannot be determined from the antibody test.

There is much heated discussion about the legal and ethical implications of mass HIV screening. On the one hand, there are societal concerns about the spread of HIV, among both high-risk groups and the general population, that stimulate interest in routine testing of all individuals. On the other hand, there are many unanswered questions about the effect of positive antibody tests on employment, housing options, and insurance status that stimulate ethical and legal concerns about routine HIV antibody testing. Individual consent and confidentiality regarding results are critical issues in HIV antibody testing (Bayer, Levine, and Wolf, 1986; Dalton et al, 1987).

Intervention

No known medical treatment eradicates HIV infection or restores cellular immunity; however, an experimental drug, zidovudine (formerly known as azidothymidine, or AZT), inhibits HIV replication. Zidovudine has been used to treat certain carefully selected adults with AIDS and HIV infection; the drug has been associated with significant reduction in mortality and reduction in occurrence of AIDS-related opportunistic infections ("Special AIDS Issue," 1987).

Kaposi's sarcoma is treated with forms of interferon (a virus-fighting protein produced by the body), surgery, radiation, and chemotherapy. *Pneumocystis carinii* pneumonia is treated with pentamidine (an experimental antibiotic provided by the Centers for Disease

Control) or sulfamethoxazole with trimethoprim. Other opportunistic infections are treated with appropriate antibiotics (*Facts about AIDS*, 1984).

The prognosis for AIDS is poor. For those diagnosed with the disease, the 2-year mortality rate approaches 75 to 80 per cent (Glover, 1984; Selwyn, 1986a).

Nursing interventions are directed toward the wide range of problems encountered by people with AIDS or HIV infection. Common problems may include the following:

- Loss of weight, strength, energy, and appetite.
- Loss of self-sufficiency (increased dependency on others).
- Change in appearance (alteration in self-concept).
- Change in usual sexual activity or behavior.
- Change in relationship with other people, including sexual partner(s).
- Lack of funding for adequate care.
- Lack of adequate housing.
- Fear and anxiety resulting from uncertainty about the future.

All health professionals need to be sensitive to their own feelings, beliefs, and attitudes toward persons with AIDS, with HIV infection, or at risk for HIV infection. Professionals who are uncomfortable about treating persons in any of these categories need to seek colleagues to whom they can refer such clients. Health professionals such as nurses can promote accurate understanding and perceptions by educating people in communities about HIV, its transmission, and methods for preventing HIV infection and AIDS.

Transmission

AIDS and HIV infection are transmitted primarily by sexual intercourse with a person who is infected with HIV or by transferring HIV-infected blood from one person to another. Transmission may also occur during pregnancy through placental exchange, at delivery, or by artificial insemination (Krim, 1987; Selwyn, 1986b). Isolated cases of HIV transmission have been associated with occupational exposures to contaminated secretions or blood via needle stick, mucous membrane splash, or open wound contamination among those not practicing strict barrier precautions ("Update: HIV in Health Care Workers," 1987). Spread of HIV merely through routine household contact (sharing bathrooms, kitchens, or eating utensils) or nonsexual physical contact (hugging and kissing) has not been documented ("Update: Acquired Immunodeficiency," 1986; Selwyn, 1986b).

Sexual spread of HIV among lesbians is theoretically possible, since HIV can be cultured from cervical secretions and can be spread through oral-genital sex. Nevertheless, the likelihood of such transmission appears quite small among lesbians.

Cases of HIV infection associated with blood or blood product transfusions given before 1985 have occurred. Since 1985, all donated blood has been screened for HIV antibodies. In addition, a method of heat treatment that inactivates HIV has been used since 1984 in producing blood concentrates for treating coagulation disorders. These measures currently make the chance of contracting HIV infection through blood or blood product transfusion very slight (Selwyn, 1986b).

To prevent misconceptions and anxiety about the spread of HIV and AIDS, professionals need to be aware of, inform others about, and act consistently with known principles for preventing HIV transmission. At work, professionals need to take special precautions in handling blood and body excretions and secretions from all clients. Such precautions include (1) avoiding direct contact with any body fluids; (2) wearing gloves for drawing blood, for starting or caring for IV lines and venous access lines, and for any anticipated contact with blood and body fluids; and (3) labeling and bagging all contaminated objects appropriately and observing strict handwashing practices. Masks are only necessary if a client is coughing profusely or has an active pulmonary infection (e.g., tuberculosis). Protective eye covering is recommended for situations likely to produce splashes of blood or body fluids into a caregiver's eyes ("Recommendations," 1987).

No special precautions are necessary for clothing, dishes, eating utensils, and bathrooms that are not visibly contaminated. Those articles that are visibly contaminated with blood or body fluids need to be disinfected. An effective disinfectant for home and hospital use is a chlorine bleach solution (one part household bleach to nine parts water) made daily and allowed to sit on contaminated surfaces for 10 minutes.

Principles of personal hygiene should be

followed for people sharing a household with a person who has AIDS or HIV infection. For example, people with AIDS or HIV infection should use their own toothbrushes and razors. Used razor blades need to be placed in a puncture resistant container (Campbell, 1986; Dhundale and Hubbard, 1986).

Health professionals and family members need not shy away from social visits, casual physical contact, shared meals, or kitchen or bathroom facilities shared with a person with AIDS or HIV infection. Maintaining usual social and physical interactions helps to avoid arousing unnecessary feelings of stigma and rejection in people with AIDS or HIV infection.

Prevention

These actions are recommended to prevent spreading AIDS and HIV infection:

- Engage in sex with one mutually faithful partner.
- Engage in safe sex (discussion follows).
- Avoid sexual contact with persons known or suspected of having AIDS or HIV infection.
- Avoid having sex with partners who are in high-risk groups.
- Avoid sexual contact with persons who have sexual partners in high-risk groups.

Physicians are encouraged to use blood transfusions only when medically necessary. Women of childbearing age who are at risk for infection by HIV should be screened for HIV antibodies prior to pregnancy. Antibody-positive women are discouraged from pregnancy not only to prevent HIV infection in their offspring but also to minimize complications for themselves, since both pregnancy and AIDS alter cell-mediated immunity. Antibody-positive mothers who have delivered are discouraged from breastfeeding (Minkoff, 1986).

SAFE SEX

Guidelines for safe sex are influenced by the HIV antibody status of sexual partners. For partners who are absolutely monogamous, do not use IV drugs, and are HIV antibody negative, any sexual activity is considered to be safe. For partners whose HIV antibody status is unknown, mutual masturbation is

considered safe. For partners who are HIV-antibody positive, safe sex measures include using birth control and avoiding sexual intercourse with partners whose HIV antibody status is negative or unknown. Risk reduction measures include using condoms, avoiding anal intercourse, and, for HIV antibody–positive individuals, avoiding partners with secondary infections (Goedert, 1987).

Because using condoms is such an important risk reduction measure, principles for using condoms should be reviewed with clients as necessary (see Chapter 11, Contraception and Sexuality). In order to be most effective, condoms should be used from start to finish of sexual intercourse (Goedert, 1987). The most effective condoms for preventing HIV transmission during sexual intercourse are made of latex, are lubricated with a spermicide, and have an adhesive strip at the base that prevents the condom from coming off prematurely (Dhundale and Hubbard, 1986; "Antibody to HIV in Female Prostitutes," 1987). Latex condoms block HIV transmission; natural membrane condoms do not ("Condoms," 1988). In one small laboratory study, lubricated condoms were ruptured to determine how their lubricants affected HIV. Lubricants containing nonoxynol-9 inhibited HIV in surrounding media more than did those not containing it (Reitmeijer et al, 1988). Using nonoxynol-9 in condom lubricant is suggested in order to offer relative, but not absolute, protection in the event of condom breakage.

UP-TO-DATE INFORMATION

The United States Public Health Service has established a toll-free AIDS hotline that provides a recorded message on AIDS and recent developments of major importance. The telephone number is 800-342-AIDS; further information is available at a second telephone number, 800-342-7514.

REFERENCES

Antibody to HIV in Female Prostitutes. MMWR 36:157–161, 1987.

Aria L, Lindley C: Chlamydia infections of the human genital tract. Med Update 3:1–3, 1980.

Baker D: Herpesvirus. Clin Obstet Gynecol 26:165–172, 1983.

Barnes RC, Holmes KK: Epidemiology of gonorrhea: Current perspectives. Epidemiol Rev 6:1–30, 1984.

Bates B: A Guide to Physical Examination. 3rd ed. Philadelphia, JB Lippincott, 1983.

Bayer R, Levine C, Wolf S: HIV antibody screening: An

ethical framework for evaluating proposed programs. JAMA 256:1768–1774, 1986.

Bell TA, Grayston JT: CDC guidelines for prevention and control of *Chlamydia trachomatis* infections. Ann Intern Med 104:524–526, 1986.

Bennett J: What we know about AIDS. AJN 86:1016–1020, 1986.

Berman M, Ballon SC, Gerek JS, et al: Carcinoma of the uterine cervix. In Haskill CM (ed): Cancer Treatment. Philadelphia, WB Saunders, 1985.

Blockstein WL (Moderator, CDC Conference): Conference on preventing disease/promoting health: Sexually transmissible diseases. Sex Trans Dis 6:273–277, 1979.

Bourcier K, Seidler A: Chlamydia and condylomata acuminata: An update for the nurse practitioner. JOGNN 16:17–22, 1987.

Campbell B: Precautions for the home care of patients with AIDS. Can Med Assoc J 134:51–52, 1986.

Carlton J, Mayes S: Gonorrhea: Not a "second class" disease. Health Soc Work 7:301–313, 1982.

Centers for Disease Control: Personal conversation with Brenda Garzo, Staff, Weekly Surveillance, May 6, 1988.

Classification system for HTLV III/lymphadenopathy—associated virus infections. MMWR 35:334–339, 1986.

Condoms for prevention of sexually transmitted diseases. MMWR 37:133–137, 1988.

Corey L, Adams H, Brown Z, Holmes K: Genital herpes simplex virus infections: Clinical manifestations, course, and complications. Ann Intern Med 98:958–972, 1983.

Corey L, Holmes K: Genital herpes simplex virus infections: Current concepts in diagnosis, therapy and prevention. Ann Intern Med 98:973–983, 1983.

Curran JW: Management of gonococcal pelvic inflammatory disease. Sex Trans Dis April/June:174–180, 1979.

Dalton H, et al: AIDS and the Law: A Guide for the Public. New Haven, Yale University Press, 1987.

Deitch K, Smith J: Cervical dysplasia and condylomata acuminata in young women. JOGNN 12:155–158, 1983.

Dhundale K, Hubbard PM: Home care for the AIDS patient: Safety first. Nursing 86 16:34–35, 1986.

Douglas J, Corey L: Fomites and herpes simplex viruses: A case for nonvenereal transmission. JAMA 250:3093–3094, 1983.

Emmons J, Courter P: Towards control of chlamydia infections. Nurse Pract 10:15–22, 1985.

Eschenbach D: Recognizing chlamydia infections. Contemp Obstet Gynecol 16:15–31, 1980.

Facts about AIDS: US Department of Health and Human Services, Public Health Service, June 1984.

Felman Y: STDs in women: An agenda for action. J Fam Pract 13:289–290, 1981.

Felmar E, Payton C, Smietanka M: Primary care office procedures: Treatment of genital lesions via cryocautery. Primary Care Cancer June:16–21, 1988.

Fiumara N: Pictorial Guide to Sexually Transmitted Diseases. Secaucus, Hospital Pub, 1987.

Fiumara N: Sexually transmissible diseases. Presentation at Ob-Gyn Update. Boston University School of Medicine, Cambridge, Massachusetts, March 23, 1982.

Fiumara N: Sexually transmitted diseases treatment guidelines. Boston, Commonwealth of Massachusetts, 1983.

Fleming WL et al: National survey of venereal disease treated by physicians in 1968. JAMA 2211:1827–1830, 1970.

Fogel CI, Woods NF: Sex in historical and cross-cultural perspective. *In* Fogel CI, Woods NF (eds): Health Care of Women: A Nursing Perspective. St. Louis, CV Mosby, 1981.

Francis D, Chin J: The prevention of acquired immunodeficiency syndrome in the U.S. JAMA 257:1357–1366, 1987.

Gaisin A, Heaton CL: Chancroid: Alias the soft chancre. Int J Dermatol 14:188–197, 1975.

Gibbs R: Sexually transmitted disease in the female. Med Clin North Am 67:221–234, 1983.

Glover ED: Acquired immune deficiency syndrome (AIDS): Number one priority. Health Values: Achieving High Level Wellness 8:3–12, 1984.

Goedert JJ: What is safe sex? Suggested standards linked to testing for HIV. N Engl J Med 316:1339–1341, 1987.

Guinan M, Hardy A: Epidemiology of AIDS in women in the U.S. JAMA 257:2039–2042, 1987.

Handsfield H: Sexually transmitted diseases. Hosp Pract 17:99–109, 113–6, 1982.

Handsfield H, Stamm W, Holmes K: Public health implications and control of sexually transmitted chlamydial infections. Sex Trans Dis 8:85–86, 1981.

Hare M, Thin RN: Chlamydial infection of the lower genital tract of women. Br Med Bull 39:138–144, 1983.

Hart G: Sexual Maladjustment and Disease. Chicago, Nelson-Hall, 1977.

Hatcher R, Stewart G, Stewart F, et al: Contraceptive Technology. New York, Irvington Publishers, 1982.

Hatcher R, Stewart G, Stewart F, et al: Contraceptive Technology. New York, Irvington Publishers, 1980.

Hoke AW: Chancroid. *In* Felman YM (ed): Sexually Transmitted Diseases. New York, Churchill Livingston, 1986.

Holmes K: Chlamydia. Sexually Transmitted Disease Conference. University of North Carolina, Chapel Hill, May 21, 1982.

Holmes K, Bell T, Berger R: Epidemiology of sexually transmitted diseases. Urol Clin North Am 11:3–13, 1984.

Holmes KK, Mardh P (eds): International Perspectives on Neglected Sexually Transmitted Diseases. New York, McGraw-Hill, 1983.

Holmes K, Stamm W: Chlamydia genital infections: A growing problem. Hosp Pract 14:105–117, 1979.

Hook E, Stamm W: Sexually transmitted diseases in men. Med Clin North Am 67:235–251, 1983.

Jaffe W, et al: Acquired immune deficiency syndrome in the United States: The first 1,000 cases. Infect Dis 148:339, 1983.

Karchmer AD: Sexually transmitted diseases. *In* Rubenstein E, Federman D (eds): Scientific American Medicine. Vol 2. New York, Scientific American, 1983.

Kellum M, Loucks A: Genital herpes infections: Diagnosis and management. Nurse Pract 7:14–21, 1982.

Klein E, Fisher L, Chow A: Anorectal gonococcal infection. Ann Intern Med 86:340–346, 1977.

Krim M: The challenge to science and medicine. Diagnosis 9:33–55, 1987.

Laurence J: Diagnostic tests for HIV infection. Infect Med May–June:187–191, 228, 1987.

Leo J: The new scarlet letter. Time Aug 2, 1982, pp 62–66.

Litt I, Edberg S, Finberg L: Gonorrhea in children and adolescents: A current review. J Pediatr 85:595–607, 1974.

Manne S, Sandler I: Coping and adjustment to genital herpes. J Behav Med 7:391–410, 1984.

Margolis S: Genital warts and molluscum contagiosum. Urol Clinics North Am 11:163–170, 1984.

Marmar JL: The management of resistant chancroid in Viet Nam. J Urol 197:807–808, 1977.

McCormick WM: Diagnosis and Treatment of Sexually Transmitted Disease. Littleton, PSG Publishing (John Wright), 1983.

McMaster A: Sexually transmitted disease. *In* Romney S, et al (eds): Obstetrics and Gynecology: Health Care of Women. New York, McGraw-Hill, 1981.

Mead P, Faro S, Gibbs R, Gomel V: Modern management protocols for PID. Contemp Obstet Gynecol 23:225–244, 1984.

Meisels A, Morin C: Human papillomavirus and cancer of the uterine cervix. Gynecol Oncol 12:S111–123, 1981.

Mertz G, Corey L: Genital herpes simplex virus infections in adults. Urol Clin North Am 11:103–119, 1984.

Minkoff H: Acquired immunodeficiency syndrome. J Nurse Midwif 31:189–193, 1986.

Minkoff H: Confronting AIDS: What every woman's physician should know. Female Patient 12:49–74, 1987.

Neeson JD, Stockdale CR: The Practitioner's Handbook of Ambulatory Ob/Gyn. New York, John Wiley & Sons, 1981.

Newton W, Keith L: Role of sexual behavior in the development of pelvic inflammatory disease. J Repro Med 30:82–88, 1985.

Noble RC: Sexually Transmitted Diseases: Guide to Diagnosis and Therapy. New York, Medical Examination Publishing Company, 1982.

Oriel J, Ridgway G: Genital infection in men. Br Med Bull 39:133–137, 1983.

Peacock J: Personal conversation. Sexually Transmitted Diseases Conference. University of North Carolina, Chapel Hill, May 21, 1982.

Popovic M, et al: Detection, isolation, and continuous production of cytopathic retroviruses (HTLV-III) from patients with AIDS and pre-AIDS. Science 224:497–500, 1984.

Public Health Service guidelines for counseling and antibody testing to prevent HIV infection and AIDS. MMWR 36:509–515, 1987.

Raab B, Lorincz A: Genital herpes simplex—concepts and treatment. Am Acad Dermatol 5:249–263, 1981.

Rapp F: Summary of discussion session I of conference of early cervical neoplasia. Gynecol Oncol 12:S88–S89, 1981.

Recommendations for prevention of HIV transmission in health care settings. MMWR 36(Suppl):1–18, 1987.

Reid R, Crum C, Herschman B, et al: Genital warts and cervical cancer. Cancer 53:943–95, 1984.

Rein M: Recent developments in sexually transmitted chlamydia infections. Med Times 109:29–35, 1981.

Reitmeijer C, Krebs J, Feorino P, Judson F: Condoms as physical and chemical barriers against human immunodeficiency virus. JAMA 259:1851–1853, 1988.

Romney SL et al: Gynecology and Obstetrics: The Health Care of Women. New York, McGraw-Hill, 1975.

Roseman DS, Ansell JS, Chapman WH: Sexually transmitted diseases and carcinogenesis. Urol Clin North Am 11:27–43, 1984.

Sarngadharan MG, et al: Antibodies reactive with human T-lymphotropic retroviruses (HTLV-III) in the serum of patients with AIDS. Science 224:506–508, 1984.

Schietinger H: A home care plan for AIDS. AJN 86:1021–1028, 1986.

Schneider A: HPV infection in women and their male partners. Contemp Obstet/Gynecol 33:131–144, 1988.

Schofield CB: Sexually Transmitted Diseases. 3rd ed. New York, Churchill Livingstone, 1979.

Selwyn PA: AIDS: What is now known. I. History and immunovirology. Hosp Pract 21:67–82, 1986a.

Selwyn PA: AIDS: What is now known. II. Epidemiology. Hosp Pract 21:127–164, 1986b.

Selwyn PA: AIDS: What is now known. III. Clinical aspects. Hosp Pract 21:119–153, 1986c.

Sexually transmitted diseases treatment guidelines 1982. MMWR (Suppl) 31:505–555, 1982.

Sexually transmitted diseases treatment guidelines 1985. MMWR (Suppl) 34:1–35, 1985.

Special AIDS issue. Food Drug Bul 17:14–24, 1987.

Spence M: Gonorrhea. Clin Obstet Gynecol 25:111–124, 1983.

Stamm WE, et al: Diagnosis of *Chlamydia trachomatis* infections by direct immunofluorescence staining of genital secretions. Ann Intern Med 101:638–641, 1984.

Sweet R, Schachter J, Landers D: Chlamydia infections in obstetrics and gynecology. Clin Obstet Gynecol 26:143–164, 1983.

Thompson S, Washington E: Epidemiology of sexually transmitted *Chlamydia trachomatis* infections. Epidemiol Rev 5:96–123, 1983.

Trachtenberg A, Washington A, Halldorson S: A cost-based decision analysis for chlamydia screening in California family planning clinics. Obstet Gynecol 71:101–108, 1988.

Treatment of sexually transmitted diseases. Med Lett Drugs Ther 26:5–10, 1984.

Treatment of sexually transmitted diseases. Med Lett Drugs Ther 30:5–10, 1988.

Update: Acquired immunodeficiency syndrome—US. MMWR 35:757–766, 1986.

Update: HIV in health care workers exposed to blood of infected patients. MMWR 36:285–289, 1987.

Update: Serologic testing for antibody to human immunodeficiency virus. MMWR 36:833–840, 1988.

US Department of Health and Human Services, Public Health Service: Public Reports 98:559, 1983.

US Department of Health and Human Services, Public Health Service, Centers for Disease Control: STD Fact Sheet. Pub no (CDC 81-8995) 2-27, edition 35.

Venereal disease surges. Philadelphia Inquirer Jan 23, 1989, pp 1–4A.

24: Drugs and Disturbed Sexual Functioning

Audrey Rogers

The human sexual response is a complex interplay of physiological, psychological, and social functions that can be presented in four phases. In the first, there is the experience of interest in or *desire* to engage in sex, traditionally referred to as libido. Given stimulation, response progresses to the second stage, *excitement*, which is marked by vaginal lubrication in the woman, penile erection in the man. This phase progresses to the next, *orgasm or climax* for both sexes, characterized in the man by ejaculation. The last phase, *satisfaction*, follows and is marked by clear physiological relief and relaxation, often in conjunction with deep emotional bonding. Of these four phases, desire, excitement, orgasm, and satisfaction, the least susceptible to pharmacological influence is the last, since it is the one most dominated by the quality of the relationship and, when preceded by successful passage through the former phases, the least affected by physiological performance. Discussion in this chapter, therefore, will be limited to the influence of drugs on the sexual response at the first three levels of the sexual response.

For some drugs, there is a clear physiological basis to their production of sexual dysfunction; for others, the mechanisms have not been elucidated, if indeed they even exist. Such drugs remain implicated on the evidence of case reports in the literature, "popular" wisdom, or the clinical experience of the health professional. The scientific evaluation of drug-induced sexual dysfunction presents methodological issues that are difficult to resolve. These issues involve biases from selection, information, and confounding factors.

METHODOLOGICAL CONCERNS

Selection Bias

In some populations, individuals with unsatisfactory sexual relationships may be over-represented, creating a selection bias. There is a substantial literature supporting the use of medical care for reasons other than illness (Barsky, 1981; Mechanic, 1972, 1976a, 1976b, 1978). Psychic distress and disordered personal relationships may motivate individuals to enter the medical care system, where they are often pharmacologically assaulted by personnel ill-equipped to recognize or treat their social problems. Disordered and stressful relationships are not associated with satisfying sexual performances. In these circumstances, and often as a result of faulty interviewing, inadequate histories, and poor interaction, drugs can frequently be blamed for pre-existing sexual dysfunction.

Information Bias

Information about sexual functioning may be biased by discomfort in exchanging such information. There is a significant background level of sexual dysfunction in the general population. Job-related stress and family crises can contribute to cyclic fluctuations in interest and performance. Since sexual performance is intricately involved in self-concept and may be mixed with feelings of shame and embarrassment, it is the rare individual who can fully share these concerns until rapport is established. Thus, there may be substantial delayed- or underreporting until the individual feels comfortable enough to broach the subject. Drug therapy may be initiated in the interim, and without an adequate evaluation by the health professional, sexual dysfunction may be attributed to the drug.

Since there is a remarkable relationship between psychological status and sexual performance, repeated questioning regarding sexual function once therapy has been initiated can increase anxiety and produce a self-fulfilling prophecy of dysfunction. In this circumstance, the drug per se does not produce the dysfunction, but the questioning process intervenes to start a cycle that culminates in a performance-anxiety dysfunction. Monitoring for drug-related sexual dysfunction requires much interpersonal sensitivity and skill.

Confounding Bias

As a rule, healthy persons do not take drugs. People with specific medical problems are most likely to receive prescriptions. The separation of drug effect from disease effect is most difficult, creating a confounding bias. In conducting a study, it is not enough to examine sexual performance in the ill at baseline before drug therapy is instituted because (1) most chronic diseases are progressive in nature and produce slowly cumulative damage and (2) the effect of perceiving oneself as ill enough to require therapy (i.e., labeling) may be sufficiently important to be a contributing factor in its own right.

In one study (Bulpitt et al, 1976), 6.9 per cent of normal subjects reported erectile dysfunction, while 24.6 per cent of the treated hypertensives did. However, 17.1 per cent of the untreated hypertensives also reported erectile dysfunction. Croog and associates (1988) reported that 40 per cent of newly or previously diagnosed and currently un-

treated hypertensive white men expressed distress with one or more sexual symptoms (i.e., difficulty with achieving or maintaining an erection or with ejaculation). In addition, there may be other agents besides a prescription drug that the individual is ingesting: over-the-counter medications, and particularly alcohol, can influence sexual functioning.

Study Strategies

Information on sexual dysfunction in the literature takes the form of case reports, study groups, or controlled clinical trials. There are advantages and disadvantages to each method of gathering information. Case reports are communications regarding isolated client experiences and represent the weakest form of evidence. They are obviously strengthened if baseline sexual performance is well documented, specific dysfunction with the drug is outlined, and performance ability is regained when the drug is discontinued (dechallenge) and is again lost when the individual is re-treated with the drug (rechallenge). The dechallenge-rechallenge process is a reasonable one and is often employed to ascertain true adverse reactions. However, it is more reliable when the adverse event is relatively free from psychological influence and can be more objectively measured (e.g., allergic dermatitis).

In a study group, the outcomes of persons with the same disease treated with the same drug over a period of time are examined. The advantage of this method over the isolated case report is its ability to generate a proportion for the occurrence of the outcome among persons with the disease (e.g., 10 per cent of all male hypertensives treated with this drug for 6 months develop erectile dysfunction).

The controlled clinical trial is a preferred method of gathering information because while it employs the same strategy as the study group, it adds a control group that does not receive the drug but is comparable in other aspects. Such comparability can never be guaranteed, but the best ensurance is the randomization of study subjects to the treated or the control group in what is called the randomized controlled trial. The addition of a control group confers the potential (1) to establish the background level of sexual dysfunction in the untreated control group,

TABLE 24–1. Therapeutic Agents Associated with the Loss of Sexual Desire

Antianxiety agents
  Diazepam (Valium)
  Doxepin (Sinequan)
Antidepressants
  Amitriptyline (Elavil, others)
  Amoxapine (Ascendin)
  Desipramine (Norpramin)
Anticonvulsants
  Phenytoin (Dilantin)
Antihypertensives
  Guanethidine (Ismelin)
  Methyldopa (Aldomet)
  Reserpine (Serpasil, others)
Antipsychotics
  Chlorpromazine (Thorazine)
Beta blockers
  Propranolol (Inderal)
  Timolol (Blocadren)
Cardiotonics
  Digoxin (Lanoxin)
Diuretics
  Chlorthalidone (Hygroton)
  Hydrochlorothiazide (Oretic, HydroDIURIL, others)
  Spironolactone (Aldactone)
Hormonal preparations
  Anabolic steroids (Dianabol)
  Estrogens in men
  Progesterone
Miscellaneous
  Carbonic anhydrase inhibitors (Diamox)
  Cimetidine (Tagamet)
  Clofibrate (Atromid-S)
  Ranitidine (Zantac)

(2) to compare that with the level of dysfunction in the treated group, and (3) to derive a risk estimate of sexual dysfunction attributable to drug therapy. Data from these randomized controlled trials represent the strongest evidence. Tables 24–1 to 24–4* list drugs that have been implicated in producing sexual dysfunction. The quality of the data supporting these claims varies from the simple case report to information from randomized controlled trials.

The Potential Contribution of the Nursing Process

Most of the literature relating to the association between sexual dysfunction and drug use suffers from the methodological flaws outlined in the previous sections. The application of a scientific process, the discussion

*Tables 24–1 to 24–4 include representatives of major categories of drugs that can affect sexual functioning but are not inclusive. For additional information, the reader is referred to *The Medical Letter of Drugs and Therapeutics*, in which drugs that can cause sexual dysfunction are reviewed on a regular basis.

of clinical findings with other members of the health care team, and appropriate and comprehensive recording in the client's health record would do much to remedy the literature, which relies on properly collected and recorded data. Nurses can take the initiative to make and record a careful baseline assessment of current drug use and any associated side effects.

REVIEW OF THE LITERATURE

The following review of the literature is not intended to be an all-inclusive presentation

TABLE 24–2. Therapeutic Agents Associated with Excitement, Diminution, or Erectile Dysfunction

Antiarrhythmics
  Disopyramide (Norpace)
Anticholinergics
  Homatropine methylbromide (Homapin)
  Mepenzolate bromide (Cantil)
  Methantheline bromide (Banthine)
  Propantheline bromide (Pro-Banthine)
Antidepressants
  Amoxapine (Ascendin)
  Clomipramine (Anafranil)
  Desipramine (Norpramin)
  Imipramine (Tofranil)
  Isocarboxazid (Marplan)
  Lithium (Eskalith)
  Nortriptyline (Aventyl, Pamelor)
  Phenelzine (Nardil)
  Protriptyline (Vivactil)
  Tranylcypromine (Parnate)
Antihypertensives
  Clonidine (Catapres)
  Guanethidine (Ismelin)
  Hydralazine (Apresoline)
  Methyldopa (Aldomet)
  Prazosin (Minipress)
  Reserpine (Serpasil, others)
Antipsychotics
  Chlorpromazine (Thorazine, others)
  Haloperidol (Haldol)
  Thioridazine (Mellaril)
Beta blockers
  Atenolol (Tenormin)
  Propranolol (Inderal)
  Timolol (Blocadren)
Cardiotonics
  Digoxin (Lanoxin, others)
Diuretics
  Chlorthalidone (Hygroton)
  Hydrochlorothiazide (Oretic, HydroDIURIL, others)
  Spironolactone (Aldactone)
Hormonal preparations
  Hydroxyprogesterone
  Progesterone
Miscellaneous
  Carbonic anhydrase inhibitors (Diamox)
  Cimetidine (Tagamet)
  Nonsteroidal anti-inflammatory agents—naproxen (Naprosyn)

TABLE 24–3. Therapeutic Agents Associated with Orgasmic and Ejaculatory Dysfunction

Orgasmic Dysfunction in Women
Antianxiety agents
    Alprazolam (Xanax)
Antidepressants
    Clomipramine (Anafranil)
    Desipramine (Norpramin)
    Imipramine (Tofranil)
    Phenelzine (Nardil)
Antipsychotics
    Chlorprothixene (Taractan)
Ejaculatory Dysfunction
Delayed Ejaculation
Antianxiety agents
    Alprazolam (Xanax)
    Diazepam (Valium)
    Doxepin (Sinequan)
Antidepressants
    Clomipramine (Anafranil)
    Imipramine (Tofranil)
    Isocarboxazid (Marplan)
    Phenelzine (Nardil)
Antihypertensives
    Clonidine (Catapres)
    Labetalol (Normodyne)
    Methyldopa (Aldomet)
    Reserpine (Serpasil; others)
Antipsychotics
    Chlorprothixene (Taractan)
    Perphenazine (Trilafon)
    Thioridazine (Mellaril)
Ejaculatory Failure
Alpha blockers
    Phenoxybenzamine (Dibenzyline)
Antidepressants
    Amoxapine (Ascendin)
    Clomipramine (Anafranil)
    Pargyline (Eutonyl)
    Phenelzine (Nardil)
Antihypertensives
    Guanethidine (Ismelin)
    Methyldopa (Aldomet)
    Reserpine (Serpasil, others)
Antipsychotics
    Mesoridazine (Serentil)
    Perphenazine (Trilafon)
    Piperacetazine (Quide)
    Thioridazine (Mellaril)
Nonsteroidal anti-inflammatory agents
    Naproxen (Naprosyn)
Painful Ejaculation
Antidepressants
    Amoxapine (Ascendin)
    Desipramine (Norpramin)
Antipsychotics
    Haloperidol (Haldol)
    Thioridazine (Mellaril)

tion in the context of a particular condition. (See Chapter 11, Contraception and Sexuality, for a discussion of estrogen and progesterone preparations; also see Chapter 29, Mental Illness, Substance Abuse, and Sexuality.) Any discussion of teratogenesis or the inappropriate use of prescription drugs is beyond the scope of this chapter.

Prescription Drugs

ANTIANXIETY AGENTS

Antianxiety drugs (barbiturates, benzodiazepines) are generally prescribed for individuals who are undergoing stress and who either are coping inadequately or require additional support in their coping efforts. These drugs appear to be most useful in allaying the anxiety associated with inhibition and self-deprecation. Indeed, in therapeutic doses, their main effect is one of disinhibition, eliminating some of the strong accompanying anxiety. This disinhibition process allows subsurface emotions to emerge. For example, if the anxiety is secondary to suppressed rage, the use of these agents may produce a violent episode. On the other hand, their use in small doses may be indicated in sex therapy when strong inhibitions prevent arousal. Obviously, an appropriate assessment and supportive counseling must occur in conjunction with their use. These agents usually have an effect similar to that of alcohol. At lower doses, there is the disinhibitory effect, but as the dosage increases, generally there is a depression of all behaviour, including sexual interest (Munjack, 1979). Additionally, if the dose is sufficiently large to induce general peripheral muscle relaxation, the orgasmic phase of sexual response may be attenuated (Renshaw, 1980).

Benzodiazepine use can affect the endocrine system, resulting in menstrual irregularities, premenstrual tension, breast engorgement, gynecomastia, and galactorrhea

TABLE 24–4. Drugs Associated with Priapism

Prescription
    Chlorpromazine (Thorazine)
    IV fat emulsion infusion
    Labetalol (Normodyne)
    Mesoridazine (Serentil)
    Prazosin (Minipress)
    Trazodone (Desyrel)
Social
    Cantharides (Spanish Fly)

of adverse sexual events associated with drug use. Rather, its purpose is to describe types of sexual dysfunction that have been reported to occur with commonly used classes of drugs. In certain instances, more detailed information about specific agents can be found in other chapters about sexual func-

(Ashton, 1986). One report of sexual precocity (enlarged uterus, fine pubic hair, vaginal discharge, and increased serum prolactin) associated with the use of clonazepam (Clonopin) for seizure control in an 11-month-old girl was attributed to clonazepam's capacity to either increase sex hormone levels or alter the sex hormone binding proteins (Choonara, Rosenbloom, and Smith, 1985).

ANTICHOLINERGIC AGENTS

Anticholinergic agents (e.g., atropine) block the activity of the parasympathetic nervous system and have been used clinically to treat disorders of the eye, the heart, and the gastrointestinal tract; to treat parkinsonism, and to prepare clients preoperatively. Since the excitement phase of the sexual act is mediated through the action of the parasympathetic nervous system, the blocking action of these drugs may produce difficulty, particularly in the male desiring erection. Indeed, any drug with strong anticholinergic properties has the potential to interfere with sexual functioning; these drugs include the antiarrhythmic disopyramide (Norpace), many of the antidepressants, antispasmodics, and the antipsychotics.

ANTIDEPRESSANT AGENTS

In general, changes in sexual function occur during the course of depressive illness as a common manifestation of the disease; however, the extent of this occurrence is unknown. There are two types of antidepressants currently available in the United States to treat unipolar depression. One type is the monoamine oxidase inhibitor (MAOI), whose action blocks the degradation of biogenic amines. The other is the tricyclic antidepressant (TCA), whose action, while not totally elucidated, enhances the activity of these biogenic amines. There is a case report (Rapp, 1979) of one dechallenge-rechallenge positive experience of retarded ejaculation with phenelzine (Nardil, an MAOI) and another of orgasmic and ejaculatory incompetence without impaired erection with the same agent. In another report (Barton, 1979), an MAOI was associated with orgasmic inhibition in a woman whose preorgasmic sexual arousal remained normal.

The tricyclic antidepressants have strong anticholinergic properties; thus, they may produce erectile dysfunction. However, other sexual problems more frequently occur as a result of their interaction with the sympathetic nervous system. Women may experience orgasmic inhibition. This can be managed successfully by changing therapy to another TCA or, alternatively, by manipulating dose in anticipation of sexual activity (Quirk and Einarson, 1982).

In men, there may be retrograde ejaculation or ejaculatory inhibition with TCA use. There are two processes to normal ejaculation: emission and ejaculation itself. Emission results from sympathetically mediated peristaltic movement of the smooth musculature of the vas deferens, seminal vesicles, and the prostate. Ejaculation itself is a parasympathetically mediated tonic-clonic contraction of the bulbocavernous and ischiocavernous muscles. As part of these processes, the internal sphincter at the base of the bladder, under sympathetic control, closes, and the parasympathetically controlled external sphincter opens. Retrograde ejaculation has been reported with amoxapine (Ascendin) (Schwarcz, 1982) and results in a dry orgasm, with the ejaculate propelled backward into the bladder, since the internal sphincter, sympathetically blocked, remains open. This same case report also studied ejaculatory inhibition, and such an occurrence has been reported elsewhere with amoxapine (Kulik and Wilbur, 1982) as well as with imipramine (Tofranil), protriptyline (Vivactil), and desipramine (Norpramin) (Simpson et al, 1965). In this situation, sexual desire remains intact, but the muscular contractions associated with emission and ejaculation are slowed or delayed and become abnormally protracted. Any associated pleasure is lost; a burning, tearing suprapubic pain is experienced; and there may be a residual feeling of intolerable muscle tension. This experience seems to be undeniably associated with TCA antidepressant use, being dechallenge-rechallenge positive. Unfortunately, it has been reported only in the case report format, so no estimate of its frequency has been generated.

A newer antidepressant, trazodone (Desyrel), has been associated with the production of priapism in men (Patt, 1985) and increased sexual desire in women (Gartrell, 1986).

Antidepressant agents, in general, can influence the function of both the sympathetic and the parasympathetic nervous systems and thus affect sexual function in multiple ways.

ANTICONVULSANT AGENTS

One report (Toone et al, 1980) demonstrated an increase in sex hormone–binding globulin during anticonvulsant therapy, particularly with the agent phenytoin (Dilantin). The increase in this specific globulin resulted in a lowered free testosterone level secondary to the increase in binding capacity. Subsequently, there was noted a decrease in the level of sexual activity among treated persons over normal male volunteers. The implications of these findings remain unclear, and any risk of sexual dysfunction attributable to anticonvulsant therapy has yet to be established.

ANTIPSYCHOTIC AGENTS

Schizophrenics in the early stages of their illness may exhibit an increased sexual drive with a preoccupation with sexual behavior; chronic schizophrenics generally demonstrate a complete lack of sexual interest. There is, therefore, the potential for confounding of the drug-dysfunction association by the progression of the disease itself.

Pimozide (Orap) is a neuroleptic that is a selective dopamine antagonist. There is a case report (Ananth, 1982) of erectile dysfunction associated with its use that was dechallenge-rechallenge positive. There have been five reports (Freyhan, 1961; Heller, 1961; Singh, 1961) of male ejaculatory failure with thioridazine (Mellaril); in four women treated with this agent, three reported no change in sexual function, the fourth described herself as less pleasurably aroused, with orgasms of diminished quality. Painful ejaculation similar to that described with antidepressant use has also been reported with thioridazine (Kotin et al, 1976). A total of 92 cases of ejaculatory dysfunction associated with thioridazine use have been reported to its manufacturer (Mitchell and Popkin, 1982).

One case has been reported (Ditman, 1964) of ejaculatory inhibition without emission and orgasm of diminished intensity with chlorprothixene (Taractan), which was dechallenge positive (no rechallenge). Berger (1979) reports a patient who experienced ejaculatory pain with trifluoperazine (Stelazine), which recurred with a subsequent trial of haloperidol (Haldol); both occurrences remitted when the drug was withdrawn. There has been a case report of ejaculatory inhibition with chlorpromazine (Thorazine) that

was dechallenge positive without rechallenge (Greenberg, 1971). Chlorpromazine has been blamed for six cases of priapism (Dawson-Butterworth, 1969, 1970), which is a prolonged, painful erection considered a medical emergency requiring immediate intervention.

A more detailed discussion of the antipsychotic agents can be found in Chapter 29, Mental Illness, Substance Abuse, and Sexuality.

CARDIOVASCULAR AGENTS
Antiarrhythmic Agents

Disopyramide (Norpace) is an antiarrhythmic agent with parasympathetic properties used to suppress and prevent ectopic ventricular contractions. Two case reports (McHaffie et al, 1977; Ahmad, 1980) have appeared: One concerned a 35-year-old white male who developed sexual dysfunction that was dechallenge-rechallenge positive; the other involved a 47-year-old white male in whom the drug was discontinued at first complaint without rechallenge. It appears that the sexual dysfunction may be secondary to anticholinergic interruption of parasympathetic sacral outflow resulting in erectile difficulty without change in sexual desire.

Antihypertensive and Diuretic Agents

Drug classes used in the treatment of hypertension include diuretics, alpha receptor agonists, adrenergic neuron blockers, alpha receptor blockers, beta receptor blockers, peripheral vasodilators, calcium antagonists, and angiotensin-converting enzyme inhibitors (ACE inhibitors). Some of these agents (diuretics, beta receptor blockers, peripheral vasodilators, and calcium antagonists) are also employed in the treatment of coronary artery disease or congestive heart failure.

There does not appear to be any clear physiological basis for the production of sexual dysfunction by the thiazide diuretics (HydroDIURIL, Oretic, Esidrix) or structurally related chlorthalidone (Hygroton). Some have suggested volume depletion as a mechanism for the sexual dysfunction, but a pronounced volume depletion does not persist beyond 3 to 4 weeks with continued treatment. This hypothesis therefore cannot explain the dysfunction beyond the time of the initial treatment period. Although reports document erectile dysfunction, their estimates range from 4 to 32 per cent. Other reported effects include diminished sexual desire, failed ejaculation, and decreased vaginal lubrication (Smith and Talbert, 1986). One case series of five men (Stressman and Ben-Ishay, 1980) treated with chlorthalidone reported decreased sexual desire in three and erectile dysfunction in all five.

The only diuretic with a known biological basis for producing dysfunction is the aldosterone antagonist spironolactone (Aldactone). Because of its steroidal structure, it competes for binding sites and, in the process, promotes gynecomastia, menstrual irregularities, and decreased desire.

All antihypertensives belonging to the class of sympatholytics, whether their action is central (é.g., alpha agonists) or peripheral (e.g., alpha, beta, or adrenergic neuronal blockers), by virtue of their interference with sympathetic functioning can theoretically produce sexual difficulty. This possibility has been confirmed consistently in the literature.

Antihypertensive agents belonging to the peripheral vasodilator class (e.g., hydralazine [Apresoline]) are associated with a relatively low incidence of sexual dysfunction (Smith and Talbert, 1986). The calcium antagonists and the ACE inhibitors (captopril [Capoten], enalapril [Vasotec]) are relatively new to the market, and experience and exposure may not yet be adequate to assess their association (if any) with sexual dysfunction. One case of gynecomastia has been reported with the use of nifedipine (Procardia), a calcium antagonist (Clyne, 1986). In a clinical trial, the effects of propranolol (beta receptor blocker), methyldopa (sympatholytic), and captopril (ACE inhibitor) on the level of distress over sexual symptoms in white men also receiving a diuretic were compared; Croog and associates (1988) found no change in sexual symptom scores from baseline for the captopril group alone and an increase in sexual symptoms from baseline in the other two groups.

In a study of 88 treated hypertensives (Laver, 1974), 40 complained of diminished sexual potency, and 13 of these spontaneously attributed their complaint to therapy. All 13 were treated with hydrochlorothiazide (10 received hydrochlorothiazide and methyldopa [Aldomet], two received hydrochlorothiazide and clonidine [Catapres], and one received hydrochlorothiazide and reserpine [Serpasil]). All 13 presented with erectile dysfunction without loss of sexual desire, and this complaint represented the single most important one attributed to therapy.

Newman and Salerno (1974) reported a sample of hypertensive males (N = 27) treated with methyldopa who were age 43 to 64. One third of this group complained of diminished sexual desire, erectile dysfunction, and difficulty with ejaculation. Their complaints began after therapy was instituted and abated after the agent was discontinued. There was no reported sexual dysfunction in a comparable group of men treated with hydrochlorothiazide alone.

Johnson (1966) treated 114 hypertensives with methyldopa. In 14, therapy was discontinued within 6 months secondary to side effects in general; of the remaining 100 (37 men, 63 women), three fourths also reported tolerable side effects; however, erectile dysfunction only accounted for two of these reports. An estimate of decreased desire with methyldopa use is 15 per cent, and for erectile dysfunction estimates range from 20 to 80 per cent (Smith and Talbert, 1986).

Hogan (1980) gave 861 male hypertensives a questionnaire to determine the incidence of sexual dysfunction over time (the incidence in 117 controls were 4 per cent). The frequency of sexual dysfunction for each therapeutic regimen was as follows: hydrochlorothiazide alone, 9 per cent (N = 287); hydrochlorothiazide and methyldopa, 13 per cent (N = 381); hydrochlorothiazide and clonidine, 15 per cent (N = 133); and hydrochlorothiazide, propranolol, and hydralazine, 23 per cent (N = 60). Thirty six per cent of those responding affirmatively did not do so consistently, thereby suggesting that sexual dysfunction in conjunction with antihypertensive use may have had a variable pattern. Also, these data suggest that dysfunction may be related to the particular drug combination being used. .

In a clinical trial ("Medical Research Council," 1981) of bendrofluazide versus propranolol versus placebo in the treatment of hypertension, individuals were assessed at 12 weeks and again at 2 years for the presence of sexual dysfunction with therapy. For bendrofluazide, the percentages of affirmative answers for the two consecutive assessments were 16.2 and 22.6, respectively; for propranolol, 13.8 and 13.2, respectively; and for placebo, 8.9 and 10.1, respectively. All complaints dissipated when treatment was stopped. In a clinical trial ("Veterans Administration," 1977) of 1070 men, approximately 5 per cent complained of erectile dysfunction with different therapeutic regimens, ranging from a low of 2.6 per cent with propranolol alone to a high of 6.6 per cent when propranolol, hydralazine, and hydrochlorothiazide were prescribed in concert.

In summary, available research supports a positive association between sexual dysfunction, particularly erectile difficulty, and antihypertensive drug therapy with diuretic and sympatholytic agents.

Beta-Blocking Agents

Drugs that can selectively block the beta receptors of the sympathetic nervous system have been employed in the management of angina pectoris as well as hypertension. A commonly used beta blocker in the United States is propranolol (Inderal). Warren and Warren (1977) reported five cases of erectile dysfunction in 95 men treated with a 120 mg or higher per day dose over a 2-year period. Subsequently, there were two case reports: one (Knarr, 1976) of penile erectile dysfunction with a decrease in sexual desire and one (Miller, 1976) of a dechallenge-rechallenge positive erectile difficulty. In a case series of individuals who had had their renin profile defined (Hollifield et al, 1976), seven of the 13 high-renin individuals received high doses of propranolol, with three complaining of diminished desire and two of erectile dysfunction.

In a study of propranolol management of chronic angina (Warren et al, 1976), 63 treated clients were followed for 5 to 8 years. Of the 49 males, three complained of erectile dysfunction. In another study group (Burnett and Chanine, 1979) of 50 men treated with propranolol, seven developed erectile dysfunction, with an additional 13 complaining of diminished potency (eight of these also had decreased sexual desire), while two others experienced decreased desire alone. The occurrence of these symptoms appeared to be dose related.

In another study (Forsberg et al, 1979) four participants (two smokers, and two others treated with propranolol) had baseline measurements obtained while smoking or taking propranolol to serve as control value for subsequent measurements after smoking or the drug had been discontinued. Serum hormone levels were estimated, and blood

pressure values and Doppler recordings were taken in the arm, the leg, and the penis. All values were essentially normal, and slight intersubject variability diminished after smoking and the drug were terminated. Overall, data from case reports and study group research suggest that a substantial number of men who use propranolol will experience some degree of erectile dysfunction. Estimates for this occurrence range from 5 to 43 per cent (Smith and Talbert, 1986).

Another adrenergic-blocking agent, labetalol (Normodyne), has been associated with delayed ejaculation, delayed detumescence, and priapism. All effects are attributed to its alpha$_1$-blocking properties (Smith and Talbert, 1986).

One controlled study with atenolol (Tenormin) versus placebo (Douglass-Jones and Cruickshank, 1976) found one case of erectile dysfunction among 11 placebo-treated persons and only one case of erectile dysfunction in the group (N = 27) treated with active drug.

Timolol (Timoptic), a beta-blocking agent used topically (eyedrops), has been associated with 28 reports of sexual dysfunction (erectile dysfunction, 18; decreased desire, 9; and decreased ejaculate volume, 1) received by the National Registry of Drug-Induced Ocular Side Effects. Therapeutic blood levels can be reached through ocular and nasal mucosal absorption (Fraunfelder and Meyer, 1985).

In summary, erectile dysfunction has been associated with the use of beta-blocking agents. It is not clear, however, to what extent other factors contribute to its occurrence, since most reports are uncontrolled studies.

MISCELLANEOUS AGENTS
Carbonic Anhydrase Inhibitors

Carbonic anhydrase inhibitors (CAI) are systemically administered drugs used in the treatment of glaucoma. In one study (Epstein and Grant, 1977) of 92 individuals treated with acetazolamide (Diamox) or methazolamide (Neptazane), 44 complained at interview of a syndrome of malaise, fatigue, weight loss, depression, anorexia, and loss of desire. Of these 44, 24 were significantly acidotic; when treated with sodium bicarbonate, 10 of these 24 had their symptoms reversed. In another study (Wallace et al, 1979) of 39 persons (33 men, 6 women) there were similar reports of malaise, depression, and loss of desire. Twelve persons were dechallenge-rechallenge positive. Three cases of erectile dysfunction reversed when the drug was discontinued.

Clofibrate

Clofibrate (Atromid-S) is a lipid-lowering agent. In a controlled clinical trial ("Coronary Drug Project," 1975) there was a 14 per cent occurrence of decreased desire or erectile function in the clofibrate-treated group versus a 10 per cent occurrence in the placebo controls. In a controlled clinical trial ("Committee of Principal Investigators," 1978) involving 15,745 subjects, there were twice as many cases of erectile dysfunction associated with clofibrate therapy than in the control groups.

H₂-Receptor Antagonists

Cimetidine (Tagamet) is a histamine receptor blocking agent used in the treatment of duodenal ulcer disease and hyperacidic states. Twenty-three cases of erectile dysfunction in men 37 years of age or older after 0 to 7 months of therapy have been reported to the British Committee on the Safety of Medicines (Peden et al, 1979). No denominator is available and so no estimate of frequency can be made. In a postmarketing study of cimetidine (Gifford et al, 1980), 9,907 individuals were followed. Eighteen men developed gynecomastia but only one complained of sexual inhibition. Two others (one man, one woman) complained of a decrease in desire and another reported "poor sexual performance." There is some evidence that cimetidine displays an antiandrogenic effect. Animal studies in rats and dogs treated with cimetidine have demonstrated a decrease in the weight of the prostate and seminal vesicles. In a study (Jensen et al, 1983) of 22 men (20 patients with Zollinger-Ellison syndrome and two with idiopathic gastric hypersecretion), 50 per cent developed adverse sexual reactions within 2 months of the initiation of therapy, and all cases did so within 5 months. Of the 11 with symptoms, nine had erectile dysfunction, nine had breast changes (eight with tenderness, five with gynecomastia), and seven had both erectile dysfunction and breast changes. In three of these men, nocturnal penile tumescence was measured (this examination permits a differentiation be-

tween organic and psychogenic erectile dysfunction). Erections were less frequent and less full in men treated with cimetidine; there was a reversion to a normal nocturnal erectile pattern both in frequency and fullness when another histamine-receptor blocker was substituted for the cimetidine. This antiandrogenic side effect of cimetidine, which may result in erectile dysfunction and gynecomastia, occurs considerably less than 1 per 100 exposures unless the clients are receiving very high doses of the drug for conditions like gastrinoma. Cimetidine is a drug that has received extensive population-based safety evaluation. Another newer H₂-receptor antagonist, ranitidine (Zantac), has been associated with reports of reduced sexual desire and gynecomastia.

Sulfasalazine

Sulfasalazine (Azulfidine), a common and effective treatment for ulcerative colitis, is associated with the production of changes in sperm motility, morphology, and concentration that may result in infertility. Fertility has been re-established when the drug has been withdrawn (Steeno, 1984).

Anabolic Steroids, Endogenous Androgens, and Testosterone

The appropriate use of these agents is limited to replacement therapy in men with deficiency or absence of endogenous testosterone and, in women, to adjunctive therapy in inoperable metastatic mammary cancer. The abuse of these agents is currently in vogue with male athletes because of the drug's protein anabolic effects, which increase muscle mass.

Androgens produce gynecomastia, persistent penile erections, and, in high doses, oligospermia in men and amenorrhea, other menstrual irregularities, and virilization in women. Both sexes may experience changes in sexual desire; both increases and decreases have been reported.

OVER-THE-COUNTER, NONPRESCRIPTION DRUGS

In general, over-the-counter agents are used for the symptomatic relief of self-limited conditions such as headache, nausea, vomiting, diarrhea, and constipation. In this regard and when used appropriately, their effect on sexual functioning should be negligible. Those that may have an adverse effect on sexual performance are agents with strong anticholinergic properties that are used on a chronic basis. Nonprescription drugs with anticholinergic properties include, but are not limited to, antidiarrheal agents (e.g., atropine sulfate), antiemetics (e.g., cyclizine, an antihistamine), antihistamines (e.g., chlorpheniramine maleate), and antitussives (e.g., diphenhydramine hydrochloride, an antihistamine). Many decongestant and cough mixtures contain antihistamines (e.g., chlorpheniramine maleate) that exert anticholinergic properties. Of these, the only class that possibly meets both conditions (anticholinergic properties and chronicity of therapy) is the antihistamines. Individuals who have allergies for which they require prolonged antihistamine therapy may experience some difficulty with sexual dysfunction, particularly if they are exceptionally sensitive to the anticholinergic effects of these drugs.

SOCIAL DRUGS

Alcohol

Alcohol taken on occasion in small to moderate amounts will produce disinhibition. The pattern is similar to that observed with the use of antianxiety agents (e.g., diazepam). In low to moderate amounts, the effect may be paradoxical, in fact, having a very positive influence on desire by lifting inhibitions in an otherwise desirous person but, at the same time, dulling sensation and delaying arousal and excitement. In large doses, its effect is simply one of depression, even somnolence.

Prolonged chronic alcohol abuse produces erectile dysfunction that is neither psychologically nor hormonally mediated (although in chronic liver disease, endogenous estrogens are not degraded and a feminizing effect may occur). Rather, alcohol has a direct destructive effect on the neurogenic reflex that produces erection. This damage is irreversible. Sexual desire remains unaffected. Lemere and Smith (1973) report a study of 17,000 alcoholics (methodology not detailed) in which 8 per cent complained of erectile dysfunction. Furthermore, this erectile dysfunction did not reverse in 50 per cent of the sample even after 5 years of sobriety.

Amyl Nitrate

Amyl nitrate is a vasodilator sometimes used clinically in the treatment of angina pectoris but is popularly believed to be an aphrodisiac. These claims seem to result from the transient feeling of hypotensive giddiness and a peripheral shunting of blood, perhaps with some genital vasocongestion. The drug is not innocuous: sudden death, myocardial infarction, and methemogloblinemia have been reported with its use (Munjack, 1979; Renshaw, 1980).

Cantharides (Spanish Fly)

Cantharides has been used by lay people to promote a vague pelvic and genital feeling of priapism, since its toxic nature irritates the bladder and urethra. Some reports of permanent penile damage associated with its use have been made (Munjack, 1979).

Stimulants

Generally, men tend toward the use of stimulants, while women prefer depressants. For amphetamines, it appears that the sexual effect they promote bears a close relationship to the sexual adjustment of the individual concerned (Bell and Trethowan, 1961), and the effect, therefore, can be a highly variable one. Cocaine, while socially stimulating, is reported to divert attention from sexual interest (Parr, 1976).

Hallucinogens: Lysergic Acid (LSD)

Reported experiences with this drug indicate that sexual thoughts and behavior become irrelevant. When sex would occur, the experience could be intense and mystical; and because of the time-expanding property of the drug, it would seem prolonged. Unfortunately, there is wide variability in individual experiences with this drug and in the same individual from time to time or dose to dose (Parr, 1976); the effect of this drug on sexual behavior is, therefore, quite unpredictable.

Marijuana

Kolodny and associates (1974) report a study of 20 heterosexual males who were chronic marijuana users compared with 20 male controls who never used marijuana. While sexual function remained unimpaired in all marijuana users but one, they did exhibit a statistically significant decrease in plasma testosterone levels. In two subjects who discontinued marijuana use, these levels subsequently and dramatically reverted to normal. The implications of these findings are unclear.

Methadone, Heroin

In one study (Cicero et al, 1975) of 29 methadone-treated persons, 16 heroin addicts, and 43 narcotic-free controls, ejaculatory volume (secretions from seminal vesicles and prostate) was diminished by 50 per cent in narcotic users. Likewise, serum testosterone levels were decreased by 43 per cent. Sperm motility was lower than normal in the narcotic users. The study sample was small; with the exception of the measurement of sperm motility, the observed differences were not statistically significant.

Forty consecutive admissions of female heroin addicts to a gynecological service were reported (Bai et al, 1974). Amenorrhea was noted in 45 per cent, oligomenorrhea in 15 per cent, polymenorrhea in 12 per cent, hypomenorrhea in 7.5 per cent, and menorrhagia in 2 per cent.

Addicts report that heroin tends to depress sexual desire and interfere with performance in males and diminish sensation in females (Parr, 1976). Some men may complain of erectile dysfunction or retarded ejaculation while taking heroin and report difficulty with premature ejaculation when "off" heroin. Since heroin withdrawal may be characterized by a genital excitation, the premature ejaculation may be a symptom of withdrawal from the drug rather than represent an occurrence in the drug-free state (Mintz et al, 1974).

More information on social drugs can be found in Chapter 29, Mental Illness, Substance Abuse, and Sexuality.

THE NURSING PROCESS

The initial sexual assessment of the client should include any past history of sexual dysfunction that the client may attribute to the use of drugs (See Chapter 2, Sexual Health Care). This assessment should extend to an assessment of nonprescription drug use, particularly chronic abuse (e.g., laxative abuse), and an estimate of the nature and frequency of recreational drug use. (Nonjudgmental interviewing techniques are presented in Chapter 29, Mental Illness, Substance Abuse, and Sexuality.) All documented drug use, prescription, nonprescription, or recreational, should have an associated list of side effects or problems that the client attributes to them.

These data should be used in consultation with other health professionals who are involved in determining therapeutic interventions. This information is important for the nurse in formulating individualized, appropriate, and effective interventions. The most important of these interventions specific to drug use is client education.

The questionable quality of the data on sexual dysfunction attributable to drugs, which is so often lacking vital information on actual risk, and the biological variability inherent in our species, suggest a prudent course of action in determining client education strategies. The style and content of this education should reduce client anxiety about drug therapy yet leave the person intellectually equipped to anticipate events that may occur. The key component of this education is to impart to the client a sense of control of the situation.

In all cases, there should be an emphasis on the quality of the professional relationship, the degree of rapport, the necessity of the therapy being acceptable to the individual in all aspects (with a spoken contract to change therapy if it is not), and a subtle and sensitive monitoring of drug effect on sexual behavior.

SUMMARY

The literature on drug-associated sexual dysfunction is extensive. It ranges from isolated case reports that lack denominator data and therefore estimates of frequency to study groups with proportions of sexual dysfunction that fail to convey a proper perspective on the level of sexual dysfunction attributable to drug use, and to clinical trials that, because they test different hypotheses, fail to evaluate fully the occurrence of sexual dysfunction side effects.

The crucial factor in understanding drug-induced sexual dysfunction is an appreciation of the variability that exists not only from person to person but also in the same individual at different times and at different doses. Certain people are exquisitely sensitive to a particular drug effect, while others remain functional regardless of dose. Therefore, no indictment of a drug should remain absolute; the decision to prescribe it must always reflect a careful balance of its risk versus its benefit.

REFERENCES

Abramowicz M (ed): Drugs that cause sexual dysfunction. Med Lett Drugs Ther 25:641, 1983.

Abramowicz M (ed): Drugs that cause sexual dysfunction. Med Lett Drugs Ther 29:65–67, 1987.

Ahmad S: Disopyramide and impotence. So Med J 73:958, 1980.

Ananth J: Impotence associated with pimozide. Am J Psych 139:1374, 1982.

Ashton H: Adverse effects of prolonged benzodiazepine use. Adv Drug React Bull 118:440–443, 1986.

Bai J, et al: Drug related menstrual aberrations. Obstet Gynecol 44:713–719, 1974.

Barsky A: Hidden reasons some patients visit doctors. Ann Int Med 94:492–498, 1981.

Barton JL: Orgasmic inhibition by phenelzine. Am J Psych 136:1616–1617, 1979.

Bell DS, Trethowan WH: Amphetamine addiction and disturbed sexuality. Arch Gen Psych 4:74–78, 1961.

Berger SH: Trifluoperazine and haloperidol: Sources of ejaculatory pain? Am J Psych 136:350, 1979.

Bulpitt CJ, et al: Change in symptoms of hypertensive patients after referral to hospital clinic. Br Heart J 38:121–128, 1976.

Burnett WC, Chanine RA: Sexual dysfunction as a complication of propranolol therapy in men. Cardiovasc Med 4:811–815, 1979.

Choonara IA, Rosenbloom L, Smith CS: Clonazepam: Sexual precocity. N Engl J Med 312:185, 1985.

Cicero TJ, et al: Function of the male sex organs in heroin and methadone users. N Engl J Med 292:882–887, 1975.

Clyne CAC: Gynaecomastia: First report. Br Med J 292:380–388, 1986.

Committee of Principal Investigators, WHO: A cooperative trial in the primary prevention of ischaemic heart disease using clofibrate. Br Heart J 40:1069–1118, 1978.

Coronary Drug Project Research Group: Clofibrate and niacin in coronary heart disease. JAMA 231:360–381, 1975.

Croog SH, et al: Sexual symptoms in hypertensive patients: A clinical trial of antihypertensive medications. Arch Intern Med 148:788–794, 1988.

Dawson-Butterworth K: Idiopathic priapism associated with schizophrenia. Br J Clin Pract 23:125–126, 1969.

Dawson-Butterworth K: Priapism and phenothiazines. Br Med J 4:118, 1970.

Ditman KS: Inhibition of ejaculation by chlorprothixene. Am J Psych 120:1004–1005, 1964.

Douglass-Jones AP, Cruickshank JM: Once-daily dosing with atenolol in patients with mild or moderate hypertension. Br Med J 1:990–991, 1976.

Epstein DL, Grant WM: Carbonic anhydrase inhibitor side effects. Serum chemical analysis. Arch Ophthalmol 95:1378–1382, 1977.

Fagan TC, Johnson DG, Grosso DS: Metronidazole: Gynaecomastia: First report? JAMA 254:3217–3218, 1985.

Forsberg L, et al: Impotence, smoking, and beta-blocking drugs. Fertil Steril 31:589–591, 1979.

Fraunfelder FT, Meyer SM: Sexual dysfunction associated with timolol eyedrops. JAMA 253:3092–3093, 1985.

Freyhan F: Loss of ejaculation during mellaril treatment. Am J Psych 118:171–172, 1961.

Gartrell N: Trazodone: First report of increased libido in women: 3 cases. Am J Psych 143:781–782, 1986.

Gifford LM, et al: Cimetidine postmarket outpatient surveillance program: Interim report on phase I. JAMA 243:1532–1535, 1980.

Greenberg HR: Inhibition of ejaculation by chlorpromazine. J Nerv Mental Disorder 152:364–366, 1971.

Heller J: Another case of inhibition of ejaculation as a side effect of mellaril. Am J Psych 118:173, 1961.

Hogan MJ, et al: Antihypertensive therapy and male sexual dysfunction. Psychosomat 21:234–237, 1980.

Hollifield JW, et al: Proposed mechanisms of propranolol's antihypertensive effect in essential hypertension. N Engl J Med 295:68–73, 1976.

Jensen RT, et al: Cimetidine-induced impotence and breast changes in patients with gastric hypersecretory states. N Engl J Med 308:883–887, 1983.

Johnson P, et al: Treatment of hypertension with methyldopa. Br Med J 1:133–137, 1966.

Klein EA, Montague DY, Steiger E: Fat emulsion: Priapism with IV infusion: 2 case reports. J Urol 133:857–859, 1985.

Knarr JW: Impotence from propranolol? Ann Int Med 85:259, 1976.

Kolodny RC, et al: Depression of plasma testosterone levels after chronic intensive marihuana use. N Engl J Med 290:872–874, 1974.

Kotin J, et al: Thioridazine and sexual dysfunction. Am J Psych 133:82–85, 1976.

Kulik FA, Wilbur R: Case report of painful ejaculation as a side effect of amoxapine. Am J Psych 139:234–235, 1982.

Laver MC: Sexual behaviour patterns in male hypertensives. Austr New Zeal J Med 4:29–31, 1974.

Lazarus A: Mesoridazine: Priapism. J Clin Psychopharmacol 6:60–61, 1986.

Lemere F, Smith JW: Alcohol induced sexual impotence. Am J Psych 130:212–213, 1973.

McHaffie DJ, et al: Impotence in patient on disopyramide. Lancet 1:859, 1977.

Mechanic D: Social psychologic factors affecting the presentation of bodily complaints. N Engl J Med 286:1132–1139, 1972.

Mechanic D: Stress, illness, and illness behaviour. J Human Stress (June)a:2–6, 1976.

Mechanic D: Sex, illness, illness behaviour, and the use of health services. J Human Stress (Dec)b:29–40, 1976.

Mechanic D: Effects of psychological distress on perceptions of physical health and the use of medical and psychiatric facilities. J Human Stress (Dec):26–32, 1978.

Medical Research Council Working Party on Mild to Moderate Hypertension: Adverse reactions to bendrofluazide and propranolol for the treatment of mild hypertension. Lancet 2:539–542, 1981.

Mintz J, et al: Sexual problems of heroin addicts. Arch Gen Psych 31:700–703, 1974.

Miller RA: Propranolol and impotence (Letter). Ann Int Med 85:682–683, 1976.

Mitchell J, Popkin M: Antipsychotic drug therapy and sexual dysfunction in men. Am J Psych 139:633–637, 1982.

Munjack D: Sex and drugs. Clin Toxicol 15:75–89, 1979.

Munjack DJ, Crocker B: Alprazolam: Inhibition of ejaculation: First report. J Clin Psychopharmacol 6:57–58, 1986.

Newman RJ, Salerno HR: Sexual dysfunction due to methyldopa. Br Med J 4:106, 1974.

Parr D: Sexual aspects of drug abuse in narcotic addicts. Br J Addict 71:261–268, 1976.

Patt N: Trazodone: Priapism. Am J Psych 142:783–784, 1985.

Peden NR, et al: Male sexual dysfunction during treatment with cimetidine. Br Med J 1:659, 1979.

Quirk KC, Einarson TR: Sexual dysfunction and clomipramine. Can J Psych 27:228–231, 1982.

Rapp MS: Two cases of ejaculatory impairment related to phenelzine. Am J Psych 136:1200–1201, 1979.

Renshaw DC: Pharmacotherapy and female sexuality. Mod Prob Pharmacopsych 15:145–157, 1980.

Russell JM, MacGregor RJ, Watson I: Prazosin: priapism: 2 case reports. Med J Austr 143:321, 1985.

Sangal R: Alprazolam: Inhibited female orgasm. Am J Psych 142:1223–1224, 1985.

Schwarcz G: Case report of inhibition of ejaculation and retrograde ejaculation as a side effect of amoxapine. Am J Psych 139:233–234, 1982.

Simpson GM, et al: Effects of antidepressants on genitourinary function. Dis Nerv Sys 26:787–789, 1965.

Singh H: A case of inhibition of ejaculation as a side effect of mellaril. Am J Psych 117:1041–1042, 1961.

Smith PJ, Talbert RL: Sexual dysfunction with antihypertensive and antipsychotic agents. Clin Pharm 5:373–384, 1986.

Steeno OP: Male infertility associated with sulphasalazine treatment. Eur J Obstet Gynecol Reprod Biol 18:361–364, 1984.

Stressman J, Ben-Ishay D: Chlorthalidone-induced impotence. Br Med J 281:714, 1980.

Toone BK, et al: Sex hormone changes in male epileptics. Clin Endocrinol 12:391–395, 1980.

Veterans Administration Cooperative Study Group on Antihypertensive Agents: Propranolol in the treatment of essential hypertension. JAMA 237:2303, 1977.

Wallace TR, et al: Decreased libido—A side effect of carbonic anhydrase inhibitors. Ann Ophthalmol 11:1563, 1979.

Warren SC, Warren SG: Propranolol and sexual impotence. Ann Int Med 86:112, 1977.

Warren S, et al: Long-term propranolol therapy for angina pectoris. Am J Cardiol 37:420–426, 1976.

25: Body Image Concerns, Surgical Conditions and Sexuality

Camille Stern

BODY IMAGE

All persons have an internal perception and subjective belief about the way they see themselves and the way in which they believe other persons see them. Body image is a reflected patterning of thoughts, impressions, and individual beliefs about appearance and presentation. It incorporates the total personal realm of physical and emotional experiences. Body image attainment is cumulative and subject to constant change. It is entirely subjective, as we do not have the capacity to view our bodies with the total detachment necessary for complete objectivity. The development of body image begins in infancy and continues throughout the life span. Change results from personal and interpersonal inspections of the self with an identified need for reorganization.

It is important for health professionals to be aware of the significance of body image in their clients. An individual's body image is closely tied to feelings of sexuality. Thus, in severe medical or surgical conditions or trauma in which body image is threatened or actually altered on a temporary or permanent basis there is a resultant impact on the client's feelings of sexuality. If the nurse is to define the total care needs of the client, the nursing process must be extended to cover the alterations in body image that may affect the client's total feeling of self and sexual capacity.

Definition

Roberts defines body image as "the image that an individual holds in the mind of his or her own body . . . [and is] concerned with the individual's subjective experience with his body and the manner in which he has organized these experiences" (Roberts, 1978, p 267–268). This definition recognizes the subjectivity with which body image is viewed and the individual variance that is necessarily a result of human perception. Castledine further defines body image as "a psychological entity deriving from past experiences, social interactions and current sensations, which is gradually built up through the years from physiological, psychological and social components, organized and integrated by the central nervous system" (Castledine, 1981, p 16). Castledine's interpretation adds both the perspectives of depth of development and of complexity, as body image is noted to evolve from the entire environmental exchange. He further notes that body image is "a central concept of the human experience" (Castledine, 1981, p 16).

One aspect of body image to consider is its role in developing individual uniqueness and personality traits (Van der Velde, 1985). Part of our ability to differentiate ourselves from others is the recognition of our singular and particular abilities and talents that make us distinct. These are in turn influential in the development of personality traits. Our own perception of our uniqueness and whether it is positive or negative in part determine the effectiveness of self-presentation. If we perceive ourselves and our potential contributions as worthy and special, then our self-image is more likely to be valued than if we do not visualize those unique talents or abilities within ourselves.

Rubin (1968) notes the high value of the ability to control one's functioning within the confinement of time and space. This relates to the prediction of ability based on the time to carry out a specific activity, the personal space needed to perform the task, *and* the judgment of one's capability to carry out the activity. She further notes that "it is possible to consider a sense of personal success or personal failure in terms of the congruence between intent or expectation of self and the effectiveness of functional control" (Rubin, 1968, p 21–22). The element of control is a critical feature of body image. Judging our ability correctly or incorrectly can strengthen or seriously weaken self-perception and therefore affect body image.

A concept central to the understanding of body image is the body boundary, which is defined differently for each individual person. Although varying in importance to individuals, body image perception includes the entire physical appearance. Selections of a particular style of clothing or jewelry, hairstyles, and make-up for women are reflections of attempts to express a certain outward appearance of the perceived body image.

The definiteness of our body boundaries is expressed by such outward appearances. Some persons have well-defined body borders, which are often demonstrated by an outward image that is immaculate, demonstrating body control. Other persons have less defined borders, demonstrated by less control in their outward appearance. McCloskey offers an example related to the relative importance of fingernails: "Though some people think nothing of biting their nails short, others feel a sense of tragedy when they break a long fingernail" (McCloskey, 1976, p 69). Boundaries are defined

differently for each person and may be defined differently by the same person for particular situations.

Van der Velde proposes a new interpretation and definition of body image, based on several premises:

1. There are multiple and innumerable body images present since humans are not able to view the entire self at any one time.
2. Body images incorporate our interpretations of others' appraisals and evaluations, as well as their reactions to our appearances.
3. The formation of body image includes the perceptions of the physical appearances of others.
4. Body image is important in its necessity for the interaction with others. Any contact with other people, whether verbal, tactile or physical, requires an image of self to be projected. (Van der Velde, 1985, p 527–528).

The framework provided within these premises allows a comprehensive view of the formation and development of individual body image. It reflects the constancy of change and the social elements of body image as other persons help us to determine our own body images and as we try to interact with others.

Of these premises proposed by Van der Velde the most unique is the concept of multiple body images existing simultaneously, which is consistent with the notion of the comprehensive list of factors that are a part of the overall perception of self-image. Because we cannot view our full-body image at one time, it may well be that the constant shifting of images may in fact be composed of many different images, blending into a composite frame.

Van der Velde further elaborates on body image and social management:

Body images thus provide three social functions. They enable man to project how others see him by means of his appearances and actions; they enable him to selectively control the establishment and preservation of a desirable view of himself; and they enable him to create within others impressions that do not precisely reflect his actual self. (Van der Velde, 1985, p 533)

Thus, humans are aware of their image projection in interactions with others and may make an attempt to control the display of that image. The projected image may or may not reflect what the individual considers to be his or her true or ideal self. The difficulties that persons with alterations in body image experience are a result of the loss of ability to control the projected body image. As a result, individuals are no longer able to understand their own body image as it is projected, nor are they able to predict reactions of other persons to the altered body image.

Development

The development of body image begins in early childhood and continually grows and changes with maturational aging. Since body image is a subjective determination, it is open to constant examination based on our perceptions of events. Because perceptions can be easily distorted, and are only partially reality based, an ongoing scrutiny must certainly bring about changes. Our perception of body image grows out of our full realm of experience, including personal, physical, cultural, social, and biological. Because increasing complexity occurs during personality development, individuals encounter more difficulty when changes in body image occur during adulthood (Wassner, 1982). The rapidity with which the circumstances of individual lives are altered will also influence the rate of body image change.

As the learning of body image is a process of interaction, a young child's first perceptions arise from parents, siblings, and other family members. The early recognition of the separation of self from the mother and father is one of the first steps in the formation of body boundaries for the infant.

For the very young child, mastery of physical and motor tasks becomes the foundation for the feelings of control of the self and environment. Gaining mastery of independent mobility within the infant's surroundings is a major step toward positive feelings of self and toward body boundary development. Sex role identification and differentiation also takes place in early childhood. The child begins to recognize maleness or femaleness without any real recognition of the physical attributes of the sexes. This is not to say that traditional sex role stereotypes are essential for recognition to occur. Instead, the child simply must correctly identify sex awareness and a clear self-recognition and differentiation. Hogan defines gender or role behavior as "all we do to disclose ourselves as male or female to others—the external behavior that identifies us. Gender role is not established at birth but is built up cumula-

tively through experience . . . ." (Hogan, 1985, p 4). Further, Hogan notes that acceptance and value of the self as male or female requires a positive sexual self-concept. This sex differentiation and beginning role identification must develop prior to any further boundary expansion.

Adolescence carries with it a special and unique set of body image experiences. At the onset of puberty and the development of actual physical changes, the adolescent is forced to constantly change the body image. During this period, interactions with peers or selected significant others may assume more importance to the adolescent than parental reinforcement. They are not only aware of the changes being experienced within their own bodies, but they are aware of the changes in friends and peers. Carroll (1981) states that awareness of the external body changes will shift as the individual begins to perceive internal changes and to respond to interactions with their peers.

Adolescents' awareness of others leads to a realization that the changes within their own bodies are visible to other persons. They may feel threatened with feelings of insecurity or fear as they compare their own perceived body image to the changing body images of their peers. The process of interaction with the environment and significant others is quite strong during this period. Whether or not the physical changes and the feedback that is received from others is perceived as positive or negative will determine to a large degree whether adolescents emerge with a strong positive body image. Peer acceptance, or the lack of it, heavily influences self-acceptance.

In adulthood, the body image becomes more stable but again is never fully constant or formed. Past experiences provide the foundation of our self-perceptions. As our environment changes, or as we perceive changes in ourselves, the image that we carry must also change. As maturity increases, the adult faces the recognition of physiological adaptation in the body due to age—wrinkles, changes in body hair, and changes in body fat deposition. Reactions to these changes will depend in part on the degree of comfort the person has with the total self. Perceptions of worth, which are most strongly and clearly linked to the physical self, will be profoundly affected by changes that are perceived as less than attractive.

Altered Body Image

Certain physical conditions, trauma, and major illnesses or injuries can cause the need for changes in body image. Often this need for change is sudden, and the client may have to deal with feelings of extreme stress in crisis situations. Part of the difficulty that arises in dealing with body image changes is an awareness on the part of the patient of the loss of uniqueness of the self. The body boundaries must be examined, shuffled, redetermined, and reintegrated into a complete sense of self. Because body image includes all aspects of the environment in which an individual functions, those abilities or attributes that the person may consider to be special are placed highly within the organization of the body image. The loss of those characteristics to which uniqueness and individuality are attributed carries the weight and threat of a psychological crisis.

Castledine notes that there "seems to be a human need to build up some ideas of wholeness" (Castledine, 1981, p 16). Individual wholeness is severely threatened by the sudden appearance of illness or injury that carries some form of disfigurement. Even though body image normally undergoes constant change, there is still a need to maintain a stable and familiar mental picture that is intact from sudden or extreme disruption.

McCloskey (1976) feels that the actual or threatened loss of control as related to body image is very frightening to clients. This is especially true when viewed in terms of the potential loss of control of body functions due to unexpected illness or injury. Further, some losses that may strongly affect the client's body image may be equated (by the client) with loss of life (McCloskey, 1976; Rubin, 1968).

When considering the strength of the need to maintain an intact image, it is important to consider the role played by the media and advertising. Generally, models and actors are seen as perfect or ideal images and demonstrate no visible flaws of face or figure. This provides the client with what may be an unrealistic picture for comparison and an expectation that since the persons seen in the advertisements are both normal and whole, anything less is unacceptable to society. The client will be especially sensitive to comparison when a physiological impairment of a body part or function necessitates a reorganization of body image.

McCloskey (1976) suggests two types of disturbances in body boundaries that may be seen in hospitalized persons. First, difficulty may be experienced when the body wall changes, but the client preserves only an awareness of the original body boundary. Examples of problems that might fall under this type of alteration include colostomies or amputations. There have been actual changes in the body wall that require corresponding changes in the perceived body boundaries. Second, disturbances may happen after changes in body boundaries when the body wall has remained intact. A client might experience this problem after a cerebrovascular accident renders half of the body immobile. The body boundaries are not changed, even though the functional abilities within those boundaries are drastically different.

A sudden and unexpected alteration in body image forces the client to tear down and rebuild images that have been accumulating over a lifetime. As with the expression of any loss, there is naturally a period of grieving through which the client must pass before a healthy reconstruction of the self and the body image can begin.

STAGES OF ALTERED BODY IMAGE

One of the most accepted frameworks identifying stages of altered body image adaptation was described originally by Lee (1970). Using these stages, a client's struggle for adjustment to an altered body image can be viewed with a greater perspective for understanding. Adaptation to an altered body image in a client can be traced through recognition of the disfigurement, distancing, grieving, and reorganization. The stages of adaptation discussed by Lee are impact, retreat, acknowledgment, and reconstruction. Each of these stages are discussed below.

Impact. Lee describes the impact phase as representative of the client's initial encounter with the illness or injury in which awareness develops of the change in the body or body functions. The client may, for a period, enter a state of shock as the reality of the irreversibility of the impairment becomes evident. Sudden alterations create a much stronger impact, as the individual has had no opportunity to begin dealing with the changes.

The dominant expression becomes anxiety, which may result in behavioral expressions poorly controlled by the client. A sense of depersonalization may be assumed as feelings are pushed away to another level, allowing numbness, strangeness, and feelings of unreality to dominate thought patterns. The client becomes very self-centered owing to the situational loss of personal control. Behaviors in this stage, which would not be permitted under normal circumstances, are often allowed and excused. Developmental regression may take place as the client seeks the comfort of dependence on other persons.

Regarding the impact phase, Roberts notes that as the client realizes the injury or illness, "the resulting behavior is a projection onto others of the guilt and shame they feel for themselves. Each might feel a sense of failure in his or her own body" (Roberts, 1978, p 282). Some clients may see the impairment as a deserved and just punishment or as a singular personal injustice.

Retreat. Eventually, the client's anxiety will become so uncomfortable that retreat is necessary. Retreat represents an attempt to return to the stable feelings of the self that existed before the critical event. During this stage, clients may indulge in wishful thinking and try to avoid reality through fantasy. However, as the client has experienced a loss and ultimately must respond to it, this stage provides a needed period of rest, which may be used for beginning the process of reorganization and strengthening. Denying the situation is merely an avenue of escape from what may be an overwhelming situation. The psychological burden of body image reconstruction is enormous. Retreat allows the client to begin sorting and reorganizing a shattered self-image as well as new energy to deal with a problem that ultimately must be handled if the process of daily life is to continue.

Acknowledgment. During acknowledgment, the client actively mourns the loss. Lee states that the client experiences a sense of profound hopelessness. The hopelessness results from the loss of control and the loss of individual uniqueness.

During this stage, Lee describes a sensation of self-not-self, which persons may experience as they attempt to work through a changed body image. Even though illness or injury has resulted in impairment and a new body image is forcibly recognized, there is still a strong image of the "old" body, to which the client clings. Thus, the client has the feelings and sensations of two body images while also knowing that neither one of them is a good "fit." Familiar components of the self will be recognized in the old body image, while the reality of the new body image intrudes on the old images. This results in confusing and distorted feelings as the client seeks to resolve the conflicts of an altered self.

During the acknowledgment phase, clients continue to be very self-centered, focusing primarily on the needs of the self. The client may feel that relationships with family and significant others are threatened and may fear abandonment. Indeed, the family or significant others may be experiencing similar feelings of grieving for the client's lost body image. They too must adapt to the changes if they are to continue providing support to the client.

Reconstruction. Gradually, "the need to mourn is replaced by the decision to try new approaches to living" (Lee, 1970, p 585). It is essential that the cycle be broken if the client is to resume a productive and healthy life. Although grieving is both natural and essential, it must end. The energy required to maintain a crisis state is exhaustive, and the client must seek relief. The major task of this period is for the client to reintegrate positive life forces. During this period, the client must reintegrate altered body image, reorganize social values, and adjust to technical devices or procedures.

Roberts (1978) observes that whether or not a person successfully passes through each of the four stages depends on the person's perception of the actual alteration, the physiological status of the individual, age, nature of the illness or injury, the duration of disability, and previous coping abilities. As is true of the client's original body image development, every area and facet of life must be considered in adaptation.

Body Image and Sexual Function

Acknowledgment of the relationship of body image and sexuality reflects the understanding and acceptance of the interdependence of the mind and body. Change to the body cannot occur without resulting changes to all aspects of the self and self-image. Wassner (1982) notes that the relationship of body image and sexuality is inseparable.

Savage (1981) regards body image and self-concept as interrelated components of the sexual self. Littlefield notes that "high self-esteem is necessary for good sexual relations because this allows an individual freedom to receive pleasure, to search for individual tastes and pleasures, and to ask another to help satisfy his or her needs" (Littlefield, 1977, p 649). Hogan states that "sexuality involves not only gender identity but also sexual self-image or self-concept. Positive sexual self-concept is characterized by acceptance of, comfort with, and value of oneself as male or female. . . . Change or disturbance in body image may negatively affect sexual self-concept" (Hogan, 1985, p 4). However, persons sexually naive prior to a major alteration in body image will probably have a less difficult time in adjustment, as they do not have existing patterns of sexual behaviors to change (McRae and Henderson, 1975). Sexuality as a part of body image is clearly part of the overall self-concept of the individual. How the body image is viewed will directly affect an individual's feelings of sexuality. In order for the total health care needs of clients to be met, sexual health must be addressed as a significant factor in the overall plan of care (Fisher and Levin, 1983).

Effect of Acute Care Settings on Body Image and Sexuality

Hospitalizations for any reason usually cause some degree of anxiety and discomfort on the part of the patients. They are entering unfamiliar surroundings and surrendering a certain amount of control to health professionals who they do not know and may not trust. The client may be concerned and worried about the condition for which admission was necessary and about being separated from family members and significant others. They have been placed in a little hospital room, given a sexless patient gown, and removed from family and friends. Often, only a minimum of personal possessions are allowed, making it difficult for the client to establish a sense of preservation of uniqueness of self or belongingness. Surgical procedures cause discomfort, injury, and fatigue as well as an altered body image. The scars are often seen as disfiguring, and clients may

fear rejection and abandonment if a partner's response to their appearance is negative.

Surgical procedures in particular are troubling. "Surgery is an intense experience, . . . a planned physical assault on the person's body" (Gruendemann, 1975, p 635). Clients must deal with the fear related to the surgery, the anxiety related to the condition requiring the surgery, and the resultant change in body image from the scarring at the incision line. Gruendemann (1975) notes that a client's anxiety over the loss of a body part will depend on the individual's feelings of significance regarding that part as well as on the psychic energy that is focused on the loss.

The unnatural change necessitated by surgery is disruptive (Wassner, 1982). However, it should also be noted that some clients view surgery with positive anticipation, expecting very successful changes in image from the surgical procedure (Gruendemann, 1975). Regardless of whether it is seen by the clients as having positive or negative results, planning of care for these persons must include aspects of body image alterations that the client will definitely experience.

Surgeries that bring about the greatest threat to body image are those directly or indirectly affecting sexual functioning or the client's view of him- or herself as a sexual being (Hogan, 1985). Surgeries involving the sexual organs or those that interrupt the client's self-view of wholeness are especially threatening to body image and sexuality. Many of these clients may feel a sense of abandonment, as a silence on the subject of sexuality is imposed by health care workers (Alexander, 1976).

CANCER

Atwell states that "cancer patients may present a dual set of symptoms: those of physical illness and those of a depressive disorder" (Atwell, 1984, p 123). The care of cancer patients is extremely complex, and both physiological and psychological sets of symptoms must be considered in the planning and delivery of care (the reader is also referred to Chapter 15, Cancer and Sexuality). The impact upon body image and sexuality is closely bound to the symptomatology and effects of the physical illness. The resultant alterations due to treatment create a potential stage for increased depression. Recognition of the interrelatedness of these aspects of care is essential. MacElveen-Hoehn and McCorkle (1985) note that whether or not interventions are successful is in part dependent on the care given to the client during the entire recovery period.

Cancer and Sexual Function

Fisher (1983) lists several elements of cancer that can affect sexuality. First is the biological process of the disease itself. The client may experience distress from the symptoms and may also have fatigue and lowered levels of energy. Second, the personal process of acceptance must be considered—the client has fears of death, mutilation, and pain. Third, cancer treatments often have unsettling side effects on the client's physical as well as psychological comfort. Fourth, the permanent alteration caused by the disease and treatment necessitates changes in sexuality. Last, the family process of accepting the diagnosis of cancer affects the client's adaptability because of the need for a strong support system.

MacElveen-Hoehn and McCorkle (1985) address similar areas of concern related to the sexuality of persons with cancer. Loss and grief are often ongoing owing to recurrence and metastasis. The client may need to be given "permission" to grieve. Symptoms affect not only physical functioning but also psychological adaptation. Alopecia directly affects body image, while pain affects ongoing comfort. The development of rapid fatigue necessitates that careful planning be carried out before engaging in strenuous sexual activity. The impact of cancer on body image and sexuality requires understanding and careful assessment.

Assessment

PSYCHOLOGICAL FACTORS

In assessing the impact of cancer on sexuality, it is important to evaluate the client's personal perspective of sexuality (Williams et al, 1986). This will help determine the emphasis of both assessment and planning and establishing goals and interventions. Fisher (1983) considers it necessary to examine the organic dysfunctions and the psychological impacts when planning care for the sexual effects of cancer treatment. The assault to body image is tremendous. The client faces single or multiple surgeries, alteration or removal of body parts or limbs, altered ability or loss of function, disfigurement and scarring, and the possibility of metastasis and repeated therapies. Fisher (1983) also states that a major outcome in treating cancer patients today is a loss of gender identity. Clients may lose an individual sense of masculinity or femininity. Cancers of the sexual organs directly affect the sexual body image and the patient's feelings of gender and role identity.

Role Function

MacElveen-Hoehn and McCorkle (1985) feel that whether or not couples are able to adapt to the physical and psychosexual traumas involved with cancer treatments is related to the strength and stability of the relationship prior to the diagnosis and onset of symptoms. Because of this variable, it is extremely important to assess both the relationship and the feelings of sexuality that exist between the client and the partner. Whether or not the client chooses to disclose sexual information is a personal matter, but the opportunity should be available. These authors further state that "for the person with cancer, the expression of sexuality may be a treasured part of a relationship signifying love, support and acceptance despite change in bodily appearance or functions" (MacElveen-Hoehn and McCorkle, 1985, p 56). This is especially important when family and sex roles are altered and the client needs to feel valued. Intimate sharing through expressive sexuality can be extremely beneficial in preventing feelings of worthlessness. In addition to a general assessment of the impact of cancer on body image and sexuality, careful assessment and planning based on the type and location of cancer are needed. Alterations in body image will be addressed in the following sections related to radical face and neck surgeries, mastectomies, and ostomies. Specific nursing care will also be discussed.

Radical Head and Neck Surgeries

EFFECT ON ADAPTATION
Physiological Function

Cancers that involve the face, neck, mouth, and throat require aggressive surgeries that excise large amounts of tissue and, as a result, are often extensively disfiguring to the client. Frequently, large portions of bony and soft tissue are removed from the face or neck, such that normal appearance is permanently altered (Dropkin, 1985). Obviously, clients become recognizably different and often fear revealing their face to a new person. Surgeries of the head and neck create alterations in body image that will require an enormous amount of coping, adjustment, and adaptation (Denning, 1982).

Metcalfe and Fischman (1985) discuss an increased incidence of alcohol abuse with clients requiring face and neck surgery for cancer. This in turn can lead to difficulties for male clients in achieving and maintaining erections. Also, they feel that the normal process of physiological aging is an important factor to consider in dealing with the psychological issues of sexuality because this group of clients tends to be older than those experiencing other types of cancers.

Psychological Function

The body image undergoes tremendous assault as the client loses facial features central to self-concept. Dropkin notes that the resulting disfigurement and dysfunction creates "considerable emotional upheaval as defects in the head and neck area are particularly threatening to senses of identity and self-concept" (Dropkin, 1985, p 130). When we consider those attributes that make us unique and different from other people, our faces become the most distinctive and primary attribute of the differentiation of self. Loss or alteration of that facial uniqueness requires almost total rebuilding of the body image. The client suffers body image disturbances within the defined boundaries and may concurrently be forced to extend the boundaries with the presence of a permanent tracheostomy or feeding tube. The difficulties that the client will experience in altering the body image serve to compound the problems of dealing with sexuality. Metcalfe and Fischman relate the following experience:

> A 50-year-old male with a 25-year history of alcohol abuse began to cry when asked about his sexual functioning since his hemimandibulectomy and radical neck dissection. Because he had not been able to have an erection since his surgery 2 years before, he had abruptly ended his relationship with his girlfriend. He exclaimed that he wasn't even able to kiss her because of his feeding tube. His distress was magnified by the fact that no health professional had ever asked him about his sexual concerns. He had suffered alone. (Metcalfe and Fischmann, 1985, p 23)

Interdependence

In addition to the physical disfigurement, cancers in the area of the face and neck may affect three vital structures: larynx, esophagus, and vocal chords. The client must cope not only with severe alterations in facial appearance but also with altered abilities for breathing, eating, and speaking. Loss of the ability to communicate verbally can severely impede relationships with significant others if adequate preparation is not carried out by the health professional.

ASSESSMENT

Metcalfe and Fischman (1985) note that it is the right of a client and the partner to expect that their sexual concerns and needs will be cared for in the same professional manner as their other health needs. Application of the nursing process is essential to the successful outcomes of clients with head and neck cancers. A baseline sexual history and assessment as a part of the total history will provide initial information and make the client realize that sexuality is not a closed subject.

Preoperative assessment of the potential impact on body image and sexuality of the client provides the nurse with the opportunity to establish a relationship based on open communication. Problem areas identified can then be further evaluated prior to and reassessed following surgery.

There is no way that the client can anticipate the visual impact of the injury resulting from the surgical procedure. Reactions must be closely observed in order to plan care. Depending on the nature of the deficit, the client may be a candidate for facial prosthetics or reconstruction. If the client's physician determines that reconstruction or prosthetics are appropriate, this may certainly aid the client in re-establishing body image.

INTERVENTION

Although indirectly related to body image, the client's teaching needs include communication, nutrition, self-care, and suctioning, if a tracheostomy was performed (Patry-Lahey, 1985). Clients' ability and willingness to care for themselves are major steps toward reintegration of the body image because desire to assume this responsibility signifies that they have come to recognize the changes in their body and to want to deal with them.

In all interactions with clients it is important to help them look beyond the surgery to recognize their individuality and importance as persons. Dropkin (1985) recommends that the nursing staff repeatedly express (1) that the surgery was necessary as a life-saving measure; (2) that the disfigurement is confined to a limited area; and (3) that the client's worth as a person has not changed. Each of these measures will help clients to begin to restore their body image and to reinforce it as time passes.

Communication between the client and the partner must be encouraged in order to resume a healthy sexual relationship. The nurse should work with both persons in performing counseling or carrying out interventions that directly or indirectly affect body image. The client and partner need to be aware of the effects that current cancer treatments may have on sexual energy and response, so that they are not alarmed by any changes that may be experienced. Alternative methods of sexual expression, including simply touching and caressing, may be encouraged to relieve any tension that the couple feels toward sexual intercourse.

Mastectomy

The incidence of breast cancer is a major threat to women today. Malignant tumors of the breast are one of the leading causes of death from cancer in North American women aged 35 to 54 and the primary cause of death from all causes in women aged 40 to 44 years (Scott, 1983). The ramifications of this diagnosis are profound, as it impacts both psychological and physiological functioning. Fear will be manifested as the multiple unknown while unpredictable factors are examined. Schain (1985) notes that the actual or potential threat of the loss or mutilation of a woman's breast may create several concerns, including the possibility of a premature death, concern about breast amputation, and anxiety about body image and self-esteem.

MASTECTOMY AND SEXUAL FUNCTION

In American society, the importance of women's breasts becomes apparent from the aspects of both nurturance and appearance. Breasts are seen as symbolizing motherhood and childrearing, emphasizing the traditional feminine role. But perhaps more important to the impact on body image and sexuality is the view of breasts as an essential body part for seduction and the achievement of sexual pleasure. Schain thinks that "we live in a mammocentric era where breasts are glamorized, idealized, and sensationalized" (Schain, 1985, p 200). As a result of this perception, a woman's feelings about her breasts are in part due to an integration of societal values and in part due to the importance that a woman and her partner assign to the breasts (Scott, 1983). Lambert and Lambert (1985) note that the client may feel she is no longer acceptable to society and to significant others and that she may feel especially unacceptable to her sex partner.

The interruption of the body image, and the sexuality of the woman, thus becomes apparent. Since many women equate their attractiveness or sense of worth with their body image and sexuality (Schain, 1985), the possibility of surgical interruption or removal of the breast threatens a part of the body image that the woman may feel is the very core of her femininity. Breast cancer is a disease of all women, not just elderly women, and "psychosexual morbidity is an outgrowth of the woman's stage of life, stage of disease, the type(s) of treatment she must undergo, and the psychologic makeup and coping strategies she characteristically employs" (Schain, 1985, p 200).

Schwartz-Applebaum and colleagues (1984) note that the relationship of the nurse and client is both close and unique. Nurses "have the opportunity to help women identify and adapt to the potential alterations in sexual self-concept, sexual relationships and sexual functioning that may accompany breast cancer treatment" (Schwartz-Applebaum, 1984, p 16). This can only be accomplished through skillful use of the nursing process in the assessment of the client and in the planning of specific interventions.

ASSESSMENT

There are three areas of assessment to consider that strongly affect the woman's self-image: body image, sexuality, and the strength of the client and partner's relationship, if one currently exists.

Body image assessment should begin prior to the surgery by noting the woman's concern for and attention to her appearance. This will provide visible clues to understanding her individual body boundaries and the importance that she may consequently attach to an intact body image and sexual image. Understanding the client's body image before surgery creates a clearer picture of the client's needs in the postoperative state.

After surgery, the nurse should analyze the severity of the body image disruption and plan for interventions to increase the client's adaptation to the altered image (Carroll, 1981). Removal of the breast creates a distortion between the body image that has been created and stored over time and the new reality of the altered appearance and sensations (Kriss, 1981). The distortion must be eliminated before a healthy body image can be re-established. The client must learn to accept herself. She should be able to learn to view her nude body without awkward or negative feelings (Kriss, 1981).

Frank (1981) offers a simple yet comprehensive plan for the sexual assessment of mastectomy clients. Basically, she suggests a three-part program, with each counseling session divided into assessment (asking questions and evaluating answers), information sharing (giving the patient information about the way in which the mastectomy may affect sexuality), and discussion (answering questions and offering suggestions). This process is best begun during the early admission period, as it establishes an open atmosphere for the patient to express her concerns and feelings.

Frank (1981) also lists some guidelines that will help ensure the success of the interviews:

- Ensure privacy.
- Create a relaxed atmosphere.
- Allow plenty of time for the client to answer questions.
- Use language that can be understood rather than technical jargon.
- Begin with general questions.
- Do not overreact by expressing shock or underreact by appearing bored.
- Preface questions with "how" or "when" instead of "did you."
- If the client does not have a regular sexual

partner, hypothetical questions may be asked.
- Encourage the client to discuss her concerns with her partner, and to let him attend the counseling sessions.

The sexual history should be brief, with general questions (Frank, 1981). This will create an open atmosphere of communication and introduce the subject of the client's sexuality. It will also provide the opportunity to evaluate the type and intensity of counseling that the client may need after the mastectomy. The actual questions to be asked in the assessment should include frequency of intercourse, frequency of orgasm, and the client's overall satisfaction with her sexual relationship.

Schain provides pointers for identifying high-risk clients who may require additional or special assistance. Women who might fall in this category include those who exhibit the following:

1. Have a hypertrophic investment in or are displeased with their breasts (especially those who have had augmentation mammoplasty).
2. Have negative views of self or femininity.
3. Reveal a history of frustrated or unpleasant sexual experiences.
4. Have been sexually abused.
5. Are apprehensive about finding a new sexual partner.
6. Acknowledge the absence of a significant support system.
7. Are uncomfortable when disclosing personal concerns, especially about sexual practices or reactions.
8. Experience serious physical disability associated with pain, arm edema, chest wall discomfort, or side effects associated with treatment. (Schain, 1985, p 203)

It is important to assess the strength of the relationship between the client and her sexual partner. Wellisch (1985) describes several variables on which to assess the closeness of the relationship: (1) the status of the relationship before the cancer developed; (2) the longevity of the marriage or relationship; (3) the stage of the breast cancer, especially as this influences the treatment that will be required; (4) the point in the course of the illness, i.e., primary treatment or recurrent or progressive disease; and (5) the interpersonal skills available to the partners, especially their ability to empathize and communicate. Schain (1985) notes that a single woman who may not have easy access to a partner may have more difficulty testing sexual feelings than a woman who already has a trusted partner. Obviously, the assessment of the presence or absence of a strong relationship will help to guide the planning and interventions that may be necessary for the individual patient.

INTERVENTION

The reintegration of body image is one of the primary factors surrounding the psychological and sexual selves of the woman undergoing mastectomy. Scott (1983) lists several goals for the postoperative period: (1) restoring feelings of attractiveness and desirability as a woman; (2) obtaining correct fit and using with comfort a breast prosthesis; (3) feeling a sense of balance in body movement; (4) experiencing minimal or no phantom sensation; (5) being able to participate in normal pleasurable activities (e.g., swimming, wearing pretty clothes, going out socially); (6) resuming normal, pleasurable sexual relations; and (7) being able to make decisions about breast reconstruction. Preoperative assessment and the establishment of a therapeutic relationship will aid the progression of these goals.

The client should be protected from comments implying that she has merely a problem of vanity as she selects a prosthesis or attempts to deal with the possibility of reconstructive surgery (Kriss, 1981; Winder and Winder, 1985). Other persons may attempt to tell the woman that she should be thankful for her life and to forget about the lost breast. Statements such as these reflect a lack of understanding of the relationship of body image and the sexual self to the overall self-esteem of the woman. The loss of a breast is the loss of a sexual organ. Adequate time and support must be given to the woman during the inevitable period of grief that follows such a traumatic assault on the central core of the self.

The reintegration of body image continues until the woman is able to view comfortably the incision or scar and to touch and accept the appearance of her anatomy after surgery (Scott, 1983). Accomplishing these actions is a major step toward the re-establishment of a new body image.

To foster communication and understanding between the client and her partner, the woman should be encouraged to ask him to participate in the teaching and counseling sessions. An atmosphere should be established that is comfortable for the couple and that allows and promotes question and answer periods. Of course, the amount of information regarding the surgery itself, the resultant alterations in shared sexual experiences, and the need for structured counseling will vary greatly. The nurse working with the couple should be prepared for open communication on a variety of levels in order to best meet their individual needs.

The client and her partner should be counseled about sexual positions to assume after surgery. Early after surgery and the return home, the woman will be more comfortable if the incision area is relieved from pressure, which may occur from a male partner's weight if he assumes the superior position. Also, phantom pain and discomfort may be relieved by gently rubbing the area. The patient may have difficulty fully undressing to reveal the incision site. This is a matter that must be worked out by the couple in a comfortable manner. Finally, the couple should understand that there is no real rush to resume a sexual relationship that includes intercourse until they are both ready. Initially, more comfort may be derived for both the client and her partner by shared closeness and more gentle or alternative expressions of their sexuality. Regardless of the direction selected by the couple, it is essential that they understand the importance of open and direct communication to solve problems and concerns. "Successful sexual adaptation is the result of desire, persistence, and allowing feelings to mature" (MacRae and Henderson, 1975, p 595).

ENTEROSTOMAL SURGERIES

Cancers of the colon and rectum are often referred to as the cancers that no one talks about. Our society regards the functions of elimination as personal and private. Because of this, a person undergoing ostomy surgery may harbor preconceived ideas that may actually be based on erroneous assumptions. Ostomies create an actual physical change in the body and alter elimination patterns. This requires an alteration in body image and thus strongly affects sexual functioning (Dobkin and Broadwell, 1986).

Effects on Adaptation
PHYSIOLOGICAL FUNCTION

Very real concerns may be expressed by the male regarding erectile difficulties. In some cases of rectal or intestinal surgeries that are quite extensive, there may be some damage to the nerves that control erection and ejaculation (Penninger, Moore, and Frager, 1985; Renshaw, 1983). Preoperatively, the client should be given accurate information regarding the potential for loss. At the same time, although he should not be given false hope, the nurse should not allow all hope to fade.

PSYCHOLOGICAL FUNCTION

Reactions to the surgery are varied, depending on the underlying problem prompting the surgery. Renshaw (1983) notes that "the asymptomatic person, in whom a silent cancer has been found, faces this bodily invasion with a complex reaction of disbelief and denial; yet a client whose chronic bowel disease causes constant pain, fatigue, and invalidism welcomes surgical creation of a stoma as a dreamed of relief" (Renshaw, 1983, p 113).

Clients experiencing enterostomal surgery often experience profound disturbances in body image. Although the stoma, beneath the clothing, cannot be seen by other persons, the ostomate may worry about it constantly. There are almost constant fears of odor and leakage. Although these occurrences are rare, the client's worry and fear during an ordinary day is usually much worse than if leakage actually occurred (Renshaw, 1983).

Because the body image must be extended to include the ostomy, the body boundaries must be altered. Gloeckner (1984) notes that this body image disturbance concerns the client's sexuality, especially when viewed against the societal norms of youth, beauty, and wholeness.

Assessment

While assessments are being performed, the nurse should take advantage of the opportunity to establish rapport and to plan for continuity of care. The client is more likely to respond to questions of sexuality if there is not a new face asking the questions or performing the counseling sessions each time. Assessment of the client and his or her feelings of the self should continue throughout preoperative interactions.

There are two studies regarding ostomy surgery that can be helpful in determining patient needs for assessment. In the first study, conducted by Gloeckner (1984), perceptions of sexual attractiveness following surgery were measured. Of the client responses, 60 per cent felt a decrease in feelings of sexual attractiveness from before surgery to the year following ostomy surgery. There were also many negative comments related to the change in body image, disfigurement, and ugliness associated with the stoma. The second study, conducted by Rolstad, Wilson, and Tebbitt (1982), was designed to determine the sexual concerns of individuals with an ileostomy after physical recovery from surgery. A total of 66 per cent responded that sex was not more physically difficult, while 50 per cent stated that sex was more psychologically difficult after surgery. Of the male respondents, 24 per cent noted that their ability to obtain and sustain an erection had been negatively affected. Finally, 60 per cent of the women and 52 per cent of the men felt less sexually desirable after surgery. These studies point to the dramatic changes in body image and sexuality that clients feel as the result of ostomy surgery.

Prior to the surgery, it is important to take a sexual history to determine the client's feelings about the surgery and to begin to evaluate the potential impact upon body image and sexuality. Even though placement of the ostomy is not visible to the general public, and the surgery does not directly involve sexual organs, the impact on body image may be quite intense. The client may feel that following the surgery and the resultant change in their outward appearance they are no longer attractive or desirable (Dobkin and Broadwell, 1986).

One of the reasons the impact of this surgery is so strong on body image stems from the loss of personal control (Rubin, 1968). Rubin feels that any loss of control will result in the appearance of shame in the client. Although there is nothing shameful about any function of the body, clients may experience feelings of shame owing to the inability to control for appropriateness in time and place (Rubin, 1968). The loss of control in this case relates to the ability to control elimination, which is a very basic developmental task accomplished in childhood. The client may feel some sense of developmental regression, which increases the sense of loss of control.

The reaction of the client may well be related to the length of time since diagnosis. Someone who has suffered from long-term and chronic bowel disease will probably not have as difficult an adjustment as someone who has been living with the diagnosis for only a short period of time. Another important factor in assessment is how the client views body functions. To elicit this information, it may be helpful to ask whether they have known someone with an ostomy and how they responded to that person. Negative impressions may become more obvious through this indirect assessment than through direct questioning. In this assessment, as in all done of body image and sexuality, it is important to be sensitive to the clients' values and to respect their sensitivity to the discussion of areas that they regard as extremely personal (Penninger, Moore, and Frager, 1985).

Intervention

Re-establishing a firm body image should begin in the immediate postoperative period. Although clients should not be forced into participating in ostomy care before they are ready, regaining recognition of the self can be encouraged through careful planning and communication. Allowing participation is not equivalent to forcing it, and the client should be encouraged to assist only when it is appropriate. Handling the appliance items may be a first step. The nurse may want to place a mirror so that the client can observe the procedure. Although clients may express reluctance to view the procedure, a mirror allows them to take first glimpses covertly and to begin to extend their body image boundaries.

In the postoperative period, the nurse can encourage the beginning of body image reintegration. Penninger, Moore, and Frager (1985) offer suggestions for helping the person with an ostomy overcome feelings of depersonalization and loss of sexuality. Although these suggestions were written for males, they may be easily adapted to be of value for female ostomates. First, clients should be encouraged to wear their own clothing, even if it creates slight difficulty with ostomy management. Even a familiar old bathrobe will be better than remaining in a hospital gown. Second, clients should use their own toiletries, especially aftershaves, colognes, and perfumes. Familiar and personal scents help to restore the body image and thus sexuality. Privacy should be provided whenever clients wish to be alone, by themselves or with a significant other. Finally, the nurse might offer to discuss sexual concerns with the partner.

Resuming a sexual relationship is dependent on the condition of the healing wound and the client's overall feeling of well-being (Penninger, Moore, and Frager, 1985). Before the client has received medical permission to resume sexual activities, it is important that sexual counseling be offered. After talking with the client, the nurse might offer to talk with the partner or to talk with them together. Three points that will help the couple as they re-establish intimacy are open and honest communication, good personal hygiene, and a good sense of humor (Penninger, Moore, and Frager, 1985; Renshaw 1983). The couple should be advised not to feel rushed to resume intercourse but to take the time to enjoy the closeness and comfort they draw from each other and to seek sexual fulfillment in alternate ways. In all phases of re-establishing the sexual relationship, it is essential that communication between the patient and partner be preserved. They must be able to discuss their fears and concerns with each other before a healthy relationship can be resumed.

There are several concerns about sexual intercourse frequently expressed by ostomates: problems with odor, emptying the pouch, drainage and leakage, and positional comfort (Simmons, 1983). Prior to any sexual activities, it is a good idea for the client to check the appliance for placement and to empty any accumulated fecal material. If the pouch is firmly secured, it should remain in place without any difficulty. There should not be any odor if the appliance is secure, but additional deodorant or colognes may help the client to feel more comfortable. If leakage does occur, the appliance should be changed. The client should simply state to the partner that the appliance is leaking and that it must be changed. Both client and partner should be encouraged to experiment with sexual positions to determine which are most comfortable and satisfying. The only restrictions would be related to comfort at the site of the stoma, especially with sexual intercourse in the early postoperative period, and the position of the appliance interfering with closeness or causing psychological distress.

The ostomate who is single and may not currently have a sexual partner may express concerns about beginning a relationship. There may be questions regarding whether or not to tell the potential partner about the ostomy and the best time to do so. In general, it is better to tell the partner before beginning sexual activities. In doing so, Renshaw (1983) cautions that clients carefully consider their motives and timing. Some clients may set themselves up for rejection by blurting out the information without any sensitivity or by telling the other person too early in the relationship. Simmons (1983) offers the advice that if the person rejects the ostomate, then perhaps that person probably was not someone with whom a healthy sexual relationship would have developed anyway.

The last area of consideration in planning interventions will be specifically addressed to male clients. If after attempting to resume sexual relationships, men find that achieving erection has become a problem, they should seek advice from their physician. An option for these men is a penile prosthesis, silicone or inflatable, which is inserted into the penis and will again make sexual intercourse possible. Counseling and testing is required prior to this surgical intervention, however, to ensure that the erectile disorder is physiological and not psychological in origin.

AMPUTATIONS

Effect on Adaptation

PHYSIOLOGICAL FUNCTION

The need for amputations may be caused by many different traumas, diseases and surgical conditions. The client experiences a loss of control in some aspects of mobility. For upper extremity amputees, the loss is the ability to manipulate their environment as effectively as before the amputation. Lower extremity amputees lose the ability to ambulate without assistive devices. All amputations carry significant impact on body image and sexuality.

PSYCHOLOGICAL FUNCTION

Comfort notes that a "sense of castration or mutilation is a predominant problem in both sexes" (Comfort, 1978, p 229). With the loss of lower extremities, men may equate the loss with castration, while women fear the mutilation of body parts that often draw admiring

glances and appreciation from men. Losses of upper extremities are often more visible, thus creating additional anxieties about coming in contact with unfamiliar people. In contrast, Comfort states that "concealed disability may produce more serious psychosexual difficulties than overt, because it has at some time during intimacy to be revealed" (Comfort, 1978, p 230).

Assessment

Two areas that require assessment preoperatively are the client's current level of sexual functioning and communication patterns between the client and partner. Establishing a sexual history is important in identifying the existing relationship in order to help the couple return to a similar level of sexual satisfaction. Open communication is essential for both the patient and the partner to be able to express their fears and concerns openly.

The intensity of experiences surrounding alterations in body image are varied. Whether or not the client has time prior to the surgery to begin to prepare psychologically will certainly affect the length of time required for adjustment. In traumatic amputations, the loss is quite sudden and extremely difficult for the person to deal with. An overall feeling in an amputee of being unattractive or unlovable may create similar feelings in a sexual relationship (Lambert and Lambert, 1985).

Intervention

The problems that amputees most frequently describe as interfering with sexual activities include upsetting established patterns of coital behaviors, interference with balance, phantom pain, and depression (Comfort, 1978; Conine and Evans, 1982). If in the past the client has been the more active participant in sexual activities, then "the need to change may be threatening, not only to sexual expression, but to the individual's view of the sex role" (Hogan, 1985, p 403). Thus, it may be helpful to work with the client and partner in discussing and exploring ways in which accustomed roles in the relationship, and in sexual activities, may change.

Difficulties with balance will be primarily experienced by lower extremity amputees.

The mechanics of sexual positioning may need to be altered (Lambert and Lambert, 1985). The couple should be advised to experiment with various positions until adequate balance is obtained. Upper extremity amputees may need to alter sleeping positions to relieve pressure on the affected arm. Likewise, in side-lying positions of intercourse, the unaffected arm would need to be superior in order for the client to have more control over sexual activities and intercourse.

Phantom pain is a very real phenomenon that can be greatly distressing to the client during sexual activity and intercourse. For some reason, unrelated healthy parts of the body may act as trigger zones, setting off episodes of pain (Conine and Evans, 1982). The client should be forewarned of the possibility of this occurrence. Appropriate measures of pain relief from phantom sensation can be prescribed by the physician or surgeon. The phantom pain may be particularly intense for either male or female clients during orgasm.

Depression may occur as a result of the surgery, pain, alteration in body image, and sexual disturbances. If severe enough, erectile dysfunction and loss of desire appear in the amputee. Counseling should be provided to prevent the circular relationship of depression, erectile dysfunction, and further depression.

THERMAL INJURIES

Thermal injuries constitute one of the most psychologically and physiologically devastating injuries known. Clients suffer through the process of recovery for many months, and for some, years. They are separated from family and friends and placed in a world that brings mostly pain and discomfort as health professionals attempt to promote healing and recovery of the damaged skin and underlying tissues.

Effects on Adaptation

The shock to the body image is enormous, especially for persons with burn injuries that involve the face, head, and neck. The client experiences a great deal of pain and altered sensation in the body. The system for environmental exchange between the body and its surrounding area has been altered.

The body image boundaries undergo continuous contractions and expansions (Lambert and Lambert, 1985). The process of dressing changes and whirlpool debridements alter the body boundaries, while the application of fresh dressings may represent new body boundaries to the client. With the loss of skin and accompanying sensation, the client is not able to feel where his body stops and the environment begins. Thus, the application of dressings may serve as a protective barrier and as a separation of the self from the world, since the damaged skin can no longer serve this function.

Sexuality does not become a concern for the client in the early postburn period. The first few days and weeks are occupied with physiological stabilization of the patient and promoting and protecting growth of skin. As the client begins to realize the extent of the injuries, there may be concern over rejection from both new persons and family members (Lambert and Lambert, 1985).

Clients may begin to believe that their disability threatens their capacity to be loved by others. Lambert and Lambert (1985) note that minor burns of the genitalia may cause more emotional distress than more serious burns elsewhere on the body. Men may fear castration from burns involving the perineum and penis.

Assessment

Assessment of the body image and sexuality of clients experiencing thermal injuries represents a major challenge to the nurse and other health professionals because there is no opportunity for assessment of stability of these areas prior to the injury. The period for assessment must be one of rebuilding and planning for the reintegration of the new body image.

As soon as stabilization has occurred, initial sexuality assessments can be carried out. The nurse will usually have to begin the discussion, as the client may not be comfortable initiating a conversation on the subject. Providing for open communication and discussion of the client's concerns and fears will be extremely valuable as the client tries to work through feelings. There must be appropriate counseling for sexual partners of the burned victims, who may be so overwhelmed by the enormity of the injuries that they are uncomfortable even considering the return to a sexual relationship.

Intervention

One of the most important interventions to utilize in working with the thermally injured client is to continue to reinforce the individual's worth as a person. The threat to body image and sense of self is extremely profound, and yet the needs in this area can be overlooked because of the intensity of physical nursing care required.

A returning sense of sexuality for the client and partner can only be provided when each person is allowed to express their individual concerns and appropriate counseling has been provided. There should be time planned for the client and partner to be alone to talk in order to begin working through their changed perceptions of the individual's appearance.

Encouragement should be given for allowing expressions of closeness and tenderness without having to feel pressured to perform sexual intercourse until the client and partner are ready. Especially in severe and extensive burns, the partner may fear hurting the client. In order for a healthy relationship to resume, the couple must allow adequate time for adjustment and must develop open communication.

OBESITY

Obesity is considered one of the most severe health problems in the United States today. Being overweight not only creates psychological problems but also can lead to serious health impairments, such as hypertension, cardiovascular disease, and diabetes mellitus. In general, more women than men are found to be overweight or obese. The normal values for measuring height and weight are usually taken from insurance tables, which offer a fairly wide range of values within any given value set. Weight exceeding the normal range by 10 per cent is classified as overweight; by 20 per cent obese; and by 100 per cent, morbidly obese. Pietrantuono (1983) states that adolescence and pregnancy are associated with definite changes in health norms and behaviors and may indeed be triggers for the development of obesity.

The origins of obesity—whether from physiological or psychological causes—are widely debated. Current theories describe an interaction between physical and emotional causes. "The interaction of a possible predisposition to obesity with socioenvironmental influences and a probable developmental or psychological basis, rather than a single cause is the accepted etiology of obesity today" (White, 1982, p 195). Complex interactions exist between the stress in the individual's life and society's reactions to the person (McBride, 1982). Contributing factors cited by Pietrantuono (1983) include the relationship of energy intake exceeding energy expenditure and the possibility that obesity represents insecurity in the obese persons, who eat to console themselves. Food has emotional connotations stemming from family background and interactions. Because this may be problematic, eating behavior lends itself to distortion (Gentry, 1984).

Society and its expectations have a tremendous responsibility for both the development of obesity and the lack of compassion for those persons who suffer from it. Contributing to the development of obesity is what Gentry (1984) describes as the irrational way our society deals with food. This in itself is a double-sided issue: Foods are used to symbolize great rewards and temptations in advertisements, yet it is the rare individual who can freely indulge in highly caloric foods and not experience an unsettling weight gain. Society idolizes slimness, just as advertisements flaunt it. This combination can contribute to an overweight person's setting unrealistic goals for behaviors.

In addition to its contributing role in the development of obesity, society also has an impact on obese persons through its ability for cruelty and lack of tolerance for their overweight condition. Gentry (1984) notes serious social complications, as job and school opportunities are impaired. Obese persons also must pay more for their oversized clothing. Pietrantuono (1983) states that negative attitudes are especially prevalent during adolescence, hindering normal psychological adjustment and creating devastating effects. Obese adolescents are seen as less attractive, with fewer opportunities for dating and acceptance among peers. In young women especially, this leads to lowered self-esteem and self-hatred. "This social attitude, implying that the obese suffer from a moral weakness, generates a kind of 'shame' therapy that is often justified by the known medical hazards of overweight" (Fitzgerald, 1985, p 154). There is a general failure on the part of the public and health professionals to allow that obesity is anything more than a failure of the individual's will power.

This devaluation of self creates cyclical problems with body image. The obesity creates intense feelings of decreased self-esteem and self-worth, which in turn can lead to an increase in obesity (White, 1982). This cycle can be extremely difficult to break. Morbidly obese patients often have conflicts between their actual physical appearances and their perceived body images (Stout, 1982). The image that they would like to see is quite different from the one that actually exists. The subjectivity with which body image is viewed prevents a full recognition of true self-image.

Obesity and Sexual Function

Relationships among obesity, body image, and sexuality are far more elusive to uncover. "In our culture slenderness is equated with attractiveness to such an extent that one might conclude that obesity and sexual enjoyment are mutually exclusive. The relationship between obesity and sex is far from simple and direct. Weight increase may be the response to sexual frustration or serve as a defense against sexuality" (Jacobson, 1974, p 51). Decreased self-esteem coupled with societal rejection creates a difficult barrier for the obese person to overcome in the search for sexual fulfillment. Certainly a need to have a more positive self-image is one of the reasons why obese persons seek surgical treatment for weight reduction. Whichever method is selected by the client and physician, counseling will probably increase the likelihood of success for weight reduction and maintenance.

Assessment

Whether the client is seeking surgical intervention for weight reduction or is undergoing other medical or surgical procedures, the presence of obesity may impede the delivery of care. Adequate assessment of the client's needs is imperative. One of the first steps is to validate that the state of obesity is troublesome for the client (White and Schroeder,

1981). This in turn may lead to a discussion of the motivation for eating, which is a highly individualized matter. Without self-initiated motivation and the validation of the need for weight loss, no interventions for weight loss will be successful. It is important during this period for health professionals to be aware of their interactions with the obese client. As society is highly prejudiced against obesity, so also are health professionals involved in the direct care. Prejudices that may further damage the client's body image should not be allowed to affect the care a health professional provides. Clients do not need lectures on obesity but may need instead simple compassion and reassurance of their worth as a person.

Intervention

In setting goals for the obese individual, McBride notes the importance of being realistic:

To the extent that treatment goals reinforce the limited cultural designation of what is an appropriate weight, a woman may not be able to savor her success in losing 12 pounds if nothing less than 50 will do. Depressed by her failure, she may eat herself into feeling good; whereas, if she could feel very successful about losing 12 pounds, she might consider losing another 12 when she next feels able to make a sustained effort (McBride, 1982, p 224).

Setting unrealistic goals is more likely to cause failure as the individual becomes frustrated with the inability to lose weight. Smaller goals will allow a sense of victory and a renewed effort for the next step. Pietrantuono (1983) believes that the changes in eating patterns must also include achieving a healthy emotional adjustment. Therapeutic counseling may be needed to deal with the full psychological impact of lowered self-esteem, self-hatred, and insecurity.

The outcome of working carefully with the obese individual in identifying a desire to lose weight and the motivation behind the willingness can ultimately result in a person who has a healthy self-concept and body image. To the point that major weight losses are accomplished, the nursing process will again have to be applied in helping the person adapt to the new body image. Although the weight may be gone, the image retained in the mind, and the one that forms the basis for social interactions, is that of the obese self. For healthy self-images and a renewed sexuality, an accurate body image of the new self must be firmly reintegrated.

Obesity is thought to be at one end of the continuum of eating disorders, with anorexia at the other. Chapter 29, Mental Illness, Substance Abuse, and Sexuality, discusses this condition.

CONCLUSION

In summary, the careful assessment of body image in clients facing threatening surgeries or conditions should be an integral part of all evaluation. In addition, the close relationship between sexuality and body image demands that the client also receive appropriate assessment and planning to restore sexual functioning. This is especially true in extreme medical and surgical conditions affecting the sense of wellness or wholeness the client may be experiencing. In planning holistic care for the individual, body image and sexuality must be considered as integral parts of the overall assessment.

Interventions that are applicable to all clients are listed as follows:

1. It is absolutely crucial that the nurse explore feelings of self and sexuality before attempting to provide assessment and counseling for clients (Littlefield, 1977; McRae and Henderson, 1975). It is important for nurses to avoid projection of their own feelings or values and moral concerns surrounding sexuality (Hogan, 1982). Clients experiencing dramatic alterations in body image must feel comfortable in discussing sensitive areas with the nurse. Feelings of disapproval or shock will terminate the subject without successful intervention.

2. Assessment of body image and sexuality should be integrated into total assessment, as this conveys to the client that self-image and sexuality are essential parts of care (Littlefield, 1977). It may be helpful to elicit information concerning the client's predisease level of sexual functioning (Bachers, 1985). This baseline information will be useful in helping clients recover the depth of their sexual intimacy.

3. The nurse performing the assessment must have an open mind in approaching the subject of sexuality. Respect must be demonstrated for the cultural values and standards that the client demonstrates. Keeping a broad and objective frame of reference in discussions will facilitate accuracy of information and understanding.

4. An action closely related to keeping an open mind is providing open communication between the nurse and the client. The atmosphere should remain free and relaxed without the client's feeling discomfort about discussing sexual issues. It is important for the nurse to pay attention to any nonverbal language, as this can provide clues to information the client is reluctant to share. Appropriate sexual terminology should be used. Common or lay terms may be used initially, which the client may be more familiar with, gradually introducing medical terms and phrases (Bachers, 1985). Finally, in considering open communication, it is essential that the nurse remember that no one should feel forced to participate in a discussion in which they are not comfortable (Carey, 1975). Often, opening the subject will be enough to encourage clients to participate at a later time when they are more comfortable.

5. Planning for client education should be comprehensive, including teaching for basic self-care and counseling for altered body image and sexuality. Clients should be encouraged to set realistic goals, as unrealistic expectations can be very threatening when they are not accomplished (Carey, 1975). Breaking goals down into smaller steps may be easier for the client to accomplish and can promote a sense of success and mastery.

6. Family members, significant others, and the client's spouse or partner should be included in all teaching, especially regarding self-care needs. In matters regarding sexuality, both the client and the partner should be counseled simultaneously. It may also be helpful to counsel them separately, as one or the other may express concerns or fears that they were not comfortable expressing in front of the other (Moore, Folk-Lighty, and Nolen, 1984).

7. Role changes may be particularly difficult for the client to acknowledge (McRae and Henderson, 1975). Anticipation of alteration should be explored carefully to determine the amount of sensitivity associated with the issue.

8. The nurse should be knowledgeable about community referral to provide follow-up and/or to direct the client toward one of the self-help groups associated with loss of a particular function (for example, Lost Chords or Reach to Recovery). Referrals can provide continued support and assistance to

the client after the period of hospitalization has ended.

With support and a caring attitude, clients experiencing altered body image can emerge with a new sense of themselves and a feeling of having conquered the disease or condition. The client's sexuality can be adapted to meet the challenge of physical impairment through sensitivity and creativity on the part of the client and partner or spouse and by comprehensive use of the nursing process.

REFERENCES

Alexander C: Nurses ignore importance of sexuality in OR. AORN J 23:743–746, 1976.

Atwell BM: Sex and the cancer patient: An unspoken concern. Pat Ed Counsel 5:123–126, 1984.

Bachers ES: Sexual dysfunction after treatment for genitourinary cancers. Semin Oncol Nurs 1:18–24, 1985.

Carey P: Temporary sexual dysfunction in reversible health limitations. Nurs Clin North Am 10:575–586, 1975.

Carroll RM: The impact of mastectomy on body image. Oncol Nurs Forum 8:29–32, 1981.

Castledine G: In the mind's eye. . . . Nurs Mirror 153:16, 1981.

Comfort A: Sexual Consequences of Disability. Philadelphia, George F. Stickley, 1978.

Conine TA, Evans JH: Sexual reactivation of chronically ill and disabled adults. J Allied Health 11:261–270, 1982.

Denning DC: Head and neck cancers: Our reactions. CA Nurs 5:269–273, 1982.

Dobkin KA, Broadwell DC: Nursing considerations for the patient undergoing colostomy surgery. Semin Oncol Nurs 2:249–255, 1986.

Dropkin MJ: Rehabilitation after disfigurative facial surgery. Plast Surg Nurs 5:130–134, 1985.

Fisher SG: The psychosexual effects of cancer and cancer treatment. Oncol Nurs Forum 10:63–68, 1983.

Fisher SG: The sexual knowledge and attitudes of oncology nurses: Implications for nursing education. Semin Oncol Nurs 1:63–68, 1985.

Fisher SG, Levin MD: The sexual knowledge and attitudes of professional nurses caring for oncology patients. CA Nurs 6:55–61, 1983.

Fitzgerald FT: The cure may be worse than the disease. Consultant 25:153–158, 1985.

Frank DI: You don't have to be an expert to give sexual counseling to a mastectomy patient. Nursing 81 11:64–67, 1981.

Gentry K: Introduction to eating disorders. Phys Assist 8:33–39, 1984.

Gloeckner MR: Perceptions of sexual attractiveness following ostomy surgery. Res Nurs Health 7:87–92, 1984.

Gruendemann BJ: The impact of surgery on body image. Nurs Clin North Am 10:635–643, 1975.

Hogan RM: Influences of culture on sexuality. Nurs Clin North Am 17:365–376, 1982.

Hogan RM: Human Sexuality: A Nursing Perspective. 2nd ed. Norwalk, Appleton-Century-Crofts, 1985.

Jacobson L: Illness and human sexuality. Nurs Outlook 22:50–53, 1974.

Kriss R: Self-image and sexuality after mastectomy. In Bullard DG, Knight SE (eds): Sexuality and Physical Disability. St. Louis, CV Mosby, 1981.

Lambert VA, Lambert CE: Psychosocial Care of the Physically Ill: What Every Nurse Should Know. 2nd ed. Englewood Cliffs, Prentice Hall, 1985.

Lee JM: Emotional reactions to trauma. Nurs Clin North Am 5:577–587, 1970.

Littlefield V: The surgical patient's sexuality. AORN J 26:649–658, 1977.

MacElveen-Hoehn P, McCorkle R: Understanding sexuality in progressive cancer. Semin Oncol Nurs 1:56–62, 1985.

MacRae I, Henderson G: Sexuality and irreversible health limitations. Nurs Clin North Am 10:587–597, 1975.

McBride AB: Obesity of women during the childbearing years: Psychosocial and physiologic aspects. Nurs Clin North Am 17:217–225, 1982.

McCloskey JC: How to make the most of body image theory in nursing practice. Nursing 76 6:68–72, 1976.

Metcalfe MC, Fischman SH: Factors affecting the sexuality of patients with head and neck cancer. Oncol Nurs Forum 12:21–25, 1985.

Moore K, Folk-Lighty M, Nolen MJ: Counseling the cardiac patient. Nursing 84 14:104–111, 1984.

Patry-Lahey R: Helping a laryngectomy patient go home. Nursing 85 15:63–64, 1985.

Penninger JI, Moore SB, Frager SR: After the ostomy: Helping the patient reclaim his sexuality. RN 48:46–50, 1985.

Pietrantuono M: The scale of obesity. Nurs Mirror 157:45–47, 1983.

Renshaw DC: How to help ostomates and partners achieve satisfaction. Consultant 23:113–119, 1983.

Rolstad BS, Wilson G, Tebbitt BV: Long-term sexual concerns in the client with ileostomy. J Enterostomal Therapy 9:10–13, 1982.

Roberts SL: Behavioral Concepts and Nursing Throughout the Life Span. Englewood Cliffs, Prentice Hall, 1982.

Rubin R: Body image and self-esteem. Nurs Outlook 16:20–23, 1968.

Savage JS: Effect of crisis on female identity. Issues Health Care Women 3:151–160, 1981.

Schain WS: Breast cancer surgeries and psychosexual sequelae: Implications for remediation. Semin Oncol Nurs 1:200–205, 1985.

Schwartz-Applebaum J, Dedrick J, Jusenius K, Kirchner W: Nursing care plans: Sexuality and treatment of breast cancer. Oncol Nurs Forum 11:16–24, 1984.

Scott DW: Quality of life following the diagnosis of breast cancer. Top Clin Nurs 4:20–37, 1983.

Simmons KN: Sexuality and the female ostomate. Am J Nurs 83:409–411, 1983.

Stout K: The surgical treatment of morbid obesity: Implications and interventions. Nurs Clin North Am 17:245–250, 1982.

Van der Velde CD: Body images of one's self and of others: Developmental and clinical significance. Am J Psychiatry 142:527–537, 1985.

Wassner A: The impact of mutilating surgery or trauma on body image. Int Nurs Rev 29:86–90, 1982.

Wellisch DK: The psychologic impact of breast cancer on relationships. Semin Oncol Nurs 1:195–199, 1985.

White JH: An overview of obesity: Its significance to nursing. Nurs Clin North Am 17:191–198, 1982.

White JH, Schroeder MA: When your client has a weight problem: Nursing assessment. AJN 81:550–553, 1981.

Williams HA, Wilson ME, Hongladarom G, McDonell M: Nurses' attitudes toward sexuality in cancer patients. Oncol Nurs Forum 13:39–43, 1986.

Winder AE, Winder BD: Patient counseling: Clarifying a woman's choice for breast reconstruction. Pat Ed Counsel 7:65–75, 1985.

26: Sexual Assault

Nancy Sharts Engels

In this chapter sexual assault of adults and children is examined. The sociocultural context in which these offenses occur is explored, including the basic values underlying the relationships of men and women in Western societies. Spousal assault is included, as it, too, is an act of violence, even though in most states spousal assault, particularly marital rape, is viewed differently and is ignored by the criminal justice system. Characteristics of assailants and of victims are enumerated. Finally, strategies for intervening in the assault of both adults and children are identified.

Readers are likely to encounter clients with a history of sexual assault no matter what their area of practice. Additionally, this chapter should serve to reinforce that readers themselves are potential victims if they do not take steps toward prevention on an individual level and in the area of community action.

RAPE

From the standpoints of promoting public awareness, of prevention of sexual abuse, and of assisting its victims, the broad term *sexual coercion* does more to convey the problem than the more technical labels of specific sexual acts. There are many forms of sexual coercion; some are more blatant than others. What they have in common is that some kind of sexual activity is being sought from a person who is an unwilling participant.

Definitions

The term *rape* evokes intuitive understanding, but there are various definitions. To *feminists*, rape is "the use of threat, physical force, or intimidation in obtaining sexual relations with another person against his or her will" (Foley and Davies, 1983, p 3). Brownmiller (1975) would add that consent could not be obtained by the use of drugs or intoxicants and that the person must be capable of consenting.

Legal definitions vary from state to state. In general, common elements to states' definitions include (1) the use of threat, duress, force, intimidation, or deception; (2) sexual relations or penile-vaginal penetration, however slight; and (3) nonconsent. In some states, but not all, forced anal and oral intercourse or penetration by something other than the penis does not constitute rape (Masters, Johnson, and Kolodny, 1982). A more complete discussion of legal definitions is found in Chapter 8, Sex and the Law.

Other coercive acts include *indecent exposure, simple* or *aggravated assault, offensive touching,* and *forced performance of deviant acts. Incest* and *sexual abuse of children* will be described indepth in a later section. The problem with some of these offenses is that standards of sexual acceptability vary among individuals (Allgeier, 1983), and it may be difficult to determine what will constitute deviant acts in a given community.

Another area of concern is *sexual harassment*. This has gained attention primarily as it occurs in the work place, although no social setting is immune. The victim—and one survey suggests that nine out of ten working women have been sexually harassed at work (MacKinnan, 1979)—is put in a position of helplessness regarding promotions, raises, job evaluations, future recommendations, even the job itself. Harassment can be verbal or physical. Because it is often so vague, most women are coerced into tolerance.

In all of these situations, the central issue is coercion. Such acts degrade, punish, or subjugate their victims.

Historical Perspective

It is a major tenet of patriarchal values systems that women are property, fathered and traded by men. It is striking that the tenth commandment (Deuteronomy 5:21) likened coveting one's neighbor's wife to coveting his house, his land, his slaves, his domestic animals, or anything else that belonged to him. Vestiges of this perspective may be found in the general obligation, honored by our court system, that marriage involves an exchange of domestic service and sexual consortium for financial support (Millett, 1978).

Rape is the clearest enactment of patriarchal force, according to feminists such as Millett (1978). Traditionally, it has been viewed as an offense of one man having injured or abused the property of another man. This concept is clear in Mosaic law (Deuteronomy 22:13–30), in which if a woman is falsely accused after her wedding night of not being a virgin, her father shall be paid 100 pieces of silver and her husband shall be forbidden to divorce her. A virgin who is raped, if she is not betrothed, is given in marriage to the rapist, since she is unsuitable for anyone else, and he must pay her father 50 pieces of silver. It is interesting to note that the father's compensation is greater when his word is unjustly questioned than when his property is seized, illustrating that virginity in the Old Testament context was prized as a sign of quality goods.

In ancient times rape was an acceptable way to procure a wife (Masters, Johnson, and Kolodny, 1982), and the word itself comes from the Latin, *rapere*, which means to steal, seize, or carry away. An example from Roman mythology is the abduction of Proserpine by Pluto, King of the Underworld (Fuller, 1959).

Once a man seized a wife he had to protect his property and his honor by preventing others from seizing or raping her; thus, laws evolved in which rape was cast as a crime against property (Brownmiller, 1975). According to Hammurabi's Code, a set of laws established in Babylonia about 2000 B.C., a man who raped a betrothed virgin was put to death. If a man raped a married woman, both rapist and victim were executed by drowning. Later laws were increasingly specific on circumstances under which rape was judged more or less serious. For example, in eleventh century England, raping a woman of lower social status might bring *no* punishment, while rape of an upper-class woman, particularly a virgin, brought heavy penalties. Guilt was determined by armed combat between the woman's father or husband and the rapist. If the victim had no one to fight for her, she had no case.

Jury trials replaced armed combat by the twelfth century. Yet rapists could pass blame on to their servants. By the thirteenth century the distinction between raping a virgin or a married woman was dropped, and the old custom of requiring a rapist to marry his victim was banned. Thus, basic elements of the definition of rape were established and have persisted to the present day (Brownmiller, 1975). Even in our modern society there have been circumstances under which rape was acceptable. In wartime it is acceptable, perhaps expected, that soldiers rape enemy women. Status differences also affect how rape is viewed; for example, in the South white males raping black females was ignored if not tacitly sanctioned.

The women's liberation movement of the 1960s and 1970s has been a major catalyst in changing public attitudes and the forensic and legal system's responses toward rape. Early responses included establishment of rape crisis centers, shelters for battered women, and telephone hot lines. Now, feminists have come, in the last decade, to focus on prevention by identifying and eliminating factors in the social climate that make rape possible (Lederer, 1982a). It is the feminist perspective that violence and pornography in the media are major factors associated with sexual violence against women. Women Against Pornography is an organization that educates women on the sex industry in America's large cities.

An incident that served to increase public awareness of the scope of the problem was the widely publicized gang rape of a young woman in a New Bedford, Massachusetts, bar as other patrons cheered (Beegan, 1983; Blakely, 1983; Goodman, 1983a; Ranzel, 1984; Simon, 1983). The woman went into the local bar to buy cigarettes, and she stayed to have a drink with a friend. When she tried to leave, a man grabbed her and dragged her to a pool table, where she was raped by four men. The bartender claimed to have given a patron a dime to call the police, but the man called the wrong number. Finally, the victim broke free and ran out, naked from the waist down.

The rapists were found guilty. But the victim's past was laid open for scrutiny, even though defendants are protected from public review of their prior misdeeds. The defense attorney accused the victim of being a liar, a welfare cheat, a person with mental problems, promiscuous, and a profiteer (Ranzel, 1984).

What is incredible about the incident is that the rapists were still in the bar when the police came a half hour after the victim left (Blakely, 1983). They did not expect to be arrested and did not believe that they had committed a crime. This incident served to remind citizens that apathy on this topic is a dangerous response.

Several key issues can be identified from this incident: (1) Many people, aware that women have become sexually liberated, cannot accept that rape is still rape regardless of past sexual experiences. (2) The incident was not an isolated one but rather exemplified a fairly common occurrence. (3) Women are still dichotomized as virgins or whores. (4) Women do not have the power to define their sexual interactions. (5) Finally, the incident may have been carried out in imitation of a recent *Hustler* magazine article that featured a woman being assaulted by four men on a pool table and appearing to enjoy it.

Contemporary Issues

The crime of rape is surrounded by a number of social issues having to do with the question: What is the meaning of rape in our culture?

BLAMING THE VICTIM

The assumption that women participate willingly in rape dates back to the Old Testament. If a virgin was raped in a town, Mosaic law dictated that both she and the rapist be put to death, since she supposedly could have screamed for help (Deuteronomy 22:23–24). Warner reported that Herodotus, the Father of History, commented in 500 B.C. that "abducting young women is not, indeed, a lawful act; but it is stupid after the event to make a fuss about it. The only sensible thing is to take no notice; for it is obvious that no young woman allows herself to be abducted if she does not wish to be" (Warner, 1980).

Bohmer (1974) interviewed judges on their attitudes toward rape. They divided rape victims into three categories. First, *genuine victims* were those about whom there was no doubt that a forcible rape had taken place. The second category was termed *consensual intercourse*, in which the judges perceived that the woman had allowed the situation by being picked up in a bar. Some of them called this "friendly rape." The third category they identified was termed *female indictiveness*, in which a woman accused a known individual of rape in order to get even with him.

Conservative activist Phyllis Schlafley made media headlines in 1981 when she testified to a Senate subcommittee that "virtuous women are seldom accosted. . . ." (Masters, Johnson, and Kolodny, 1982). One recent survey of 762 men and women revealed a direct relationship between traditional views about women and the belief that women are primarily responsible for avoiding rape (Costin, 1985).

The myth that most victims provoke rape is not substantiated by research. Amir (1971) found that in 87 per cent of reported rapes the rapist carries a weapon or threatens to kill the victim. In Philadelphia over a 2-year period, in only 15 per cent of cases was there no physical brutality whatsoever. Many victims are elderly women or young children, and about 80 per cent of victims are able to substantiate a virtuous reputation.

Nonetheless, in one study, respondents within the forensic and health care systems, rapists, and citizens at large agreed with the statement, "A woman should feel guilty following a rape" (Feild, 1978). Similar findings were reported by Williams and Holmes (1981). Often partners tend to blame spouses who have been raped (McCahill, Meyer, and Fischman, 1979).

Rape as a Political Act

Rape does not occur among lower primates and has been characterized by Brownmiller

(1975) as an invention of men designed to keep women in a state of fear. Because women learn and live with this fear, termed *learned vulnerability* (Radloff, 1975), they may seek the protection of being officially associated with a man. Women who lack this protection may be considered open targets for violence.

Millett's (1978) theory of sexual politics points out that while indirect means of control of women are most prevalent in Western societies, force, particularly rape, has been a major deterrent to women expanding their power. Feminists once believed that when greater sexual equality was achieved, rape would diminish in incidence (Brownmiller, 1975). In fact, the reverse has occurred, lending credence to Millett's theory (Ellis and Beattie, 1983).

Pornography is a major type of propaganda in a patriarchal system, and rape is a major act of subjugation. The two are related in that most women fear rape and alter their behaviors to some degree in response to this fear (Russell, 1982a). Thus, the patriarchy maintains the balance of power.

LaBelle (1982) further elucidated the dynamics of this view in her discussion of pornography as distinct from erotica as the "propaganda of misogyny." Erotica depicts "mutually pleasurable sexual expression between people who have enough power to be there by positive choice . . . and has been widely enjoyed by both sexes throughout recorded history. In contrast, pornography depicts violence, dominance, and control. It is sex being used to reinforce some inequality or to create one or to tell us that pain and humiliation . . . are the same as pleasure" (Steinem, 1982, p 33). Pornography *stereotypes* women as carnal, promiscuous, and submissive, to be conquered via the phallus. Women are referred to in derogatory terms such as "cunts," "a piece," or "chick." Women's sexuality is selectively presented; for example, a common theme is that rape victims actually enjoy being conquered. Victims of sexual violence are portrayed as enjoying the experience. The editorial content of the mass media and advertising also contribute to this view with the message that women are to be used for pleasure.

Date Rape

Date rape is a frequent, although underreported, occurrence in the United States.

Masters, Johnson, and Kolodny (1982) found that of 300 young women whom they surveyed, one in five had been forced into some form of unwanted sexual activity on a date or at a party and one woman in 25 had been raped under such circumstances. Kanin (1969) reported on date rape among 348 unmarried male college students and found that 25 per cent of his sample admitted having performed at least one act of sex aggression (defined as making a forceful attempt at coitus to the point of being disagreeable), with the woman responding by fighting or crying. While in some instances the basic problem seemed to be miscommunication or misreading of cues, in others the behavior reflected a male belief that "when she says 'no,' she really means 'yes.' " Ageton (1983) suggests that nonviolent assaults by dates or boyfriends are construed as something other than legitimate sexual assaults. This underscores the imbalance of power in male-female relationships.

Greer (1977) and others (Dull and Giacopassi, 1987) observed that many men believe they have a *right* to sex after they have paid for a woman's dinner. At least one study of college males suggested a normative attitude that sexual aggression on dates is necessary to prove manliness (Smeaton and Byrne, 1987).

Historically, men have paid for dates, and women may have felt some pressure to reciprocate (Korman and Leslie, 1982). Among a group of 400 women at a large southeastern university, 63 per cent reported that they had experienced offensive acts of sexual aggression on dates during their senior year of high school. Women who *shared* dating expenses experienced significantly more sexual aggression. In another study, 71 volunteer self-disclosed date rapists revealed that they were hypersexually socialized—unusually sexually active young men with exaggerated levels of sexual aspiration—who used coercion in response to relative deprivation. They differed from a control group in that they were generally more sexually active as young adolescents and viewed their fathers three times more disapproving of premarital sex (Kanin, 1985).

Gang rapes continue to be part of the university milieu. One client reported that she became quite intoxicated and "went along" with what was going on. One Ivy League fraternity lost its charter because of such an incident (Associated Press, 1983b).

Intoxication of the victim is common. These cases are rarely reported, and charges are rarely filed probably because of shame on the victim's part. One university with which this author is familiar established a peer counseling team to deal with victims of date rape, but rate of use was low.

McCahill, Meyer, and Fischman (1979) found that victims of date rape typically experience a worsened self-concept, see themselves as "bad," and develop an increased fear of male acquaintances. This is explained by their feeling that they never know when a male friend may become aggressive with them. Ageton (1983), in a national study of adolescent rape victims, found reactions to date rape included anger, depression, and embarrassment. Additionally, guilt, reflecting ambivalence about the victim's role in the incident, was common. The seriousness of the assault and the victim's negative feelings increased with age. Intensity of feelings declined considerably by 6 months after the rape. By up to 2 years later depression and guilt were less, but victims were more fearful of being alone than they had been right after the assault, and their feelings of embarrassment and anger were greater. By 3 years after the incidents, more respondents reported depression than had done so in the first 6 month follow-up. Thus, certain reactions may have incubation periods or may be initially suppressed, and a 6- to 12-month follow-up period may be inadequate. No characteristics of the assaults or demographic variables could be related to the pattern of response over 3 years in Ageton's study.

The *New York Times* featured a fashion article several years ago that promoted the "bruised" look (Weir, 1982). Designer Claude Montana's fall preview included 35 models displaying what was described as a battered appearance. In this way violence is glamorized.

The 1970 Commission on Obscenity and Pornography recommended that all restrictions on pornography, both soft and hard, be removed. They emphasized that most pornographic material is geared to the male heterosexual market—predominantly white, middle-class, middle-aged, and married—and that most graphic depictions are of the naked female body and acts done to that body. This was regarded as harmless.

Russell (1982a) reported that of 933 women interviewed, nearly 10 per cent had been upset at least once by a man trying to coerce them to do something he had seen in a pornographic movie. Examples included urinating in the victim's mouth, group sex, hitting, sadomasochistic acts including bondage, anal intercourse, bestiality, branding the woman, and inserting objects into the woman's vagina. Russell's findings cast doubt on the conclusion that pornography is harmless.

There is a growing body of research to support the belief that exposure to sexual violence in pornography can have antisocial effects, such as increased acceptance of rape myths and violence against women (Malamuth and Check, 1981), increased laboratory aggression against a female confederate (Donnerstein and Berkowitz, 1981), decreased perception of rape victims' suffering (Malamuth, Haber, and Feshback, 1980), and increased violent sexual fantasies (Malamuth, 1981). More recently, Freund and associates (1986) observed that while some men rape only when sexually deprived, others are rape prone, that is, they prefer to rape even when they have access to willing partners. These individuals are preoccupied by rape urges or fantasies. In a Canadian sample of rape-prone men and controls, rape-prone men responded with penile erection more often to narratives of sexual encounters in which the women were afraid than to narratives in which the women participated freely. In contrast, the control group was aroused more by the narratives in which the women participated freely and rated them more erotic. Such a study suggests that there might be a link between violent pornography and acts of sexual violence.

Another Canadian study involving 36 college men showed that a videotape of a gang rape was rated more pornographic if it was accompanied by rock music and less pornographic if it was accompanied by an easy listening soundtrack. One implication is that the context in which pornography is viewed can alter its perceived acceptability (Pfaus, Myronuk, and Jacobs, 1986).

Male domination and female subjugation has been a central theme in literary descriptions of sexual activity (Millett, 1978). With increased sexual permissiveness in this century came greater latitude for the expression of violent encounters. Diamond (1982) observed that the President's Commission on the Causes and Prevention of Violence in 1969 concluded that media violence can induce individuals to act aggressively.

Response of the Criminal Justice System

Reported rape is the most frequent violent crime in the United States; the number of reported rapes has increased throughout the 1970s and 1980s. Further, rapes that are reported may be only a small percentage (less than 10 per cent) of those that do occur. The Federal Bureau of Investigation recommends that in order to obtain an accurate picture of the incidence of rape, it is necessary to multiply reported rape figures by a factor of at least 10 and possibly 20 (Griffin, 1971). Factors that contribute to underreporting include a sense of humiliation or futility, concern regarding possible retribution by the rapist, and ignorance of the criminal justice system and how to use it.

That rape is so underreported may reflect the sluggish response of the legal-forensic system and the low rate of rape convictions.

Often, the rape victim experiences numerous police interrogations, protracted legal *negotiations*, and a lengthy trial. This route can be expensive and drawn out, thus delaying the victim's putting it all behind her. Holmstrom and Burgess (1978) found that the time between assault and trial is easily 2 years. Because the courts seek to demonstrate guilt "beyond the shadow of a doubt," the victim's character comes under scrutiny.

The first decisions the rape victim must make while she is still likely to be in a state of shock are to seek emergency care and to report the incident to the police. If she pursues these options, she is likely to encounter male authority figures. In some instances, cultural values will cause her survival within her own reference group to be jeopardized (Ours, 1986). Holmstrom and Burgess (1978) found that emergency room staff tended to make judgments whether or not the rape was "legitimate," whether or not the victim had "asked for it," and the perceived moral character of the victim. This may have an impact on the quality and quantity of data gathered on a specific case. Moreover, the treatment a victim receives in this setting may influence her decision to seek police intervention.

The first contact with police represents a major hurdle. They may make insensitive remarks, particularly if the women is unattractive, such as "Who'd want to rape you?" (Jacobson and Popovich, 1983). Other biases that have been documented include the as-

sumed personal role in the rape of women who are attractive and the meaning and definition of resistance (Dietz, Littman, and Bentley, 1984; Masters, Johnson, and Kolodny, 1982). Additionally, humiliating questions commonly asked include "Are you a virgin?" "Did you like it?" or "What were you wearing?" The woman may be expected to demonstrate resistance or provide corroboration of her statements. The reader is referred to Chapter 8, Sex and the Law for a complete discussion of the issue of consent.

It is often alleged that women make unfounded accusations. In fact, a New York City experiment showed that if police women instead of men were placed in charge of interviewing complainants, the number of unfounded cases dropped from 20 to 2 per cent, a figure comparable to the incidence of false reports of other violent crimes (Brownmiller, 1975). Barshis (1983) suggested, based on results of another New York City study, that better-designed complaint forms could elicit additional data to strengthen women's cases.

Needs in the criminal justice system identified by Holmstrom and Burgess (1978) include better court-witness liaison, including education of witnesses about their role and improved efforts to keep them abreast of changes in court schedules, stricter criteria for court continuances, early screening of cases' chances of success, simplification of the trial procedure, greater sensitivity toward the victim, consideration of the victim's sexual history as irrelevant, controls on the type of statements made by defense attorneys during cross-examination, and greater compensation for victims.

Rape Myths

A number of myths have been identified in the rape literature (Amir, 1971; Foley and Davies, 1983; Masters, Johnson, and Kolodny, 1982). Some of the most prevalent include the following:

1. The primary motivation is sexual. Rape is not sexually motivated, but is rather an act of violence. Most rapists have regular sexual partners, although a significant portion have sexual problems, including erectile dysfunction or premature or retarded ejaculation (Groth, 1979).

2. Rapists are crazy. While rape is symptomatic of psychological distress, rapists do

not differ significantly from normal men on personality variables, nor are they different in intellectual ability. Situations in which otherwise respectable men rape include fraternity parties or date situations (Griffin, 1971).

3. Rape is an impulse act. The proportion of rapes that are planned range from 58 to 71 per cent (Amir, 1971; Griffin, 1971). Often the rapist may plan to rape a particular victim, or he may plan to rape a passer-by.

4. Rape occurs only among strangers. Though 66 per cent of the cases in one study (Amir, 1971) occurred among strangers, the study dealt only with *reported* cases. Brownmiller (1975) stated that women are far less likely to report rape in which the rapist is known. Several studies (Masters, Johnson, and Kolodny, 1982; Kanin, 1985; Korman and Leslie, 1982) have shown that date rape is a common occurrence. DiVasto and associates' (1984) study of Albuquerque women showed that of those who were raped, 75 per cent had been raped by acquaintances or relatives.

5. Women who let themselves get raped really want it. Burgess and Holmstrom (1976) found that most rape victims are paralyzed by fear or else hope that by cooperating they can avoid injury or murder. Amir (1971) found that 87 per cent of rapists threatened the woman with death or carried a weapon, while only 15 per cent of rapists used no force whatsoever. Various degrees of brutality occur in 74 per cent of rape cases.

6. Women provoke rape. The Federal Commission on Crimes of Violence (Griffin, 1971) found only 4 per cent of rapes were attributable to behaviors of the victims. This myth fails to take into account the high incidence among children and elderly women. The related idea that women want to be raped has been perpetuated in pornography and in such popular media as the film *Gone With The Wind*. While Hite (1981a) observed that many women experience rape fantasies, that does not mean that they actually want rape to occur. Most modify their daily routines to some extent in order to avoid rape, for example glancing in the back seat of their parked car before getting in, avoiding city streets after dark, and double- or triple-locking their residence. This myth is related to the stereotypical gender role expectation that healthy men are supposed to see how far they can get sexually while nice women are supposed to resist.

7. Rape occurs in dark alleys. Most rapes occur in the victim's or rapist's home (Foley and Davies, 1983).

8. A rapist will flee if the woman resists. Many rapists are armed and most use some degree of brutality (Amir, 1971). Provoking a rapist may cost the woman her life.

9. Rape is usually interracial. In fact, Amir (1971) found in his study of reported rapes that most occurred between members of the same race.

The Rapist

Based on indepth interviews with rapists, Groth (1979) identified three categories of rape, each of which represents unique psychodynamics. The most common type of rape is *power rape*, accounting for 55 per cent of cases. Characteristics of power rapists include an intention to possess rather than harm their victims and the use of physical aggression to subdue the woman. These men reported having obsessional fantasies about sexual conquest and rape. Their victims tended to be the same age as they were or younger. Power rapists experience the incident as a reaffirmation of their manhood. While sexual gratification is a part of power rape, sex is more a means of demonstrating control.

Anger rape accounts for about 40 per cent of cases. This is the use of several behaviors for nonsexual motives. The rapist is venting hostility, rage, or hatred on the victim and uses sex as a weapon. Humiliation or degradation of the victim is important to this type of rapist, as he is often seeking revenge for perceived hurts by women in his past. The victim is more likely to experience injury as more physical violence is used than needed merely to subdue her. The violence is important for its own sake, whereas sexual gratification is not. Anger rapes are frequently of short duration.

Sadistic rape occurs in only about 5 per cent of cases. Sexuality and aggression are transformed so that violence itself becomes erotic to the rapist. He engages in bizarre abusive acts, including mutilation, particularly of the victim's breasts or genitalia. Such cases often end in homicide and necrophilia. Prostitutes are particular targets. This rapist thrives on feelings of omnipotence and gains pleasure by inflicting pain on his victims. He may demonstrate a ritualistic nature, even psychosis, but he is often able to hide this in daily interactions. His intent is to abuse and torture his victims in order to punish them, and they rarely survive. If the victim does live, she is at particular risk for depression and suicide.

Additional categories that have been identified include sexual gratification rape, which generally includes the phenomena of date and marital rapes. Sexual gratification is the primary goal and force is the means, similar to power rape. The impulse or predatory rapist (Selkin, 1975) sees the opportunity for rape, and he takes advantage of the situation.

Pair or group rape (Holmstrom and Burgess, 1980) may be similar to above classifications in terms of motivation. An important difference is the sense of camaraderie, even competition, among peers that characterizes this type of rape. The interaction among the rapists is as important as that between rapists and victims. Sometimes other females act as confederates to the rapists. Group rape may be one way to affirm status within a peer group. Common examples include hiring prostitutes for bachelor parties or gang rape at college parties. In 23 per cent of common rape situations there are multiple assailants (McDermott, 1979). Part of the "turn-on" is the opportunity to watch others engaging in sex.

It should be noted that in one to six per cent of reported rapes the victims are males. Also, females have been convicted of rape in cases in which they colluded with male rapists. No information is available on actual sexual coercion toward men or women by women.

Characteristics of rapists vary widely, and studies generally focus on convicts, ignoring the large number of individuals who are never identified or arrested. Amir (1971) found the largest cohort of accused rapists to be 15 to 19 years old, with 20 to 25 years being second. In general, the older the rapist, the younger his victim. Of Amir's sample, 66 to 75 per cent were unmarried, and most were from the lower end of the socioeconomic scale. This may reflect bias in reporting or bias within the criminal justice system. More blacks than whites have been convicted of rape, although again, that may reflect biases in reporting and conviction (Foley and Davies, 1983). Over half of reported rapes occur on weekends, peaking between 8:00 p.m. to 2:00 a.m. Among Amir's sample, half had previous arrest records; 9 per cent had been convicted of rape in the past, and four

per cent had been arrested for other sexual offenses.

Forty per cent of booked rapists have a history of chronic drinking, often dating from adolescence (Groth, 1979). In Groth's sample, 45 per cent had been sexually assaulted, 18 per cent had experienced sexual pressure by an adult, 18 per cent had experienced sexually stressful situations (such as circumcision in adolescence), 3 per cent had witnessed upsetting sexual activity, and 2 per cent had a sexual injury or other physical handicap.

Sexual dysfunction is common among rapists, affecting as many as 58 per cent (Groth and Burgess, 1977). One potentially important difference between rapists and nonrapists seems to be that rapists are sexually aroused by observing rape, whereas nonrapists are not (Wydra et al, 1983). However, the rapists also appear to be capable of identifying inappropriate sexual cues in tapes and in inhibiting sexual arousal when instructed to do so as nonrapists (Wydra et al, 1983). A more recent study suggested that rapists are actually more accurate in interpreting nonverbal behavioral cues than nonrapists, a skill which they use in selecting victims (Giannini and Fellows, 1986). It was suggested that this ability is developed in response to a pathological experience of intimacy within the family of origin.

While traumatic sexual events, painful experiences with women, socialization into violence within the family of origin, and exposure to violence in the media as well as general societal values about women all contribute to the occurrence of rape, increased current life stress, job pressures, or other trigger events may catalyze specific episodes (Groth, 1979).

The Victim

Females of any age from infancy to senescence are raped (Horos, 1981). The incidence is highest among 16 to 24 year olds. Black women are nearly twice as likely to be raped by a stranger as white women, but among both blacks and whites, rape by a stranger is twice as likely among those with little education and income as it is among middle- and upper-class women (McDermott, 1979). In cases of rape by a stranger the victim and offender tend to share demographic characteristics, namely age, class, and ethnicity.

Women who are victims of repeated incidents tend to be of lower socioeconomic status, are often unemployed, and have disclosed a higher than usual frequency of seeking professional help for emotional problems (Foley and Davies, 1983).

Do rape victims share distinctive qualities? Sanford and Fetter (1979) have identified characteristics that they feel women who are more likely to be raped exhibit, such as a disheveled appearance, resigned hapless manner, appearing disorganized, and sending out "victim vibrations." They suggest that this type of woman sends a message of inability to cope and that her fearful manner practically assures the success of the rapist's attack.

These authors assert that femininity has guaranteed the victim status of women. Women are afraid of being rude, so they do not flee from suspicious strangers or cause a "scene" if accosted. If a stranger detains them on some pretext, women generally seek to accommodate his needs and thus place themselves in a vulnerable position. Their term for the degree to which given women exhibit these tendencies is compliance quotient.

Measures of a woman's compliance quotient include a gracious smile, answering questions when asked, deferring to the protection and judgment of men when in difficulty, accepting casual touching and suggestive comments in social settings, allowing men to pay for social outings, avoiding shows of superiority in sports or games, accepting the assistance of strangers, acting graciously toward service personnel who come to the door, and demonstrating helpfulness and compassion toward those less fortunate (all part of an American etiquette). Such a woman is easily manipulated.

Sanford and Fetter (1979) further maintain that the "victim type," or this aspect of all women, is identifiable by gestures and language of self-deprecation and that poor self-concept enhances one's chances for being victimized. In contrast, a brisk, purposeful stride with head held high gives a distinctively different message.

In most cases (72 per cent) the victim makes some effort to protect herself (McDermott, 1979). The most common response is to try to attract attention or help, followed by attempts at physical force, resistance, and efforts to argue, reason with, or threaten the rapist.

Ninety-two per cent of the victims of completed rape and 62 per cent of victims of attempted rape in McDermott's sample received injuries besides forced vaginal penetration. Most frequent were cuts, bruises, black eyes, and scratches. Next were internal injuries or broken bones or teeth. Two to three per cent experienced knife or gunshot wounds. Women who tried to protect themselves generally experienced greater injury.

Physiological Consequences of Rape

The occurrence of physical trauma during sexual assault has already been described. Injury represents the most serious result in the immediate post-rape period. One caveat would be that not all genital trauma indicates sexual assault. Sexual activity between consenting adults can result in penile, vaginal, anorectal, or oral injury and even fatal air embolism resulting from air blown into the vagina of pregnant women (Aftermath of Love, 1987).

Holmstrom and Burgess's victims experienced a high incidence of physical damage or injury (defined as "objective evidence of injury that could be seen by a person other than the victim" [Holmstrom and Burgess, 1978, pp 87–88]). At least one sign of general trauma was found among 63 per cent of adult and 73 per cent of young victims; and at least one sign of gynecological injury was noted among 43 per cent of adults and 59 per cent of young victims. While most victims experienced minor injury, almost one third suffered moderate or severe gynecological trauma.

Another potential problem is sexually transmitted disease. This is a major concern of rape victims and health professionals, although the incidence is unknown (Holmstrom and Burgess, 1978; Kolodny, Masters, and Johnson, 1979). Police tend to urge victims to seek prophylactic treatment, and it is a routine part of emergency room intervention.

Pregnancy is a third potential physical consequence of rape. Conception occurs in about 5 per cent of cases (Foley and Davies, 1983). For most of Holmstrom and Burgess's sample this was the primary concern. It was an especially difficult issue for those women who were unable to accept abortion or for those who might have been pregnant by their husbands at the time of the rape.

Means of preventing pregnancy after rape will be described in a following section. Effectiveness is not guaranteed, side effects may be problematic, and, for some women, such measures are not acceptable. Therefore, the decision of what to do in case of pregnancy is a major one among fertile women, and the first menstrual cycle after the rape often represents an important step in the woman's recovery.

One social issue that has arisen in regard to this problem is that of the government's refusal to pay for abortions even in cases of rape or incest. Thus, one solution to the problem of pregnancy resulting from rape is out of reach of a segment of the population (Hatcher et al, 1986).

Psychological Consequences of Rape

The effects of rape on its victims are profound and often long-lasting. Metzger (1976), who herself was a victim of rape, described the rape victim's reaction as a total loss of self, leading to a sense of emptiness and isolation from self and society. The fact that rape is an isolating experience has been noted elsewhere (Griffin, 1971).

The general pattern of reactions consists of the following (Kolodny, Masters, and Johnson, 1979): The impact or acute-reaction phase lasts from several days to several weeks and is characterized by gross anxiety, disorganization, shock, and disbelief. During the post-traumatic or recoil phase, the woman exhibits outward adjustment that may entail denial of the impact of the rape. While the victim may appear to be well-integrated, suppression is occurring at a deeper level. The post-traumatic reconstitution phase is a time of integration and resolution sometimes at great psychological expense. Self-concept may be lessened. This phase may be characterized by recurring depression and the need to talk.

Somatic symptoms in the acute phase include soreness and pain in body areas that were the focus of the rapist's force. Disorganized sleep patterns are prevalent, and both falling asleep and staying asleep are difficult. Nightmares are common. Most victims experience anorexia to some degree. Some complain of stomach pain or nausea. Specific symptoms may reflect the nature of the sex act.

Burgess and Holmstrom's sample did not immediately express shame and guilt; rather, fear was the primary reaction in the majority of cases. Most felt they were lucky to be alive. However, guilt, shame, self-blame, and anger did emerge early on. Mood swings were frequent. Victims noted that their feelings were often out of proportion to daily situations. They exhibited frequent irritation with others and caution with all people. Victims' thoughts focused on trying to block the assault from their minds and on undoing what had happened.

During the long-term reorganization process, victims often modified their life styles. For example, becoming reclusive, returning to the family of origin for awhile, or moving away from the locale of the rape.

Nightmares often persist over time. In one type, victims experience dreams similar to the attack itself. A second type, which occurs as time progresses, often involves the victim dreaming that she is committing acts of violence.

Phobias tend to develop in reaction to circumstances such as being in crowds, being alone, or being exposed to specific odors or physiognomies associated with the attack. Paranoia and suspicion are common, and often for a long time afterward women cannot tolerate being touched even by friends.

Rape has also been observed to impair seriously developmental task achievement (Holmstrom and Burgess, 1978). For children, this involved school attendance and performance, while for adults task disruption most commonly occurred in the areas of housewifery and parenting, employment, and schooling, in which independence and dependability must be exercised. Many women needed assistance from their husbands, mothers, sisters, or others in coping with daily routines.

Stopping work is often a response to phobic reactions. Many women are afraid that if they remain accessible their assailants will return. Others have a hard time explaining what has happened to co-workers. Sometimes employers have reacted negatively and have not wanted the victim to let anyone else at work know what happened (Pekkanen, 1976).

Rape is an emotionally hazardous event. Most women experience the preceding progression of reactions, but, for some, psychological equilibrium is *not* regained (Forman, 1983). These individuals require referral to intensive treatment with a therapist trained in rape trauma intervention. Others suppress the whole experience, never telling anyone. For them, a later crisis may bring the unresolved trauma back to the surface. These individuals are known as silent reactors. Victims' patterns of sexual activity are usually disrupted following rape. Burgess and Holmstrom (1979) observed this in 81 per cent of cases. Even when behaviors are unchanged, feelings profoundly differ. Masters, Johnson, and Kolodny (1982) cited one example of a woman who believed that she needed to resume intercourse as quickly as possible but was totally devoid of feeling.

Becker and associates (1982) found that 56 per cent of a group of 83 rape victims experienced sexual dysfunction afterward. Common sexual problems include sexual aversion, which may occur abruptly or gradually, impaired vaginal lubrication, loss of genital sensations, dyspareunia, vaginismus, and anorgasmia (Kolodny, Masters, and Johnson, 1979). Underlying causes of such reactions are complex but often involve induced self-esteem, guilt, fear of rejection by the mate, anger toward men in general, depression, and reinforced feelings of learned helplessness. Women who continue sexual intercourse with the same frequency may suffer from reduced sexual satisfaction.

The victim's partner is not immune from strong emotional reactions, and his response influences the victim's long-term adjustment. He may feel anger and a desire for revenge as though he personally had been attacked. Or, he may be disgusted or revolted by his partner, acting as though she had willingly participated and had been tainted by the rape. Whereas some men respond with sensitivity and kindness, others may be defensive. Some partners of rape victims experience erectile dysfunction, diminished sexual interest, or ejaculatory disturbance (Kolodny, Masters, and Johnson, 1979).

Those dimensions of sexuality that do not seem to be affected by rape include activities that were not part of the rape experience, such as masturbation, holding hands with, or hugging one's partner (Feldman-Summers, Gordon, and Meagher, 1979).

Burgess and Holmstrom (1979) noted that while it is not necessarily true that sexual adjustment after rape is easier for sexually experienced women than for virgins, it is true that rape will dramatically influence a woman's view of heterosexual activity if it is her first experience. One client was sexually inexperienced when she was raped while babysitting during high school. Several years later she described herself as "changed" by it, much more compliant and fearful than before. When she became engaged, she felt that she had to experience intercourse with her fiance, even though she and her family generally did not condone premarital sex, to see if she could accept it. She felt that it would be unfair to marry if sex were impossible for her. Fortunately, her significant others have all been extremely supportive of her, and she found her sexual experience with her fiance to be very positive. This young woman gained a tremendous amount of weight after being raped, and she was unable to lose it. It may represent her armor against further assault.

The implications of these findings for helping rape victims return to a satisfactory sexual life include the woman's taking her time and engaging in activities that have not become fear stimuli. Communication with her partner is essential, so that positive feelings can once again be associated with sexual interaction. But a return to normalcy may take a long time.

Factors that have an impact on recovery after rape are numerous. Burgess and Holmstrom (1978) followed a sample for 4 to 6 years after rape to assess the impact of life stressors. They found that different life events demonstrated different effects. Stressors that delayed recovery included prior victimization and the chronic stressors of poverty, lack of social support, and pre-existing physical or psychological problems. On the other hand, the loss of a family member prior to the rape was associated with hastened recovery. A possible explanation for this is that the rape was perceived as less traumatic than the death of a loved one or divorce. A surprising result of this research was that current life stress, 6 months before the rape or less, had no statistically significant impact on recovery from the rape, although there were clinical exceptions. One explanation may be that most victims had experienced only one life event in that time-span, thus providing a narrow range of variance of that factor.

McCahill, Meyer, and Fischman (1979) in their study of 1401 Philadelphia assault victims found that adults were more likely to face adjustment problems than adolescents or children. This may have had to do with their difficulty with some regression to a dependent state. Married women experienced more difficulty following rape than singles, probably reflecting the complex responses of their mates. Women experienced significantly less distress if they lived with their parents or siblings; presumably, this arrangement enhanced their feelings of security. Women who had consulted psychotherapists before their rape tended to feel more pessimistic than those who had not. Working women and women with more education demonstrated greater difficulty interacting with men, but both groups experienced less sexual dysfunction than unemployed and less educated women. As was noted earlier, women who experienced less trauma and women who responded sexually suffer from greater guilt following rape.

While this discussion has focused on the experiences of female rape victims, male victims also are subject to the rape trauma syndrome (Collins, 1982). In addition, they must bear the burden of wondering why they were selected. There is the expectation in our society that males should be able to fight and defend themselves. Victims perceive that they have failed at this.

Prevention of Rape

No one can know what triggers a particular rapist, and research has not discussed facilitating or inhibiting factors. However, resources such as the handbook by Sanford and Fetter (1979) have suggested precautionary behaviors that may make the difference between being victimized or not. Health professionals have a responsibility to inform their clients regarding measures that may protect them.

Securing one's home is critical, since many rapes occur in the victim's home (Horos, 1981). Routes of entry should be strong, snugly fitted, and securely locked. Dead bolts and peepholes should be installed *and used*. Service personnel should not be admitted until they show proper identification. Strangers who need to make a telephone call can wait outside while the number is called for them. Children should be instructed *never* to open the door, and they should never give out information over the telephone. Women and children should avoid giving the impression that they are alone at home.

Good lighting in and around one's home

and parking area is essential. Telephone listings should exclude a woman's first name. Women should get to know their female neighbors. They should not release apartment keys to building personnel nor leave them under doormats. Laundry rooms and elevators are high-risk areas. They should be used quickly and avoided when strange men appear. Dogs are good protection, and self-defense training is a good investment.

Women need to exercise caution in going out alone in isolated areas, particularly at night. Clothing should allow maximum mobility. For example, flat shoes and full skirts permit one to run, arms should not be restricted, and no hair, chains, or scarves that can be used to restrain the woman should protrude. Communities often offer rape prevention education.

Spousal Assault

Spousal assault is consistent with the tenets of a patriarchal ideology. It may or may not entail coercive sexual activity, but the dynamics of rape and wife abuse are similar enough that the issue needs to be explored here. Reports on the extent of the problem vary from roughly 33 per cent (Gelles, 1974) to 60 per cent (Steinmetz, 1984) of American families having engaged in some degree of physical violence, ranging from hitting to attack with a weapon. Episodes of severe beatings at least once per year may occur in nearly 5 per cent of American marriages (Barden, 1981). Affluent families are at equal or even greater risk than lower class families (Gelles, 1974; Stark and McEvoy, 1970).

The cycle of violence includes three phases. The *initial* or *build-up* phase consists of relatively minor incidents of violence that gradually escalate in severity to culminate in phase two, an *acute battering incident*. Phase three is the *honeymoon*, characterized by remorse, promises, tranquility, peace offerings, affection, and intimacy. If the cycle is repetitive, the relationship may be deemed a "battering relationship" (Cook and Frantz-Cook, 1984).

Bowlby (1984) notes that relationships with a sexual partner, when threatened, are likely to generate anxiety and anger because of the strength of emotion underlying them. Indeed, a person's whole emotional life may be determined by the state of this relationship. Anger is often functional in bringing about compromise or in shaping behaviors. The problem with batterers and their victims is that although often committed to one another, they failed to learn appropriate caregiving and attachment behaviors when growing up. Such people often enter into a relationship with the first person who comes along and frequently have a child right away.

Many times the pattern may be evident in a relationship before marriage occurs. One study of 461 college students showed that 30 per cent either had abused or had been abused in a partner relationship. It was striking that the forms that abuse took were often those experienced or observed in the family of origin (Bernard and Bernard, 1983).

Until recently, many jurisdictions followed the rule of spousal immunity, which prevented a woman from suing her husband for assault and battery or for sexual assault (Langley and Levy, 1977). Some feminists describe wife beating as another form of rape, with the striking difference that in this case, the woman is expected to continue to fraternize with her attacker. Some judges, police officers, lawyers, and psychotherapists have expressed the bias that "any woman dumb enough to marry such a jerk deserves what she gets."

Russell (1982b) reported that at least 14 per cent of American women who have ever been married have been raped by their husband or exhusband; this finding was based on her study of about 930 San Francisco women. A key characteristic of relationships in which rape occurs is that the husband is the breadwinner and the wife is the homemaker and rearer of children. The economic imbalance may lead the men to believe that their wives do not have the right to refuse to have sex with them.

The concept of spousal rape is currently undergoing close scrutiny by feminists, legal scholars, and possibly the criminal justice system. Complete discussion of the controversy is found in Chapter 8, Sex and The Law.

Strauss (1976) identified eight ways in which male domination of the family has perpetuated a high level of family violence, including marital rape: (1) the need to defend the presumption of male authority; (2) compulsive masculinity; (3) economic discrimination against women; (4) the burden of child care being placed on women; (5) the myth that a single parent is inadequate; (6) the pre-eminence of the wife role for women; (7) the common perception of women as childlike; and (8) the male orientation of the criminal justice system.

Family violence experts consistently report that the pattern often escalates to homicide (Star, 1982). Violence that goes unchecked spreads; over time the frequency and severity increase, while the amount of provocation necessary decreases.

Spousal Abusers

Most marital abusers are 26 to 35 years of age, with many in the 36- to 50-year-old group. Most have children between 1 and 13 years of age. Typically, their relationship with their partner has lasted from late adolescence or early adulthood. In most cases both partners work outside the home. There is a greater known incidence among blue collar families. Most abuse occurs within the first 15 years of the relationship; 70 per cent abuse soon after the partnership begins. Ninety per cent of abusers do not have a criminal record.

Flanzer (1982) identified several characteristics of marital abusers: their behavior is learned, usually in the family of origin; they project blame onto their victims; they are possessive and jealous of their victims; they have inappropriate expectations of their victims; and they generally cannot recall the details of specific incidents.

Alcohol increases the odds that an individual will cross the line of violence (Flanzer, 1982; Steffen, 1982). A predisposing factor to spousal violence is the abuser's learned belief that under certain circumstances violence is the only answer to problems, and alcohol distorts the perception of these circumstances. In about 16 per cent of cases drugs play a role (Roy, 1982).

There is an unusually high incidence of spousal abuse among military personnel (Raiha, 1978). This may reflect factors such as economic stress, job stress, the prevalence of intercultural marriages, separation from traditional support systems, the military philosophy that "might equals right," and marital separations, which frequently go with the job.

Abusers have learned to repress most feelings; in particular, they believe that men should not show affection or cry (Adams, 1977). They may not have ever learned to relate to others, including their wives. These men may often feel a deep sense of power-lessness (Roy, 1982).

Schauss (1982) pointed out that in some cases the abuser is suffering from a physio-logical problem, such as lead or other heavy metal toxicity; cerebral allergic response to wheat, corn, or potato products; or extreme responses to fatigue. Once treated, the abuse may stop.

Spousal abusers cannot be dismissed as "crazy." Steinmetz (in Langley and Levy, 1977) is quoted as saying that wife beaters are found among every type of man and differ little from anybody else, although they are less skilled at conflict resolution.

Spousal Abuse Victims

Abused wives are often socially isolated. They withdraw over time because of feelings of humiliation, because they are too over-whelmed to carry on the pretext of a happy family, or because their significant others do not appreciate what is occurring.

They tend to be very loyal. Many abused wives are committed to saving their mar-riages, and often they love their husband (Strube and Barbour, 1983). They tend to internalize blame, guilt, and shame for what is going on. And some wives may manipulate significant others by taking on the helpless role; this may be the only role they have learned for interacting with others.

Giles-Sims (1983) studied a group of 31 women in a women's shelter. A high per-centage of these women were cohabiting with a partner, and many were much younger than their partners. Three fourths of these women had been violent themselves. Some had divorced abusive partners but then re-married or moved back in with them. More than a third felt anger at themselves. Ninety per cent felt anger toward their partner, and 93 per cent said they had "forgiven and forgotten" after the first beating. This rate dropped to 20 per cent after the third inci-dent. Overall they saw the man as responsi-ble. Of this group two thirds did not seek help after the first incident. Unfortunately, the sample is too small to be considered typical, but their responses to the abuse might represent a pattern.

It has been commonly believed that victims are as disturbed as their abusers, but this is probably one more instance of blaming the victim (Pogrebin, 1974). Most victims do not like being abused or want to be abused. Rather, due to early socialization they accept the violence and may even agree that they deserve it. These women suffer from ex-tremely diminished self-concept, and they may play a reciprocal role to maintain some sort of balance in the family (Steffen, 1982), such as carrying out the pretense of domestic tranquility for outsiders.

Why do women stay in such relationships? There are themes in our culture that rein-force rape or battery as the norm. Often, they are reinforced with humor, e.g., the saying, "There's nothing wrong with her that a good lay wouldn't cure," or joking refer-ences to wife beating. Some women have grown up in families in which marital vio-lence was usual. Many women in abusive relationships accept that if their loved one treats them in this manner, they must deserve it. The self-concept of many abuse victims is low. The term "loved one" is used advisedly; abusive relationships are usually punctuated by good times, and the woman can experi-ence genuine affection as well as false re-assurances that the problem will not recur.

It is humiliating to admit to one's parents, friends, or even oneself that one is the victim of abuse. Many women hold on to the idea that if they could only change their own behavior in some elusive way, their spouse would not abuse them. Another significant reason for staying in an abusive relationship, perhaps the most salient, is economic de-pendence (Strube and Barbour, 1983). Fear of the unknown is enough to entrap many individuals. If the wife falls into the pattern of trying very hard not to arouse her mate's violent temper, she will blame herself if he becomes violent. Other reasons cited include commitment to making the marriage work, the presence of children, and the lack of a place to go (NiCarthy, 1982; Strube and Barbour, 1983). Even though women's shel-ters have emerged in many cities over the past few years, they are not readily available in rural areas, some cannot accommodate children, and many are very limited in space. Still, they offer some women escape, support, and appropriate referrals.

One client remained in a violent marriage because of the man's threat to kill himself if she left. When she finally did leave, he car-ried out his threat. Other women have elected to stay because they believed they could help their mates deal with emotional problems.

The reasons women remain in these relationships serve to underscore stereotypical gender role differences promulgated in our culture. Women are socialized as passive, weak caregivers; compliance with this social norm works against them.

Women who do seek to prosecute abusive mates generally find the justice system inadequately responsive, and the system often wears them down before the defendant is due to stand trial (Ford, 1983). Most salient is the lack of economic resources (Strube and Barbour, 1983).

Factors That Precipitate Violence

Domestic violence is more likely to occur when couples experience increased life stress. Giles-Sims' (1983) sample of women reported the following problem areas in association with their latest attacks: Ninety per cent reported problems regarding the children; 90 per cent reported jealousy on the part of their mates; 86 per cent reported economic stress; 83 per cent observed that sex was a problem area; 76 per cent observed that allocation of household tasks was an issue; 72 per cent cited the man's drug or alcohol problem; 69 per cent cited their own jobs as an area of conflict, whereas 59 per cent cited the man's employment; and in 55 per cent of cases the woman was jealous.

These situations, commonly reported in the literature on family violence, are characterized by frustration. Other changes often associated with domestic outbursts include pregnancy, the wife's becoming financially independent or assuming the position of financial head of household, and the wife's resuming her career or education. Another time in the family life cycle when marital violence is especially likely is when children reach adolescence (Langley and Levy, 1977).

Because violence is an ill that spreads, domestic abuse can culminate in homicide or suicide.

The Sexual Assault Victim and the Health Care System

Foley and Davies (1983) discuss the need for health professionals who come into contact with victims of rape to clarify or identify their own values about rape. Their attitudes will fall on a continuum from denial of rape facts through anger. Intermediary attitudes on this continuum include cognitive dissonance, or the tension between subscribing to rape myths yet seeing that they are not accurate, and anxiety, probably in recognition of one's own vulnerability. These authors maintain that anger is an informed, logical, and appropriate response to an insane, violent, culturally determined crime, which serves to oppress women.

The goal of providing nonjudgmental care remains an ideal. Holmstrom and Burgess (1978) noted that the vast majority of emergency room personnel maintain a professionally polite demeanor toward rape victims; that is, they are pleasant, but they focus on accomplishing their technical tasks and do not go out of their way to express sympathy. Neither do they express overtly negative feelings. However, exceptions were noted. In their study of 146 rape victims, Holmstrom and Burgess (1978) followed them through the health care and criminal justice systems and found that physicians were especially positive toward women who were pretty and articulate and toward children. Those who elicited particularly negative responses included especially inarticulate individuals, e.g., persons with obvious psychiatric disorders, or individuals with "discrediting" moral backgrounds, such as prostitutes, or circumstances under which they were raped, such as women who were intoxicated.

A great deal of staff energy went into trying to decide whether or not the case was "legitimate." One physician was able to identify his bias against women whose response to rape was defensiveness. Other themes included whether or not the victim had "asked for it" and the victim's perceived moral character. The staff were particularly unsettled by rape victims who were also psychotic.

A basic problem for victims, according to Holmstrom and Burgess (1978), is that the emergency room's two main duties, *to provide medical care* and *to collect legal evidence*, are somewhat contradictory. Health professionals face the duty of helping patients no matter what they have done; on the other hand they must collect data to either legitimate or cast doubt on the patient's claim.

On the whole the victims in the Holmstrom and Burgess study felt that they were treated well at the hospital; however, they often reported feeling that they had to prove that their rape had occurred, perhaps sensing the staff's behind-the-scenes judging. Most thought that the style of interaction of the staff was acceptable. The sex of the physician (male) was not a problem among this group. Victims responded negatively to the pelvic examination, injections, and other further violations of their bodies, although they recognized their importance.

Other issues for victims in the health care system included depersonalization, being kept in ignorance, and the lack of privacy in emergency rooms.

Nursing Process

When a rape victim goes to a health care facility, she should immediately be acknowledged as a person who has experienced a crisis situation (Kolodny, Masters, and Johnson, 1979). She should be made to feel that she is in control of the interaction, so that the role of victim is not reinforced. The nurse's response should be reassuring and not patronizing or judgmental. Outrage on the part of the staff, while a legitimate emotional reaction, is not helpful for the client; neither is sympathy. The victim should be offered support and encouragement to talk about her feelings and about what has happened. While staff in busy emergency rooms may be pressed for time, victims must be offered an opportunity to talk without pressure. Most important in helping the victim talk about the rape are a nonthreatening, genuine demeanor toward the victim and a measure of privacy, the latter a serious problem in emergency rooms (Holmstrom and Burgess, 1978).

The support and sensitivity of staff are of great importance. Staff need to be flexible in terms of the age range, sociocultural background, educational level, marital status, and personalities of their clients. Active communication techniques to draw the victim out are needed. The victim needs to be assured that her response to the rape and her behaviors afterward have been appropriate to help reduce guilt feelings she may have.

A health professional's caring for rape victims needs to create an atmosphere of warmth, safety, and caring. Touch may be appropriate if it is not forced. Offering a cup of tea or coffee may convey concern. Discussion should proceed from least to most threatening aspects. For example, the first

question should *not* be, "Did he penetrate you?" Rather, a general open-ended question such as, "Can you tell me what happened?" may prod the victim to share her story. A victim may *not* spontaneously share that rape occurred during her assault. In that case she needs to be asked. Details about the experience need to be elicited with tact. Legal jargon should be avoided.

Ideally, one staff member and/or volunteer will coordinate care for this client throughout her contact with the health care system. If she is immediately referred to a rape counselor, it should be one who will offer continuity throughout follow-up.

Initially, the caregiver needs to explain to the victim step by step in quantities of information that she can handle what will be done for her and to her in the health care setting.

Many hospitals have provided for staff to receive special training in dealing with rape victims. In a number of cities health care agencies or police departments sponsor rape crisis teams, which often include volunteers who can go to victims as they make initial contact with the police or emergency departments. Such a person can sit with the victim as she waits for attention or until she can collect herself enough to talk about the incident.

Assessment

A general medical and sexual history should be taken from every rape victim. This should include a full menstrual and reproductive history, the date of the last menstrual period, contraceptive use, and the date and type of the last sexual contact prior to the rape. If the victim is or might be pregnant at the time of the rape, this should be noted, as should any reproductive health problems that she may have experienced in the past.

Information about the assault should be documented in the victim's own words when possible. The assault needs to be reconstructed in as much detail as possible. This includes the date, time, place, and circumstances under which the rape occurred; the name of or identifying information about the assailant(s); whether or not she was restrained; the nature of threats or physical force, including the presence of a weapon; the type and extent of injury; the type and amount of sexual or other forced acts; whether the rapist ejaculated, used a condom, or experienced sexual dysfunction; whether or not there were witnesses; whether or not the rapist was under the perceptible influence of drugs or alcohol; whether, and in what way, the victim resisted; whether or not the victim lost consciousness; whether or not the victim injured the rapist; and the victim's post-rape behaviors such as bathing, voiding, having a bowel movement, gargling, douching, changing clothes, or other behaviors that could alter evidence (Foley and Davies, 1983; Kolodny, Masters, and Johnson, 1979). Tactful inquiry might be made as to the client's response at the time of the rape. If she experienced orgasm, guilt may be very intense. Male victims should be asked whether or not they experienced erection. These individuals need reassurance and information about the role of reflexes in sexual responsiveness.

Assessment of the signs and symptoms of physical assault and injury are crucial, both for the treatment of the client and for evidence to be presented if there is a trial.

First, the victim's clothing should be collected, examined for stains that may have resulted from the assault and tagged. It should be explained to the client that forensic laboratories can analyze such stains to better document what has happened and to assist in identifying the offender.

Evidence of trauma should be carefully noted. Instantly developing photographs of bruises, cuts, scratches, or other signs of trauma provide useful documentation. Common sites of injury include the breasts, the head and neck, the extremities, and the rectum, and trauma may take the form of contusion, abrasion, laceration, concussion, stab wounds, or fractures. Gynecological injuries may include abrasion, laceration, or contusion of the external genitalia, the perineum, and the urethra. Sadistic rape will often entail much more extensive damage to the perineal and internal tissues (Kolodny, Masters, and Johnson, 1979).

A pelvic examination is important in order to assess the presence of pregnancy and extent of trauma and to obtain appropriate smears and cultures; however, the examination should never be forced on the victim, lest she be twice traumatized. Rather, the procedure should be explained, along with reasons for performing it, and the woman's consent obtained. The victim should be able to stop this procedure at any time. The speculum should be warmed, and every effort should be made to perform the examination in a gentle manner, with explanations of what will happen next at each step.

Smears, for sperm, seminal fluid, and gonorrhea, should be obtained from the vulva, the vagina, and the cervix; washings should be made of dried secretions on the thighs, perineum, or buttocks. A fluid specimen should be obtained from the posterior fornix. The anus should also be examined, and if the client indicates the need, swabbed. A urethral swab may be required in the case of male victims.

The victim's oral pharynx should be examined and swabbed. Urine should be collected for a pregnancy test, to determine pregnancy prior to the rape, and a blood sample should be taken for serological testing for syphilis. Cultures for gonococci and serological testing for syphilis taken at this time will indicate whether or not the victim had an infection at the time of the assault. However, follow-up tests after 4 to 6 weeks and again at 6 months are needed to see if venereal disease resulted from the rape. Rape victims should have two negative cultures for gonorrhea before they can be considered disease free.

All data should be recorded, and specimens must be labelled immediately. Descriptions should be complete and in terms that non–medically oriented legal personnel can understand whenever possible.

Other evidence to be collected during the physical examination includes combings of the victim's pubic hair, using a new comb and a clean paper towel, and scrapings from under each fingernail as well as nail clippings. All of these specimens should be placed in plastic bags or in test tubes and labelled. A few of the victim's own pubic hairs should be obtained, to differentiate the rapist's from her own (Kolodny, Masters, and Johnson, 1979).

Thorough data collection is tedious and time consuming, but it may make the difference between success or failure in prosecuting the offender.

Initially, for the client's safety, the extent of physical injury needs to be assessed. Severe trauma requires immediate emergency treatment. Every effort must be made to explain what is going on and to reassure the victim.

If trauma is not so extensive, the victim's psychosocial needs will take greater precedence. Her emotional status should be reassessed. Rape is a crisis, and the victim has lost temporary control of her life. Fear is a usual response in the immediate post-rape period, more so than agitation.

It is likely that the victim will be afraid to be alone and afraid to return to her home if that was the scene of the incident. Thus, an immediate need will be the identification of someone to whom the victim can turn, such as a friend or family member willing to take her home with them. This may mean giving emotional support to the victim as she contacts someone and relates what has happened to her, or as significant others arrive on the scene and learn what has happened. It is important to determine the response of close family members or friends to this news. The nurse is in a position to provide support to them as well as to clarify misinformation they may have about sexual assault and to give instructions on how they can be most helpful to the victim in the immediate post-rape phase.

If possible, data on the victim's prior patterns of coping should be obtained and used to compare her current state with previous crisis states as well as to help in identifying supports she may need.

Generally, the nurse will need to make a determination of resources available to the victim, both those identified by the victim in the history and other conversation and those known by the nurse, of which the client may be unaware, such as community shelters, counseling centers, or rape crisis facilities.

The safety of the victim is of primary importance. Assessment of physical safety includes the extent of injury, the victim's competence to drive home, the degree to which her home is rape-proofed, and the likelihood that a rapist might return, particularly if he knows she has sought help. Assessment of psychological safety includes her risk for self-destructive behavior.

Intervention

Based on a theoretical understanding of the experience of assault victims, the nurse can anticipate many of their needs. Clearly, physical injuries need treatment and follow-up.

Pregnancy is a concern among fertile women who have been raped. It is particularly worrisome to women who might have been pregnant already at the time of the assault and to women who for reasons of conscience cannot consider termination of a pregnancy. Pregnancy occurs in about 5 per cent of cases.

Methods of preventing pregnancy include the use of postcoital hormonal contraception, menstrual extraction, or abortion if pregnancy occurs (Foley and Davies, 1983; Kolodny, Masters, and Johnson, 1979).

Although postcoital contraceptive methods have not been approved by the U.S. Food and Drug Administration (FDA), physicians have used them for several years, particularly to treat rape victims. Diethylstilbestrol, the original "morning after pill," was so likely to cause serious side effects that it is no longer used in the United States for that purpose. Currently, combined birth control pills containing 50 mcg of ethinyl estradiol and 0.5 mg of norgestrel are favored: Two tablets are taken within 72 hours (preferably within 12 to 24 hours) of coitus and two more tablets are taken 12 hours later (Hatcher et al, 1988). No data are available regarding harm to the woman or her offspring if she is already pregnant when she takes it.

This regimen may cause nausea; vomiting within an hour of taking the pills necessitates taking a replacement dose. The next menstrual period should occur within 2 to 3 weeks. The client should be told of the following danger signs: severe abdominal pain, severe chest pain or dyspnea, severe headache, sudden visual disturbance, and severe pain in the calf or thigh. Contraindications to the use of estrogen-containing drugs are numerous and must be reviewed with the client before giving them. Some institutions require that clients sign a consent form stating that they have read and understood the package insert before this type of drug is administered.

Higher dose oral estrogens are used, but nausea is a greater problem. Higher dose progestins are also used, but they must be taken within 24 hours of intercourse.

Postcoital insertion of an intrauterine device after rape is *not* advisable because of the increased risk of sexually transmitted disease, which could lead to pelvic inflammatory disease (Hatcher, 1986).

Menstrual extraction may be performed if the menstrual period is 1 or 2 days late. It is advisable to wait until pregnancy is confirmed in order to avoid performing unnecessary procedures. However, some women prefer not to know that they were pregnant so that the ethical dilemma is avoided.

Therapeutic abortion is the final alternative for terminating pregnancy. Some women will choose to carry the pregnancy to term either because termination of pregnancy is unacceptable to them or because the infant might be their spouse's. Such women still have the option of placing the child for adoption after it is born. A minority of women will keep their babies.

Generally, the rape victim will be treated prophylactically for gonorrhea. Procaine penicillin G boosted by the use of probenecid is the drug regimen of choice (Kolodny, Masters, and Johnson, 1979). The client must return for follow-up culture and serology in 4 to 6 weeks. As a result of this treatment, the victim might get vaginitis.

The woman should be counseled to undergo AIDS screening now and at 6 months. She and her partner are advised to use condoms during sexual intercourse and to avoid other high-risk sexual practices until it is confirmed that she was not infected by the human immunodeficiency virus.

Often the health professionals with whom the victim has initial contact are not those who follow-up on her progress, but they are in a position to make appropriate referrals for long-term care. Staff of every emergency department should be aware of rape crisis resources in the community and should offer it to every victim. Either they may tell the victim about the service, and even help her to initiate contact, or they may routinely provide the names and telephone numbers of all victims to the service, so that its personnel can initiate follow-up. Some emergency departments call victims a few days after the rape to see how they are doing and to express concern. This relieves the victim of taking the initiative in seeking help. Burgess and Holmstrom (1974) advocate the counselor taking the initiative in establishing the relationship, making the initial phone call and going to see the victim. The victim is viewed as a normal person whose life has been temporarily disrupted in the physical, emotional, social, and sexual areas. The goal of counseling is to get the victim back into her previous life style as quickly as possible. Previous problems that are not associated with the rape are not considered priority issues. This approach is not viewed by the authors as psychotherapy. If other issues are identified that impede resolution of this crisis, referral for more intense therapy is warranted.

Even in the absence of psychopathology, individuals may need more extensive intervention if they resolve the crisis in a maladaptive way, ending up with a less advanced level of functioning than they had before the rape and thus more vulnerable to future stressors (Forman, 1983). Also, a minority of clients develop no symptoms after the rape, but they may have repressed the situation; they may later develop phobias or other difficulties that necessitate treatment.

Another common type of intervention with rape victims is telephone crisis counseling. This type of counseling is easier for the client to use, since she does not have to seek help physically. Her privacy is respected while reality orientation and reassurance are provided. Finally, it affords the client more control over the interaction (Foley and Davies, 1983).

Victims should be urged to report their assaults to police and to pursue prosecution if it is a criminal offense. This reinforces the feelings that the victim has regained control and that she has done everything possible about the assault (Pekkanen, 1976; Towson and Zanna, 1983). If the victim chooses this route, a long-term supportive relationship with a rape counselor or other such person is particularly desirable, since the legal process will be drawn out over many months or even years.

Some victims may benefit from referrals to clergy; however, it should be known to the staff before making such referrals whether or not individual clergy will respond in a supportive manner. Some, regretably, still express the view that women are seductresses.

Victims of spousal assault should be referred to a women's shelter, if there is one available, or at the very least, to marital counselors. Most city or county health departments offer mental health services with fees on a sliding scale. Assessing the safety of returning home is of paramount importance if the spouse abuse victim has no alternative.

SEXUAL ABUSE OF CHILDREN

A 6-year-old girl and her 8-year-old brother testified that the 31-year-old man who was babysitting them forced them to perform oral sex on him and raped and sodomized them (Greer, 1984).

A mother of five made half a million dollars per year by supplying 80 per cent of the national market for child pornography. Her titles included "Little But Lewd" and "Kinder Orgy" ("Los Angeles Presenting," 1984c).

A middle school science teacher turned himself in after two adolescent girls reported to their mothers incidents of offensive touching in the classroom during regular hours; their mothers in turn contacted state police (Brown, 1984).

A 40-year-old man discovered four teenagers raping a 12-year-old girl in a shed in his backyard during school recess. His response? He got in line and participated (Associated Press, 1983a).

The attorney who successfully prosecuted the mass murderer "Son of Sam" admitted that he sexually molested the 10-year-old daughter of a colleague (Associated Press, 1983c).

Detroit citizens were alarmed by 50 known rapes of students on their way to school during 1983 (Blum, 1984).

This is but a sampling of the many news items on the topic of child sexual abuse that have appeared in the media. The problem is awesome in its scope.

Incidence

Of the 4000 American women interviewed by Kinsey and his associates (1953), 25 per cent had experienced a sexual encounter with an adult before they were 13 years old, which because of the developmental and age differences would, by most authorities, be considered child sexual abuse. Extrapolation of this figure suggests that 25 million American women have been abused to some degree as children (Rush, 1980). Most sexual abuse of children involves a male offender and a female victim (Taubman, 1984).

More recent surveys corroborate that the incidence is high. Estimates range from 50,000 to 336,000 cases of sexual abuse per year (Burgess et al, 1978; Finkelhor, 1978; Sarafino, 1979; Summit and Dryso, 1978), not including the more than 1 million runaways annually. Finkelhor (1979a), surveying 796 students at the University of New Hampshire, found that 19.2 per cent of the females and 8.6 per cent of the males had experienced in childhood sexual contact with an adult. A survey of 267 West Virginia students showed that 43.8 per cent had experienced one or more such episodes before the age of 12 (Schultz and Jones, 1983). A survey of over 500 Boston families indicated that one in ten parents knew that their child had been the victim of actual or attempted sexual abuse ("1 in 10 children," 1983).

Even with studies such as these, it is hard to know the real extent of sexual abuse involving children, since much is unreported (Russell, 1983) and since social problems such as running away are often related to rape and juvenile prostitution (Engel and Lau, 1983).

Definitions

Groth and Burgess (1977) distinguish between sexual pressure and sexual force in the sexual assault of a child. Sexual pressure involves enticement or entrapment of the child into feeling obligated to perform sexually, whereas sexual force is exploitative, involving threat or force. Sexual force may be sadistic, in that the use of physical violence is itself sexually gratifying for the offender.

Sexual abuse of children is defined as the involvement of dependent, developmentally immature children and adolescents in sexual activities that they do not fully comprehend, to which they are unable to give informed consent, or that violate social taboos of family roles (Kempe, 1982). Incest is broadly defined as sexual intercourse between persons so closely related that marriage is illegal. Usually, incest refers to blood relationships such as parent-child, grandparent-grandchild, uncle-niece, or sibling-sibling, but legal authorities have generally included adoptive and stepparent-stepchild relationships as well (Burgess et al, 1978). Pedophilia is an adult's preference for sexual relationships with children (Jones, 1982).

Terminology in this area is confusing. The incest literature includes all possible situations in which partners are related by blood or marriage as if they were a single type of incident. Yet, for example, incest can involve adults mutually consenting to sexual relations or young cousins or siblings playing doctor as well as the adolescent girl who is raped by her father.

Types of sexual abuse of children are varied. Coercive rape certainly occurs to children of both sexes, as does the crime of statutory rape. Sexual assault, voyeurism, sodomy, indecent exposure, and offensive touching are frequent.

Armstrong (1978), herself a victim of incest, interviewed informants about their experiences and identified nine types of incest. *Incidental incest* occurs among related individuals, who are about the same age, as a matter of course during exploration and growing up. Contact may be fleeting and instances may be isolated. A parent may inadvertently fondle and be aroused by fondling his or her child, or siblings may explore each others' bodies. These instances are rarely traumatic to the child. *Ideological incest* represents the minority of cases of adult-child relations in which parents espouse total sexual freedom of expression. In one example of this, parents on a commune thought it was fine that their adult male friend engaged in coitus with their 4-year-old daughter, since they believed both were freely expressing natural feelings. *Psychotic incest* is characterized by other signs of behavioral deviance, such as alcohol or drug abuse, violence, or otherwise diagnosible conditions. *Rustic incest* is characterized by its setting. These are isolated, rural communities, particularly in the mountains, in which incest is a social norm. No particular harm results, although such communities often demonstrate signs of inbreeding. True *endogamous incest* is most typical. The incest, a sign of communications breakdown within the family system, persists over time. Physical battery does not take place; in fact, the father probably feels strong affection for his child, and although there is tremendous conflict, the child probably feels affection for him. In all other respects this family may appear "normal." One of the problems that Renshaw (1982) identified, particularly in step-families, is that feelings among related individuals have not been desexualized.

Misogynistic incest is characterized by the offender's feelings that all women, including his wife and his daughters, are whores; therefore, what one does with them does not matter. *Imperious incest* is characterized by a father figure who exercises total control of the women in his family; he may pick a favorite daughter for sexual relations. However, her siblings may contend for the "honor" or inherit it when she leaves the home. *Pedophilic incest* occurs when the offender prefers children as sexual partners. Child rape is an act of violence like other cases of rape described previously. It may occur in response to stress or anger but rarely typifies a family pattern. *Perverse* or *pornographic incest* entails getting children to perform deviate acts, perhaps with each other,

to be filmed or photographed or to engage in prostitution.

The lack of clear, consistent definitions in the area of sexual abuse of children represents a methodological obstacle in this body of research (Bixler, 1983; Finkelhor and Hotaling, 1984). For example, the National Incidence Study of Child Abuse and Neglect limited its definition of sexual abuse to those cases in which the offender is a caretaker. This excluded cases in which the perpetrator was a stranger, a family friend, an acquaintance, or a relative, although the definition can be construed to include teachers, coaches, and others who work with children.

While incest is the focus of most of the literature in this area, terms are often interchanged, and the type of sexual abuse being discussed is often unclear. It is important for future research that classification of sexual abuse of children be clarified and standardized.

Historical and Transcultural Perspectives

There are both Biblical and mythical references to incest. In the Old Testament, the widower Lot settled in a cave in the hills with his two virgin daughters. Recognizing that their family would die out under such isolated circumstances, the daughters gave their father enough wine to intoxicate him and then engaged in sexual relations with him. In that way each bore a son (Genesis 19).

Classical references include the fact that Jupiter, king of the Roman gods, gave his daughter Venus to his son Vulcan, Venus's half brother, as his wife (Fuller, 1959). Sophocles' tragic hero Oedipus was ruined when he lived out the prophesy, albeit unknowingly, that he would marry his mother and slay his father. One version of the death of King Arthur is that his kingdom, Camelot, was destined to be destroyed by Arthur's son Mordred, who was born of the teenage Arthur's sexual union with his sister, Morgane le Fay. A Japanese Shintoist informant shared other examples with the author—the winter season is the unhappy result of attempted incest from which the Sun Goddess fled; and less traumatically, the Japanese people are reported to have descended from the union of ancient sibling gods.

Historically, sibling pairing has been prevalent in some societies. During the Ptolemaic dynasty in Egypt, full-sibling marriages were common among royalty. During the first two or three centuries after Christ in Roman Egypt, sibling marriages were frequent among commoners. There is some evidence that sibling marriages were common in the royal families of Peru and Hawaii as well.

In certain open societies in which young girls and boys freely interact, sexual experimentation among siblings or cousins is quite usual during preadolescence (Tannahill, 1982). There are cultures, such as the traditional society of Crete, in which it is not only a father's right, but it is his parental duty to introduce his daughters to coitus before they marry. Among the Mormons, incest was permitted until 1892 (Renvoize, 1982).

In regard to the age at which youngsters were expected to become sexually active, it is interesting to reflect that Mary was about 12 years old when she became the mother of Jesus in Christian tradition, and Juliet was no more than 14 when she died with her beloved Romeo. These observations reflect their cultural context and the relatively shorter life-expectancies of those times. Today, in traditional Moslem societies a prized bride is about 14 years old, although her husband is much older, and the most desirable marriage is made between first cousins in order to keep wealth, in the form of dowries, within the clan. In 1880 sexual abuse of children comprised 10 per cent of cases reported in the Boston social service agencies (Gordon and O'Keefe, 1984); yet Sigmund Freud was unable to accept that Viennese men could be guilty of sexual abuse to the extent that his female patients reported (Taubman, 1984). In an act that probably undermined efforts to deal with this problem from his time to the present, Freud renounced his earlier public position that incestuous sexual exploitation was common and attributed reports to his patients' wishful fantasies.

Legal Issues

The criminal justice system has generally responded more sympathetically and more actively toward children who are victims of sexual abuse than toward women. At the same time, society's response to incest is hampered by laws that vary widely among the 50 states in terms of definitions and sanctions (Renshaw, 1982). Chapter 8, Sex and the Law, provides an indepth discussion of the legal complexities surrounding sexual abuse of children.

Several authors (Renshaw, 1982; Renvoize, 1983; Thorman 1983) have questioned whether the criminal justice system is the appropriate resource for handling incest, that it is better viewed as a clinical family-system problem rather than as a crime. Renvoize (1983) observed that it is peculiar that incest offenders may routinely be sentenced to seek psychotherapy; yet in no other criminal case does this happen, thus exemplifing society's confusion as to the nature and meaning of incest.

Most intervention with incest offenders is carried out jointly by mental health personnel and the courts (Stark, 1984). In one large intervention program in Santa Clara, California, offenders must face charges within the criminal justice system. However, it is believed that if the offender does not have the threat of a prison sentence hanging over his head, he will be better motivated to deal constructively with the problem. The goal of this program is to reunite the family, and they achieve this in 80 per cent of cases, with less than a 1 per cent incidence of relapse.

The Sociocultural Context of Sexual Abuse in Children

In our society there is an increased sexualization of children. Examples abound in advertising, films, and popular music, such as an adolescent Brooke Shields modeling her designer jeans while posed suggestively and making verbal innuendos or the popular film *The Hotel New Hampshire*. The latter, based on John Irving's novel, chronicled the sexual awakening of two adolescent siblings. Ultimately, the girl was gang raped by schoolmates and then consummated her sexual desire for her brother. A recent advertisement for another manufacturer of designer apparel featured preschoolers dancing the "bump" to the jingle, "You've got the look to make things happen." Young people and educators report that pressure to begin dating is well established in many social groups by the time children are 12 years old. Part of the increasing sexualization of adolescents and children is in response to the sexual revolution of the 1960s, when it became passé to draw boundaries in terms of sexual behaviors, and limits were expanded. Columnist Ellen Goodman (1983b) observed that as a result of this social upheaval sex educators today have trouble defining developmentally appropriate sexual behaviors for young people.

While all of this was taking place the child pornography business was booming. Following a 1970 Presidential Commission conclusion that there was no evidence that exposure to sexually explicit materials resulted in social or individual harm (Associated Press, 1984b), pornographers became more blatant in the use of children.

The traditional ideal of femininity has been the infantilized woman (Rush, 1982), and helplessness has been her key characteristic. Over that past 100 years, numerous authors have portrayed young girls as sirens, from Dostoyevsky in *The Possessed* to Nabokov in *Lolita*. Advertisers have capitalized on men's erotic attraction to little girls, such as when Bell Telephone's advertisement for its telephone directory featured a little girl standing on a telephone book with her buttocks exposed. Numerous examples of children having been sexually assaulted in response to the offender's exposure to pornography have been reported (Rush, 1982). In one case a 15-year-old boy attempted to rape a 9-year-old girl. He admitted when he was caught that he had done the same thing in three other cities and attributed the urge to do so as a result of poring over his father's pornography.

One factor that makes it easy to lure children into sexually abusive situations is their fear of refusing adults. Other significant ones are the enticement of money, records and tapes, clothing, drugs, or alcohol. The sex industry is cloaked in a veneer of glamor. Youngsters who are enticed into the sex industry are attracted to this. One young client of the author's was taking home $750 per week for performing in a live sex act. It was extremely difficult to talk with this girl about giving up the money to enter school, even though she was very unhappy and was mixing a large daily intake of alcohol with assorted psychotropic drugs. Sometimes the promised reward never materializes, but by the time children realize it, they are under the control of a pimp.

The sex industry pushes a life style that is free of responsibility. It is not a big step from portraying women as "bunnies," youthful playthings, to acceptance of children as sex objects (Lederer, 1982b).

Taubman (1984) clearly delineates a broad multifactorial approach to the cause of incest in particular, emphasizing that incest is better viewed as a process than as an event. Taubman suggests that all people experience incestuous tensions, particularly within the family context. Many parents exhibit incestuous feelings in the form of possessiveness or jealousy, for example, a father's feelings of indignation regarding his daughter's boyfriend. In this context, incest is part of the process of living. However, experiencing feelings is very different from acting on them, and Taubman does not excuse consummation of incestuous feelings.

Four aspects of American society can be examined in order to better understand incest. These are cultural attitudes toward sex, the patriarchy system, depersonalization within the culture, and compartmentalization of life styles.

The social context in which incest occurs in America is one in which attitudes toward sex are contradictory. Taubman notes that Americans are either obsessive or repressive about sex. Sex education is still controversial in most communities, although newstands across the country openly sell soft- and hard-core pornography.

Western societies are clearly patriarchal (Taubman, 1984; Millet, 1978). Women are sex objects, while men are production or achievement objects. In this way both men and women are depersonalized. Such depersonalization will occur in any postindustrial nation in which people are valued more for their ability to contribute to the economic system than for their intrinsic worth (Taubman, 1984); depersonalization is reinforced by the breakup of extended families and communities.

Finally, factors that have contributed to perpetuation of the problem of sexual abuse of children are denial of the extent of the problem and stereotyping of child molesters. Most citizens would probably be shocked if they thought someone in their social circle were either a perpetuator or a victim of this problem; yet, either situation is likely. The broadcast of the television movie "Something About Amelia" was an important consciousness-raising event, even though some experts have criticized the film for oversimplifying the situation. In contrast, a pro-pederasty lobby has recently emerged (Renvoize, 1982).

These individuals idealize adult-child sex and seek to abolish prohibitions ostensibly on the basis that children should not be denied this pleasure. In fact, at the time when leaders of a large sex ring in Boston were tried, the first openly publicized conference on man/boy love was held in Boston, and 30 adults and minors established an organization entitled the North American Man Boy Love Association (Burgess & Birnbaum, 1982).

Incest

CHARACTERISTICS OF OFFENDERS AND VICTIMS

In a study by Finkelhor (1979a), coercive sexual experiences recalled by female college students involved family members in 43 per cent of cases, acquaintances in 33 per cent of cases, and strangers in only 24 per cent of cases. For male victims the incidence of abuse by a family member was 17 per cent; by acquaintances, 53 per cent; and by strangers, 30 per cent. Offenders averaged 32 years of age in the case of female victims and 27 years of age in the case of male victims. The average age of male victims at the time of the offense was 10.2 years and of females, 11.2 years. About half were victimized between the ages of 4 and 6. Females between 6 and 12 years were twice as likely as males to be abused, while the reverse was true during the early teen years. A substantial number of perpetrators were often the adolescents' relatives. Offenders were most often males (84 per cent of cases involving boys and 94 per cent of cases involving girls). Coitus was rare, whereas fondling and exhibitionism were common.

In another study Finkelhor (1980) found that 13 per cent of college students had experienced sexual activity with a sibling. (Cousins were also common participants.) These activities were primarily heterosexual, and most instances occurred after age 8. Genital fondling and touching were the most frequent activities, although the incidence of intercourse and attempted intercourse rose with age. In only one third of cases was it an isolated experience. Nearly one third continued their relations longer than 1 year. Coercive incidents were relatively rare, but most involved a female victim. In most cases in which there was an age span greater than 5 years, the younger sibling was usually female. Thirty per cent of these respondents found their sexual experience with a sibling to be positive, whereas 30 per cent found it negative, and 40 per cent were neutral. Negative feelings were nearly all reported by females, particularly when coercion and a wide age span were factors.

Once incestuous relationships begin, they generally continue until some specific event stops them, such as marriage of the victim or her leaving home, divorce of the parents, pregnancy, or the daughter's reporting the incest (Revoize, 1982). Victims are the most frequent reporters of incest, followed by school authorities and parents.

Incest is rarely accompanied by physical abuse, and in almost all cases the parents are living together. In about a third of cases, in a study cited by Renvoize (1982), there were four or more children in the family. Many of the fathers were extremely religious; among religious groups Roman Catholics were most represented.

Three types of incestuous males are described by Renvoize (1982): the rigid and isolated promiscuous male, the pedophile, and the male in the endogamic family, who is fairly law abiding, and whose family appears apparently normal. The last type, the most prevalent, may be paranoid or may experience unusually intense unconscious homosexual urges, according to Renvoize. He often has transferred his hostility toward his mother to his wife. It is likely that he grew up on a farm or otherwise experienced social isolation during childhood, and he is often immature. She observed that such men not only have sexual desire but also emotional needs that they seek to satisfy via their daughters. They often romanticize their daughters in a manner evocative of adolescent crushes. They tend to behave in an authoritarian manner toward their families.

Renvoize claims that most of these men do not venture outside the family for sexual relations, although others have claimed that the opposite is true (Gebhard et al, 1965). They tend to be inexperienced and uninformed regarding sexual matters, and while they blame their wives for unsatisfactory sex, they often do not know how to satisfy women. Some studies suggest that this group of men tends to have poorer employment records than most, and alcohol plays a role in about a third of cases. Offenders tend to see their wives as stronger than they actually are. Stepfathers are more likely than biological fathers to commit incest, and incestuous men tend to be older than other fathers of the same age children.

Mothers in these families have often been victims of physical or sexual abuse in childhood. These women are often withdrawn or emotionally distant from their spouses. Daughters are much more vulnerable to incest in families in which the mother has scolded them for asking about sex or for masturbating; that is, sex is not an acceptable topic for communication.

There tend to be strict rules to keep these family systems intact, and the children follow them blindly. Daughters who are victims often suspect that their mothers know what is going on, but the mothers do not broach the topic. It may be that they are too horrified to do so (Cohen et al, 1987). Communication is generally poor. There tend to be fused boundaries, the members of these families seem to experience more physical ailments than in other families, and children are parentalized. Role reversal between mother and daughter may relieve her of sexual duties, although Renvoize (1982) believes these women generally are not conscious of the situation in their homes. These mothers are often quite independent, and they rarely leave the marriage.

In a classic study Gebhard and associates (1965) found that the average age of prepubescent female victims was 9, and that in over one third of cases the incest had been going on from 1 to 3 years. The victim was typically the eldest daughter. Coitus was rarely involved. However, when the daughter was in her early teen years, intercourse was usual, alcohol was commonly involved, and most incidents were premeditated. Armstrong (1978) observed that often a daughter's reaching menarche precipitated or escalated incestuous activity. More recent work (Cohen et al, 1987) demonstrates that the same vulnerability or "special child" quality that places children at risk for other forms of abuse increases their risk for sexual abuse.

In cases in which daughters were in late adolescence, the relationships resembled adult patterns of sexual activity. Most incidents were not planned, alcohol was generally not a factor, and among the 20 per cent of cases in which the daughter was between 20 and 25 years of age, most had begun their incestuous relationships before the age of 16.

INCEST MYTHS

Several myths, particularly in regard to incest, have been perpetuated, including the following:

1. Incest occurs primarily in poor, uneducated families. It *is* true that lower-class families may be subject to more frequent reporting of incest to legal authorities, but incest is not bound by socioeconomic status or professional level (Renvoize, 1982).

2. Incest is usually committed by a father figure who is crazy or degenerate. It is generally held that incest is a symptom of a dysfunctional family system, and it is often the case that offenders grew up in families in which they did not learn appropriate expressions of intimacy and caring. It is also true that many offenders abuse alcohol. However, only a small minority appear psychologically abnormal to outsiders or experience deviant sexual preferences, such as pedophilia. Most do not batter their victims, and they are generally law-abiding (Renvoize, 1982).

3. Most claims of incest are fabricated by the child. This myth may underly the legal requirement of corroboration of the child's testimony. It probably began with Freud, who suggested that reports of incest were actually cases of wishful thinking, symptomatic of unresolved Oedipal desires (Stone, Tyler, and Mead, 1984; Taubman, 1984). In fact, most children's reports are true.

4. The child provokes or actively participates in the relationship. It *may* be that youngsters occasionally behave seductively as they try new aspects of their gender roles and test significant others. This is not done with full awareness of its meaning or potential outcome. Piagetian theory of cognitive development has provided the understanding that youngsters do not develop the ability to abstract about possible outcomes of actions until late adolescence.

5. Mothers of incest victims know that it is occurring or even actively collude. While in hindsight many mothers recognize signs that the incest was occurring, they are rarely consciously aware of the situation at the time. Communication is generally poor in these families (Armstrong, 1978; Taubman, 1984). In cases in which the mother *is* aware, reasons that she tolerates it include economic dependency, fear, lack of knowledge of resources, lack of a support system, and the inability to identify alternatives (reasons sim-

ilar to those cited by battered wives for remaining in an abusive situation).

BREAKING THE CYCLE OF ABUSE

Sooner or later in most cases of incest some event breaks the cycle: discovery, pregnancy, rebellion by the victim, the victim's leaving home, divorce, a change in victim, or more rarely, reporting of the problem to authorities (Taubman, 1984).

Victims tend not to seek exposure of the problem. They generally feel love for their fathers even when they are angry with them. They may feel pain and guilt for humiliating and degrading their father, and the threat of break-up of the family and home is real. After reporting the situation, the child may grieve the loss of her father or her intact family.

The mother of an incest victim who reports the problem often doubts her child, preferring to believe her husband instead. The mother, too, is threatened by the possible break-up of the family system. Families fear that the child is playing a hoax or manipulating family members. However, false accusations are very rare. Stone, Tyler, and Mead (1984) noted that if a child knows enough about sexual abuse to make the accusation, he or she has probably experienced some sort of trauma.

Even when family members believe the child, they often condemn the child for publicizing their problem. A vicious cycle of blaming is established, and often the child who may already be feeling guilty bears the brunt of this. Mothers who become aware of incest in their families are often ashamed that they failed to protect their child or that they failed to see the signs and act on them. They blame themselves in addition to lashing out at their child and dealing with their husband's guilt. Public admission of incest in the family system forces the mother to acknowledge that she had been sexually rejected for a younger woman.

The father, after a period of denial, may rationalize his behavior by blaming the child for seducing him or for seeking sex, by calling his behavior "sex education," by noting that others do it, or by criticizing his spouse for withholding sex and/or affection.

All of these pressures within the family result in a high proportion of cases in which accusations are retracted before offenders can be prosecuted. There is also pressure from outside the family to hold the mother and daughter responsible for the man's behavior (Taubman, 1984).

Sexual Abuse Outside the Family

Burgess and associates (1984) in studying youngsters who were victims of sex rings and pornographic exploitation, found that the children were socialized in such a way as to convince them that the behaviors were normal. Threat and peer pressure were used, and children were often locked up. Perpetrators were often respected members of the community who had legitimate contact with children, such as teachers, coaches, or scout leaders. Not only did adult leaders abuse the youngsters, but they also pitted them against each other. A hierarchy was established in which it was acceptable for older or larger youths to harass younger or smaller ones. The sex rings often existed over a period of time; 61 per cent of the youths in the Burgess study had been in such rings for at least 1 year. Activities, often photographed, included sodomy, sadism, exhibitionism, and degradation such as urinating into a victim's mouth. Adult pornography books were used for instruction. While the youths were paid, in money, alcohol, or drugs, they were also victims of blackmail or extortion. Often, ring members recruited other, younger children. In Burgess and associates' study, half the respondents (49 boys and 17 girls) had two parents in the home. Their ages ranged from 6 to 16 years at the time of disclosure.

Sex rings maintain children's collusion by positive motivators such as money, alcohol, and drugs and by negative motivators such as threats of harm, blackmail, and extortion. This control over the children is intense. Therefore, disclosure is most often indirect. Ring leaders may be caught dealing in pornography, or parents' suspicions that something is wrong may be aroused by problems such as genital or anal complaints, an increase in common childhood complaints such as headache or anorexia, sudden alterations in social or school behavior, and an increase in acting out. Community responses may include detailed media coverage, which the victims find humiliating, and ridicule and stigmatization by classmates. Parents who support the child with counseling and the opportunity to make a fresh start with new peers in a new school offer the best chance of their child's integrating the event and focusing on the future.

When the perpetrator is a stranger or even an acquaintance outside the family, parents are the ones who typically report the offense to authorities. They initially feel blame and guilt for not having protected their child adequately. But as in the case of incest, blame may shift to the child as the crisis develops. For example such beliefs may be expressed as, "If he came home when I told him to, it would not have happened," or "If she had told me about this, I could have stopped it."

Effect of Sexual Abuse on Its Victims

Much has been written on the impact of sexual abuse on children. The act of abusing a child causes the child to be sexualized before it is developmentally appropriate. Under normal circumstances, when family communications are open, children seek information as they are ready. In early dating situations young people generally engage in a gradual progression of sexual behaviors in which they have consented to participate. In instances of sexual coercion, the child does not consent and has no control over what is going on. Children's trust in adults has been betrayed. They are generally ignorant of the consequences of sexual behavior because of their immaturity and inexperience. They participate out of fear or because they may have been offered bribes (Finkelhor, 1979b).

In his study of college students who had been sexually assaulted as children, Finkelhor (1979a) found that females viewed the majority of experiences as negative even when there was no physical brutality. Only 7 per cent found it to be positive. In contrast, only about a third of males viewed the experience as a negative one. The salient variables for both genders were the amount of force used and the age of the offender. The more brutal the experience and the older the perpetrator, the worse the perception of the child. Surprisingly no significant relationships were found among the sex of the offender, duration of the relationship, the child's age, whether or not the experience was reported, whether or not coitus was involved, or the nature of the relationship between victim and

offender and perceived trauma. This finding is in contrast to more recently reported clinical findings that the ability to form close relationships is permanently impaired when the offender is an adult family member (Cohen et al, 1987).

Initially, victims may repress the incident, and many years later it can be the underlying source of depression, feelings of worthlessness, and sexual problems such as promiscuity. Realizing this after a long struggle to come to terms with her own experience, United States Senator Paula Hawkins of Florida disclosed that she had been abused as a 5 year old ("Dark Memory," 1984b). It was her hope that her story would serve as a lesson for parents and children on the need to communicate openly about sexual abuse. At least one youngster was inspired by Hawkins' report to share what had happened to her (Associated Press, 1984a). Hawkins said that she now makes it a practice to ask youngsters to whom she is close if anything "spooky" ever happens to them in order to promote an open environment for their sharing incidents.

Clinicians and researchers in the area of sexual abuse of children have noted high incidences among abuse victims of problems such as psychiatric illness in childhood or later years and running away. Perhaps half of runaway girls have been sexually abused by relatives or other known adults (Goodwin, 1982). It was a common factor in histories of clients of one New York City shelter for runaway youths. In one case of an extremely disturbed young woman, the client reported that her mother, a bisexual, had assaulted her during childhood. This youngster fled at age 17 and was in an extreme state of confusion regarding her own sexuality. She was supporting herself by performing in live sex acts in the Times Square sex industry.

Young people who are sexually abused learn that sexual behavior is devoid of feeling and trust and leads to material gratification (Burgess et al, 1981). Prostitution is a natural, frequent outcome for them. Several studies of prostitutes have found that they were initiated into sex earlier than most young people, with more partners and with less emotional involvement. In as many as one third of cases, they have been victims of rape or incest. They are likely to begin working as prostitutes while in their teens (James and Meyerding, 1977; Marieskind, 1980; Winick and Kinsie, 1971). Once initiated into sexual behavior with adults, it is difficult to return to a more developmentally appropriate level of sexuality.

It has been suggested that sexual abuse is more damaging the later in childhood it occurs and the more emotionally reactive parents and significant others are to disclosure (Goodwin, 1982). Additionally, in the case of assault by strangers, and perhaps also when the offender is known, a critical factor in the outcome for the child is whether or not his or her parents believe the accusation. Stone, Tyler, and Mead (1984) stress the importance for the victim of law enforcement officers' behaving with tact and empathy toward the family during interviews and later contacts. They note that the victims typically exhibit fear, embarrassment, guilt, confusion, and shame. Children may cling to their parents and exhibit shock manifested by agitation or crying. Girls in particular may behave in a fearful manner toward male officers. When the accused offender is a family member, generally a father figure, it is crucial to remember that most often the child has love for him, and therefore it may be more upsetting to refer to this person as being punished than to stress that he needs help. It is not the man that the child dislikes, but having sex with him.

Betrayal by family members or friends is a major theme for victims of abuse. In Erikson's theory of growth and development it is emphasized that the very first developmental task to be mastered is trust in one's family and environment. The child learns that its needs will be met as long as it remains in a state of dependency. The Freudian model portrays the child learning in the preschool years that parents are not appropriate sex objects for children and that in general children cannot successfully compete with them. It would make a fascinating research project to assess mastery of these tasks by children in abusive families. Assuming that children have progressed beyond these points, abuse renders these fundamental principles false. The child *cannot* trust parents, and the child-parent boundary in regard to sexual relations does *not* exist. This reversal is anxiety producing; children often present to health professions with a sudden onset of behavioral problems, sleep disturbances, depression, or other manifestations of anxiety.

From the child's perspective, the betrayal is committed not only by the offender but also, in the case of father-daughter abuse, by the mother as well. She failed to stop the abuse and upon being confronted with it, she may deny the child's accusation or vent anger toward the child for threatening the stability of the home.

An additional lesson learned by victims is that sex becomes equated not with affection but with power. They were powerless in the abuse situation, and they may continue to be victims in relationships, as in cases in which they marry abusers, become prostitutes under the control of abusive pimps, or proceed from one heart-breaking sexual relationship to the next. Or they may seek to control others with sex (Renshaw, 1982). Many victims, as the favored child in the family, have been granted rewards or privileges in exchange for sex. They learn that love is a response to what they *give* rather than to what they *are* (Rosensweig-Smith, 1982).

Consistent with Sanford and Fetter's (1979) contention—that there are victim types who wear their low self-esteem for prospective offenders to see—incest victims experience a higher incidence of rape later on than do nonvictims (Renvoize, 1982). They are more vulnerable because they do not react aggressively.

One family systems theorist suggests that the father has actively intervened to prevent a close mother-daughter relationship, since a strong alliance of women in the family would vastly diminish his power (Taubman, 1984). The daughter may feel guilty for humiliating or displacing her mother. Where there are female siblings they may be pitted against one another in competition for the father's attention and rewards. Victims often withdraw from social relationships with peers because they perceive that they are different. Additionally, a jealous father may restrict his victim's activities as much as possible. Rewards may be the means for preventing the daughter's leaving as well as disclosing the activity.

With such intense negative emotions so pervasive in the family, everyone is at risk for self-destructive behaviors. These may include suicide, prostitution, or dropping out of school as well as drug or alcohol abuse or children's fleeing into early pregnancy and/or marriage. Delinquent behaviors may be a mechanism for attracting attention or for punishment of the parents.

Not only do victims lack support because of role confusion in the home or restrictions made by the father, but also they tend to believe that incest is much rarer than it is and that they are the only persons in their community who have undergone this experience. They lack someone with whom they can talk about the experiences and a peer group to help them deal with the usual traumas of adolescence.

After disclosure, the whole family may experience rejection by the community and, perhaps, financial hardships. The victim may feel responsible for bringing this about. If she is removed to a foster home, she may perceive that *she* is being punished for what happened (Stark, 1984).

Incest victims usually have cooperated with their abusers. Physical force is rare, and sometimes the incestuous relationship develops so subtly that the child does not realize that it is abnormal. Abusers generally reinforce the naturalness of it, although a conflicting message is given when they swear their victims to secrecy or blackmail them. Later, victims may believe that they were willing participants, thus reinforcing guilt feelings. On the other hand they may believe that by participating they are holding their families together, or they may be grabbing for affection in whatever form it comes.

Renvoize (1982) proposed that incest victims feel less badly about themselves than children who have been physically brutalized by abusive parents. But there is no support for this view, and it certainly contradicts research of rape victims, in which their guilt feelings are found to be greater the less physical violence they endured. Decreased self-confidence and increased social isolation have been documented in one follow-up investigation of 49 children who were sexually assaulted an average of 2.6 years prior (Tong, Oates, and McDowell, 1987).

Female incest victims often have sexual difficulties throughout life relating to an inability to trust men or to their own feelings of guilt (Becker et al, 1986). These women report numerous instances of multiple divorces, marriages to abusers, an inability to enjoy sexual relations, or a lesbian life style (Armstrong, 1978). Many experience flashbacks and nightmares for years after the abusive situation ends. Stark (1984) found that one third of a group of incest victims in California had become lesbians. In contrast, another study reported that many victims over-valued and idealized men, seeking to recreate the same special relationship they had had with their fathers. Perceiving other

women as rivals or as powerless, they tended to be generally hostile toward them.

Victims may get involved with men whom they do not respect because they feel they deserve no better (Taubman, 1984). They may vacillate between promiscuity and celibacy, as it is difficult for them to maintain relationships without letting them become sexual, owing to their confusion regarding the nature of affection, sex, and power.

In a survey of nearly 1000 university students, Fritz, Stroll, and Wagner (1981) noted that 1.8 per cent of all females and 25 per cent of those who had been incest victims had sexual problems relating to childhood molestation. While 4.8 per cent of males in the sample had been molested, they tended not to relate any sexual difficulties they were experiencing to their prior abusive experiences. The authors observe that whereas women are taught that sex must occur within the context of affection, males are taught to "score," and they suggest that men could be objective about their initiation into sex, whereas young women felt violated. Their sexual difficulties were most often related to feelings of guilt.

Many victims display *dysfunctional sexual arousal*, formerly termed frigidity (McGuire and Wagner, 1978; Renvoize, 1982; Wallace, 1981). They relate sexual contact to their molestation. If that experience was pleasurable, guilt will often persist. Additionally, victims may feel the need to be in control of sensual contact, and they may maintain strict self-control in order to repress their feelings of anger at having been violated. Furthermore, since most molestation of girls occurs in relationships in which there was prior trust that was subsequently abused, it becomes difficult to trust one's sexual partner.

It is often sexual dysfunction, decades after the fact, that brings a victim into therapy, in which she is finally able to share her secret and to deal with it (Summit and Dryso, 1978).

Burgess and associates (1984), in studying children involved in sex rings, identified several types of symptoms that were common before disclosure. Physical signs included urinary tract infections, genital soreness, and anal irritation. Children tended to complain more of headaches, stomachaches, loss of appetite, and vomiting. There was also an increase in insomnia, fantasizing, and daydreaming. Many experienced a decline in grades, withdrawal from peer group activities, increased argumentativeness at home and with friends, and such acting-out behaviors as stealing, setting fires, and using sexually focused language, mannerisms, and dress. Upon disclosure, most of the children demonstrated signs of post-traumatic stress, including intrusive thoughts, flashbacks, nightmares, and withdrawal. The children were less trusting of others and felt they did not need significant others in their lives. Truancy and getting in trouble at school increased. The children were ambivalent about whom to talk to about the incident and felt pressure due to media coverage of the disclosure. Some experienced ridicule at school. They tended either to distance themselves from or to align themselves more closely with other members of the ring. Some became suicidal, and others increased their use of drugs or alcohol.

Most developed symptoms that had not been present prior to disclosure, including hyperalertness and increased fist fighting and risk-taking behaviors. Others demonstrated general malaise, bed wetting, moodiness, or guilt.

Specific behavioral patterns were also identified during follow-up of these children (Burgess et al, 1984). Integration of the event was defined as mastery of anxiety about it. The child developed objectivity about the event, saw the adult leaders as wrong and responsible, and hoped for their punishment. The child who integrated the experience was future oriented and demonstrated age-appropriate adjustments to family, peers, and schools, often in a new setting. Avoidance of the event occurred in those children who repressed their anxiety about it, consciously or unconsciously. They denied that the event occurred or reacted stoically but still feared the offender and tended to be present oriented. When life stress increased, these children were thrown back into the crisis reaction, which typified disclosure, although they could manage when life stress was low. These children felt guilty and often were unable to break cycles of failure or self-destructiveness.

Repetition of symptoms entailed feelings of anxiety and powerlessness and the belief that they were personally responsible for what happened. These children were generally unable to establish stable family, peer, or school relationships. Many of this group tended to continue in sexually abusive relationships, such as prostitution or as abusers of others, or to drop out of school.

Identification with the exploiter entailed

dealing with anxiety by transformation of one's self into the person making the threat. These children became antisocial, minimized the event, had difficulty dealing with authorities, and often perpetuated acts of sexual abuse, such as child molestation, rape, or pimping.

Children who were able to integrate the experience, about 25 per cent of the group, tended to be those who were involved in the sex rings for less than a year and who were not directly involved in pornography.

In the clinical experience of this author prognosis for victims' rebuilding their lives is poor. Most clients were unable to break out of the cycle, and many died soon after contact because of drug overdose or alcohol toxicity, physical illness resulting from their overall run-down state, or brutality by customers or pimps.

There may be instances in which victims of sexual abuse or incest in particular are not traumatized by it. One of Armstrong's (1978) informants described her affair with her father, beginning when she was 19 years old and continuing up to the time she wrote to Armstrong, about 8 years, in glowing terms. It had been satisfying to her, and she had no desire to terminate it or to seek another partner. A few studies have suggested that some victims can become well-integrated adults (Masters, Johnson, and Kolodny, 1982). But generally an incestuous relationship between a child and an adult creates major conflicts for the child (Briere and Runtz, 1988).

The Health Care System and the Sexually Abused Child

Anger and revulsion are typical responses of most health professionals who come into contact with families in which adult-child incest occurs. This response is not necessarily the healthiest for the child who feels conflicted enough in regard to her father. The child does not want her loved one to be publicly humiliated. She primarily wants him to stop what he has been doing to her (Stone, Tyler, and Mead, 1984).

Holmstrom and Burgess (1978) observed that health professionals are generally quite sympathetic to juvenile rape victims. But adolescents may be at risk to be viewed more negatively if they are perceived to have put themselves in jeopardy. Youngsters often experiment with dress, mannerisms, and interactions with the opposite sex as they struggle to come to terms with their sexual identity and may often put themselves in vulnerable situations (Goodman, 1983b). Typically, young girls are attracted to boys a few years older because of the girls' faster rate of maturation. High school or even junior high school students may experiment with drugs or alcohol. Therefore, it is easy for health professionals to become exasperated with young girls who are sexually assaulted if it appears that they contributed to the incident to any extent.

Sexual abuse of children is an emotional issue for health professionals and often for the community at large. Thus, advocates for these victims need to be especially sensitive to the issue of privacy for the child and his or her family. Attention from various personnel in the health care agency, community leaders, and the media is often traumatic for youngsters (Burgess et al, 1984). It could jeopardize the family even further if the father is the offender and if he loses his job as a result of publicity; additionally, the odds of a fair trial, should he be prosecuted, are reduced. Confidentiality is critical.

Assessment

Disclosure is often indirect in the case of sexual abuse of children; it may not come immediately after an abusive act. The health professional needs to collect the same type of information as in the case of rape, but communication may be impeded by the child's level of cognitive development. One method of drawing children out that has worked well in this context is the use of expressive art (Miller, Veltkamp, and Janson, 1987). The child might be asked to draw a picture of her family, her house, the inside of her body, her dreams, or the person who assaulted her (Goodwin, 1982). These drawings can be analyzed for overt information, such as the addition of a very large phallus to the picture of the perpetrator, or for more subtle cues, such as the spatial relationships among people in the family drawings. Other useful expressive techniques are doll play or story completion. The child might be given a pair of dolls with the same name as herself and her abuser; she is then asked to show how

they interact. Or, the nurse can start a story featuring a little girl such as herself, with the same name, who has had a scary experience. The child is then asked to finish the story.

Health professionals need to listen carefully to the language children use. It may be indirect, as in, "Daddy hurt my pee-pee," or "My brother tickles me between my legs." Comments regarding the mother's inadequacy may take the form, "Mommy is never here." Older children may make more bold statements, particularly when abuse has occurred over time, such as, "Dad uses us in bed." They can give fairly detailed descriptions of what has occurred. By adolescence children fear pregnancy or internal damage. They are particularly likely to blame their mothers for what has happened, in the case of incest. Older adolescents may express self-blame or guilt for not revealing the situation sooner.

It is essential that health professionals treat seriously all reporting by youngsters of sexual experiences in order to assess the magnitude of stress and the significant developmental issues at risk (Burgess and Birnbaum, 1982). Health professionals should believe what the child says about the situation unless there is evidence to the contrary; even then, there is justifiable concern for the child's situation. Goodwin (1982) observed that the more articulate children, especially older ones, are in describing their sexual abuse, the less likely they are to be believed.

Historical data to be collected include whether or not the child has verbalized concerns about sex or pregnancy or has displayed regression, withdrawal, increased fears, sleep disturbance, irritability, withdrawal from peers, sudden disruptiveness or inattention in school, seductiveness, or inappropriate displays of affection (Foley and Davies, 1983).

PHYSIOLOGICAL FACTORS

While genital examination is not essential on the first contact with health professionals, important physical data are obtained from a rectovaginal examination, which must be done at some point. Whenever the examination is done, it is critical that it be performed with gentleness and include much explanation. A speculum examination should be avoided if possible. If it is necessary, a test tube or pediatric speculum should be used on a young girl. Anesthesia or sedation might be used, although some authorities view this use as further violation of the individual.

Cervical gonorrheal cultures and sperm and semen smears should be obtained. The hymen can be examined for intactness, old scarring, recent trauma, or absence. If the hymen is intact, a genital examination can be deferred.

Other physical data needed include evidence of physical abuse, anal and oral cultures for gonococci, serology for syphilis, oral swabbings, and combing of head hair. If the girl has reached puberty, a pregnancy test should be done.

Health professionals should remember that not all suspicious signs indicate sexual abuse. Vaginal bleeding can result from cervical pinworms or from insertion of foreign bodies by the child or her agemates. Monilia can occur in a diabetic child. What appear to be bruises can be birthmarks. And animals can bite children on their rumps (Goodwin, 1982).

PSYCHOLOGICAL FACTORS

In order to assess the impact of sexual abuse, it is useful to obtain a developmental history of the child as a measure of comparison. A general health history will also be useful. Both of these may offer clues as to when the sexual abuse began.

The health professional should also assess the structure and interaction of the family system, especially if the perpetrator is a close relative. The child will have to cope with the assault within the context of its family and abuse of a child is likely to precipitate a crisis.

Intervention

The physical safety of the child and risk of retribution by the perpetrator are major concerns. If there has been serious physical injury, emergency treatment is a priority. Treatment of injuries and sexually transmitted disease is similar to that described for rape.

The long-range goals of intervention with children are to help them develop as individuals who care about themselves and to help them grow up to enjoy fulfilling sexual relationships. Short-term goals include the return to a developmentally appropriate life style, with competency in school and in family and peer relationships. The goal for the family is to learn to communicate with one another, to redistribute power equitably, and to cease incestuous behavior.

Peer counseling for assault victims is often a way to help them realize that they are not alone in this situation and that others have shared the experience and to provide an environment for sharing feelings (Renvoize, 1982). This can be an effective strategy for children, particularly adolescents, since they are more articulate than younger children, as well as for silent victims who disclose their stories in adulthood. For younger children therapeutic play or other expressive techniques can help them express their feelings. Some communities have incest hot lines, which help victims disclose and later deal with their problem.

Taubman (1984) observes that most sexual abuse within the family is reported on impulse in the heat of a family argument. Once the situation cools down, the accusation may be withdrawn. And even though an offender may actually feel relief when disclosure occurs, he may be pressured into cooperating with his defense attorney's instructions to remain silent or to deny the charges. Thus, it is extremely difficult to engage incestuous families in a counseling program. It must be rapid, and the program must be credible to the family if success is to be achieved. Counseling is most successfully offered via another offender, spouse, or victim who can communicate with the family from experience and convince them of the merit of a full confession by the offender and of family treatment. Mutual self-help groups for offenders and for spouses of offenders are also beneficial, helping members to reduce feelings of shame and anger and instilling hope. Helping free family members from rigid role expectations can open communications among them.

The daughter of an incestuous family needs to increase her self-concept and reduce her feelings of guilt, isolation, and identity confusion. In addition, a mother-daughter bond needs to be developed. Taubman (1984) advocates putting the spouse and victim in contact with women's support groups, so that the family can come to understand the patriarchal values that contributed to their destructive patterns of interaction.

Parents of children who have been abused outside the family and the victims themselves may also benefit from support groups and by family counseling as they cope with the crisis and their individual feelings of guilt and blame.

It is not necessarily best for incestuous families to be broken up and for fathers to be jailed over extended periods. They are likely to be the financial support of the family, and removal of that support can intensify the crisis. The victim may experience heightened guilt for having caused this. Removal of the child from her home may be perceived as punishment (Stark, 1984). When the child's safety from physical abuse or further sexual assault is in jeopardy, temporary placement outside the home is necessary. If efforts to control violence are not successful, the spouse may need to remove herself and the children from the situation.

Children who have been sexually abused need privacy after the disclosure. Their chance of returning to a developmentally appropriate level of functioning may be improved by transfer to a new school and peer group in which they can experience a fresh start, particularly if media coverage or gossip has exposed them to the community. They need to remaster or work through developmental tasks of a younger age, such as development of trust and a sense of autonomy, so that they can begin to come to terms with their own identity and exert control over their environment and their future. They cannot hope to become healthy adults until they work through the lower level needs of developing a sense of security and of being loved, or lovable.

The road to health is a long one for victims of childhood sexual assault. Some never overcome the trauma (Armstrong, 1978). But as health professionals and the community at large become increasingly aware of the problem, more sources of assistance are emerging. It should be noted that increased community awareness and prevention strategies aimed at children, are not without cost. Well-intended teachers can unduly frighten children and, in their zeal, cause breaches in ethics (Trudell and Whatley, 1988). In one case known to this author, one third grader wanted to report her victimization to school authorities but she would not unless her friend came along and said something also. The friend fabricated a similar story, resulting in an investigation over a period of months of her own family. Although the investigation was ultimately dropped, the family's experience was horrendous.

SUMMARY

Sexual assault is a rapidly growing problem even as strides are made in promoting equality regardless of gender. The areas for intervention are many. In addition to direct assistance to victims and their families, action is needed in a variety of other areas. Women need to exert control over what is said about them in the media, and much work is needed with young children in the areas of sex education, values clarification, appropriate social interaction that acknowledges the worth of each person, and stress reduction. Parent education is a growing field; it should include content addressed at debunking myths about rape, sexual assault, spousal abuse, and incest. Political action is necessary to bring about legal reforms, such as facilitating prosecution of offenders and protecting victims of marital rape.

The human rights violations in need of action are numerous, and health professionals often feel overextended and stressed by such demands. While all cannot become active in the community, health professionals can be sensitized to the likelihood of dealing with sexual assault in their own practice or in their personal lives.

REFERENCES

Adams DC: Men Unlearning Violence. Boston, Emerge Collection, 1977.

Aftermath of Love: Emerg Med, pp. 24–28, 30, 32, 41, 1987.

Ageton SS: Sexual Assault Among Adolescents. Lexington, D.C. Health/Lexington, 1983.

Allgeier ER: Violent erotica and the victimization of women. SIECUS Report 9:7–8, 10, 1983.

Amir M: Patterns in Forcible Rape. Chicago, University of Chicago Press, 1971.

Amy's story. New York Times Jan 15, 1984, p E22.

Armstrong L: Kiss Daddy Goodnight: A Speak-Out on Incest. New York, Hawthorne Books, 1978.

Associated Press: Nursery cited for sex abuse. The Morning News (Wilmington, DE) July 30, 1981, p A2.

Associated Press: Man finds four teens raping girl, then gets in line and participates! The Morning News (Wilmington, DE) March 23, 1983a, p A10.

Associated Press: Penn fraternity loses fight. The Morning News (Wilmington, DE) April 8, 1983b, p B6.

Associated Press: Son of Sam's prosecutor admits to child molesting, gets probation. The Morning News (Wilmington, DE) October 21, 1983c, p A6.

Associated Press: Child molestation story on t.v. helps girl to reveal own secret. Evening Journal (Wilmington, DE) May 3, 1984a, p A8.

Associated Press: Child porno study revived. Evening Journal (Wilmington, DE) May 22, 1984b, p A2.

Barden JC: Violence in the family assessed at conference. New York Times July 26, 1981, p A43.

Barshis VRG: The question of marital rape. Women's Studies Int Forum 6:383–393, 1983.

Bart PB, Jozsa M: Dirty books, dirty films and dirty data. In Lederer L (ed): Take Back the Night: Women on Pornography. New York, Bantam, 1982, pp 201–215.

Becker JV et al: Incidence and types of sexual dysfunction in rape and incest victims. J Sex Marital Therapy 8:65–74, 1982.

Becker JV et al: Level of post assault sexual functioning in rape and incest victims. Arch Sex Behav 15:37–49, 1986.

Beegan D: 2500 march to protest gang rape at tavern. The Morning News (Wilmington, DE) March 15, 1983, p A8.

Bernard ML, Bernard JL: Violent intimacy: The family as a model for love relationships. Fam Relations 32:283–286, 1983.

Bixler RH: Sibling incest in the royal families of Egypt, Peru, and Hawaii. J Sex Res 18:264–281, 1982.

Bixler RH: The multiple meanings of "incest." J Sex Res 19:197–201, 1983.

Blakely MK: The New Bedford gang rape: Who were the men? Ms 12:50–53, 100–101, 1983.

Blum H: Detroiters alarmed over rapes of students on the way to and from school. New York Times Feb 5, 1984, p 19.

Bohmer C: Judicial attitudes toward rape victims. Judicature 57:303–307, 1974.

Bowlby J: Violence in the family as a disorder of the attachment and caregiving systems. Am J Psychoanalysis 44:9–27, 1984.

Briere J, Runtz M: Symptomatology associated with childhood sexual victimization in a nonclinical adult sample. Child Abuse Neglect 12:51–59, 1988.

Brown R: Science teacher cited for fondling students. Evening Journal (Wilmington, DE) April 4, 1984, p B3.

Brownmiller S: Against Our Will. New York, Simon and Schuster, 1975.

Burgess AW, Birnbaum HJ: Youth prostitution. AJN 82:832–834, 1982.

Burgess AW, Holmstrom LL: Rape: Victims of Crisis. Bowie, RJ Brady, 1974.

Burgess AW, Holmstrom LL: Coping behavior of the rape victim. Am J Psychiatry 133:413–418, 1976.

Burgess AW, Holmstrom LL: Recovery from rape and prior life stress. Res Nurs Health 1:165–174, 1978.

Burgess AW, Holmstrom LL: Rape: Sexual disruption and recovery. Am J Orthopsychiatry 49:648–657, 1979.

Burgess AW et al: Sexual Assault of Children and Adolescents. Lexington, Lexington Books, 1978.

Burgess AW et al: Child sex initiation rings. Am J Orthopsychiatry 51:110–119, 1981.

Burgess AW et al: Response patterns in children and adolescents exploited through sex-rings and pornography. A J Psychiatry 141:656–662, 1984.

Cohen ML et al: The psychology of rapists. Semin Psychiatry 3:307–327, 1979.

Cohen TB, Galenson E, Van Leeuwen K, et al: Sexual abuse in vulnerable and high risk children. Child Abuse & Neglect 11:461–474, 1987.

Collins G: Counseling male rape victims. New York Times January 18, 1982, p A15.

Collins G: Sex abuse: The child's word isn't enough. New York Times July 11, 1983, p B5.

Cook DR, Frantz-Cook A: A systematic treatment approach to wife battering. J Marital Family Therapy 10:83–93, 1984.

Costin F: Beliefs about rape and women's social roles. Arch Sex Behav 14:319–325, 1985.

Dark memory. New York Times April 29, 1984, p E9.

Deuteronomy. The New English Bible with Apocrypha. London, Oxford and Cambridge University Presses, 1970.

Diamond I: Pornography and repression: A reconsideration of "who" and "what." In Lederer L (ed): Take Back The Night: Women on Pornography. New York, Bantam, 1982.

Dietz SR, Littman M, Bentley BJ: Attribution of responsibility of rape: The influence of observer empathy, victim resistance, and victim attractiveness. Sex Roles 10:261–280, 1984.

DiVasto PV et al: The prevalence of sexually stressful events among females in the general population. Arch Sex Behav 13:59–67, 1984.

Donnerstein E, Berkowitz L: Victim reactions in aggressive erotic films as a factor in violence against women. J Personal Soc Psychol 41:710–724, 1981.

Dull RT, Giacopassi T: Demographic correlates of sexual and dating attitudes: A study of date rape. Criminal Justice Behav 14:175–193, 1987.

Ellis L, Beattie C: The feminist explanation for rape: An empirical test. J Sex Res 19:74–93, 1983.

Engel NS, Lau AD: Nursing care of the adolescent urban nomad. MCN 8:74–77, 1983.

Feild HS: Attitude toward rape: A comparative analysis of police, rapists, crisis counselors and citizens. J Personal Soc Psychol 36:156–179, 1978.

Feldman-Summers S, Gordon P, Meagher JR: The impact of rape on sexual satisfaction. J Abnormal Psychol 88:101–105, 1979.

Finkelhor D: Psychological, cultural and family factors in incest and family sexual abuse. J Marriage Fam Counsel October:41–49, 1978.

Finkelhor D: Sexually Victimized Children. New York, Free Press, 1979a.

Finkelhor D: What's wrong with sex between adults and children? Am J Orthopsychiatry 49:692–697, 1979b.

Finkelhor D: Sex among siblings: A survey on prevalence, variety and effects. Arch Sex Behav 9:171–194, 1980.

Finkelhor D, Hotaling GT: Sexual abuse in the national incidence study of child abuse and neglect: An appraisal. Child Abuse Neglect 8:23–33, 1984.

Flanzer JP (ed): The Many Faces of Family Violence. Springfield, Charles C Thomas, 1982.

Foley TS, Davies MA: Rape: Nursing Care of Victims. St. Louis, CV Mosby, 1983.

Ford DA: Wife battery and criminal justice: A study of victim decision-making. Fam Relations 32:463–475, 1983.

Forman BD: Assessing the impact of rape and its significance in psychotherapy. Psychotherapy Theory Res Pract 20:515–519, 1983.

Freund K et al: Males disposed to commit rape. Arch Sex Behav 15:23–35, 1986.

Fritz GS, Stoll K, Wagner NN: A comparison of males and females who were sexually molested as children. J Sex Marital Therapy 7:54–59, 1981.

Fuller E (ed): Bullfinch's Mythology. New York, Dell, 1959.

Gebhard PH et al: Sex Offenders. New York, Harper & Row, 1965.

Gelles RJ: The Violent Home, A Study of Physical Aggression Between Husbands and Wives. Beverly Hills, Sage, 1974.

Genesis. The New English Bible with Apocrypha. London, Oxford and Cambridge University Presses, 1970.

Giannini AJ, Fellows KW: Enhanced interpretation of nonverbal facial cues in male rapists—A preliminary study. Arch Sex Behav 15:153–156, 1986.

Giles-Sims J: Wife Battering: A Systems Theory Approach. New York, Guilford Press, 1983.

Goodman E: Confusion rampant in reaction to rape. The Morning News Wilmington, DE April 4, 1983a, p D3.

Goodman E: The turmoil of teenage sexuality: Parents' mixed signals. Ms 12:37–41, 1983b.

Goodwin J: Sexual Abuse: Incest Victims and Their Families. Boston, John Wright, 1982.

Gordon L, O'Keefe P: Incest as a form of family violence: Evidence from historical case records. J Marriage Fam 10:27–34, 1984.

Greer G: Seduction is a four letter word. In Chappell D et al (eds): Forcible Rape: The Crime, The Victim and The Offender. New York, Columbia University Press, 1977.

Greer T: Man guilty of rape, sodomy. Evening Journal (Wilmington, DE) May 30, 1984, p B4.

Griffin S: Rape: The all American crime. Ramparts 10:26–33, 1971.

Groth NA: Men Who Rape. New York, Plenum Press, 1979.

Groth NA, Burgess AW: Sexual dysfunction during rape. N Engl J Med 297:764–766, 1977.

Hatcher RA et al: Contraceptive Technology 1988–1989. 14th ed. New York, Irvington, 1988.

Hite S: The Hite Report. 2nd ed. New York, Dell, 1981a.

Hite S: The Hite Report on Male Sexuality. New York, Ballantine, 1981b.

Holmstrom LL, Burgess AW: The Victim of Rape: Institutional Reactions. New York, John Wiley & Sons, 1978.

Holmstrom LL, Burgess AW: Sexual behavior of assailants during reported rapes. Arch Sex Behav 9:427–439, 1980.

Horos CV: Rape. New York, Dell, 1981.

Jacobson MB, Popovich PM: Victim attractiveness and perception of responsibility in an ambiguous rape case. Psychol Women Quart 8:100–104, 1983.

James J, Meyerding J: Early sexual experience and prostitution. Am J Psychiatry 134:1381–1385, 1977.

Jones JG: Sexual abuse of children. Am J Dis Child 136:142–146, 1982.

Kanin E: Selected dyadic aspects of male sex aggression. J Sex Res 5:12–28, 1969.

Kanin EJ: Date rapists: Differential sexual socialization and relative deprivation. Arch Sex Behav 14:219–231, 1985.

Kempe CH: Sexual abuse, another hidden pediatric problem. Pediatrics 62:382–389, 1982.

Kinsey AC et al: Sexual Behavior in the Human Female. Philadelphia, WB Saunders, 1953.

Kolodny RC, Masters WH, Johnson VE: Textbook of Sexual Medicine. Boston, Little, Brown & Co, 1979.

Korman SK, Leslie GR: The relationship of feminist ideology and date expense sharing to perceptions of sexual aggression in dating. J Sex Res 18:114–129, 1982.

Labell LS: Wife abuse: A sociological study of battered women and their mates. Victimology 4:258–267, 1979.

LaBelle B: The propaganda of misogyny. In Lederer L (ed): Take Back the Night: Women on Pornography. New York, Bantam, 1982.

Landers A: Judge's warning to rape victim injudicious. Evening Journal (Wilmington, DE) May 21, 1984, p D6.

Langley R, Levy RC: Wife Beating: The Silent Crisis. New York, Pocket Books, 1977.

Lederer L: Introduction. In Lederer L (ed): Take Back the Night: Women on Pornography. New York, Bantam, 1982a.

Lederer L: "Playboy isn't playing," an interview with Judith Bat-Ada. In Lederer L (ed): Take Back the Night: Women on Pornography. New York, Bantam, 1982b.

Los Angeles presenting inquiry into sexual abuse of child. New York Times April 1, 1984, p A24.

MacKinnon CA: Sexual Harassment of Working Women. New Haven, Yale University Press, 1979.

Malamuth NM: Rape fantasies as a function of exposure to violent sexual stimuli. Arch Sex Behav 10:33–47, 1981.

Malamuth NM, Check JVP: Debriefing effectiveness following exposure to pornographic rape depictions. J Sex Res 20:1–13, 1981.

Malamuth NM, Haber S, Feshback S: Testing hypotheses regarding rape: Exposure to sexual violence, sex differences and the "normality" of rapists. J Res Personal 14:121–137, 1980.

Marieskind HI: Women in the Health System. St. Louis, CV Mosby, 1980.

Masters WH, Johnson VE, Kolodny RC: Human Sexuality. Boston, Little, Brown & Co, 1982.

McCahill TW, Meyer LC, Fischman AM: The Aftermath of Rape. Lexington, Lexington Books, 1979.

McDermott J: Rape Victimization in 26 American Cities. Washington, DC, U.S. Department of Justice, Law Enforcement and Assistance Administration, 1979.

McGuire LS, Wagner NN: Sexual dysfunction in women who were molested as children: One response pattern and suggestions for treatment. J Sex Marital Therapy 4:11–15, 1978.

Metzger D: It is always the woman who is raped. Am J Psychiatry 133:405–408, 1976.

Miller TW, Veltkamp LJ, Janson D: Projective measures in the clinical evaluation of sexually abused children. Child Psychiatry Human Develop 18:47–57, 1987.

Millett K: Sexual Politics. New York, Ballantine, 1978.

NiCarthy G: Getting Free: A Handbook for Women in Abusive Relationships. Seattle, The Seal Press, 1982.

Oliver M: Civil damages sought for incest. The Morning News (Wilmington, DE) March 17, 1983, p A12.

1 in 10 children suffers sex abuse, study reports. Am Med News Feb 25, 1983, p 35.

Ours J: An empty promise. AJN 86:782, 1986.

Pekkanen J: Victims: An Account of Rape. New York, Dial Press, 1976.

Pfaus JG, Myronuk LDS, Jacobs WJ: Soundtrack contents and depicted sexual violence. Arch Sex Behav 15:231–237, 1986.

Pogrebin LC: Do women make men violent? Ms 3:49–52, 1974.

Radloff L: Sex differences in depression: The effects of occupation and marital status. Sex Roles 1:249–265, 1975.

Raiha NK: Spouse abuse in the military community: Factors influencing incidence and treatment. In Eekelar JM, Katz SN (eds): Family Violence: An International and Interdisciplinary Study. Toronto, Butterworth, 1978.

Ranzel J: Rape trial keeps Massachusetts area on an

emotional edge. New York Times March 4, 1984, p A22.

Renshaw DC: Incest: Understanding and Treatment. Boston, Little, Brown & Co, 1982.

Renvoize J: Incest: A Family Pattern. London, Routledge & Kegan Paul, 1982.

Rosensweig-Smith J: Human sexuality concerns in the treatment of child sexual abuse and incest. In Flanzer JP (ed): The Many Faces of Family Violence. Springfield, Charles C Thomas, 1982.

Roy M: The Abusive Partner: An Analysis of Domestic Battering. New York, Van Nostrand Reinhold, 1982.

Rush F: The Best Kept Secret: Sexual Abuse of Children. New York, McGraw Hill, 1980.

Rush F: Child pornography. In Lederer L (ed): Take Back the Night: Women on Pornography. New York, Bantam, 1982.

Russell DEH: Pornography and violence: What does the new research say? In Lederer L (ed): Take Back The Night: Women on Pornography. New York, Bantam, 1982a.

Russell DEH: Rape in Marriage. New York, Macmillan, 1982b.

Russell DEH: The incidence and prevalence of intrafamilial and extrafamilial sexual abuse of female children. Child Abuse Neglect 7:133–146, 1983.

Sanford LT, Fetter A: In Defense of Ourselves: A Rape Prevention Handbook for Women. Garden City, Dolphin/Doubleday, 1979.

Sarafino EP: An estimate of nationwide incidence of sexual offenses against children. Child Welfare 58:127–134, 1979.

Schauss AG: Effect of environmental and nutritional factors on potential and actual batterers. In Roy M (ed): The Abusive Partner: An Analysis of Domestic Battering. New York, Van Nostrand Reinhold, 1982.

Schultz LG, Jones P: Sexual abuse of children: Issues for social service and health professionals. Child Welfare 62:99–107, 1983.

Selkin J: Rape. Psychology Today 8:70, 1975.

Simon J: Patrons cheer as woman is raped in Massachusetts bar. The Morning News (Wilmington, DE) March 14, 1983, p A1.

Smeaton G, Byrne D: The effects of r-rated violence and erotica, individual differences, and victim characteristics on acquaintance rape proclivity. J Res Personal 21:171–184, 1987.

Star B: Characteristics of family violence. In Flanzer JP (ed): The Many Faces of Family Violence. Springfield, Charles C Thomas, 1982.

Stark E: The unspeakable family secret. Psychology Today 18:38–46, 1984.

Stark R, McEvoy J: Middle class violence. Psychology Today 4:52–54, 110–112, 1970.

Steffen JJ: Social competence, family violence, problem drinking. In Flanzer JP (ed): The Many Faces of Family Violence. Springfield, Charles C Thomas, 1982.

Steinem G: Erotica and pornography: A clear and present difference. In Lederer L (ed): Take Back The Night: Women on Pornography. New York, Bantam, 1982.

Steinmetz S: Personal communication. May 3, 1984. University of Delaware, Newark, Delaware.

Stone LE, Tyler RPT, Mead JJ: Law enforcement officers as investigators and therapists in child sexual abuse: A training model. Child Abuse Neglect 8:75–82, 1984.

Strauss M: Sexual inequality, cultural norms, and wife beating. Victimology 1:54–70, 1976.

Strube MJ, Barbour SL: The decision to leave an abusive relationship: Economic dependence and psychological commitment. J Marriage Fam 45:785–793, 1983.

Summit R, Dryso J: Sexual abuse of children: A clinical spectrum. Am J Orthopsychiatry 48:237–251, 1978.

Tannahill R: Sex in History. New York, Scarborough Books, 1982.

Taubman S: Incest in context. Social Work 29:35–40, 1984.

Thorman G: Incestuous Families. Springfield, Charles C Thomas, 1983.

Tong L, Oates K, McDowell M: Personality development following sexual abuse. Child Abuse Neglect II:371–383, 1987.

Towson SMJ, Zanna MP: Retaliation against sexual assault: Self-defense or public duty? Psychol Women Quart 8:89–99, 1983.

Trudell B, Whatley M: School sexual abuse prevention: Unintended consequences and dilemmas. Child Abuse Neglect 12:103–113, 1988.

Wallace DH: Affectional climate in the family of origin and the experience of subsequent sexual-affectional behaviors. J Sex Marital Therapy 7:296–306, 1981.

Warner CG: Rape and Sexual Assault. Germantown Aspen, 1980.

Weir J: What's behind the mask. The New York Times Magazine July 18, 1982, pp 36–38.

Williams JE, Holmes KA: The Second Assault: Rape and Public Attitudes. Westport, Greenwood Press, 1981.

Winick C, Kinsie P: Prostitution in the United States. Chicago, Quadrangle Books, 1971.

Wydra A et al: Identification of cues and control of sex by rapists. Behav Res Therapy 21:469–476, 1983.

27: Psychosomatic Sexual Dysfunction

Mary Lyn Field

Current knowledge about sexual dysfunction indicates that pathophysiological causes of dysfunction are probably more common that psychogenic ones. Nonetheless, it is important to consider both causes in the initial assessment of sexual dysfunction.

This chapter focuses on the psychogenic explanations for sexual dysfunctions. The term *psychogenic* does not imply the lack of any possible relationship between the dysfunction and organic factors; it simply means that a single organic factor is not identifiable as the immediate cause of the dysfunction although psychogenic factors can be demonstrated. Health professionals believe that the somatic and psychic causes always interact in some way. It is crucial that this philosophy be conveyed in counseling the client with a sexual dysfunction.

INHIBITED SEXUAL DESIRE

Inhibited sexual desire can be defined as some degress of loss of interest or desire in sexual activity. The problem may be primary or lifelong, or it may occur after a period of normal sexual desire. Primary inhibition of sexual desire is much less common than the secondary form. When primary lack of desire does occur, is it usually in women.

A lack of sexual desire may not be perceived as a problem unless it is prolonged and the partner, still interested in sexual contact, is frustrated: A conflict emerges, and there is stress in the relationship (Livingston, McIntyre, and Fogel, 1982).

Patients with low sexual desire fall into two groups: those in whom a reduction in sexual responsiveness accompanies the loss of desire and those in whom responsiveness remains intact. Obviously, the effect of each of these conditions resides in the dynamics of sexual initiation between the partners. If the partner who usually initiates sexual activity is dysfunctional and consequently does not initiate sexual activity, the effect is less activity, unless there is a role reversal. If a role reversal occurs and the affected partner is still responsive, sexual activity might continue despite a decrease in sexual desire. When the affected partner suffers a decrease in responsiveness along with a decrease in desire, the sexual relationship is likely to be profoundly affected.

Effect of Inhibited Sexual Desire on Adaptation

PSYCHOLOGICAL FUNCTION

The effect of inhibited sexual desire on psychosocial adaptation is complex and often difficult to determine. A common cause of inhibited sexual desire detectable during assessment is depression. Through its effect on the autonomic nervous system, depression leads to decreased desire for sex. As with other activities, there is a general decrease in pleasure, which is called anhedonia. This eventually is manifested as a decrease in being able to experience pleasure with any activity, including sexual interaction (Livingston, McIntyre, and Fogel, 1982).

Guilt and anxiety associated with early sexual learning continue to have an effect on sexual attitudes and behavior, especially in women, leading to inhibited desire in adulthood. In men, the performance anxiety associated with sexual activity leads to an association of discomfort with sexual activity, and the effect is a lack of sexual desire.

Patients with dysfunction in other phases of the sexual response cycle, besides initiation, are likely also to lose desire. Those whose partners suffer from a sexual dysfunction may have learned to suppress their desires rather than to seek other outlets. This is likely to lead to anger, which they also suppress. These negative feelings can stimulate the "natural physiologic inhibitory mechanisms which suppress sexual desire" (Kaplan, 1979, p 83). The effect of religious, social, and family taboos sometimes creates an inhibition of desire. Fetishism, paraphilias, and a same-sex orientation can also result in a lack of sexual desire for an opposite-sex partner.

ROLE FUNCTION

Relationship problems are often the cause of low or absent desire. Dynamics such as power struggles, sibling rivalry, and the fear of being overwhelmed or exploited by the partner's needs have the potential to inhibit sexual desire.

Intervention

Treatment of inhibited sexual desire includes elements found in the treatment of other sexual dysfunctions, such as sensate focus exercises with a blend of behavioral and psychosocial approaches (Livingston, McIntyre, and Fogel, 1982). The partner's commitment is a prerequisite to the success of these methods.

SEXUAL AROUSAL DISORDERS
Male Erectile Disorder

In the past, the term *impotence* has been used to refer to erectile difficulty. Because it is a pejorative term, erectile disorder has replaced impotence as the preferable term. Erectile disorder is the persistent or recurrent, partial, or complete failure to attain or maintain an erection of sufficient firmness to permit coitus to be initiated or completed. Erectile disorder is present when a conscious intention or attempt at intercourse fails for involuntary reasons. Loss of desire and ejaculatory difficulty may accompany erectile disorder.

In primary erectile disorder the man has never been able to have intercourse. A period of inability to have intercourse preceded by a period of normal functioning is referred to as secondary erectile dysfunction. In erectile disorder, whatever its cause, the vascular reflex mechanism fails to pump enough blood into the cavernous sinuses of the penis to make the penis firm and erect. While the man may even feel aroused and excited, his penis does not become erect. Because the erectile and ejaculatory responses are dissociable, the man may ejaculate despite the flaccid penis.

It is important to note that isolated, transient episodes of inability to obtain or maintain an erection are normal and do not require assessment or intervention. A pattern that is persistent warrants intervention.

Approximately one half of the male population has occasional transient episodes of erectile failure (Kaplan, 1974). While most of the literature attests to the fact that more clients seek treatment for erectile difficulties than for other sexual problems (e.g., loss of desire or ejaculatory difficulty), the actual prevalence of erectile dysfunction is uncertain, owing to inconsistencies in research methodology and in differentiating types of sexual complaints. Also, clinicians often fail to allow for age factors. The development of erectile difficulty as a part of the aging process is well documented. Studies have shown that 75 per cent of men are unable to sustain an erection by age 80, whereas only 2 per cent of men experience difficulty before age 40 (Karacan, Aslan, and Williams, 1983).

The incidence of erectile disorder does not seem to be affected by sex or social class. The problem may have its onset in adolescence, adulthood, or old age (Kaplan, 1974). In recent years it has been suggested that an increase in the assertiveness of women in economic and social interactions has led to an increased incidence of erectile disorder in men. A flaw in this reasoning is evidenced by the fact that in societies in which traditionally there was an explicit recognition of the female sexual role and in which female sexuality was actively encouraged, such as in ancient China and especially in India, there does not seem to have been an increasing incidence of erectile disorders.

ERECTILE DISORDER AND SEXUAL FUNCTION

There are a number of theories about the causes of psychogenic erectile disorder. No one specific psychodynamic pattern has been correlated with erectile disorder, yet each has validity in some cases. Psychological factors associated with erectile disorder fall into three major categories.

1. Intrapsychic factors develop over years of interaction with the family and external social structures. These factors include a fear of intimacy, hostility toward women, sexual guilt, a weak masculine image, and sexual aggression. These negative effects can all be exacerbated in vulnerable adults in sexual interactions. If effects such as guilt and hostility are sufficiently strong, they interfere with the ability to function sexually and inhibit the erectile reflex.

2. Interpersonal factors thought to be causative of erectile dysfunction are often related to disturbed marital or partnership relations. Examples include unmet dependency needs that result in the overdependency of one partner on the other and competitive struggles between the partners. Chronic anger and resentment between couples often precedes the onset of erectile dysfunction.

If a female partner is chronically ill, the male partner might feel guilty about his sexual desires if they seem to necessitate disregard of his partner's disability. On the other hand, the ill partner may be experiencing such an impairment of her sexual interest and attractiveness that her partner loses his erection during sexual interactions. Life crises can sap physical and emotional energy of one or both partners; one result of this could be the inability to have an erection.

3. Experiential behavioral factors might also account for erectile disorder. While anxiety is often a part of the dynamic operating with the intrapsychic factors, there is a particular type of performance anxiety that interferes with erectile capability as well. Spectatoring is the process by which one becomes an observer of one's own performance by psychologically removing oneself from the situation. The placement of the self psychologically out of the experience precipitates a loss of the tactile, visual, auditory, and olfactory stimuli that maintain arousal.

The man who is intensely concerned with his sexual performance can lose track of the sensations he is experiencing and hence the sexual arousal that produces an erection.

The man who lacks knowledge about sexual arousal and what works for him is also vulnerable to erectile disorder. If he has been in a situation unfavorable to stimulating an erection but is not aware that the situation is not conducive to arousal, he might experience a first episode of erectile failure and subsequently experience anxiety that blocks the erectile reflex.

Psychosomatic theory holds that the events themselves do not induce erectile disorders; rather, the resultant anxiety either motivates the man to avoid sexual activity or interferes with the physiological reflex that produces erection. Underlying the hypothesis that anxiety can induce failure of the physiological reflexes is the presupposition of an organic vulnerability to stress. The cause of this vulnerability is not fully understood but might include both experiential and constitutional factors, such as familial experiences or a sexual response style that is extremely sensitive to emotions and environmental factors. A good example of a similar process is the child who develops gastrointestinal symptoms in response to stress.

The man who is reactive or vulnerable to emotional arousal reacts to an episode of erectile disorder with acute anxiety, which is re-experienced in similar situations. This is often how an acute episode results in a persistent problem. Sometimes a traumatic initial failure during a first attempt at intercourse precipitates the problem.

The psychoanalytic theory of erectile disorder, to which most health professionals give little credence, suggests that the erectile disorder is the result of unresolved oedipal conflicts. This theory postulates that the man fears his sexual impulses toward his mother will be detected and will lead to castration. Psychoanalytic theory claims that if these conflicts are not successfully resolved in childhood, the associated anxiety and guilt are re-evoked when the man is sexually excited, resulting in inhibition of the erectile reflex, a defense against castration anxiety by guaranteeing a man's inability to compete with his father.

A common sequel to erectile disorder is depression. It is important to determine whether the depression precedes or follows the erectile disorder. Marital discord may be either a precipitating or a resulting factor.

ASSESSMENT

The primary consideration in diagnosing erectile disorder is the determination of whether the origin of the problem is primarily organic or primarily psychological. Even when there is an identifiable organic etiology, it is common for psychological or behavioral changes to then affect sexual function. Men with psychological problems that might contribute to the development of erectile disorder may also have organic causes for the problem. There are also cases in which men with a marginal sexual dysfunction become more acutely dysfunctional because of the onset of an illness that may require medications that cause erectile disorder or because of physical changes that occur with aging (Kolodny, Masters, and Johnson, 1979). Consequently, the clinician's assessment must take into account both organic and psychological aspects of erectile disorder.

There are probably more than 100 conditions of the cardiovascular, endocrine, genitourinary, hematological, neurological, and respiratory systems, as well as certain drugs and various psychological conditions, that can produce erectile disorder. Also, nearly every psychological condition—psychosis, depression, anxiety, personality characteristics—has been associated with erectile disorder, yet only functional psychoses and inverted sex drive have been clinically assigned definite etiological significance.

In many studies, nocturnal penile tumescence (NPT) monitoring has been used to determine erectile disorder. While this technology can be costly and at times inconvenient, the findings of studies using tumescence monitoring have contributed significantly to our understanding of erectile functioning.

The purpose of nocturnal penile tumescence monitoring is to establish whether the basic neurophysiological mechanisms involved in the erectile reflex are intact. The healthy male has five to six erections per night. These occur during REM sleep and are unrelated to emotional states. The technique of NPT involves intensive study of nocturnal erections, EEG recordings, and electroculographic recordings for a minimum of two nights. The electroculographic recordings detect REM sleep.

A summary of some conclusions from one research team's (Karacan et al, 1983) clinical experience follows. The findings of other studies in the literature are consistent:

1. Most men with erectile dysfunction in whom the probability of organogenic dysfunction was high had impaired NPT tests.

2. Most men with erectile dysfunction in whom the probability of organogenic dysfunction was low had normal NPT tests.

3. Dysfunctional men with impaired NPT tests benefited from corrections of contributory physiological deficits.

4. Behavioral or psychiatric treatment of erectile disorders did not improve the erectile functioning of men with deficits in NPT monitoring.

5. Dysfunctional men with normal NPTs did not respond well to medical treatment, but behavioral or psychiatric treatment did result in an improvement in erectile functioning.

6. General or acute psychological factors did not significantly alter the results of NPT monitoring.

7. NPT was not affected by either REM sleep irregularities or the frequency and proximity to sexual activity.

Based on these principles, the results of NPT monitoring can be used to guide decisions about which studies and tests should be done to determine specific causes of erectile dysfunction. A history may reveal the use of drugs or psychological factors that contribute to the dysfunction. Points to be aware of when collecting data are lack of a long-term sexual relationship; sudden onset of persistent erectile difficulty in the absence of any traumatic condition or relevant medical complaint, especially when discord in the relationship is also evident; a report of decreased desire; the presence of erections on awakening; wide variation in erectile capacity with different partners; and successful masturbation.

Another factor that often distinguishes psychogenic from organic erectile disorder is mode of onset. When the cause of the disorder is primarily organic, the onset is usually slow or insidious. In contrast, psychogenic erectile disorder is characteristically sudden in onset. There may be a precipitating stressful event that causes the initial episode of failure, but then subsequent anxiety and fear about performance ability become the perpetuating mechanism. Some propose that psychogenic erectile disorder is a diagnosis of exclusion; that is, it becomes the diagnosis after organic factors are eliminated.

INTERVENTION

Treatment approaches to erectile disorder are generally based on the premise that nonorganically caused erectile disorder is primarily related to the interference of anxiety with erectile capacity. The achievement of a successful experience is the primary goal. In most cases the man will begin to have erections both during nongenital or genital sensate focus exercises (Hawton, 1985). A crucial point to be made to the male client and his partner is that he is *not* to try to have an erection during the exercises. This removes any pressure that raises his anxiety level, interfering with the normal cycle. This approach is referred to as paradoxical intention. Sensate focus exercises are described in greater detail in Chapter 2, Sexual Health Care.

Once the man has erections during these exercises, a waxing and waning approach should be suggested. This approach involves allowing erections to subside once they occur and then resuming caressing to the point of erection. This sequence should be repeated two or three times a session. It is useful in helping to eliminate the man's fear that if he loses an erection it will not return. Another helpful suggestion is to tell the man to ejaculate extravaginally, so that he does not feel pressured to maintain an erection once intercourse begins. Initially, vaginal containment should be brief, with little movement, and achieved with the woman partner's help. A few failures are common at this stage. Once the man has been successful at maintaining an erection during containment several times he can proceed with the program (Hawton, 1985).

ORGASMIC DISORDERS
Inhibited Female Orgasm

Inhibited female orgasm is the most prevalent sexual problem among women. Prior to 1970 the term *frigid* was used to describe the woman who did not respond with orgasm when stimulated sexually. Because this term is pejorative, it is no longer used. Persistent or recurrent delay in or absence of orgasm following the sexual excitement phase during sexual activity is now referred to as inhibited female orgasm. The condition is considered primary if a woman has never experienced orgasm and secondary if the disorder developed after a period of being able to reach orgasm. The problem may be absolute, if it occurs in all situations, or situational, if it occurs only under specific circumstances. The failure to experience orgasm can be defined as a problem only if the woman has received what she considers effective stimulation.

Many women experiencing inhibited female orgasm are not generally sexually inhibited. They often desire, enjoy, and initiate sexual activity. Most attain the excitement and plateau stages but then do not progress from plateau to orgasm.

Because of differences in the definitions of orgasmic disorders, incidence reports vary. It has been estimated that 8 to 15 per cent of all American women have never experienced orgasm at any time other than during sleep. Situational inhibited female orgasm has been experienced by as many as 50 per cent of all women (Munjack and Oziel, 1980).

Organic precipitants of orgasmic dysfunction, such as the effects of alcohol, barbiturates and narcotics, and inflammatory or infectious conditions, are responsible for the problem in less than an estimated 10 per cent of cases (Munjack and Oziel, 1980).

INHIBITED FEMALE ORGASM AND SEXUAL FUNCTION
The Orgasmic Response

The stimuli necessary to produce an orgasm and the intensity of the orgasm vary tremendously among women. The continuum of sufficient stimuli ranges from fantasy only to minimum stimuli and fantasy, intense foreplay, a few penile thrusts, male superior position, female superior position, clitoral stimulation and intercourse, direct oral or manual stimulation, and lengthy and intense clitoral stimulation. The range of sufficient stimuli varies from little direct stimulation to intense direct stimulation. Variability in the intensity of the orgasm can only be surmised from subjective description.

There has been much controversy in recent

years about what is considered a normal orgasmic response. In the past many psychologists and psychoanalysts considered orgasm induced by intercourse the sole "authentic" female sexual response, and climax induced by any other form of stimulation was viewed as a symptom of neurotic conflict. In the past, the clitoral versus vaginal orgasm debate dominated discussions of female sexual function. It is now generally accepted that the dichotomy of clitoral and vaginal orgasm is mythical.

Three very important facts about the relationship between intercourse and female orgasm are presented here:

1. Evidence suggests that stimulation of the clitoris is important and probably crucial to the production of female orgasm. In most women vaginal stimulation plays a lesser role in triggering the orgasmic reflex.

2. The intensity of clitoral stimulation varies with the particular form of sexual activity. Direct tactile stimulation of or pressure on the clitoris is the most intense physical stimulus.

3. The amount of stimulation required to elicit the female orgasm varies tremendously, not only among different individuals but also in the same woman under different circumstances.

It is interesting to note that Hite (1976) reported that of all women who are orgasmic through noncoital means only 30 per cent are able to regularly have orgasms from intercourse alone.

EFFECTS OF INHIBITED FEMALE ORGASM ON ADAPTATION

Psychological Function

There are several hypotheses about the psychogenic sources of orgasmic disorders, with a restrictive home environment seemingly the most prevalent cause. The environment is usually one that taught the female child to associate sexual pleasure with anxiety, guilt, and shame. Other characteristics of this environment include infrequent references to sex, little nudity, sparse factual sex education, a lack of affectionate display by parents, disturbed interaction between parents, and the association of sex with dirtiness and sin. For women raised in a restrictive environment, orgasm may engender fear, as it appears to represent rebellion and an assertion of independence. Other historical features

sometimes characteristic of these women include an absent father and a bitter mother, a situation that often fosters distorted perceptions about men. A current power struggle with the partner or fear of rejection by the partner may contribute to the withholding of orgasm.

Women raised with a negative self-concept protect themselves from anticipated hurt by holding back (Munjack and Oziel, 1980). An association of orgasm with loss and, more dramatically, with death, stimulates fear and withholding. In some women self-punishment may be a desired effect of inhibiting this pleasurable reflex, which would explain why some women who do not feel they deserve to feel pleasure inhibit the reflex. Fear of losing control also interferes with the experience of orgasm. This fear limits a woman's ability to allow herself to experience the intensity of emotion associated with orgasm.

Unrealistic expectations about sexual performance is another basis for orgasmic disorder. Women who feel that simultaneous orgasm only via coitus constitutes adequate performance may believe that they (or their partners) are inadequate when this does not occur.

Women who feel sex and orgasm are best associated with commitment have difficulty allowing themselves to experience orgasm with a person to whom they do not want to be committed. In this sense orgasm is equated with commitment, and the logic is extended that to avoid orgasm is to avoid commitment.

The woman's historical factors are important to the extent that they evoke emotions, thoughts, and perceptions. Emotional states are the immediate stimuli that mediate inhibition of the orgasmic response. These states include sexual anxiety, guilt, anger, hostility, or indifference toward her partner; depression; and excessive and distracting intrusive thoughts (Munjack and Oziel, 1980). Some sources of anxiety include fear of looking silly, urinating, or becoming pregnant. Women involved with men who are premature ejaculators may be trying to avoid stimulating their partner's rapid ejaculation. Also, there are women who fear promiscuity once they experience orgasm.

In secondary inhibited female orgasm, depression is often a prominent factor. Treatment of the depression will often result in return of the ability to experience orgasm. A woman's level of self-esteem affects her experience of sexuality. A woman with low self-esteem may not allow herself to experience the pleasure of orgasm because she does not think she deserves it. A negative body image can also contribute, playing a large role in her experience or lack of experience with orgasm. Partner-related problems include ineffective communication, hostility between partners, distrust, divergent sexual preferences, and boredom or monotony. If the male or female partner is ignorant about what constitutes adequate stimulation, it may be difficult for the woman to communicate this. The women who seek treatment for orgasmic disorder are those who are unhappy about the problem.

Reactions to orgasmic difficulties vary. Some women adapt to the problem by lowering their expectations of pleasurable experiences, some deny the importance of orgasm, and others may seek satisfaction by trying different partners. Another way in which some women deal with the problem is to pretend to have orgasms, so that their partners will not be hurt or angry. Because of the deception and lack of pleasure involved, this can decrease the woman's interest in sexual activity and may even lead to more severe orgasmic difficulties. The woman whose partner reacts negatively if she fails to reach orgasm often experiences anger if she feels pressured to pretend. This anger can interfere significantly with the relationship in all aspects as well as with efforts at remedying the orgasmic disorder.

ASSESSMENT

To differentiate situational orgasmic disorder from absolute inhibited female orgasm, it is important to ask the woman about her sexual responsiveness with different partners. Patterns of success in achieving orgasm should be explored. If it becomes apparent that a woman has orgasms with some men and not with others, characteristics of the men and the relationships in which orgasm occurs can be explored and compared with the characteristics of the men and the relationships in which orgasm does not occur.

Important points in a client's history that help establish a diagnosis include information about contraceptive practices and reproductive goals. Questions to be asked include the following: Is there a fear of pregnancy? Are adequate contraceptive methods being used? Is there a desire to be pregnant, and is this a shared or one-sided goal? Also important

to assess are the sexual attitudes of both partners. Confirmation of whether or not the woman has truly not experienced orgasm is important. Because some women have unrealistic expectations of what orgasm should feel like and others are simply misinformed about the experience, very specific questions must be asked to elucidate the woman's understanding of the orgasmic response and, in turn, her experience during sexual stimulation. All types of sexual stimulation should be determined, for example, masturbation and vibrator use. Also, historical points pertinent to etiology are vital to developing the diagnosis.

The presence of concurrent psychopathology is an important factor to consider. For example, depression may contribute to orgasmic disorders. If the client has previously been in psychotherapy, the nature and outcome of treatment should be documented.

INTERVENTION

Approaches to treatment of the woman with inhibited female orgasm must take into consideration whether the orgasmic disorder is primary or secondary and whether the woman has a current sexual partner. Treatment in all of these cases varies but shares the common element of increasing self-awareness and teaching effective self-stimulation.

In primary orgasmic disorder, the woman has never experienced orgasm. One recommended approach for these women is to begin with masturbation training and progress to sensate focus exercises with a partner. Masturbation is considered especially therapeutic for the woman who has never experienced an orgasm from any source of physical stimulation. It is the most probable way of producing an orgasm and, according to many women, produces the most intense orgasm (LoPiccolo and Lobitz, 1978). Frequent orgasms produce an increase in vascularity, enhancing orgasmic potential. The increased number of orgasms can lead to a psychological anticipation of pleasure in sex (Bardwick, 1971).

A program in masturbation instruction can be used as an adjunct to behavioral treatment involving both husband and wife. Prior to beginning the program it is important to assess the couple's attitudes toward masturbation. Many married couples underestimate the prevalence of masturbation among married people and, for this reason, believe it is abnormal. Providing cognitive information prior to masturbation training can increase the woman and her partner's acceptance of masturbation as a legitimate and helpful practice. Provision of facts, including Kinsey and associates' findings (1953) that 94 per cent of men and 58 per cent of women have masturbated to orgasm at some point, may support the couple's attempts. Dearborn's survey (1967) is more impressive, finding that 100 per cent of men and 85 per cent of women studied had masturbated to orgasm at some point.

The therapist can help the woman's partner in masturbation training to learn to make supportive statements and should suggest that he masturbate and, if he already does, that he should tell his partner about it. This can help in firmly establishing the acceptability of the practice.

The steps in masturbation training include the following:

1. Increase self-awareness by using a mirror to view the genital region and practice Kegel's exercises, tensing and relaxing the pubococcygeal muscle 10 times three times a day.

2. Tactually explore the genitals without trying to achieve arousal.

3. Continue to view and feel the genital area, locating sensitive areas that produce pleasurable sensations, specifically the clitoral shaft, hood, major and minor labia, vaginal opening, and the whole perineum.

4. Manually stimulate the pleasure-producing area. The woman should be given specific instructions regarding clitoral manipulation, using stroking and pressure with lubrication.

5. If no orgasm occurs with step 4, the woman is instructed to increase the intensity and duration of the masturbation. Thirty to forty-five minutes is the suggested upper limit of duration. Reading erotic material and fantasizing during masturbation can also be helpful.

6. If no orgasm occurs with step 5, the woman can try using a vibrator, such as the ones sold for use in facial massage.

7. Once orgasm through self-masturbation is achieved, the woman may choose to focus on achieving orgasm through stimulation by the partner. The woman is then instructed to masturbate while the partner observes.

8. The partner then does what the woman has been doing for herself.

9. Heterosexual couples may now engage in intercourse while the male stimulates the female's genitals. It is easiest to achieve simultaneous clitoral stimulation in the female superior sitting position or the lateral or rear entry positions.

Figure 27–1 illustrates two coital positions in which the woman's position allows the man to stimulate her genitals and affords maximum clitoral contact.

Orgasm achieved at step 9 deems the therapy a success. For the woman with secondary orgasmic disorder, the problem is usually one of a decreased frequency of coital orgasms. The masturbation training may help to reestablish a higher degree of sensitivity to pleasurable sensations, clarify what is indeed most stimulating to the woman, and establish the effectiveness of self-stimulation or genital manipulation during coitus.

For the woman without a current sexual partner, the first six steps of masturbation training will help her provide her own sexual pleasure and subsequently feel capable of reaching orgasm if and when she chooses to have a partner in the future.

Some have recommended group rather than couples therapy for preorgasmic women (Barbach, 1975). The suggested advantages of a group therapy approach are that it is significantly less expensive than couples' treatment and does not eliminate those women without partners or women who have partners who do not wish to participate.

Studies about the efficacy of group therapy when compared with individual therapy do not consistently show the superiority of group therapy but do support the advantage of either of these therapies over no therapy at all (Spence, 1985). These groups generally include a series of sessions in which women share their sexual difficulties; participate in discussions of the physiology of the sexual response, female anatomy, and sexuality; and do homework assignments that include genital exploration and self-stimulation as described in the discussion of masturbation training (Barboch, 1975).

Premature Ejaculation

Premature ejaculation has been defined in a variety of ways: if a man reached orgasm before his partner more than 50 per cent of the time or if he ejaculated before 10 thrusts or within 30 seconds of vaginal penetration. A major problem with these definitions is

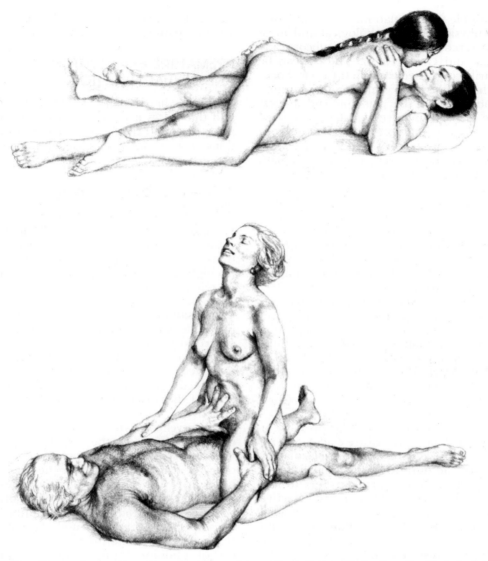

FIGURE 27–1. Woman-above positions. (Reproduced by permission of Crooks R, Baur K: Our Sexuality. Menlo Park, Benjamin/ Cummings, p 327. Copyright 1980.)

that they do not take into account variations in female orgasmic response (Kaplan, 1979): For example, suppose a woman has difficulty reaching orgasm unless she experiences 2 hours of penile thrusting. If her male partner ejaculated within 1 hour of penetration more than 50 per cent of the time, he would be labeled a premature ejaculator according to these definitions. Another difficulty in defining premature ejaculation is that there is no specific "normal" time interval after intro-

mission during which ejaculation should occur.

It is helpful to review briefly the neurophysiology of the ejaculatory reflex. Ejaculation is activated and controlled by the lumbar area of the spinal cord. Mediated by the sympathetic nervous system, ejaculation, once activated, cannot be terminated (Tollison, 1979). Sexual stimulation that exceeds an individual's biological threshold for orgasmic response triggers the spinal reflex that is responsible for ejaculation. The stimulation is both physical and psychological and must be registered cortically and subcortically (Munjack and Oziel, 1980). Thus, it can be voluntarily controlled early in the cycle. Some researchers base their definition of premature ejaculation on this principle and suggest that the term premature ejaculation be used when a man, unable to exert voluntary control over the ejaculatory reflex, reaches orgasm very quickly once aroused (Kaplan, 1974). This definition applies no specific time frame and does not assume a uniformity of female response. The American Psychiatric Association defines premature ejaculation as "persistent or recurrent ejaculation with minimal sexual stimulation or before, upon, or shortly after penetration and before the person wishes it (APA, 1987, p 245). It is important to take into account factors that affect duration of the excitement phase, such as age, novelty of the partner or situation, and frequency of sexual activity, when diagnosing premature ejaculation. Some researchers have said that it is easier to define what is not premature ejaculation: when the partners agree that the quality of their sexual encounters is not influenced by the need for efforts to delay ejaculation (LoPiccolo, 1975).

Premature ejaculation may be primary or secondary. Primary premature ejaculation refers to lack of control over the ejaculatory reflex since the onset of sexual activity. Secondary premature ejaculation refers to loss of control after a period of more effective sexual functioning. In some men, erectile dysfunction may occur simultaneously with premature ejaculation, and when the erectile dysfunction is resolved, the presence of premature ejaculation is then evident. Situational premature ejaculation may be primary or secondary. It refers to premature ejaculation that is selective or intermittent.

Premature ejaculation occurs in postpubertal men of all ages and social classes with and without psychological disorders. Premature ejaculation seems to be reported more often in recent years because of either an actual increase in the prevalence of the problem or an increase in the frequency of reporting due to a greater sense of acceptance of such reporting by the medical community (Munjack and Oziel, 1980).

Premature ejaculation has not been found to correlate directly with either specific or general sexual conflicts. The quality of the marital relationships of men with premature ejaculation varies and is not characterized by any one pattern or problem.

PREMATURE EJACULATION AND SEXUAL FUNCTION

It is only when a man has ejaculatory control and then loses it that it is important to consider organic causes and perform examinations to rule out urological or neurological problems.

Behavioral and Learning Theories

Some researchers have proposed that anxiety is the basic cause of premature ejaculation in that when anxiety is experienced at the point of high erotic arousal, an involuntary orgasmic response is triggered (Kaplan, 1974). Anxiety may interfere with the perception of the sensations of excitement, thus distracting the male and resulting in a lack of actual control over ejaculation. Ironically, methods that decrease anxiety are not the most effective means of treatment, whereas methods that focus on enhancing the man's perceptions of the sensations preceding orgasm are effective.

Nonpsychoanalytic theories about premature ejaculation see the symptoms as somewhat less serious than do psychoanalytic theories. Learning and behavior theories do not necessarily see premature ejaculation as a symbolic symptom or a way of resolving a specific conflict. Rather, the involuntary ejaculation is viewed as a learned response. The premature ejaculation is acquired as a function of conditions requiring rapid ejaculation. The classic example is sex in the back seat of a parked car or on the couch in the family living room when the parents are due to arrive at any moment. In these situations, anxiety becomes a factor. The result is that the young male gets a lot of good practice at ejaculating rapidly and being rewarded for it by not getting caught. It is doubtful that the young woman in this situation complains about the rapid ejaculation. Rather, she is probably relieved and may in some sense reward the behavior, reinforcing the premature ejaculation.

Questions have been raised about the adequacy of this theory (Kaplan, 1974): While many men have the rushed sexual experiences described, only a small percentage go on to become premature ejaculators. An alternate hypothesis about the dynamics involved in premature ejaculation has been proposed by Kaplan. This hypothesis incorporates knowledge of the neurophysiology of ejaculation as well as the concepts of anxiety and conflict.

A listing of the main points in a logical order is helpful:

1. A clear perception of sexual feelings is indispensable for the development of ejaculatory continence.

2. Because treatment techniques that focus the man's attention on the sensations preceding orgasm are effective, it can be concluded that the absence of voluntary control is the central problem.

3. The absence of control is secondary to impaired perceptions of preorgasmic erotic sensations.

4. The impaired perception is due to conflict and anxiety surrounding sexuality, which the man with premature ejaculation avoids by erecting defenses against the perception of the intense sensations that precede orgasm.

5. Treatment of premature ejaculation does not require knowledge of the underlying conflict.

Psychoanalytic Theories

As with other psychoanalytic theories, most sex therapists do not find those pertaining to premature ejaculation particularly helpful. Psychoanalytic theorists have considered premature ejaculation to be a serious symptom. It has been related to hysteria in people of predominantly homosexual orientation. Some have theorized that men with premature ejaculation have guilt over masturbation, others associate premature ejaculation with a denial of aggressive impulses toward women, and some describe it as a masochistic wish to be refused (Munjack and Oziel, 1980). Other psychoanalytic theorists consider premature ejaculation a neurotic symptom. They suggest that men with premature ejaculation harbor intense unconscious sadistic feelings toward women, with the purpose of rapid ejaculation being to defile the woman. Some researchers report difficulty actually demonstrating in studies that these men are indeed hostile toward women (Kaplan, 1974).

EFFECTS OF PREMATURE EJACULATION AND ADAPTATION

Psychological Function. Reactions to premature ejaculation range from unaware-ness—until the frustrated partner seeks help—to guilt about the problem. This sometimes leads to avoidance of sexual encounters or to the development of erectile dysfunction.

Interdependence. A woman's reaction depends on her own expectations of the sexual relationship. Some women are pleased because the time required for a given sexual encounter is brief. Those expecting little satisfaction from intercourse per se may not be affected by their partner's premature ejaculation. On the other hand, many women respond to a persistent pattern of premature ejaculation by seeing their partner as selfish. This perception may be openly expressed or silently resented. Depending on the woman's level of self-esteem, she may begin to doubt her own femininity (Munjack and Oziel, 1980). Some may have affairs as a way of satisfying their needs of expressing anger.

INTERVENTION

Premature ejaculation is treated by helping the man achieve ejaculatory control. Techniques commonly employed include more frequent ejaculation, variation in coital positions, striving for a subsequent orgasm shortly after a preceding one, communicating during coitus to prolong the experience, and the stop-start and squeeze techniques (Crooks and Baur, 1983).

More frequent orgasms help some men delay ejaculation more easily when they want to. If sex with a partner is not a viable option, frequent masturbation to orgasm can be helpful (Crooks and Baur, 1983).

The recommended coital position for men who have trouble controlling their ejaculations is the relaxed supine position with the woman on top. The decrease in muscle tension during coitus can result in greater ejaculatory control.

Because of the presence of a male refractory period, sexual activity that follows initial male orgasm is unlikely to result in rapid ejaculation.

The stop-start technique was developed by Semans in 1956. It is designed to prolong the sensations prior to orgasm, increasing the man's awareness and potential for control of ejaculation. The partner is instructed to stimulate the man's penis, either manually or orally, to the point of impending orgasm and then stop until the pre-ejaculatory sensations subside. Practice of this technique may take weeks or months. Couples should be forewarned about the likelihood of initial failure (Crooks and Baur, 1983).

Inhibited Male Orgasm

Inhibited male orgasm is described as the persistent or recurrent delay in or absence of orgasm in a male following a normal sexual excitement phase during sexual activity that is adequate in focus, intensity, and duration (APA, 1987). Some lay terms that have been used include "dry runs," "blue balls," "not being able to do any damage," or "having a hard time coming." As with other sexual dysfunctions, inhibited male orgasm may be primary or secondary or absolute or situational. The rarest and most severe form is absolute inhibited male orgasm. This term indicates that ejaculation takes place only with nocturnal emissions. Primary inhibited orgasm exists when intravaginal ejaculation has never occurred. Secondary inhibited male orgasm exists when a period of dysfunction begins after a period of healthy functioning (Munjack and Oziel, 1980).

Secondary inhibited male orgasm may be mild, moderate, or severe. In the most common form (situational inhibition), the man can ejaculate intravaginally but only in certain circumstances, with the classic example being the man who voluntarily ejaculates with a prostitute but is unable to do so with his wife. A mild form of inhibited male orgasm involves ejaculation in another's presence but not during intercourse, the moderate form occurs even when the man is alone and attempting mechanical manual stimulation, and the most severe form involves the inability to ejaculate under any condition.

Inhibited male orgasm may be intermittent, occurring sometimes, but not always, in a given situation. Alcohol ingestion and anxiety are two factors that may be involved (Schull and Sprenkle, 1980).

There is also a form of ejaculation referred to as incomplete partial. In this condition there is a gathering of sperm but only emission occurs. Because of the absence of an actual orgasm, there is a seepage of semen and slow detumescence.

Retrograde ejaculation, often associated with surgical procedures and the use of certain medications, involves ejaculatory travel back into the bladder rather than forward through the urethra.

The incidence of inhibited male orgasm is not well studied. Some authors (Munjack and Oziel, 1980) have noted that Masters and Johnson reported that out of 510 couples treated, 17 men suffered from inhibited male orgasm. As the general public develops increased awareness of sexual behavior and therapy, therapists can anticipate more requests for help with retarded ejaculation difficulties (Tollison and Adams, 1979). In the past, patients rarely presented with this problem. As of 1973 there was no paper in the literature regarding inhibited male orgasm, giving further support to the claim that while this may seem like but not truly be a rare problem, it is certainly not well studied (Tollison and Adams, 1979).

There is no definite conclusion about the etiology of inhibited male orgasm. Physiological causes are not common but include the effects of drugs that impair the sympathetic nervous system (e.g., thioridazine and antihypertensives) and neurological diseases such as atropic lateral sclerosis and multiple sclerosis.

Suggested causes of inhibited male orgasm include marital conflict, relationship ambivalence, and environmental causes. In the case of marital conflict, no single dynamic is identified, but the outcome of the conflict seems to be the man's fear of rejection if he ejaculates, and thus he withholds ejaculation. Another hypothesis is that the withholding is a form of rebellion.

The lack of ejaculation may be symptomatic of relationships in which there is a lack of commitment or in which there are major power struggles. The "holding back" involved in inhibited orgasm functions as a part of the man's defense system (Schull and Sprenkle, 1980).

The anxiety associated with inhibited male orgasm is based on some actual or threatened unpleasant consequence of ejaculation in the recent or remote past. A traumatic event associated with ejaculation in the past results in an involuntary, unconscious conditioned inhibition.

In psychoanalytic thought inhibited male orgasm is viewed as a variant of erectile dysfunction. It develops out of a fear of physical injury, such as castration, and the conflict that exists as the man seeks the pleasure of an activity that he fears will do him physical harm.

There is also the possibility that satisfying orgasm has become associated with very specific stimuli that the man provides for himself during masturbation. When the man stimulates himself successfully and repeatedly in ways that are difficult to duplicate in intercourse, the behavior becomes reinforced, and a conditioned response exists. Thus, it is not always true that a painful event associated with intervaginal ejaculation is the inciting event. It may be that no negative contingency is involved but rather that the ejaculatory response is so conditioned to a very specific stimulus that it does not occur in other circumstances such as intercourse. The problem is further reinforced because the man with inhibited male orgasm during intercourse often continues to masturbate successfully with the same frequency (Dow, 1981).

INTERVENTION

As with erectile dysfunction, the treatment of ejaculatory difficulty involves behavioral reconditioning. Psychotherapy to reduce relationship conflicts may also be indicated. Treatment begins with sensate focus exercises, during which there is no attempt to complete the act. In other words, the man should not try to ejaculate during this time. The next phase involves the man's experiencing ejaculation by whatever means work. He may begin with self-masturbation after being stimulated to an aroused state by his partner. For some it is acceptable at this point for the partner to be responsible for stimulating the man rather than his masturbating himself. The next phase involves the partner trying to bring the man to orgasm with manual or oral stimulation. During this phase, communication is crucial. The man should be instructing his partner in what feels most pleasurable and stimulating. Once the man is able to be stimulated to orgasm by his partner, the couple can move to the last phase, in which ejaculation occurs during penetration. Inserting the penis at the moment of highest excitement is a good initial technique that can be abandoned later, opting for insertion at any point followed by prolonged coital contact prior to intravaginal ejaculation (Crooks and Baur, 1983).

Referral Considerations

Clients in need of basic information can gain much even from providers who are not specially trained in sex therapy. The basic mechanisms of sexual arousal, the phases of the sexual response cycle, the frequency of sexual dysfunction, a hopeful attitude, and information about treatment options are all areas within the counseling role of the primary care provider. When a relationship is already established with the client, the primary care provider is in an ideal position to influence the client's attitude positively toward treatment. This can significantly influence both the client's attitude as well as the follow through with the referral. For the problems listed below it is best to refer the client to a counselor or sex therapist:

1. Clinical depression underlying the sexual complaint.
2. Significant past psychiatric history.
3. Problems complicated by homosexual conflict or gender confusions, overt or latent.
4. Patients who present with marked personality or character disorders.
5. Primary sexual dysfunctions.
6. Lack of commitment to the relationship by one or both partners.
7. Lack of commitment to therapy by one or both partners.
8. Significant secrets, such as ongoing infidelities, kept by one partner.
9. Major reality concerns, such as family or work problems, at the time therapy is sought.
10. Major difficulties in a relationship with a partner.

The referring provider can bridge the client's transition into therapy by sending a note or calling the client's therapist. If the provider will continue to follow the client for primary care, it might be helpful if the sex therapist occasionally communicates progress reports back to the provider. This is contingent on the therapist's policies and the client's wishes.

SEXUAL PAIN DISORDERS

Vaginismus

Vaginismus is the recurrent or persistent involuntary spasm of the musculature of the outer third of the vagina that interferes with coitus (APA, 1987). The musculature of the pelvis, perineum, and thigh are also affected (Kolodny, Masters, and Johnson, 1979). Unlike the other sexual dysfunctions, vaginismus is not related to a specific sexual phase of the sexual response cycle but occurs whenever vaginal entry is attempted. The analogy in males is psychogenic ejaculatory and post-ejaculatory pain (Kaplan, 1979).

Primary vaginismus refers to vaginismus that has been present since a woman's first attempts at intercourse. Secondary vaginismus refers to vaginismus that occurs after a period of intercourse without a vaginismic response. Situational vaginismus occurs sometimes but not other times and is rare.

Vaginismus can be very traumatic to the heterosexual couple that prefers intercourse to other forms of sexual activity. It is important that health professionals remember that vaginismus is not a willful response. It is a conditioned, involuntary response and must be treated as such.

Vaginismus is thought to be relatively uncommon and can affect women of any age. While there are several possible causes of vaginismus, the process is basically the same whatever the cause: negative connotations become associated with the act or fantasy of vaginal penetration and a conditioned reflex is established. Subsequently, affected women may avoid onset of pain by avoiding sexual encounters. The relief this affords reinforces the avoidance pattern (Fertel, 1977).

The original or remote cause of penetration fear and spasm is highly variable (Kaplan, 1974). Because clients are often unable to recall traumatic events, it is difficult to make a case for conscious fear as a determinant in the formation of the symptom. Excessively severe control, such as is characteristic of religious orthodoxy, has been found to characterize many vaginismic women. A high association with primary erectile dysfunction in the partner has been proposed as well. Secondary erectile dysfunction may occur as a result of repetitive failure at intromission (Fertel, 1977).

Another possible etiological factor is prior sexual trauma. Women who have been raped or molested may understandably develop a phobic response to vaginal contact. Attempted heterosexual activity in women with prior same-sex identification may also be causative of vaginismus. Early childhood physical trauma, most commonly rectal, can be an important etiological factor in vaginismus. Others have noted painful, unhappy first experiences with intercourse. Women with any one of these events in their history often develop an anxiety-fear-guilt cycle that perpetuates the problem.

Adult behavioral patterns associated with the development and maintenance of vaginismus include fear of pregnancy, venereal disease, pain, and the assumption of an adult role. Fears of pain and punishment then operate actively to maintain vaginismus. The fears may stem from misinformation, ignorance, or guilt. Vaginismic women unfailingly report that they are fearful of intercourse. One study reported that a disproportionate number of vaginismic women, when compared with orgasm-inhibited women, described their fathers as threatening figures.

The psychoanalytic explanation of vaginismus is not accepted by most sex therapists. According to this explanation, vaginismus is a hysterical or conversion symptom that is the symbolic expression of a specific unconscious intrapsychic conflict. Psychoanalysts have postulated that women with vaginismus experience penis envy and that the vaginismus is an expression of a castration desire. These theories are not helpful in practice and can interfere with attempts to help the woman with vaginismus.

Immediate factors contributing to vaginismus include the role of the passive male, who can contribute as much to the problem as an aggressive partner. The passive man, who backs off at the first hint of anxiety, reinforces the notion that sex is painful. The pairing of sexually fearful men and women can allow the couples mutually to protect themselves from their fear of aggression in sex (Munjack and Oziel, 1980).

EFFECTS OF VAGINISMUS ON ADAPTATION

Physiological Function. It is common for women with vaginismus to have no problem with sexual arousal. Lubrication may occur normally, and noncoital sexual activity may well be pleasurable even to the point of orgasm. It is only at the point of vaginal penetration that the problem ensues. The reaction to imminent vaginal penetration is not limited to sexual encounters but also occurs with any attempt at vaginal penetration, such as a pelvic examination.

Psychological Function. Vaginismus makes intercourse impossible. The effect is often devastating. To avoid the painful feelings associated with sexual interactions, many women try to avoid all sexual encounters. By achieving a level of psychological comfort without curing the vaginismus, an avoidance pattern is reinforced. The implications of this pattern for a heterosexual marriage are all too obvious.

ASSESSMENT

Clinicians are more likely to detect vaginismus if they are aware that most vaginismic women do not present with vaginismus as their chief complaint. One study (Ellison, 1972) found that in 38 per cent of cases of severe psychogenic vaginismus, the primary physical complaint was not vaginismus but one of the following: difficulty breathing, abdominal pain, vomiting, or diarrhea. An open-ended approach to the interview, with specific attention to sexual function, is the key to eliciting a history of vaginismus.

The histories of women with vaginismus also often include one or more of the following: an unconsummated marriage, primary erectile failure, the woman's complaint of low desire, and inability to use a tampon. The practitioner should take a careful history that includes questions about menstruation, contraception, pregnancy, therapeutic abortion, pelvic trauma, and masturbatory patterns.

The diagnosis of vaginismus can be established only by pelvic examination with a chaperon present. Each step should be explained before proceeding. Because vaginismus cannot be diagnosed if there is voluntary guarding, the client must be assisted in relaxation by talking or by special breathing techniques. Insertion of a single lubricated finger into the introitus may be enough to stimulate the muscle spasm characteristic of vaginismus. This involuntary spasm is diagnostic.

It is important to distinguish dyspareunia, or pain with intercourse, from vaginismus. There are many organic causes of dyspareunia. In contrast, an estimated 90 per cent of vaginismus is considered psychogenic in origin. While vaginismus may be reported as pain with intercourse, it may be distinguished from dyspareunia by performing a physical examination. In women with dyspareunia, guarding occurs if contact is made with the painful area, whereas in women with vaginismus there is an involuntary spasm that makes it very difficult if not impossible to perform a bimanual examination. Dyspareunia often results from physical causes such as infection, bleeding, or neoplasm, whereas these conditions rarely result in vaginismus. If they do, vaginismus persists even after the physical problem resolves. In contrast, dyspareunia resolves when the physical problem improves.

INTERVENTION

The treatment of vaginismus usually begins during the pelvic examination. The health professional should be the person involved in a counseling relationship with the woman. Initially, the goal is to help the woman understand more precisely and objectively what is occurring anatomically and physiologically. This information is provided in a gentle way by having the counselor demonstrate vaginal spasm when one finger is partially inserted at the introitus. Some therapists then use graduated dilators. An alternative or additional approach is to have the woman practice relaxation and self-awareness exercises at home. Soothing warm baths and manual exploration of the vagina, aided by use of a lubricant such as K-Y jelly, are some approaches that can be helpful. Gradually, the partner is included in home treatment. He can follow the same gradual, gentle steps described above. The couple progresses from finger insertion by the male with assistance and direction from the female to vaginal-penile penetration. Initially, no movement should occur during penetration; with time the couple progresses to pelvic movement. Throughout the process, open communication is important. Varying degrees of success have been reported with use of this treatment approach. One variable seems to be whether couples previously achieved penile-vaginal penetration (Crooks and Baur, 1983).

REFERENCES

APA: Diagnostic and Statistical Manual of Mental Disorders. 3rd ed rev. Washington, DC, American Psychiatric Association, 1987.

Barbach LG: For Yourself: The Fulfillment of Female Sexuality. New York, Doubleday, 1975.

Bardwick JM: Psychology of Women: A Study of Biocultural Conflicts. New York, Harper & Row, 1971.

Crooks R, Baur K: Our Sexuality. Menlo Park, Benjamin/Cummings, 1983.

Dearborn LW: Autoeroticism: In Ellis A, Abarbanel A (eds): The Encyclopedia of Sex Behavior. Dallas, Hawthorn, 1967.

Dow MG: Retarded ejaculation as a function of non-aversive conditioning and discrimination: A hypothesis. J Sex Marital Ther 7:49, 1981.

Ellison C: Vaginismus. Med Asp Human Sex 6:34, 1972.

Fertel NS: Vaginismus: A review. J Sex Marital Ther 3:13, 1977.

Hite S: The Hite Report: A Nationwide Study of Female Sexuality. New York, Dell, 1976.

Hawton K: Sex Therapy: A Practical Guide. Oxford, Oxford University Press, 1985.

Kaplan HS: The New Sex Therapy. New York, Brunner/Mazel, 1974.

Kaplan HS: Disorders of Sexual Desire and Other Concepts and Techniques In Sex Therapy. New York, Brunner/Mazel, 1979.

Karacan I, Aslan C, Williams RL: Diagnostic evaluation of male impotence: Problems and promises. In Fann WE et al (eds): Pharmacology and Treatment of Sexual Disorders. Jamaica, SP Medical and Scientific Books, 1983.

Kinsey AC et al (eds): Sexual Behavior in the Human Female. Philadelphia, WB Saunders, 1953.

Kockott G et al: Symptomatology and psychological aspects of male sexual inadequacy: Results of an experimental study. Arch Sex Behav 9:457, 1980.

Kolodny RC, Masters WH, Johnson VE: Textbook of Sexual Medicine. Boston, Little, Brown & Co, 1979.

Livingston CA, McIntyre MC, Fogel CI: Sexual dysfunction: Etiology and treatment. In Woods NF (ed): Human Sexuality in Health and Illness. 3rd ed. St. Louis, CV Mosby, 1982.

LoPiccolo J: Review of *The New Sex Therapy* by HS Kaplan. Behav Ther 6:136, 1975.

LoPiccolo J, Lobitz CL: The role of masturbation in the treatment of orgasmic dysfunction. In LoPiccolo J, LoPiccolo L (eds): Handbook of Sex Therapy. New York, Plenum Press, 1978.

Meyer JK: Diagnosis and diagnostic techniques. In Meyer JK, Schmidt CW, Wise TN (eds): Clinical Management of Sexual Disorders. Baltimore, Williams & Wilkins, 1983.

Munjack DJ, Oziel LJ: Sexual Medicine and Counseling in Office Practice. Boston, Little, Brown & Co, 1980.

Nash EM, Louden LM: The premarital medical examination and the Carolina Population Center. JAMA 210:2365, 1969.

Schull GR, Sprenkle DH: Retarded ejaculation: Reconceptualization and implications for treatment. J Sex Marital Ther 6:234, 1980.

Spence SH: Group versus individual treatment of primary and secondary female orgasmic dysfunction. Behav Res Therapy 5:539, 1985.

Tollison C, Adams HE: Sexual Disorders: Treatment, Theory and Research. New York, Gardner Press, Inc, 1979.

28: Developmental Disability and Sexuality

Victoria Shea

This chapter discusses issues pertaining to the sexual health and development of people with developmental disabilities. This is a population whose sexual needs and rights have traditionally been forgotten or even discounted generally by society, and often, even by health professionals. Some have perceived the sexuality of the developmentally disabled as dangerous to society, on the grounds that it would lead to promiscuous and criminal public behavior and would increase the population of defective individuals. Others have thought of the developmentally disabled as perpetual children who do not have the same sexual nature as normally developing people and should be protected from learning about the subject (Morgenstern, 1973). Over the past 20 years, however, the principle of "normalization" has emerged as a guiding philosophy for the lives of people with developmental disabilities (Baroff, 1974). This principle suggests that the developmentally disabled should be permitted and encouraged to live as much like normal people as possible. Normalization implies having normal daily routines of work and recreation, living in communities, and obtaining services from community businesses and agencies, including private and public health care providers. Leading a normal life also includes sexual development and feelings, usually accompanied by some sexually related behaviors. It is therefore important for health professionals to be educated about developmental disabilities and their impact on a variety of health-related issues, including sexuality.

Because so few health professionals are trained in developmental disabilities, it is essential to present a brief overview of types of developmental disabilities before turning to a discussion of the normal development of sexuality, the impact of the various disabilities on sexuality, and the potential contributions of health professionals.

THE DEVELOPMENTALLY DISABLED

The term "developmentally disabled" refers to a broad category of persons with mental or physical limitations. The current federal definition of developmental disabilities is a "severe, chronic disability that is attributable to a mental or physical impairment or combination of mental and physical impairments; is manifest before age 22; is likely to continue indefinitely; results in substantial functional limitations in three or more of the following areas of major life activity: self-care, receptive and expressive language, learning, mobility, self-direction, capacity for independent living, or economic self-sufficiency; and reflects the need for a combination and sequence of special, interdisciplinary, or generic care, or of other services which are of a lifelong or extended duration and individually planned and coordinated" (Thompson and O'Quinn, 1979, p 14).

This definition replaces earlier versions that designated as developmental disabilities five specific diagnoses: mental retardation, autism, cerebral palsy, epilepsy, and a learning disorder with characteristics similar to mental retardation. Thus, the current conceptualization potentially includes more handicapping conditions, for example, hearing loss and chronic childhood illnesses, but includes them only when they result in impaired ability to function in an age-appropriate fashion.

Mental Retardation

The most frequently occurring developmental disability is mental retardation, which refers to "significantly subaverage general intellectual functioning existing concurrently with deficits in adaptive behavior, and manifested during the developmental period" (Grossman, 1983, p 11). The estimated prevalence of mental retardation in the United States is 3 per cent, or approximately 7 million persons. Within the mentally retarded population, approximately 89 per cent are *mildly retarded*, with IQs ranging from −2 to −3 standard deviations below the mean of 100. Thus, their IQs are in the range of the mid 50s to 70. As children, their cognitive development generally proceeds at approximately two thirds the average rate, so that as adults their mental age equivalent ranges from approximately 8 1/2 to 11 years. Mildly retarded people are frequently able to master basic academic skills such as reading with comprehension, addition and subtraction, spelling, and legible handwriting, up to the third to fourth grade level. With appropriate education and support, most mildly retarded adults can live and work independently.

Moderately mentally retarded children generally develop cognitively at approximately half the normal rate, with IQs in the range of the mid 30s to mid 50s, (−3 to −4 standard deviations). Their mental age equivalents as adults range from 6 to 8 1/2 years. Although some moderately mentally retarded adults live independently in the community, they tend to function poorly in terms of social judgment, money management, and self-care. Most moderately mentally retarded people need supervision and support from relatives, social service agencies, or structured living situations such as group homes to function adequately in modern society. Within sheltered employment and living settings, most moderately mentally retarded people can be productive and well-adjusted citizens.

Severely mentally retarded persons can also function well within the community, given appropriate support services and stimulation. With a developmental rate of approximately one third normal and adult mental age equivalents from 3 1/2 to 6 years (IQs mid 20s to mid 30s), the severely mentally retarded cannot live independently, although many are capable of independent semi-independent self-help skills, such as dressing, simple food preparation and housekeeping, and bathing and personal hygiene. The *profoundly mentally retarded* (IQs below 25, mental age equivalent below 3 1/2 years) make extremely slow developmental progress through childhood and are likely to have other developmental disabilities in addition to mental retardation, such as epilepsy, cerebral palsy, and/or sensory losses. Functional abilities within the population of the profoundly mentally retarded vary greatly, ranging from persons with infant-level perceptual and cognitive abilities to persons with the ability to understand and speak some words.

Autism

Autism is a disorder characterized by delayed development, severe communication handicaps, and abnormal ways of relating to people, objects, and events (Ritvo and Freeman, 1977). The prevalence of autism is 4 per 10,000 people, making it a relatively rare developmental disability affecting approximately 100,000 Americans. Although early conceptualizations of autism considered it a psychogenic illness, it is now widely accepted to be an organically based developmental disability. Most autistic people are significantly mentally retarded (DeMyer, 1979), with particular difficulty in language skills. Thus, although their nonverbal cognitive skills might be quite good, their functional abilities on tasks that require understanding or use of language are usually significantly limited. Most autistic persons require supervised living and vocational arrangements throughout life.

Cerebral Palsy

The most common developmental disabilities that result in motor handicaps are cerebral palsy and meningomyelocele (spina bifida). The term cerebral palsy describes a variety of abnormal motor patterns due to an insult to the developing brain. Common features are abnormally high or low muscle tone, increased or abnormal reflexes, and limitations of voluntary movement. Cerebral palsy affects approximately 5 per 1000 babies, so that over 500,000 Americans have this disorder. Approximately 50 per cent of people with cerebral palsy are mentally retarded, and another 25 per cent function cognitively in the borderline or "slow learner" range. The incidence of mental retardation varies significantly with the type of cerebral palsy, however; individuals with the athetoid form, for example, are frequently of average or above average intelligence.

Meningomyelocele

Meningomyelocele (spina bifida) is a malformation during gestation of the neural tube, which results in sensory and/or motor paralysis of areas innervated below the level of the spinal cord lesion. Frequent complications of this condition include hydrocephalus, recurrent urinary tract infections, orthopedic problems, and absent bowel and bladder control. Mental retardation can, but does not necessarily, accompany this condition.

Epilepsy

Epilepsy (seizure disorder) is a symptom of central nervous system dysfunction rather than an independent disease process. Seizures result from abnormal patterns of electrical activity in the brain. This activity can remain localized in one area of the brain and produce focal seizures, usually consisting of a repetitive involuntary motor behavior or unusual sensory experience. If the abnormal electrical activity generalizes through the brain, a common result is a grand mal or tonic-clonic seizure followed by loss of consciousness. Although almost 6 in 100 persons in the United States have a seizure at some time in their lives, the prevalence of a recurrent seizure disorder is only 6 per 1000. Most seizure disorders can be well controlled with medication and rarely have any effect on sexuality. Epilepsy is not necessarily accompanied by any other developmental disability.

NORMAL DEVELOPMENT OF SEXUALITY

The development of human sexuality includes both the mastery of concrete facts and skills and the integration of abstract concepts, values, and psychological needs. It may be helpful to consider both the concrete and abstract issues in normal developing sexuality before looking at the effects of a developmental disability.

Childhood—Concrete Issues

Young children are expected to learn many facts and behaviors related to their bodies, some of which are broadly associated with sexuality. Concrete skills generally mastered by young children include names of body parts (including genitals) and abilities to dress and use the bathroom independently and privately. In addition, since most children masturbate, they soon learn their families' rules about where, when, or even whether this activity is permitted. They learn other social rules, too, such as acceptable and unacceptable ways of touching other people, words and subjects that are not to be used or brought up in public, and the standards of privacy and modesty followed by their household and community.

Childhood—Abstract Issues

In addition to learning facts and rules, children are developing ideas about issues related to sexuality. The abstract concepts they attempt to master mainly have to do with family relationships and procreation. Children come to understand that their parents had parents, that they themselves will age and perhaps marry and have children, and that they were once babies. This line of thinking eventually leads to the question, "Where did I come from?" although many children do not ask this question directly.

Early Adolescent—Concrete Issues

With the onset of puberty, young adolescents are confronted with the need to learn a new repertoire of practical skills. In the area of hygiene, for example, they learn about deodorants, frequent bathing, shaving, and the use of medication for acne. Young women must also learn the practical and social aspects of managing their menstrual periods. Concrete social behaviors that most adolescents master include techniques for expressing interest in the opposite sex, for example, flirting and telephoning, and specific sexual behaviors, such as holding hands and kissing.

Early Adolescent—Abstract Issues

One of the most significant abstract issues that young adolescents must face in the area of sexuality concerns self-esteem and feelings of acceptance or rejection. Adolescents often have strong physical and psychological feelings of attraction that may not be returned, or even noticed, by the object of their affection. One of the developmental tasks of adolescence is to learn to deal with these feelings and thus to develop a realistic and comfortable sense of self-esteem and identity in the area of sexuality.

Late Adolescent— Concrete Issues

Late adolescent/adult developmental tasks of sexuality concern responsible genital sexuality. Concrete issues that must be mastered include the use of contraception and protection against venereal disease. In addition, adults learn the distinction between acceptable public acts, for example, holding hands, hugging, and kissing goodnight, and private sexual behavior, such as foreplay and intercourse. They also learn ways of arranging for privacy.

Late Adolescent—Abstract Issues

Abstract issues at this stage involve the issue of responsibility for and relationship with the sexual partner. Adults learn to integrate physical desires with emotional intimacy, and most adopt the abstract value that sexual behavior requires concern for the partner's feelings and needs. Most adults form committed relationships, usually heterosexual, although some adults face decisions and conflicts about same-sex behavior.

EFFECTS OF DEVELOPMENTAL DISABILITIES ON ADAPTATION

Since there are many different developmental disabilities and many aspects of sexuality, the interactions of the two areas are complex. As a general rule, the main effect of developmental disabilities involving cognitive impairments (i.e., mental retardation and autism) is to limit the developmental level and abstractness of the individual's sexual concerns. Conversely, the physical/motor disabilities in some way affect the concrete issues of sexuality but do not diminish the individual's abstract psychological needs, interests, and desires.

Mental Retardation

PSYCHOLOGICAL FUNCTION

The sexual issues for moderately, severely, and profoundly mentally retarded people are most likely to be similar to the issues facing young children in addition to the concrete issues of mature bodies. Like young children, significantly mentally retarded persons may not have learned rules related to privacy and modesty of activities such as dressing, using the bathroom, and masturbation; unfortunately, mistakes or uninformed behavior in these domains are often upsetting to the general public when performed by physically mature people. There is some evidence that the onset of puberty is delayed in some individuals with severe mental retardation, although other studies have found no such effect (Saunders, 1981). The literature also suggests that females with brain damage begin their menstrual periods earlier than average (Craft and Craft, 1981). At the time of puberty and the development of secondary sex characteristics, significantly mentally retarded persons may need instruction and/or supervision in personal hygiene tasks such as shaving or changing sanitary napkins. Those individuals who experience attraction and sexual feelings toward other people may not have the social skills to express their interest and form a mutually enjoyable relationship.

In terms of sexual health, moderately to profoundly mentally retarded people may not recognize or be able to describe symptoms of disease, such as painful urination or unusual discharges.

The mildly mentally retarded generally confront the entire range of concrete and abstract issues related to sexuality (Kempton, 1977). They are capable of learning the skills involved in hygiene and contraception but tend to learn best through repeated practice and concrete demonstration rather than through abstract verbal explanations. The major effect of their cognitive impairment is greater than average difficulty dealing with the conceptual and psychological issues of adolescence and adulthood. Most mildly retarded people identify themselves with the general population and want to be like everyone else. However, especially during their school years, they are the least successful students and are often socially rejected or isolated because of their limited competence at school tasks. These individuals struggle with their sense of being different, although usually they do not understand (and are not taught) why they are different. Mildly mentally retarded teenagers will express strong desires to be popular, date, and marry and are often frustrated by their lack of popularity. This frustration, especially when compounded by a poor self-image because of academic failures, may make the individual vulnerable to sexual exploitation or impulsive sexual behavior. Other potential problems found among the mildly retarded are limited social judgment and poor ability to make long-range plans and to understand future consequences. Clearly, these deficiencies can contribute to significant sexual health problems, such as unwanted pregnancies, venereal disease, and sexual exploitation. With specific instruction, however, many mildly retarded persons are capable of functioning at a much healthier and safer level. They can learn to consider others' feelings, form intimate commitments with their partners, and make reasonable, responsible decisions about sexual behavior and contraception.

Autism

PSYCHOLOGICAL FUNCTION

Because the majority of individuals with autism are also significantly mentally retarded,

the sexual problems and needs of the two groups are similar. Many autistic persons have limited ability to interact with other people and function at an extremely young developmental level, so that their sexual activity is usually limited to masturbation; their health care and educational needs are very basic. Abstract psychological and conceptual issues are generally beyond their understanding.

Cerebral Palsy and Meningomyelocele

PHYSIOLOGICAL FUNCTION

These two disorders will be discussed together because they have many similar effects on the development of sexuality, as both can involve significant disorders of movement. As described previously, cerebral palsy varies in severity, ranging from a slight limp or limitation of arm function to total dependence in activities of daily living (e.g., bathing and dressing). People with meningomyelocele generally have adequate hand and upper extremity function, but gross motor skills such as sitting unsupported or standing alone may be compromised. With both disorders, specific motor movements related to personal hygiene, such as bathing, shaving, and changing sanitary napkins, may be limited. In addition to these problems, toileting functions may be disrupted by the spinal lesion and require procedures such as catheterization and suppositories. Girls with meningomyelocele may have early onset of puberty (Stewart, 1979). Toileting and menstrual hygiene can eventually be performed independently by individuals with normal intelligence or mild cognitive handicaps, but significant mental retardation decreases the likelihood of independent self-care.

Many people with meningomyelocele have decreased or absent sensation in the genital area, depending on the level of the spinal lesion. Men may have erectile problems, although some have reported themselves capable of erections and ejaculation (Dorner, 1977). Sexual feelings and sexual pleasure are still possible for all affected individuals, however, even if conventional intercourse is not (Stewart, 1979).

PSYCHOLOGICAL FUNCTION

Both disorders may significantly limit the individual's experience of privacy and independence. Occasionally, persons with severe cerebral palsy have had such distorted experiences of lack of privacy that they attempt to obtain sexual gratification from persons providing personal care such as bathing.

In adolescence, the developmental tasks of establishing a positive body image and sexual desirability are more difficult (although not impossible) for motorically impaired youngsters, who must often struggle to maintain their self-esteem in the face of social isolation or rejection by their peers. Even when peers are friendly, the logistics of arranging recreational activities are much more complicated than for able-bodied teenagers. As adults, people with cerebral palsy often require special counseling and equipment to aid in activities such as masturbation, intercourse, and conception (Stewart, 1979).

ADDITIONAL EFFECTS OF DEVELOPMENTAL DISABILITY

There are at least three significant but indirect effects of developmental disabilities on sexuality. These are limited access to information about sexuality, increased vulnerability to sexual abuse and exploitation, and the likelihood of spending significant amounts of time in institutions of various sorts.

Limited Information

Unfortunately, the developmentally disabled are often tremendously ignorant about normal sexual development and about their own sexual capabilities. As mentioned previously, the sexual needs of the developmentally disabled may not be dealt with by parents who are uncomfortable with the child's developing sexuality or who are unsure of what information to give their handicapped offspring. Similarly, sex education is much less likely to be included in special education classes than in regular education. Other potential sources of information may also be unavailable to the developmentally disabled if they cannot read, use a library, or purchase books or magazines. Even information from peers may not be available to the developmentally disabled in the same way that it is

to nonhandicapped youth, or the peers may be especially poor sources of accurate information.

Sexual Abuse and Exploitation

There are several risk factors for sexual abuse and exploitation to which developmentally disabled persons are more vulnerable than normally developing individuals. Because of limited information and education, some developmentally disabled persons have less understanding about what kinds of behavior are generally considered inappropriate and should be refused, for example, removing clothes on request and allowing fondling. Unfortunately, the less clear the potential victim is about what is or is not appropriate, the less likely he or she will be to protest. Furthermore, because of developmental delays or physical handicaps, the developmentally disabled may have been dependent on adults as caretakers for more time and more activities than normally developing children. Thus, they may have very strong habits of compliance with adult directions and less practice in refusing to follow directions, even inappropriate ones. Another risk factor is that developmentally disabled persons may be seen as relatively safe victims for abusers, since they are less likely to be believed if they complain.

Institutionalization

Although most children and adults with developmental disabilities live in normal communities, many of them have spent a significant portion of time living in institutions of some kind—medical hospitals, residential schools, group homes, or state facilities for the retarded. Although these settings vary greatly in mission and quality, they tend to have in common several features that may influence the development of sexuality. First, in institutions the developmentally disabled person has multiple caretakers who are likely to have different, and even conflicting, attitudes about sexuality. For example, some caretakers may ignore masturbation, some may punish it, and some may encourage it as a normal outlet for sexual feelings. Under such circumstances it would be very difficult for the developmentally delayed person to develop a clear understanding of social norms and of personal ideas and values. Second, in most institutions privacy is lacking; this can lead to public displays of behaviors, such as masturbation, that should be private. Further distortions occur when these behaviors are either punished for being displayed in public, even though there is no privacy, or ignored because privacy is not possible. Third, many institutions do not provide opportunities to observe and practice normal heterosexual development and behavior. Many institutions discourage dating and attempt to keep men and women separated or tightly supervised. This, at times, leads to situational same-sex behavior. Even enlightened residential programs run the risk of serious legal and community relations problems if they allow more liberal sexual behaviors than the surrounding community; therefore, they may attempt to supervise or limit sexual behavior. Developmentally disabled persons who are in institutions often find themselves with significantly more intrusions into their sexual behavior than do normally developing people (Carruth, 1973; Deisher, 1973).

INTERVENTION

Sexual health promotion for the developmentally disabled takes a variety of forms, including medical and well-child care in pediatric settings, preventive services and consultation in schools, and direct services in adult medicine and obstetrical/gynecological clinics and offices.

The importance of sexual health promotion in pediatric settings cannot be overemphasized. Children who are developmentally disabled, for whatever reason, need more help, rather than less, in developing appropriate sexual behaviors. Too often this area of their development is forgotten or ignored. Parents and teachers, who may be uncomfortable with their own sexuality, are frequently unprepared to deal explicitly and at length with teaching skills that normally developing children pick up rapidly or learn from remote sources such as books, movies, or friends. Thus, health professionals can make a major contribution to the care of developmentally disabled children by using anticipatory guidance with families about the sexual issues that their youngsters will face at various stages of development. Discussing

these issues in a health care setting, openly and before the issue has become a problem, can be extremely useful in making sexuality a normal part of the child's development, in spite of the presence of a developmental disability. Of course, explanations and instruction must be individualized according to the child's level of understanding and physical ability.

Young children should be taught the names their families want them to use for body parts, including sexual ones. Families should begin explicitly to teach them their standards of privacy and modesty, for example, by closing the bathroom door, limiting nudity, or not discussing certain topics in public. Children can be introduced to the concept of aging from infancy to adulthood and learn that there are different relationships between persons, for example, mother and father, sister and brother, husband and wife, grandchildren and grandparents. Young children need to learn appropriate ways of touching other people (e.g., shaking hands with a stranger, kissing a relative) and need to learn that certain ways of touching may not feel good to the receiver (e.g., being touched too hard, being tickled too long, having sexual parts touched). Families should also be helped to understand that masturbation and sexual exploration are normal behaviors for young children. During childhood, it is appropriate to explain that babies grow inside adult women during pregnancy.

Before entering puberty, children should be prepared for the changes their bodies will undergo. This includes knowing that they will have a growth spurt, which begins at different ages for different individuals. They should be prepared for the development of secondary sex characteristics such as breasts, pubic hair, and facial and leg hair. Girls need instruction about the blood flow and hygiene involved in menstruation, and boys should be helped to understand nocturnal emissions. Once puberty begins, youngsters may need help with new hygiene techniques, such as shaving, the use of deodorants, and frequent bathing. Adolescents should also be helped to understand that their strong new sexual feelings are normal, as are masturbation and orgasm. In adolescence the mechanics of sexual intercourse can be described, if this has not already been done. Parents of adolescents should be encouraged to talk openly with their youngsters about family and religious values about the relationship of sexuality and love. This discussion would be appropriate for all developmentally disabled people except those who are so mentally retarded that they cannot understand the abstract concepts involved.

Suggested readings for parents of developmentally disabled children and adolescents include the following books:

An Easy Guide for Caring Parents: Sexuality and Socialization. Lyn McKee and Virginia Blackridge. Champaign, Research Press, 1984.

Raising a Child Conservatively in a Sexually Permissive World. Sol and Judith Gordon. New York, Simon and Schuster, 1983.

Sex Education and the Intellectually Handicapped: A Guide for Parents and Caregivers. Wendy McCarthy and Lydia Fegan. Sydney, Australia, ADIS Health Science Press, 1984. (Available in U.S. through John Wright/PSG, Inc., 545 Great Road, Littleton, Massachusetts 01460.)

The Family Book About Sexuality (revised edition). Mary Calderone and Éric Johnson. New York, Bantam Books, 1983.

There are also a number of books available for parents to read to and look at with their children:

Did the Sun Shine Before You Were Born? A Sex Education Primer. Sol and Judith Gordon. New York, Joseph Okapu Publishing Company, 1974.

Facts About Sex for Today's Youth. Sol Gordon. Fayetteville, Ed-U-Press, 1978.

Girls are Girls and Boys are Boys, So What's the Difference? A Nonsexist Sexuality Education Book for Children Age 6 to 10 (revised edition). Fayetteville, Ed-U-Press, 1983.

Growing Up: A Social and Sexual Education Picture Book for Young People with Mental Retardation. Victoria Shea and Betty Gordon. Chapel Hill, Division for Disorders of Development and Learning, University of North Carolina, 1984.

Where Do Babies Come From? Margaret Sheffield. New York, Knopf, 1973.

Particular attention should be paid to the issue of sexual abuse prevention for all children, not just the developmentally disabled. Excellent materials for young children are available; many of these could be used with older, cognitively delayed children. The following materials are recommended:

A Better Safe Than Sorry Book: A Family Guide for Sexual Assault Prevention. Sol and Judith Gordon. Fayetteville, Ed-U-Press, 1984.

It's My Body: A Book To Teach Young Children

How To Resist Uncomfortable Touch. Tory Freeman. Seattle, Parenting Press, 1982.

My Very Own Book About Me. Jo Stowell and Mary Dietzel. Spokane, Lutheran Services of Washington, 1982.

No More Secrets: Protecting Your Child From Sexual Assault. Caren Adams and Jennifer Fay. San Luis Obispo, Impact Publishers, 1981.

Health professionals can also have a significant impact on sexual health promotion through consultation with school systems. Offering sex education in regular classes has been controversial in many communities but has become fairly common nationally. However, sex education for handicapped children is often forgotten or ignored. Several special education curricula are available, however, and health professionals can often facilitate their use in school. Readily available materials are listed as follows:

Being Me . . . : A Social/Sexual Training Guide for Those Who Work with the Developmentally Disabled. Jean Edwards and Suzan Wapnick. Portland, ASIEP Education Company, 1979.

Developing Responsible Sexuality. Book 5 of A Comprehensive Skills Program for the Handicapped. Mary Moore. New York, Walker Educational Book Corporation, 1984.

Essential Adult Sex Education for the Mentally Retarded. David Zelman and Kathie Tyser. Santa Monica, James Stanfield Film Associates, 1979.

Education for Adulthood: A Curriculum for the Mentally Retarded Who Need a Better Understanding of Life's Processes and a Training Guide for Those Who Will Teach the Curriculum. Madeline Greenbaum and Sandra Noll. Staten Island, Staten Island Mental Health Society, Inc., 1982.

Sex Education for Persons with Disabilities That Hinder Learning: A Teacher's Guide. Winifred Kempton. Chicago, Stoelting Co., 1980.

Health professionals who deal with developmentally disabled adults should be aware that many of their clients may not have had access to the same kinds of information and experience as their normally developing peers. They may have numerous misconceptions and areas of ignorance, so that simple, basic explanations of procedures would be appropriate, even for people of normal intelligence. Physically handicapped and mildly mentally retarded adults might also appreciate suggestions of pamphlets and books they could read themselves. Good sources of information about sexuality and various disabilities include the following:

"Sexuality and Disability: A Bibliography of Resources Available for Purchase" (available from The Sex Education and Information Council of the U.S., Inc., 80 Fifth Avenue, Suite 801-2, New York, NY 10011).

Who Cares?: A Handbook on Sex Education and Counseling Services for Disabled People (second edition). Debra Cornelius, Sophia Chiporas, Elaine Makas, Susan Daniels. Baltimore, University Park Press, 1982.

Not Made of Stone: The Sexual Problems of Handicapped People. K. Heslinga. Springfield, Charles C Thomas, 1974.

Mentally retarded women seen in obstetrical and/or gynecological clinics and offices generally have special needs for explanations and reassurance. The pelvic examination, for example, might seem extraordinarily awkward, uncomfortable, and frightening. Slow, calm explanations are important, and practice sessions might be helpful in teaching the woman appropriate positions and behavior.

The issue of contraception for mentally retarded women involves behavioral and legal issues in addition to standard medical concerns (Chamberlain et al, 1984). If oral contraceptives are used, the mentally retarded woman or her caretaker must ensure regular use. Similarly, condoms would only be effective if the mentally retarded man or his partner understood the importance of using them regularly and properly. Intrauterine devices are often not indicated because of the dangers that expulsion or serious side effects would not be noticed or communicated by the woman. Injections of Depo-Provera have not been approved by the FDA for contraception. In many jurisdictions, sterilization requires a court order or other legal procedures to ensure the protection of the woman's rights.

The sexual health needs of developmentally disabled people are more similar to than different from the needs of the general population. In spite of our cultural stereotypes, sexuality does not depend on intellectual process or physical beauty and strength. Sexual development, feelings, and behaviors are normal parts of human development. The task for health professionals is to adapt general health care principles and practices to the developmentally disabled and to meet their special needs for education and support.

REFERENCES

Baroff GS: Mental Retardation: Nature, Cause, and Management. New York, Hemisphere, 1974.

Carruth DG: Human sexuality in a halfway house. In De la Cruz FF, La Veck GD (eds): Human Sexuality and the Mentally Retarded. New York, Brunner/Mazel, 1973, pp 153–156.

Chamberlain A et al: Issues in fertility control for mentally retarded female adolescents: 1. Sexual activity, sexual abuse, and contraception. Pediatrics 73:445, 1984.

Craft A, Craft M: Sexuality and mental handicap: A review. Br J Psychiatry 139:494, 1981.

Deisher RW: Sexual behavior of retarded in institutions. In De la Cruz FF, La Veck GD (eds): Human Sexuality and the Mentally Retarded. New York, Brunner/Mazel, 1973, pp 145–152.

DeMyer MK: Parents and Children in Autism. New York, Halstead Press, 1979.

Dorner S: Sexual interest and activity in adolescents with spina bifida. J Child Psychol Psychiatry 18:229, 1977.

Grossman HJ (ed): Classification in Mental Retardation. Washington, DC, American Association on Mental Deficiency, 1983.

Kempton W: The sexual adolescent who is mentally retarded. J Ped Psychol 2:104, 1977.

Morgenstern M: Community attitudes toward sexuality of the retarded. In De la Cruz FF, La Veck GD (eds): Human Sexuality and the Mentally Retarded. New York, Brunner/Mazel, 1973, pp 156–162.

Ritvo ER, Freeman BJ: National Society for Autistic Children definition of the syndrome of autism. J Ped Psychol 2:146, 1977.

Saunders EJ: The mental health professional, the mentally retarded, and sex. Hosp Comm Psychiatry 32:717, 1981.

Stewart WFR: The Sexual Side of Handicap. Cambridge, Great Britain, Woodhead-Faulkner, 1979.

Thompson RJ, O'Quinn AN: Developmental Disabilities: Etiology, Management, Diagnosis, and Treatment. Oxford, Oxford University Press, 1979.

29: Mental Illness, Substance Abuse and Sexuality

Elizabeth M. Munsat

The relationship between sexual functioning and mental illness is complex. Since sexual behavior represents an interrelationship among an individual's "intrapsychic, intrapersonal, biological, and social factors," (Woods, 1981, p 199), all of these aspects affect sexual functioning. Emotional state can influence sexual behavior in a number of ways, such as mood changes that affect interest in sex, increased or decreased energy state, and/or interpersonal aspects that affect ability to form and maintain relationships. It is also evident that sexual problems or changes in sexual interest or behavior can contribute to emotional problems; stress from an individual's experience of sexuality can cause exacerbations in a chronic mental illness or cause or increase depression or anxiety. There is then a reciprocal relationship between sexuality and emotional state. The possibility that physiological mechanisms may concurrently affect both sexual behavior and emotional state is under investigation.

Not every psychiatric diagnosis implies a sexual dysfunction. Woods notes that "there is no *consistent* relationship between any specific psychiatric illness and disordered sexuality." (Woods, 1981, p 200, [italics author's]) Emotional problems may or may not be expressed in sexual symptoms. Problems in the area of sexuality can affect interest/desire, pleasure/satisfaction, and/or performance/functioning. Instead of directly affecting a client's sexuality, an individual's mental illness may have an effect on the partner's sexual satisfaction, interest, or behavior.

In assessing a disturbance in sexual functioning, the problem must be comprehensively evaluated. A history and physical examination are essential to rule out possible organic causes—physical problems or effects of drugs or medications. A client with a known psychiatric illness may have sexual symptoms unrelated to this diagnosis. In taking a sexual history, the health professional needs to determine whether a sexual dysfunctional problem is primary or secondary, that is, whether the client has always had this particular sexual problem or whether this represents a change in sexual performance. Assessment of the psychogenic component should include obtaining information about the client's attitudes and early sexual experience, the client's knowledge about technique, performance expectations, beliefs pertaining to sexuality, and situational factors such as family or work stress that may be causing sexual dysfunction. As already noted, there is frequently an interaction between organic and psychogenic components in producing sexual symptoms. It is important that the health professional be aware of the many and varied causes of disturbances in sexual functioning and the potential for interaction of causal components in order to proceed with appropriate assessment and intervention.

This chapter will discuss disturbances in sexual functioning associated with mood disorders (formerly called affective disorders), anxiety and somatoform disorders, schizophrenia, organic mental syndromes and disorders, anorexia nervosa, substance use, gender identity disorder, some sexual disorders, and the effects of medications used in treatment of mental illness. Terminology and classifications used are based on the American Psychiatric Association's DSM-III-R (Diagnostic and Statistical Manual of Mental Disorders, Third Edition, Revised). The sexual aspects of these diagnoses will be described, and interventions relevant to each will be presented.

MOOD DISORDERS: DEPRESSION AND BIPOLAR DISORDER (MANIC-DEPRESSIVE ILLNESS)

Depression

Depression can be either the result or cause of sexual dysfunctions. Kolodny, Masters, and Johnson (1979) report that approximately 70 per cent of depressed clients have decreased sexual desire. Other authors note that this decreased sexual desire may be part of the general decreased energy level, withdrawal, and decreased capacity for pleasure seen in depression. Depressed individuals have few sexual fantasies or thoughts about sex; they also show a decrease in initiating sexual behavior. Their diminished sexual desire and decreased orgasmic capacity may also be viewed as a form of self-deprivation, an acting out of "self-punitive impulses in patients who are depressed and guilt-ridden" (Spencer and Raft, 1977, p 59).

Depression can be a reaction to diminished sexual desire or diminished sexual performance of any etiology. Depression and decreased performance are interrelated; as one worsens, the other is affected, drawing the client into a downward spiral that needs intervention to be broken. The health professional must compare the time of onset and duration of both the depressive and sexual symptoms in order to determine the sequential relationship between the two. Once it is determined which symptom came first, the health professional can intervene appropriately.

Biochemical changes in depression may have a direct effect in decreasing sexual responsivity. Kaplan states that depression "is probably best viewed as a genetically transmitted psychosomatic disorder of brain metabolism" (Kaplan, 1974, p 477). If this is the case, one must treat the depression, both its chemical and psychic causes.

Primary depression is one of the most common causes of loss of interest in sex and decreased frequency of intercourse. Frequency of intercourse is most often decreased in depressed men; depressed women seem to participate in sex but with less enjoyment. Munjack and Oziel (1980) describe one study of 500 psychiatric outpatients in which 42 per cent of depressed men and 33 per cent of depressed women showed decreased sexual drive beginning after the onset of the depression. In another study of outpatient depressed men, subjects reported significantly lower sexual interest and satisfaction than did the healthy controls (Howell et al, 1987). In inpatients hospitalized for primary depression, up to 80 per cent of men and 96 per cent of women reported decreased desire. Sexual dysfunction in depressed women has not been adequately studied. There is disagreement in the literature about whether depression affects the orgasmic capacity of women. Paykel and Weissman (1972) studied depressed women in an outpatient setting and found that the most impairment was in sexual interest and satisfaction; they also noted some complaints of dyspareunia, increased hostile behavior toward spouses, and a disproportionate amount of guilt over previous sexual involvement. Several authors report depressed men experiencing erectile failure to varying degrees: 23 to 28 per cent of outpatients and 23 to 50 per cent of inpatients (Kolodny, Masters, and Johnson, 1979; Woodruff, Murphy, and Herjanic, 1967).

In the initial phase of primary depression, clients sometimes exhibit increased sexual activity in an attempt to counteract or overcome the depression. This is generally seen as an effort to increase self-esteem, to obtain reassurance, or to decrease loneliness, "[rather] than a genuine increase in sexual desire or response" (Bancroft, 1983, p 361).

Secondary depressions are depressive syndromes that develop in the course of another illness (e.g., in clients with schizophrenia). Munjack and Oziel (1980) note that the sexual symptom most reported is decreased desire in 25 per cent of such depressed male outpatients, in 41 per cent of depressed female outpatients, and in 56 per cent of all depressed inpatients.

Depression also has an effect on the client's relationship with a spouse or significant other. The depressed client has increased needs and demands, hostility and resentment toward the partner, and worries about ability to function in the marriage or relationship. Often such clients are withdrawn and unable to talk to their spouse or partner about their feelings. Weissberg (1982) describes the stress that depression imposes on a marriage or serious relationship: because of the depressed client's inability to experience pleasure, the partner's pleasure-providing role is blocked. This is an important part of the relationship that is often not verbalized. In their study of depressed women, Paykel and Weissman (1972) found problems with interpersonal communication, submissiveness and dependency on the spouse, ambivalence in feelings of affection toward the spouse, guilt and a sense of failure in the marriages, and interpersonal friction in the marital relationship.

ASSESSMENT

In assessing a client's depression, it is important to ask questions about whether sexual interest or activity has changed. If you do not bring up the subject, the client may not. This is an early intervention in the course of assessment because it makes it more likely that the client will bring up any sexual concerns in the future. It makes it clear that the health professional is comfortable discussing such concerns and open to hearing about them. Involve the partner in the assessment as well as in the treatment.

Sometimes when interviewing depressed clients and their partner, the health professional discovers that it is the partner who is having a sexual problem. If this is the case, it may not be advisable to begin treatment of the sexual problem—if sexual therapy involving the depressed partner is the recommended treatment—until after the depression is resolved. A depressed individual cannot participate in a giving, loving way, which is necessary for successful sexual therapy. In fact, instituting sexual therapy while one member of the couple is depressed could increase the depression, as this would replace unrealistic demands on the depressed individual.

INTERVENTION

Treatment depends on whether the sexual dysfunction is a cause of or the result of depression. If the depressed client has a sexual problem that is caused by depression, the general rule is to treat the depression rather than the sexual problem initially. Treatments most commonly used are antidepressant medication (see Table 29–1) and psychotherapy, usually on an outpatient basis, although at times hospitalization and sometimes electroconvulsive therapy (ECT) are needed. Treatment of the sexual dysfunction as an isolated symptom is contraindicated in acute depression. Kaplan states that the exceptions to this are treatment of the symptoms of premature ejaculation and vaginismus, which do not seem to be substantially influenced by depression; therefore, treatment of these symptoms does not need to be deferred. Sexual therapy may be used to treat these symptoms while concurrently treating the client's depression. (See Chapter 27, Psychosomatic Sexual Dysfunction, for discussion of these treatments.)

Providing information about depression and the time needed for medication to work is an important intervention that must include the client and the partner. The health professional should provide information about the relationship between depression and sexual symptoms and should reassure the client that this is not a permanent state. Psychotherapies used in treating depression include cognitive therapy, psychodynamically oriented psychotherapy, and behavior modification for decreasing nonproductive thoughts and activities. Psychodynamically oriented psychotherapy is based on a theory of human personality development and focuses on understanding the interaction of the conscious and unconscious aspects of the mind with reality and of past, present, and future. Behavior modification focuses on the symptoms or troublesome behaviors and is based on the assumption that most behavior is learned, is shaped by the environment, and is maintained by consequences. Since behavior is learned, different, more adaptive behaviors can be learned (and maladaptive behaviors modified, reduced, or eliminated) by changing the reinforcers or consequences. Cognitive therapy is designed to refute the irrational ideas and beliefs that people tell themselves, thereby unintentionally causing themselves stress and emotional disturbance.

Through such therapy, irrational internal statements are converted to more rational ones. After treating the depression, clients with marital or sexual problems may need marital therapy, sexual therapy, or psychotherapy. It is important for clients to be aware that the marital disturbances subside much more slowly than do the clinical symptoms of depression.

If depression is the result of a sexual dysfunction, then it would be appropriate to treat the sexual problem with sexual therapy. As the sexual problem is successfully treated, the depression should decrease.

Bipolar Disorder (Manic-Depressive Illness)

Clients diagnosed as having bipolar disorder show a range of variations in sexual interest and activity. Kolodny, Masters, and Johnson (1979) report increased sexual activity in 30 to 65 per cent of hypomanic and manic clients. Woods (1981) notes that an increased energy state, such as with mania, makes more energy available for sexuality. The increased sexuality seen in manic clients may reflect the general increase in feelings of well-being and energy, or "the biochemical basis may have a parallel effect on sexuality" (Bancroft, 1983, p 361).

Hypersexuality may be the first symptom of a manic episode. Manic individuals have decreased sexual inhibitions, they often impulsively choose sexual partners or begin extramarital affairs, and they may display inappropriate sexual behavior (e.g., disrobing in public or masturbating publicly) or may act seductively or flirtatiously. They often have sexual preoccupations or delusions; female manic individuals commonly wish to be pregnant.

A smaller percentage (13 to 15 per cent) of manic individuals show decreased sexual interest. Erectile dysfunction has been occasionally observed in manic males, although there is some question whether this is related to the lithium medication treatment.

Mania usually has a deleterious effect on an individual's relationship with a spouse or significant other. In one study, 42 manic-depressive inpatients and their spouses were compared with 30 healthy pairs. The marriages of the manic-depressive patients were higher in levels of expressed conflict than those of the control group (Hoover and Fitzgerald, 1981). Another reported stress on the marital relationship is that the sexual demands of a hypomanic/manic partner may be exhausting to a spouse or significant other. These relationship stresses indicate the necessity of including the partner in both the assessment and intervention aspects of working with bipolar disorder clients.

INTERVENTION

It is important to work with bipolar disorder clients in counseling to prevent their engaging in promiscuous sexual activity that they may later regret. It is especially important to protect clients under 20 years of age from engaging in such behavior because the impact of promiscuous sexual acts seems to be greater on these younger clients: Many continued to engage in sexual activity "to a degree not acceptable in their community even after they were well" (Tsuang, 1975, pp 88–89).

Because of the effect of manic behavior on interpersonal relationships, it is important to include the spouse or significant other in the treatment. Providing information to the client and family about bipolar disorder is an important aspect of treatment. It is helpful to family members to know that changes in sexual behavior are probably related to the illness and that aberrant sexual behavior will most likely not continue after the illness is successfully treated. In addition to providing education about characteristics of bipolar illness, the health professional should educate the client and family to recognize warning signs of relapse, such as increased sexual activity or spending sprees.

Rather than treating the sexual dysfunction, treatment of the bipolar illness is indicated. Such clients often need hospitalization to help control their behavior. Lithium carbonate and/or antipsychotic medication to control the manic excitement is usually used; lithium is continued on a maintenance level on an outpatient basis, usually for an indefinite period of time. Sometimes ECT is indicated to control acute manic symptoms that do not respond to medication. Success of treatment is increased if the client continues with follow-up mental health care and has available a support system that can help with treatment compliance and recognition of signs of relapse.

ANXIETY AND SOMATOFORM DISORDERS

Anxiety

"Anxiety" per se is not a psychiatric classification or diagnosis, although there are DSM-III-R classifications of anxiety disorders. Even when an individual is not classified as having an anxiety disorder, the presence of anxiety can cause alterations in sexual behavior, such as erectile dysfunction in males or lack of sexual response or pleasure in females. Underlying anxiety sometimes causes individuals to engage in sexual activity as a tranquilizer to relieve the symptoms of anxiety. Such underlying anxiety could be from various causes: fears of being homosexual ("homosexual panic"), increased anxiety from stress such as college examinations, times of transition, reaction to guilt or rejection, rebellion in adolescence, or fears of sexual inadequacy. It is not clear why anxiety increases sexual interest and activity in some individuals and inhibits it in others.

ASSESSMENT

Any assessment of problems with or alterations in a client's sexual behavior must include assessing the psychogenic component. If anxiety is a factor contributing to sexual problems, interventions aimed at decreasing the anxiety are in order.

INTERVENTION

If the client's sexual behavior is a result of underlying anxiety, often all that is needed is for the health professional to provide information and education. For example, the client reacting to a dream reflecting a latent homosexual wish will find it reassuring to know that such dreams or thoughts are a normal part of human sexuality and do not indicate that one is homosexual. Individuals contemplating beginning a sexual relationship may be afraid or feel inadequate because of lack of knowledge or experience; often providing them with information about anatomy, technique, or even interpersonal aspects of a sexual relationship is sufficient to decrease their anxiety. Recommending reading material on the subject may be helpful to certain clients. Often it is enough for the health professional comfortably to open the topic of sexuality for discussion; conveying to the client an accepting attitude is an anxiety-decreasing intervention in itself.

It is frequently helpful to involve the partner in treatment. If one member of a couple is experiencing anxiety that affects the sexual relationship, the partner will also be affected. Helping the partner to understand the source of the anxiety and encouraging participation in discussion of the situation usually increase the couple's comfort with each other and decrease the anxiety about their sexuality. If the client is reacting with anxiety only to his sexual partner, it is appropriate to proceed with sexual therapy.

Anxiety Disorders: Phobic Disorders and Anxiety States

At an unconscious level, the anxiety disorders may be caused by conflicts over unacceptable or frightening sexual impulses. Woods notes that the symptoms may be a "defensive attempt to ward off unacceptable sexual impulses" (Woods, 1981, p 206). Specific sexual problems or complaints, however, may not be part of the client's symptomatology.

In this group of disorders anxiety is either the predominant disturbance (as in panic disorder or generalized anxiety disorder), or anxiety is experienced if the individual attempts to master the symptoms (as in phobic disorder or obsessive-compulsive disorder). Under the DSM-III-R classification of anxiety disorders, phobic disorders and anxiety states (panic disorder, generalized anxiety disorder, obsessive-compulsive disorder, and post-traumatic stress disorder) are included.

PHOBIC DISORDERS

Individuals with phobic disorders exhibit an irrational fear of a specific object, situation, or activity that they therefore attempt to avoid. The individual recognizes that the fear is excessive or unreasonable but nevertheless experiences extreme anxiety when exposed to the object, situation, or activity.

The majority of such clients function sexually without difficulty. Exceptions are those clients who are phobic about some aspect of sexual activity.

ANXIETY STATES: PANIC DISORDER, GENERALIZED ANXIETY DISORDER, OBSESSIVE-COMPULSIVE DISORDER, POST-TRAUMATIC STRESS DISORDER

Panic disorder clients experience recurrent panic anxiety attacks that occur at times unpredictably, although they may occur in certain predictable situations, such as driving a car. The condition occurs more commonly in women. In some cases the panic could be related to a sexual situation.

Generalized anxiety disorder features an anxious mood with associated symptoms occurring for at least 1 month. Some clients may experience erectile dysfunction and/or a lack of warmth in their sexual relationships.

Individuals with obsessive-compulsive disorder are plagued by obsessive thoughts and/or compulsive rituals, which may or may not be specifically related to areas of sexual behavior or thought. Acute anxiety is experienced if the compulsive ritual is not carried out. Obsessive individuals confuse sexuality and aggression, which results in their strong need to be in control of themselves and others. This fear of loss of control affects their sexual experience, since part of sexual pleasure and orgasm involves "giving oneself up to sensation and allowing oneself to relinquish control" (Woods, 1981, p 207). Sexual problems in obsessive-compulsive individuals include mechanization of sex, erectile dysfunction, and/or premature ejaculation in males, retarded orgasm, compulsive genital acts, and upsetting fantasies of carrying out some "unacceptable" sexual behavior.

Post-traumatic stress disorder involves development of symptoms following a psychologically distressing event outside the range of usual human experience, for example, serious threat to one's life, serious threat or harm to a close friend or relative, sudden destruction of one's home or community, and seeing someone seriously injured or killed. Characteristic symptoms include re-experiencing the traumatic event, numbing of responsiveness to the external world, and increased arousal. "Psychic numbing" may result in the person feeling detached or estranged from other people. The ability to feel emotions, especially those associated with intimacy, tenderness, and sexuality, is markedly decreased.

INTERVENTION

In clients with anxiety disorders and accompanying sexual difficulties, it is advisable to treat the anxiety disorder rather than the sexual dysfunction. Kolodny, Masters, and Johnson note that sexual therapy is unlikely to cure the sexual difficulties related to these disorders.

The partner should be included in the treatment plan, and the health professional should provide information about the illness. It is reassuring to clients to know that although uncomfortable, such disorders do not lead to severe mental illness. Reid (1983) suggests telling the client that the illness has predictable patterns and is thus potentially understandable and also that it is separate from the psychotic illnesses; the patient will not "go crazy." Family or marital therapy may be indicated if the relationship is contributing to the anxiety disorder.

Medications can be a useful adjunct to other forms of therapy. Antianxiety medications can be used to treat the anxiety symptoms, although they do not block the occurrence of panic attacks. Tricyclic antidepressants, in doses lower than those used for treating depression, are sometimes helpful, especially for panic disorder and agoraphobia with panic attacks. To prevent the need for extensive use of medication in the more chronic generalized anxiety disorder, the formation of a therapeutic relationship usually provides reassurance. Simply having medications available symbolically allows the client to "carry the therapist" (or other supportive health professional) (Reid, 1983).

Behavioral therapy is the recommended treatment for most phobias. Gradual exposure to the anxiety-producing object or situation, a form of systematic desensitization used in fantasy and in real life, is frequently used. Flooding or implosion, another behavioral technique that involves rapid exposure to phobic material and causing high levels of anxiety initially, is also used with phobic clients.

Other methods often successful in counteracting anxiety include relaxation techniques, biofeedback, or regular transcendental meditation. Supportive psychotherapy is a useful accompaniment to helping the client give up the symptom via any of the methods discussed. This support can be provided by any health professional working in a therapeutic relationship with the client. Reassurance is helpful when it is specific, not vague, for example:

I understand that you feel that your heart might be damaged or break down when it beats so fast. Fortunately, the EKG shows that your heart is strong enough to endure that. I think it is useful to talk about when you have these palpitations though, because we may be able to identify what is contributing to your anxiety response. (Leigh, 1983, p 165)

Some clients who may not respond to the briefer symptomatic treatments, or whose symptom removal results in other problems, may need more indepth psychodynamically oriented psychotherapy. Hospitalization may be considered for severe anxiety states and for disabling obsessive-compulsive behavior, either of which may be severely restricting the client's ability to function in daily life.

Somatoform Disorders: Somatization Disorder (Hysteria) and Conversion Disorders

This classification includes those clients with physical symptoms suggesting a physical disorder for which there are no demonstrable organic findings or known physiological mechanisms *and* for which there is strong evidence that the symptoms are linked to psychological factors. It is important to note that the symptom formation is not under voluntary control.

SOMATIZATION DISORDER

Clients with this disorder (formerly referred to as hysteria) have had recurrent and multiple somatic complaints of several years' duration for which medical attention has been sought but which are apparently not due to any physical disorder. Common complaints involve psychosexual symptoms (e.g., sexual indifference, lack of sexual pleasure, or dyspareunia) or female reproductive symptoms (e.g., painful menstruation). Such clients often appear seductive, which masks their underlying passive-dependent need for help, protection, and nurturance (APA, 1987).

Intervention

Such clients can be trying to the health professional on an ongoing basis, as they are often very demanding, yet no cause can be found for their symptoms. However, they are very needy individuals; understanding the dynamics underlying their disorder helps the health professional to provide a consistent relationship as well as support, empathy, and understanding. The health professional must be well informed about the client's illness and should relate to the client as a medically ill individual. Once a trusting relationship is established, it is useful to encourage the client to express feelings toward the somatic symptoms and to explore with the client the possibility that the feelings could be related to the physical symptom. It is extremely important not to be confrontational when using this approach, as such clients express their feelings in terms of physical symptoms and are least accepting of a psychological approach. Group therapy is helpful because it provides support as well as tolerable confrontations from a peer group.

It is important to maintain continued contact with the client, even at times when the symptoms decrease. Consistent brief visits decrease the need for escalation of symptoms to secure attention. Discontinuation of appointments can be perceived by the client as rejection.

CONVERSION DISORDER (HYSTERICAL NEUROSIS, CONVERSION TYPE)

Clients with this disorder show a loss of or alteration in physical functioning that suggests a physical disorder but actually is apparently an expression of a psychological conflict or need. Sex-related symptoms are frequently reported. Purtell, Robins, and Cohen (1951) reported that 98 per cent of their 50 clients with conversion disorder had sexual problems (sexual indifference, no sexual pleasure, or dyspareunia) compared with 52 per cent of a control group. In conversion disorder the symptom is often a defense against unacceptable sexual or aggressive impulses (e.g., hysterical seizures can be a response to unacceptable sexual excitement). If the disorder is limited to a disturbance in sexual functioning, it is classified as a sexual dysfunction in the DSM-III-R. For many of the sexual dysfunctions, it is difficult to determine whether the symptom represents a physiological reaction to anxiety or a direct expression of a psychological conflict or need (conversion symptom).

Intervention

Involvement of the partner and/or important family members in the client's care can improve communication, which may decrease the need for future conversion symptoms; that is, if clients can express their feelings directly, they would not need to express them via bodily symptoms. Changing this behavior, however, should not be expected to occur rapidly; it takes time, patience, and persistence for all concerned, health professionals and family members as well as the client, in order to improve the communication patterns.

Behavior therapy or hypnosis can often successfully remove the symptoms, although this may result in only temporary improvement. Reid (1983) suggests that these techniques should be used in a broader context than "mere symptom alleviation": the health professional should include techniques that increase the probability of continued improvement. Sexual therapy is unlikely to provide a cure for sexual problems that are conversion symptoms, since it does not address the underlying conflict. Long-term intensive psychotherapy may be indicated.

OTHER EMOTIONAL ILLNESSES: SCHIZOPHRENIA, ORGANIC MENTAL SYNDROMES AND DISORDERS, AND ANOREXIA NERVOSA

Schizophrenia

Schizophrenia is a mental illness that affects thinking, mood, and behavior. The relationship between schizophrenia and sexual problems is complex. Kaplan (1974) notes that sexual dysfunctions are not symptoms of schizophrenia per se and that the two conditions are independent and dissociable. There is a wide range of clinical manifestations of schizophrenia, depending on the severity of the illness, its acuteness or chronicity, whether it develops early or late in life, and the extent of the disruption in overall social functioning. If schizophrenia occurs early, such as in childhood or adolescence, the development of normal sexual relationships is likely to be seriously impaired. Sexual

disturbances in schizophrenia may result either from distorted interpersonal relationships or as a direct consequence of the acute psychosis. The quality of a schizophrenic's relationships often deteriorates, from withdrawal or sometimes from participating sexually with a partner in a detached manner. An essential characteristic of schizophrenia is a confused preoccupation with one's own body, its boundaries, and therefore one's relationship to others. It is thought that the sexual behavior of schizophrenics results from their anhedonia (inability to experience pleasure) and their distorted body awareness (Woods, 1981).

Most commonly seen in schizophrenia is a great preoccupation with sex—either normal or reduced frequency of sexual activity. The sexual preoccupation includes many sexual delusions, for example, delusions of being a member of the opposite sex, being homosexual, being pregnant, having lovers, delusions about one's sex organs (e.g., that one's vagina is filled with concrete, that one's penis is becoming smaller), or delusional fears about sex organs of the opposite sex (e.g., "dentate vagina"—the idea that a woman's vagina has teeth in it) (Goldberg, 1975).

Hypersexuality can occur during an acute schizophrenic psychosis. There are differing reports on sexuality in the early stages of the illness: Some report increased sexual desire and increased masturbation, while others have found decreased sexual drive. One study of male outpatients with schizophrenia found sexual dysfunctions reported by 63 per cent of the patients; 31 per cent reported difficulty achieving or maintaining erections (Lukoff et al, 1986). Skopec, Rosenberg, and Tucker (1976) note that in acute schizophrenia, masturbation may be used to control painful anxiety instead of for pleasure. Chronic schizophrenics are often socially withdrawn and isolated, so that there is almost no sexual activity except for solitary masturbation.

Kaplan emphasizes that actual sexual dysfunction, such as erectile dysfunction or premature ejaculation, in schizophrenic clients may either be intimately associated with their distortions and defenses or may be "relatively independent of the schizophrenic process" (Kaplan, 1974, p 490). This means that it is imperative that the health professional evaluating sexual dysfunctions in such clients be aware that the two problems can be either related or independent and evaluate them accordingly.

INTERVENTION

Treatment of acute schizophrenia with antipsychotic medications may reverse the sexual problems; however, it is important to be aware that such medications can cause other sexual problems. (See the section on "Medications Used To Treat Mental Illnesses: Effects on Sexuality.")

The client's significant other should be included in the treatment plan. This allows for additional support for the client as the problem is being addressed by any of several treatment modalities. Couple therapy may be indicated if problems within the relationship itself are contributing to the sexual problem. It is important to provide a nonjudgmental relationship in which clients can discuss their concerns and/or fears regarding sexuality as well as their current interpersonal relationships. The client may need education about sexuality, developmental issues, interpersonal relationships and what a partner might need or want, and sexual techniques. At times it may be appropriate to provide such education to the client and partner together. A long-term supportive relationship is helpful in maintaining the functioning of schizophrenic clients in the community.

Group therapy may help increase the client's degree of comfort with other individuals of both sexes and may provide support, help develop social skills, and help begin or sustain relationships.

Schizophrenic patients can benefit from a sex education program, such as that described in a study on male schizophrenic outpatients (Lukoff et al, 1986). The program was introduced because of patients' problems of sexual dysfunction and of inappropriate sexual behavior. Patients were invited to participate in an 8-session series of group sex education sessions, which included role playing and discussions. Patients participated in exercises and brought up relevant questions for discussion. The authors recommend that clients recuperating from a recent decompensation not be included in such a group until their clinical condition stabilizes. Topics covered included sexual identity and self-esteem, viewing sexual partners as persons, male and female reproductive anatomy, strengths as a partner, dating behavior, pleasure instead of performance as

the focus in sex, birth control and prevention of sexually transmitted diseases, open communication with sexual partners, and human sexual response and sexual dysfunction. Sex education needs to be included in comprehensive rehabilitation programs for schizophrenic patients to prevent deterioration of sexual functioning. The group program described above benefited the participants. No exacerbations or relapses occurred among the participants during the program.

Sexual therapy is possible during the stable phase of the schizophrenic illness, although as Kaplan (1974) states, it is contraindicated in the acute (psychotic) stage of the illness as well as in the recovery phase. It is important to ascertain what role the sexual symptom is playing in the schizophrenic person's "total psychic structure." Sexual therapy may be a real hazard to the schizophrenic's compensation; the same applies when the spouse of the client with sexual problems is schizophrenic. The schizophrenia may be exacerbated if the sexual symptom is removed or if sexual therapy results in a rapid change in the relationship with the partner. Kaplan points out that often a schizophrenic employs the defense of emotional detachment; closeness may be terrifying, and the sexual symptom may offer protection. Thus, the closeness and openness that are an integral part of sexual therapy may be extremely threatening to the defensively isolated schizophrenic client and in fact could cause exacerbation of an acute psychosis.

Organic Mental Syndromes and Disorders

In DSM-III-R, a distinction is made between organic mental syndromes and organic mental disorders. Organic mental syndrome has no reference to etiology, whereas organic mental disorder designates particular organic brain syndromes in which the etiology is known or presumed. The disorder may result from primary disease of the brain, from a systemic illness that secondarily affects the brain, or from a psychoactive substance or toxic agent. One of the most common organic mental syndromes and disorders is dementia. Dementias involve global cognitive deficits occurring in a normal state of consciousness. These may result from neurological disease (examples are Alzheimer's disease, Pick's disease, Huntington's chorea, and multi-infarct dementia) or from substances such as alcohol, barbiturates or sedatives/hypnotics, opioids, cocaine, amphetamines, or hallucinogens. The impairment of brain function may be transient or permanent, depending on the cause. Changes in cognitive function resulting from this impairment include losses of attention, memory, orientation, and logical thought.

Associated with these organic mental syndromes or disorders are some specific features related to sexuality. These include decreased control over sexual impulses, which may accompany cognitive impairment as well as impaired social judgment. The combination of impaired social judgment and decreased sexual impulse control often results in inappropriate sexual behavior, including inappropriate sexual advances or exhibitionistic acts. However, Mace and Rabins (1981) note that inappropriate sexual behaviors in persons with dementia are uncommon. They state that sometimes accidental self-exposure, aimless masturbation, or fidgeting with clothing do occur. Much of such behavior that at first seems sexual is really a result of disorientation and confusion.

INTERVENTION

Many authors have emphasized the biopsychosocial approach to clients with organic mental syndromes and disorders, which includes treatment aimed at removing the cause, symptomatic treatment if the cause cannot be removed or is unknown, and client management and support of the client's family.

The only specific treatment for an organic mental disorder is proper correction of the underlying cause. Therefore, it is crucial that every effort be made to identify the etiology of the disorder and reverse the problem by medical or surgical intervention. Often, such clients may be misdiagnosed and may be taking antianxiety medications or sedatives, which do not help; in fact such medications often increase the client's agitation because they further depress the client's sensorium (Leigh, 1983).

Client management interventions depend on the severity of the disorder, whether the setting is home or institution, and the degree of involvement of family members. The client needs reassurance that the health professional understands what is happening and is

handling the treatment aspects. Complicated explanations should be avoided, since they only increase the client's confusion. It is important to maintain a stable and familiar environment; if the client must be hospitalized, the use of familiar objects from home, such as photographs, and frequent family visits make a strange environment more familiar and comforting. Use of orienting aids, such as television viewing and a calendar, will help the client with dementia. Sensory input should be kept at a low level, such as a quiet single-bed room with soft lighting. The number of health personnel should be limited in order to increase the client's familiarity with them. Frequent or constant supervision and protection from accidents should be provided. Physical restraints should only be used when absolutely necessary and then only for brief periods; control of agitation is better managed by appropriate use of medication and personal contact and supervision by a family member or familiar staff person.

Staff and family member reactions to clients' inappropriate sexual behaviors should be calm and matter-of-fact. Often, simply moving the client to a more private location, such as his bedroom or bathroom, or assisting him to get dressed is the most helpful intervention. Often, buying clothes that the client cannot easily remove (trousers without zippers, blouses that button in back) is helpful. Sometimes distracting the client from socially unacceptable behaviors is successful, such as giving him something else to do. Inappropriate sexual advances to staff or others can be controlled by setting firm limits in a nonpunitive manner. Clients who rub their genitals may be doing this not for sexual pleasure but to communicate distress from a painful urinary tract or vaginal infection. When such behavior occurs as a sudden change, it is important to consider the possibility of such an infection and run the appropriate tests. Because these clients are vulnerable to infection, their status should be monitored every 6 months.

Involvement with and support of the client's family has recently been increasingly emphasized. An essential intervention is explanation to the family of the cause of the client's behavior, especially if the behavior is socially inappropriate. If the client will be at home, keeping the setting as familiar as possible will help decrease the client's disorientation. If the client's deterioration is so severe that his behavior becomes dangerous to himself or others, such as wandering away from home or turning the stove on, the family needs support for placing the client in an institution. Family members often feel guilt about making such a decision; it often helps to let them know that such placement is for the client's as well as the family's well-being.

The partner of a client with an organic mental syndrome or disorder often needs support, counseling, and information regarding the couple's sexual relationship. Introduce sexual questions as part of the medical history: "I'd like to know how you communicate with each other, how well you get along, and about your sleeping and sexual patterns" ("Alzheimer's Disease," 1984, p 8). It is often useful to interview the couple together as well as the partner alone, in case there are issues or concerns that need to be discussed privately. Sometimes a client may feel unloved and angry because the partner does not want to have frequent sexual relations. If partners are exhausted from the demands of care, it is helpful to discuss this with the couple and explain that the love is still there but cannot be expressed sexually as frequently. The partner of a client who cannot respond as a lover or companion may choose to become intimately involved in another relationship and needs to be supported in this, although the client need never be involved in this arrangement. Partners may need help in examining sexual options and support for their choices—masturbation, celibacy, or another relationship.

Teusink and Mahler (1984) discuss ways of helping families cope with the onset and progression of an organic mental disorder. They note that in a sense clients with such disorders are intellectually dying, so reactions of families may be similar to those coping with dying family members. Thus, families may go through a series of responses, consisting of initial denial, then overinvolvement with the client in an effort to compensate for their losses, followed by anger, guilt, and finally acceptance. Families must be helped to deal with unrealistic expectations regarding the current and future capacity of the client to function. In order to make the best decisions for their family member, they need education about the disorder and the progression of the illness and about available resources; they may also need to be advised to seek legal advice or to take legal responsibility for the client in order to be able to continue to make the best decisions for the client, who may not be capable of doing so. There are support groups available in many communities for families of Alzheimer's disease clients, which many family members find extremely helpful. Adjustment to reversal in roles is often difficult for a family member; often family members must become a "parent" to their own parents and make decisions for them. The health professional should help the family members recognize the occurrence of role reversal; help them express their feelings about it; discuss the normalcy of feeling fear, anger, and disappointment; and help them accept this change in their concepts of themselves and the client. Counseling is often recommended to help family members reduce stress and resolve conflicts within the family, which often surface as a family member is ill.

Anorexia Nervosa

Anorexia nervosa is an eating disorder characterized by an intense fear of becoming obese, significant weight loss (at least 25 per cent of the original body weight), disturbed body image, and amenorrhea (in females). This disorder most frequently occurs in adolescent females and is correlated with disturbances in sexual feeling and activity. Individuals with this disorder are believed to be retreating from issues of independence and perhaps sexuality; their preoccupation with control of their bodily impulses and appetites is reflected in their food-related behavior. Sexual behavior in individuals with anorexia nervosa is frequently constrained. Low levels of desire are reported in both men and women. Volunteer subjects in one study described by Garfinkel and Garner (1982) reported loss of sexual interest, avoidance of the opposite sex, and greatly reduced masturbation, sexual fantasies, and dreams. A lack of orgasmic response has also been noted in such patients.

A frequent accompaniment to anorexia is delayed psychosexual development. Female adolescents with anorexia nervosa often look like "little girls"; as Neuman and Halvorson (1983, p 14) note, "They are totally out of touch with the sexual part of their being." Developmental tasks other than sexuality are avoided by remaining a child: issues of intimacy and issues of responsibility that accompany the adult role.

Anorexia nervosa is not a sexual disorder

per se, and the sexual behavioral manifestations are only part of the disturbance. Therefore, it is important to treat the total illness and not simply focus on one aspect, such as a sexual dysfunction.

INTERVENTION

A variety of treatment modalities have been used with anorexia nervosa: nutritional, pharmacological, and various psychotherapeutic approaches. The recommended approach is a long-term combined medical and psychiatric treatment. Acute inpatient treatment may be needed for severe metabolic disturbances, suicidal depression, psychosis, or infection, although these are not common occurrences. Research done to date makes comparison of treatment methods difficult.

The initial goal of treatment is necessarily restoration of adequate nutrition. Choice of intervention depends on the severity of the illness. It is important to include the client in decision-making as much as possible. If one begins treatment before the client's weight loss is extreme, education is an important early intervention: explanation of nutritional needs of the body and the effects of starvation, explanation of the purposes the illness can serve and discussion of common fears and anxieties associated with it, and contracting for stabilization of weight (including setting a limit below which hospitalization will occur).

Establishing a relationship of trust and partnership is important in working with anorectics. It is helpful to reassure the client that you do not want to see fatness develop and that you will be careful not to encourage excessive or rapid weight gain.

In addition to attention to nutritional issues, attention should also be focused on individual emotional and family issues. Psychotherapeutic modalities used with anorexic clients include specialized groups for weight control, behavior modification, individual psychotherapy, and family therapy. The major goal of individual psychotherapy is to help the client modify dysfunctional eating behavior and become more effective in managing personal life situations. Psychotherapeutic issues often include looking at the client's personal experience and that of parents, autonomy and self-control, recognition and acceptance of impulses (including sexual ones), differentiation between internal physical sensations and emotional states, and attitudes about closeness/dependence/independence. In a setting that promotes expression of thoughts and feelings, the client can be encouraged to develop self-initiated behaviors that lead to a sense of autonomy. If the client experiences a greater sense of control, personal and environmental, the struggle for control of the body through dieting might become less important. Teaching assertiveness skills—how to express thoughts and feelings in a direct manner—is another important component of individual work with anorectic clients. Behavior modification therapy manipulates the client's eating behavior and therefore may heighten the client's sense of ineffectiveness and lack of control, which Drossman (1983) notes is a disadvantage of this therapeutic approach. He notes that a combination of behavior modification and long-term psychotherapy may avoid this problem.

Family therapy is especially important for those clients living with their family of origin. A major aim of therapy with anorectic clients is to facilitate separation from the family and the development of autonomy. The anorectic needs help in establishing an identity as an individual. Parents often need help in allowing and encouraging their child to become independent, in permitting the child to have thoughts and feelings independent from theirs. Some family theorists have described characteristic interactional patterns typical of families of anorectics: overprotectiveness, rigidity, enmeshment, and conflict avoidance. Systems theorists assume that the anorexic symptoms fulfill some role in maintaining the family equilibrium. Therefore, the goal of family therapy would be to disrupt and alter the dysfunctional patterns of communication so that the client could "let go" of symptoms. The younger the client, the more likely it is that family therapy will be helpful.

Group therapy is also a useful treatment approach for anorexia nervosa clients. In a group composed of eating-disordered clients, sharing the common experience of these disorders helps members provide support, understanding, and encouragement to each other. Another useful group approach is use of self-help groups, such as those modeled after Overeaters Anonymous, which can be used as an adjunct to other treatment modalities.

GENDER IDENTITY DISORDER: TRANSSEXUALISM

The essential feature of gender identity disorders is an incongruence between anatomic sex and gender identity, that is, the sense of knowing to which sex one belongs (e.g., "I am a female"). Disturbance in gender identity is rare. The two subcategories of this disorder are transsexualism and gender identity disorder of childhood (not discussed here).

Clients with transsexualism experience a persistent sense of discomfort and inappropriateness about their anatomic sex and a persistent wish to be rid of their genitals and to live as a member of the other sex. Sometimes they engage in cross-dressing; often their behavior and mannerisms are also those of the other sex. Both male and female transsexuals are likely to seek medical help to alter their bodies to be consistent with their psychological gender; that is, they seek anatomical change in the form of hormone effects or surgery.

Intervention

There are several gender identity clinics in the United States that provide an interdisciplinary approach to such clients by such health professionals as psychologists, psychiatrists, endocrinologists, and surgeons. Transsexual clients often seek unrealistic and immediate solutions and may move from one clinician to another if they fail to obtain what they demand. It is important to realize that sex-reassignment surgery does not automatically solve all the problems of transsexual clients. It is useful to point out to such clients that most of the problems of sex reassignment—being accepted as a member of that sex, working and living from day to day as that sex—will not be solved by surgery. Most sex-reassignment clinics do require that the client live as a member of the other sex for a reasonable period of time—sometimes as much as 12 to 18 months—before surgery is performed. Working with such a client requires a long-term relationship, during which a sense of trust can develop and the client can continue to try out new behaviors, and the client and health professional can determine whether a more permanent sex change is likely to be helpful.

SEXUAL DISORDERS

The diagnostic class sexual disorders includes disorders of sexual functioning in which psychological factors are assumed to be of major etiological significance. The category discussed below is sexual deviations (paraphilias).

Sexual Deviations (Paraphilias)

Clients with a paraphilia find that unusual or bizarre imagery or acts are necessary for sexual excitement. These clients often have impairment in the capacity for reciprocal affectionate sexual activity, and sexual dysfunctions are common. Social and sexual relationships may suffer if others, such as a spouse, become aware of the unusual sexual behavior. In addition, if the individual engages in sexual activity with a partner who refuses to cooperate in the unusual behavior, such as fetishistic or sadistic behavior, sexual excitement may be inhibited, and the relationship may suffer.

Fetishism. The essential feature in fetishism is the use of nonliving objects (fetishes) as a preferred or exclusive method of achieving sexual excitement. Often the fetishes tend to be articles of clothing, often associated with someone with whom the individual was intimately involved during childhood, such as a caretaker. Usually, the disorder begins by adolescence.

Transvestic Fetishism. This disorder includes recurrent and persistent cross-dressing by a heterosexual male that is for the purpose of sexual excitement, at least during the initial phase of the disorder. The individual with transvestic fetishism considers himself to be basically male and predominantly heterosexual. The client experiences intense frustration when the cross-dressing is interfered with.

Pedophilia. This refers to the act or fantasy of engaging in sexual activity with prepubertal children as a preferred or exclusive method of achieving sexual excitement. This disorder most frequently begins in adolescence. Most incidents are initiated by individuals who are in the intimate interpersonal environment of the child.

Exhibitionism. The essential feature is repetitive acts of exposing the genitals to an unsuspecting stranger for the purpose of achieving sexual excitement, with no attempt at further sexual activity with the stranger. The wish to surprise or shock the observer is often conscious. The condition apparently occurs only in males.

Voyeurism. This involves repetitive looking at unsuspecting people, usually strangers who are naked, in the act of disrobing, or engaging in sexual activity, as the preferred or exclusive method of achieving sexual excitement. No sexual activity with the person being observed is sought.

Sexual Masochism. Sexual masochism refers to a preferred mode of producing sexual excitement that requires the individual's own suffering, that is, being humiliated, bound, beaten, or otherwise made to suffer, *or* that requires the individual's intentional participation in an activity in which physical harm or threat to life occurs.

Sexual Sadism. This involves the infliction of physical or psychological suffering on another person in order to achieve sexual excitement. This can involve a nonconsenting partner on whom an individual has repeatedly and intentionally inflicted suffering in order to achieve sexual excitement, or it can involve a consenting partner on whom one has inflicted bodily injury (extensive, permanent, or possibly mortal) or on which one has inflicted humiliation with simulated or mildly injurious bodily suffering.

Other Paraphilias (Zoophilia, Necrophilia). These include sexual urges and arousal from other sources, for example animals (zoophilia) or corpses (necrophilia).

INTERVENTION

The most important aspect of treatment of clients with a paraphilia is a therapeutic orientation rather than a punitive one. Of note is the distinction among paraphilias that do not intrude on the wishes of others, those that do intrude on the wishes of others, and those that intrude on others and are also aggressive and potentially injurious. The client may be self-referred because of discomfort with sexual orientation, a family member may be uncomfortable or unhappy with the client's sexual orientation, or the client may be referred through the criminal justice system. If the client is sent for treatment by the court, or by a lawyer in order to avoid prosecution, the issues of motivation, coercion, and manipulation need to be considered.

Such clients may not be good candidates for psychotherapeutic treatment.

Long-term insight-oriented psychotherapy may be the treatment of choice for many clients with paraphilias. Behavior modification has also been used successfully with such clients. It is important to include the client's family (spouse or significant other) in the treatment, often in concurrent individual therapy or in couples therapy. Bancroft (1983) states that often a fetishistic or sadomasochistic pattern increases because of difficulties in the couple's sexual relationship. If the couple focuses in therapy on their basic sexual relationship and this improves, often the deviant preference will decrease.

For fetishism, transvestic fetishism, and zoophilia, important interventions are education about the condition, helping the client handle anxiety, and being accepting of the client and comfortable giving permission for the client's sexual orientation, which then helps decrease the client's degree of guilt. Of course zoophilia, like other paraphilias to be discussed, involves some exploitation or even cruelty in some instances, so the issues of sadism need to be explored.

Some of the paraphilias have criminal implications, since participating in zoophilia, pedophilia, exhibitionism, voyeurism, or certain degrees of sexual masochism or sadism is against the law. Frequently, such clients come to the attention of health professionals because of the client's attempt to avoid prosecution or as a means of reducing the severity of the legal punishment for criminal actions. Psychological treatment of these clients is only likely to be successful if it is desired by the client, not forced by someone else. A therapeutic relationship, voluntary on the part of the client, is necessary for such treatment to work. There are several problem areas that may need focus in the counseling: "problems in establishing satisfactory sexual relationships; problems in established relationships of a sexual or general kind; problems of lowered self-esteem; lack of assertiveness or lack of rewarding activities; inadequate sexual arousal to 'normal' sexual stimuli; problems of self-control and inappropriate sexual arousal to 'deviant' stimuli" (Bancroft, 1983, p 433). Bancroft notes that it is desirable to reinforce or help the client build new, more adaptive behaviors rather than simply eliminate undesirable ones. Social skills training, methods of self-assertion, modeling and rehearsal of new behaviors, and role playing of relevant social situations are all techniques that have been used successfully, either in groups or individually. Aversive conditioning is another approach that is sometimes used. Desire-lowering drugs can be used in conjunction with other counseling approaches; since these reduce the strength of the deviant urge, it may be more possible for the offender to learn more appropriate alternative behaviors. Desire-lowering drugs include cyproterone acetate, an antiandrogen, and medroxyprogesterone acetate (Depo-Provera, Provera), a progestin, which is being used experimentally in the United States as an antiandrogen for the treatment of sex offenders (Buffum, 1982). Three studies using cyproterone acetate noted no gynecomastia or other side effects (Bancroft et al, 1974; Cooper et al, 1972; Laschet et al, 1967). A study using medroxyprogesterone acetate lists as major side effects weight gain and mild lethargy, cold sweats, hyperglycemia, hypogonadism, and leg cramps (Berlin and Meinecke, 1981). One hopes that prescribing medication does not decrease the client's sense of responsibility for his own behavior, often a problem when prescribing a pharmacological treatment.

In looking at treatment interventions for pedophilia, the basic principles of psychotherapeutic treatment are similar to those for the other paraphilias "except for not giving the patient permission to continue the symptoms" (Reid, 1983, p 162). Insight-oriented psychotherapies are not widely used for this disorder because they are not effective in changing the behavior. Behavioral conditioning is the most widely used treatment, specifically aversive conditioning such as electric shock and induction of vomiting. Milder techniques have been developed, such as the client snapping a rubber band against his skin; this is one type of self-management program, recently more popular than the more passive types of aversion therapy.

There are no data that demonstrate successful treatment of exhibitionism and voyeurism through verbal psychotherapy. Group psychotherapy and participation of the spouse or significant other has been used by many. Involvement of the spouse or significant other is likely to provide more support and understanding for the client as he is working on changing his behavior. Blair and Lanyon (1981) review outcome studies of behavioral treatment of exhibitionism, including 12 controlled studies. Treatment methods used were aversive conditioning, assisted covert sensitization (ACS), and covert sensitization. Subjects receiving ACS (and 40 per cent also receiving another treatment, such as booster sessions at 3-, 6-, and 12-month intervals) showed 86 per cent improvement to the extent of eliminating all overt exhibitionist behaviors at follow-up 1 to 9 years later. The studies on covert sensitization, the most popular treatment, had a reported success rate of almost 100 per cent.

Clients who appear for treatment for sexual masochism may be helped with assertiveness training to increase their self-image and self-worth. The masochism may also be masking a depression, in which case psychotherapeutic or pharmacological treatment for depression is in order. Some clients may be candidates for more intensive insight-oriented psychotherapy to resolve their underlying conflicts and to develop less destructive defense mechanisms.

Sexual sadism may be inflicted on consenting or nonconsenting others, which may influence how such clients come to the attention of a health professional. Social and legal issues are important when partners are nonconsenting. Even if partners are "consenting," if they receive severe injury, legal issues may arise, and control of the sadistic behavior is especially important. A behavioral technique called fading, described by Marks (1981), has been used. It is a method of decreasing deviant sexual arousal: clients are gradually shifted toward more conventional sexual stimuli during periods of sexual arousal by use of fantasy, visual techniques, or conditioning orgasm.

MEDICATIONS USED TO TREAT MENTAL ILLNESS: EFFECTS ON SEXUALITY

Sexual response is a complex interaction between the physiological and psychological aspects of sexuality. A drug that modifies a person's physiology may also affect perception of sexual activity, which in turn may affect performance. This section will discuss medications used to treat mental illness that have direct physiological effects on sexuality. Most such drug-induced changes in sexuality are a result of chemical alterations of nerves regulating sexual response (Bianchine and Lubbers, 1983). It is of note that all psychotropic drugs affect sexuality indirectly in a positive way, owing to their calming effect; they also affect sexuality directly in a dose-related way that may impede either the arousal or orgasmic phase of the sexual response by autonomic effects.

Studies and reports concerning drug-induced effects on sexual function are rare in the literature. Buffum and associates (1981) note that reports often do not specify the gender or age of the patients, other medications being taken, how the data were obtained (interview, questionnaire, or patient volunteering the information), any history of sexual problems before the patient began taking the drug, or at what dosage the dysfunction occurs. This makes it difficult, if not impossible, to evaluate any results reported.

The categories of medications discussed here include the antipsychotics (major tranquilizers), antianxiety medications and sedatives/hypnotics, and the antidepressants, including lithium carbonate. A summary of the effects of these medications is included in Table 29–1.

Antipsychotic Drugs (Major Tranquilizers)

Since the pharmacological action of these drugs is to block dopamine in the central nervous system, sexual desire may be adversely affected and the sex-related drives inhibited owing to the reduced intensity of perceived stimuli. Large doses may also reduce such drives because of the associated drowsiness and slowed reactions in the client. Buffum and associates (1981) state that the antiadrenergic action of most major tranquilizers can interfere with innervation of the internal genital organs, which can cause ejaculatory problems in males. Some erectile problems may be caused by the vasodilating action of the drugs, which shunts blood away from the genitals; vaginal lubrication can be decreased (Sarrel and Sarrel, 1983). Endocrine effects reported in both men and women include galactorrhea and gynecomastia. Women can experience amenorrhea or menstrual cycle alteration with long-term high-dose treatment.

The sexual effects of the antipsychotic drugs do tend to be dose related and generally disappear as the dosage is reduced. It is also of note that there has been very little

study or reporting on the problem of sexual dysfunction in women secondary to antipsychotic drug therapy. Also, no studies have specifically addressed how sexual drive is affected by such drugs. Mitchell and Popkin state that changes in desire "could conceivably be more of a problem with the newer neuroleptics that possess more potent dopamine-blocking properties" (Mitchell and Popkin, 1982, p 635).

The most common sexual effects of the phenothiazines are erectile (35 to 54 per cent) and ejaculatory (30 to 57 per cent) disturbances in males (Mitchell and Popkin, 1982). Total inhibition of ejaculation is the most frequent ejaculatory dysfunction with thioridazine, although delayed ejaculation is also reported. Erectile dysfunction occurs usually at doses equivalent to greater than 400 mg of chlorpromazine per day; there are no reports of chlorpromazine affecting ejaculation (Segraves, 1977). Tennent, Bancroft, and Cass (1974) in a well-designed double-blind study of 15 patients taking chlorpromazine found no effect on erectile capacity; however, the dosage per day was low—125 mg.

Priapism, a prolonged painful erection of the penis, is an infrequent but serious possible side effect of antipsychotic drugs, especially thioridazine and chlorpromazine.

The most frequently reported sexual effects of the butyrophenones (e.g., haloperidol) include decreased desire, galactorrhea, and gynecomastia. In addition, 10 to 20 per cent of males report erectile dysfunction, while others report decreased or no ejaculation. Some females report menstrual irregularities.

Although the antipsychotic drugs do have certain pharmacological characteristics that affect sexuality, there is the possibility that certain schizophrenic clients may function better sexually while taking such medications, possibly because of alleviation of psychotic anxiety, thought disorganization, fear of physical intimacy, and other symptoms that could interfere with their sexual functioning (Nestoros, Lehmann, and Ban, 1980).

Sedative/Hypnotics and Antianxiety Drugs (Minor Tranquilizers)

These drugs are central nervous system depressants. Low doses may decrease a client's

TABLE 29–1. Medications Used to Treat Mental Illnesses: Effects on Sexuality

Medication	Libido	Orgasm	Erectile Capacity (M) (Erectile Dysfunction)	Ejaculation (M)	Vaginal Lubrication (F)	Others
Aspect of Sexual Dysfunction						
Antipsychotics (major tranquilizers) Phenothiazines	↓	↓	↓ ↓ (especially from thiorizadine)	↓ ↓ (from thiorizadine) ↓ (from others)	↓	Retrograde ejaculation Painful ejaculation Priapism Gynecomastia Menstrual irregularities
Butyrophenones	↓	ND	↓	↓	ND	Priapism Galactorrhea Gynecomastia Menstrual irregularities
Sedatives/hypnotics and antianxiety drugs (Minor tranquilizers) Benzodiazepines	↑ or ↓	↓	↓	↓	ND	
Buspirone	↑	↑	(see "other" column)	(see "other" column)	ND	Increased sexual interest, arousability, performance
Barbiturates	↓	↓ (males)	↓	ND	ND	
Antidepressants Tricyclics/tetracyclics	↑ or ↓	↓	↓	↓	ND	Testicular swelling (from desipramine) Painful ejaculation
Trazodone	↑ (F)	ND	ND	↓	ND	Priapism
MAOIs	↑ or ↓	↓ (especially from phenelzine)	↓ ↓ (especially from phenelzine)	↓ ↓	ND	Priapism
Lithium carbonate	↓	ND	↓	ND	ND	

M = males; F = females; ↓ low incidence (below 20%); ↓ ↓ = higher incidence; ND = no data reported. Unless specified, effect was seen in both men and women.

inhibition temporarily and therefore enhance sexual behavior, while larger doses depress all behavior, including sexual. Since these drugs are used to lower anxiety and since decreased anxiety generally enhances sexual performance, it is difficult to assess the effect these drugs have on sexual function.

There is little data relevant to meprobamate, although it may alter desire or sexual functioning, since it appears to affect the limbic system.

The benzodiazepines may produce increased or decreased desire, owing to decreased anxiety and sedation, respectively. Rare instances of sexual dysfunctions have been reported with use of the benzodiazepines: erectile dysfunction (several cases; Lydiard et al, 1987), ejaculatory failure (two cases; Munjack and Crocker, 1986), inhibited orgasm in women (two cases; Sangal, 1985), and infrequently decreased desire.

Side effects of barbiturates seem to be similar to those of other depressants. Males have reported decreased desire, erectile dysfunction, or loss of orgasmic response. Many clients report no alteration in sexual function.

Antidepressants

Sexual side effects are not common with the tricyclic and tetracyclic antidepressants. There have been infrequent reports of erectile dysfunction and ejaculatory problems in males, and delayed orgasm in males and females, probably due to the anticholinergic effects of such drugs. The erectile insufficiency that occurs does not appear to be dose related. Several cases of anorgasmia have been reported, especially from clomipramine use (Monteiro et al, 1987). There have also been infrequent reports of testicular swelling associated with desipramine (Deicken and Carr, 1987; Thienhaus and Vogel, 1988). Frequently, when a client is taking an antidepressant medication, as the depression decreases, the client experiences increased sexual drive and improved sexual performance.

Trazodone is a newer antidepressant drug with antianxiety effects. Increased desire has been reported in three women receiving trazodone (Gartrell, 1986). Scher, Krieger, and Juergens (1983) report that in the first year of the availability of trazodone in the United States, 11 cases of priapism were reported, five of which required surgical procedures to correct. More than 60 cases have been reported since then (Patt, 1985; Raskin, 1985; Warner et al, 1987). The health professional should watch for an increase in the duration and frequency of a client's erections due to the possible priapism. Male patients should be informed of the potential occurrence of priapism and should be instructed to discontinue trazodone if unusual erectile problems develop.

The monoamine oxidase inhibitors (MAOIs) are another type of antidepressant often associated with decreased sexual activity. Kolodny, Masters, and Johnson (1979) reported erectile dysfunction in 10 to 15 per cent of men receiving moderate to high doses of an MAOI and delayed ejaculation or loss of ability to ejaculate in 25 to 30 per cent of men. Other authors have reported anorgasmia in both men and women taking an MAOI (Lesko, Stotland, and Segraves, 1982; Christenson, 1982; Moss, 1983; Pohl, 1983; Rabkin et al, 1985; Harrison et al, 1986; Jacobson, 1987; Nurnberg and Levine, 1987). One case of priapism during MAOI therapy has also been reported (Yeragani and Gershon, 1987).

Lithium Carbonate

Lithium carbonate is used in treating mania and hypomania as well as bipolar (manic-depressive) illness. The drug has not been studied systematically, and it is difficult to assess its specific effects on sexual behavior and function, since mania itself can produce both hypersexual and hyposexual behavior. There have been reports of erectile dysfunction or decreased or absent desire in males; some females have reported decreased sexual desire. Renshaw (1978, p 19) states that lithium "reduces the symptom of undifferentiated sexual urgency in manic-depressive males or females."

Assessment

Before the client begins taking medication, it is important to obtain a sexual history, especially information about any previous sexual problems. This provides a baseline against which to measure any subsequent change.

The first intervention of the health professional is to identify the problem—to assess whether the client taking psychotropic medication is indeed having any changes in sexual behavior. Since clients are often reluctant to volunteer information about sexual problems spontaneously, it is the responsibility of the health professional to ask the right questions as well as to provide appropriate information to the client. A comfortable permissive approach is basic to facilitating the expression of sexual concerns.

Intervention

If the prescribed medication is known to disturb sexual function, it is important to mention this possibility, although not in a way that suggests problems will probably occur. For example, let male clients know the particular medication causes some men to not have as firm erections as they have had. Of course, it is important to let them know that this occurs in only a small percentage of clients and that sexual behavior alterations are not medically serious and are easily reversible with decreased dosage or a change to another medication. This reassurance decreases anxiety if the problem should in fact occur, and it also makes it acceptable for the client to discuss sexual problems or changes at future visits.

It is important to counsel clients about drug-related side effects because such effects can decrease compliance with the medication regimen. The client's sexual partner should be included in such discussions, since the partner's response to a client's altered sexuality may significantly affect the client's acceptance or rejection of the drug treatment. Health professionals must be alert to subtle clues that clients are experiencing changes in their sexuality and that they may believe the medication is responsible. Client statements such as "I've been feeling different since I started taking those pills," "I'm not as good as I used to be," or "My husband (wife) thinks the medicine is making me worse" should lead the health professional to further exploration of the difficulties the client is experiencing. The health professional needs to get a description of what is different or what the client sees as the problem, when it started, and what the client thinks is causing the changes. It may be difficult to determine whether a client's complaint of sexual difficulties or changes is drug related, since other biopsychosocial factors may also cause the problem, including the client's set or expectations regarding his illness or the treatment as well as the setting or psychosocial environmental elements (family, job, interpersonal relationships, or other stressors). When sexual symptoms arise, it is important to inquire about other etiological possibilities, such as drug or alcohol use, marital difficulties, or physical illness. After a thorough assessment at each visit, the health professional may decide that a change in the medication dosage or a change to another medication is warranted. Even if the dosage is not reduced, there is sometimes a spontaneous reversal of sexual side effects after several weeks, especially with tricyclic and MAOI antidepressants, and patients may be willing to continue the medication to see if the side effects will abate.

If a change in the medication regimen is not advisable, the health professional needs to counsel the client and sexual partner about adjustments in their sexual relationship in order to help them cope with the sexual dysfunction. Patience and understanding on the part of the spouse or significant other may be crucial to maintenance of a satisfactory sexual relationship.

Priapism is one side effect that should be regarded as a medical emergency requiring immediate urological consultation to avoid permanent physiological impairment. Mitchell and Popkin (1982) state that needle aspiration of the corpora cavernosa or a surgical shunting procedure may be indicated. The health professional should be alert to the possibility of impending priapism if the client is experiencing an increase in the duration and frequency of erections.

An accepting, comfortable attitude on the part of the health professional, providing the client with information, and assessment of the client's sexual function at each visit should result in prevention of severe sexual side effects from psychotropic medications. Such interventions will also aid in adjusting the medication type and dosage to best treat the client's emotional illness, yet not cause additional problems by causing sexual impairment.

SUBSTANCE USE: ALCOHOL AND RECREATIONAL DRUGS

Alcohol

Ethyl alcohol (ethanol) is a central nervous system depressant that has both short- and long-term adverse effects on sexual functioning. Its effects are dosage dependent. Low levels depress the brain centers governing fear and inhibition, resulting in temporary increase in desire in men and women. Small to moderate levels may impair a male's ability to maintain erection; this almost invariably generates anxiety, which persists long after the alcohol has been excreted. This, in fact, is one way that secondary erectile dysfunction is frequently caused (Bancroft, 1983). A similar effect may occur in women who experience sexual difficulties with alcohol use and then observe themselves to monitor their responsiveness, which usually produces the opposite effect to that desired; their "performance anxieties create physical and emotional tension, loss of spontaneity, and impaired sexual sensations" (Kolodny, Masters, and Johnson, 1979, p 242).

Large single-dose quantities of alcohol decrease the extent of and maintenance of a male's erection. Long-term usage causes damage to the hypothalamus, resulting in decreased testosterone levels in males; the effects are often irreversible. Return to normal sexual functioning has been found in only about 50 per cent of cases after abstention from alcohol use for months or years (Lemere and Smith, 1973). There is a deterioration of functioning in both men and women, but especially in men, which is presumably a consequence of neurological damage. Sexual effects of long-term alcohol usage in males include decreased ability to attain or maintain an erection, delayed ejaculation, lowered sex drive, infertility, and feminization. If there are no morning erections and difficulty in masturbatory erections, the erectile dysfunction in recovered alcoholics is probably physical, that is, caused by neurological damage produced by prolonged heavy drinking (Lemere, 1976). Long-term usage in females results in decreased interest in sexual relationships, decreased sexual activity, and disturbed physiological functioning of the reproductive system (menstrual irregularity and infertility). Alcoholic women also report difficulties in arousal (30 to 40 per cent) and/or loss of orgasmic response or reduced frequency or intensity of orgasm (15 per cent). A recent study found that 56 per cent of the alcoholic women studied had various degrees of "inadequate sexual response" (Kolodny, Masters, and Johnson, 1979).

In addition to the psychological factors of expectation, set, or performance anxiety, the effects of alcohol on tumescence and ejaculation are a result of the direct physiological action of alcohol on the spinal reflex centers controlling erectile and ejaculatory processes (Abel, 1980). A similar physiological effect in women may interfere with a woman's ability to respond sexually, indicated by a lack of vaginal lubrication. A study by Wilson and Lawson (1976) showed that although the women subjects had a decreased vaginal response with increasing blood alcohol levels, they tended to predict and then report high levels of sexual arousal with increasing alcohol levels. It seems while a man's expectation of a sexual enhancing effect of alcohol is challenged by a visible failure of erection, such an expectation in women is not as challenged because her genital responses are "less tangible" (Bancroft, 1983).

Recreational Drugs

The sexual impact of recreational drug use varies with the dosage and frequency of use. It is difficult to assess a drug's specific effect on sexual behavior because of complications of the setting in which a drug is used as well as the individual's expectations of the drug's effects (such as expectations of enhanced sexual experience). The drugs that will be discussed below include marijuana, cocaine and amphetamines, opiates and methadone, and psychedelics (e.g., LSD, PCP).

MARIJUANA

Marijuana's effects on sexuality have not been scientifically studied in a controlled experiment. Although use of the drug does increase suggestibility, and alterations in perception of the sexual experience are expected and reported, in fact "sexual performance may be unaltered or even impaired" (Kolodny, Masters, and Johnson, 1979, p 340).

Interviews with 800 men and 500 women between ages 18 and 30 at the Masters and Johnson Institute about the effects of marijuana on sex have provided interesting information about this drug. The majority of all subjects (81 to 83 per cent) reported enhanced enjoyment of sex. However, men and women stated that marijuana did *not* increase their sexual interest, desire, or intensity of orgasm. Males stated that it did not increase their ease of attaining or maintaining erections, nor did it increase their control over ejaculation. In fact, 20 per cent of males using marijuana on a daily basis reported erectile dysfunction. Females stated that marijuana use did not increase their arousability, their amount of vaginal lubrication, or their frequency of orgasm. Both men and women attributed the positive effect of marijuana on sex to factors such as increased sense of touch, greater relaxation, and "being in tune with one's partner" (Kolodny, Masters, and Johnson, 1979).

There are discrepancies in the results of studies on the effect of marijuana use on males' testosterone levels. Two studies reported that both acute administration and chronic frequent use of marijuana caused decreased levels of testosterone in healthy young men (Cohen, 1976; Kolodny, Masters, and Johnson, 1974). Other studies found no significant differences in testosterone levels after 3 to 4 weeks of high-dose marijuana use in either "casual" or "heavy" users (Hembree, Zeidenberg, and Nahas, 1976; Mendelson, 1976). Other studies comparing control groups with both casual and chronic marijuana smokers found no differences in the plasma testosterone levels between the groups (Coggins et al, 1976; Cushman, 1975). Another study comparing the testosterone levels of occasional and habitual marijuana users 30 and 90 minutes after one high dose found a small decrease in but no abnormally low testosterone level (Schaeffer, Gunn, and Dubowski, 1975). Some possible reasons for the discrepancies in the results could be study design ("between subjects" design, as Kolodny, Masters, and Johnson used, is likely to be less sensitive than "within subject" design used by Schaeffer, Gunn, and Dubowski and Mendelson); Kolodny, Masters, and Johnson's subjects' possible ingestion of testosterone-lowering substances other than marijuana, such as alcohol or narcotics; dosage and purity of marijuana used; and normal episodic variation in testosterone levels (Abel, 1981; Mendelson, 1976). Mendelson also notes that if any changes in testosterone levels do occur in some marijuana smokers, "such changes are probably not biologically significant since they are well within the wide range found in the control group of adult male nonusers" (Mendelson, 1976, p 24). Marijuana does inhibit male sexual behavior in animals, although this may not be especially relevant, as the social factors are eliminated in any animal studies. Some studies report that sperm count is decreased during the 2-week period after marijuana use. Gynecomastia has been noted in males who are chronic users of marijuana, possibly related to endocrine disturbances due to undernutrition.

Several survey studies indicate that marijuana is associated with increased sexual activity and enjoyment for many people. However, some individuals report becoming lethargic and sleepy, with decreased sexual interest, after marijuana use. "Set" and "setting" are more important when drug potency is low, and with increasing drug potency, pharmacological effects become increasingly important in affecting sexual responsiveness.

COCAINE AND AMPHETAMINES

Both cocaine and amphetamines are centrally acting brain stimulants that have been reputed to enhance sexual interest and performance. There has been very little research on the sexual effects of these drugs. Small doses of cocaine, usually inhaled through the nose, produce a feeling of euphoria, loss of fatigue, delayed ejaculation, and heightened sensory awareness, all of which may enhance a sexual experience. Spontaneous erections and multiple orgasms have been reported following intravenous use. Occasionally "acute doses" of cocaine cause "heightened libido, undifferentiated sexual urgency,

frenzy, loss of control, and mania" (Bianchine and Lubbers, 1983, p 131). High doses cause distracting psychic effects that result in a loss of the aphrodisiac effect. Ball (1980) describes the effect of high doses as somewhat "orgasmic" in quality and notes that this may serve as a substitute for rather than enhancing sexual pleasure. Other reports of adverse sexual effects from cocaine use include loss of erection (reported in 36 per cent of 39 men studied); priapism has also occurred.

Amphetamines produce effects similar to those of cocaine. The effect on sexual functioning appears to be related to dose, route of administration, and frequency of use. Smaller doses generally seem to enhance sexual experience, increasing desire in both men and women and sustaining erections but delaying ejaculation in males. There have been variable reports of the effect on orgasm in women; some say the drug increases their ability to achieve orgasm, while others report decreased ability. Higher doses of amphetamine more consistently cause sexual dysfunction in both males and females: There is a higher incidence of men reporting erectile dysfunction and of both men and women reporting failure to achieve orgasm. Other studies show both increases and decreases in sexual desire and enjoyment, indicating that the drug has different effects on different individuals. The episodic user reports more positive effects on sexual activity and experience than does the habitual user.

Amphetamines may enhance male sexual behavior but inhibit female sexuality (Bancroft, 1983). Individuals severely dependent on amphetamines may experience physical discomfort and psychotic delusions and may have minimal or no interest in sex. A study by Greaves (1972) indicated that chronic amphetamine use is neither a sexual substitute nor direct contribution to sexual disturbances, although female amphetamine users expressed negative feelings about sex. Both drug use and sexual problems associated with such use result from common personality variables as yet unidentified. Smith, Buxton, and Dammann, (1979), however, report that use of high doses intravenously produces a "pharmacogenic orgasm," and in couples in whom both individuals are using amphetamines, sexual activity frequently ceases and is replaced by mutual injection of the drug.

OPIATES AND METHADONE

The most consistently abused opiates include morphine, codeine, meperidine, and heroin.

Such drugs suppress basic drives, including the sex drive, and impair sexual experience in a high percentage of both men and women. Males report decreased desire, erectile difficulties, and delayed ejaculation or anorgasmia. Females also report decreased desire and anorgasmia, as well as decreased frequency of sexual activity, diminished or absent menstrual periods, infertility, or spontaneous abortion. Chronic use may seriously impair sexual function. As the individual is withdrawn from the drug, sexual problems usually disappear, and sexual activity and enjoyment increases; however, erectile dysfunction from chronic use may be permanent owing to neurological damage.

Methadone is a synthetic narcotic analgesic pharmacologically similar to morphine. Methadone has been reported to cause decreased desire (6 to 38 per cent), erectile failure (6 to 50 per cent), retarded ejaculation (5 to 22 per cent), and failure of orgasm (5 to 88 per cent). Female methadone users report diminished sexual activity and desire. It appears that dosage is an important factor influencing incidence of side effects from methadone (Buffum, 1982; Rosenbaum and Murphy, 1987). Improvement in sexual function is often reported in individuals switching from heroin use to methadone maintenance, although delayed ejaculation frequently persists.

PSYCHEDELIC DRUGS

Since psychedelic drugs cause perceptual and psychic effects, they also affect sexual experience. Psychedelic drugs most often used recreationally include lysergic acid diethylamide, or "acid" (LSD), psilocybin, and phencyclidine, or "angel dust" (PCP). Reports of the sexual side effects of these drugs are conflicting, and systematic research has not been done. Some reports of sexual experiences under the influence of these drugs indicate that sexual effects are dose related, with lower doses having aphrodisiac effects in some individuals, while larger doses often detract from sexuality as the individual may lose bodily control and be distracted psychically.

One study of 140 LSD users found less than 15 per cent of such users reporting enhanced sexuality (Kolodny, Masters, and Johnson, 1979). PCP does not seem to be used for sexual purposes; in fact, recreational users report a decrease in sexual feelings following PCP use. Heavy abusers coming down from a PCP high frequently experience depression and decreased desire. Chronic use of large doses of PCP has been associated with adverse effects on sexuality, specifically on erection and ejaculation.

INTERVENTION

Intervention with drug-related sexual dysfunction depends on identification of the substance abuse problem. Every case of sexual dysfunction should be assessed for alcohol or drug use. The health professional should take the alcohol and drug history as part of the medical history, asking questions using nonjudgmental terms such as "use" instead of "abuse." If the client gives vague responses, the health professional should try to elicit more specific responses regarding substances used as well as amount and frequency. It is often the health professional's accepting matter-of-fact attitude that makes it possible for the client to respond to such potentially embarrassing or incriminating questions.

Assisting a client with sexual problems who is also abusing drugs or alcohol involves several treatment approaches, including providing information, pharmacological methods when indicated, counseling, or referral. However, basic to a therapeutic relationship with such clients is a nonjudgmental or nonmoralistic attitude. Poor self-image and low self-esteem are common characteristics of substance abusers, and feelings about their sexual functioning affect their sense of self and their self-esteem. Judgmental attitudes on the part of the health professionals and failure to focus on the healthy and satisfying sexual functioning of the clients can interfere with the treatment process (Smith, Buxton, and Dammann, 1979). It is imperative that health professionals not add to clients' negative feelings about themselves by projecting a judgmental attitude about the client's sexual orientation or behaviors or about their choice of using substances to alter their sexual feelings or behaviors.

Pharmacological treatment is sometimes indicated when withdrawing a client from alcohol or drugs. If an underlying depression is causing the sexual dysfunction, then tricyclic antidepressant medications may be helpful. Disulfiram (Antabuse) has been used successfully in helping alcoholics refrain from drinking. Benzodiazepines or low doses of neuroleptics may be used on a short-term basis for control of anxiety as needed following detoxification. Methadone maintenance is an effective method to help the opioid abuser reduce illicit drug use and reintegrate into the community; methadone is available in special clinics under federal supervision and involves close monitoring of the client.

Provision of accurate information is essential. This includes giving information about the sexual effects of substances as well as the toxic effects associated with certain drugs. Mendelson (1976) discusses informing the client of the "risk-benefit ratio associated with use of any drug to modify sexual function," noting that although LSD may enhance a client's sexual enjoyment, the toxicity of this substance is so great and continued use may so adversely affect brain function that the client should be informed of these harmful effects.

The client must abstain from substance use and may need detoxification before any treatment program is likely to be effective. It is important to provide accurate information about the effects of abstinence on sexuality. Often clients have been told erroneously that their sexual function will return to normal upon cessation of the drug, whereas this is not always true; providing inaccurate information can impair the treatment process. The health professional must be aware of and provide the correct information about the physiological effects of stopping the use of the drug. In addition, the client will also need information about and support in dealing with psychological and emotional problems that may emerge as a result of abstinence. The client has been abusing alcohol or other drugs as a means of defensively coping with stresses, lack of interpersonal social skills, low self-esteem, or even underlying sexual problems. Therefore, as the client abstains from the drug, the underlying problems are likely to emerge. If clients are not helped with these underlying problems, they will be tempted to again begin using the alcohol or drug.

Therefore, counseling is a necessary adjunct to prescribing abstinence or pharmacological treatment. Since substance-abusing clients are "used to rapid relief of distressing emotional states by means of chemicals and usually have little tolerance for the slow, often frustration-evoking process, of the in-sight-oriented therapeutic approach," the most successful counseling techniques are "reality-oriented and focus[ing] on the here and now" (Kleber, 1983, p 282). The client may need help with relations with friends or family or with job or school problems. Although the health professional cannot support the substance use, treating clients judgmentally will cause them either to lie and distort facts or to leave treatment. A useful alliance is more likely to result from an attitude of accepting the client but questioning the need for such destructive behavior.

Involvement of the family, especially a partner if the client is having sexual problems, is important in both the assessment and treatment phases. If the substance abuse has been masking underlying sexual problems, these will re-emerge and will need discussion and intervention involving both partners. Family members need the same accurate information that is provided to the client.

In the abstinence phase, the client is relearning how to function sexually without the use of drugs or alcohol. Even if such functioning is re-established, clients may have problems with their social skills. Often, the substance abuse occurred as a means of dealing with anxiety about rejection or fear of intimacy and simply eliminating the substance use will not solve the underlying problems. Therefore, couple and/or group therapy is often helpful. An improved sexual relationship often accompanies improved couple communication skills. It is important for both the client and the partner to know that stopping drug use will not immediately restore sexual and reproductive function to normal. The couple needs to know each other without using drugs or alcohol and to work on improving their communication patterns relationship; the sexual aspect should be deemphasized during the initial abstinence phase. Teaching the couple relaxation techniques may help them decrease their anxiety and be more comfortable with each other.

Since erectile dysfunction and decreased desire may persist even after discontinuation of alcohol or drug use, health professionals should be sensitive to this possibility and, if it occurs, work with the client and partner to find alternatives to intercourse for sexual satisfaction. Such clients "need to be given the necessary information, permission, and encouragement to explore a variety of ways to be sensual and sexual with their partners"

(Redl, 1982, p 139). Since these clients often have low self-esteem, it is especially important to let them know that their continued problems of sexual functioning are not a reflection of failure as a person but are a direct result of the alcohol or drug use. Additionally, recovering alcoholic male clients often believe that their partners are extremely dissatisfied or unhappy if they are unable to perform sexually. Often the partner is happier to have him sober rather than sexually active, and encouraging the couple to discuss their feelings about their sexual relationship openly is usually very helpful to both partners.

Often a family member may need support for any confrontation that may have to occur, such as a spouse of a substance abuser, who may need to say, "I'll leave if you don't get treatment." Any such confrontation has to be thoroughly thought out, and the spouse should only make such a statement when prepared to carry out possible consequences. The health professional may need to provide short-term crisis-oriented help to families and focus on improving communication, setting realistic goals, negotiation, limit setting, and sometimes referral, if necessary.

Referral is indicated any time the health professional's evaluation indicates that the client needs more intensive treatment, either inpatient or outpatient, than the practitioner has the time or skills to provide. For an effective referral, the health professional must be aware of the resources available, including Alcoholics Anonymous, drug treatment centers, therapeutic communities, halfway houses, or other health professionals (psychiatrists, psychiatric nurses, psychologists, or social workers) who are experienced in working with substance-abusing clients. Often, local mental health centers have drug- or alcohol-treatment programs.

Reinforcement of abstinence seems to occur best in peer group settings. There are various drug-free therapeutic communities, such as Synanon and Phoenix House, that use group confrontation and milieu therapy techniques. There has not been systematic research on such programs to assess their success. There is probably a very high initial dropout rate, and there may be a high success rate among those who remain. One of the major problems with such communities is development of dependence, perhaps for life, on the community. Self-help groups, such as Alcoholics Anonymous and Narcotics Anonymous, have also been successful, and many communities have such groups available.

SUMMARY

Due to the complex relationship between sexual functioning and mental illness, it is not easy to specify a causative relationship between mental illnesses and sexual problems. It is necessary to evaluate all the factors which may be affecting the client's experience of sexuality—the intrapsychic, intrapersonal, biological, and social aspects of that individual. It is important to note that emotional problems may or may not be expressed in sexual symptoms. A client's mental illness may affect sexuality, or it may affect the partner's sexual behavior or satisfaction.

Some emotional problems, such as anxiety or depression, may be either the result or cause of sexual dysfunction. Other mental illnesses, such as schizophrenia, organic mental syndromes or disorders, or anorexia nervosa, may more indirectly affect sexual behavior because of the symptoms specific to the illness. There may be a biochemical component affecting sexuality associated with certain mood states. Treatment of mental illness pharmacologically can cause sexual problems because of medication side effects, which only complicates the client's life and perception of his illness. Other drugs, such as those used recreationally, can affect sexuality to varying degrees. There is still much research needed on the reciprocal effects of mental illness and sexuality.

Interventions should be directed to any aspect of the client's problem that may help alleviate it: biological, intra- or interpersonal, or social. It is important to include the family, spouse, or significant other in the assessment and intervention. Especially in matters of sexual functioning, the partner is an important component, both being affected by the problem and being able to participate in support of the client and in improvement of the problem. It is important that the health professional be well-educated about the various factors that may interrelate and affect a client's sexuality. The health professional must establish a nonjudgmental therapeutic relationship when helping a client come to terms about sexuality. While sexuality is an important concern of any client, clients with emotional problems especially need attention and intervention in this area.

REFERENCES

Abel EL: A review of alcohol's effects on sex and reproduction. Drug Alcohol Dependence 5:321–332, 1980.

Abel EL: Marihuana and sex: a critical survey. Drug Alcohol Dependence 8:1–22, 1981.

Alzheimer's disease: Sexual manifestations require understanding. Sex Med Today 8:6–9, 1984.

American Psychiatric Association: Diagnostic and Statistical Manual of Mental Disorders. 3rd ed. revised (DSM-III-R). Washington, DC, American Psychiatric Association, 1987.

Ball W: Drugs that affect sexuality. In Hogan R (ed): Human Sexuality: A Nursing Perspective. Norwalk, Appleton-Century-Crofts, 1980.

Balon R, Berchou R, Han H: Priapism associated with thiothixene, chlorpromazine, and thioridazine (letter). J Clin Psych 48:216, 1987.

Bancroft J: Human Sexuality and Its Problems. New York, Churchill Livingstone, 1983.

Bancroft J, et al: The control of deviant sexual behaviour by drugs: I. Behavioural changes following oestrogens and anti-androgens. Br J Psychol 125:310–315, 1974.

Barnett J: Sex and the obsessive-compulsive person. Med Asp Human Sex 5:34–45, 1971.

Berlin FS, Meinecke CF: Treatment of sex offenders with anti-androgenic medication: Conceptualization, review of treatment modalities, and preliminary findings. Am J Psychol 138:601–607, 1981.

Bianchine JR, Lubbers JR: Drugs and sexual dysfunction. In Pariser SF, et al (eds): Clinical Sexuality. New York, Marcel Dekker, Inc, 1983.

Blair CD, Lanyon RI: Exhibitionism: Etiology and treatment. Psychol Bull 89:439–463, 1981.

Buffum J: Pharmacosexology: The effects of drugs on sexual function—a review. J Psychoactive Drugs 14:5–44, 1982.

Buffum J et al: Drugs and sexual function. In Lief HI (ed): Sexual Problems in Medical Practice. Chicago, American Medical Association, 1981, pp 211–242.

Christenson R: MAOI's, anorgasmia, and weight gain (letter). Am J Psychol 140:1260, 1982.

Coggins WJ et al: Health status of chronic heavy cannibis users. Ann NY Acad Sci 282:148–161, 1976.

Cohen S: Cannabis and sex: Multifaceted paradoxes. J Psychoactive Drugs 14:55–58, 1982.

Cohen S: The 94-day cannibis study. Ann NY Acad Sci 282:211–219, 1976.

Cooper AJ: Antidepressant medication and sexual function (letter). J Clin Psychopharmacol 7:120, 1987.

Cooper AJ, et al: Antiandrogen (cyproterone acetate) therapy in deviant hypersexuality. Br J Psychol 120:59–63, 1972.

Cushman P: Plasma testosterone levels in healthy male marijuana smokers. Am J Drug Alcohol Abuse 2:269–275, 1975.

Decastro RM: Reversal of MAOI-induced anorgasmia with cyproheptadine (letter). Am J Psychol 142:783, 1985.

Degen K: Sexual dysfunction in women using major tranquilizers. Psychosomatics 23:959–961, 1982.

Deicken RF, Carr RE: Testicular swelling associated with desipramine. J Clin Psychol 48:251–252, 1987.

DeLeo D, Magni G: Sexual side effects of antidepressant drugs. Psychosomatics 24:1076–1082, 1983.

Drossman DA: Anorexia nervosa: A comprehensive approach. In Stollerman GH (ed): Advances in Internal Medicine. Vol 28. Chicago, Year Book Medical Publishers, 1983.

Drugs that cause sexual dysfunction. Med Lett Drugs Therap 29:65–70, 1987.

Dudek F, Turner DS: Alcoholism and sexual functioning. J Psychoactive Drugs 14:47–54, 1982.

Duncan D, Gold R: Drugs and the Whole Person. New York, John Wiley and Sons, 1982.

Fahrner EM: Sexual dysfunction in male alcohol addicts; prevalence and treatment. Arch Sex Behav 16:247–257, 1987.

Fishbain DA: Priapism resulting from fluphenazine hydrochloride treatment reversed by diphenhydramine. Ann Emerg Med 14:600–602, 1985.

Garfinkel PE, Garner DM: Anorexia Nervosa: A Multidimensional Perspective. New York, Brunner/Mazel, 1982.

Gartrell N: Increased libido in women receiving trazodone. Am J Psychol 143:781–782, 1986.

Goldberg M: Quiz. Med Asp Human Sex 9:77–78, 1975.

Gomez EA: Neuroleptic-induced priapism. Texas Med 81:47–48, 1985.

Greaves G: Sexual disturbances among chronic amphetamine users. J Nerv Ment Dis 155:363–365, 1972.

Greenberg M, Lee KK: Priapism treated with benztropine (letter). Am J Psychol 144:383–385, 1987.

Griffith SR, Zil JS: Priapism in a patient receiving antipsychotic therapy. Psychosomatics 25:629–631, 1984.

Harrison WM: Response to Dr. Cooper (letter). J Clin Psychopharmacol 7:120, 1987.

Harrison WM, et al: Effects of antidepressant medication on sexual function: A controlled study. J Clin Psychopharmacol 6:144–149, 1986.

Hembree WC, Zeidenberg P, Nahas GG: Marihuana effects on human gonadal function. In Nahas GG (ed): Marihuana: Chemistry, Biochemistry, and Cellular Effects. New York, Springer-Verlag, 1976.

Hoover CF, Fitzgerald RG: Marital conflict of manic-depressive patients. Arch Gen Psychol 38:65–67, 1981.

Howell JR, et al: Assessment of sexual function, interest and activity in depressed men. J Affect Disord 13:61–66, 1987.

Jacobson JN: Anorgasmia caused by an MAOI (letter). Am J Psychol 144:527, 1987.

Jeffries JJ, Walker C: Cyproheptadine and drug-induced anorgasmia (letter). Can J Psychol 32:79, 1987.

Jones SD: Ejaculatory inhibition with trazodone. J Clin Psychopharmacol 4:279–281, 1984.

Kaplan HS: The New Sex Therapy. New York, Brunner/Mazel, 1974.

Klassen AD, Wilsnack SC: Sexual experience and drinking among women in a U.S. national survey. Arch Sex Behav 15:363–392, 1986.

Kleber HD: Drug dependence. In Leigh H (ed): Psychiatry in the Practice of Medicine. Menlo Park, Addison-Wesley, 1983.

Kogeorgos J, deAlwis C: Priapism and psychotropic medicine. Br J Psychol 149:241–243, 1986.

Kolodny RC, Masters WH, Johnson VE: Textbook of Sexual Medicine. Boston, Little, Brown & Co, 1979.

Kristensen E, Jorgensen P: Sexual function in lithium-treated manic-depressive patients. Pharmacopsychiatry 20:165–167, 1987.

Kulik FA, Wilbur R: Case report of painful ejaculation

as a side effect of amoxapine. Am J Psychol 139:234–235, 1982.

Laschet U, et al: Results in the treatment of hyper- or abnormal sexuality of men with antiandrogens. Acta Endocrinol (Suppl)119:54, 1967.

Leigh H (ed): Psychiatry in the Practice of Medicine. Menlo Park, Addison-Wesley, 1983.

Lemere F: Sexual impairment in recovered alcoholics. Med Asp Human Sex 10:69–70, 1976.

Lemere F, Smith JW: Alcohol-induced sexual impotence. Am J Psychol 130:212–213, 1973.

Lesko LM, Stotland NL, Segraves RT: Three cases of female anorgasmia associated with MAOI's. Am J Psychol 139:1353–1354, 1982.

Lukoff D, et al: Sex education and rehabilitation with schizophrenic male outpatients. Schizophrenia Bull 12:669–677, 1986.

Lydiard RB, et al: Sexual side effects of alprazolam (letter). Am J Psychol 144:254–255, 1987.

Mace NL, Rabins PV: The 36-Hour Day. Baltimore, The Johns Hopkins University Press, 1981.

Marks IM: Review of behavioral psychotherapy. II: Sexual disorders. Am J Psychol 138:750–756, 1981.

Marks R, Fuentes RJ, Rosenberg JM: Sexual side effects: What to tell your patients, what not to say. RN 46:35–41, 1983.

Mendelson JH: Marihuana and sex. Med Asp Human Sex 10:23–24, 1976.

Mitchell JE, Popkin MK: Antipsychotic drug therapy and sexual dysfunction in men. Am J Psychol 139:633–637, 1982.

Monteiro WO, et al: Anorgasmia from clomipramine in obsessive-compulsive disorder: A controlled trial. Br J Psychol 151:107–112, 1987.

Moss HB: More cases of anorgasmia after MAOI treatment (letter). Am J Psychol 140:266, 1983.

Munjack DJ, Crocker B: Alprazolam-induced ejaculatory inhibition. J Clin Psychopharm 6:57–58, 1986.

Munjack DJ, Oziel LJ: Sexual Medicine and Counseling in Office Practice: A Comprehensive Treatment Guide. Boston, Little, Brown & Co, 1980.

Nestoros NN, Lehmann HE, Ban TA: Neuroleptic drugs and sexual dysfunction in schizophrenia. Med Probl Pharmacopsychol 15:111–130, 1980.

Neuman PA, Halvorson PA: Anorexia Nervosa and Bulimia: A Handbook for Counselors and Therapists. New York, Van Nostrand and Reinhold, 1983.

Nurnberg HG, Levine PE: Spontaneous remission of MAOI-induced anorgasmia. Am J Psychol 144:805–807, 1987.

Othmer E, Othmer SC: Effect of buspirone on sexual dysfunction in patients with generalized anxiety disorder. J Clin Psychol 48:201–203, 1987.

Patt N: More on trazodone and priapism (letter). Am J Psychol 142:783–784, 1985.

Paykel ES, Weissman MM: Marital and sexual dysfunction in depressed women. Med Asp Human Sex 5:73–101, 1972.

Pfaus JG, Borzalka BB: Opioids and sexual behavior. Neurosci Behav Rev 11:1–34, 1987.

Pohl R: Anorgasmia caused by MAOI's (letter). Am J Psychol 140:510, 1983.

Pollack MH, Rosenbaum JF: Management of antidepressant-induced side effects: A practical guide for the clinician. J Clin Psychol 48:3–8, 1987.

Purtell JJ, Robins E, Cohen ME: Observations on clinical aspects of hysteria: A quantitative study of 50 hysteria patients and 156 control subjects. JAMA 146:902–909, 1951.

Rabkin JG, et al: Adverse reactions to monoamine oxidase inhibitors. Part II. Treatment correlates and clinical management. J Clin Psychopharm 5:2–9, 1985.

Raskin DE: Trazodone and priapism (letter). Am J Psychol 142:142–143, 1985.

Redl M: Sexual interaction among recovering chemically dependent couples. J Psychoactive Drugs 14:137–141, 1982.

Reid WH: Treatment of the DSM-III Psychiatric Disorders. New York, Brunner/Mazel, 1983.

Renshaw DC: Drugs and sex: A study of the effect of drugs on human sexuality. Nurs Care 11:16–19, 1978.

Riley AJ, Riley EJ: Cyproheptadine and antidepressant-induced anorgasmia (letter). Br J Psychol 148:217–218, 1986.

Rosenbaum M, Murphy S: Not the picture of health: Women on methadone. J Psychoactive Drugs 19:217–236, 1987.

Sangal R: Inhibited female orgasm as a side effect of alprazolam (letter). Am J Psychol 142:1223–1224, 1985.

Sarrel PM, Sarrel LJ: Sexual dysfunctions. In Leigh H (ed): Psychiatry in the Practice of Medicine. Menlo Park, Addison-Wesley, 1983.

Schaeffer CF, Gunn CG, Dubowski KM: Normal plasma testosterone concentrations after marihuana smoking. N Engl J Med 292:867–868, 1975.

Scher M, Krieger JN, Juergens S: Trazodone and priapism. Am J Psychol 140:1362–1363, 1983.

Schwarz G: Case report of inhibition of ejaculation and retrograde ejaculation as side effects of amoxapine. Am J Psychol 139:233–234, 1982.

Segraves RT: Pharmacological agents causing sexual dysfunction. J Sex Marital Ther 3:157–176, 1977.

Segraves RT: Reversal by bethanechol of imipramine-induced ejaculatory dysfunction (letter). Am J Psychol 144:1243–1244, 1987.

Skopec HM, Rosenberg SD, Tucker GJ: Sexual behavior in schizophrenia. Med Asp Human Sex 10:32–47, 1976.

Smith DE, Buxton ME, Dammann G: Amphetamine abuse and sexual dysfunction: Clinical and research considerations. In Smith DE, et al (eds): Amphetamine Use, Misuse, and Abuse: Proceedings of the National Amphetamine Conference, 1978. Boston, GK Hall & Co, 1979.

Sovner R: Treatment of tricyclic antidepressant-induced orgasmic inhibition with cyproheptadine (letter). J Clin Psychopharm 4:169, 1984.

Spencer RF, Raft D: Depression and diminished sexual desire. Med Asp Human Sex 11:57–61, 1977.

Tennent G, Bancroft J, Cass J: The control of deviant sexual behavior by drugs: A double-blind controlled study of benperidol, chlorpromazine, and placebo. Arch Sex Behav 3:261–271, 1974.

Teusink JP, Mahler S: Helping families cope with Alzheimer's disease. Hosp Commun Psychol 35:152–156, 1984.

Thienhaus OJ, Vogel N: Desipramine and testicular swelling in two patients. J Clin Psychol 49:33–34, 1988.

Tsuang MT: Hypersexuality in manic patients. Med Asp Human Sex 9:83–89, 1975.

Warner MD, et al: Trazodone and priapism. J Clin Psychol 48:244–245, 1987.

Weissberg JH: Commentary (on Appleton's article). Med Asp Human Sex 16:163–167, 1982.

Weissman MM, Paykel ES: The Depressed Woman: A

Study of Social Relationships. Chicago, University of Chicago Press, 1974.

Wilson GT, Lawson D: Effects of alcohol on sexual arousal in women. J Abnorm Psychol 85:489–497, 1976.

Woodruff RA, Murphy GE, Herjanic M: The natural history of affective disorders. I. Symptoms of 72 patients at the time of index hospital admission. J Psychiatr Res 5:255–263, 1967.

Woods SM: Sexuality and mental disorders. In Lief H (ed): Sexual Problems in Medical Practice. Chicago, American Medical Association, 1981.

Yager J: Bethanechol chloride can reverse erectile and ejaculatory dysfunction induced by tricyclic antidepressants and mazindol: Case report. J Clin Psychol 47:210–211, 1986.

Yeragani VK, Gershon S: Priapism related to phenelzine therapy (letter). N Engl J Med 317:117–118, 1987.

Index

Note: Numbers in *italics* refer to illustrations;
numbers followed by (t) indicate tables.